ENDOCRINE

SECRETS

SEVENTH EDITION

ENDOCRINE

EDITOR:

MICHAEL T. McDERMOTT, MD
Professor of Medicine and Clinical Pharmacy
University of Colorado Denver School of Medicine
Director, Endocrinology and Diabetes Practice
University of Colorado Hospital
Aurora, Colorado

ELSEVIER

ENDOCRINE SECRETS, SEVENTH EDITION

ISBN: 978-0-323-62428-2

Notice

Practitioners and researchers must always rely on their own experience and knowledge in evaluating and using any information, methods, compounds or experiments described herein. Because of rapid advances in the medical sciences, in particular, independent verification of diagnoses and drug dosages should be made. To the fullest extent of the law, no responsibility is assumed by Elsevier, authors, editors or contributors for any injury and/or damage to persons or property as a matter of products liability, negligence or otherwise, or from any use or operation of any methods, products, instructions, or ideas contained in the material herein.

Previous editions copyrighted 2013, 2009, 2005, 2002, 1998, and 1994.

Library of Congress Control Number: 2019937967

Content Strategist: Marybeth Thiel
Content Development Specialist: Angie Breckon
Publishing Services Manager: Shereen Jameel
Senior Project Manager: Umarani Natarajan
Design Direction: Bridget Hoette

Printed in the United States of America

Last digit is the print number: 9   8   7   6   5   4

3251 Riverport Lane
St. Louis, Missouri 63043

  Working together to grow libraries in developing countries

www.elsevier.com • www.bookaid.org

This book is dedicated to Libby, whose strength, courage, and love of life are a daily inspiration, and to Katie Cohen, Emily Cohen, Hayley McDermott, and Henry McDermott, for making life fun.

LIST OF CONTRIBUTORS

Abdurezak A. Abdela, MBBS
Internal Medicine
Addis Ababa University
Addis Ababa, Ethiopia

Veena R. Agrawal, MD, FRCPC
Assistant Professor
Department of Internal Medicine
University of Manitoba
Winnipeg, MB, Canada

Maria B. Albuja-Cruz, MD
Assistant Professor
Department of Surgery
University of Colorado Anschutz Medical Campus
Aurora, CO, United States

Sarah L. Anderson, PharmD
Associate Professor
Department of Clinical Pharmacy
University of Colorado Skaggs School of Pharmacy and
    Pharmaceutical Sciences
Aurora, CO, United States
Clinical Pharmacy Specialist
Ambulatory Care Services
Denver Health Medical Center
Denver, CO, United States

Harris M. Baloch, MD
Department of Endocrinology
Walter Reed National Military Medical Center
Bethesda, MD, United States

Linda A. Barbour, MD, MSPH
Professor
Medicine and Obstetrics and Gynecology
University of Colorado School of Medicine
Aurora, CO, United States

Brenda K. Bell, MD
Clinical Endocrinologist
Private Practice
Lincoln, NE, United States

Helen Y. Bitew, MD
Assistant Professor of Medicine
Internal Medicine
Addis Ababa University
College of Health Sciences
Addis Ababa, Ethiopia

Mark Bridenstine, MD
Banner Health Clinic
Loveland, CO, United States

Tamis M. Bright, MD
Associate Professor
Chief, Division of Endocrinology
Texas Tech University
El Paso, TX, United States

Henry B. Burch, MD, FACE
Program Director
Division of Diabetes, Endocrinology, and Metabolic
    Diseases
National Institute of Diabetes and Digestive and Kidney
    Diseases
Professor of Medicine
Endocrinology Division
Uniformed Services Health Sciences University
Bethesda, MD, United States

Anne-Marie Carreau, MD, MSc
Faculty of Medicine
Université Laval
Division of Endocrinology and Nephrology
Centre de Recherche du CHU de Québec-Université
    Laval
Quebec, Canada

Ana Chindris, MD
Endocrinology
Mayo Clinic
Jacksonville, FL, United States

Melanie Cree-Green, MD, PhD
Assistant Professor
Division of Endocrinology
Department of Pediatrics
University of Colorado Anschutz Medical Campus
Director, Multi-Disciplinary PCOS Clinic
Children's Hospital Colorado
Aurora, CO, United States

Mark M. Cruz, MD
Fellow
Department of Endocrinology
Walter Reed National Military Medical Center
Bethesda, MD, United States

Shanlee M. Davis, MD, MSCS
Assistant Professor
Pediatric Endocrinology
Children's Hospital Colorado
University of Colorado
Aurora, CO, United States

Stephanie Davis, MD
General Surgery Resident
University of Colorado Anschutz Medical Campus
Aurora, CO, United States

Meghan Donnelly, MD
Assistant Professor
Obstetrics and Gynecology
University of Colorado School of Medicine
Denver, CO, United States

William E. Duncan, MD, PhD, MACP
Professor of Medicine
Department of Medicine
Uniformed Services University
Bethesda, MD, United States

Oliver J. Fackelmayer, MD
Surgical Resident
University of Colorado Anschutz Medical Campus
Department of Surgery
Aurora, CO, United States

Shari C. Fox, BS, MS, MD, FACE
Department of Endocrinology
Colorado Permanente Medical Group
Denver, CO, United States

Michele B. Glodowski, MD
Clinical Instructor
New York University School of Medicine
New York, NY, United States

Bryan R. Haugen, MD
Professor of Medicine and Pathology
Head, Division of Endocrinology, Metabolism
    and Diabetes
Mary Rossick Kern and Jerome H. Kern Chair of
    Endocrine Neoplasms Research
University of Colorado School of Medicine
Aurora, CO, United States

Matthew R. Hawkins, BSW, MMSc
Senior Instructor/Physician Assistant
Division of Endocrinology, Metabolism and Diabetes
University of Colorado School of Medicine
Aurora, CO, United States

James Vincent Hennessey, MD
Clinical Director
Endocrinology
Beth Israel Deaconess Medical Center
Associate Professor
Medicine
Harvard Medical School
Boston, MA, United States

Thanh Duc Hoang, DO, FACP, FACE
Director, NCC Endocrinology Fellowship Program
Department of Endocrinology
Walter Reed National Military Medical Center
Associate Professor, Internal Medicine
Director, Endocrinology Division
Uniformed Services Health Sciences University
Bethesda, MD, United States

Sean J. Iwamoto, MD
Instructor of Medicine
Endocrinology, Metabolism and Diabetes
University of Colorado School of Medicine
Rocky Mountain Regional VA Medical Center
Aurora, CO, United States

Thomas Jensen, MD
Assistant Professor
University of Colorado Denver
Aurora, CO, United States

Janice M. Kerr, MD
Associate Professor
Endocrinology, Metabolism and Diabetes
University of Colorado, Denver
Denver, CO, United States

Pratima Kumar, MD, FACE
Assistant Professor, Division of Endocrinology
Department of Medicine
Dell Medical School
The University of Texas at Austin
Austin, TX, United States

Helen M. Lawler, MD
Assistant Professor
Division of Endocrinology, Metabolism, and Diabetes
University of Colorado
Aurora, CO, United States

Homer J. LeMar Jr., MD
El Paso Veterans Affairs Health Care System
El Paso, TX, United States

Vinh Q. Mai, DO, FACP, FACE
Chief and Associate Professor
Endocrinology, Diabetes and Metabolism
Walter Reed National Military Medical Center
Bethesda, MD, United States

Ayesha F. Malik, MD
Fellow
Endocrinology
Mayo Clinic
Jacksonville, FL, United States

Roselyn I. Mateo, MD, MSc
Endocrinology
Beth Israel Deaconess Medical Center
Boston, MA, United States

Sarah E. Mayson, MD
Assistant Professor
Division of Endocrinology, Department of Medicine
University of Colorado School of Medicine
Rocky Mountain Regional Veterans Affairs Medical Center
Aurora, CO, United States

Michael T. McDermott, MD
Professor of Medicine and Clinical Pharmacy
University of Colorado School of Medicine
Director, Endocrinology and Diabetes Practice
University of Colorado Hospital
Aurora, CO, United States

Robert C. McIntyre Jr., MD
Professor
Department of Surgery
University of Colorado Anschutz Medical Campus
Aurora, CO, United States

Logan R. McKenna, MD
Surgical Resident
University of Colorado Anschutz Medical Campus
Aurora, CO, United States

Shon Meek, MD, PhD
Assistant Professor
Endocrinology Division
Mayo Clinic
Jacksonville, FL, United States

Richard Millstein, DO
University of Colorado Health Endocrinology
Greeley, CO United States

Kerrie L. Moreau, PhD
Professor
Division of Geriatrics
University of Colorado Anschutz Medical Campus
Aurora, CO, United States
Research Health Scientist
Geriatric Research Education Clinical Center (GRECC)
Denver Veterans Administration Medical Center
Denver, CO, United States

Wesley Nuffer, PharmD
Associate Professor
Department of Clinical Pharmacy
University of Colorado Skaggs School of Pharmacy &
   Pharmaceutical Sciences
Aurora, CO, United States

John J. Orrego, MD
Endocrinologist
Endocrinology and Metabolism
Colorado Permanente Medical Group
Denver, CO, United States
Endocrinology Department Chair
Endocrinology and Metabolism
St. Joseph Hospital
Denver, CO, United States

Roger A. Piepenbrink, DO, MS, MPH, FACP, FACE
Staff Physician
Departments of Adult Endocrinology and Sleep Medicine
Mike O'Callaghan Federal Medical Center
Nellis Air Force Base
Las Vegas, NV, United States

Christopher D. Raeburn, MD
Associate Professor
Department of Surgery
University of Colorado Anschutz Medical Campus
Aurora, CO, United States

Aziz Ur Rehman, MD
Assistant Professor
Division of Endocrinology
Texas Tech University
El Paso, TX, United States

Richard O. Roberts III, MD, MPH
Fellow Physician
Children's Hospital Colorado
Department of Pediatrics
Section of Endocrinology and Diabetes
University of Colorado Anschutz Medical Campus
Aurora, CO, United States

Kevin B. Rothchild, MD
Assistant Professor
GI, Tumor, and Endocrine Surgery
University of Colorado Hospital
Aurora, CO, United States

Micol Sara Rothman, MD
Associate Professor of Medicine
Endocrinology, Diabetes and Metabolism
University of Colorado School of Medicine
Aurora, CO, United States

Shauna Runchey, MD, MPH
Fellow
University of Colorado Anschutz Medical Campus
Denver, CO, United States

Mary H. Samuels, MD
Professor of Medicine
Program Director, Clinical and Translational Research
   Center
Oregon Health & Science University
Portland, OR, United States

Leonard R. Sanders, MD, FACP, BC-ADM, CDE, CLS
Director of Diabetes Care
Endocrinology
Montage Medical Group
Monterey, CA, United States

Virginia Sarapura, MD
Associate Professor
Medicine-Endocrinology
University of Colorado Anschutz Medical Campus
Aurora, CO, United States

David Saxon, MD, MSc
Assistant Professor
Division of Endocrinology, Metabolism, and Diabetes
University of Colorado
Aurora, CO, United States

Jonathan A. Schoen, MD
Associate Professor of Surgery
GI, Tumor, and Endocrine Surgery
University of Colorado Hospital
Aurora, CO, United States

Emily B. Schroeder, MD, PhD
Clinician Investigator
Institute for Health Research
Kaiser Permanente Colorado
Assistant Professor
Division of Endocrinology, Metabolism and Diabetes
University of Colorado School of Medicine
Aurora, CO, United States

Stacey A. Seggelke, DNP, APRN, ACNS-BC, BC-ADM
Senior Instructor of Medicine
Department of Medicine, Division of Endocrinology
University of Colorado Denver
Aurora, CO, United States

Kenneth J. Simcic, MD[†]
Formerly Assistant Professor
Division of Endocrinology
Department of Medicine
University of Texas Health Science Center at San Antonio
San Antonio, TX, United States

Robert H. Slover, MD
Director of Pediatrics
The Barbara Davis Center for Diabetes
Professor of Pediatrics
Wagner Family Chair in Childhood Diabetes
University of Colorado Denver
Anschutz Medical Campus
Aurora, CO, United States

Robert Smallridge, MD
Professor of Medicine
Endocrinology Division
Mayo Clinic
Jacksonville, FL, United States

Christine M. Swanson, MD, MCR, CCD
Assistant Professor
Division of Endocrinology, Metabolism and Diabetes
University of Colorado
Aurora, CO, United States

Elizabeth A. Thomas, MD
Assistant Professor
Division of Endocrinology, Metabolism and Diabetes
University of Colorado School of Medicine
Rocky Mountain Regional Veterans Affairs Medical
    Center
Aurora, CO, United States

Carlos A. Torres, MD
William Beaumont Army Medical Center
El Paso, TX, United States

Sharon H. Travers, MD
Associate Professor
Pediatric Endocrinology
Children's Hospital Colorado
University of Colorado
Aurora, CO, United States

Jennifer M. Trujillo, PharmD
Associate Professor
Clinical Pharmacy
University of Colorado
Aurora, CO, United States

Amy M. Valent, DO
Assistant Professor
Obstetrics and Gynecology
Oregon Health and Science University
Portland, OR, United States

Nicole Odette Vietor, MD
Department of Endocrinology, Diabetes, and Metabolism
Walter Reed National Military Medical Center
Bethesda, MD, United States

Robert A. Vigersky, MD
Professor of Medicine
Endocrinology Service
Walter Reed National Military Medical Center
Bethesda, MD, United States

Katherine N. Vu, DO
Assistant Professor
Endocrinology Service
Naval Medical Center San Diego
San Diego, CA, United States

Cecilia C. Low Wang, MD, FACP
Associate Professor of Medicine
Associate Director, Fellowship/Education
Division of Endocrinology, Metabolism and Diabetes
University of Colorado School of Medicine
Aurora, CO, United States

Matthew P. Wahl, MD
Assistant Professor of Medicine (Clinical)
Division of Endocrinology Metabolism, and Diabetes
University of Utah School of Medicine
Salt Lake City, UT, United States

Katherine Weber, MD
Endocrinology
Kaiser Permanente
Denver, CO, United States

Margaret E. Wierman, MD
Professor of Medicine
University of Colorado School of Medicine
Aurora, CO, United States

Majlinda Xhikola, MD
Fellow
Endocrinology Division
Mayo Clinic
Jacksonville, FL, United States

Adnin Zaman, MD
Clinical/Research Fellow
Division of Endocrinology, Metabolism and Diabetes
University of Colorado
Aurora, CO, United States

Philip Zeitler, MD, PhD
Professor
Pediatrics
University of Colorado Denver Anschutz Medical Campus
Chair
Endocrinology
Children's Hospital Colorado
Aurora, CO, United States

†Deceased

PREFACE

Medical and scientific investigations are progressing at an astounding pace. It is difficult for any provider, at whatever level, to keep up with the enormous volume of primary research, case reports, review articles, and clinical practice guidelines that are published daily in printed and online forms. The authors of the chapters in this book have carefully reviewed and summarized each specific assigned area and have added their own opinions, based on their extensive clinical experience, to give readers the best possible coverage of these topics in a well-organized and concise form. I thank each author, from mentored fellows to seasoned faculty and practitioners, for their selfless and painstaking efforts to educate our readers with their own unique blends of knowledge, experience, and humanism.

The question-and-answer format, intended to mimic the interchanges between mentors and trainees on rounds, has been preserved and carried on from the 1st Edition (1994) to the current 7th Edition (2019) of *Endocrine Secrets*. But the original goal of 20 questions followed by short and to-the-point answers has been eclipsed by the ever-expanding volume of research discoveries and evidence-based clinical practice guidelines for the multiple conditions and issues in our field. As a result the chapters are necessarily longer now, with more questions and answers than before.

I have also added numerous chapters to cover areas that were not covered in previous editions. One chapter is devoted to case-based practical exercises in carbohydrate counting and insulin dose calculations; another tackles the rapidly expanding field of diabetes technology; and yet another details the causes of spontaneous hypoglycemia, including the cause and management of postbariatric surgery hypoglycemia. There are interesting new chapters on pituitary stalk lesions, adrenal incidentalomas, and polycystic ovary syndrome. There is a specific chapter that covers the emerging field of endocrinopathies resulting from the use of immune checkpoint inhibitors. There are now four separate chapters on endocrine surgery. The new chapter on the care and management of transgender patients is one of the highlights of this edition. Finally, I have included a unique and fascinating chapter detailing the state of Endocrinology in Africa, authored by my valued colleagues from Ethiopia, Dr. Helen Y. Bitew and Dr. Abdurezak A. Abdela.

I hope the readers of this book will find it readable, enjoyable, educational, and sufficiently comprehensive to enable them to practice Endocrinology at the highest possible level for the benefit of all the patients who entrust their care to them. Never stop learning. And I hope that all your patients reap the benefits of your expanding knowledge, devotion to lifelong learning, and continuing compassion for them.

Michael McDermott, MD
Editor, *Endocrine Secrets,* 7th Edition

CONTENTS

TOP SECRETS   **1**

I   FUEL METABOLISM

CHAPTER 1   DIABETES MELLITUS: ETIOLOGY, CLASSIFICATION, AND DIAGNOSIS   8
Adnin Zaman and Cecilia C. Low Wang

CHAPTER 2   DIABETES MELLITUS: ACUTE AND CHRONIC COMPLICATIONS   12
Cecilia C. Low Wang and Adnin Zaman

CHAPTER 3   TYPE 1 DIABETES MELLITUS   21
Jennifer M. Trujillo

CHAPTER 4   TYPE 2 DIABETES MELLITUS   31
Sarah L. Anderson and Jennifer M. Trujillo

CHAPTER 5   DIABETES TECHNOLOGY: PUMPS, SENSORS, AND BEYOND   43
Adnin Zaman and Cecilia C. Low Wang

CHAPTER 6   CARBOHYDRATE COUNTING–GUIDED INSULIN DOSING: PRACTICE EXERCISES   50
Michael T. McDermott

CHAPTER 7   INPATIENT MANAGEMENT OF DIABETES AND HYPERGLYCEMIA   61
Stacey A. Seggelke and R. Matthew Hawkins

CHAPTER 8   DIABETES IN PREGNANCY   67
Amy M. Valent and Linda A. Barbour

CHAPTER 9   HYPOGLYCEMIC DISORDERS   87
Helen M. Lawler

CHAPTER 10   LIPID DISORDERS   92
Emily B. Schroeder and Michael T. McDermott

CHAPTER 11   OBESITY   100
Elizabeth A. Thomas and David Saxon

II   BONE AND MINERAL DISORDERS

CHAPTER 12   OSTEOPOROSIS AND OTHER METABOLIC BONE DISEASES: EVALUATION   110
Michael T. McDermott

CHAPTER 13   MEASUREMENT OF BONE MASS   116
Christine M. Swanson

CHAPTER 14   OSTEOPOROSIS MANAGEMENT   123
Michael T. McDermott

CHAPTER 15   OSTEOMALACIA, RICKETS, AND VITAMIN D INSUFFICIENCY   134
William E. Duncan

CHAPTER 16   PAGET'S DISEASE OF BONE   140
Matthew P. Wahl and Christine M. Swanson

CHAPTER 17   HYPERCALCEMIA   144
Leonard R. Sanders

CHAPTER 18   HYPERPARATHYROIDISM   153
Leonard R. Sanders

CHAPTER 19   HYPERCALCEMIA OF MALIGNANCY   161
Michael T. McDermott

CHAPTER 20   HYPOCALCEMIA   164
Shari C. Fox

CHAPTER 21   NEPHROLITHIASIS   170
Leonard R. Sanders

III   PITUITARY AND HYPOTHALAMIC DISORDERS

CHAPTER 22   PITUITARY INSUFFICIENCY   182
John J. Orrego

CHAPTER 23   NONFUNCTIONING PITUITARY TUMORS AND PITUITARY INCIDENTALOMAS   188
Janice M. Kerr and Michael T. McDermott

CHAPTER 24   PITUITARY STALK LESIONS   196
Janice M. Kerr

CHAPTER 25   PROLACTIN-SECRETING PITUITARY TUMORS   203
Virginia Sarapura

CHAPTER 26   GROWTH HORMONE–SECRETING PITUITARY TUMORS   208
Mary H. Samuels

CHAPTER 27   CUSHING'S SYNDROME   213
Mary H. Samuels

CHAPTER 28   GLYCOPROTEIN-SECRETING PITUITARY TUMORS   219
Majlinda Xhikola, Shon Meek, and Robert C. Smallridge

CHAPTER 29   WATER METABOLISM   225
Leonard R. Sanders

CHAPTER 30   DISORDERS OF GROWTH   243
Philip Zeitler

CHAPTER 31   GROWTH HORMONE USE AND ABUSE   253
Carlos A. Torres and Homer J. LeMar, Jr.

IV   ADRENAL DISORDERS

CHAPTER 32   PRIMARY ALDOSTERONISM   258
John J. Orrego

CHAPTER 33   PHEOCHROMOCYTOMAS AND PARAGANGLIOMAS   265
John J. Orrego

CHAPTER 34   ADRENAL INCIDENTALOMAS   271
Michael T. McDermott

CHAPTER 35   ADRENAL MALIGNANCIES   275
Michael T. McDermott

CHAPTER 36   ADRENAL INSUFFICIENCY   281
Emily B. Schroeder and Cecilia C. Low Wang

CHAPTER 37   CONGENITAL ADRENAL HYPERPLASIA   288
Harris M. Baloch, Nicole Vietor, and Robert A. Vigersky

V THYROID DISORDERS

CHAPTER 38 THYROID TESTING 300
Michael T. McDermott

CHAPTER 39 HYPERTHYROIDISM 304
Thanh D. Hoang and Henry B. Burch

CHAPTER 40 HYPOTHYROIDISM 311
Katherine Weber and Bryan R. Haugen

CHAPTER 41 THYROIDITIS 315
Ayesha F. Malik, Robert C. Smallridge, and Ana Chindris

CHAPTER 42 THYROID NODULES AND GOITER 321
Michele B. Glodowski and Sarah E. Mayson

CHAPTER 43 THYROID CANCER 327
Veena R. Agrawal and Sarah E. Mayson

CHAPTER 44 THYROID EMERGENCIES 335
Michael T. McDermott

CHAPTER 45 EUTHYROID SICK SYNDROME 341
Michael T. McDermott

CHAPTER 46 THYROID DISEASE IN PREGNANCY 345
Meghan Donnelly and Linda A. Barbour

CHAPTER 47 PSYCHIATRIC DISORDERS AND THYROID DISEASE 359
Roselyn I. Mateo and James V. Hennessey

VI REPRODUCTIVE ENDOCRINOLOGY

CHAPTER 48 DIFFERENCES (DISORDERS) OF SEXUAL DIFFERENTIATION 372
Richard O. Roberts, III and Robert H. Slover

CHAPTER 49 DISORDERS OF PUBERTY 382
Shanlee M. Davis and Sharon H. Travers

CHAPTER 50 MALE HYPOGONADISM 393
Katherine N. Vu, Vinh Q. Mai, and Robert A. Vigersky

CHAPTER 51 ERECTILE DYSFUNCTION 404
Mark M. Cruz, Thanh D. Hoang, and Robert A. Vigersky

CHAPTER 52 GYNECOMASTIA 413
Mark Bridenstine, Brenda K. Bell, and Micol S. Rothman

CHAPTER 53 AMENORRHEA 417
Micol S. Rothman and Margaret E. Wierman

CHAPTER 54 POLYCYSTIC OVARIAN SYNDROME 422
Melanie Cree-Green and Anne-Marie Carreau

CHAPTER 55 HIRSUTISM AND VIRILIZATION 427
Tamis M. Bright and Aziz Ur Rehman

CHAPTER 56 MENOPAUSE 433
Wesley Nuffer

CHAPTER 57 GENDER-AFFIRMING TREATMENT FOR ADULTS WITH GENDER INCONGRUENCE
AND GENDER DYSPHORIA 438
Micol S. Rothman and Sean J. Iwamoto

CHAPTER 58 USE AND ABUSE OF ANABOLIC–ANDROGENIC STEROIDS AND ANDROGEN PRECURSORS 446
Carlos A. Torres and Homer J. LeMar, Jr.

VII MISCELLANEOUS TOPICS

CHAPTER 59 AUTOIMMUNE POLYGLANDULAR SYNDROMES 452
Richard Millstein

CHAPTER 60 MULTIPLE ENDOCRINE NEOPLASIA SYNDROMES 455
John J. Orrego

CHAPTER 61 PANCREATIC NEUROENDOCRINE TUMORS 462
Michael T. McDermott

CHAPTER 62 CARCINOID SYNDROME 467
Michael T. McDermott

CHAPTER 63 AGING AND ENDOCRINOLOGY 473
Kerrie L. Moreau, Sean J. Iwamoto, and Shauna Runchey

CHAPTER 64 ENDOCRINOPATHIES CAUSED BY IMMUNE CHECKPOINT INHIBITORS 487
David Saxon and Thomas Jensen

CHAPTER 65 SLEEP AND ENDOCRINOLOGY 493
Roger A. Piepenbrink

CHAPTER 66 THYROID AND PARATHYROID SURGERY 510
Logan R. McKenna, Maria B. Albuja-Cruz, Robert C. McIntyre Jr., and Christopher D. Raeburn

CHAPTER 67 ADRENAL SURGERY 518
Oliver J. Fackelmayer, Chris Raeburn, Robert McIntyre Jr., and Maria Albuja-Cruz

CHAPTER 68 PANCREAS AND OTHER ENDOCRINE TUMOR SURGERY 523
Stephanie Davis, Maria Albuja-Cruz, Chris Raeburn, and Robert McIntyre, Jr.

CHAPTER 69 BARIATRIC SURGERY 527
Jonathan A. Schoen and Kevin B. Rothchild

CHAPTER 70 ENDOCRINOLOGY IN AFRICA 532
Helen Y. Bitew and Abdurezak A. Abdela

CHAPTER 71 FAMOUS PEOPLE WITH ENDOCRINE DISORDERS 535
Pratima Kumar, Kenneth J. Simcic, and Michael T. McDermott

CHAPTER 72 INTERESTING ENDOCRINE FACTS AND FIGURES 539
Michael T. McDermott

CHAPTER 73 ENDOCRINE CASE STUDIES 542
Michael T. McDermott

INDEX 551

TOP SECRETS

Michael T. McDermott

1. Diabetes mellitus results from absolute or relative insulin deficiency. In type 1 diabetes (T1D), the beta cells are destroyed, resulting in complete insulin deficiency. In type 2 diabetes (T2D), the beta cells cannot produce enough insulin to compensate for the underlying insulin resistance and excess hepatic glucose production.
2. The basic principles of diabetic ketoacidosis (DKA) management are: (1) volume repletion, (2) correction of electrolyte abnormalities, (3) insulin therapy for hyperglycemia and ketonemia, and (4) identification and treatment of the precipitating event(s).
3. Hypoglycemia unawareness occurs when a patient has had recurrent hypoglycemia, since repeated episodes of hypoglycemia lower the glucose level that triggers release of counterregulatory hormones. It is reversible with strict avoidance of hypoglycemia for an extended period of time (weeks to months). Hypoglycemia-associated autonomic failure (HAAF) consists of hypoglycemia unawareness and impaired counterregulatory hormone responses.
4. Diabetic kidney disease (DKD) may manifest in various ways. These include albuminuria (urinary albumin excretion), decreased glomerular filtration rate, glomerular hematuria, other abnormalities of the urinary sediment, or abnormalities on imaging studies. Not all individuals with DKD and reduced eGFR have increased albuminuria.
5. The diabetic neuropathies have 2 distinct patterns of progression. Sensory and autonomic neuropathies generally progress gradually with increasing duration of diabetes. In comparison, mononeuropathies, radiculopathies, and acute painful neuropathies present acutely, are short-lived, and resolve completely.
6. An individualized hemoglobin A1C (A1C) target should be established for each patient with T2D. A target A1C < 7% is reasonable for most patients but should be individualized. A more stringent A1C target may be appropriate for young, otherwise healthy patients with newly diagnosed T2D. A less stringent A1C target may be appropriate for older patients with short life expectancies and/or serious comorbidities.
7. Second-line options to add to metformin include glucagon-like peptide receptor 1 agonists (GLP-1 RAs), sodium glucose transporter 2 (SGLT-2) inhibitors, dipeptidyl peptidase 4 (DPP-4) inhibitors, sulfonylureas, thiazolidinediones (TZDs), and basal insulin. The decision about which to add should depend on whether the patient has atherosclerotic cardiovascular disease (ASCVD), heart failure, chronic kidney disease and other patient and drug considerations, such as glycemic efficacy, risk of hypoglycemia, effect on weight, ease of use, mechanism of delivery, cost, and side effects.
8. Women who develop gestational diabetes have a 30-74% risk of developing T2D within 5 to 10 years.
9. Insulin requirements often decrease in the first trimester of pregnancy placing the mother at high risk of severe hypoglycemia, especially at night, but insulin requirements may double or triple in the late second and third trimesters due to the insulin resistance of pregnancy.
10. Hyperinsulinemic hypoglycemia suggests the presence of islet beta-cell hyperfunction (insulinoma, non-insulinoma pancreatogenous hypoglycemia syndrome, or post-gastric bypass hypoglycemia), the surreptitious use of insulin or oral hypoglycemic agents, or insulin autoimmune hypoglycemia.
11. Non-insulin mediated hypoglycemia may be secondary to critical illness, starvation, alcohol abuse, adrenal insufficiency, non-islet cell tumors, glycogen storage diseases, or consumption of an unripe ackee fruit.
12. Food and Drug Administration–approved medications to help overweight and obese patients lose weight are phentermine, orlistat, lorcaserin, phentermine/topiramate ER, naltrexone/bupropion SR, and liraglutide 3.0 mg.
13. Disorders causing secondary bone loss are present in approximately 1/3 of women and 2/3 of men who have osteoporosis.
14. If a patient has a fragility fracture, this establishes the diagnosis of osteoporosis regardless of the patient's bone mineral density (BMD) or FRAX risk score.
15. T-scores are preferentially used to diagnose low BMD and osteoporosis in postmenopausal women and men ≥ 50 years old, but Z-scores can provide additional insight on possible underlying causes of low BMD and osteoporosis.
16. Dual energy x-ray absorptiometry (DEXA) cannot establish why BMD is low – an appropriate medical evaluation to exclude secondary causes of osteoporosis (e.g., osteomalacia) should be performed.
17. Pharmacological therapy should be offered to patients who have had a fragility fracture, a BMD T-score ≤ −2.5, or a FRAX-derived 10-year risk of ≥ 3% for hip fractures and ≥ 20% for other major osteoporosis fractures.
18. Osteonecrosis of the jaw (ONJ) and atypical femoral fractures (AFF) are uncommon complications that can result from the use of anti-resorptive agents to treat osteoporosis, but these complications do not occur with the osteoanabolic agents.

19. The causes of osteomalacia and rickets fall into three categories: (A) deficient vitamin D and/or calcium intake in children or disorders associated with abnormal vitamin D metabolism or action; (B) disorders associated with abnormal phosphate metabolism; and (C) a small group of disorders with normal vitamin D and mineral metabolism.

20. Paget's disease of bone (PDB) is a chronic condition characterized by focal areas of abnormal osteoclast activity that causes excessive bone resorption, followed by abnormal bone formation resulting in disorganized, weak bone.

21. The treatment of choice of PDB is IV zoledronate; treatment is indicated in PDB patients with symptomatic bone pain, hypercalcemia, and those at high risk of developing complications from PDB or undergoing surgery at or near a Pagetic site.

22. Although there are more than 30 different causes of hypercalcemia, hyperparathyroidism and hypercalcemia of malignancy account for more than 90% of cases.

23. Recommendations for surgery in patients with asymptomatic primary hyperparathyroidism include any one of the following: serum calcium more than 1.0 mg/dL above the normal upper limit; decreased estimated GFR < 60 mL/min; calcium nephrolithiasis or nephrocalcinosis; 24-h urine calcium > 400 mg/d and increased stone risk by biochemical analysis; reduced bone density with T-score ≤ -2.5; fragility fracture; or increased fracture assessment risk; and age less than 50 years.

24. Humoral Hypercalcemia of Malignancy (HMM) usually results from solid tumor production of parathyroid hormone–related peptide (PTHrp), which binds to parathyroid hormone (PTH) and PTH/PTHrp receptors to stimulate bone resorption and renal tubular calcium reabsorption.

25. Calcitriol Mediated Hypercalcemia occurs when granulomatous disorders (especially sarcoidosis) or marrow/hematologic malignancies express 1 alpha hydroxylase, resulting in production of high levels of 1,25 (OH)2 Vitamin D.

26. Hypocalcemia is a frequent problem in trauma and intensive care settings and is often a result of intravenous agents.

27. Kidney stone prevalence has increased in the US and likely relates to dietary and lifestyle changes associated with increased obesity and the metabolic syndrome; increased sodium and animal protein intake; and decreased intake of fiber, fruits, vegetables and water.

28. Kidney stones form because of supersaturation of urinary stone precursors (such as calcium and oxalate), insufficient stone inhibitors (such as citrate), abnormal urine pH, or low urine volume.

29. Traumatic brain injury and subarachnoid hemorrhage are increasingly recognized as causes of hypopituitarism.

30. The best biochemical indicator of optimal thyroid hormone replacement therapy in patients with central hypothyroidism is a serum free T4 concentration in the mid- to upper-half of the reference range.

31. Silent and pluri-hormonal pituitary adenomas are characteristically aggressive, invasive, and frequently recurrent tumors that may later transform to functionally-active tumors.

32. A serum prolactin level higher than 200 ng/mL is almost always indicative of a prolactin-secreting tumor, except during pregnancy.

33. Dopamine agonist treatment of patients with prolactinomas is well tolerated and quickly effective in normalizing the serum prolactin level and shrinking the tumor mass of even very large prolactin-secreting tumors.

34. Acromegaly causes damage to bones, joints, the heart, and other organs and is associated with considerable morbidity and excess mortality.

35. The best screening test for acromegaly is a serum insulin-like growth factor type 1 (IGF-1) level.

36. Screening biochemical tests for Cushing's syndrome can be misleading, and repeated testing or more extensive confirmatory testing is often necessary.

37. Hyperthyroid patients with detectable serum TSH levels should always be evaluated for inappropriate TSH secretion (either a TSH tumor or thyroid hormone resistance), but assay interference is a more common cause.

38. Hypothyroidism can produce thyrotroph hyperplasia and pituitary pseudotumors with hyperprolactinemia.

39. Hypophysitis can be divided into primary (autoimmune mediated) and secondary (systemic inflammatory and infectious mediated) etiologies.

40. A biopsy of pituitary stalk lesions is recommended for: stalk lesions > 6.5 mm, progressive growth, hypopituitarism, unclear diagnosis, and lack of alternative tissue sites for biopsy. Transsphenoidal surgical resection can also be considered for a presumed pituitary stalk neoplasm.

41. Effective correction of water balance disorders requires addressing abnormalities of plasma sodium (P_{Na}) and a clear understanding of changes in plasma and urine osmolality, urine sodium and potassium, and effective circulating volume (ECV). A thorough assessment of neurologic symptoms is also essential.

42. If neurologic symptoms occur rapidly or are severe, correction of P_{Na} toward normal should be rapid; if symptoms are absent, there is no urgency, and P_{Na} correction should occur more slowly to avoid osmotic demyelinating syndrome in the brain.

43. An abnormal growth velocity for age generally distinguishes growth abnormalities from normal growth variants, which are the most frequent causes of apparent growth abnormalities; poor growth secondary to chronic medical illness is the next most frequent cause, while hormonal disorders are less common.

44. Growth hormone abuse is used by athletes to enhance performance, but little evidence supports meaningful performance enhancement, except for some increase in anaerobic exercise capacity.

45. Spontaneous hypokalemia in a hypertensive patient should suggest the possibility of primary aldosteronism – but normokalemic hypertension is the most common presentation.

46. The best test for primary aldosteronism case detection is a plasma aldosterone to renin ratio.
47. The best screening tests for pheochromocytomas and paragangliomas are fractionated urinary or plasma free metanephrines.
48. About 30-40% of pheochromocytoma and paraganglioma patients have a disease causing germline mutation.
49. Incidentally discovered adrenal masses are most often benign non-functioning adrenal cortical adenomas; the most common hormonal abnormality seen with adrenal incidentalomas is autonomous cortisol secretion, which is best detected with a 1 mg overnight dexamethasone suppression test.
50. Features suggesting that an adrenal tumor is malignant are size > 6 cm, heterogeneity, calcifications, irregular borders, local invasion, lymphadenopathy, decreased lipid content (Hounsfield Units > 20), or elevated levels of serum androgens or urinary or plasma dopamine.
51. Surgery is the treatment of choice for all malignant adrenal tumors; mitotane with or without chemotherapy and tumor bed radiation therapy is recommended as adjuvant therapy for adrenocortical carcinomas.
52. Adrenal insufficiency should be suspected in outpatients who have received supraphysiologic doses of glucocorticoids for > 1 month, intensive care unit (ICU) patients, especially those with septic shock who are hemodynamically unstable despite aggressive fluid and pressor resuscitation, and any patient with signs or symptoms suggesting adrenal insufficiency.
53. Adrenal crisis should be treated aggressively using IV saline and dextrose, IV glucocorticoids (dexamethasone if treating before drawing random cortisol and ACTH, hydrocortisone afterwards), other supportive care, and a search for the precipitating illness.
54. Congenital adrenal hyperplasia (CAH), the most common inherited disease, is a group of autosomal recessive disorders, the most frequent of which is 21-hydroxylase deficiency.
55. Serum thyroid-stimulating hormone (TSH) measurement is the best overall test to screen and evaluate patients for thyroid disease. Serum free thyroxine (T4) should be measured in all patients whose TSH is elevated, and serum free T4 and total triiodothyronine (T3) should be measured in patients whose TSH is suppressed.
56. Biotin supplements and human anti-mouse antibodies (HAMA) can cause significant interference with assays used to evaluate the thyroid system and multiple other hormones.
57. Once hyperthyroidism is diagnosed based on clinical features and testing with TSH, free T4 and total T3, the etiology can be determined with a radioiodine uptake (RAIU) measurement and thyroid radionuclide scanning, measurement of TSH-receptor antibodies, or with the use of color-flow Doppler in experienced hands.
58. The major treatment choices for hyperthyroidism are antithyroid drugs (usually methimazole), radioiodine ablation and thyroidectomy. Beta-blockers can significantly improve adrenergic symptoms of thyrotoxicosis and do not interfere with testing or later treatment.
59. Levothyroxine (LT_4) is the preferred initial treatment for hypothyroidism; a full replacement dose of 1.6 mcg/kg/day can be started in healthy young patients but patients over age 60 years or with known coronary artery disease should be started on 25-50 mcg daily, to avoid precipitating myocardial ischemia, with gradual dose titration until the serum TSH is within the target range.
60. Many, but not all, experts consider the goal serum TSH level on treatment in most younger patients with primary hypothyroidismto to be 0.5-2.0 mU/L but current recommendations state that a target serum TSH level of 4.0-6.0 mU/L may be preferable in patients over age 70-75 years.
61. Approximately 10% of premenopausal women are TPO-antibody positive and many develop postpartum thyroid dysfunction.
62. The decision to biopsy a thyroid nodule depends on its size and sonographic features.
63. Molecular testing can be useful in the management of thyroid nodules with indeterminate cytology, specifically for Bethesda III and IV cytology.
64. Prognosis in DTC is determined by initial staging, risk stratification, and ongoing assessment of response to therapy.
65. Pregnant women with current Graves' disease or a history of Graves' disease (regardless of history of thyroid ablation or thyroidectomy) should be evaluated for TRAb and TSI. If levels are ≥ 3 times elevated at 18 weeks or beyond, the fetus should be monitored for the development of fetal and neonatal Graves' disease.
66. Thyroid hormone requirements usually increase in pregnancy, beginning in the 1st trimester, and it is reasonable to increase thyroid hormone doses by 25% in athyreotic women as soon as pregnancy is confirmed. Only LT4 (not T3) should be used for thyroid hormone replacement during pregnancy and a full replacement dose is estimated at ~ 2 mcg/kg in pregnancy.
67. Euthyroid sick syndrome (non-thyroidal illness syndrome) appears to be an adaptive response to reduce tissue metabolism and preserve energy during systemic illnesses; therefore, treatment with thyroid hormone is not generally recommended but may be beneficial in patients with chronic heart failure.
68. Normalization of the serum TSH level with levothyroxine (LT4) therapy may completely reverse the neuropsychiatric features of overt hypothyroidism but is far less likely to be effective if the symptoms are not due to the under-lying hypothyroidism.
69. When thyroid storm is diagnosed or suspected, treatment with antithyroid drugs, cold iodine, beta-blockers, and stress doses of glucocorticoids, along with management of any precipitating factors, should be promptly initiated.

70. When myxedema coma is diagnosed or suspected, management should include rapid repletion of thyroid hormones, stress glucocorticoid doses, and treatment of any precipitating causes.

71. Evaluation of sexual ambiguity must consider the major categories of children presenting with this problem: virilized 46XX females, under-virilized 46XY males, disorders of gonadal differentiation including chromosomal abnormalities, and unclassified forms (cryptorchidism, hypospadias, developmental anomalies).

72. Central precocious puberty occurs more frequently in girls than boys. Boys with central precocity, however, have a much higher incidence of underlying central nervous system pathology.

73. Children with delayed puberty and normal linear growth will most likely have constitutional growth delay.

74. Monitor patients on testosterone replacement for polycythemia, sleep apnea, gynecomastia, psychological difficulties, prostate size, prostate symptoms and PSA increases.

75. The cause of impotence can be identified in 85% of men. Besides diabetes mellitus, the three most common endocrine causes of impotence are primary hypogonadism, secondary hypogonadism and hyperprolactinemia.

76. Rapid breast enlargement, size > 4 cm, pain, and age < 10 years or between 20 and 50 years correlate with a systemic illness/pathological cause for gynecomastia; these men should be evaluated thoroughly if the cause is not apparent after the history and physical examination.

77. Hyperprolactinemia and hypothalamic amenorrhea are the most common causes of acquired (secondary) amenorrhea with low estrogen and low follicle-stimulating hormone (FSH) levels.

78. Premature ovarian insufficiency is an autoimmune disease; affected patients are at risk for other autoimmune disorders, such as adrenal and thyroid disease, pernicious anemia, celiac sprue, and rheumatologic disorders.

79. Polycystic ovarian syndrome (PCOS) is the most common type of hyperandrogenic amenorrhea, and is associated with risks of infertility, endometrial cancer, metabolic syndrome, and type 2 diabetes

80. The common causes of hirsutism are PCOS, nonclassical CAH (NCCAH), idiopathic or familial hirsutism, and medications; the common causes of virilization are ovarian tumors, adrenal tumors, and CAH.

81. While having an excellent study design, the Women's Health Initiative (WHI) trial results may not accurately translate to all women in menopause due to the wide age range of enrollment up through age 79.

82. Autoimmune polyglandular syndrome type 1 (APS 1), which results from mutations in the autoimmune regulator (AIRE) gene, consists of mucocutaneous candidiasis, hypoparathyroidism, and adrenal insufficiency as well as other autoimmune conditions; autoimmune polyglandular syndrome type 2 (APS 2), a polygenic HLA related disorder, consists of adrenal insufficiency, type 1 diabetes mellitus, and thyroid disorders as well as other autoimmune conditions.

83. Multiple Endocrine Neoplasia Type 1 (MEN1), due to germline mutations in the Menin gene, consists of neoplastic transformation in at least two of these three glands: parathyroid glands, pancreas, and anterior pituitary; testing for the mutation is currently available.

84. Multiple Endocrine Neoplasia Type 2A (MEN2A) consists of neoplastic transformation of parathyroid glands, thyroid parafollicular C cells, and adrenal medullae while MEN2B consists of neoplastic transformation of thyroid parafollicular C cells and adrenal medullae, with mucosal neuromas and marfanoid habitus; germline mutations in the Ret gene are responsible for both disorders and genetic testing is available to identify these mutations.

85. Suspected insulinomas are investigated by measuring serum glucose, insulin, C-peptide, proinsulin, beta hydroxybutyrate and a sulfonylurea screen during a symptomatic episode or a supervised fast.

86. Gastrinomas are diagnosed by finding a markedly elevated serum gastrin level or a prominent increase in gastrin after intravenous secretin administration in a patient with significant gastric acidity.

87. Carcinoid syndrome results from metastatic neuroendocrine tumors (NETs) that produce multiple humoral mediators that cause flushing, diarrhea, bronchospasm, and fibrosis of the endocardium, heart valves, pleura, peritoneum and retroperitoneal spaces; carcinoid syndrome is best diagnosed by demonstrating markedly increased urinary excretion of 5-hydroxyindoleacetic acid (5-HIAA).

88. Carcinoid crisis is best treated with intravenous octreotide and hydrocortisone and avoiding the use of adrenergic and sympathomimetic agents for the hypotension.

89. Sleep-wake regulators and neuroendocrine controllers are co-located in the hypothalamus and are responsible for functional integration to accomplish and protect homeostasis; this likely underlies the overlap of sleep maladies and endocrine disorders.

90. The endocrine diseases associated with abnormal sleep include: type 2 diabetes mellitus, obesity, acromegaly, hyperthyroidism, hypothyroidism, and polycystic ovarian syndrome.

91. Gender incongruence can lead to gender dysphoria, which is the distress and unease that may occur when a person's gender identity and/or gender expression differs from that which was assigned at birth.

92. Gender-affirming hormone therapy is associated with many benefits for patients. Hormone preparations that allow for monitoring of serum levels are preferred, with dose adjustments made to keep estradiol and testosterone levels within the desired ranges and to balance risks with benefits.

93. The use of immune checkpoint inhibitors (ICPis) to treat advanced cancers is growing and these agents have the potential to cause a variety of endocrinopathies. The most common endocrinopathies associated with ICPis are acute hypophysitis (with accompanying central adrenal insufficiency, central hypothyroidism, and hypogonadotropic hypogonadism) and thyroid dysfunction.

94. Most hormonal axes are associated with a gradual decline over time, beginning at about age 30, with the exception of the relatively rapid decline in estradiol associated with the menopause transition in women.

95. Low-risk thyroid micro-carcinomas (< 1 cm, no invasion or evidence of nodal/distant metastasis) can sometimes be managed by active surveillance if both the patient and physician agree; otherwise, a thyroid lobectomy should be performed unless there is a clear indication to remove the contralateral lobe.
96. Current guidelines recommend that the initial surgical procedure for unifocal thyroid tumors 1-4 cm in size without extrathyroidal extension and without nodal/distant metastases can be *either* thyroidectomy *or* thyroid lobectomy.
97. Insulinomas are the most common functional pancreatic neuroendocrine tumor (PNET), are usually benign, and in most cases can be treated by enucleation; gastrinomas are usually malignant and can occur in the pancreas, duodenum (most common), and lymph nodes.
98. PNETs in patients with multiple endocrine neoplasia type 1 (MEN-1) are most commonly gastrinomas, are frequently multifocal, and are usually treated medically. Tumors > 2 cm should be resected.
99. Biopsy of an adrenal mass is only indicated if a metastatic deposit in the adrenal gland is suspected and the biopsy results will alter management of the primary malignancy. Pheochromocytoma must be ruled out prior adrenal biopsy.
100. Surgery is the only therapy that consistently results in significant, long-term weight loss in morbidly obese patients. Laparoscopic Sleeve Gastrectomy is now the most common bariatric operation performed in the U.S., followed by the Laparoscopic Roux-en-Y gastric bypass. These procedures typically result in loss of 60-80% of excess weight (weight above ideal body weight).

I

FUEL METABOLISM

CHAPTER 1

DIABETES MELLITUS: ETIOLOGY, CLASSIFICATION, AND DIAGNOSIS

Adnin Zaman and Cecilia C. Low Wang

1. What is diabetes mellitus?

   Diabetes mellitus is a term that encompasses a heterogeneous group of metabolic disorders, all of which are characterized by elevated blood glucose levels.

2. What is the origin of the term *diabetes mellitus*?

   Although diabetes has been described in literature as ancient as the Ebers Papyrus of Egypt by Hesy-Ra (1552 BCE), the word *diabetes* comes from Arateus and the Greek word "diabainein" which means "siphon," because affected people excreted excessive amounts of urine. The term *diabetes mellitus* was coined by Thomas Willis of Oxford, England, in 1675, when it was discovered that the urine of people with diabetes was sweet rather than tasteless (insipidus).

3. What is the epidemiology of diabetes?

   Approximately 1.5 million Americans are diagnosed with diabetes each year. Thirty million Americans, or nearly 9% of the population, had diabetes mellitus in 2015. Of this, 1.25 million children and adults had type 1 diabetes. However, evidence suggests that out of the 30 million adults with diabetes, 7.2 million remain undiagnosed. The number of individuals with prediabetes is roughly 84 million. American Indians and Alaskan Natives have the highest rate of diabetes (15.1%), whereas non-Hispanic whites have the lowest prevalence.

4. What is the underlying pathophysiology of the two most common types of diabetes?

   Type 1 diabetes results from autoimmune destruction of pancreatic beta cells causing complete or nearly complete insulin deficiency. Type 2 diabetes is characterized by excessive hepatic glucose production, tissue insulin resistance, and relative insulin deficiency, resulting in insufficient beta cell insulin production to compensate for the increased insulin requirements. In both cases, it is ultimately the absolute or relative insulin deficiency that results in elevated blood glucose levels.

5. Why do people get diabetes?

   Type 1 diabetes occurs in people who have an inherited susceptibility (genetic—HLA related) and later a superimposed environmental trigger (theories have focused on food exposures, viral infections, and alterations of the intestinal microbiome). Type 2 diabetes has an even stronger genetic influence (polygenic, but not yet well defined) and more established environmental triggers (obesity, physical inactivity, glucocorticoid therapy).

6. How is diabetes diagnosed?

   Diabetes is diagnosed through laboratory testing; there are several criteria for the diagnosis of diabetes. Ideally, two tests on different occasions are needed to confirm the diagnosis:

   a. Hemoglobin A_{1c} (HbA_{1c}) $\geq$ 6.5% (HbA_{1c} of 5.7%–6.4% establishes a diagnosis of prediabetes
   b. Fasting plasma glucose $\geq$ 126 mg/dL. *Fasting* is defined as no caloric intake for at least 8 hours
   c. Random plasma glucose $\geq$ 200 mg/dL in a patient with classic symptoms of hyperglycemia
   d. Oral glucose tolerance test with a 2-hour plasma glucose $\geq$ 200 mg/dL after a 75-g load of anhydrous glucose dissolved in water

7. What is the current classification for different types of diabetes?

   Previously, diabetes was classified as type 1, type 2, gestational, or "secondary" diabetes. The most current classification of diabetes includes type 1, type 2, type 3c (pancreatogenous), gestational (type 4), latent autoimmune diabetes of adulthood (LADA), and maturity-onset diabetes of the young (MODY), among many others.

   European investigators have recently proposed that types of diabetes be divided into five relatively distinct groups, which may offer greater predictability for diabetes-related outcomes:

   Cluster 1 (severe autoimmune diabetes)—early-onset disease, low body mass index (BMI), poor metabolic control, insulin deficiency, glutamic acid decarboxylase antibody (GAD Ab) positive
   Cluster 2 (severe insulin-deficient diabetes)—similar to cluster 1, but GAD Ab negative
   Cluster 3 (severe insulin-resistant diabetes)—high BMI and insulin resistance
   Cluster 4 (mild obesity-related diabetes)—high BMI, but no insulin resistance
   Cluster 5 (mild age-related diabetes)—similar to cluster 4, but higher age at diagnosis, and with modest metabolic derangements

Table 1.1. Classification of Diabetes Based in Antibody Status and Beta Cell Function.

	A+	A−
β+	A+/β+ Presence of autoantibodies but preserved β-cell function (ex. LADA)	A−/β+ Absence of autoantibodies and preserved β-cell function (ex. type 2 DM)
β−	A+/β− Presence of autoantibodies and absent β-cell function (ex. type 1 DM)	A−/β− Absence of autoantibodies with absent β-cell function (ex. type 3c DM)

DM, Diabetes mellitus; *LADA,* latent autoimmune diabetes of adulthood.

Another way to classify diabetes is to consider antibody status and beta cell function (Aβ±), which places all forms of diabetes along a spectrum. In this system, for example, type 1 diabetes would be reclassified as autoimmune positive and beta cell negative (A+/β−) to indicate that it is a disease of hyperglycemia in the presence of autoimmunity with no beta cell production of insulin. Similarly, one might think of LADA as A+/β+ (autoimmune disorder of pancreas but with continued beta cell function) and type 2 diabetes as A−/β+ and postpancreatectomy diabetes as A−/β− (Table 1.1).

8. What is the natural history of type 1 diabetes?

The natural history of type 1 diabetes involves lifelong requirement for insulin therapy. Soon after the diagnosis of type 1 diabetes is made, there is often a "honeymoon phase," during which beta cells are still able to produce small amounts of insulin. Patients usually still require insulin during this time but at generally smaller doses than later in the course of their diabetes. Without insulin therapy, patients develop a life-threatening condition known as *diabetic ketoacidosis* (DKA; see Chapter 2). If hyperglycemia is not adequately controlled, patients may suffer from chronic complications of diabetes, such as retinopathy, diabetic kidney disease, and neuropathy.

9. What is the natural history of type 2 diabetes?

In individuals with type 2 diabetes, generally there is some degree of insulin resistance in the initial stages, but eventually, insulin deficiency develops and worsens over time. Diabetes (with hyperglycemia) does not develop until pancreatic beta cells become incapable of producing enough insulin to compensate for the individual's insulin resistance. Noninsulin medications are often effective in restoring euglycemia initially, but multiple agents are often needed over time to maintain glycemic control. If patients are on several noninsulin agents but have not achieved their goal HbA$_{1c}$, insulin can be added to the regimen. Some patients with type 2 diabetes may ultimately require basal-bolus insulin therapy (as with type 1 diabetes) to achieve glycemic control. Weight loss is an effective strategy to reduce insulin resistance and usually allows patients to reduce the number of medications needed to achieve and maintain their goal HbA$_{1c}$.

10. Who develops ketosis-prone diabetes?

A less commonly encountered form of diabetes is characterized by a temporary lack of insulin production by pancreatic beta cells. Ketosis-prone diabetes disproportionately affects nonwhite individuals. Patients with DKA require insulin therapy to manage this condition and for a short time after resolution of DKA. However, in most individuals, beta cell function is eventually recovered, and insulin therapy can be tapered off within a few months. In fact, patients tend to become hypoglycemic within weeks of hospital discharge if maintained on their original basal-bolus regimen unless the clinician and patient closely monitor blood glucose values to scale back the insulin regimen. Once the immediate post-DKA period of glucose toxicity is overcome and beta cell function is regained, patients can typically be maintained on one or more noninsulin agents. Without lifestyle modifications and medication adherence, patients are at risk for a repeating cycle of DKA–glucose toxicity–insulin dependence–possible hypoglycemia–recovery.

11. What is LADA?

LADA is a form of autoimmune diabetes with onset later in life compared with typical type 1 diabetes. This was previously thought to be a rare cause of diabetes, and individuals were often misdiagnosed as having type 2 diabetes because of the later age of presentation. However, unlike patients with type 2 diabetes, patients with LADA have positive antibodies (usually GAD Ab). After their initial presentation, they may go through a "honeymoon phase," during which noninsulin agents are sufficient to achieve and maintain glycemic control. However, as beta cell failure progresses, patients eventually require insulin and ultimately experience a course similar to those with type 1 diabetes.

12. What other causal factors should I be thinking about when I see a patient with high glucose?

When evaluating a patient with high blood glucose, a new diagnosis of diabetes or existing poorly controlled diabetes should always be at the forefront of consideration. However, there are other causes of hyperglycemia that ought to be considered. The most common non–diabetes-related cause is glucocorticoid administration. Although most individuals do not develop hyperglycemia while on steroids, these medications (given via any route) may precipitate hyperglycemia in those with underlying glucose intolerance. Critical illnesses and medical conditions, such as infections, may also cause hyperglycemia because of stress-induced increase in cortisol production. Similarly, hyperglycemia may develop in patients with endogenous hypercortisolism (Cushing syndrome)—either from overproduction of adrenocorticotropic hormone (ACTH) by a pituitary tumor or ectopic tumor or from overproduction of cortisol by an adrenal tumor. Other rare causes of hyperglycemia include acromegaly resulting from a growth hormone–secreting pituitary adenoma or a catecholamine-producing tumor, such as a pheochromocytoma or paraganglioma. In the inpatient setting, patients with glucose intolerance receiving intravenous dextrose as either maintenance fluid or with IV medications may also develop hyperglycemia. Those receiving enteral nutrition or total parenteral nutrition are at particularly high risk for developing hyperglycemia when nutrition is delivered in this nonphysiologic manner.

13. **What is type 3c diabetes?**

Also known as *pancreatogenic* or *pancreatogenous diabetes*, type 3c diabetes is a form of diabetes that develops when nonautoimmune disorders of the pancreas compromise pancreatic endocrine function, resulting in decreased insulin production. Patients who have had recurrent acute pancreatitis or chronic pancreatitis; those who have sustained abdominal trauma, such as from a motor vehicle accident; and those who have undergone partial or complete pancreatectomy are most likely to develop type 3c diabetes.

14. **Who should be screened for diabetes?**

The United States Preventive Services Task Force (USPSTF) recommends screening for abnormal fasting plasma glucose levels in overweight and obese adults ages 40 to 70 years. People who have a family history of diabetes, those who have a history of gestational diabetes or polycystic ovarian syndrome, and those who are members of certain racial/ethnic groups (African American, American Indian or Alaskan Native, Asian American, Hispanic or Latino American, or Native Hawaiian/Pacific Islander in origin) may develop diabetes at a younger age or at a lower BMI and, therefore, should be screened earlier. The American Diabetes Association (ADA) has made similar recommendations and suggests screening every 3 years starting at age 45 years with a fasting plasma glucose test.

15. **Can diabetes be prevented?**

The Diabetes Prevention Program (DPP) has demonstrated the significant beneficial effects of intensive lifestyle modifications in patients with prediabetes to prevent progression to diabetes. Randomized controlled trials have shown that pharmacotherapy may also reduce the rates of progression to overt diabetes in individuals at high risk for type 2 diabetes, but the risks of these medications may outweigh their benefits in some patients. The ADA recommends pharmacotherapy for patients who are at high risk for progression to diabetes because of multiple risk factors at baseline and for those who have a persistently elevated $HbA_{1c} > 6\%$ despite lifestyle modifications.

Although numerous strategies have been evaluated in controlled clinical trials, no therapies have been demonstrated to effectively prevent the progression of type 1 diabetes.

16. **What is monogenic diabetes?**

Unlike type 1 and type 2 diabetes, which are multifactorial in etiology, monogenic diabetes results from single gene mutations causing pancreatic beta cell dysfunction or insulin signaling defects. Patients are typically young at the time of diagnosis, do not require insulin, and lack autoantibodies. Monogenic diabetes is often inherited in an autosomal dominant pattern, and it is common to have multiple generations of family members affected. Neonatal diabetes and MODY are the two more common forms of monogenic diabetes. Identification of the affected genes is beneficial from a therapeutic standpoint because the various forms of monogenic diabetes are treated differently. For example, MODY3 is caused by a mutation in the hepatocyte nuclear factor-1 alpha and is most effectively treated with sulfonylureas, whereas MODY2 results from a defect in the glucokinase gene and is best treated with dietary changes alone.

17. **How can insulin resistance be assessed clinically?**

Insulin resistance has a wide array of clinical manifestations, including acanthosis nigricans, skin tags, hirsutism, ovarian hyperandrogenism, and androgenic alopecia. Of these, acanthosis nigricans is the most commonly recognized sign and is described as symmetric, velvety, light brown to black, thickened plaques and accentuated skin marks that appear on knuckles and in intertriginous areas. The pathophysiology is thought to be stimulation of insulin growth factor-1 receptors in fibroblasts and keratinocytes by extremely high insulin levels, resulting in proliferation of these skin cells. Insulin resistance can be estimated in patients without diabetes by using the Homeostatic Model Assessment of Insulin Resistance (HOMA-IR) score after measuring fasting blood glucose and serum insulin levels. Measurements of insulin resistance, such as the hyperinsulinemic euglycemic clamp, are used in the research setting but not in the clinical setting.

18. **What is metabolic syndrome?**

The diagnosis of metabolic syndrome requires at least 3 out of 5 of the following: hyperglycemia, hypertension, hypertriglyceridemia, low levels of high-density lipoprotein (HDL), or increased abdominal circumference. When present, metabolic syndrome is associated with significantly increased risk of heart disease, stroke, and diabetes (if not already present). Treatment to reduce the risk for cardiovascular events requires intensive lifestyle modification with dietary changes, exercise, and weight loss. Often, medications are needed to treat each individual component of metabolic syndrome.

KEY POINTS

- Diabetes results from absolute or relative insulin deficiency. In type 1 diabetes, beta cells are destroyed, resulting in complete insulin deficiency. In type 2 diabetes, beta cells cannot produce enough insulin to compensate for the underlying insulin resistance.
- Diabetes is diagnosed via blood testing and requires abnormal results on two separate occasions to confirm the diagnosis. The diagnostic criteria include $HbA_{1c} \geq$ 6.5%, fasting plasma glucose $\geq$ 126 mg/dL, random plasma glucose $\geq$ 200 mg/dL in addition to the typical symptoms of diabetes, or plasma glucose $\geq$ 200 mg/dL 2 hours after receiving a 75-g glucose load during an oral glucose tolerance test (OGTT).
- There are several ways to classify the types of diabetes. The first method involves classifying diabetes as type 1, type 2, type 3c, gestational (type 4), and "other." Diabetes can also be conceptualized as falling on a spectrum of autoimmunity and beta cell function (A $+/\beta-$). More recently, some investigators have proposed that the types of diabetes be divided into five distinct groups, which may be more helpful in predicting diabetes-related outcomes.
- Patients with type 1 diabetes require lifelong insulin therapy, although there is often a short-lived initial "honeymoon phase" during which pancreatic beta cells are still able to produce a small amount of insulin. In comparison, the natural history of type 2 diabetes involves insulin resistance that develops before beta cell dysfunction, at which stage patients can be managed with noninsulin agents, but progressive insulin deficiency ensues. Approximately half the patients with type 2 diabetes in the United States are on insulin therapy with or without noninsulin agent(s).
- When evaluating a patient with hyperglycemia, a new diagnosis of diabetes or preexisting diabetes should be at the forefront of consideration. However, glucocorticoids, critical illness, or medical therapies, such as enteral or parenteral nutrition, may cause stress hyperglycemia. Acromegaly and pheochromocytoma are rare causes of hyperglycemia and diabetes.

BIBLIOGRAPHY

Ahlqvist, E., Storm, P., Käräjämäki, A., Martinell, M., Dorkhan, M., Carlsson, A., … Groop, L. (2018). Novel subgroups of adult-onset diabetes and their association with outcomes: a data-driven cluster analysis of six variables. *Lancet Diabetes & Endocrinology, 6,* 361–369.

American Diabetes Association. (2018). Classification and diagnosis of diabetes: standards of medical care in diabetes—2018. *Diabetes Care, 41*(Suppl. 1), S13–S27.

Balasubramanyam, A., Nalini, R., Hampe, C. S., & Maldonado, M. (2008). Syndromes of ketosis-prone diabetes mellitus. *Endocrine Reviews, 29,* 292–302.

Duggan, S. N., & Conlon, K. C. (2017). Pancreatogenic type 3c diabetes: underestimated, underappreciated and poorly managed. *Practical Gastroenterology, 163,* 14–23.

Fajans, S. S., & Bell, G. I. (2011). MODY: history, genetics, pathophysiology, and clinical decision making. *Diabetes Care, 34*(8), 1878–1884.

González-Saldivar, G., Rodríguez-Gutiérrez, R., Ocampo-Candiani, J., González-González, J. G., & Gómez-Flores, M. (2017). Skin manifestations of insulin resistance: from a biochemical stance to a clinical diagnosis and management. *Dermatologic Therapy, 7*(1), 37–51.

U.S. Preventive Services Task Force. (2018, April). *Final recommendation statement: abnormal blood glucose and type 2 diabetes mellitus: screening.* Rockville, MD: U.S. Preventive Services Task Force.

CHAPTER 2

DIABETES MELLITUS: ACUTE AND CHRONIC COMPLICATIONS

Cecilia C. Low Wang and Adnin Zaman

1. What are the acute complications of diabetes?
   Diabetic ketoacidosis (DKA), hyperglycemic hyperosmolar state (HHS), and hypoglycemia.

2. What symptoms are characteristic of hyperglycemia?
   Patients are often asymptomatic, but when the hyperglycemia is severe, individuals may report the "3 P's"—polyuria, polydipsia and polyphagia—along with blurry vision and fatigue. Patients may note more frequent urinary tract or genitourinary infections and/or delayed healing of skin infections or ulcers. With insulin deficiency, patients become catabolic and experience weight loss. Some patients report feeling agitated or confused, although this is not common.

3. What is DKA, and how common is it?
   DKA stands for diabetic ketoacidosis. Three elements are required for the diagnosis: uncontrolled hyperglycemia (blood glucose usually > 250 mg/dL), metabolic acidosis (pH $\leq$ 7.3), and increased ketone concentrations. It occurs more often in patients with type 1 diabetes and is the first presentation of type 1 diabetes in about 25% of patients. DKA accounts for 140,000 hospital admissions in the United States each year. The age-adjusted rate declined by 1.1% per year from the years 2000 to 2009 but then increased dramatically by 54.9% between 2009 and 2014, from 19.5 to 30.2 per 1000 persons (an increase of 6.3% per year), with the highest rates in adults < 45 years old. This group of younger adults also had a 27-fold higher rate of hospitalization for DKA compared with adults $\geq$ 65 years of age. The T1D Exchange Network reports that young adults, ages 18 to 25 years, have the overall highest occurrence of DKA.

4. What is the mortality rate for DKA?
   Before the discovery of insulin in 1921, the mortality rate in DKA was > 90%. The mortality rate for DKA in the United States and in the European countries is currently < 2% but is > 10% in countries with limited resources for acute care. DKA is the leading cause of death in children and young adults with type 1 diabetes ($\approx$ 50% of all deaths in individuals with diabetes < 24 years of age). The case fatality rate for mortality in the hospital decreased from 1.1% to 0.4% during the years 2000 to 2014.

5. Do all patients who develop DKA have type 1 diabetes?
   No. Patients with type 2 diabetes may also develop DKA if the relative insulin deficiency is severe enough, such as with severe stress or concurrent illness. Patients with ketosis-prone diabetes (KPD), which is described in Chapter 1, are diagnosed when they present with DKA.

6. What causes DKA?
   The two key factors leading to DKA are insulin deficiency and elevated levels of counterregulatory hormones (epinephrine, glucagon, cortisol, growth hormone). These factors promote hepatic glycogenolysis and gluconeogenesis, resulting in increased hepatic glucose production. Glucose uptake into skeletal muscle is reduced as a result of insulin deficiency. Catabolism of fat stores increases serum concentrations of free fatty acids, which are then oxidized to ketone bodies (beta-hydroxybutyrate and acetoacetate) in the liver; this also consumes bicarbonate, resulting in metabolic acidosis.

7. What are the common precipitating factors for DKA?
   A new diagnosis of diabetes, omission of insulin doses, infection, myocardial infarction, pancreatitis, stroke, alcohol use, and insulin pump malfunction may all precipitate DKA. Risk factors include psychiatric disorders, eating disorders, substance abuse, and homelessness. In the United States, the most common precipitating factor is failure to adhere to insulin therapy. Elsewhere in the world, infections are the most common precipitating factors.

8. What are the symptoms and signs of DKA?
   Patients often present with nausea and vomiting, abdominal pain, polyuria, polydipsia, fatigue, and weight loss. They may have decreased mental status but < 25% present with coma. Signs of volume depletion, such as hypotension, tachycardia, dry mucous membranes, and decreased skin turgor, are usually apparent. Patients with severe DKA may have Kussmaul respirations (respiratory compensation for metabolic acidosis) and a "fruity" breath resulting from acetone production.

9. How is DKA diagnosed?

The following laboratory findings are also needed for the diagnosis of DKA:

- Hyperglycemia (blood glucose usually $\geq$ 250 mg/dL)
- Anion gap metabolic acidosis (pH $\leq$ 7.3; $HCO_3 \leq$ 18 mEq/L; anion gap $>$ 15)
- Positive serum or urine ketones

    Blood glucose levels are usually over 250 mg/dL but may be lower than this (termed "euglycemic DKA") in the following situations: pregnancy, starvation, alcohol use, insulin therapy, and use of sodium-glucose cotransporter-2 (SGLT-2) inhibitors. A definitive determination of anion gap metabolic acidosis can only be made with simultaneous measurement of blood gases (partial pressure of carbon dioxide [$PaCO_2$] and pH are decreased) and serum chemistries (basic metabolic panel). Ideally, arterial blood gas measurement is done for the diagnosis, but venous blood gas measurements may be used to monitor therapy. The anion gap is calculated using the equation: sodium [Na^+] $-$ chloride [Cl^-] $-$ bicarbonate [HCO_3^-]. Ketonemia may be documented by using the serum beta-hydroxybutyrate method, but it may be underestimated if ketones are measured by using the nitroprusside method.

10. What are the basic principles of DKA management?

Key measures for treating DKA include:

1. Volume repletion
2. Correction of electrolyte abnormalities
3. Insulin therapy to correct hyperglycemia and ketonemia
4. Identification and treatment of the precipitating event(s)

    DKA often resolves within 10 to 18 hours if appropriate treatment is instituted promptly. Patients must be monitored every 1 to 2 hours initially and then every 2 to 4 hours, with assessment of serial vital signs, physical examination to determine volume status and mental status, urine output, basic metabolic panels (for bicarbonate, potassium, anion gap) and venous blood gas measurements (pH) to assess the effectiveness of treatment. Changes in the rate of intravenous fluid administration and insulin doses are often needed.

11. Should ketones be monitored in the management of DKA?

When point-of-care beta-hydroxybutyrate measurements are available, these can be used to diagnosis ketosis and to monitor therapy. However, measurement of ketones by using the nitroprusside method helps detect acetoacetate and acetone but not beta-hydroxybutyrate, which is the main ketone body produced in DKA. Serial measurement of ketones in DKA, therefore, is not accurate if the nitroprusside method is used.

12. When can patients be transitioned off intravenous insulin infusion after treatment for DKA?

Intravenous insulin can be discontinued when the patient's acidemia (determined by both the absolute bicarbonate concentration and the elevated anion gap) has resolved, the patient shows clinical improvement (off vasopressors), the patient is able to tolerate oral intake, and the precipitating cause(s) have been addressed. Factors that predict successful transition from intravenous insulin to a subcutaneous regimen include a stable infusion rate of $<$ 2.0 to 2.5 units/hr with blood glucose levels consistently $<$ 130 mg/dL.

13. What is HHS?

HHS is an abbreviation for hyperglycemic hyperosmolar state.

14. Who develops HHS?

HHS generally occurs in elderly patients with type 2 diabetes who have an impaired thirst mechanism or are unable to access free water for any reason.

15. What are symptoms and signs of HHS?

Patients often report typical symptoms of hyperglycemia, including polyuria, polydipsia, blurred vision, and weakness. They may have decreased mental status and often will have signs of dehydration, such as dry mucous membranes and decreased skin turgor. Patients with HHS are often hemodynamically unstable with significantly decreased blood pressure and tachycardia.

16. Why do people with HHS generally not have ketoacidosis?

Patients with HHS have sufficient insulin production to suppress lipolysis and subsequent generation of ketones. In addition, these patients usually have lower circulating levels of the counterregulatory hormones.

17. How does one distinguish between DKA and HHS? (Table 2.1)

Patients with DKA have increased acidemia with ketonemia, whereas patients with HHS have little to no ketones, normal serum bicarbonate levels, and elevated serum osmolality of $>$ 320 mOsm/kg. Patients with HHS also usually have more severe hyperglycemia compared with those with DKA (occasionally presenting with blood glucose levels $>$ 1000 mg/dL) and have a more severe volume deficit.

18. Can a patient present with both DKA and HHS?

Yes. Patients may have features of both ketoacidosis and hyperosmolarity. Patients with HHS may have mild to moderate ketonemia and may have a concomitant metabolic acidosis caused by lactic acidosis, uremia, or alcoholic ketoacidosis.

Table 2.1. Diagnostic Criteria for DKA and HHS.

MEASURE	MILD	MODERATE	SEVERE	HHS DKA
Plasma glucose (mg/dL)	> 250	> 250	> 250	> 600
Arterial pH	7.25–7.30	7.00 to < 7.24	< 7.00	> 7.30
Serum bicarbonate (mEq/L)	15–18	10–15	< 10	> 18
Urine to serum ketones[a]	Positive	Positive	Positive	Small
Urine or serum β-hydroxybutyrate (mmol/L)	> 3.0	> 3.0	> 3.0	< 3.0
Effective serum osmolality[b]	Variable	Variable	Variable	> 320 mOsm/kg
Anion gap	> 10	> 12	> 12	Variable
Mental status	Alert	Alert/drowsy	Stupor/coma	Stupor/coma

[a]Nitroprusside reaction.
[b]Effective serum osmolality: 2[measured Na^+(mEq/L) + glucose (mg/dL)/18.
DKA, Diabetic ketoacidosis; *HHS*, hyperglycemic hyperosmolar state.
Adapted from Kitabchi, A. E., Umpierrez, G. E., Miles, J. M., & Fisher, J. N. (2009). Hyperglycemic crises in adult patients with diabetes. *Diabetes Care, 32*(7), 1335–1343. With permission.

19. What is needed for the diagnosis of HHS?
    The diagnosis of HHS is made by the following findings:
    • Serum glucose of > 600 mg/dL
    • Serum osmolality > 320 mOsm/kg
    • Ketones absent

    Effective osmolality ≡ sodium ion (mEq/L) × 2 + glucose (mg/dL)/18 + blood urea nitrogen (BUN) (mg/dL) ÷ 2.8

20. What is key to the treatment of HHS?
    Patients with HHS are extremely volume depleted; therefore, the key to treatment is adequate volume repletion.

21. What role does insulin play in the treatment of HHS?
    Insulin therapy is important but is secondary. Unlike the treatment for DKA, in which insulin deficiency is the most important driving factor, correction of volume loss is the critical element in the management of HHS.

22. Describe the signs and symptoms of hypoglycemia
    Common symptoms of hypoglycemia include shakiness, diaphoresis, irritability, hunger, and fatigue. Neuroglycopenic symptoms, such as confusion, unusual behavior, visual disturbances, and loss of consciousness, may also occur. Patients with severe hypoglycemia may appear to be intoxicated, with slurred speech and clumsiness, and seizures can develop. Hypoglycemia can be fatal, with recent reports indicating that 4% to 10% of deaths in type 1 diabetes were caused by hypoglycemia.

23. What are common reasons patients with diabetes become hypoglycemic?
    Hypoglycemia in patients with diabetes most often results from missed or delayed meals after taking rapid-acting insulin, a sulfonylurea, or a meglitinide; excessive prandial and/or correctional insulin; too much basal insulin; physical activity without medication or nutritional adjustments; and renal disease resulting in decreased insulin clearance and loss of renal gluconeogenesis. Other causes are similar to those in patients with diabetes and in those without diabetes: liver failure, cardiac failure, sepsis, critical illness, untreated adrenal insufficiency, untreated hypothyroidism, and starvation or malnutrition. Patients with diabetes rarely have insulinomas, but this is still in the differential diagnosis for hypoglycemia.

24. Which diabetes medications are most commonly associated with hypoglycemia?
    Insulins, sulfonylureas, and meglitinides (repaglinide, nateglinide) account for the vast majority of cases of hypoglycemia in patients with diabetes.

25. What diabetes medications are associated with a low risk of hypoglycemia?
    Metformin, acarbose, thiazolidinediones, dipeptidyl peptidase-4 inhibitors, glucagon-like peptide-1 receptor agonists, and SGLT-2 inhibitors rarely cause hypoglycemia, unless used in combination with one of the medications listed in question 24. Two of the more recently approved, but less often used, "old drugs for a new indication" (bromocriptine and colesevelam) may occasionally lead to mild hypoglycemia.

26. Do patients with type 1 diabetes and type 2 diabetes have the same risk of hypoglycemia?
    Patients with type 1 diabetes are two to three times more likely to develop hypoglycemia compared with patients with type 2 diabetes, and the risk increases with increasing duration of diabetes. Other risk factors for hypoglycemia include advancing age, intensive glycemic control, renal disease, and decreased cognitive function.

27. What is "hypoglycemia unawareness"?

Patients with diabetes typically develop adrenergic symptoms of hypoglycemia when blood glucose levels drop below 70 mg/dL; lower glucose levels may also be associated with neuroglycopenic symptoms. "Hypoglycemia unawareness" (absence of hypoglycemic symptoms when blood glucose levels decrease into the hypoglycemic range) typically occurs when a patient has had multiple, recurrent episodes of hypoglycemia, resulting in lowering of the glucose threshold that triggers counterregulatory hormone release. Affected patients often need assistance from others to recognize and treat hypoglycemia. Hypoglycemia-associated autonomic failure (HAAF) is a term that is used to describe hypoglycemia unawareness and impaired counterregulatory hormone responses.

28. Is hypoglycemia unawareness reversible?

Yes. With strict avoidance of hypoglycemia for a certain period (weeks to months), patients often regain hypoglycemia awareness.

29. How is hypoglycemia treated in a conscious patient?

Hypoglycemia in a conscious patient should be treated with 15 g of oral carbohydrates (glucose tablets or gel; half cup, or 4 ounces, of juice or regular soda; 1 cup, or 8 ounces, of milk; 1 tablespoon of honey; three 3-packs of SweeTARTS; or $\approx$ 3 rolls of Smarties).

30. What should be done if a patient is unconscious and severe hypoglycemia is suspected?

For severe hypoglycemia, when a patient is unconscious or otherwise unable to take anything by mouth, glucagon (available as a glucagon kit) should be injected subcutaneously or intramuscularly to stimulate immediate glycogenolysis in the liver. Because glucagon is injected in these situations by a family member, friend or coworker, individuals who may potentially need to administer glucagon should be trained on when and how to inject this hormone. An emergency 911 call should also be made.

31. What are the key elements of education needed to prevent and avoid hypoglycemia?

Patient education is essential to decrease the risk of iatrogenic hypoglycemia. Key elements of patient education include recognizing the symptoms of hypoglycemia, proper treatment of hypoglycemia, and being familiar with situations in which one might anticipate a higher risk for hypoglycemia. These elements need to be reviewed at every visit. In addition, patients may require guidance on dietary and exercise modifications, medication adjustments, and sensible glucose monitoring methods. Meticulous surveillance by the health care provider is imperative.

32. What are the common long-term complications of diabetes mellitus?

The long-term complications of diabetes are often divided into microvascular and macrovascular types; the former include retinopathy, diabetic kidney disease (DKD), and neuropathy, whereas the latter includes atherosclerotic cardiovascular disease (coronary heart disease, cerebrovascular disease, and peripheral arterial disease presumed to be of atherosclerotic origin). Macrovascular disease is the leading cause of morbidity and mortality among individuals with diabetes and is the largest contributor to the direct and indirect costs of diabetes, but microvascular disease also causes significant morbidity and decreased quality of life. Diabetic foot ulcers are multifactorial and cannot be classified neatly into a "microvascular versus macrovascular" complication.

Diabetes is associated with a number of comorbid conditions, including obesity, obstructive sleep apnea, fatty liver disease, fractures, pancreatitis, hearing loss, certain cancers (liver, pancreas, endometrium, colon/rectum, breast, bladder), depression, anxiety, cognitive impairment and dementia, eating disorders, and periodontal disease; these will not be discussed in this section.

33. Why do these complications develop in individuals with diabetes?

The basic mechanisms underlying the development of microvascular and macrovascular complications are complex and are under intensive investigation by researchers around the world. Uncontrolled hyperglycemia, insulin resistance, and hyperinsulinemia, as well as associated conditions, such as dyslipidemia, hypertension, and obesity, conspire to create a "perfect storm" leading to increased oxidative stress and inflammation and promoting the development of these complications. With microvascular complications, hyperglycemia leads to activation of protein kinase C and reactive oxygen species and to the generation of toxic products of abnormal glucose metabolism (e.g., advanced glycation end-products and methylglyoxal).

34. What fundamental factors need to be managed to prevent microvascular complications?

Hyperglycemia, hypertension, and dyslipidemia must all be well controlled to prevent the development and/or progression of these conditions.

35. How common is diabetic retinopathy?

Diabetic retinopathy is the most common microvascular complication of diabetes. Globally, diabetic retinopathy affects almost 100 million people. In developed countries, it is the most common cause of new cases of blindness among adults 20 to 74 years of age. Glaucoma and cataracts also occur earlier and at a higher frequency in patients with diabetes.

36. How does diabetic retinopathy manifest?

Patients are asymptomatic in the earlier stages, and therefore, without routine ophthalmologic screening, retinopathy can be missed. The different types include nonproliferative diabetic retinopathy (NPDR), proliferative diabetic retinopathy (PDR), and diabetic macular edema (DME). NPDR is the earliest detectable stage and includes a number of findings on retinal examination, such as microaneurysms, retinal hemorrhages, intraretinal microvascular abnormalities (IRMAs), and venous caliber changes. PDR, which indicates a more advanced stage, is characterized by preretinal neovascularization. Evolving technologies are allowing for the detection of more subtle abnormalities, such as alterations of retinal function and of the neural layer. DME can occur at any stage of diabetic retinopathy and is the most common cause of visual loss in this disorder. In DME, the blood–retina barrier breaks down with leakage of circulating fluid and proteins into the neural retina, leading to abnormal retinal thickening and cystoid macular edema.

37. How is diabetic retinopathy managed?

Treatment options include focal and panretinal laser photocoagulation, intravitreal injections of anti–vascular endothelial growth factor (VEGF), intravitreal steroids, and vitreoretinal surgery. The eye-specific therapeutic paradigm is designed to treat advanced disease (PDR and/or DME).

38. How common is DKD?

Approximately 35% of adults with diabetes develop chronic kidney disease. DKD disproportionately affects middle-aged African Americans, Native Americans, and Hispanic Americans; these groups also have significantly higher rates of progression to end-stage renal disease (ESRD).

39. Is there more than one manifestation of DKD?

Yes. Albuminuria, decreased glomerular filtration rate (GFR), glomerular hematuria, other abnormalities of the urinary sediment, and abnormalities on imaging studies are all manifestations of DKD. Not all individuals with DKD and reduced estimated GFR (eGFR) have increased albuminuria. The United Kingdom Prospective Diabetes Study (UKPDS) reported that only about 50% of people who developed an estimated creatinine clearance of < 60 mL/min/1.73 m^2 ever tested positive for albuminuria.

40. What is the treatment for DKD?

Good control of blood glucose and blood pressure, especially with an angiotensin-converting enzyme (ACE) inhibitor or an angiotensin receptor blocker (ARB) can prevent or slow the progression of established DKD. When DKD progresses to ESRD despite these measures, dialysis or kidney transplantation becomes necessary.

41. What types of diabetic neuropathies are there?

Multiple types of neuropathies occur in people with diabetes; these include distal symmetric sensorimotor polyneuropathy (the most common); autonomic neuropathy; focal limb neuropathies; mononeuropathies; entrapment syndromes, such as carpal tunnel syndrome; diabetic amyotrophy (proximal motor neuropathy); diabetic truncal radiculopathy; and acute sensory neuropathy. Diabetic neuropathies have two distinct patterns of progression: sensory and autonomic neuropathies generally progress gradually with increasing duration of diabetes, whereas mononeuropathies, radiculopathies, and acute painful neuropathies may be quite severe at onset but are short-lived and often resolve completely. Diabetic neuropathies encompass heterogeneous clinical presentations, and the incidence, prevalence; however, the natural histories of diabetic neuropathies have not been well defined. This can be attributed to variable diagnostic criteria, lack of standardized methods for evaluation, and lack of recognition by clinicians.

42. What is the pathogenesis of the diabetic neuropathies?

Metabolic abnormalities within the nerves and/or Schwann cells, as well as microvascular injuries contribute to diabetic neuropathies. In distal symmetric polyneuropathy, progressive axonal degeneration occurs in different fiber types, usually preceded by segmental demyelination.

43. What are the symptoms of distal symmetric polyneuropathy, and what is the usual pattern of progression?

Numbness, the sensation of a toe or part of the foot "falling asleep," prickling, tingling, stabbing, burning, electrical-like shocks, or aching pains may all occur. Symptoms start in the toes or the plantar surface of the foot in a symmetric pattern and travel proximally. Patients usually do not develop symptoms in the upper extremities until lower extremity symptoms have reached the knees ("stocking–glove distribution"). Distal symmetric polyneuropathy is a diagnosis of exclusion; other causes that must be considered include chronic inflammatory demyelinating polyneuropathy, vitamin B$_{12}$ deficiency (particularly in patients on metformin therapy for longer than a year), hypothyroidism, and uremia.

44. How is diabetic neuropathy treated?

Tight glycemic control prevents progression of neuropathy but does not reduce the pain in distal symmetric polyneuropathy. Therapies for painful diabetic neuropathy approved by the U.S. Food and Drug Administration (FDA) are pregabalin and duloxetine, which are also recommended by the American Diabetes Association (ADA) as first-line therapies. Other potentially beneficial treatments include gabapentin, sodium valproate, venlafaxine, amitriptyline, dextromethorphan, topical capsaicin, isosorbide dinitrate spray, and typical opioids. Nonpharmaco-logic therapies, other than percutaneous electrical nerve stimulation (PENS), lack data to support their use. These therapies all target the symptoms, and not the underlying mechanisms.

45. What foot problems can patients with diabetes experience?
Diabetic foot ulcers; insensate feet; foot infections; foot deformities, including Charcot foot; peripheral artery disease; and amputations can all occur in patients with diabetes.

46. What are the important strategies for preventing diabetic foot ulcers?
Patients should be aware of the risk factors for diabetic foot ulcers and amputations; these include poor glycemic control, peripheral neuropathy with loss of protective sensation, cigarette smoking, foot deformity, preulcerative calloses and corns, peripheral artery disease, history of previous foot ulcers, prior amputations, visual impair-ment, and DKD (particularly ESRD on dialysis). Proper foot care includes daily assessment of skin and nails, palpa-tion or visual surveillance (including use of an unbreakable mirror, if needed) to monitor the condition of the feet, use of well-fitting shoes (custom-fitted in select circumstances), and proper wound care if an ulcer develops.

47. What are the clinical features of diabetic autonomic neuropathy?
Autonomic neuropathy can cause a variety of clinical manifestations, including hypoglycemia unawareness, resting tachycardia, orthostatic hypotension, gastroparesis, constipation, diarrhea, fecal incontinence, erectile dysfunction, neurogenic bladder, and sudomotor dysfunction with either increased or decreased sweating.

48. How do you detect cardiac autonomic neuropathy?
Early cardiac autonomic neuropathy is usually asymptomatic and only manifests as decreased heart rate variabil-ity with deep breathing. Later, it causes resting tachycardia and orthostatic hypotension. Cardiac autonomic neuropathy is independently associated with mortality.

49. When do patients with diabetes develop gastroparesis, and when should it be suspected?
Patients with type 1 diabetes generally do not develop gastroparesis until 10 to 15 years after diabetes is diag-nosed; the condition takes even longer to develop in those with type 2 diabetes. Gastrointestinal neuropathies can manifest along any portion of the gastrointestinal tract, resulting in esophageal dysmotility, gastroparesis, diarrhea with or without fecal incontinence, and constipation. Patients who have poorly controlled blood glucose (especially a pattern of frequent postprandial hypoglycemia, followed by prolonged hyperglycemia) and unexplained gastric or esophageal symptoms should be suspected of having gastroparesis.

50. How is gastroparesis diagnosed?
Gastric-emptying scintigraphy is the gold standard for diagnosis but mechanical obstruction, and gastric or peptic ulcer must first be excluded. Patients must discontinue any drugs that might affect gastric emptying, fast overnight, and then consume a standard low-fat radiolabeled meal within 10 minutes. Imaging is performed at baseline and then 1, 2, and 4 hours later with the patient in the standing position. Glucose values should be < 275 mg/dL for a valid result because hyperglycemia itself acutely inhibits gastric emptying. Delayed gastric emptying is defined as > 60% retention at 2 hours or > 10% retention at 4 hours. Limitations include low sensitivity for detecting mild or moderate gastroparesis, potential for overdiagnosis in women who have a physiologic delay of gastric emptying, and intraindividual variation of up to 24%. Furthermore, the low-fat, low-fiber test meal used to standardize testing conditions may not be similar to actual meals that patients normally consume and may, therefore, lead to underdi-agnosis of gastroparesis. An alternative is a gastric emptying breath test with use of a radiolabeled carbon-containing test meal (carbon13–labeled *Spirulina platensis* or octanoic acid). After consuming this meal, radiola-beled carbon is released during digestion and is detected as exhaled radiolabeled carbon dioxide 4 to 6 hours later. Comparative studies suggest that the breath test may be as accurate as scintigraphy. Another approach is a wire-less motility capsule (a "smart pill"), but evidence supporting its use is of low quality.

51. What is diabetes-related distress?
This is relatively new term for an increasingly recognized affective state resulting from constant worry about ad-herence to a strict regimen of diet, exercise, and frequent blood glucose monitoring, while feeling afraid, anxious, overwhelmed, at times angry, and eventually burned out. There is no standard definition for this condition, but it may be defined simply as "decreased quality of life resulting from a combination of the medical and psychological burden of diabetes as a complex and chronic condition creating emotional distress often hidden from providers and sometimes from the sufferer." Diabetes-related distress can negatively impact diabetes management and outcomes. The level of diabetes-related distress does not appear to be associated with the duration of diabetes but has been noted to be much higher in younger patients, females, nonwhite patients, those with a higher body mass index (BMI), and patients treated with insulin compared with those not treated with insulin.

52. How common is depression in people with diabetes?
Depression is two to three times more common in people with diabetes than in the general population. There is now emerging evidence that depression may actually be a risk factor for the development of diabetes (up to 60% increased risk). Conversely, the pooled relative risk (RR) for developing depression in individuals with preexisting diabetes is 1.15.

53. How can macrovascular disease be prevented in persons with diabetes?

Standard measures for the prevention of atherosclerotic cardiovascular disease (ASCVD) include smoking cessation and lowering of blood pressure and low-density lipoprotein (LDL) cholesterol levels. The recommended intensity of LDL lowering is greater for individuals with diabetes compared with those of low to moderate ASCVD risk without diabetes. Regular physical activity and a healthy dietary pattern that emphasizes intake of fruits and vegetables, reduced saturated fat, and low-fat dairy products is recommended; the Mediterranean diet and the Dietary Approaches to Stop Hypertension (DASH) diet are both consistent with those recommendations. Low-dose aspirin (75–162 mg per day) in those individuals with a 10-year ASCVD risk of $\geq$ 10%, avoidance of hypoglycemia, and prevention of DKD are additional important preventive measures.

54. Should people with diabetes be screened for coronary artery disease and peripheral arterial disease?

Resting electrocardiography, ankle-brachial index, and electron beam computed tomography (CT) for measurement of the coronary artery calcium (CAC) score are reasonable choices to assess for the presence of coronary artery disease (CAD) and peripheral arterial disease (PAD). Stress myocardial perfusion imaging, however, is not indicated in asymptomatic individuals at low or intermediate ASCVD risk, unless there is a strong family history of CAD or if previous risk assessment testing suggests a high individual risk of CAD (e.g., high CAC).

55. What is the best strategy for the secondary prevention of ASCVD in individuals with diabetes?

Smoking cessation, regular physical activity, and a heart-healthy diet, with weight loss, if needed, are the cornerstones of secondary ASCVD prevention. In addition, patients should maintain good blood pressure control, and most should take a statin and aspirin. Glucose-lowering therapy with an agent indicated for reduction of ASCVD risk (glucose-dependent insulinotropic peptide-1 [GLP-1] analogues, SGLT-2 inhibitors) should also be considered.

56. How important is glycemic control in preventing the chronic complications of diabetes mellitus?

The Diabetes Control and Complications Trial/Epidemiology of Diabetes Interventions and Complications (DCCT/EDIC) and the UKPDS are landmark trials that demonstrated the importance of good glycemic control in prevention of diabetic microvascular complications; long-term follow-up of these studies (DCCT/EDIC and UKPDS) also showed a legacy effect, demonstrating a beneficial impact on macrovascular complications. More recent trials (Action to Control Cardiovascular Risk in Type 2 Diabetes [ACCORD] and Action in Diabetes and Vascular Disease: Preterax and Diamicron MR Controlled Evaluation [ADVANCE]) also confirmed the importance of good glycemic control for the prevention of microvascular complications (particularly kidney disease).

57. What are the clinical implications of the ACCORD, ADVANCE, and VADT trials?

The ACCORD trial was published in 2008 and was the first of three large contemporary randomized controlled trials designed to determine whether intensive glycemic control would further reduce the risk of major adverse cardiovascular events in individuals with diabetes. The study population consisted of patients with type 2 diabetes of long duration and mostly with established ASCVD. There was no difference in the primary outcome of three-point major adverse cardiovascular event (MACE; nonfatal myocardial infarction, nonfatal stroke, or death from cardiovascular causes; $P = 0.13$) between the intensive treatment group and the conventional treatment group. However, the trial was stopped early by the Data Safety Monitoring Board because all-cause mortality was increased (driven primarily by cardiovascular-related death, especially congestive heart failure) in the intensive treatment group. Because the trial was stopped early, there was insufficient power to draw other definitive conclusions, but much has been learned from post hoc analyses of data, including differential relationships between hemoglobin A_{1c} (HbA_{1c}) and mortality in the intensive versus conventional treatment groups, and the relationships between hypoglycemia and cardiovascular events and mortality. For example, in the intensive-treatment group only subjects with a baseline HbA_{1c} > 8.5% were at higher risk for mortality. Increased mortality was also associated with history of neuropathy and higher on-treatment HbA_{1c} (i.e., those unable to achieve the target glycemia).

The ADVANCE and VADT (Veterans Affairs Diabetes Trial) studies were two other large randomized controlled trials of intensive versus conventional glycemic control in subjects with longstanding type 2 diabetes that were published around the same time. These trials did not show increased mortality or adverse cardiovascular outcomes but also did not show improved cardiovascular outcomes with intensive glycemic control targeting HbA_{1c} < 7% in patients with longer duration (> 10–15 years) type 2 diabetes with or without established or high risk for ASCVD.

KEY POINTS

- The basic principles of diabetic ketoacidosis (DKA) management are (1) volume repletion, (2) correction of electrolyte abnormalities, (3) insulin therapy for hyperglycemia and ketonemia, and (4) identification and treatment of the precipitating event(s).
- Patients may be transitioned off the intravenous insulin infusion after resolution of DKA (the acidemia and elevated anion gap have resolved, the patient is clinically improved and able to tolerate oral intake, and the precipitating cause(s) have been addressed) AND when the insulin infusion rate has been stable for at least 6 hours at 2-3 units/hr or lower, and glucose is well-controlled.
- Patients with DKA are significantly acidemic and have ketonemia, while patients with hyperglycemic hyperosmolar state (HHS) have little to no ketones, normal serum bicarbonate levels, and serum osmolality

KEY POINTS—cont'd

of $\geq$ 320 mOsm/kg. Patients with HHS often have more severe hyperglycemia (occasionally presenting with blood glucose levels > 1000 mg/dL) compared with patients with DKA and have a more severe volume deficit. To diagnose HHS, the patient should have serum osmolality $\geq$ 320 mOsm/kg, serum glucose > 600 mg/dL, and no (or only small) ketones. A significant proportion of individuals may have components of both HHS and DKA.

- Hypoglycemia unawareness occurs when a patient has had recurrent hypoglycemia because repeated episodes of hypoglycemia lower glucose levels, triggering the release of counterregulatory hormones. It is reversible with strict avoidance of hypoglycemia for a period (weeks to months). Hypoglycemia-associated autonomic failure (HAAF) consists of hypoglycemia unawareness and impaired counterregulatory hormone responses.
- Diabetic kidney disease (DKD) may manifest in various ways. These include albuminuria (urinary albumin excretion), decreased glomerular filtration rate (GFR), glomerular hematuria, other abnormalities of the urinary sediment, or abnormalities on imaging studies. Not all individuals with DKD and reduced estimated GFR (eGFR) have increased albuminuria.
- Diabetic neuropathies have two distinct patterns of progression. Sensory and autonomic neuropathies generally progress gradually, with increasing duration of diabetes. In comparison, mononeuropathies, radiculopathies, and acute painful neuropathies present acutely, are short-lived, and resolve completely.
- The best strategy for both primary and secondary prevention of ASCVD in patients with diabetes includes smoking cessation, regular physical activity, and a heart-healthy diet, with weight loss, if needed. Patients should also take a statin, aspirin, and maintain good blood pressure control; for high-risk patients or those with established ASCVD, use of a glucose-lowering agent is indicated for the reduction of CVD risk in diabetes.

BIBLIOGRAPHY

American Diabetes Association. (2019). 11. Microvascular complications and foot care: standards of medical care in diabetes - 2019. *Diabetes Care, 42*(Suppl. 1), S124–S138.

Barrett, E. J., Liu, Z., Khamaisi, M., King, G. L., Klein, R., Klein, B. E. K., … Casellini, C. M. (2017). Diabetic microvascular disease: an endocrine society scientific statement. *Journal of Clinical Endocrinology and Metabolism, 102*(12), 4343–4410.

Benoit, S. R., Zhang, Y., Geiss, L. S., Gregg, E. W., & Albright, A. (2018). Trends in diabetic ketoacidosis hospitalizations and in-hospital mortality - United States, 2000-2014. *Morbidity and Mortality Weekly Report, 67*(12), 362–365.

Beulens, J. W., Patel, A., Vingerling, J. R., Cruickshank, J. K., Hughes, A. D., Stanton, A., … Stolk, R. P. (2009). Effects of blood pressure lowering and intensive glucose control on the incidence and progression of retinopathy in patients with type 2 diabetes mellitus: a randomised controlled trial. *Diabetologia, 52*(10), 2027–2036.

Bril, V., England, J., Franklin, G. M., Backonja, M., Cohen, J., Del Toro, D., … Zochodne, D. (2011). Evidence-based guideline: treatment of painful diabetic neuropathy: report of the American Academy of Neurology, the American Association of Neuromuscular and Electrodiagnostic Medicine, and the American Academy of Physical Medicine and Rehabilitation. *Neurology, 76*(20), 1758–1765. (Erratum in: *Neurology,* (2011). *77*(6), 603. Dosage error in article text.)

Cefalu, W. T., Kaul, S., Gerstein, H. C., Holman, R. R., Zinman, B., Skyler, J. S., … Riddle, M. C. (2018). Cardiovascular outcomes trials in type 2 diabetes: where do we go from here? Reflections from a diabetes care editors' expert forum. *Diabetes Care, 41*(1), 14–31.

Desai, D., Mehta, D., Mathias, P., Menon, G., & Schubart, U. K. (2018). Health care utilization and burden of diabetic ketoacidosis in the U.S. over the past decade: a nationwide analysis. *Diabetes Care, 41*(8), 1631–1638. doi:10.2337/dc17-1379.

Duh, E. J., Sun, J. K., & Stitt, A. W. (2017). Diabetic retinopathy: current understanding, mechanisms, and treatment strategies. *JCI Insight, 2*(14), 93751.

Fayfman, M., Pasquel, F. J., & Umpierrez, G. E. (2017). Management of hyperglycemic crises: diabetic ketoacidosis and hyperglycemic hyperosmolar state. *Medical Clinics of North America, 101*(3), 587–606.

Fox, C. S., Golden, S. H., Anderson, C., Bray, G. A., Burke, L. E., de Boer, I. H., … Vafiadis, D. K. (2015). Update on prevention of cardiovascular disease in adults with type 2 diabetes mellitus in light of recent evidence: a scientific statement from the American Heart Association and the American Diabetes Association. *Circulation, 132*(8), 691–718.

Hingorani, A., LaMuraglia, G. M., Henke, P., Meissner, M. H., Loretz, L., Zinszer, K. M., … Murad, M. H. (2016). The management of diabetic foot: a clinical practice guideline by the Society for Vascular Surgery in collaboration with the American Podiatric Medical Association and the Society for Vascular Medicine. *Journal of Vascular Surgery, 63*(Suppl. 2), 3S–21S.

Iqbal, Z., Azmi, S., Yadav, R., Ferdousi, M., Kumar, M., Cuthbertson, D. J., … Alam, U. (2018). Diabetic peripheral neuropathy: epidemiology, diagnosis, and pharmacotherapy. *Clinical Therapeutics, 40*(6), 828–849.

Ismail-Beigi, F., Craven, T., Banerji, M. A., Basile, J., Calles, J., Cohen, R. M., … Hramiak, I. (2010). Effect of intensive treatment of hyperglycaemia on microvascular outcomes in type 2 diabetes: an analysis of the ACCORD randomised trial. *Lancet, 376*(9739), 419–430. (Erratum in: *Lancet,* (2010). *376*(9751), 1466.)

Kumar, M., Chapman, A., Javed, S., Alam, U., Malik, R. A., & Azmi, S. (2018). The investigation and treatment of diabetic gastroparesis. *Clinical Therapeutics, 40*(6), 850–861.

Lee, A. K., Warren, B., Lee, C. J., McEvoy, J. W., Matsushita, K., Huang, E. S., … Selvin, E. (2018). The association of severe hypoglycemia with incident cardiovascular events and mortality in adults with type 2 diabetes. *Diabetes Care, 41*(1), 104–111.

Low Wang, C. C., Hess, C. N., Hiatt, W. R., & Goldfine, A. B. (2016). Clinical update: cardiovascular disease in diabetes mellitus: atherosclerotic cardiovascular disease and heart failure in type 2 diabetes mellitus - mechanisms, management, and clinical considerations. *Circulation, 133*(24), 2459–2502.

National Center for Chronic Disease Prevention and Health Promotion, Division of Diabetes Translation, & Centers for Disease Control and Prevention. *Chronic kidney disease: kidney disease and diabetes.* Retrieved from https://www.cdc.gov/diabetes/pdfs/programs/fact-sheet-chronickidneydiseasekidneydiseasediabetes.pdf. Accessed March 30, 2019.

Regensteiner, J. G., Golden, S., Huebschmann, A. G., Barrett-Connor, E., Chang, A. Y., Chyun, D., … Anton, B. (2015). Sex differences in the cardiovascular consequences of diabetes mellitus: a scientific statement from the American Heart Association. *Circulation, 132*(25), 2424–2447.

Seaquist, E. R., Anderson, J., Childs, B., Cryer, P., Dagogo-Jack, S., Fish, L., … Vigersky, R. (2013). Hypoglycemia and diabetes: a report of a workgroup of the American Diabetes Association and the Endocrine Society. *Journal of Clinical Endocrinology and Metabolism, 98*(5), 1845–1859.

Tareen, R. S., & Tareen, K. (2017). Psychosocial aspects of diabetes management: dilemma of diabetes distress. *Translational Pediatrics, 6*(4), 383–396.

Tuttle, K. R., Bakris, G. L., Bilous, R. W., Chiang, J. L., de Boer, I. H., Goldstein-Fuchs, J., … Molitch, M. E. (2014). Diabetic kidney disease: a report from an ADA Consensus Conference. *Diabetes Care, 37*(10), 2864–2883.

van den Berge, J. C., Constantinescu, A. A., Boiten, H. J., van Domburg, R. T., Deckers, J. W., & Akkerhuis, K. M. (2018). Short- and long-term prognosis of patients with acute heart failure with and without diabetes: changes over the last three decades. *Diabetes Care, 41*(1), 143–149.

CHAPTER 3

TYPE 1 DIABETES MELLITUS

Jennifer M. Trujillo

1. What is the general approach to the treatment of type 1 diabetes mellitus?

Type 1 diabetes mellitus is caused by autoimmune destruction of the pancreatic beta cells, and this leads to an absolute deficiency of insulin. Therefore, the mainstay of treatment of type 1 diabetes is insulin, administered in a way that mimics normal physiologic insulin secretion. The goals of therapy are to prevent or delay the onset of long-term complications of diabetes, including retinopathy, kidney disease, neuropathy, and cardiovascular disease; to prevent treatment induced hypoglycemia; and to maintain quality of life. For most patients, the target hemoglobin A_{1c} (HbA_{1c}) is < 7%, but this goal should be individualized on the basis of patient-specific factors. A fasting plasma glucose (FPG) target of 80 to 130 mg/dL and a postprandial glucose (PPG) target of < 180 mg/dL correlate with a target HbA_{1c} of < 7%. The American Diabetes Association (ADA) recurrently recommends a PPG target of < 180 mg/dL, whereas the American Association of Clinical Endocrinologists (AACE) recommends a PPG target of < 140 mg/dL.

Achieving good glycemic control in type 1 diabetes usually requires intensive insulin therapy (IIT). IIT is the use of multiple daily injections (MDIs) of insulin (both long-acting and rapid-acting formulations) or an insulin pump in an effort to mimic the normal insulin secretion pattern by the pancreas. IIT may also be referred to as *physiologic, multiple-component,* or *basal-bolus insulin therapy.* IIT is only one aspect of comprehensive, intensive diabetes therapy to achieve tight glycemic control. IIT is complex because it requires multiple injections or pump boluses each day in addition to basal insulin delivery, routine monitoring, and collaborative decision making. The most successful IIT is delivered and adjusted on the basis of changes in nutritional intake, glucose levels, stresses, and physical activity.

2. List the critical components of intensive insulin therapy.

- Frequent self-monitored blood glucose (SMBG) or a continuous glucose monitoring (CGM)
- Defined and individualized target blood glucose (BG) levels
- Use of SMBG data or sensor data and glucose patterns to meet treatment goals
- Dose modifications according to the individual's response to therapy
- Understanding of diet composition, specifically carbohydrate content
- Careful balance of food intake, activity, and insulin dosage
- Use of accurate carbohydrate-to-insulin (C:I) ratios according to food intake
- Use of correction factors (CFs) for the adjustment of insulin according to glucose levels
- Patient education, motivation, and ongoing interaction between patient and health care team

3. Summarize the studies evaluating optimal glycemic control to decrease chronic diabetes complications

The Diabetes Control and Complications Trial (DCCT), evaluating patients with recent-onset type 1 diabetes, showed that improved glycemic control (HbA_{1c} < 7%) not only significantly reduced the rates of microvascular complications, including progression of retinopathy, nephropathy, and neuropathy, but also increased the rates of hypoglycemia. IIT was a key part of achieving glycemic control in the DCCT. The Kumamoto Study and the United Kingdom Prospective Diabetes Study (UKPDS) extended these findings to show that improved glycemic control (HbA_{1c} < 7%) was associated with significantly reduced rates of microvascular complications in patients with recent-onset type 2 diabetes. The long-term extensions of the DCCT and the UKPDS showed significant reductions in cardiovascular complications, as well as good glycemic control, and demonstrated that the microvascular benefits of good glycemic control persisted for decades. Subsequent studies (Action to Control Cardiovascular Risk in Diabetes [ACCORD], Action in Diabetes and Vascular Disease: Preterax and Diamicron Modified Release Controlled Evaluation [ADVANCE], and VADT) in patients with more advanced type 2 diabetes failed to show that more aggressive glycemic targets (HbA_{1c} < 6%–6.5%) reduced cardiovascular complications, and one study (ACCORD) showed an increase in mortality. Rates of hypoglycemia with more aggressive glucose control were significant in all three trials.

4. Which patients are candidates for IIT?

All people with type 1 diabetes should be considered potential candidates for IIT. However, the degree of intensification must be based on each patient's personal situation and abilities. Patient characteristics that predict greater success with IIT include motivation, willingness to perform frequent SMBG and record results or use a continuous glucose monitor, time available to spend with a diabetes educator, the ability to recognize and treat hypoglycemia, sick days, and a supportive network of family or friends. In addition, implementation of IIT requires a cohesive diabetes team that is available for frequent interaction and discussion about results from monitoring, insulin adjustments, and other issues.

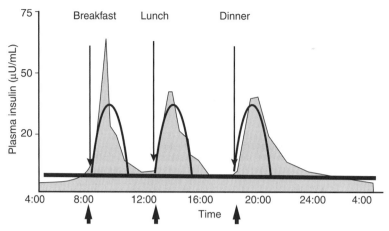

Fig. 3.1. Intensive insulin therapy pattern with multiple daily injections (MDIs).

5. What are the risks of IIT?

Hypoglycemia and weight gain are the most common adverse effects of insulin therapy. IIT in the DCCT resulted in a threefold increased risk of severe hypoglycemia compared with conventional treatment (62 episodes per 100 patient-years of therapy). Since the completion of the DCCT, newer rapid-acting and long-acting insulin analogues have been developed and are associated with less hypoglycemia compared with the short-acting and intermediate-acting human insulin products used in the DCCT. Frequent episodes of hypoglycemia can lead to loss of clinical warning symptoms (e.g., palpitations, sweating, hunger) with hypoglycemia (known as *hypoglycemia unawareness*). A unique risk of insulin pump therapy is diabetic ketoacidosis (DKA) as pump malfunctions or infusion site problems can interrupt insulin delivery. Finally, IIT requires time and commitment from the patient and may have negative psychosocial and economic implications.

6. What is the difference between basal insulin coverage and bolus insulin coverage?

IIT is designed to mimic the normal insulin secretion pattern, which includes continuous basal coverage in addition to bursts of insulin to regulate the rise in glucose after food intake (Fig. 3.1). Basal insulin secretion suppresses hepatic glucose production to control blood glucose levels in the fasting state and premeal periods. Normal basal insulin secretion from the pancreas varies slightly throughout the day, responding to changes in activity, blood glucose levels, and regulatory hormones. Basal insulin coverage in IIT is usually accomplished with injections of long-acting insulin analogues or with the basal infusion function on the insulin pump. Bolus insulin doses consist of two components, the *nutritional dose,* which is the amount of insulin required to manage glucose excursions after meals, and the *correction dose,* which is the amount of insulin required to reduce a high glucose level detected before a meal. Bolus coverage is accomplished by administration of rapid-acting or short-acting insulin preparations or using the bolus function on the insulin pump. Physiologic insulin secretion requirements are approximately 50% basal and 50% bolus.

7. How are basal and bolus insulins used with an MDI regimen?

A long-acting insulin is injected either once or twice daily to provide the basal insulin portion of an MDI regimen, which is approximately 50% of a patient's total daily dose. Ideally, basal insulin should cover background insulin needs only, independent of food intake. A rapid-acting or short-acting insulin is injected before meals to provide the bolus insulin portion of an MDI regimen (see Fig. 3.1). Rapid-acting insulin is preferred because of the rapid onset and short duration of action. A patient can adjust each bolus dose to match the carbohydrate intake and to correct for high glucose levels before the meal, whereas the basal dose remains constant from day to day. Premixed "biphasic" insulin preparations combine either a rapid-acting insulin analogue or regular human insulin with a crystalline protaminated form of the analogue or regular human insulin in an attempt to imitate basal or bolus therapy with fewer injections.

8. What are the currently available bolus insulin preparations?

Bolus insulin options include rapid-acting analogues (aspart, glulisine, and lispro), short-acting regular human insulin, and ultrarapid-acting agents (faster-acting insulin aspart and inhaled insulin). See Table 3.1 for a complete list of products and their pharmacodynamic profiles. All bolus insulin agents are effective at lowering PPG levels and HbA$_{1c}$. Rapid-acting agents have a faster onset of action and shorter duration of action compared with short-acting insulin. Because of this, current guidelines recommend the use of rapid-acting agents over short-acting agents in patients with type 1 diabetes to reduce the risk of hypoglycemia; however, cost may necessitate the use of regular insulin in some patients. Ultrarapid-acting agents may be an option for patients who have rapid rises

Table 3.1. The Pharmacodynamics of Insulin Preparations.

PREPARATIONS (U-100 UNLESS OTHERWISE NOTED)	ONSET	PEAK[a]	DURATION[a]
Bolus Insulin Products			
Ultra-rapid acting			
Insulin aspart (Fiasp)	15–20 min.[b]	90–120 min.	5–7 hours
Insulin human—inhaled (Afrezza)	12 min.	35–40 min.	90–180 mins.
Rapid-acting analog			
Insulin aspart (NovoLog)			
Insulin lispro U-100, U-200 (Humalog)	10–20 min.	30–90 min.	3–5 hours
Insulin glulisine (Apidra)			
Short-acting			
Regular (Humulin R, Novolin R)	30–60 min.	2–4 hours	5–8 hours
Basal Insulin Products			
Intermediate-acting			
NPH (Humulin N, Novolin N)	2–4 hours	4–10 hours	10–24 hours
Long-acting analog			
Insulin detemir (Levemir)	1.5–4 hours	6–14 hours[c]	16–20 hours
Insulin glargine U-100 (Lantus, Basaglar)	2–4 hours	No peak	20–24 hours
Insulin glargine U-300 (Toujeo)	6 hours	No peak	36 hours
Insulin degludec U-100, U-200 (Tresiba)	1 hour	No peak	42 hours
Combination Products			
70% NPH/30% regular (Humulin 70/30, Novolin 70/30)	30–60 min.	Dual	10–16 hours
75% NPL, 25% lispro (Humalog 75/25)	5–15 min.	Dual	10–16 hours
50% NPL, 50% lispro (Humalog 50/50)	5–15 min.	Dual	10–16 hours
70% insulin aspart protamine, 30% insulin aspart (Novolog 70/30)	5–15 min.	Dual	15–18 hours

[a]The peak and duration of insulin action are variable, depending on injection site, duration of diabetes, renal function, smoking status, and other factors.
[b]Onset of appearance is 2.5 minutes compared to 5.2 minutes for insulin aspart (NovoLog)
[c]Long-acting insulins are considered "peakless" although they have exhibited peak effects during comparative testing.
NPH, neutral protamine Hagedorn; *NPL,* insulin lispro protamine suspension

in glucose after meals and desire a bolus insulin with a faster pharmacokinetic onset. Faster-acting insulin aspart (Fiasp) is insulin aspart formulated with niacinamide, which aids in speeding the initial absorption of insulin.

9. What are the currently available basal insulin preparations?

Basal insulin options include long-acting analogues (detemir, glargine U-100, glargine U-300, degludec) and neutral protamine Hagedorn (NPH) insulin. See Table 3.1 for a complete list of products and their pharmacodynamics profiles. All basal insulin agents are effective at lowering FPG levels and HbA$_{1C}$. The pharmacodynamics of NPH insulin make it a less ideal basal insulin because it has a distinct peak effect and does not last a full 24 hours. It must be administered twice daily in patients with type 1 diabetes. Insulin detemir and glargine U-100 have improved pharmacodynamic profiles compared with NPH, but they may still exhibit a peak effect and may not last a full 24 hours in all patients. Insulin glargine U-300 and insulin degludec are newer basal insulins without peak effects and have durations of action that exceed 24 hours. These pharmacodynamic benefits are appealing because they permit once-daily dosing without the effect wearing off, allow for more dosing flexibility, and are less likely to cause hypoglycemia. Studies have shown that these agents result in similar reductions in FPG and HbA$_{1C}$ but result in less nocturnal hypoglycemia compared with insulin glargine U-100.

10. When should bolus insulin be taken?
   - Rapid-acting insulin should be taken 5 to 10 minutes before meals and snacks.
   - Rapid-acting insulin can be taken:
     - 15 to 30 minutes before meals if the premeal BG is higher than 130 mg/dL
     - Immediately after eating, if gastroparesis or a concurrent illness is present
     - Upon arrival of food, if unfamiliar with meal size, content, or timing (i.e., in a restaurant or hospital)
   - Fast-acting insulin aspart (Fiasp) should be taken at the beginning of the meal or within 20 minutes after starting the meal.

- Inhaled insulin should be taken at the beginning of the meal.
- Human regular insulin should be taken 15 to 30 minutes before meals.

11. When should basal insulin be taken?
- Insulin glargine U-100, detemir, glargine U-300, and degludec should be taken once a day at the same time each day.
- Insulin glargine U-100 or detemir may be taken at bedtime if the "dawn phenomenon" is present.
- Basal insulin analogues (glargine, detemir, or degludec) cannot be mixed with other insulins.
- If nocturnal hypoglycemia results from taking a full dose of glargine or detemir at bedtime, an option would be to split the dose so that 50% is taken in the morning and the other 50% is taken in the evening, approximately 12 hours apart.
- NPH insulin is taken in the morning and at bedtime to avoid nocturnal hypoglycemia.
- Doses of insulin glargine U-300 and insulin degludec should not be adjusted more frequently than every 3 to 4 days because of their longer half-lives.

12. What is the role of SMBG?
Optimal diabetes control requires frequent SMBG (or CGM) to permit well-informed adjustments in insulin doses. Patients on IIT, who do not use CGM, should perform SMBG at least four times daily, before meals, and at bedtime. Patients should also test if symptoms of hypoglycemia occur and should always test before driving if frequent hypoglycemia or hypoglycemia unawareness is present. SMBG is crucial during times of intercurrent illness or stresses for early detection and potential prevention of hyperglycemic emergencies, such as DKA. Patients may also benefit from occasional testing 1 to 2 hours after meals. Patients using CGM may perform SMBG with less frequent use of the glucometer, but the glucometer should still be easily accessible in case of emergencies or device failure. The role of CGM is described below.

13. What is an insulin pump?
An insulin pump is a small, lightweight, portable, battery-operated device, which is either attached directly to the body (patch pump) or worn on clothing or a belt similar to a pager (traditional pump). A traditional pump is composed of a pump reservoir (which holds a 2- to 3-day supply of rapid-acting or short-acting insulin), connected to an infusion set, which ends in a cannula that is inserted into the skin and changed every 2 to 3 days. A patch pump is tubing free and consists of a disposable reservoir that attaches directly to the body with self-adhesive backing and a built-in infusion set in the device for insertion into the subcutaneous tissue. The patch pump is controlled by a handheld personal digital assistant (PDA). Insulin is delivered through either system in microliter amounts continuously over 24 hours. The user is responsible for setting the basal rates and determining the bolus doses, depending on the meal ingested and the results of SMBG. Currently, three companies offer insulin pumps in the United States. Each pump has special features and functions that are unique and help with the flexibility of pump use. To learn more about each of these pumps, contact the companies listed in Table 3.2.

14. What are the patient's responsibilities before insulin pump therapy can be initiated?
- Commit at least 2 to 3 months to pump initiation and training, including multiple meetings with the diabetes team before, during, and after the pump is initiated.
- Demonstrate the ability to monitor BG values at least 4 to 10 times per day, keep logs of BG readings, insulin doses and food consumed, and communicate information to the team.

Table 3.2. Currently Available Insulin Pumps and Continuous Glucose Monitors.

	PRODUCT	COMPANY AND WEBSITE
Insulin pumps	MiniMed Paradigm Revel	Medtronic Diabetes (www.medtronicdiabetes.com)
	Omnipod	Insulet Corporation (www.myomnipod.com)
	t:slim X2	Tandem Diabetes Care (www.tandemdiabetes.com)
Continuous glucose monitors	G4 Platinum	Dexcom (www.dexcom.com)
	G5	
	G6	
	Guardian Connect	Medtronic Diabetes (www.medtronicdiabetes.com)
	FreeStyle Libre Flash system	Abbott (www.freestylelibre.us)
Combination insulin pump/continuous glucose monitor	MiniMed 530G with Enlite sensor	Medtronic Diabetes (www.medtronicdiabetes.com)
	MiniMed 630G with Enlite sensor	
	MiniMed 670G with Guardian Sensor	

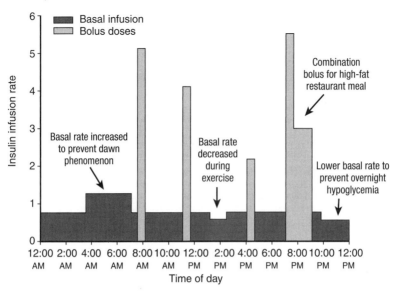

Fig. 3.2. Insulin delivery pattern with pump therapy.

- Review pump training materials and practice pump functions at least two to three times before wearing the pump.
- Be willing to test basal rates or agree to wear a CGM system to ensure that the basal rates are set appropriately.

15. What are the benefits of insulin pump therapy?

Currently, insulin pump therapy is the dosing strategy that most closely mimics physiologic insulin secretion. Benefits include better, more precise glucose control with less glycemic variability, a reduction in frequency and severity of hypoglycemia, ability to adjust basal rates throughout the day (Fig. 3.2), ability to extend bolus dose durations to better cover high-fat meals (see Fig. 3.2), improved flexibility of lifestyle, ability to administer small amounts of insulin (as little as 0.025 units), protection from overcorrection by tracking active insulin, and ability to integrate with CGM technology.

16. What are the limitations of insulin pump therapy?

The cost of an insulin pump and supplies is higher compared with that of an MDI regimen. The device must be worn 24 hours a day, and optimal use requires highly motivated, competent patients and a higher level of training. A strong support system from a diabetes team is beneficial. Other limitations include infusion site infections and risks of DKA if insulin delivery is interrupted.

17. What is CGM?

Currently, three companies offer CGM devices in the United States. To learn more about CGM products, contact the companies listed in Table 3.2. CGM devices report interstitial glucose levels in real time and provide an insight into glucose trends. Traditional systems consist of a sensor, which is placed just under the skin and senses the glucose level in interstitial fluid; a transmitter, which is attached to the sensor and collects the glucose data; and a separate receiver, which collects the data from the transmitter and displays current and stored glucose readings. The receiver updates the user's glucose levels in real time, providing values every 5 minutes, and displays glucose trends with a graph and arrows. With some CGM devices, a smartphone or an insulin pump can be used as the receiver. Some newer CGM devices have received approval from the U.S. Food and Drug Administration (FDA) for the data to be used for treatment decision making without verification by SMBG. Some CGM devices require routine calibration with SMBG to maintain accuracy; some newer systems do not. Traditional CGM devices also provide alerts to the patient when glucose levels are too high or too low or are falling or rising rapidly. A new intermittent or "flash" CGM system differs from the traditional CGM devices in that it only communicates readings on demand (not continuously), does not have alarms, and does not require calibration with SMBG.

Some CGM devices are integrated with an insulin pump in one system. To date, we do not yet have an integrated insulin pump/CGM system that truly functions as an artificial pancreas (a system that reads glucose levels and automatically delivers the right amount of basal and bolus insulin doses to maintain glycemic control), but the technology is getting closer. The MiniMed 530G and 630G systems include the Enlite CGM device with a low glucose threshold suspend feature, which automatically stops insulin delivery for up to 2 hours when glucose levels fall below a predetermined threshold and the user does not respond to the alert. The MiniMed 670G system is the first hybrid closed-loop system. The system provides automated insulin delivery by automatically adjusting basal insulin delivery every 5 minutes on the basis of CGM data. It can also suspend insulin delivery up to 30 minutes before low glucose levels are predicted to occur. Integrated systems with either a t:slim X2 (Tandem) or Omnipod insulin pump combined with a Dexcom CGM are expected in the near future as well.

CGM use with IIT can reduce HbA$_{1C}$, hypoglycemia, and glucose variability in patients with type 1 diabetes. Current guidelines recommend CGM when patients with type 1 diabetes are not meeting glycemic targets. Traditional CGM may also be useful for patients with hypoglycemia unawareness and/or frequent hypoglycemic events.

18. What is carbohydrate counting, and how is it used with IIT?
Currently, carbohydrate counting is considered the "gold standard" for estimation of meal-time insulin doses. Carbohydrate counting is a tool used to match bolus insulin doses to food intake because carbohydrates have the greatest effect on BG levels. The peak of bolus insulin analogues should match the peak of BG following carbohydrate digestion and absorption ($\approx$ 1–3 hours, depending on the fat and fiber content of the meal).

19. List the common foods that contain dietary carbohydrates.
- Starch: cereals, grains, beans, bread, rice, pasta, and starchy vegetables
- Sugar: lactose (milk and yogurt), fructose (fruit, juice, and honey), and sucrose (table sugar and desserts)
- Fiber: cellulose and hemicellulose, lignins, gums, or pectins found in fruits, vegetables, legumes, and whole grains

20. How are carbohydrates counted?
Calculating the number of carbohydrates may initially require measuring and weighing commonly eaten foods. Nutrition labels on the package state the number of grams of carbohydrates based on the serving size. Carbohydrate reference books are available at bookstores or through the American Dietetic Association (http://www.eatright.org) or the American Diabetes Association (ADA; http://www.diabetes.org). Software programs are available for PDAs or online. Many restaurant chains provide nutrition brochures. See Chapter 6 for practical exercises in carbohydrate counting and insulin dosing.

21. What is the C:I ratio?
The C:I ratio is used to estimate how many grams of carbohydrate each unit of rapid-acting insulin will cover (e.g., 20:1 = 20 g of carbohydrate consumed requires 1 unit of bolus insulin).

22. How do you determine an initial C:I ratio?
Ratios are based on a patient's weight and the total daily dose (TDD) of insulin, which usually indicates the patient's sensitivity to insulin. An MDI regimen of basal insulin and premeal injections of rapid-acting insulin must be previously (or concurrently) implemented before establishing a C:I ratio. A person must be taught to count carbohydrates before using a C:I ratio safely.
1. Add up the patient's TDD of insulin on current therapy.
2. Consider the HbA$_{1C}$ value (ADA target is < 7%), frequency of hypoglycemia, and comorbidities.
3. The initial C:I ratio is estimated in our practice by dividing 550 by the TDD. Example: 550 divided by 30 units = 18:1 C:I ratio.
    In clinical practice, the constant in the C:I formula may range from 350 to 550. The initial calculated C:I must then be adjusted on the basis of each patient's records and is, therefore, only a starting point.

23. What is an example of an initial C:I ratio when changing to basal and bolus insulins?
- 40 units of Humulin 70/30 premixed insulin in the morning
- 17 units of Humulin 70/30 premixed insulin before the evening meal
- TDD = 57 units (HbA$_{1C}$ of 8.5% with 2–3 nocturnal hypoglycemic episodes per week)
- 550 ÷ 57 = 9.6
- Begin with a C:I = 10:1
    In this example, 1 unit of rapid-acting insulin will be given for every 10 g of carbohydrate eaten.

24. How do you adjust the C:I ratio once the initial ratio has been established?
Fine-tuning of a C:I ratio is based on BG records before meals and 2 hours after meals. The desired premeal BG is typically 80 to 130 mg/dL for most patients using IIT. A C:I ratio is correct if the BG increases by approximately 30 to 50 mg/dL over the premeal value at the 2-hour postprandial reading and returns to the range of 80 to 130 mg/dL by about 4 to 5 hours after the bolus insulin is given (Fig. 3.3). If 2-hour PPG level increments exceed 50 mg/dL, the C:I ratio should be adjusted and testing repeated with further adjustments until the desired excursion is consistently achieved.

25. What are the common causes of high BG?
- Missing an injection or bolus dose of insulin
- Menstrual cycle
- Decreased activity
- Stress, illness, or infection
- Underestimating carbohydrates
- Steroids or other medications

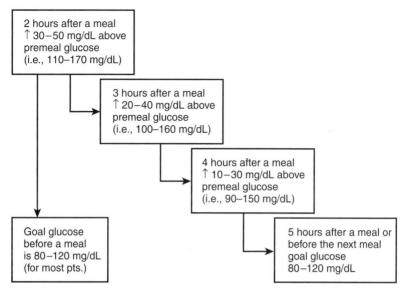

Fig. 3.3. Expected postprandial blood glucose (BG) range with rapid-acting bolus insulin.

26. What are other factors to consider when troubleshooting high BG readings?
    - Dawn phenomenon: a rise in BG occurs in predawn hours because of increased growth hormone and cortisol production.
    - Bad insulin: high BG occurs when insulin denatures if exposed to moderate-to-extreme temperatures or agitation, is beyond expiration date, or vial or pen device has been used for longer than the manufacturer's storage recommendations.
    - Insulin pump or infusion set technical problems: settings programmed incorrectly; battery depleted; pump malfunctions; tubing incorrectly primed; air bubbles in the tubing; dislodged, bent or kinked cannula; occlusion at infusion site; infusion set in place > 72 hours.

27. What causes high postprandial BG readings that are difficult to explain?
    - Coffee (caffeine): a rise in BG after drinking coffee (including drinking it black, without cream or sugar) is seen in many patients' records and likely results from increases in epinephrine or free fatty acid mobilization and subsequent worsening insulin resistance.
    - Cereal: a rise in BG is seen by patients consuming cereal, often requiring a lower C:I ratio (more insulin) and may be related to the glycemic index of most cereals combined with greater insulin resistance in the morning.
    - Food-on-the-fingers: high BG readings occur from residual food or dextrose on fingers when testing (patients must wash hands or wipe off first drop of blood).
    - Restaurant meals: Chinese food, Mexican food, pizza, and fried foods are high in fat and may require more insulin because of insulin resistance. A delay in digestion following a high-fat meal may require a split or extended bolus dose.

28. How is correctional insulin added for high BG before meals?
    Correctional or supplemental insulin (high BG CF) is used to reduce high BG detected before meals. A high BG CF is the expected amount that one unit of insulin will decrease the BG under normal circumstances. It is determined by using a formula based on the person's insulin sensitivity. The initial CF is estimated in our practice by dividing 1650 by the TDD. In clinical practice, the constant in the CF formula may range from 1500 to 1800. The initial calculated CF must then be adjusted on the basis of each patient's records and is, therefore, only a starting point.

29. What is an example of determining an initial CF?
    - 17 units of insulin glargine at noon and 5 units insulin lispro before each meal
    - TDD = 32 units (HbA$_{1C}$ of 7.2% with 1–2 hypoglycemic episodes per week)
    - 1650 ÷ 32 = 52
    - Begin with a CF of 50:1
        In this example, 1 unit of rapid-acting insulin will lower the BG about 50 mg/dL; therefore, 1 extra unit will be taken (in addition to the meal insulin dose) for each 50 mg/dL that the premeal BG is over the premeal goal of 100 mg/dL.

30. What is an example of C:I and CF usage?

To determine the amount of insulin needed before a meal, start with calculating the amount of bolus insulin needed to cover the meal. Example:
- C:I ratio is 20:1
- Meal consists of 80 g of carbohydrates
- Calculation: 80 ÷ 20 = 4 units of insulin to cover the meal

     Next, determine the amount of correctional insulin needed. If the BG is out of the target range before a meal, subtract the goal BG (100 mg/dL) from the actual BG and divide by the CF. Example:
- CF is 60:1
- Preprandial BG is 220 mg/dL
- Calculation: 220 − 100 mg/dL = 120 mg/dL above target
- Calculation: 120 (mg/dL) ÷ 60 = 2 units of insulin

     In this example, the patient should take 6 units of bolus insulin before the meal—4 units to cover the carbohydrates in the meal and 2 units to return the premeal high BG to the target range.

31. When is a CF used?
- It is recommended that high BG corrections be taken before meals or at least 5 hours after the last bolus because of the duration of action of the bolus insulin analogues.
- Hypoglycemia may occur from the accumulation of active insulin if BG corrections are performed too frequently (stacking).

32. What can be done for a high postprandial BG reading?
- If a postprandial BG is dangerously high (i.e., > 300 mg/dL) or a patient insists on making high BG corrections < 5 hours since the last bolus or during the night, he or she should be instructed in how to take a partial correction for safety.
- Using one half of the usual premeal CF to lower the BG to the target level is safest between meals.
- A target level of 150 mg/dL (expected BG level 2 hours postprandial) rather than a target BG of 100 mg/dL is used as the correction target between meals.

33. What is an example of using a half CF?
- BG before dinner = 100 mg/dL
- BG 2 hours after dinner = 300 mg/dL
- "Expected" BG 2 hours after dinner = ≈130 to 150 mg/dL
- Calculation: 300 minus 150 mg/dL = 150 mg/dL above target
- CF is 60:1
- Calculation: 150/60 = 2.5 units (full CF)
- The premeal insulin is still active for about 3 more hours; therefore, use a half CF
- Calculation of half CF: 2.5 (units) ÷ 2 = 1.3 units

     In this example, 1.3 units with an insulin pump or 1 unit with a syringe or insulin pen should be given 2 hours after the meal to bring the postprandial BG into the target range. BG should be rechecked within 2 hours to avoid a severe low glucose.

34. How do you calculate an initial basal rate for insulin pump therapy?
- An established C:I ratio and CF on MDI are critical for a smooth transition to pump therapy.
- To calculate an initial basal rate, take the current TDD of insulin on MDI, and reduce it by 25% (or other appropriate reduction, depending on current HbA_{1c} and number of hypoglycemic episodes).
- Use 50% of this reduced dose as the new total basal dose to be given over 24 hours.
- Start with one basal rate for 24 hours (divide the total basal dose by 24). [Initial basal rate per hour = (TDD × 0.75) ÷ (2 × 24).]
- The remaining 50% will be used as bolus doses for meals on the basis of carbohydrate counting.

35. Calculate an example of an initial basal rate for insulin pump therapy
1. Current TDD of insulin is 50 units. 25% reduction of TDD = 37.5 units
2. 50% of reduced dose = 37.5 ÷ 2 = 18.75 units as total basal
3. Total basal insulin = 18.75 ÷ 24 = 0.78 U/hr

     In this example, the initial basal rate will be 0.8 U/hr. Basal rate adjustments will then be made on the basis of testing and recording BG profiles throughout the day.

36. When are nighttime basal rate adjustments made?

Nighttime basal rates should be adjusted before the daytime basal rates are verified. Testing is typically performed during the first week of insulin pump therapy. Be aware that patients transitioning from injected long acting insulins (glargine, detemir, or degludec) may have overlapping insulin activity, which may cause hypoglycemia during the first week. Testing is then repeated if a significant weight change occurs, if an exercise routine is begun or altered, following hormonal changes (e.g., puberty, menopause), or as needed.

37. List the recommendations to follow during the nighttime basal rate verification process
Here are the instructions for the patient to use when verifying overnight basal rates:
- Assess basal rate accuracy on three nights.
- Eat the evening meal early, preferably before 5 PM (or begin the test period ≈ 5 hours after eating), and take the usual insulin bolus for dinner and correction, if needed.
- Choose a meal that you frequently eat or one for which you are confident of the carbohydrate amount.
- Avoid meals with > 15 to 20 g of fat, 10 g of fiber, and alcohol on testing nights.
- Avoid any food or insulin bolus after the evening meal.
- Avoid exercise other than typical activity.
- Monitor BG before and 2 hours after the evening meal, at 9 PM, 12 midnight, 3 AM, 6 AM, and before breakfast (or use CGM during this time).
- Stop the test if BG is < 70 mg/dL or > 250 mg/dL during the basal test and treat the abnormal BG.

38. How are nighttime basal rate adjustments made?
- If BG levels change by > 20 to 30 mg/dL during overnight monitoring, adjust the basal rate for the next night by 0.1 U/hr, starting 1 to 3 hours before the BG change was seen.
- Changes are made until the FBG level in the morning is within the target range (80–130 mg/dL).
- Daytime basal rates are verified next, usually 1 to 2 weeks after pump initiation or as necessary.

39. Describe the procedure for making daytime basal rate adjustments
- Have patients skip breakfast and check their BG levels every hour from 7 AM to 12 noon (or use a CGM) to verify the morning basal rate.
- If BG levels change by > 20 to 30 mg/dL during this time, adjust the basal rate for the next day by 0.1 U/hr, starting 1 to 3 hours before the glucose change was seen.
- After the morning basal rate is set, have patients skip their other meals (on separate days), and follow the same monitoring and adjustment procedures to confirm the afternoon and evening basal rate(s).

40. What is the role of noninsulin medications in the treatment of type 1 diabetes?
Pramlintide, an amylin analogue, delays gastric emptying, decreases inappropriate glucagon secretion from the pancreas after a meal, and increases satiety. It is approved for use as an adjunct to insulin therapy in patients with type 1 diabetes who have failed to achieve desired glycemic control despite optimal insulin therapy. Pramlintide has been shown to induce weight loss and lower insulin doses. It is administered before meals and concurrent reduction of meal-time bolus insulin dosing is required to reduce the risk of hypoglycemia.

Metformin, glucagon-like protein-1 (GLP-1) receptor agonists, and sodium-glucose cotransporter-2 (SGLT-2) inhibitors may reduce insulin requirements and improve metabolic control in patients with type 1 diabetes. Several medications in these classes have been or are being studied in patients with type 1 diabetes, but none has been approved by the FDA for use in type 1 diabetes.

41. What is the recommended treatment of hypoglycemia?
Dextrose should be taken for a BG of < 70 mg/dL. The patient should take 15 g of a quick-acting carbohydrate: fruit juice, glucose tablets or gel, or dextrose-based candy (SweetTARTS, Smarties, Spree). Pure glucose (without added fat or protein) is preferred. The patient should wait 15 minutes and test the BG again. If the repeat BG is < 70 mg/dL, additional dextrose should be taken. Once glucose returns to normal, the patient should eat a meal or snack to prevent recurrent hypoglycemia.

42. Why does rebound hyperglycemia occur after hypoglycemia?
- Overtreatment with an inappropriate amount of carbohydrate may occur.
- No treatment (i.e., sleeping through a low glucose episode) may result in counterregulatory hormone release and increased hepatic glycogenolysis.
- Treatment with a food that contains fat will delay digestion and absorption, thereby prolonging hypoglycemia and causing counterregulatory hormone release with subsequent hepatic glycogenolysis.

43. Discuss the use of glucagon to treat severe hypoglycemia
All patients using MDI or pump therapy should be given a glucagon emergency kit prescription and a demonstration. Glucagon is used to raise BG when a person is unable to swallow. This may occur either as a result of a seizure or unconsciousness. Family members should receive instruction, and the patient should be able to demonstrate the procedure to a third party (coworker or neighbor).

KEY POINTS

Intensive Insulin Therapy

1. Studies have demonstrated that optimal diabetes management decreases chronic complications.
2. Intensive insulin therapy, or basal-bolus therapy, is required to mimic normal pancreatic insulin secretion.
3. Basal insulin is physiologic insulin required to manage blood glucose (BG) fluctuations due to hepatic glucose production.
4. Bolus insulin is matched to carbohydrate intake using a carbohydrate-to-insulin ratio.
5. Correctional bolus insulin reduces the BG to within normal limits when a high glucose correction factor is used.

BIBLIOGRAPHY

American Diabetes Association. (2018). Standards of medical care in diabetes – 2018. *Diabetes Care, 41*(Suppl. 1), S1–S159.

Aschner, P., Horton, E., Leiter, L. A., Munro, N., & Skyler, J. S. (2010). Practical steps to improving the management of type 1 diabetes: recommendations from the Global Partnership for Effective Diabetes Management. *International Journal of Clinical Practice, 64,* 305–315.

Chamberlain, J. J., Kalyani, R. R., Leal, S., Rhinehart, A. S., Shubrook, J. H., Skolnik, N., & Herman, W. H. (2017). Treatment of type 1 diabetes: synopsis of the 2017 American Diabetes Association Standards of Medical Care in Diabetes. *Annals of Internal Medicine, 167*(7), 493–498.

Danne, T., Nimri, R., Battelino, T., Bergenstal, R. M., Close, K. L., DeVries, J. H., ... Phillip, M. (2017). International consensus on use of continuous glucose monitoring. *Diabetes Care, 40*(12), 1631–1640.

Davidson, P. C., Hebblewhite, H. R., Steed, R. D., & Bode, B. W. (2008). Analysis of guidelines for basal-bolus insulin dosing: basal insulin, correction factor, and carbohydrate-to-insulin ratio. *Endocrine Practice, 14,* 1095–1101.

DeWitt, D. E., & Hirsch, I. B. (2003). Outpatient insulin therapy in type 1 and type 2 diabetes mellitus: scientific review. *JAMA, 289,* 2254–2264.

Diabetes Control and Complications Trial Research Group. (1993). The effect of intensive treatment of diabetes on the development and progression of long-term complications in insulin-dependent diabetes mellitus. *New England Journal of Medicine, 329,* 977–986.

Duckworth, W., Abraira, C., Moritz, T., Reda, D., Emanuele, N., Reaven, P. D., ... Huang, G. D. (2009). Glucose control and vascular complications in veterans with type 2 diabetes. *New England Journal of Medicine, 360,* 129–139.

Harris, K., Boland, C., Meade, L., & Battise, D. (2018). Adjunctive therapy for glucose control in patients with type 1 diabetes. *Diabetes Metabolic Syndrome and Obesity, 11,* 159–173.

Heinemann, L. (2009). Insulin pump therapy: what is the evidence for using different types of boluses for coverage of prandial insulin requirements? *Journal of Diabetes Science and Technology, 3,* 1490–1500.

Nathan, D. M., Cleary, P. A., Backlund, J. Y., Genuth, S. M., Lachin, J. M., Orchard, T. J., ... Zinman, B. (2005). Intensive diabetes treatment and cardiovascular disease in patients with type 1 diabetes. *New England Journal of Medicine, 353,* 2643–2653.

Ohkubo, Y., Kishikawa, H., Araki, E., Miyata, T., Isami, S., Motoyoshi, S., ... Shichiri, M. (1995). Intensive insulin therapy prevents the progression of diabetic microvascular complications in Japanese patients with non-insulin-dependent diabetes mellitus: a randomized prospective 6-year study. *Diabetes Research and Clinical Practice, 28,* 103–117.

Patel, A., MacMahon, S., Chalmers, J., Neal, B., Billot, L., Woodward, M., ... Travert, F. (2008). Intensive blood glucose control and vascular outcomes in patients with type 2 diabetes. *New England Journal of Medicine, 358,* 2560–2572.

Pickup, J. C. (2012). Insulin-pump therapy for type 1 diabetes mellitus. *New England Journal of Medicine, 366,* 1616–1624.

Skyler, J. S., Bergenstal, R., Bonow, R. O., Buse, J., Deedwania, P., Gale, E. A. ... Sherwin, R. S. (2009). Intensive glycemic control and the prevention of cardiovascular events: Implications of the ACCORD, ADVANCE, and VA diabetes trials: a position statement of the American Diabetes Association and a scientific statement of the American College of Cardiology Foundation and the American Heart Association. *Diabetes Care, 32,* 187–192.

Switzer, S. M., Moser, E. G., Rockler, B. E., & Garg, S. K. (2012). Intensive insulin therapy in patients with type 1 diabetes mellitus. *Endocrinology and Metabolism Clinics of North America, 41*(1), 89–104.

The Action to Control Cardiovascular Risk in Diabetes Study Group. (2008). Effects of intensive glucose lowering in type 2 diabetes. *New England Journal of Medicine, 358,* 2545–2559.

UK Prospective Diabetes Study (UKPDS) Group. (1998). Intensive blood-glucose control with sulphonylureas or insulin compared with conventional treatment and risk of complications in patients with type 2 diabetes (UKPDS 33). *Lancet, 352,* 837–853.

UK Prospective Diabetes Study (UKPDS) Group. (1998). Effect of intensive blood-glucose control with metformin on complications in overweight patients with type 2 diabetes (UKPDS 34). *Lancet, 352,* 854–865.

White, R. D. (2007). Insulin pump therapy (continuous subcutaneous insulin infusion). *Primary Care, 34,* 845–871.

Wolpert, H. (Ed.). (2016). *Intensive diabetes management* (6th ed). Alexandria, VA: American Diabetes Association.

CHAPTER 4

TYPE 2 DIABETES MELLITUS

Sarah L. Anderson and Jennifer M. Trujillo

1. **What are the standards of care for the management of type 2 diabetes (T2D) mellitus?**
   Both the American Diabetes Association (ADA) and the American College of Clinical Endocrinologists (AACE) have published evidence-based minimum standards of diabetes care. Both sets of standards include recommendations on the screening, diagnosis, classification, prevention, and management of diabetes, including lifestyle modifications, glycemic treatment, cardiovascular (CV) risk management, prevention and treatment of complications, and glycemic management in specific populations and practice settings. Both recommend that patients have a comprehensive medical evaluation and assessment of comorbidities at each visit. The standards from both organizations are evidence based, frequently updated, and easily accessible. The ADA Standards of Care are available at: https://professional.diabetes.org/content-page/standards-medical-care-diabetes, and the AACE guidelines are available at: https://www.aace.com/files/dm-guidelines-ccp.pdf.

2. **What should be included in a comprehensive evaluation of a patient with T2D?**
   At the initial visit, a complete diabetes and medical history, family history, and personal history of complications and common comorbidities should be completed. Lifestyle and behavior patterns, as well as glucose monitoring, need to be assessed initially and at every visit. A medication history is essential and should include medication-taking behaviors, intolerances, complementary and alternative medicine use, and vaccination history. A complete physical examination, including vital signs, thyroid palpation, skin examination, and comprehensive foot examination, should be performed. Referral for an ophthalmologic examination and, if appropriate, smoking cessation counseling, are also recommended. Overall glycemic control, including a glycosylated hemoglobin (HbA_{1C}) should be assessed initially and every 6 months in patients with adequate glycemic control and every 3 months in patients with uncontrolled glucose levels.

   Laboratory data that are recommended at the initial visit and annually thereafter include a lipid panel, liver function tests, spot urinary albumin-to-creatinine ratio, serum creatinine and estimated glomerular filtration rate (eGFR), vitamin B_{12} (if on metformin), and serum potassium (if on an angiotensin-converting enzyme [ACE] inhibitor, angiotensin receptor blocker [ARB], or diuretic). Screening for psychosocial conditions, self-management education needs, hypoglycemia, and pregnancy planning should be performed. Atherosclerotic cardiovascular disease (ASCVD) risk assessment and staging of chronic kidney disease (CKD) are also recommended. Patient-specific, individualized goals should be set for HbA_{1C}, blood pressure (BP; for those with hypertension [HTN]), and self-management behaviors.

3. **What are the goals of therapy for people with T2D mellitus?**
   The primary goals of therapy for T2D are to prevent or delay the progression of long-term microvascular and macrovascular complications, including retinopathy, neuropathy, diabetic kidney disease (DKD) and ASCVD. Additional goals of therapy are to alleviate symptoms of hyperglycemia, minimize hypoglycemia and other adverse medication effects, minimize treatment burden, and maintain quality of life. To achieve these goals, several organizations, including the ADA and the AACE, recommend surrogate targets for glycemic control. The ADA Standards of Care indicate that an A1C target should be established for each patient; $HbA_{1C} < 7\%$ is reasonable for most nonpregnant adults, but the HbA_{1C} goal should be individualized on the basis of patient-specific factors (see Section 5, How should glycemic targets be established?). A fasting plasma glucose (FPG) target range of 80 to 130 mg/dL and a postprandial glucose (PPG) target of < 180 mg/dL (1–2 hours after the beginning of a meal) correspond with an HbA_{1C} target of $< 7\%$. The AACE guidelines are more aggressive and indicate that $HbA_{1C} \leq 6.5\%$ is optimal if it can be achieved in a safe and affordable manner. A FPG target of < 110 mg/dL and a 2-hour PPG target of < 140 mg/dL correspond with this recommendation (Table 4.1).

4. **What is the evidence to support tight glycemic control?**
   The United Kingdom Prospective Diabetes Study (UKPDS) was a landmark trial evaluating the impact of intensive glucose control on the incidence of long-term complications in patients with T2D. Investigators recruited 5102 patients with newly diagnosed T2D in 23 centers within the United Kingdom between 1977 and 1991. Patients were followed up for an average of 10 years to determine the impact of intensive versus conventional glycemic control. The results showed that the intensive glycemic control arm achieved an HbA_{1C} of 7% compared with 7.9% in the conventional group. This translated into a 12% reduction in the primary composite endpoint of any diabetes-related complication ($P = 0.029$). Most of this resulted from a 25% reduction in microvascular complications in patients assigned to the intensive treatment arm compared with those in the conventional arm. There was

Table 4.1. Glycemic Target Recommendations for Most Nonpregnant Adults with Diabetes.[a]

	ADA	AACE
HbA$_{1C}$	< 7.0%	≤ 6.5%
Fasting plasma glucose (FPG)	80–130 mg/dL	< 110 mg/dL
Postprandial glucose (PPG)	< 180 mg/dL	< 140 mg/dL

[a]Glycemic targets should be individualized. More or less stringent goals may be appropriate for some patients.
AACE, American Association of Clinical Endocrinologists; *ADA*, American Diabetes Association; *HbA$_{1C}$*, glycosylated hemoglobin.

also a 16% reduction in ASCVD events in the intensive group, but this did not quite reach statistical significance ($P = 0.052$). The microvascular benefits of early glucose control persisted 10 years after the end of the original trial. The 10-year follow-up report also showed a significant long-term reduction in myocardial infarction (MI) and all-cause mortality.

Three additional large-scale studies were performed after the UKPDS to compare the effects of different intensities of glycemic control on the risk of macrovascular complications. These studies included patients who had longstanding, advanced T2D and were at high risk for ASCVD; in contrast, the UKPDS included subjects with newly diagnosed T2D. The Action to Control Cardiovascular Risk in Diabetes (ACCORD) study (n = 10,251) showed that lower HbA$_{1C}$ levels (achieved mean HbA$_{1C}$ 6.4% versus 7.5%) reduced the risk of some microvascular complications but did not reduce the risk of macrovascular complications. The risk of hypoglycemia was significantly higher in the intensive treatment group. Most importantly, this study was stopped early because of an increase in mortality in the intensive treatment arm. The Action in Diabetes and Vascular Disease: Preterax and Diamicron Modified Release Controlled Evaluation (ADVANCE) study (n = 11,140) similarly showed no significant differences in ASCVD outcomes between two levels of glycemic control (achieved mean HbA$_{1C}$ 6.3% versus 7%) but did show that more intensive glucose control reduced microvascular complications. The Veterans Affairs Diabetes Trial (VADT; n = 1791) also suggested reduced microvascular complications but reported no significant reduction in ASCVD outcomes with more intensive glycemic control (HbA$_{1C}$ 6.9% versus 8.5%). On the basis of the results of these studies in aggregate, the relatively intense effort required to achieve more stringent glucose control should be considered when setting targets.

5. How should glycemic targets be determined?
Glycemic targets must be individualized for each patient based on patient-specific factors and the potential risks and benefits of treatment. Ideally, glycemic targets should be established at the time of diagnosis and should be reviewed and reevaluated at each visit. When possible, these decisions should be made in collaboration with the patient. Patient or disease factors to consider include the following: treatment-related risks, such as hypoglycemia and other adverse medication effects; disease duration; life expectancy; comorbidities; established vascular complications; patient attitude and expected treatment effort; resources; and a support system. Although an HbA$_{1C}$ < 7% is recommended by the ADA for most nonpregnant adults with T2D, a more stringent goal (e.g., < 6.5%) may be appropriate for some patients if it can be achieved without significant adverse effects, particularly hypoglycemia. Those patients might be younger, have a longer life expectancy, have a short duration of diabetes, be treated only with lifestyle modifications or metformin, or be without significant comorbidities. Less stringent goals (e.g., < 8%) may be appropriate for older patients, those with a limited life expectancy, those with a long duration of diabetes, those with a history of severe hypoglycemia, and those with extensive serious comorbidities or advanced complications. A higher HbA$_{1C}$ goal may also be appropriate when it is difficult to achieve the goal despite appropriate education, monitoring, and drug therapy. For those treated with complex medication regimens, especially those that include insulin, the risks in attempts to achieve stringent glycemic goals may outweigh the benefits.

Higher HbA$_{1C}$ goals should be considered in patients > 65 years of age. An HbA$_{1C}$ goal of < 7.5% is reasonable for healthy older adults, whereas an HbA$_{1C}$ goal of < 8% is reasonable for older adults with multiple coexisting chronic diseases, multiple impairments of activities of daily living (ADLs), or mild-to-moderate cognitive impairment. An HbA$_{1C}$ goal of < 8.5% is reasonable for older adults with end-stage chronic diseases, multiple dependencies for ADLs, or moderate-to-severe cognitive impairment or for those who live in long-term care facilities. Clinicians should consider adjusting the FPG and PPG target ranges to correspond with a higher target HbA$_{1C}$.

6. What lifestyle modifications are recommended for patients with T2D?
All patients with T2D should participate in diabetes self-management education (DSME) to acquire the knowledge, skills, and abilities needed for self-care. DSME should occur at the time of diagnosis, annually, when complicating factors arise, and when transitions of care occur. Goals of nutrition therapy are to promote and support healthy eating patterns; achieve and maintain body weight goals; achieve individualized glycemic, blood pressure, and lipid goals; and delay or prevent the complications of diabetes. Nutrition recommendations should be individualized on the basis of needs, personal and cultural preferences, health literacy and numeracy, and willingness and ability to make changes. Healthy eating and meal plans should follow the Dietary Guidelines for Americans and

focus on eating more nutrient-dense foods (e.g., vegetables), eating less saturated fat and added sugar, eating a variety of foods, decreasing empty calories (e.g., candy, sweets, sugar-sweetened beverages), making half of grain consumption be from whole grains, and shifting to lower-fat dairy products.

Weight loss of at least 5% of body weight should be recommended for any patient who is overweight or obese. Evidence supports focusing on a reduction in calorie intake instead of macronutrient distribution. Studies have shown that reduced calorie interventions reduce HbA_{1c} by 0.3% to 2% in patients with T2D. Weight loss can be attained by reducing portion sizes, reducing calorie intake by 500 to 750 kcal/day, or by targeting daily caloric intake goals to less than 1200 to 1500 kcal/day for women and 1500 to 1800 kcal/day for men.

Carbohydrate counting can be a useful tool for minimizing postmeal glucose excursions. Patients should be educated about which foods are sources of carbohydrates and that carbohydrates are the nutrient group that increases blood glucose (BG) levels. The diabetes plate method can be used to help patients identify a reasonable amount of carbohydrate intake per meal and to encourage them to limit their starch or grain consumption to one fourth of a 9-inch plate per meal. A common, but more complex, approach is to provide more specific carbohydrate serving limits to patients: limit carbohydrates to three to four servings (45–60 g) per meal for women or four to five servings (60–75 g) per meal for men and 1 serving (15 g) per snack. Individuals with T2D who are taking mealtime insulin may be instructed on how to count carbs to determine their premeal insulin dose. Although this is a more common practice in type 1 diabetes (T1D), it may be beneficial in patients with T2D who are on intensive insulin regimens.

Adults with T2D should engage in 150 minutes or more of moderate-to-vigorous intensity aerobic activity per week with no more than two consecutive days without activity. Patients should decrease the amount of sedentary time and avoid prolonged periods of sitting. Adults with T2D who are overweight or obese and have achieved short-term weight loss goals should participate in 200 to 300 minutes of physical activity per week as part of a comprehensive, long-term weight maintenance program.

7. What is the first-line medical treatment for T2D?

First-line medical therapy for T2D, in the absence of contraindications, is metformin. Metformin is a biguanide, which is an oral agent that decreases glucose production by the liver, reduces the amount of glucose absorbed from the intestines, and improves the body's sensitivity to insulin. Metformin is recommended as a first-line agent because it is effective and there is good evidence to support its use, including a reduced risk of CV outcomes, as shown by the UKPDS trial. Metformin is inexpensive, carries no long-term safety issues, and causes neither hypoglycemia nor weight gain. Metformin is indicated either as monotherapy or in combination with other oral agents or injectables, including insulin and glucagon-like peptide-1 receptor agonists (GLP-1 RAs). Changes to the renal dosing recommendations for metformin based on the eGFR, instead of serum creatinine levels, have appropriately extended the use of metformin in patients in whom it would previously have been contraindicated. Metformin is now indicated for patients with an eGFR $\geq$ 30 mL/min/1.73m^2, although starting metformin in a patient with an eGFR between 30 and 45 mL/min/1.73 m^2 is not recommended; if done, the dose should not exceed 1000 mg daily in those patients. This is largely because of the potential for further renal function decline that would necessitate stopping the medication.

Metformin is also available as fixed-dose combination products with several other oral agents, including the following: sulfonylureas, thiazolidinediones (TZDs), dipeptidyl peptidase-4 (DPP-4) inhibitors, sodium glucose cotransporter-2 (SGLT-2) inhibitors and meglitinides. Fixed dose combination products can increase adherence and minimize pill burden.

8. How can adverse effects of metformin be minimized?

The most common side effects of metformin are gastrointestinal (GI) in nature and include diarrhea, nausea, vomiting, and flatulence. To minimize these side effects, metformin should be initiated at a low dose and titrated up in a stepwise fashion. The target dose of metformin is 2000 mg/day (usually given in two divided doses); however, this is not the starting dose. Metformin should be initiated at 500 mg orally daily and titrated up by 500 mg each week until a maximum tolerated dose or 2000 mg daily is achieved. Other strategies for minimizing GI-related side effects of metformin include taking metformin with food and using an extended-release (ER) preparation; an important patient counseling point when using the ER preparations is that patients may see parts of the ER tablets in their stool.

Metformin also reduces intestinal absorption of vitamin B_{12} and may lower serum B_{12} concentrations. The longer the duration of metformin use, the more likely it is that B_{12} deficiency will occur. Because of the insidious onset of B_{12} deficiency, it is recommended that serum B_{12} levels be monitored every 2 to 3 years and treated accordingly. Severe vitamin B_{12} deficiency may present as peripheral neuropathy (PN). If the symptoms of PN are present and the patient is taking metformin, the B_{12} level should be checked to determine whether the symptoms are caused by B_{12} deficiency or by the progression of diabetes or another cause.

9. What are second-line medical options for the treatment of T2D?

If metformin monotherapy is not successful in getting a patient to the glycemic goal or if metformin therapy is not tolerated or contraindicated, a number of second-line agents are available. These include SGLT-2 inhibitors, GLP-1 RAs, DPP-4 inhibitors, sulfonylureas, TZDs, and basal insulin. These will be individually discussed in the sections below. Mechanisms, physiologic actions, and renal dosing recommendations of each drug category are summarized in Table 4.2.

Table 4.2. Mechanisms and Physiologic Actions of Common Glucose-Lowering Agents to Treat Type 2 Diabetes.

CLASS	COMPOUND(S)	RENAL DOSING RECOMMENDATIONS	CELLULAR MECHANISM(S)	PRIMARY PHYSIOLOGIC ACTION(S)
Biguanides	Metformin	Do not initiate if eGFR 30–45; Do not use if eGFR < 30. If eGFR drops to < 45 and metformin is continued, consider a maximum of 1000 mg daily	Activates AMP kinase (? Other)	↓ Hepatic glucose production
Sulfonylureas; second generation (SU)	Glyburide Glipizide Glimepiride	Avoid use in renal impairment (glyburide); initiate conservatively to avoid hypoglycemia	Closes K_{ATP} channels on beta cell plasma membranes	↑ Insulin secretion
Thiazolidinediones (TZD)	Pioglitazone Rosiglitazone	No dose adjustment required	Activates the nuclear transcription factor PPAR-gamma	↑ Insulin sensitivity
Dipeptidyl peptidase (DPP)-4 inhibitors	Sitagliptin Saxagliptin Linagliptin Alogliptin	Adjust dose if eGFR ≤ 50 (sitagliptin, saxagliptin); eGFR ≤ 60 (alogliptin); no dose adjustment needed (linagliptin)	Inhibits DPP-4 activity, increasing postprandial incretin (GLP-1, GIP) concentrations	↑ Insulin secretion (glucose dependent); ↓ glucagon secretion (glucose dependent)
Sodium-glucose cotransporter (SGLT)-2 inhibitors	Canagliflozin Dapagliflozin Empagliflozin Ertugliflozin	Adjust dose if eGFR < 60 (canagliflozin); avoid use if eGFR < 60 (dapagliflozin, ertugliflozin), eGFR < 45 (canagliflozin), eGFR < 30 (empagliflozin)	Inhibits SGLT-2 in the proximal nephron	Blocks glucose reabsorption by the kidney, increasing glycosuria
Glucagon-like peptide (GLP)-1 receptor agonists	Dulaglutide Exenatide Exenatide XR Liraglutide Lixisenatide Semaglutide	Limited experience with severe renal impairment; avoid use if eGFR < 30 (exenatide, exenatide XR), eGFR < 15 (lixisenatide); no dose adjustment recommended (dulaglutide, semaglutide)	Activates GLP-1 receptors	↑ Insulin secretion (glucose dependent); ↓ Glucagon secretion (glucose dependent); Slows gastric emptying; ↑ Satiety
Basal Insulin	Degludec Detemir Glargine	Lower insulin doses may be required with decreased eGFR	Activates insulin receptors	↑ Glucose disposal; ↓ Hepatic glucose production; Suppresses ketogenesis

AMP, Adenosine monophosphate; *eGFR*, estimated glomerular filtration rate; *GIP*, glucose-dependent insulinotropic polypeptidase; *PPAR*, peroxisome proliferator-activated receptor; *XR*, extended release.

10. **What is a sulfonylurea?**

Sulfonylureas that are most commonly in use today are glipizide, glyburide, and glimepiride. Sulfonylureas—also known as insulin secretagogues—are oral agents that work by stimulating endogenous insulin secretion by the pancreatic beta cells. Because of this, sulfonylureas are only useful in patients with some residual beta cell function. These agents predominantly lower PPG but also positively affect FPG. Side effects of sulfonylureas include weight gain and hypoglycemia. Although sulfonylureas contain a sulfonamide structure, the cross-reactivity between this type of sulfonamide and an antibiotic sulfonamide is significantly low.

Glipizide and glimepiride are shorter acting than glyburide and, therefore, may cause less hypoglycemia. In addition, glyburide is excreted renally and its active metabolites may accumulate in patients with renal dysfunction, again leading to hypoglycemia. Glipizide and glimepiride, in contrast, are metabolized by the liver and primarily excreted via urine as inactive metabolites, making them a preferred choice in patients with diabetes and CKD. Of note, micronized products are not bioequivalent, and retitration may be needed when switching between products.

11. **What is a GLP-1 RA?**

GLP-1 RAs are also known as *incretin mimetics*. These agents mimic the effects of endogenous incretins (specifically, GLP-1) in the body by (1) stimulating insulin secretion after eating, (2) inhibiting glucagon release, and (3) slowing gastric emptying, which increases satiety earlier and slows glucose absorption into the blood. GLP-1 RAs cause weight loss because of their effects on gastric emptying and early satiety. These agents are administered subcutaneously with an injectable pen device. Although they are not typically used as monotherapy, they are often used in conjunction with metformin when it has not been sufficiently effective for patients to achieve their glycemic goals. Because these agents promote glucose-dependent insulin secretion (insulin secretion only occurs when BG levels are high or rising), their risk of hypoglycemia is low when used as monotherapy or with other agents, such as metformin, for which the risk of hypoglycemia is also low. However, their use in conjunction with agents known to cause hypoglycemia may increase this risk. Currently available GLP-1 RAs include dulaglutide, exenatide (twice daily), exenatide (once weekly), liraglutide, lixisenatide, and semaglutide. Liraglutide and lixisenatide are also available in fixed-ratio combinations with basal insulin (degludec and glargine, respectively).

Exenatide (twice daily) and lixisenatide are short-acting GLP-1 RAs that have more pronounced PPG-lowering effects, especially after a meal that immediately follows the injection. This contrasts with the long-acting GLP-1 RAs, liraglutide (once daily dosing), and dulaglutide, exenatide QW, and semaglutide (all once weekly dosing), which lower FPG in addition to their PPG effects.

The most common side effects of GLP-1 RAs are GI related, with nausea being the most common. This underscores the importance of titration to target doses in a stepwise fashion to minimize this risk. Fixed-ratio combinations of GLP-1 RAs and basal insulin (liraglutide plus degludec, lixisenatide plus glargine), which are appropriate for patients requiring combination therapy for better glycemic control, minimize this side effect because the titration of the GLP-1 RA dose is much more incremental than with a GLP-1 RA alone. If a long-acting GLP-1 RA dose is missed, retitration may be necessary.

These agents may also be associated with acute pancreatitis; however, there is not enough evidence to prove a cause-and-effect relationship. Nonetheless, GLP-1 RA should not be initiated in patients with active pancreatitis or a history of pancreatitis related to a GLP-1 RA. If pancreatitis is suspected while a patient is using a GLP-1 RA, the drug should be discontinued. If the patient is confirmed to have pancreatitis related to the GLP-1 RA, the patient should not be rechallenged with a drug from this class. A rare but important potential side effect of GLP-1 RAs is thyroid C-cell tumors. Patients with a personal or family history of medullary thyroid cancer or multiple endocrine neoplasia-2 (MEN-2) should not be prescribed a GLP-1 RA.

12. **What is a DPP-4 inhibitor?**

DPP-4 inhibitors work by blocking DPP-4, which is an enzyme responsible for breaking down GI incretins (including glucose-dependent insulinotropic polypeptide [GIP] and GLP-1). DPP-4 inhibitors increase the circulating levels of incretin hormones, which then promote glucose-dependent insulin secretion and inhibit glucagon secretion. However, in contrast to GLP-1 RAs, they do not affect gastric emptying or satiety and, thus, the glycemic-lowering effect of DPP-4 inhibitors is modest, and they are weight neutral as opposed to promoting weight loss. Benefits of these agents include their good tolerability, low risk of hypoglycemia, and their ability to target PPG. Examples of medications in this class include alogliptin, linagliptin, saxagliptin, and sitagliptin; all have similar glycemic efficacy.

Cardiovascular outcomes trials (CVOTs) of DPP-4 inhibitors have been largely neutral; that is, there are generally no cardiovascular disease (CVD) concerns, but no CV benefits have been reported either. Saxagliptin is the exception; the Saxagliptin Assessment of Vascular Outcomes Recorded in Patients with Diabetes Mellitus (SAVOR)–Thrombolysis in Myocardial Infarction (TIMI) 53 trial showed an increased risk of hospitalizations for heart failure. Because of this, all DPP-4 inhibitors now carry a warning about use in patients at risk for heart failure.

In general, DPP-4 inhibitors are well tolerated, and their risk of adverse effects is low. Like GLP-1 RAs, DPP-4 inhibitors have been associated with an increased risk of pancreatitis. DPP-4 inhibitors should be avoided in patients with active pancreatitis or a history of pancreatitis thought to have been caused by a DPP-4 inhibitor. If a patient develops pancreatitis while taking one of these agents, the DPP-4 inhibitor should be discontinued. If the DPP-4 inhibitor is implicated in causing the pancreatitis, a drug from this class should not be used for the patient. Additionally, DPP-4 inhibitors have been associated with an increased risk of joint pain; if this occurs, the DPP-4 inhibitor should be discontinued, and symptoms should resolve.

13. What is a SGLT-2 inhibitor?

SGLT-2 inhibitors prevent the kidneys from reabsorbing glucose from urine in the proximal tubules back into the bloodstream, leading to increased glucose excretion in urine. This results in lowering of both FPG and PPG and modest weight loss caused by the loss of glucose (4 kcal/g) in urine. Because of their mechanism of action, SGLT-2 inhibitors do not require insulin or functional beta cells to be effective. The presence of more glucose in urine causes an osmotic diuresis that can also lower BP. This may be beneficial in patients with hypertension, but in those with low baseline BP, this can lead to hypotension. The excess urinary glucose increases the risk of urinary tract and genital mycotic infections, some of the more common side effects of this class of medications. Examples of SGLT-2 inhibitors include canagliflozin, dapagliflozin, empagliflozin, and ertugliflozin.

14. What is a TZD?

TZDs are a class of agents that target the peroxisome proliferator-activated receptor (PPAR) gamma, which activates the genes that influence how glucose is metabolized and how fat is stored in the body. These agents, pioglitazone and rosiglitazone, improve insulin sensitivity in muscle and fat tissue, and protect pancreatic beta cells. TZDs predominantly improve FPG. Because of their effects on gene activation, they have a slow onset of action; it typically takes several weeks for their full glycemic effects to be realized.

The use of rosiglitazone has fallen out of favor because of a meta-analysis that showed it to be associated with a statistically significant increased risk of MI and nonstatistically significant increased risk of death. Pioglitazone has been associated with a potential increased risk of bladder cancer, although clinical trial data regarding this risk are inconsistent. Both agents are known to cause dose-related edema and should not be used in patients with symptomatic heart failure.

15. What is basal insulin?

Basal insulin, also called "background insulin," is designed to provide 24-hour glycemic control by suppressing hepatic glucose production and maintaining near-normal glucose levels in the fasting state when taken in appropriate doses. Basal insulin is used in patients with T2D to supplement their endogenous insulin production. This option may be a first-line choice for patients whose HbA_{1c} is well above the goal (e.g., $\geq$ 10%) and is an effective second-line choice if a patient does not achieve glycemic targets on maximum-dose metformin.

The currently available basal insulins include long-acting agents (degludec [U-100 and U-200], detemir, glargine [U-100 and U-300], and intermediate-acting NPH (see Chapter 3, Table 3.1 for a complete list of products and their pharmacodynamics [PD]). All basal insulins are effective at lowering FPG levels and HbA_{1c}. Each has an onset of action of approximately 2 hours, but the duration of action varies among the agents; for example, insulin degludec has a duration of over 40 hours, whereas neutral protamine Hagedorn (NPH) insulin lasts approximately 12 hours and is typically dosed twice daily. Newer agents, such as degludec and glargine U-300, have longer durations of action and minimal or no peaks, which has translated into more consistent pharmacokinetics (PK) and PD, less nocturnal hypoglycemia, and more dosing flexibility compared with older agents, such as glargine U-100 and NPH.

The main side effects associated with basal insulin are hypoglycemia and weight gain. Using basal insulin in combination with certain oral or injectable agents known to be weight neutral or to promote weight loss may both mitigate weight gain and minimize the dose of insulin required, decreasing the risk of hypoglycemia. Stepwise titration of basal insulin also minimizes the risk of hypoglycemia.

16. What are third-line classes of diabetes medications?

In addition to the agents already discussed, there are several other classes of oral diabetes medications that are less frequently used in practice. Meglitinides (repaglinide and nateglinide) enhance endogenous insulin secretion (secretagogues) and thereby reduce postprandial hyperglycemia, similar to the sulfonylureas. Meglitinides have a more rapid onset and are shorter acting than sulfonylureas. Meglitinides may have a role in patients with true allergies to sulfonylureas because they work similarly and have comparable HbA_{1c}-lowering ability; however, they are more expensive and must be taken before all meals.

Alpha-glucosidase inhibitors (miglitol and acarbose) have modest HbA_{1c}-lowering efficacy (0.5%–0.8%) and work by slowing the absorption of dietary carbohydrates. Because of their mechanism of action, the hallmark side effect of these medications is GI intolerance, including flatulence and diarrhea, and many patients do not tolerate these effects.

Colesevelam, a bile acid sequestrant, modestly improves HbA_{1c} (0.5%) by decreasing bile acid reabsorption. It is unknown how this effect on reabsorption decreases BG. An added benefit is that in addition to lowering BG, it lowers low-density lipoprotein cholesterol (LDL-C).

Last, the immediate-release dopaminergic agonist bromocriptine also lowers BG by activating central dopamine-2 receptors and increasing insulin sensitivity. Like colesevelam, its effect on HbA_{1c} lowering is modest. It is not commonly used because of its high cost and its side-effect profile (dizziness, nausea, and fatigue).

17. **What is the general approach to the treatment of T2D?**
    The general approach to glycemic management in nonpregnant adults with T2D includes prompt initiation of life-style modification, determination of appropriate glycemic targets, and initiation of pharmacologic therapy based on the initial HbA$_{1c}$ at the time of diagnosis. The ADA algorithm recommends monotherapy (metformin if no con-traindications exist) for patients with an initial HbA$_{1c}$ < 9%; dual therapy (metformin plus an additional agent) for patients with an initial HbA$_{1c}$ ≥ 1.5% above their glycemic target; and combination injectable therapy for patients with an initial HbA$_{1c}$ > 10% and BG ≥ 300 mg/dL or for those who are markedly symptomatic. When needed, the next step is to add a second-line medication; the recommended agents are GLP-1 RAs, SGLT-2 inhibitors, DPP-4 inhibitors, sulfonylureas, TZDs, and basal insulin. The ADA recommends making the choice of a second agent, initially depending on whether or not the patient has existing ASCVD, heart failure, or CKD. Patients with ASCVD should be treated with metformin plus an agent proven to reduce major adverse cardiovascular events (MACEs); these medications currently include empagliflozin, liraglutide, canagliflozin, and semaglutide. The ADA's preference currently is liraglutide or empagliflozin because both medications have been proven, in large randomized controlled trials, to reduce both MACEs and CV mortality and have stronger data than other agents in the same classes. For patients where heart failure or CKD predominates, an SGLT-2 inhibitor such as empagliflozin or canagliflozin should be added based on evidence that each agent has demonstrated reductions in HF and/or CKD progression. For patients without ASCVD, the choice of which agent to add to metformin should be based on patient-specific and drug-specific considerations, including efficacy, hypoglycemia risk, effect on weight, effect on ASCVD outcomes, renal effects, adverse effects, safety concerns, ease of use, and cost (Table 4.3). The response to therapy should be evaluated after 3 months. If the patient has not achieved his or her glycemic goals at that time, adherence should be assessed, and additional therapy should be considered.
    The AACE guidelines recommend monotherapy for patients with an initial HbA$_{1c}$ of < 7.5%. Several medica-tions are listed as potential options, in order of preferred use, with metformin highest on the list. Dual therapy is recommended for patients with an initial HbA$_{1c}$ of ≥ 7.5% with metformin or other first-line agent plus an addi-tional medication. Again, medications are suggested in a hierarchy of preference. For patients with an initial HbA$_{1c}$ of > 9%, the AACE guidelines suggest dual or triple therapy for patients without symptoms and insulin with or without other agents for those with symptoms. The response to therapy should be evaluated after 3 months. If glycemic goals have not been achieved, adherence should be assessed, and therapy should be intensified. The hierarchy of drugs listed on the algorithm is based on the benefits and risks of each medication class. Minimizing the risk of hypoglycemia and weight gain are priorities. It is also recognized that combination therapy is usually required and should involve drugs with complementary mechanisms of action.
    Both the ADA and the AACE have issued recommendations that are sequential in their approach. Some emerging research and commentaries are recognizing the limitations of this sequential approach, and some have even referred to it as a "treat to fail" approach. An alternative strategy is using early combination therapy that targets multiple pathophysiologic defects to quickly achieve and then maintain glycemic control for a longer period and to possibly salvage existing beta cell function. This approach is not currently recommended by major clinical guidelines but is an area that is under investigation.

18. **What is the evidence supporting the use of specific agents in T2D patients with ASCVD?**
    In 2008, the U.S. Food and Drug Administration (FDA) set a requirement that all new drugs developed and studied for the treatment of T2D must undergo CV safety testing. Subsequent trials have uniformly included patients with existing CVD or at high risk for CVD and studied a three-point MACE endpoint, including a composite of CV death, nonfatal MI, and nonfatal stroke. In these CVOTs, liraglutide, semaglutide, empagliflozin, and canagliflozin have been reported to have beneficial effects on CV outcomes, as demonstrated in the LEADER (Liraglutide Effect and Action in Diabetes: Evaluation of Cardiovascular Outcome Results), SUSTAIN-6 (Trial to Evaluate Cardiovascular and Other Long-term Outcomes with Semaglutide in Subjects with Type 2 Diabetes), EMPA-REG OUTCOME (Empagliflozin Cardiovascular Outcome Event Trial in type 2 Diabetes Mellitus Patients), and CANVAS (Canagliflozin Cardiovascular Assessment Study) studies, respectively.
    The current ADA Standards of Care endorse the use of a GLP-1 RA or SGLT-2 inhibitor with proven CVD benefit in patients with a history of CVD to reduce the risk of CV mortality. The ADA acknowledges that the strongest evidence for CVD benefit in the GLP-1 RA class is with liraglutide and with empagliflozin in the SGLT-2 inhibitor class. Canagliflozin reduced the three-point MACE but not CV mortality. Canagliflozin also has the disadvantages of being linked to the rare but serious increased risk of bone fractures and lower extremity amputations. The AACE guidelines acknowledge that liraglutide is FDA approved for prevention of MACEs, empagliflozin is FDA approved to reduce CV mortality, and canagliflozin has been proven to reduce MACEs, but these guidelines do not have specific recommendations for when to use these agents.

19. **How should insulin therapy be initiated and titrated?**
    Basal insulin therapy should be initiated at a low dose (10 units or 0.1–0.2 units/kg) subcutaneously daily for safety and then titrated up by 10% to 15% (or 2–4 units) once or twice a week until the patient reaches the FPG target or a basal insulin dose of 0.5 units/kg is reached. On average, people with T2D treated with insulin glargine U-100 have a daily insulin dose of around 45 units. There are several available dose titration algorithms that can achieve optimal basal insulin doses, including the 3-0-3 method (if 3-day FPG average is above goal, increase by

Table 4.3. Drug-Specific and Patient Factors to Consider when Selecting Common Drug Therapy for Type 2 Diabetes.

	EFFICACY	HYPOGLYCEMIA RISK	EFFECT ON WEIGHT	ASCVD EFFECTS	PROGRESSION OF DKD EFFECTS	COST	ORAL/ SC	ADVERSE EFFECTS AND SAFETY
Metformin	High	No	Neutral	Potential benefit	Neutral	Low	Oral	GI (diarrhea), B_{12} deficiency
SUs	High	Yes	Gain	Neutral	Neutral	Low	Oral	Hypoglycemia, weight gain
TZDs	High	No	Gain	Potential benefit (pioglitazone)	Neutral	Low	Oral	Edema, weight gain, risk of heart failure, bone fractures, bladder cancer
DPP-4 inhibitors	Intermediate	No	Neutral	Neutral	Neutral	High	Oral	Risk of heart failure, pancreatitis, joint pain
SGLT-2 inhibitors	Intermediate	No	Loss	Benefit[a]	Benefit[a]	High	Oral	GU infections, risk of volume depletion, hypotension, risk of amputations, bone fractures (canagliflozin), risk of DKA
GLP-1 RAs	High	No	Loss	Benefit[b]	Benefit[b]	High	SC	GI (nausea, vomiting), injection site reactions, risk of thyroid C-cell tumors, pancreatitis, cholelithiasis
Basal Insulin	High	Yes	Gain	Neutral	Neutral	High	SC	Hypoglycemia, weight gain, Injection site reactions

[a]Empagliflozin, canagliflozin.
[b]Liraglutide, semaglutide.
ASCVD, Atherosclerotic cardiovascular disease; DKA, diabetic ketoacidosis; DKD, diabetic kidney disease; DPP, dipeptidyl peptidase; GI, gastrointestinal; GLP, glucagon-like peptide; GU, genitourinary; RA, receptor agonist; SC, subcutaneous; SGLT, sodium-glucose cotransporter; SU, sulfonylurea; TZD, thiazolidinedione.

3 units; if at goal, no change; if below goal, decreased by 3 units). If a patient experiences hypoglycemia, the basal insulin dose should be reduced by 10% to 20% or 4 units. Doses of insulin glargine U-300 and insulin degludec should not be adjusted more frequently than every 3 to 4 days because of their longer half-lives. Patients should be educated up front about how to titrate the dose as well as the anticipated final insulin dose. If patients are unable or unwilling to self-titrate, close follow-up is needed to ensure timely and effective insulin dosing.

20. When and how should insulin therapy be intensified?
If a patient does not reach his or her HbA$_{1C}$ goal despite adequately titrated basal insulin, insulin therapy can be intensified by adding an injection of rapid-acting insulin before the largest meal or changing to premixed insulin twice daily (before the morning and evening meals). When implementing the former, a dose of 4 units should be given before the largest meal. When implementing the latter, the current basal dose should be divided as two thirds in the morning (AM) and one third in the evening (PM), or one half (AM) and one half (PM). In either case, the dose can be titrated up by 1 to 2 units or 10% to 15% once or twice a week until BG targets are achieved. If hypoglycemia occurs, the dose should be decreased by 10% to 20% or 2 to 4 units (similar to basal insulin).

In the event that the HbA$_{1C}$ goal is not achieved with either strategy, rapid-acting insulin can be given at the two largest meals or at all three meals each day or the premixed insulin can be administered three times daily (breakfast, lunch, and dinner) by using the same titration strategy as described above.

Another option to intensify insulin therapy is to add a GLP-1 RA to the basal insulin. This combination offers many potential benefits, including provision of complementary mechanisms and effects on the glucose profile. GLP-1 RAs complement basal insulin because they target PPG (short-acting GLP-1 RAs) or PPG and FPG (long-acting GLP-1 RAs). The combination is also effective at any stage of the disease process. Combination therapy may also potentially lower the risk of adverse effects. Basal insulin causes hypoglycemia and weight gain. GLP-1 RAs do not cause hypoglycemia and lead to weight loss but do cause GI-related side effects. Combining the two classes may allow patients to achieve glycemic control with lower doses of both agents, potentially reducing the risk of adverse effects. Finally, the combination offers a potentially safer and easier option compared with adding rapid-acting insulin. The addition of a GLP-1 RA to basal insulin does not require additional glucose monitoring or carbohydrate counting and carries a lower hypoglycemic risk compared with basal-bolus insulin therapy.

21. What is overbasalization?
Overbasalization is a term used to describe the continued use of escalating doses of basal insulin to target FPG, with no improvement in PPG or HbA$_{1C}$. The total daily insulin requirement in most patients with T2D is approximately 1 unit/kg/day and in more insulin-resistant patients is approximately 1.5 units/kg/day; the total daily dose (TDD) should be divided as 50% basal insulin and 50% rapid-acting insulin with meals. When this 50/50 guideline is violated by continuing to increase the basal insulin dose, overbasalization occurs. Overbasalization has the potential to alter the PK of basal insulin, leading to peaks and hypoglycemia, especially when patients miss or delay meals.

Overbasalization often occurs because of the desire to keep the insulin regimen simple and not prescribe multiple daily injections. However, many patients need medication (e.g., rapid-acting insulin) to cover their postprandial glucose excursions. Continually increasing their basal insulin dose will not correct a prandial defect in their glucose profile and will greatly increase the risk of hypoglycemia. Overbasalization can be avoided by not continuing the up-titration of basal insulin once the FPG is in the target range or the total basal dose is 0.5 units/kg/day; at this point, it is safer and more effective to add a strategy that will reduce PPG levels, such as meal-time rapid-acting insulin, a GLP-1 RA, or an SGLT-2 inhibitor.

22. When should self-monitoring of blood glucose (SMBG) be performed in T2D?
SMBG is necessary for patients with T1D on intensive insulin regimens. The role of SMBG in patients with T2D is less clear. SMBG alone does not improve glycemic control. It is only effective if the results are used to modify management strategies. However, SMBG is appropriate in certain clinical situations. SMBG should be prescribed for anyone who is taking a medication that increases the risk of hypoglycemia (insulin, sulfonylurea, meglitinide) so that testing can occur if hypoglycemia is suspected. If a patient is prescribed basal insulin, morning SMBG is required for basal insulin dose titration. If meal-time rapid-acting insulin is added, SMBG is necessary for titration of meal-time bolus doses. For all patients with T2D, SMBG may be helpful to guide treatment decisions or lifestyle modification. However, clinical evidence is mixed about whether routine SMBG improves HbA$_{1C}$ in patients who are taking noninsulin medications only. The potential benefits must be weighed against the burden and cost of testing, and an individualized approach is recommended.

23. Which medications should not be used (or require dose adjustments) in patients with CKD?
Metformin may be used in patients with an eGFR $\geq$ 30 mL/min/1.73 m^2; however, it is not recommended that metformin be initiated in a patient with a baseline eGFR between 30 and 45 mL/min/1.73 m^2. When a patient's eGFR falls below 45 mL/min/1.73 m^2, continued use of metformin should be discussed. If continued, a half-maximal dose (1000 mg daily) should be considered.

Although no specific renal dose adjustment recommendations exist for glyburide, its use in patients with impaired renal function should be minimized because of its renal metabolism, accumulation of active metabolites, and the resulting risk of hypoglycemia; glipizide is a better choice if a sulfonylurea is used in this situation. The doses of DPP-4 inhibitors alogliptin, saxagliptin, and sitagliptin need to be adjusted for patients with renal dysfunction; linagliptin is the only DPP-4 inhibitor that does not require renal dysfunction dose adjustments. These agents may be useful in patients with renal dysfunction–related contraindications to metformin. Because of their action in the kidney, SGLT-2 inhibitors are less effective in patients with renal impairment. Dapagliflozin and ertugliflozin are not recommended in patients with an eGFR < 60 mL/min/1.73 m^2; canagliflozin and empagliflozin should not be initiated in patients with an eGFR < 45 mL/min/1.73 m^2.

Renal function of patients receiving exenatide twice daily with a creatinine clearance (CrCl) of 30 to 50 mL/min should be carefully monitored when increasing from 5 to 10 mcg doses; exenatide should not be used in patients with a CrCl < 30 mL/min. There is limited experience in the use of liraglutide or dulaglutide in patients with severe renal impairment (CrCl 15–29 mL/min). Patients should not receive lixisenatide with a CrCl < 15 mL/min. The prescribing information for dulaglutide and semaglutide does not include specific renal dose adjustment recommendations.

24. Which diabetes medication classes should not be used in combination?

Because of their overlapping mechanisms of action, GLP-1 RAs and DPP-4 inhibitors should not be used in combination. Both work by enhancing circulating GLP-1 activity and are not likely to demonstrate increased efficacy when used in combination.

There is lack of data to support the use of GLP-1 RAs in combination with rapid-acting insulin because both target prandial glucose excursions. Short-acting GLP-1 RAs, such as twice-daily exenatide and lixisenatide, have a pronounced prandial effect that may be unpredictably additive when used with rapid-acting insulins or sulfonylureas. This practice is not advocated in either the ADA or the AACE guidelines. If a GLP-1 RA is initiated in a patient who is on > 30 units of rapid-acting insulin daily, it is recommended that the rapid-acting insulin dose be decreased by approximately 50%. If a patient is on a lower dose of rapid-acting insulin, consideration should be given to stopping it when a GLP-1 RA is added. Similarly, sulfonylurea doses should be lowered or discontinued when starting a GLP-1 RA.

Other combinations that should not be used in combination include sulfonylureas, meglitinides, and rapid-acting insulins (in any combination) because of their overlapping mechanisms of action and the increased risk of hypoglycemia.

25. What is clinical inertia in diabetes management?

In diabetes care, *clinical inertia* is defined as the failure to establish appropriate glycemic targets and to escalate oral or injectable treatment to achieve these glycemic goals. Clinical inertia has a negative impact on patient care, including the development of preventable complications and excess direct and indirect health care costs. Contributing factors to clinical inertia include the following: hesitation to start and optimize drug therapy early in the course of the disease, fear of side effects, and lack of provider support to properly monitor and titrate medications. Data from the 2007 to 2014 National Health and Nutrition Examination Survey (NHANES) indicate that despite the development and availability of many new antihyperglycemic medications, only 50% of patients with diabetes achieve an HbA$_{1C}$ goal of $< 7\%$. This failure to achieve glycemic targets is multifactorial, one potential reason being clinical inertia. Clinicians should appreciate the high rates of clinical inertia in T2D and consistently address glycemic control in their patients with T2D to avoid this inertia.

26. Can T2D be prevented or delayed?

Several studies have evaluated whether T2D could be prevented or delayed in individuals at high risk. The most notable of these is the Diabetes Prevention Program (DPP). The DPP was a prospective, randomized trial evaluating the impact of intensive lifestyle intervention versus metformin versus placebo on the progression to diabetes diagnosis in patients with prediabetes. The intensive lifestyle intervention arm focused on achieving and maintaining 7% weight loss and 150 minutes of physical activity per week. This intervention was administered through a 16-session structured, core curriculum followed by a maintenance program. The curriculum included sections on lowering calories, increasing physical activity, self-monitoring, healthy lifestyle behaviors, and psychological and social challenges. Results demonstrated that lifestyle intervention reduced the incidence of T2D by 58% over 3 years. Long-term follow-up in the study has shown sustained effects. Metformin reduced the incidence of T2D by 31% and, thus, was about half as effective as lifestyle modifications. Metformin, however, was as effective as lifestyle modifications in patients with a body mass index (BMI) ≥ 35 kg/m^2 and women with prior gestational diabetes. Metformin was not effective in patients over age 60 years. Clinical studies have also demonstrated the potentially beneficial effects of other pharmacologic interventions. TZDs, alpha-glucosidase inhibitors, GLP-1 RAs, and orlistat, have all decreased incident T2D in individuals with prediabetes, although none of these agents is FDA approved specifically for diabetes prevention.

Therefore, the current ADA standards of care recommend that patients with prediabetes be referred to an intensive behavioral lifestyle intervention program modeled on the DPP to achieve and maintain 7% weight loss and increase moderate-intensity physical activity to at least 150 minutes per week. Metformin has the strongest efficacy and long-term safety evidence for diabetes prevention. In addition, cost, adverse effects, and durability should also be considered. Therefore, the ADA's recommendation for pharmacologic intervention to prevent or delay diabetes is limited to metformin. Specifically, the ADA suggests that metformin therapy should be considered in those with prediabetes, especially for those with BMI ≥ 35 kg/m^2, those < 60 years of age, and women with prior gestational diabetes.

KEY POINTS

- A glycosylated hemoglobin (HbA_{1C}) target should be established for each patient with type 2 diabetes (T2D). A target HbA_{1C} of < 7% is reasonable for most patients but should be individualized. A more stringent HbA_{1C} target may be appropriate for young, otherwise healthy patients with newly diagnosed T2D. A less stringent HbA_{1C} target may be appropriate for older patients with short life expectancies and serious comorbidities.
- First-line therapy for T2D is lifestyle modifications and metformin. The metformin dose should be started low (500 mg once daily) and titrated up slowly over time to a target dose of 2000 mg per day (usually 1000 mg twice daily).
- The most common side effect of metformin is diarrhea. This side effect is usually transient and can be minimized by starting at a low dose and titrating up the dose slowly, taking the medication with food, and using an extended-release (ER) formulation.
- Major lifestyle modifications for T2D include weight loss (if overweight or obese) with an initial goal of 5% weight reduction, increased physical activity (at least 150 minutes per week of moderate to vigorous intensity exercise), and carbohydrate counting. Weight loss should focus on calorie restriction, as opposed to macronutrient content. Healthy eating strategies, such as decreasing added sugars and solid fats, reducing portions, eating more vegetables, and shifting to whole grains and lower-fat dairy choices, should be encouraged.
- HbA_{1C} levels should be checked after 3 months of therapy. If the target HbA_{1C} has not been achieved, adherence should be assessed, and additional therapy should be considered. Once the HbA_{1C} target has been achieved, HbA_{1C} levels can be measured every 6 months.
- Second-line options to add to metformin include glucagon-like peptide-1 receptor agonists (GLP-1 RAs), sodium glucose cotransporter-2 (SGLT-2) inhibitors, dipeptidyl peptidase-4 (DPP-4) inhibitors, sulfonylureas, thiazolidinediones (TZDs), and basal insulin. The decision about which to add should depend on whether the patient has atherosclerotic cardiovascular disease (ASCVD) and other patient and drug considerations, such as glycemic efficacy, risk of hypoglycemia, effect on weight, ease of use, mechanism of delivery, cost, and side effects.
- Currently, there are four available agents with positive cardiovascular outcomes trial (CVOT) data in patients with T2D and established ASCVD. In these patients, T2D therapy should begin with lifestyle modifications and metformin. If these therapies fail to achieve the glycemic targets, liraglutide or empagliflozin should be added to reduce cardiovascular (CV) mortality. Canagliflozin and semaglutide are also options, although their benefits are related to the reduction of major adverse cardiovascular events (MACEs) and not CV mortality.
- Basal insulin is an option in patients who have a markedly elevated HbA_{1C} ($\geq$ 10%) or those who cannot achieve glycemic targets despite the use of first-line therapy. Basal insulin should be initiated at a dose of 10 units (or 0.1–0.2 units/kg) once daily and titrated up to glycemic targets. If fasting plasma glucose (FPG) is controlled on basal insulin but the HbA_{1C} is not at goal, therapy should be intensified with the addition of either a GLP-1 RA or meal-time rapid-acting insulin.
- Intensive lifestyle modifications and metformin have both been proven to prevent or delay the onset of T2D in patients with prediabetes; lifestyle modification is about twice as effective as metformin. Lifestyle modification should focus on 7% weight loss and 150 minutes of moderate-intensity exercise per week. Metformin can be considered in addition to lifestyle modification, especially in those with a body mass index (BMI) $\geq$ 35 kg/m^2, those < 60 years of age, and women with prior gestational diabetes.

BIBLIOGRAPHY

Action to Control Cardiovascular Risk in Diabetes Study Group, Gerstein, H. C., Miller, M. E., Byington, R. P., Goff, D. C., Jr., Bigger, J. T., Buse, J. B., ... Friedewald, W. T. (2008). Effects of intensive glucose lowering in type 2 diabetes. *New England Journal of Medicine, 358*, 2545–2559.

ADVANCE Collaborative Group, Patel, A., MacMahon, S., Chalmers, J., Neal, B., Billot, L., Woodward, M., ... Travert, F. (2008). Intensive blood glucose control and vascular outcomes in patients with type 2 diabetes. *New England Journal of Medicine, 358*, 2560–2572.

American Diabetes Association. (2019). Standards of medical care in diabetes – 2019. *Diabetes Care, 42*(Suppl. 1), S1–S193.

Carls, G., Huynh, J., Tuttle, E., Yee, J., & Edelman, S. V. (2017). Achievement of glycated hemoglobin goals in the US remains unchanged through 2014. *Diabetes Therapy, 8*(4), 863–873.

Duckworth, W., Abraira, C., Moritz, T., Reda, D., Emanuele, N., Reaven, P. D., ... Huang, G. D. (2009). Glucose control and vascular complications in veterans with type 2 diabetes. *New England Journal of Medicine, 360*, 129–139.

Garber, A. J., Abrahamson, M. J., Barzilay, J. I., Blonde, L., Bloomgarden, Z. T., Bush, M. A., ... Umpierrez, G. E. (2018). Consensus statement by the American Association of Clinical Endocrinologists and American College of Endocrinology on the comprehensive type 2 diabetes management algorithm – 2018 executive summary. *Endocrine Practice, 24*(1), 91–120.

Handelsman, Y., Bloomgarden, Z. T., Grunberger, G., Umpierrez, G., Zimmerman, R. S., Bailey, T. S., ... Zangeneh, F. (2015). American Association of Clinical Endocrinologists and American College of Endocrinology – clinical practice guidelines for developing a diabetes mellitus comprehensive care plan – 2015. *Endocrine Practice, 21*(Suppl. 1), 1–87.

Holman, R. R., Paul, S. K., Bethel, M. A., Matthews, D. R., & Neil, H. A. W. (2008). 10-year follow-up of intensive glucose control in type 2 diabetes. *New England Journal of Medicine, 359*, 1577–1589.

Ismail-Beigi, F., Craven, T., Banerji, M. A., Basile, J., Calles, J., Cohen, R. M., ... Hramiak, I. (2010). Effect of intensive treatment of hyperglycaemia on microvascular outcomes in type 2 diabetes: An analysis of the ACCORD randomised trial. *Lancet, 376*, 419–430.

Knowler, W. C., Barrett-Connor, E., Fowler, S. E., Hamman, R. F., Lachin, J. M., Walker, E. A., & Nathan, D. M. (2002). Reduction in the incidence of type 2 diabetes with lifestyle intervention or metformin. *New England Journal of Medicine, 346*, 393–403.

LaSalle, J. R., & Berria, R. (2013). Insulin therapy in type 2 diabetes mellitus: a practical approach for primary care physicians and other health care professionals. *Journal of the American Osteopathic Association, 113*(2), 152–162.

Marso, S. P., Daniels, G. H., Brown-Frandsen, K., Kristensen, P., Mann, J. F., Nauck, M. A., … Buse, J. B. (2016). Liraglutide and cardiovascular outcomes in type 2 diabetes. *New England Journal of Medicine, 375*, 311–322.

Marso, S. P., Bain, S. C., Consoli, A., Eliaschewitz, F. G., J√≥dar, E., Leiter, L. A., … Vilsbøll, T. (2016). Semaglutide and cardiovascular outcomes in patients with type 2 diabetes. *New England Journal of Medicine, 375*, 1834–1844.

Neal, B., Perkovic, V., Mahaffey, K.W., de Zeeuw, D., Fulcher, G., Erondu, N., … Matthews, D. R. (2017). Canagliflozin and cardiovascular and renal events in type 2 diabetes. *New England Journal of Medicine, 377*(7), 644–657.

Strain, W. D., Blüher, M., & Paldánius, P. (2014). Clinical inertia in individualising care for diabetes: Is there time to do more in type 2 diabetes? *Diabetes Therapy, 5*(2), 347–354.

UK Prospective Diabetes Study (UKPDS) Group. (1998). Effect of intensive blood-glucose control with metformin on complications in overweight patients with type 2 diabetes (UKPDS 34). *Lancet, 352*, 854–865.

UK Prospective Diabetes Study (UKPDS) Group. (1998). Intensive blood-glucose control with sulphonylureas or insulin compared with conventional treatment and risk of complications in patients with type 2 diabetes (UKPDS 33). *Lancet, 352*, 837–853.

U.S. Food and Drug Administration. (2008). Guidance for industry diabetes mellitus—evaluating cardiovascular risk in new antidiabetic therapies to treat type 2 diabetes. Retrieved from https://www.fda.gov/downloads/Drugs/Guidances/ucm071627.pdf

Zinman, B., Wanner, C., Lachin, J. M., Fitchett, D., Bluhmki, E., Hantel, S., … Inzucchi, S. E. (2015). Empagliflozin, cardiovascular outcomes, and mortality in type 2 diabetes. *New England Journal of Medicine, 373*, 2117–2128.

DIABETES TECHNOLOGY: PUMPS, SENSORS, AND BEYOND

Adnin Zaman and Cecilia C. Low Wang

CHAPTER 5

1. What is a continuous subcutaneous insulin infusion (CSII) device?

   More commonly known as an "insulin pump," a CSII device is a small, wearable, portable device that delivers preprogrammed and user-adjusted doses of insulin both continuously and in boluses. This is an insulin delivery system used in lieu of multiple daily injections (MDIs).

2. What are the components of a CSII device, and how does CSII work?

   Insulin pump—the machine that is programmed to deliver insulin. Basal infusion rates are set to deliver a specific amount and pattern of continuous background insulin throughout the day. To provide insulin doses for food intake, the pump has "bolus" settings that are determined by the specific needs of each patient. These include a carbohydrate-to-insulin (CI) ratio, which is the grams of carbohydrates that will be covered by one unit of bolus insulin; a correction factor (CF; also known as *insulin sensitivity factor*), which is an estimate of how much each additional unit of bolus insulin is expected to lower an elevated premeal blood glucose; and the blood glucose targets for the correction boluses. Together, these settings allow the pump to calculate how much insulin is needed for a meal and to correct an elevated premeal blood glucose level, if present.

   ## EXAMPLE:

   A patient with type 1 diabetes will eat a meal containing 30 g of carbohydrates at noon; the blood glucose prior to the meal is elevated at 220 mg/dL. The insulin pump settings for this period include a basal rate of 0.5 units/hr, a CI ratio of 10:1, a CF of 30:1, and a blood glucose target of 100. The patient enters the premeal glucose value (220 mg/dL) and amount of carbohydrate to be consumed (30 g) into the pump. Although the pump is infusing 0.5 units/hr of basal insulin at this time, a bolus of 3 units for carbohydrate intake (30 g ÷ 10) and 4 units more ([220 mg/dL − 100 mg/dL] ÷ 30) to correct the elevated premeal glucose to the target of 100 mg/dL will be delivered (total bolus = 7 units).

   In the above scenario, if the patient had a normal blood glucose before eating the meal, the pump would still deliver the basal 0.5 units/hr and the 3 units to cover the meal, but the additional correctional insulin would not be needed.

   Reservoir—this is a cartridge that typically holds a three-day supply of rapid-acting insulin. Insulin is withdrawn from a vial and used to fill the reservoir. The reservoir fits inside the pump and is changed every 3 days when the insulin infusion site is changed.

   Infusion sets—this is the part that is inserted subcutaneously into the body. A fine needle in the infusion set cannula is used to insert the cannula into subcutaneous tissue. Once inserted, the needle is removed and the cannula is left under the skin. Tubing then connects the cannula to the reservoir inside the pump. This insertion point serves as the delivery site for both the basal insulin that is delivered continuously and the insulin boluses that are delivered periodically by the patient when consuming food and/or to correct elevated blood glucose levels.

3. What kind of insulin is used in a CSII device?

   Rapid-acting insulin is used in a CSII device. The options include lispro (Humalog), aspart (Novolog), and glulisine (Apidra). Rarely, concentrated insulin (U-500 regular insulin) is used, although this is reserved for individuals with significant insulin resistance who require very high amounts of insulin. Intermediate or long-acting insulins (often called "basal insulins") are not used in insulin pumps.

4. How does CSII improve glycemic control?

   The use of an insulin pump improves glycemic control through better matching of basal insulin delivery to basal insulin requirements and by allowing for more consistent and accurate bolus dosing for meals. Because the CI ratios and CFs are preprogrammed into the pump, patients do not need to manually calculate the amount of insulin to administer for meals or for high blood glucose corrections; this reduces the risk of math (numeracy) errors. In addition, patients are able to more easily administer insulin boluses for every meal and snack because the use of a syringe vial or pen needle with MDIs is not required. Although the same goals could be accomplished with intensive subcutaneous injection therapy, the manual calculations and multiple injections throughout the day often pose barriers to therapy adherence. Other advantages of an insulin pump include the ability to deliver varying rates of basal insulin at different time points throughout the day to more closely mimic true physiology and the ability to deliver insulin boluses in increments smaller than a half unit to allow for more accurate insulin dosing, especially in patients who are sensitive to insulin.

5. Who is a good candidate for an insulin pump?

An insulin pump is a good option for patients who have inadequate glycemic control despite intensive efforts to optimize therapy with MDIs. Those with high glucose variability throughout the day, suggesting a corresponding underlying variability in insulin requirements, may benefit from a CSII device programmed with multiple basal insulin schemes. Similarly, patients who work erratic schedules, travel frequently, desire more flexibility, or simply prefer increased convenience may benefit from a CSII device. In these patients, an insulin pump may increase adherence with an insulin regimen. A candidate for the insulin pump must have demonstrated strong motivation to use the device, as training on the device requires substantial education, trouble-shooting, and time investment. The candidate should have realistic expectations of the capabilities of pump therapy, demonstrate significant knowledge of diabetes self-management, and be able to problem-solve potential challenges with the pump. Finally, unless a patient also has a continuous glucose monitor (CGM), he or she should be willing to check finger-stick blood glucose levels multiple times per day, because this information needs to be entered into the pump so that it can deliver accurate doses of bolus insulin.

6. Are insulin delivery settings on a CSII device universal?

No, it is critical to titrate insulin delivery settings to each patient's individual needs when he or she is using an insulin pump. Every patient should monitor fingerstick glucose values frequently (at least four times a day) or use a CGM. The patient must also have consistent follow-up visits with an endocrinologist and a diabetes educator, who have the technology and expertise to download insulin pump, glucose meter, and CGM data to analyze glucose patterns and make informed insulin delivery adjustments.

7. What basic knowledge does a patient need to be started on an insulin pump?

To use insulin pumps effectively, individuals must be willing to learn and practice carbohydrate counting and be able to understand the essential insulin pump functions (basal rates, CI ratios, CFs, and blood glucose targets). Furthermore, they should be able to apply and alter these settings in response to common, but variable, real-life scenarios (carbohydrate intake, stress, exercise, and miscellaneous activities). They should also be aware of how to avoid and respond to hypoglycemia.

8. How much patient input is required to safely and effectively operate an insulin pump?

Contrary to common belief, currently available insulin pumps cannot independently control blood glucose levels and still require considerable input from patients to maximize benefits. Each patient needs to perform fingerstick blood glucose testing multiple times per day, especially before each meal and at bedtime, or the person must wear a CGM. He or she should also be able to accurately estimate the carbohydrate contents of meals and snacks to bolus the appropriate insulin dose for all types of nutrient intake. All insulin pump patients should change their infusion sites every 3 days and be able to problem-solve to prevent the development of diabetic ketoacidosis (DKA).

9. What are the major challenges for patients who use insulin pumps?

The major challenges include accurately counting carbohydrates and checking blood glucose levels frequently enough to allow the pump to deliver appropriate amounts of insulin at the right times. Other challenges often arise with the physical device itself, such as leaking of insulin if the infusion set cannula is not inserted properly, kinking of the cannula so that insulin is not delivered appropriately, or, rarely, insertion site infections.

10. What are the major complications that patients face while using a CSII device?

Inadequate glycemic control is still a major complication with insulin pumps, especially if the preprogrammed settings are incorrect. The settings are determined by the patient's needs and adjusted on the basis of patterns of blood glucose in the context of daily life. As such, patients may continue to experience hyperglycemia and/or hypoglycemia. Correcting the settings to eliminate hypoglycemia—which can be acutely life-threatening—takes priority over optimizing control of hyperglycemia.

11. What are the major differences between the insulin pumps currently available on the market?

The three major insulin pump brands in the United States (at the time of this writing) are Medtronic, T-Slim, and Omnipod. Medtronic and T-Slim pumps consist of cell phone–sized machines that are connected through a tube (or infusion set) to the body. Omnipod pumps do not require tubing and, instead, are configured as a small water-proof pod that is worn attached directly to the body; a remote-control device is used to manage the pump's functions. Some insulin pump models now have the capability to communicate with a CGM to receive glucose readings every 5 minutes or less, thereby reducing the need for multiple manual blood glucose checks throughout the day.

12. What is a CGM?

A CGM is a device that allows for real-time monitoring of glucose levels throughout the day and night every 5 minutes or even more often. CGMs rely on extracellular fluid sampled by using a subcutaneous catheter and allow patients to see real-time blood glucose values and blood glucose trends over time while reducing the need for fingerstick blood glucose testing. The three major CGM brands available in the United States (at the time of this writing) are Dexcom, Libre, and Guardian.

13. How does a CGM work?

A glucose sensor in the form of a tiny electrode is inserted under the skin and measures the glucose levels in the interstitial fluid. It is connected to a transmitter that sends the information via wireless radiofrequency to a display device, which, in some cases, can even be a i-Phone or i-Watch.

14. What are the major benefits of using a CGM?

Apart from giving the patient an easy way to know their blood glucose levels at all times, CGM systems also provide information on the rate of blood glucose change. When the blood glucose is rising, an "up" arrow is displayed alongside the glucose reading, and a "down" arrow is displayed when the blood glucose is decreasing. One arrow up or down indicates that the blood glucose level is changing in that direction by approximately 1 mg/dL/min ($\approx$60 mg/dL/hr), and two arrows up or down indicate that the blood glucose level is changing in that direction by about 2 mg/dL/min ($\approx$120 mg/dl/hr). Some CGM devices also provide audible alarms as a warning before hyperglycemic or hypoglycemic values actually occur. This information allows patients to preempt major hyperglycemic and hypoglycemic events. Data from the CGM can also be downloaded and reviewed during a visit with a diabetes care provider, allowing the provider and the patient to make more informed changes to the insulin regimen. Patterns detected on these downloads provide valuable insights to the patient and the provider that lead to improved hemoglobin A_{1c} (HbA$_{1c}$) values, less hypoglycemia, and decreased glucose variability.

15. What are the major problems with a CGM?

CGM systems have certain limitations: (1) glucose in extracellular fluid lags behind capillary blood glucose by approximately 15 minutes; so when blood glucose is changing rapidly, glucose readings on a CGM will be less accurate in real time; and (2) certain medications, such as acetaminophen or ascorbic acid, interfere with accurate assaying of blood glucose with some CGM models. Some CGM models require a patient calibrate the device with two or more fingerstick blood glucose values per day; however, some newer models are factory calibrated and do not require these frequent calibrations by the patient.

16. What is a hybrid closed-loop insulin delivery system?

Although the creation of a fully closed-loop insulin delivery system (true artificial pancreas) remains in development, one hybrid closed-loop insulin delivery system, the Medtronic 670G, is available in the United States (at the time of this writing). It consists of an insulin pump and a CGM, which are integrated and communicate with each other to allow for automated adjustments of basal insulin delivery in response to continuously monitored glucose values. Additional brands and models of hybrid closed-loop systems are anticipated to be available in the near future.

17. How does a hybrid closed-loop insulin delivery system work?

The patient wears both an insulin pump and a CGM inserted at different subcutaneous sites. The CGM senses real-time blood glucose values and trends, and transmits this information to the insulin pump. The insulin pump uses an algorithm to continuously adjust the basal insulin delivery rate to maintain glucose within a target range. If the blood glucose levels are rising, the basal rate is automatically increased. Similarly, if the blood glucose levels are dropping, the basal rate is automatically decreased; if the glucose levels continue to decline despite this, the insulin pump may temporarily suspend insulin delivery and resume once blood glucose has increased and stabilized within the goal range.

18. How much patient involvement is required to operate a hybrid closed-loop system?

Because the hybrid closed-loop system is only able to adjust basal rates, the patient must still estimate the carbohydrate content of food to be consumed and enter this information into the pump to deliver accurate mealtime insulin boluses. If the patient does not enter an estimated carbohydrate intake for a mealtime bolus, the system will detect the increasing blood glucose levels after the meal and will temporarily increase the basal insulin delivery rate. However, the system has a maximal allowable basal rate and will exit the automatic mode if this maximal rate is reached for a period without improvement in the blood glucose. The patient must then manage the insulin pump in "manual mode" and recalibrate the system before it can resume the "auto mode."

19. Do you need to titrate insulin if a patient is using a hybrid closed-loop system?

Titration of insulin settings is not as intensive in a hybrid closed-loop system but is still required. Because the hybrid closed-loop system exits the automatic mode in certain circumstances, traditional pump settings for the manual mode must be preprogrammed so that the system can be used as a traditional insulin pump during these periods. In addition, because the patient is still required to input carbohydrate content of food to be consumed, the CI ratio needs to be assessed and adjusted, as needed.

20. Are there any disadvantages to a hybrid closed-loop insulin delivery system?
    Currently, the only hybrid closed-loop system (Medtronic 670G) that has been approved by the U.S. Food and Drug Administration is designed to maintain a stable blood glucose level of 120 mg/dL. For situations in which glycemic targets are more intensive (e.g., pregnancy or patient preference), the hybrid closed-loop system may not be the ideal technology for insulin delivery.

21. What is a smart insulin pen, and how does it work?
    In a traditional insulin pen, insulin is prefilled for delivery, but a smart insulin pen goes one step further by having "memory." These pens are able to record the date, time, and amount of insulin taken. Certain pens also allow for half-unit insulin dosing. These smart pens can communicate via Bluetooth with a smartphone and corresponding smartphone app to give patients reminders or recommendations on insulin dosing.

22. Who is a good candidate for a smart insulin pen?
    Smart pens are not often used because of the wide availability of insulin pumps. However, a patient who is not a candidate for an insulin pump or who declines pump therapy but still needs more intensive insulin administration may benefit from this technology. Smart pens assist patients by providing a record of insulin administration. They do not directly attach to the body and yet can be used to deliver insulin relatively discreetly. Like regular insulin pens, they offer the benefit of portability without the disadvantages of a vial and a syringe.

23. What types of apps are available for people with diabetes?
    There are a variety of applications for smartphones to help people with diabetes. Common free apps to help with carb counting include MyFitnessPal, Calorie King, and SparkPeople. Other apps, such as Dario or Diabetes:M, are available for purchase and allow individuals to keep track of their blood glucose values, activity levels, meals, and insulin doses to help visualize one's daily routine and glucose control performance.

24. CGM Interpretation Practice: Interpret the following CGM download patterns and suggest an appropriate change in therapy.
    Download 1

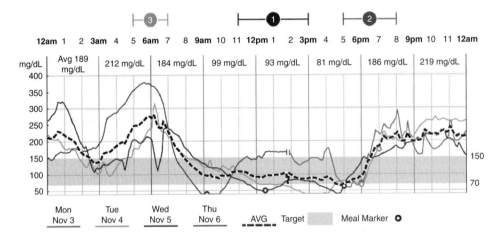

Download 2

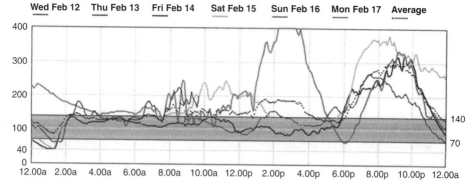

	Wed Feb 12	Thu Feb 13	Fri Feb 14	Sat Feb 15	Sun Feb 16	Mon Feb 17	Average / Total
# Sensor Values	0	182	288	288	288	116	1,162
Highest	N/A	267	322	379	400	224	400
Lowest	N/A	69	40	41	66	61	40
Average	N/A	150	138	179	202	140	166
Standard Dev.	N/A	50	62	88	81	39	75
MAD %	N/A	14.5	24.1	17.6	18.0	10.3	17.5
Correlation	N/A	N/A	N/A	0.97	0.94	N/A	0.95
# Valid Calibrations	0	3	2	4	4	1	14
Designation	S		X			X	

X: Use Clinical Judgment   S: No Sensor Data   C: No Calibration BG's

Download 3

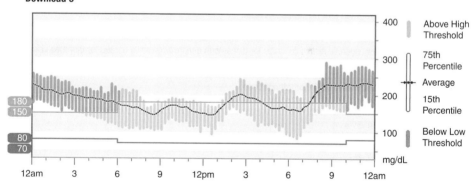

Download 4

Sensor Data (mg/dL)

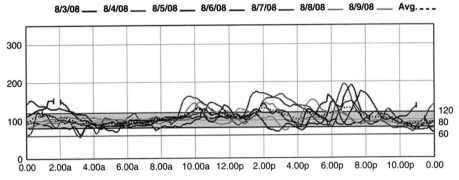

	Sun Aug 3	Mon Aug 4	Tue Aug 5	Wed Aug 6	Thu Aug 7	Fri Aug 8	Sat Aug 9	Average / Total
# Sensor Values	246	288	288	276	277	288	285	1,948
High SG (mg/dL)	152	194	174	190	174	152	146	194
Low SG (mg/dL)	66	56	72	62	72	72	84	56
Average SG (mg/dL)	103	111	107	106	110	101	106	106
Standard Dev.	18	29	22	23	25	16	14	22
MAD %	6.4	22.0	17.5	11.8	4.5	3.8	7.2	10.6
# Valid Calibrations	6	4	3	2	4	4	3	30

Download 1 Interpretation and Recommendations:
   Interpretation: elevated blood glucose after dinner caused by inadequate dinner coverage, resulting in high bedtime glucose levels that persist throughout the night, causing elevated morning fasting blood glucose levels.
   Recommendation: improve insulin coverage for dinner with a more aggressive CI ratio for that meal.
Download 2 Interpretation and Recommendations:
   Interpretation: elevated blood glucose after dinner caused by inadequate dinner coverage, necessitating evening correction doses. The evening CF is too aggressive, causing nighttime hypoglycemia.
   Recommendation: improve insulin coverage for dinner with a more aggressive CI ratio for that meal; change CF after dinner and at bedtime to make it less aggressive to avoid nighttime hypoglycemia because patients are less aware of hypoglycemic episodes while sleeping.
Download 3 Interpretation and Recommendations:
   Interpretation: elevated blood glucose levels after dinner caused by inadequate dinner coverage, resulting in high bedtime glucose levels with overnight basal insulin compensating to yield a target range morning fasting blood glucose.
   Recommendation: improve insulin coverage for dinner with a more aggressive CI ratio for that meal; reduce overnight basal rates to prevent hypoglycemia because bedtime glucose values will be lower as a result of the stronger CI ratio.
Download 4 Interpretation:
   Interpretation: morning fasting blood glucose values within goal range. Most postprandial glucose excursions after breakfast, some postprandial lunch excursions, and some postprandial dinner excursions are within goal ranges. Significant variability after lunch and dinner—cause to be determined.
   Recommendation: have the patient keep records of all meals and activities for 1 to 2 weeks and return to have another CGM download so that lifestyle issues causing the high and low blood glucose values can be determined.

KEY POINTS

- A continuous subcutaneous insulin infusion device, also known as an *insulin pump*, is a wearable, portable device that delivers preprogrammed and user-adjusted doses of rapid-acting insulin both continuously and in boluses.
- The insulin pump may help improve hemoglobin A_{1c} and glucose variability through optimized matching of basal insulin delivery to basal insulin requirements and improved meal-time insulin management. Pump settings change over time for individuals and require adjustments based on glucose patterns from multiple

KEY POINTS—cont'd

daily fingersticks or data from a continuous glucose monitor (CGM). Patients should have close follow-up with a diabetes care provider who can review glucose data and patterns and help make informed changes to the insulin pump settings.

- A CGM is a device that allows for real-time monitoring of glucose levels throughout the day and night. Readings can occur as often as every 5 minutes. The system allows patients to make changes to prevent an episode of hyper- or hypoglycemia. Because the CGM measures glucose in the interstitial fluid, there is a 15-minute lag behind blood glucose values.
- A hybrid closed-loop system consists of an insulin pump and a CGM that are integrated and communicate with each other to allow for basal insulin delivery at varying rates to maintain glucose within a target range. The user is still required to input carbohydrate content of food so that the pump can deliver mealtime insulin boluses.

BIBLIOGRAPHY

American Association of Diabetes Educators. (2018). *Continuous subcutaneous insulin infusion (CSII) without and with sensor integration.* Chicago, IL: AADE.

American Diabetes Association. (2015). How do insulin pumps work? Retrieved from http://www.diabetes.org/living-with-diabetes/treatment-and-care/medication/insulin/how-do-insulin-pumps-work.html.

Chait, J. (2006, Aug 31). Insulin pumps. Retrieved from http://www.Diabetesselfmanagement.com.

Manderfeld, A. (2018, May 28). Everything you need to know about insulin pumps. Thediabetescouncil.com. Retrieved from http://main.diabetes.org/dforg/pdfs/2017/2017-cg-insulin-pumps.pdf.

Prašek, M., Bozek, T., & Metelko, Z. (2003). Continuous subcutaneous insulin infusion (CSII). *Diabetologia Croatica, 32*(3), 111–124.

Peters, A. L., Ahmann, A. J., Battelino, T., Evert, A., Hirsch, I. B., Murad, M. H., ... Wolpert, H. (2016). Diabetes technology-continuous subcutaneous insulin infusion therapy and continuous glucose monitoring in adults: an endocrine society clinical practice guideline. *Journal of clinical endocrinology and metabolism, 101*(11), 3922–3937.

CARBOHYDRATE COUNTING–GUIDED INSULIN DOSING: PRACTICE EXERCISES

Michael T. McDermott

1. Define and explain the carbohydrate-to-insulin ratio.

   The carbohydrate-to-insulin (C:I) ratio is an estimate of the grams of carbohydrate that will be covered by each unit of insulin. A C:I ratio of X:1 means that 1 unit of insulin should be given for each X grams of carbohydrate to be consumed. The initial C:I ratio for each patient is usually calculated as follows: 500 ÷ total daily dose (TDD) of insulin. The C:I ratio must then be evaluated (see testing below) and adjusted to achieve the optimal post-prandial glucose excursions for each individual (usually 30–50 mg/dL rise from premeal value to 2-hour postmeal value).

2. How do you determine if the current C:I ratio is correct?

   The accuracy of each individual's C:I ratio is tested with the following protocol:

   A. Preparation for the test meal: consume something that is easily covered at the meal before the test meal so that your glucose level immediately before the test meal is in the target range and does not require a correction dose. If glucose before the test meal is < 70 mg/dL or > 140 mg/dL, do not proceed with the test.

   B. If the glucose just before the test meal is in the desired range (70–140 mg/dL), eat a meal that has a well-known carbohydrate content and < 20 g of fat.

   C. Test your glucose level just before the test meal, take the insulin dose calculated from your C:I ratio, and recheck your glucose 2 hours after the test meal; calculate the glucose excursion. The glucose excursion from premeal value to 2-hour postmeal value should be about 30 to 50 mg/dL.

   D. If the rise is > 50 mg/dL, the C:I ratio should be strengthened and if the rise is < 30 mg/dL, the C:I ratio should be weakened.

3. What is a high blood glucose (BG) correction factor (CF)?

   A high BG CF is an estimate of the glucose drop expected for each unit of insulin given when the glucose is elevated above the goal. A CF of N:1 means that 1 unit of insulin will drop the glucose N mg/dL; therefore, a patient will give 1 unit of insulin for every N mg/dL the current glucose level is above the glucose target. An initial CF for a patient is calculated as follows: 1650/TDD (some institutions use an initial CF of 1800/TDD, 1700/TDD or 1500/TDD). The initial CF must then be evaluated and adjusted to achieve appropriate reductions of high glucose values to the target range by 4 hours after the dose is given.

4. How do you calculate and use insulin bolus on board (BOB) and duration of insulin action (DIA) estimates.

   BOB and *insulin on board (IOB)* are similar terms used to indicate how much insulin is still active after the last short-acting insulin bolus; the term *BOB* is used in this chapter. *DIA* and *active insulin time (AIT)* are similar terms used to indicate how long an insulin bolus lasts for an individual; the term DIA is used in this chapter. DIA is often ≈ 4 hours, but some patients consider their DIA to be shorter (≈ 3 hours) or longer (≈ 5 hours) on the basis of their own experience. To calculate BOB, use the previous bolus dose, subtract from that the same dose, multiply by the time elapsed since that bolus, and divide by DIA. The formula is, therefore: BOB ≡ Bolus − Bolus × (elapsed time since bolus ÷ DIA). Example: If a 6-unit bolus was taken 2 hours ago and the DIA is 4 hours, BOB is 3 units (6 − 6 × [2 ÷ 4] ≡ 3). When a person plans to take a high blood glucose correction dose, BOB should be subtracted from the planned correction dose.

5. Do people who take basal-bolus insulin need to do these calculations before every meal and correction dose?

   Patients who administer insulin by multiple daily injections (MDIs) should be very familiar with these calculations and use them before every meal bolus and correction bolus. Insulin pumps, however, do the math to calculate the insulin dose necessary for the carbohydrate content, the correction dose, and BOB and then display the recommended dose of insulin. In either case, accurate carbohydrate counting is essential.

6. Explain what additional information is provided by a continuous glucose monitoring (CGM) system and how that affects the correction dose.

   A CGM system is a subcutaneous device that measures interstitial glucose every 3 to 5 minutes and displays this in real time. A person sees the current blood glucose value along with a trend arrow to indicate the direction the glucose is going (trend). For every trend arrow up (glucose rising ≈ 1 mg/dL/min or 60 mg/dL/hr), we recommend adding 1 unit of insulin to the CF dose (1 unit for one arrow up and 2 units for two arrows up). For one arrow down (glucose dropping ≈ 1 mg/dL/min or 60 mg/dL/hr), we recommend subtracting 1 unit of insulin from the CF dose, and if there are two arrows down, the correction dose should be omitted. Other suggested tables for adjusting correction doses based on trend arrows have been published.

7. What basic carbohydrate counting skills should every patient with diabetes and their providers know?
Carbohydrate counting is usually taught by a certified diabetes educator. However, all providers involved in managing patients with diabetes who are on insulin regimens should be familiar with the basics of carbohydrate counting. Table 6.1 is useful as an introduction to the basics of carbohydrate counting and for the practice cases used later in this chapter.

Table 6.1. Carbohydrate Counting Basics.

15 Gram (g) Carbohydrate Servings (60 kcal of Carbohydrate)
1 slice of bread ≡ 15 g carbohydrate
1 small roll ≡ 15 g carbohydrate
1 small potato (3 oz) ≡ 15 g carbohydrate
½ cup of mashed potatoes ≡ 15 g carbohydrate
½ cup of corn ≡ 15 g carbohydrate
½ cup of peas ≡ 15 g carbohydrate
⅓ cup of cooked rice ≡ 15 g carbohydrate
⅓ cup of cooked pasta ≡ 15 g carbohydrate
1 medium apple ≡ 15 g carbohydrate
½ of a 6-inch banana ≡ 15 g carbohydrate
2 Oreos ≡ 15 g carbohydrate
2 × 2 inch unfrosted cake ≡ 15 g carbohydrate
½ cup (4 oz) of fruit juice ≡ 15 g carbohydrate
1.25 cup (10 oz) of milk ≡ 15 g carbohydrate
1.5 cup (12 oz) regular beer or nonalcoholic beer ≡ 15 g carbohydrate

30 Gram (g) Carbohydrate Servings (120 kcal of Carbohydrate)
1 medium potato (6 oz) ≡ 30 g carbohydrate
1 cup of mashed potatoes ≡ 30 g carbohydrate
1 cup of corn ≡ 30 g carbohydrate
1 cup of peas ≡ 30 g carbohydrate
⅔ cup of cooked rice ≡ 30 g carbohydrate
⅔ cup of cooked pasta ≡ 30 g carbohydrate
1 6-inch banana ≡ 30 g carbohydrate
4 Oreos ≡ 30 g carbohydrate
1 cup (8 oz) wine cooler ≡ 30 g carbohydrate
1.5 cup (12 oz) microbrew beer ≡ 30 g carbohydrate
½ cup (4 oz) margarita ≡ 30 g carbohydrate
½ cup (4 oz) daiquiri ≡ 30 g carbohydrate

45 Gram (g) Carbohydrate Servings (180 kcal of Carbohydrate)
1 cup of cooked rice ≡ 45 g carbohydrate
1 cup of cooked pasta ≡ 45 g carbohydrate
6 Oreos ≡ 45 g carbohydrate

Other Gram (g) Carbohydrate Servings (1 g Carbohydrate ≡ 4 kcal)
1 small corn tortilla ≡ 10 g carbohydrate
1 cup (8 oz) milk ≡ 12 g carbohydrate
1 can (12 oz) regular soda ≡ 40 g carbohydrate
1 bottle (20 oz) regular soda ≡ 75 g carbohydrate
1 teaspoon sugar (5 mL) ≡ 4 g carbohydrate
1 tablespoon sugar (15 mL) ≡ 12 g carbohydrate
1 teaspoon honey (5 mL) ≡ 5 g carbohydrate
1 tablespoon honey (15 mL) ≡ 15 g carbohydrate

Work through the following 10 practice cases (the answers will follow). Test your skills.

CASE 1

Petunia has type 1 diabetes mellitus (T1D), which she treats with 28 units of basal insulin daily and meal-time bolus insulin by using a C:I ratio of 12:1 and a CF of 40:1, with a target premeal BG of 100 mg/dL. Her prelunch BG is 180 mg/dL. She plans to eat the following meal:

1 bologna sandwich
1 medium apple
1 6-inch banana
12-oz can of nondiet cola

1. How many grams of carbohydrate does she plan to consume?
2. How many units of short-acting insulin should she take before lunch?
   To cover carbohydrates (C:I ≡ 12:1)
   To cover high BG (CF ≡ 40:1)
   Total insulin to use
3. If a continuous glucose sensor showed one arrow up, how would this change?

CASE 2

Josephine has T1D, which she treats with an insulin pump by using 24 units of basal insulin daily and meal-time bolus insulin by using a C:I ratio of 15:1 and a CF of 50:1, with a target premeal BG of 120 mg/dL. Her predinner BG is 220 mg/dL. She plans to eat the following meal for dinner:

1 cup of cooked pasta
1 small roll
½ cup of peas
12 oz diet soda
2 Oreos
1 cup of milk

1. How many grams of carbohydrate does she plan to consume?
2. How many units of short-acting insulin should she take before lunch?
   To cover carbohydrates (C:I = 15:1)
   To cover high BG (CF = 50:1)
   Total insulin to use
3. If a continuous glucose sensor showed one arrow down, how would this change?

CASE 3

Darko has T1D, which he treats with an insulin pump by using 32 units of basal insulin daily and meal-time bolus insulin by using a C:I ratio of 10:1 and a CF of 30:1 with a target premeal BG of 100 mg/dL. His predinner BG is 220 mg/dL. He plans to eat the following meal for dinner:

12 oz steak
1 medium potato (6 oz)
12 oz microbrew beer
4 Oreos
1 cup of milk

1. How many grams of carbohydrate does he plan to consume?
2. How many units of short-acting insulin should he take before lunch?
   To cover carbohydrates (C:I = 10:1)
   To cover high BG (CF = 30:1)
   Total insulin to use
3. If a continuous glucose sensor showed one arrow up, how would this change?

CASE 4

Dagobert has T1D, which he treats with an insulin pump by using 44 units of basal insulin daily and meal-time bolus insulin by using a C:I ratio of 8:1 and a CF of 25:1, with a target premeal BG of 125 mg/dL. His prelunch BG is 200 mg/dL. He plans to eat the following meal for lunch:

1 grilled cheese sandwich
1 summer sausage
⅔ cup of rice

½ cup of fruit juice
1. How many grams of carbohydrate does he plan to consume?
2. How many units of short-acting insulin should he take before lunch?
   To cover carbohydrates (C:I = 8:1)
   To cover high BG (CF = 25:1)
   Total insulin to use
3. If a continuous glucose sensor showed one arrow down, how would this change?

CASE 5

Gertrude has T1D, which she treats with 18 units of basal insulin daily and meal-time bolus insulin using a C:I ratio of 18:1 and a CF of 60:1, with a target premeal BG of 120 mg/dL. Her predinner BG is 180 mg/dL. She plans to eat the following meal:
   8 oz tuna steak
   1 small roll
   ⅓ cup cooked pasta
   ½ cup of corn
   8 oz wine cooler
1. How many grams of carbohydrate does she plan to consume?
2. How many units of short-acting insulin should she take before lunch?
   To cover carbohydrates (C:I = 18:1)
   To cover high BG (CF = 60:1)
   Total insulin to use
3. If a continuous glucose sensor showed one arrow up, how would this change?

CASE 6

Carmello has T1D, which he treats with an insulin pump by using 48 units of basal insulin daily and meal-time bolus insulin by using a C:I ratio of 6:1 and a CF of 20:1, with a target premeal BG of 100 mg/dL. His predinner BG is 160 mg/dL. He is at a restaurant and plans to eat the following meal for dinner:
   2 beef tacos with lettuce and sour cream each on a small corn tortilla
   ⅔ cup of rice with chorizo sausage
   12 oz Margarita
1. How many grams of carbohydrate does he plan to consume?
2. How many units of short-acting insulin should he take before lunch?
   To cover carbohydrates (C:I = 6:1)
   To cover high BG (CF = 20:1)
   Total insulin to use
3. If a continuous glucose sensor showed one arrow down, how would this change?

CASE 7

Rose has T1D, which she treats with an insulin pump by using 18 units of basal insulin daily and meal-time bolus insulin by using a C:I ratio of 15:1 and a CF of 50:1, with a target premeal BG of 100 mg/dL. She took a CF bolus of 2 units 2 hours ago. Her predinner BG is 248 mg/dL. The DIA on her pump is set for 4 hours to estimate her BOB. She plans to eat the following meal for dinner:
   1 breast baked chicken
   ½ cup mashed potatoes
   ½ cup of corn
   2 × 2 inch unfrosted cake
   Unsweetened tea
1. How many grams of carbohydrate does she plan to consume?
2. How many units of short-acting insulin should she estimate before dinner?
   To cover carbohydrates (C:I = 15:1)
   To cover high BG (CF = 50:1)
   To compensate for BOB
   Total insulin to use
3. If a continuous glucose sensor showed one arrow down, how would this change?

CASE 8

Dmitri has T1D, which he treats with an insulin pump by using 16 units of basal insulin daily and meal-time bolus insulin by using a C:I ratio of 15:1 and a CF of 40:1, with a target premeal BG of 100 mg/dL. He took a CF bolus of 4 units 3 hours ago. His predinner BG is 219 mg/dL. The DIA on his pump is set for 4 hours to estimate his BOB. He plans to eat the following meal for dinner:

12 oz roast beef
1 6-oz potato
½ cup of peas
1 small roll
10 oz milk

1. How many grams of carbohydrate does he plan to consume?
2. How many units of short-acting insulin should he estimate before dinner?
   To cover carbohydrates (C:I = 15:1)
   To cover high BG (CF = 40:1)
   To compensate for BOB
   Total insulin to use
3. If a continuous glucose sensor showed one arrow up, how would this change?

CASE 9

Nadia has T1D, which she treats with an insulin pump by using 20 units of basal insulin daily and meal-time bolus insulin by using a C:I ratio of 12:1 and a CF of 40:1, with a target premeal BG of 100 mg/dL. She took a snack bolus of 2 units and a CF bolus of 2 units 2 hours ago. Her predinner BG is 179 mg/dL. The DIA on her pump is set for 4 hours to estimate her BOB. She plans to eat the following meal for dinner:

8 oz ham
⅓ cup of cooked pasta
½ cup of peas
1 medium apple
2 Oreos
Unsweetened tea

1. How many grams of carbohydrate does she plan to consume?
2. How many units of short-acting insulin should she estimate before dinner?
   To cover carbohydrates (C:I = 12:1)
   To cover high BG (CF = 40:1)
   To compensate for BOB
   Total insulin to use
3. If a continuous glucose sensor showed 1 arrow down, how would this change?

CASE 10

Cody has T1D, which he treats with an insulin pump by using 24 units of basal insulin daily and meal-time bolus insulin by using a C:I ratio of 13:1 and a CF of 35:1, with a target premeal BG of 100 mg/dL. He took a CF bolus of 4 units 3 hours ago and a snack bolus of 4 units 2 hours ago. His predinner BG is 134 mg/dL. The DIA on his pump is set for 4 hours to estimate his BOB. He is not hungry but plans to eat the following meal for dinner:

6 oz ground beef
1 small tortilla
⅓ cup cooked rice
12 oz regular beer

1. How many grams of carbohydrate does he plan to consume?
2. How many units of short-acting insulin should he estimate before dinner?
   To cover carbohydrates (C:I = 13:1)
   To cover high BG (CF = 35:1)
   To compensate for BOB
   Total insulin to use
3. If a continuous glucose sensor showed one arrow up, how would this change?

The following are the author's answers to the 10 cases above. Read them and see if you agree.

CASE 1 Answers

Petunia has T1D, which she treats with 28 units of basal insulin daily and meal-time bolus insulin using a C:I ratio of 12:1 and a CF of 40:1, with a target premeal BG of 100 mg/dL. Her prelunch BG is 180 mg/dL. She plans to eat the following meal:

    1 bologna sandwich
    1 medium apple
    1 6-inch banana
    12-oz can of nondiet cola.

    1. How many grams of carbohydrate does she plan to consume?
        2 slices bread ≡ 30 g
        1 medium apple ≡ 15 g
        1 6-inch banana ≡ 30 g
        12 oz cola ≡ 40 g
        Total carbohydrates: 115 g
    2. How many units of short-acting insulin should she take before lunch?
        To cover carbohydrates (C:I ≡ 12:1): 9 U
        To cover high BG (CF ≡ 40:1): 2 U
        Total insulin to use: 11 U
    3. If a continuous glucose sensor showed one arrow up, how would this change?
        Add 1 U for 1 arrow up (BG increasing by 1 mg/dL/min)
        Answer: 12 U

CASE 2 Answers

Josephine has T1D, which she treats with an insulin pump by using 24 units of basal insulin daily and bolus insulin with each meal by using a C:I ratio of 15:1 and a CF of 50:1, with a target premeal BG of 120 mg/dL. Her predinner BG is 220 mg/dL. She plans to eat the following meal for dinner:

    1 cup of cooked pasta
    1 small roll
    ½ cup of peas
    12 oz diet soda
    2 Oreos
    1 cup of milk

    1. How many grams of carbohydrate does she plan to consume?
        1 cup cooked pasta ≡ 45 g
        1 small roll ≡ 15 g
        ½ cup peas ≡ 15 g
        2 Oreos ≡ 15 g
        1 cup milk ≡ 12 g
        Total carbohydrates: 102 g
    2. How many units of short-acting insulin should she take before lunch?
        To cover carbohydrates (C:I ≡ 15:1): 7 U
        To cover high BG (CF ≡ 50:1): 2 U
        Total insulin to use: 9 U
    3. If a continuous glucose sensor showed one arrow down, how would this change?
        Subtract 1 U for 1 arrow down (BG decreasing by 1 mg/dL/min)
        Answer: 8 U

CASE 3 Answers

Darko has T1D, which he treats with an insulin pump by using 32 units of basal insulin daily and meal-time bolus insulin by using a C:I ratio of 10:1 and a CF of 30:1, with a target premeal BG of 100 mg/dL. His predinner BG is 220 mg/dL. He plans to eat the following meal for dinner:

    12 oz steak
    1 medium potato (6 oz)
    12 oz microbrew beer
    4 Oreos
    1 cup of milk

1. How many grams of carbohydrate does he plan to consume?
   1 medium potato (6 oz) ≡ 30 g
   12 oz microbrew beer ≡ 30 g
   4 Oreos ≡ 30 g
   1 cup of milk ≡ 12 g
   Total carbohydrates: 102 g
2. How many units of short-acting insulin should he take before lunch?
   To cover carbohydrates (C:I ≡ 10:1): 10 U
   To cover high BG (CF ≡ 30:1): 4 U
   Total insulin to use: 14 U
3. If a continuous glucose sensor showed one arrow up, how would this change?
   Add 1 U for 1 arrow up (BG increasing by 1 mg/dL/min)
   Answer: 15 U

CASE 4   Answers

Dagobert has T1D, which he treats with an insulin pump by using 44 units of basal insulin daily and meal-time bolus insulin by using a C:I ratio of 8:1 and a CF of 25:1, with a target premeal BG of 125 mg/dL. His prelunch BG is 200 mg/dL. He plans to eat the following meal for lunch:
1 grilled cheese sandwich
1 summer sausage
⅔ cup of rice
½ cup of fruit juice

1. How many grams of carbohydrate does he plan to consume?
   2 slices of bread ≡ 30 g
   ⅔ cup of rice ≡ 30 g
   ½ cup of fruit juice ≡ 15 g
   Total carbohydrates: 75 g
2. How many units of short-acting insulin should he take before lunch?
   To cover carbohydrates (C:I ≡ 8:1): 9 U
   To cover high BG (CF ≡ 25:1): 3 U
   Total insulin to use: 12 U
3. If a continuous glucose sensor showed one arrow down, how would this change?
   Subtract 1 U for 1 arrow down (BG decreasing by 1 mg/dL/min)
   Answer: 11 U

CASE 5   Answers

Gertrude has T1D, which she treats with 18 units of basal insulin daily and meal-time bolus insulin by using a C:I ratio of 18:1 and a CF of 60:1, with a target premeal BG of 120 mg/dL. Her predinner BG is 180 mg/dL. She plans to eat the following meal:
8 oz tuna steak
1 small roll
⅓ cup cooked pasta
½ cup of corn
8 oz wine cooler

1. How many grams of carbohydrate does she plan to consume?
   1 small roll ≡ 15 g
   ⅓ cup cooked pasta ≡ 15 g
   ½ cup corn ≡ 15 g
   8 oz wine cooler ≡ 30 g
   Total carbohydrates: 75 g
2. How many units of short-acting insulin should she take before lunch?
   To cover carbohydrates (C:I ≡ 18:1): 4 U
   To cover high BG (CF ≡ 60:1): 1 U
   Total insulin to use: 5 U
3. If a continuous glucose sensor showed one arrow up, how would this change?
   Add 1 U for 1 arrow up (BG increasing by 1 mg/dL/min)
   Answer: 6 U

CASE 6   Answers

Carmello has T1D, which he treats with an insulin pump by using 48 units of basal insulin daily and meal-time bolus insulin by using a C:I ratio of 6:1 and a CF of 20:1, with a target premeal BG of 100 mg/dL. His predinner BG is 160 mg/dL. He is at a restaurant and plans to eat the following meal for dinner:

2 beef tacos with lettuce and sour cream each on a small corn tortilla
⅔ cup of rice with chorizo sausage
12 oz Margarita

1. How many grams of carbohydrate does he plan to consume?
   2 small corn tortillas ≡ 20 g
   ⅔ cup rice ≡ 30 g
   12 oz Margarita ≡ 90 g
   Total carbohydrates: 140 g
2. How many units of short-acting insulin should he take before lunch?
   To cover carbohydrates (C:I ≡ 6:1): 23 U
   To cover high BG (CF ≡ 20:1): 3 U
   Total insulin to use: 26 U
3. If a continuous glucose sensor showed one arrow down, how would this change?
   Subtract 1 U for 1 arrow down (BG decreasing by 1 mg/dL/min)
   Answer: 25 U

CASE 7   Answers

Rose has T1D, which she treats with an insulin pump by using 18 units of basal insulin daily and meal-time bolus insulin by using a C:I ratio of 15:1 and a CF of 50:1, with a target premeal BG of 100 mg/dL. She took a CF bolus of 2 units 2 hours ago. Her predinner BG is 248 mg/dL. The DIA on her pump is set for 4 hours to estimate her BOB. She plans to eat the following meal for dinner:

1 breast baked chicken
½ cup mashed potatoes
½ cup of corn
2 × 2 inch unfrosted cake
Unsweetened tea

1. How many grams of carbohydrate does she plan to consume?
   ½ cup mashed potatoes ≡ 15 g
   ½ cup of corn ≡ 15 g
   2 × 2 inch unfrosted cake ≡ 15 g
   Total carbohydrates: 45 g
2. How many units of short-acting insulin should she estimate before dinner?
   To cover carbohydrates (C:I ≡ 15:1): 3 U
   To cover high BG (CF ≡ 50:1): 3 U
   To compensate for BOB: − 1 U
   Total insulin to use: 5 U
3. If a continuous glucose sensor showed one arrow down, how would this change?
   Subtract 1 U for 1 arrow down (BG decreasing by 1 mg/dL/min)
   Answer: 4 U

CASE 8   Answers

Dmitri has T1D, which he treats with an insulin pump by using 16 units of basal insulin daily and meal-time bolus insulin by using a C:I ratio of 15:1 and a CF of 40:1, with a target premeal BG of 100 mg/dL. He took a CF bolus of 4 units 3 hours ago. His predinner BG is 219 mg/dL. The DIA on his pump is set for 4 hours to estimate his BOB. He plans to eat the following meal for dinner:

12 oz roast beef
1 6-oz potato
½ cup of peas
1 small roll
10 oz milk

1. How many grams of carbohydrate does he plan to consume?
   1 6-oz potato ≡ 30 g
   ½ cup of peas ≡ 15 g
   1 small roll ≡ 15 g
   10 oz milk ≡ 15 g
   Total carbohydrates: 75 g

2. How many units of short-acting insulin should he estimate before dinner?
   To cover carbohydrates (C:I ≡ 15:1): 5 U
   To cover high BG (CF ≡ 40:1): 3 U
   To compensate for BOB: − 1 U
   Total insulin to use: 7 U
3. If a continuous glucose sensor showed one arrow up, how would this change?
   Add 1 U for 1 arrow up (BG increasing by 1 mg/dL/min)
   Answer: 8 U

CASE 9 Answers

Nadia has T1D, which she treats with an insulin pump by using 20 units of basal insulin daily and meal-time bolus insulin by using a C:I ratio of 12:1 and a CF of 40:1, with a target premeal BG of 100 mg/dL. She took a snack bolus of 2 units and a CF bolus of 2 units 2 hours ago. Her predinner BG is 179 mg/dL. The DIA on her pump is set for 4 hours to estimate her BOB. She plans to eat the following meal for dinner:

8 oz ham
⅓ cup of cooked pasta
½ cup of peas
1 medium apple
2 Oreos
Unsweetened tea

1. How many grams of carbohydrate does she plan to consume?
   ⅓ cup of cooked pasta ≡ 15 g
   ½ cup of peas ≡ 15 g
   1 medium apple ≡ 15 g
   2 Oreos ≡ 15 g
   Total carbohydrates: 60 g
2. How many units of short-acting insulin should she estimate before dinner?
   To cover carbohydrates (C:I ≡ 12:1): 5 U
   To cover high BG (CF ≡ 40:1): 2 U
   To compensate for BOB: − 2 U
   Total insulin to use: 5 U
3. If a continuous glucose sensor showed one arrow down, how would this change?
   Subtract 1 U for 1 arrow down (BG decreasing by 1 mg/dL/min)
   Answer: 4 U

CASE 10 Answers

Cody has T1D, which he treats with an insulin pump by using 24 units of basal insulin daily and meal-time bolus insulin by using a C:I ratio of 13:1 and a CF of 35:1, with a target premeal BG of 100 mg/dL. He took a CF bolus of 4 units 3 hours ago and a snack bolus of 4 units 2 hours ago. His predinner BG is 134 mg/dL. The DIA on his pump is set for 4 hours to estimate his BOB. He is not hungry but plans to eat the following meal for dinner:

6 oz ground beef
1 small tortilla
⅓ cup cooked rice
12 oz regular beer

1. How many grams of carbohydrate does he plan to consume?
   1 small tortilla ≡ 10 g
   ⅓ cup cooked rice ≡ 15 g
   12 oz regular beer ≡ 15 g
   Total carbohydrates: 40 g
2. How many units of short-acting insulin should he estimate before dinner?
   To cover carbohydrates (C:I ≡ 13:1): 3 U
   To cover high BG (CF ≡ 35:1): 1 U
   To compensate for BOB: − 3 U
   Total insulin to use: 1 U
3. If a continuous glucose sensor showed one arrow up, how would this change?
   Add 1 U for 1 arrow up (BG increasing by 1 mg/dL/min)
   Answer: 2 U

8. How do you assess if your patients are counting their carbohydrates accurately?

Numerous carbohydrate counting quizzes and other assessment tools are available on the Internet. Here is one we use, adapted from one used at the Cleveland Clinic.

University of Colorado Hospital: Carbohydrate Counting Quiz

Name:

Date:

Food	Does This Food Contain Carbohydrates? (Circle Only One Answer)		
1. Bread	Yes	No	Don't know
2. Breakfast sausages	Yes	No	Don't know
3. Baked potato	Yes	No	Don't know
4. Maple syrup, regular	Yes	No	Don't know
5. American cheese	Yes	No	Don't know
6. Low-fat milk	Yes	No	Don't know
7. Apple juice	Yes	No	Don't know
8. Soda pop (not diet)	Yes	No	Don't know
9. Apple	Yes	No	Don't know
10. Cooked dried beans (lentils, navy beans)	Yes	No	Don't know

Food	How Many Grams of Carbohydrate does this Portion Contain? (Circle)						
11. 1 Cup milk	0 g	15 g	30 g	45 g	60 g	75 g	Don't know
12. 1 Cup pasta	0 g	15 g	30 g	45 g	60 g	75 g	Don't know
13. 1 Cup cooked rice	0 g	15 g	30 g	45 g	60 g	75 g	Don't know
14. 1 Cup juice	0 g	15 g	30 g	45 g	60 g	75 g	Don't know
15. 1 Cup hot cereal	0 g	15 g	30 g	45 g	60 g	75 g	Don't know
16. 1 Cup cooked dried beans	0 g	15 g	30 g	45 g	60 g	75 g	Don't know
17. 1 Cup mashed potatoes	0 g	15 g	30 g	45 g	60 g	75 g	Don't know

For each question, circle the best answer below.

18. Read the Nutrition Facts label to the right, what is the serving size?

    Don't know   1 cup   2 cups   4 cups

19. How many grams of carbohydrate would you consume if you ate one serving?

    Don't know   228 g   5 g   31 g

20. How many grams of carbohydrate would you consume if you ate the whole package?

    Don't know   456 g   10 g   62 g

Nutrition Facts

Serving Size 1 cup (228g)
Servings Per Container 2

Amount Per Serving

Calories 260   Calories from Fat 120

	% Daily Value*
Total Fat 13g	**20**%
Saturated Fat 5g	**25**%
Cholesterol 30mg	**10**%
Sodium 660mg	**28**%
Total Carbohydrate 31g	**10**%
Dietary Fiber 0g	**0**%
Sugar 5g	
Protein 5g	

Vitamin A 4%	•	Vitamin C 2%
Calcium 15%	•	Iron 4%

*Percent daily values are based on a 2,000 calorie diet. Your daily values may be higher or lower depending on your calorie needs:

	Calories:	2,000	2,500
Total Fat	Less than	65g	80g
Sat Fat	Less than	20g	25g
Cholesterol	Less than	300mg	300mg
Sodium	Less than	2,400mg	2,400mg
Total Carbohydrate		300g	375g
Dietary Fiber		25g	30g

Calories per gram:
Fat 9   •   Carbohydrate 4   •   Protein 4

Number of correct answers:

Percent correct answers
(number correct ÷ 20 × 100):

Answers:
1. Yes   2. No   3. Yes   4. Yes   5. No   6. Yes   7. Yes   8. Yes   9. Yes   10. Yes
11. 15   12. 30   13. 45   14. 30   15. 30   16. 30   17. 30   18. 1 cup   19. 31 g   20. 62 g

BIBLIOGRAPHY

Aleppo, G., Laffel, L. M., Ahmann, A. J., Hirsch, I. B., Kruger, D. F., Peters, A., … Harris, D. R. (2017). A practical approach to using trend arrows on the Dexcom G5 CGM System for the management of adults with diabetes. *Journal of the Endocrine Society, 1*(12), 1445–1460.

Holzmeister LA. (2010). *The Diabetes Carbohydrate and Fat Gram Guide*. 4th Edition. Publisher, American Diabetes Association.

Laffel, L. M., Aleppo, G., Buckingham, B. A., Forlenza, G. P., Rasbach, L. E., Tsalikian, E., … Harris, D. R. (2017). A practical approach to using trend arrows on the Dexcom G5 CGM System to manage children and adolescents with diabetes. *Journal of the Endocrine Society, 1*(12), 1461–1476.

Walsh, J., & Roberts, R. (2000). *Pumping Insulin* (3rd ed.). San Diego, CA: Torrey Pines Press.

Warshaw HS, Bolderman KM. (2008). Practical Carbohydrate Counting: A How-To-Teach Guide for Health Professionals. Publisher, American Diabetes Association.

https://www.CalorieKing.com - Official Website
https://www.sparkpeople.com

CHAPTER 7

INPATIENT MANAGEMENT OF DIABETES AND HYPERGLYCEMIA

Stacey A. Seggelke and R. Matthew Hawkins

1. **Does evidence support intensive management of blood glucose in the hospital setting?**
   It is well established that hyperglycemia in hospitalized patients contributes to increased morbidity, mortality, and length of stay (LOS). A well-done study found that the LOS and rates of inpatient complications were four times higher in patients with diabetes or stress hyperglycemia than in those with normal blood glucose (BG) levels. Furthermore, the RABBIT 2-Surgery (Randomized Study of Basal-Bolus Insulin Therapy in the Inpatient Management of Patients With Type 2 Diabetes Undergoing General Surgery) trial demonstrated a decreased rate of inpatient complications with reduction of hyperglycemia in noncritically ill patients undergoing surgery. Extensive published literature has demonstrated that good inpatient glycemic management clearly improves patient outcomes and shortens LOS.

   However, there is controversy over what degree of glycemic control is most appropriate. The largest randomized controlled trial (RCT), the NICE-SUGAR (Normoglycemia in Intensive Care Evaluation and Surviving Using Glucose Algorithm Regulation) study, demonstrated an increased risk of mortality in patients with tight glycemic control (glucose target: 81-108 mg/dL) compared with those with standard glycemic control (glucose target: 144–180 mg/dL). The increase in mortality is thought to result partially from the high rate of hypoglycemia ($\leq$ 40 mg/dL) seen in the intensively treated group. Although this study corroborated previous evidence that glycemic control is important, it did underscore the risks of hypoglycemia and supported relaxing of the glycemic targets that had been recommended before that time.

2. **What are the glycemic targets for the critically ill patient population?**
   The American Diabetes Association (ADA) recommendations are to initiate insulin therapy for treatment of hyperglycemia at a BG threshold of $\geq$ 180 mg/dL in critically ill patients. Insulin therapy should then be titrated to maintain glycemic levels between 140 and 180 mg/dL. The BG goal can be further lowered to 110 to 140 mg/dL in select patients, as long as it can be attained without hypoglycemia.

3. **What are the glycemic targets for noncritically ill patients?**
   The ADA's current recommendations are to maintain BG targets between 140 and 180 mg/dL. In patients with a history of tighter outpatient glycemic control, the target may be lowered if this can be done with avoidance of hypoglycemia.

4. **What are the Inpatient glycemic targets for pregnant patients?**
   BG goals for pregnancy are tighter than for the general population. Hyperglycemia during pregnancy is associated with many adverse outcomes, including macrosomia, congenital abnormalities, fetal hyperinsulinemia, and fetal mortality. For patients with gestational diabetes, type 1diabetes, or type 2 diabetes, the recommendations are a fasting BG level < 95 mg/dL, 1-hour postmeal BG $\leq$ 140 mg/dL, and 2-hour postmeal BG level $\leq$ 120 mg/dL.

KEY POINTS 1: TARGET GLUCOSE LEVELS FOR HOSPITALIZED PATIENTS

- Critically ill: 140 to 180 mg/dL
- Non–critically ill: 140 to 180 mg/dL
- Pregnant: fasting < 95 mg/dL; 1 hr postprandial $\leq$ 140 mg/dL; 2 hr postprandial $\leq$ 120 mg/dL

5. **Which patients are at high risk for hyperglycemia during their hospital stay?**
   Numerous factors can contribute to inpatient hyperglycemia in patients with or without a preexisting diagnosis of diabetes. These include the severity of the underlying illness, initiation of glucocorticoid therapy, enteral nutrition (EN) or parenteral nutrition (PN), immunosuppressive agents, and/or metabolic changes associated with increased circulating counterregulatory hormones and proinflammatory cytokines. It is recommended that BG be monitored (point-of-care or laboratory testing) in all patients receiving therapies that may cause hyperglycemia. If hyperglycemia occurs, appropriate treatment should be initiated with the same glycemic goals discussed above. The ADA recommends that hemoglobin A_{1c} (HbA_{1c}) levels be measured in all patients with diabetes admitted to the hospital if the results of HbA_{1c} testing in the previous 3 months are not available.

6. What is the best treatment in the inpatient management of diabetes?
Insulin therapy, given as intravenous (IV) infusion or subcutaneous injections, is the safest and most effective way to treat hyperglycemia in the hospital setting. Insulin is effective and can be rapidly adjusted to adapt to changes in glucose levels or food intake. It is recommended that standardized insulin protocols be used, whenever available.

7. What is IV insulin infusion, and why is it used in critically ill patients?
With IV insulin infusion, 1 unit of regular human insulin per 1 mL of 0.9% sodium chloride (NaCl; normal saline) is administered. When given intravenously, regular insulin has a rapid onset and a short half-life, allowing for quick adjustment of insulin doses to achieve appropriate glycemic control.

8. At what rate should insulin infusion be started?
Insulin infusion is usually initiated at 0.1 unit/hr/kg body weight.

9. How should the IV insulin infusion rate be adjusted?
Insulin infusions should be adjusted on an hourly basis. Dosage adjustments should be made on the basis of the current BG level and the rate of change from the previous BG level. If the BG level does not change by 30 to 50 mg/dL within an hour, the insulin rate should be increased. Conversely, if the BG level drops by > 30 to 50 mg/dL in an hour, the insulin drip rate should be reduced. Many insulin infusion protocols have been published and are available for use. Additionally, computer-based algorithms to direct nursing actions are commercially available.

10. How do you transition a patient off insulin infusion?
Because of the short duration of action of IV regular insulin, it is imperative to give subcutaneous insulin before discontinuation of an insulin infusion. Basal insulin (long acting or intermediate acting) should be given at least 2 hours before discontinuation of insulin infusion. If using rapid-acting insulin, it should be given 1 to 2 hours before discontinuation of insulin infusion. To calculate the total daily dose (TDD) of subcutaneous insulin needed, add up the amount of insulin given during the past 6 hours of IV insulin infusion, and multiply by 4 for an estimate of the 24-hour requirement. Then reduce that amount by 20% for a new TDD. This TDD should then be split as 50% to 80% basal insulin (higher percentage if the patient is fasting) and 20% to 50% meal-time bolus insulin.

11. How should you select a basal insulin dose?
Basal coverage can be achieved through the use of intermediate-acting human insulin (neutral protamine Hagedorn [NPH]) given twice daily or, preferably, long-acting insulin analogues (glargine, detemir, degludec) given once or twice a day. Long-acting insulins generally provide more consistent coverage with minimal insulin peaks, whereas NPH insulin is more likely to cause hypoglycemia because of variable insulin action and peaks. Regardless of the type of insulin used, the basal insulin dose usually accounts for approximately 50% of the TDD of insulin in patients who have a normal dietary intake.

12. How should you select a prandial dose for patients on insulin?
Prandial insulin should include both nutritional (meal coverage) and correctional (treatment of hyperglycemia) components. Rapid-acting insulin analogues (lispro, aspart, glulisine) are best given 0 to 15 minutes before meals, whereas short-acting insulin (regular) should be given 30 minutes before meals. Rapid-acting analogues provide increased flexibility in dosing and have a shorter duration of action, making them the preferred agents. In general, the total bolus insulin doses each day should be about 50% of the TDD of insulin delivery. However, in the hospital setting, a reduced prandial dose may be needed because of decreased appetite or variance in oral intake. Correction insulin dosing can be calculated based on the patient's insulin sensitivity. This insulin is either added to the nutritional dose or given alone if the patient is not receiving calories. For inpatients with type 1 diabetes or for those who are insulin sensitive, a good initial correction dose is 1 unit of insulin for every 50 mg/dL the current BG is above a goal of 150 mg/dL. For patients with type 2 diabetes or insulin resistance, you can use 1 unit of insulin for every 25 mg/dL the current BG is above 150 mg/dL (See Table 7.1 for examples). To prevent hypoglycemia caused by "stacking" of insulin, correction insulin doses should not be given more often than every 4 hours.

13. How should you adjust insulin dosages?
BG levels should be assessed multiple times a day in patients receiving insulin (preferably four times daily: before breakfast, before lunch, before dinner, and at bedtime). Basal insulin dosages are assessed mainly by reviewing morning fasting BG levels. BG levels should remain relatively steady through the night if the basal dose is correct. A significant rise or drop in BG during the night would necessitate a change in basal insulin dosing. Prandial insulin doses are assessed by prelunch, predinner, and bedtime BG values. For more precise prandial dosing, a 2-hour postprandial BG check can be performed. It is expected that this postprandial value will be about 30 to 50 mg/dL higher than the preprandial reading.

14. Is "sliding scale" insulin administration still used?
"Sliding scale" insulin administration is not an effective treatment for hyperglycemia and, therefore, is no longer recommended. Traditionally, a sliding scale was a set amount of bolus insulin, usually regular insulin, which was

Table 7.1. Example of Nutritional and Correctional Insulin Dosing Chart.

BLOOD GLUCOSE (mg/dL)	☐ SENSITIVE TO INSULIN Type 1 DM Stress hyperglycemia Normal body weight		☐ RESISTANT TO INSULIN Type 2 DM Steroids Overweight/obese		☐ EXTRA RESISTANT TO INSULIN Blood glucose uncontrolled by "resistant to insulin" table		☐ CUSTOMIZED	
	Receiving Calories	No Calories	Receiving Calories	No Calories	Receiving Calories	No Calories	Receiving Calories	No Calories
≤ 70	Implement hypoglycemia orders		Implement hypoglycemia orders		Implement hypoglycemia orders		Implement hypoglycemia orders	
71–124	3 units	No insulin	6 units	No insulin	10 units	No insulin	____ units	____ units
125–149	3 units	No insulin	7 units	No insulin	11 units	No insulin	____ units	____ units
150–199	4 units	1 unit	8 units	2 units	12 units	2 units	____ units	____ units
200–249	5 units	2 units	10 units	4 units	14 units	4 units	____ units	____ units
250–299	6 units	3 units	12 units	6 units	16 units	6 units	____ units	____ units
300–349	7 units	4 units	14 units	8 units	18 units	8 units	____ units	____ units
350–399	8 units	5 units	16 units	10 units	20 units	10 units	____ units	____ units
≥ 400	Call MD		Call MD		Call MD		Call MD	

given to treat high BG levels, generally above 200 mg/dL. The insulin was given without consideration of meal times, previous dosages, carbohydrate content of meals, or the patient's insulin sensitivity. This often resulted in a wide fluctuation of BG levels because hyperglycemia was not treated preemptively but, instead, was treated after the fact.

KEY POINTS 2: INPATIENT TREATMENT OF HYPERGLYCEMIA

- Insulin is the most appropriate treatment agent for hyperglycemia in the hospital.
- IV insulin Infusion is the best therapy for critically ill patients.
- Basal-bolus (prandial and correction) insulin is the best therapy for non–critically ill patients.
- BG levels should be evaluated daily and insulin adjusted, as needed.

15. **What is hypoglycemia, and how should it be treated?**
Hypoglycemia in hospitalized patients is defined as a BG level < 70 mg/dL, because this is considered the initial threshold for counterregulatory hormone release (epinephrine, glucagon, cortisol, and growth hormone). Patients at high risk for hypoglycemia include those with renal or liver failure, altered nutrition, and a history of severe hypoglycemia. Treatment of hypoglycemia is based on the patient situation. For a patient who is able to take oral treatment, 15 to 30 g of quick-acting carbohydrates, such as juice, regular soda, or glucose tablets (5 g each) is the preferred treatment. If unconscious or unable to take oral treatment, the patient can be given 50 g (1 ampule) of dextrose 50% intravenously or 1 mg of glucagon intramuscularly. BG levels should be rechecked 15 to 20 minutes later to assess the efficacy of treatment. If the BG level is still < 70 mg/dL, treatment should be repeated.

16. **Are oral agents or noninsulin injectables appropriate to use in hospitalized patients?**
Data on the safety and efficacy of using oral agents or noninsulin injectables (glucagon-like protein-1 [GLP-1] analogues or pramlintide) in hospital settings are limited. In most cases of hyperglycemia, noninsulin treatment options are not effective in lowering BG to goal levels, especially in acute illness. Recent studies have demonstrated the safety of using dipeptidyl peptidase-4 (DPP-4) inhibitors in the hospital setting. When used alone or in combination with basal insulin or correctional bolus insulin, DPP-4 inhibitors have proven to be an effective treatment. Oral agents may be initiated or resumed in clinically stable patients in anticipation of discharge.

17. **What is the best treatment for steroid-induced hyperglycemia?**
Steroids stimulate hepatic gluconeogenesis and impair insulin action, resulting in hyperglycemia caused by increased hepatic glucose production and insulin resistance. The BG effects of steroids often present as elevated postprandial BG excursions. The extent of BG elevation is dependent on the type, amount, and duration of steroids used. Individuals who are on low steroid doses and who are insulin naive may be adequately treated with bolus insulin at meal times. If the patient is receiving higher steroid doses or has a history of insulin-treated diabetes, a good treatment option is intermediate-acting basal insulin (NPH) administered concurrently with the steroid. For patients on steroids with long durations of action, such as dexamethasone or depot steroid injections, long-acting basal insulin may be used. Insulin needs should be assessed and adjusted as the steroid therapy is tapered and discontinued.

18. **What is the best treatment for hyperglycemia resulting from EN or PN?**
There are several approaches to insulin treatment for hyperglycemia resulting from nutritional support. For total parenteral nutrition (TPN), the addition of regular insulin to the TPN bag is the safest approach to glycemic control. The initial dosing recommendation is 1 unit for every 10 to 12 g of dextrose in the TPN solution. The amount of insulin in the TPN solution can be adjusted daily or an additional rapid-acting insulin correction scale can also be used for immediate correction of hyperglycemia. Another approach to treatment is the use of a subcutaneous basal-bolus insulin regimen. However, this poses an increased risk of hypoglycemia if TPN is unexpectedly discontinued or the TPN dextrose concentration is changed without adjustment of insulin concentration.

There are many approaches to treatment for hyperglycemia caused by EN. Basal insulin can be administered once or twice daily in combination with a rapid-acting insulin correction scale every 4 to 6 hours. Regular insulin administered every 6 hours is another option. Alternatively, intermediate-acting 70/30 human insulin given every 8 hours with a correctional rapid-acting scale every 4 hours is an approach used by the authors of this chapter. Hypoglycemia is an immense concern in these patients because feeding can be interrupted unexpectedly with dislodgement of the feeding tube or discontinuation of the EN because of nausea experienced by the patient or because of diagnostic testing while the injected subcutaneous insulin is still active. If EN or TPN is unexpectedly interrupted, it is important to start IV dextrose 10% in water (D10W) at the same hourly rate as with the continuous tube feeding, PN, or TPN, and to reduce or hold the next dose of long-acting or intermediate-acting insulin. It is important to remember that these patients are in a consistent postprandial state and that glucose goals should be adjusted accordingly.

19. **Can a continuous subcutaneous insulin infusion be used in the inpatient setting?**

Continuous subcutaneous insulin infusion (CSII), also known as *insulin pump infusion,* can be safely used in the inpatient setting. It is imperative that the patient is mentally and physically able to operate his or her own insulin pump. It is also recommended that staff with CSII experience help manage these cases. Current pump settings, including basal rates, bolus settings, and bolus dosages, should be documented on a daily basis.

The use of a continuous glucose monitor (CGM), either as a standalone device or in combination with an insulin pump, is controversial because CGM has not yet been documented to be sufficiently accurate in the inpatient setting to allow for insulin dosing based on CGM BG values. CGM still provides important information about BG trends and can give audible alarms when BG levels are too high or too low. However, until CGM diagnostic accuracy has been sufficiently well documented in hospitalized patients to get approval from the U.S. Food and Drug Administration (FDA) for diagnostic use in the inpatient setting, insulin dosing adjustments should still be made on the basis of finger-stick point-of-care BG testing.

20. **How do you adjust diabetes medications before surgery?**

Hypoglycemia is a considerable risk for patients undergoing surgery because of their NPO (nothing by mouth) status. All oral diabetes medications should be held the morning of the procedure. For patients on long-acting insulin analogues (glargine, detemir, degludec), it recommended that they take about 80% of their normal dose the night before or the morning of surgery. Patients on intermediate-acting insulin (NPH) should take 50% of their typical dose on the morning of the procedure. Correction doses of rapid-acting insulin analogues can be given in the perioperative period every 4 hours to maintain BG levels < 180 mg/dL. If the procedure is lengthy or if prolonged NPO status is expected, the use of insulin infusion is recommended.

21. **How do you decide what home regimen to order at discharge?**

This is where the most recent HbA_{1C} value (obtained upon hospital admission or from the patient's records if obtained < 90 days before admission) is especially helpful. If there has been good glycemic control in the outpatient setting (HbA_{1C} at or near target), the patient can be sent home on the same regimen he or she was on previously. For patients with a new diagnosis of diabetes or for those requiring a change in previous therapy because of poor outpatient glycemic control (HbA_{1C} above target), recommendations should be based on the patient's preferences and abilities, and the costs, side effects, and benefits of additional medications. It is also recommended that medication administration instructions, especially for insulin, be given in both oral and written formats. Details of discharge medications and instructions should be communicated promptly and clearly to the patient's primary care provider.

⊕ WEBSITES

1. American Association of Clinical Endocrinologist Inpatient Glycemic Control Resource Center: http://resources.aace.com
2. Society of Hospital Medicine Glycemic Control Resource Room: https://www.hospitalmedicine.org/clinical-topics/glycemic-control/

BIBLIOGRAPHY

American Diabetes Association. (2018). Standards of medical care in diabetes, 2018. *Diabetes Care, 41,* S144–S151.

Buehler, L., Fayfman, M., Alexopoulos, A. S., Zhao, L., Farrokhi, F., Weaver, J., ... Umpierrez, G. E. (2015). The impact of hyperglycemia and obesity on hospitalization costs and clinical outcome in general surgery patients. *Journal of Diabetes and Its Complications, 29*(8), 1177–1182.

Fowler, M. J. (2009). Inpatient diabetes management. *Clinical Diabetes, 27,* 119–122.

Hsia, E., Seggelke, S. A., Gibbs, J., Rasouli, N., & Draznin, B. (2011). Comparison of 70/30 biphasic insulin with glargine/lispro regimen in non-critically ill diabetic patients on continuous enteral nutrition therapy. *Nutrition in Clinical Practice, 26*(6), 714–717.

Hsia, E., Seggelke, S., Gibbs, J., Hawkins, R. M., Cohlmia, E., Rasouli, N., ... Draznin, B. (2012). Subcutaneous administration of glargine to diabetic patients receiving insulin infusion prevents rebound hyperglycemia. *Journal of Clinical Endocrinology and Metabolism, 97,* 3132–3137.

Low Wang, C. C., & Draznin, B. (2013). Practical approach to management of inpatient hyperglycemia in select patient populations. *Hospital Practice (1995), 41,* 45–53.

Magaji, V., & Johnston, J. M. (2011). Inpatient management of hyperglycemia and diabetes. *Clinical Diabetes, 29,* 3–9.

Moghissi, E. S., Korytkowski, M. T., DiNardo, M., Einhorn, D., Hellman, R., Hirsch, I. B., ... Umpierrez, G. E. (2009). American Association of Clinical Endocrinologists and American Diabetes Association consensus statement on inpatient glycemic control. *Diabetes Care, 32,* 1119–1131.

Seggelke, S. A., Gibbs, J., & Draznin, B. (2011). Pilot study of using neutral protamine Hagedorn insulin to counteract the effect of methylprednisolone in hospitalized patients with diabetes. *Journal of Hospital Medicine, 6*(3), 175–176.

Umpierrez, G. E., Smiley, D., Zisman, A., Prieto, L. M., Palacio, A, Ceron, M., ... Mejia, R. (2007). Randomized study of basal-bolus insulin therapy in the inpatient management of patients with type 2 diabetes (RABBIT 2 trial). *Diabetes Care, 30*(9), 2181–2186.

Umpierrez, G. E., Hellman, R., Korytkowski, M. T., Kosiborod, M., Maynard, G. A., Montori, V. M., … Van den Berghe, G. (2012). Management of hyperglycemia in hospitalized patients in non-critical care setting: an endocrine society clinical practice guideline. *Journal of Clinical Endocrinology and Metabolism, 97*, 16–38.

Umpierrez, G. E., Smiley, D., Jacobs, S., Peng, L., Temponi, A., Mulligan, P., … Rizzo, M. (2011). Randomized study of basal-bolus insulin therapy in the inpatient management of patients with type 2 diabetes undergoing general surgery (RABBIT 2 surgery). *Diabetes Care, 34*, 256–261.

Umpierrez, G. E., & Pasquel, F. J. (2017). Management of inpatient hyperglycemia and diabetes in older adults. *Diabetes Care, 40*(4), 509–517.

Van den Berghe, G., Wilmer, A., Hermans, G., Meersseman, W., Wouters, P. J., Milants, I., … Bouillon, R. (2006). Intensive insulin therapy in the medical ICU. *New England Journal of Medicine, 354*, 449–446.

CHAPTER 8

DIABETES IN PREGNANCY

Amy M. Valent and Linda A. Barbour

1. How does normal pregnancy affect fuel metabolism?

   Pregnancy is a complex metabolic state that involves marked alterations in steroid and protein hormone production (increases in estrogen, progesterone, prolactin, cortisol, human chorionic gonadotropin, placental growth hormone, and human placental lactogen), increased inflammatory cytokines (tumor necrosis factor-alpha [TNF-α], interleukin-6 [IL-6], C-reactive protein [CRP]), and adipokines (leptin and adiponectin) to alter maternal fat accretion and insulin resistance, providing the necessary nutrients for the growing fetal-placental unit. There is support from cumulative data for the notion that the intrauterine metabolic environment characterized by overnutrition or undernutrition may be a risk factor for abnormal fetal growth and future risk of childhood obesity.

2. What metabolic changes occur in the first trimester of pregnancy?

   Early pregnancy is characterized as an anabolic state, fostering nutrient storage in preparation for the greater fetal demands in late gestation and lactation. Metabolic changes promote lipogenesis, reduce fatty acid oxidation, and increase adipose tissue fatty acid synthesis and lipoprotein lipase, fostering maternal fat storage in early gestation. In the setting of normal insulin sensitivity, a rise in first-phase and second-phase insulin secretion, cortisol, and leptin contribute to the increased maternal fat accretion. Between 6 and 20 weeks of pregnancy, many women demonstrate a relative increase in insulin sensitivity attributable to increased adiponectin, but this is variable, depending on pregestational insulin sensitivity. Adiponectin, at least in normal-weight women, may transiently increase before it falls with advancing gestation. Potential roles of adiponectin in pregnancy include its insulin-sensitizing effects, its influence on hepatic gluconeogenesis, lipid metabolism, and placental signaling. There is generally a net lipogenesis during early pregnancy among normal-weight individuals. In contrast, obese women with insulin resistance predating the pregnancy demonstrate relative lipolysis throughout all of gestation.

3. Describe the metabolic changes in the second and third trimesters and the immediate postpartum period.

   The placenta is responsible for maintaining a balanced and continuous supply of nutrient substrates from the mother to the fetus throughout gestation to develop a healthy and growing fetus. Because of the increased fetal–placental glucose demand during the second and third trimesters, glycogen stores are quickly depleted in the fasting state and the increased insulin resistance in skeletal muscle and the liver results in increased hepatic gluconeogenesis. Pregnant women must transition from carbohydrate to fat metabolism earlier ($<$ 12 hours) in the fasting state. Maternal insulin resistance in adipose tissue decreases the ability of insulin to suppress whole-body lipolysis, thereby increasing free fatty acid (FFA) levels for maternal energy use and sparing glucose for the placenta and the fetus. These physiologic changes describe the "accelerated starvation of pregnancy," which results in increased ketogenesis. Consequently, there is an approximately 50% decrease in insulin-mediated glucose disposal (assessed by the hyperinsulinemic euglycemic clamp technique) and a 200% to 300% increase in insulin secretion in late pregnancy. While maintaining euglycemia in the mother, these metabolic changes are necessary to meet the metabolic demands of the placenta and growing fetus, which requires 80% of its energy as glucose. By the third trimester, this is estimated to be $>$ 150 g of glucose daily. The human fetus is dependent on a steady supply of maternal glucose until late gestation because of its limited ability to oxidize fat as an energy source. In addition, there are higher metabolic needs as the maternal body mass index (BMI) increases. Immediately after delivery of the placenta, insulin sensitivity returns, with potentially increased sensitivity among breastfeeding mothers.

4. Do normal-weight women have different glycemic patterns from those of women with a BMI $\geq$ 30 kg/m^2 in pregnancy?

   Extensive reviews of glycemia patterns in normal pregnancy have reported that mean fasting glucose levels were 72 mg/dL, 1-hour postprandial values were 109 mg/dL, and 2-hour values were 99 mg/dL, with a 24-hour mean glucose of 88 mg/dL, all much lower than current therapeutic targets. Even after controlling for diet, compared with normal-weight women, obese women have higher fasting and postprandial glucose levels (averaging 5–10 mg/dL higher) and 24-hour glycemic profiles in early ($\approx$ 16 weeks) and late ($\approx$ 28 weeks) gestation, despite having higher insulin levels.

5. Is glucose the only fuel altered in normal pregnancy, and what is the role of lipids in fetal growth?

   Although glucose is the most abundant nutrient crossing the placenta and plays a significant role in fetal overgrowth in the setting of maternal hyperglycemia, major changes in maternal lipid metabolism during gestation

67

also play an important role in the development of fetal fat mass and growth. The relationship among maternal lipid metabolism, placental lipid transport, and fetal fat accretion and growth is not well understood. Serum triglycerides (TGs), cholesterol, and FFAs increase across gestation, with TGs rising two- to threefold by the third trimester. The increase in FFAs may further accentuate the insulin resistance of pregnancy. Obese mothers have higher FFAs and higher fasting and postprandial TG during early and late pregnancy compared with normal-weight women. Furthermore, maternal BMI, gestational weight gain, insulin resistance, maternal TGs and FFAs, and placental lipoprotein lipase activity are associated with higher rates of large-for-gestational age (LGA) infants (> 90th percentile for gestational age) and increased newborn adiposity. Infant adiposity is associated with long-term risks for dysmetabolism and obesity. Prior studies suggest that the 1-hour or 2-hour postprandial TG levels in early pregnancy (16 weeks) are strongly associated with infant adiposity among obese pregnant women. In contrast, in normal-weight pregnant women, a higher rise in fasting TG levels from early to late pregnancy is associated with infant adiposity. At this time, there are no formal recommendations to target maternal TG levels in pregnancy as a potential intervention to decrease the risk for newborn adiposity or macrosomia (birth weight > 4000 g), but studies are ongoing.

Amino acids are essential for protein synthesis, oxidation, and normal fetal development. They are actively transported through the placenta across a concentration gradient. Because fat is preferentially used for fuel metabolism, protein catabolism is lower during normal pregnancy. The contribution of maternal amino acids to fetal growth and fat accretion is recognized, but there is a need for more diet-controlled studies in normal pregnancy, obesity, and gestational diabetes mellitus (GDM) to determine the influence of amino acids in fetal growth and composition.

6. Explain the effect of the metabolic changes in pregnancy on diabetes management in the first trimester.
In diabetes, optimal glycemic control should be ensured before conception to decrease adverse perinatal outcomes, including miscarriage, congenital anomalies, intrauterine fetal demise, macrosomia, and developmental programming of adult metabolic disease. During the first trimester, nausea, increased insulin sensitivity, and accelerated starvation may place a woman with type 1 diabetes (T1D) at risk for hypoglycemia, and thus, insulin requirements are extremely variable at this time. This risk for hypoglycemia is especially high at night because of prolonged fasting and continuous fetal–placental glucose utilization. Severe hypoglycemia occurs in 30% to 40% of pregnant women with T1D in the first 20 weeks of pregnancy, most often between midnight and 8:00 AM. Individuals with gastroparesis or hyperemesis gravidarum are at the greatest risk for daytime hypoglycemia. With the increasing use of continuous glucose monitors and insulin pumps, hypoglycemic events can often be avoided. A bedtime snack with protein and good-quality fat, routine early-morning breakfast, and potentially lowering the evening basal insulin dose are strategies to avoid early-morning hypoglycemia. During the first trimester, improving glycemic control with lower pregnancy targets and minimizing hypoglycemic episodes are the management goals to improve overall pregnancy outcomes.

7. How do metabolic changes in pregnancy affect the management of diabetes in the second and third trimesters?
Increases in insulin resistance are similar in women with diabetes and those without diabetes during the second half of the pregnancy, although women with obesity enter pregnancy with increased insulin resistance and their greater insulin resistance persists throughout pregnancy. Because the beta cells are unable to compensate for insulin in type 2 diabetes (T2D) or unable to produce insulin (T1D), pregnant women may require two to four times as much insulin as they did before pregnancy. Fasting and postprandial hyperglycemia are risk factors for LGA infants, macrosomia, neonatal hypoglycemia, hyperbilirubinemia, polycythemia, and long-term fetal programming of childhood and adult metabolic disease. Therefore, tight glucose control in women with preexisting diabetes usually requires both basal insulin and rapid-acting insulin with meals, and premeal and postmeal glycemic monitoring to objectively assess and make insulin dosage adjustments.

8. What is the role of sleep in diabetes and pregnancy outcomes?
Adequate sleep duration and quality are important for normal physiologic functions, metabolic and appetite regulation, and hormone processes. Physiologic and anatomic changes with advancing gestation during pregnancy are associated with altered sleep quality compared with that in nonpregnant women. Disturbances in sleep duration and quality have long been associated with carbohydrate metabolism, cardiovascular function, and appetite control. Sleep-breathing disorder (SBD) encompasses a spectrum that ranges between mild and complete obstruction of airflow, and defines the etiology of the disruption during active respiratory effort (central, obstructive, and mixed events). Women with obesity and higher weight gain are at higher risk for the development and worsening of SBDs, including obstructive sleep apnea (OSA). Rates of OSA in pregnancy have been reported as 15% to 67% and can be associated with oxidative stress, pulmonary hypertension, and, in severe cases, right heart failure. SBDs and shorter sleep duration alter glycemic patterns, likely as a result of increasing insulin resistance, and are associated with significantly increased rates of GDM and preeclampsia. Moreover, SBDs have been correlated with both growth-restricted and LGA infants, suggesting the potential developmental programming influence of altered sleep during pregnancy on the long-term health of future offspring.

9. What are the key preconception counseling recommendations for women with diabetes desiring pregnancy?

Women with poorly controlled glycemia and/or poor maternal health before conception have increased risks for adverse perinatal outcomes, including, but not limited to, miscarriages, congenital anomalies, diabetic ketoacidosis (DKA), hypoglycemic events, macrosomia, stillbirth, preeclampsia, and cesarean deliveries. Women with advanced-stage nephropathy have higher risks for developing severe preeclampsia earlier in pregnancy and the need for dialysis during pregnancy. Because of increases in mitogenic growth factors, relative anemia, the hypercoagulability of pregnancy, and the rapid institution of tight glucose control, proliferative retinopathy can worsen with advancing gestation. Therefore, unplanned pregnancies should be avoided with reliable long-acting reversible contraception (LARC), especially in the presence of glycosylated hemoglobin (HbA$_{1C}$) level $\geq$ 8%, evidence of advanced renal disease, or untreated proliferative retinopathy.

Because most pregnancies among women with diabetes are unplanned, a multidisciplinary team approach, including primary, endocrinology, and obstetrics/gynecology care providers, is recommended to address precon-ception care and management of women of childbearing age who have diabetes. Preconception care has been demonstrated to improve glycemia, perinatal mortality, preterm birth, and congenital malformations. Attempts to achieve a preconception HbA$_{1C}$ of < 6.5% are critical because the majority of organogenesis is complete by postconception week 6 (8 weeks after the last menstrual period). To transition more smoothly to strict pregnancy targets, glycemic goals in the preconception period, using self-monitoring of blood glucose (SMBG) or continuous glucose monitoring (CGM), are premeal glucose values of 80 to 110 mg/dL and 2-hour postprandial levels < 155 mg/dL, while minimizing hypoglycemic events. Insulin is the recommended pharmacotherapy to achieve these targets if the woman is actively pursuing pregnancy in the near future. If metformin alone can achieve the glycemic targets, it can be continued and used safely in the first trimester.

Women should begin folic acid supplementation with 0.8 to 1 mg daily, ideally for 3 months before conception to reduce the risk of fetal neural tube defects, which form by 4 weeks after conception. Maternal screening for abnormal thyroid function, retinopathy, nephropathy, neuropathy, cardiovascular disease (CVD), and hypertension should be performed and these conditions addressed before conception, if indicated. Increased cardiac output and reduced systemic vascular resistance are physiologically demanding. Women with longstanding T1D and T2D with or without other comorbidities are at high risk for underlying coronary artery disease, and functional testing should be considered before pregnancy. Medications should be reviewed, and alternative medications that are safe in pregnancy should be prescribed. The risks of tobacco, alcohol, and marijuana use should be reviewed, with goals implemented for cessation.

Women with diabetes are at high risk for depression, anxiety, sleep disorders, and eating disorders, all of which can affect glycemic control and fetal outcomes. Untreated OSA with undiagnosed pulmonary hypertension can result in maternal or infant hypoxemia and right heart failure. The risk of fetal exposure to untreated major depression is considered a greater concern compared with the risk of fetal exposure to the selective serotonin reuptake inhibitor (SSRI) class of antidepressants. In addition, women with T1D are at risk for B$_{12}$ deficiency, celiac sprue, vitamin D deficiency, and hypothyroidism, which should be screened for, if clinically suspected.

Referral to a dietitian to review current nutritional status, as well as pregnancy challenges and expectations, is advised. Women should be encouraged to incorporate high levels of complex carbohydrates and soluble fiber and to reduce levels of saturated fats. Providers should review the recommendations by the United States Preventive Services Task Force (USPSTF) and the American College of Obstetricians and Gynecologists (ACOG) for physical activity ($\geq$ 150 minutes of cardiovascular exercise per week with no more than 2 days of inactivity and 2 to 3 days per week of resistance activity), and patient goals should be established; this may improve placentation.

10. What is the relationship between depression and diabetes?

One in 10 women in the United States suffer from symptoms of depression, but this likely an underestimation of the true prevalence. Pregnant women are challenged by the dramatic physiologic, anatomic, and emotional changes that occur throughout pregnancy and by the reality of transitioning to a new life after delivery. A diagnosis of GDM complicates the psychosocial disturbances of a "normal" pregnancy. Women with pregestational diabetes or GDM have higher rates of antenatal and postpartum depression. Anxiety and depression in early pregnancy are associated with higher rates of preterm birth among women with pregestational diabetes. As observed in non-pregnant populations, women with depression have higher rates of GDM and other adverse pregnancy outcomes. Treatment of GDM has been demonstrated to lower the rates of postpartum depression and improve health-related quality of life. Nationwide registries have suggested that diabetes combined with obesity in the pregnant woman increases the risk for childhood psychiatric and neurodevelopmental disorders in their offspring. Further studies are needed to determine effective interventions for treating depression and anxiety during pregnancy and whether treatment improves perinatal and later outcomes in the offspring.

11. Why is maintenance of glucose control essential for the well-being of the fetus and for pregnancy outcomes?

Maintenance of normal glucose control is the key to preventing perinatal complications, including congenital anomalies, miscarriage, stillbirth, macrosomia, LGA infants, neonatal metabolic abnormalities, and neonatal intensive care unit admissions, as well as long-term offspring programming of adult diseases, such as CVD and diabetes. Congenital malformations are the leading cause of infant death. Diabetes and hyperglycemia induce abnormalities of yolk sac nutrient transport and morphology and promote vasculopathy. Molecular pathways that have been proposed to contribute to these pathologies are (1) down regulation of hypoxia inducible factor-1 (HIF-1) and vascular endothelial growth factor (VEGF), both of which are important for angiogenesis; and (2) activation of apoptosis signal-regulating kinase-1 (ASK-1), which promotes apoptosis. Hyperglycemia modulates the expression of this apoptosis regulatory gene as early as the preimplantation blastocyst stage in the mouse, resulting in fetal wastage that can be prevented with insulin treatment. This finding may account for the high risk of first-trimester loss in pregnant women with poor glycemic control.

In late gestation, women with T1D have a three- to fivefold increased risk of stillbirths and perinatal deaths compared with the general population, especially if diabetes is poorly controlled or complicated by hypertension, renal disease, or vascular disease. The rates of adverse pregnancy outcomes are similar in women with T2D and those with T1D, likely because of obesity, severe insulin resistance, and comorbidities. Women with GDM may also have higher, but variable, rates of stillbirth, particularly when pregnancy is complicated by obesity and poor glycemic control. Progressively higher HbA_{1c} correlates with higher rates of LGA infants, preeclampsia, fetal growth restriction, neonatal hypoglycemia, preterm birth, and stillbirth.

12. Describe the relationship among HbA_{1c}, the teratogenic effects of hyperglycemia, and abnormal fetal growth.
    The prevalence of congenital anomalies in the general population is 2% to 3%. By using HbA_{1c} as a surrogate marker for periconception glycemic control, studies have demonstrated a linear relationship between the risk of hyperglycemia-induced anomalies and HbA_{1c}. The most common fetal anomalies include neural tube, skeletal, and cardiac defects. Formation of the neural tube is complete by 4 weeks and that of the heart by 6 weeks after conception, underscoring the critical importance of preconception glycemic control by the primary care provider or endocrinologist, optimizing nutrition, and establishing healthy lifestyle behaviors. Rarer conditions associated with hyperglycemia include caudal regression syndrome, which is characterized by severe lower spine, genitourinary, and limb defects.

    Overall, the risk of an adverse outcome is reduced by 50% with each percentage point reduction in HbA_{1c} level achieved before pregnancy. It has been demonstrated that women with a normal HbA_{1c} ($< 6\%$–6.5%) at conception and during the first trimester have risks similar to baseline population risks and that the risks progressively rise with increasing HbA_{1c}. It is generally recommended for women to aim for a preconception HbA_{1c} goal of $< 6.5\%$ if it can be achieved safely.

    The utility of HbA_{1c} measurement as a surrogate for glycemic control is limited because it is an average measurement and does not reflect glycemic patterns or fluctuations; therefore, it should not be used for advising therapeutic changes. Furthermore, because of the increased plasma volume and increased red blood cell turnover during pregnancy, HbA_{1c} is reduced by pregnancy itself (0.5%–0.8%). HbA_{1c} assessment is most useful as a tool for counseling women on their perinatal risks associated with glycemia, especially in early pregnancy.

13. How has the incidence of congenital abnormalities and macrosomia in the offspring of mothers with diabetes changed over the past decade?
    Rates of macrosomia have risen around the world over the last 2 to 3 decades, paralleling the rising prevalence of obesity and diabetes. Macrosomia is associated with adverse perinatal outcomes, such as birth trauma, cesarean delivery, postpartum hemorrhage, and long-term health consequences for the offspring. These complications have long-term implications and challenge the health care system, particularly in the resource-poor areas of the world.

    The incidence of congenital abnormalities in the offspring of mothers with T1D in the early era of insulin use was 33%. Since the mid-1990s, this has improved to $< 10\%$ with better glycemic monitoring tools, pregnancy targets, and insulin delivery systems. The randomized prospective Diabetes Control and Complications Trial (DCCT) has shown that timely institution of intensive therapy before conception is associated with rates of spontaneous abortion and congenital malformations similar to those occurring in mothers without diabetes.

14. What are the maternal/fetal risks of severe hypoglycemia?
    The fetus has minimal capability for hepatic gluconeogenesis until close to delivery. In sheep, sustained hypoglycemia reduces basal and glucose-induced fetal pancreatic insulin secretion and recovery from this inhibition is slow. Whether severe and prolonged hypoglycemia or wide fluctuations between severe hyperglycemia and hypoglycemia could have long-term adverse neurologic effects in the offspring is unknown. Hypoglycemic episodes should be prevented to reduce hypoglycemia unawareness and the risk of hypoglycemic seizures. These events can be prevented during pregnancy by establishing prolonged glycemic stability before conception. The best predictors of severe hypoglycemia during pregnancy are hypoglycemia unawareness and the occurrence of at least one episode of severe hypoglycemia the year before pregnancy. The first trimester is especially challenging because of the higher frequency of hypoglycemia when women are relatively more insulin sensitive. The risk of hypoglycemia is highest overnight and during fasting because the fetal–placental unit continues to extract glucose at these times.

15. Discuss the role of oral hypoglycemic agents and their limitations during periconception and pregnancy.
    There are nine pharmacologic subclasses of oral antidiabetes agents: sulfonylureas, biguanides, alpha-glucosidase inhibitors, dipeptidyl peptidase-4 (DPP-4) inhibitors, meglitinides, sodium-glucose cotransporter-2 (SGLT-2) inhibitors,

bile acid resins, dopamine agonists, and thiazolidinediones; in addition, there are injectable glucagon-like peptide-1 (GLP-1) agonists. In spite of limited data, if any, on the use of many of these agents in pregnancy, none of the drug subclasses has been reported to cause any structural abnormalities in the fetus. The use of all oral antidiabetes agents for the treatment of GDM is currently off-label. The most commonly used oral agents during pregnancy are glyburide (sulfonylurea) and metformin (biguanide) in GDM; however, up to half of the women with GDM taking glyburide or metformin will eventually need insulin therapy.

Insulin is the first-line agent for the treatment of diabetes in pregnancy. Although insulin is the only FDA-approved therapy for the treatment of diabetes in pregnancy, several professional groups and guidelines acknowledge the off-label use of glyburide and metformin for treatment of GDM, but *not* for pregestational diabetes during pregnancy. If a woman is taking a sulfonylurea or metformin during early pregnancy, it should be continued until she can be effectively transitioned to insulin because the risk of teratogenicity from hyperglycemia is higher than any risk posed by these agents.

16. How should women on angiotensin-converting enzyme (ACE) inhibitors or angiotensin II receptor (ATIIR) blockers be counseled before conception and after delivery?
The goal of antihypertensive treatment is to maintain blood pressure at a level that minimizes maternal cardiovascular and cerebrovascular risks. ACE inhibitors and ATIIR blockers taken in the second and third trimesters of pregnancy are both associated with increased rates of fetal growth restriction, oligohydramnios, patent ductus arteriosus, neonatal hypotension refractory to treatment, and neonatal renal failure. Exposure to these agents in the first trimester has been reported to be associated with increased cardiac and central nervous system malformations, but the findings of those studies were confounded by concurrent use of other medications and the influence of comorbidities, such as diabetes, CVD, and obesity. A recent study of women with chronic hypertension, including over 4100 pregnant women exposed to ACE inhibitors during the first trimester of pregnancy, found no significant increase in major congenital anomalies. Health care providers should discuss alternative agents to manage hypertension before pregnancy (calcium channel blockers, beta-blockers, labetalol, or hydralazine) with women who are considering pregnancy. Women who have significant renal disease and are taking ACE inhibitors may consider continuing them until pregnancy is confirmed for the renoprotective effects and then discontinuing them immediately thereafter.

During the postpartum period, women who are candidates for an ACE inhibitor can be started on either enalapril or captopril; both these agents have not been shown to appear in breast milk in appreciable concentrations. Other antihypertensives with no known adverse effects on infants receiving breast milk include labetalol, nifedipine, verapamil, and hydralazine. Diuretics should generally be avoided because of their possible suppressive effects on breast milk production.

17. How does pregnancy affect morbidity and mortality resulting from coronary artery disease in women with diabetes?
The United States has the highest incidence of myocardial infarction during pregnancy, and rates have risen over the past several decades, reflecting the contributions of advanced maternal age, obesity, hypertension, and diabetes. The cardiovascular system undergoes significant physiologic changes during pregnancy: increased plasma volume, oxygen consumption, cardiac output, and left ventricular size; decreased systemic vascular resistance; and volume, blood pressure, and catecholamine response variability during labor, delivery, and the immediate postpartum period. These changes are especially challenging in a woman with preexisting CVD, potentially leading to an inadequate oxygen supply to the myocardium. The morbidity and mortality rates of coronary artery disease are high in pregnant women with diabetes. Cardiac status should be assessed with functional testing before conception in women with diabetes who have any additional cardiac risk factors, such as hyperlipidemia, hypertension, smoking, cardiac autonomic neuropathy, and strong family history and in women with any suggestive symptoms. Resting electrocardiography (ECG) should be considered for asymptomatic women age $\geq$ 35 years. Women with longstanding diabetes and/or nephropathy are at the highest risk for coronary artery disease and would benefit from cardiac functional testing with ECG to assess baseline risks.

18. How should women with diabetes be screened and treated for thyroid disease before pregnancy?
Women with T1D have an increased risk of developing postpartum thyroiditis (3–4 times higher than in women without diabetes) and hypothyroidism from Hashimoto's thyroiditis. Therefore, screening with measurement of serum thyroid-stimulating hormone (TSH) levels is recommended. Because women with hypothyroidism have an increased risk for developing diabetes, some would support that women with T2D might also be considered for thyroid screening. Women with high serum thyroid peroxidase (TPO) antibodies should have TSH surveillance because they are at risk for developing subclinical hypothyroidism during pregnancy, and about half these women will develop postpartum thyroiditis. In one study, treating very mild subclinical hypothyroidism in pregnant women did not improve cognitive outcomes in the offspring at age 5 years, but women in this study were not randomized and they did not reach their recommended treatment goals until the second trimester. It is recommended that women with a serum TSH level > 4.0 mU/L, especially if they also have positive TPO antibodies, be treated with levothyroxine.

19. Should statins or fibrates be discontinued before conception?

Statins and fibrates have not been demonstrated to have increased teratogenicity despite the previous FDA "X" warning on statins. However, because of insufficient data regarding their safety during pregnancy, it is recommended that both drug classes be discontinued during pregnancy unless the woman has severe hypertriglyceridemia. Fibrates may be indicated for the treatment of hypertriglyceridemia to prevent pancreatitis among pregnant women whose condition is refractory to nutritional modifications and high-dose fish oil therapy. Because triglycerides increase two- to threefold during pregnancy, women are at increased risk for pancreatitis if they have fasting triglyceride levels > 400 mg/dL in early pregnancy.

Lipophilic statins, such as atorvastatin and lovastatin, have had mixed reports regarding risks for fetal malformations, but hydrophilic statins, such as pravastatin, are minimally detectable in the embryo. Pravastatin has shown promise in animal models for improving abnormal vascular profiles and preventing growth restriction. In human primary endothelial cells, purified cytotrophoblast cells, and placental explants obtained from women with preterm preeclampsia, pravastatin reduced soluble fms-like tyrosine kinase 1 (sFlt-1) secretion and improved markers of endothelial dysfunction. Clinical trials are still needed to determine the efficacy and safety of pravastatin for preeclampsia prevention, but there is no indication for statin use to reduce low-density lipoprotein cholesterol (LDL-C) during pregnancy.

20. Summarize the effect of smoking during pregnancy.

Smoking, smokeless tobacco use, and second-hand smoke continue to be the leading environmental causes of low-birth-weight infants in patients with diabetes and those without diabetes. Additionally, smoking increases the risk for fetal growth restriction, placental abruption, abnormal placentation, altered maternal thyroid function, preterm births, and perinatal mortality. Children face continued consequences of maternal gestational smoking with higher rates of asthma, infantile colic, childhood obesity, and sudden infant death syndrome. Smoking cessation counseling and goal setting are advised before conception and at every prenatal visit. There is insufficient evidence to assess the balance of benefits and harms of nicotine-replacement products (i.e., patch) or the use of alternative forms of nicotine, such as e-cigarettes and vaping, in pregnant women, but nicotine-replacement products are likely to result in less exposure of the fetus to toxins compared with cigarettes.

21. How does pregnancy affect diabetic nephropathy?

Diabetic nephropathy is a progressive disease and is the leading cause of end-stage renal disease in the United States. The glomerular filtration rate (GFR) normally increases by nearly 50% during pregnancy, and proteinuria commonly increases in pregnancy. Pregnancy is not associated with a greater decline in kidney function or impaired long-term maternal survival among women with a normal baseline serum creatinine level. Women with more severe renal insufficiency (serum creatinine > 1.5 mg/dL or estimated GFR < 30 cc/min) have a 30% to 50% risk of a permanent pregnancy-related decline in GFR and may require dialysis during pregnancy. Poor maternal and fetal outcomes are more likely among pregnancies complicated by elevated serum creatinine, severe hypertension, nephrotic range proteinuria, and preexisting CVD.

22. Does diabetic nephropathy increase the risk of preeclampsia?

Preeclampsia complicates approximately 20% of pregnancies in women with preexisting diabetes, and the risk is much higher in women with hypertension or renal disease. The risk of preeclampsia developing in women with diabetic nephropathy is $> 60\%$, and the risk is highest among women with hypertension, nephrotic range pro-teinuria, and abnormal renal function, especially those with a serum creatinine > 1.4 mg/dL. Women with signifi-cant nephropathy are also at higher risk of having preterm and low-birth-weight infants. Women with diabetic nephropathy should be counseled to have children when their diabetes is optimally controlled and preferably early in the course of their nephropathy. Continuing renoprotective antihypertensive medications, such as ACE inhibitors and ATIIR blockers, until the woman with renal disease is ready for pregnancy should be considered. However, switching to antihypertensive agents with better safety profiles in pregnancy is recommended in those without significant renal disease. It is recommended that women with diabetes and proteinuria begin taking low-dose aspirin in the first trimester and consider more intensive antihypertensive therapy to target blood pressures $< 140/90$ mm Hg to decrease or minimize the risk of hypertensive renal disease. Women with advanced renal disease, on dialysis, or with a renal transplantation can still conceive, and thus, it is critical that they are counseled and use effective long-acting reversible contraception.

23. How does renal transplantation affect pregnancy outcomes?

Women who have had a successful renal transplantation at least 1 to 2 years before pregnancy and who have good renal function, have adequate blood pressure control, and are being treated with immunosuppressive medications with appropriate safety profiles in pregnancy have more favorable outcomes compared with women with severe renal disease who have not received a transplant. Women with severe renal insufficiency who require dialysis during pregnancy have the highest risk of adverse pregnancy outcomes, including severe growth restriction, prematurity, preeclampsia, and stillbirth. With the continual developments in immunosuppressive regimens, health care providers are responsible for providing pregnancy counseling to all patients before and after transplantation. In renal transplant recipients, the rates of preeclampsia, cesarean delivery, urinary tract infections, preterm birth, and lower birth weights are higher. A multidisciplinary approach can improve outcomes and overall care.

24. Summarize the effects of pregnancy on diabetic retinopathy.

Because of its hypercoagulable state, relative anemia, and increase in growth factors, pregnancy may cause progression of diabetic retinopathy regardless of glycemic control. Therefore, it is recommended that women with retinopathy, particularly those with proliferative retinopathy, receive treatment before conception. Women with T1D rarely have retinopathy within 5 years after diagnosis, but women with T2D have higher rates of retinopathy at the time of diagnosis. Therefore, all pregnant women with preexisting diabetes should have an ophthalmologic examination in the first trimester; the frequency of follow-up visits depends on severity of disease and the risk of vision loss. Nonproliferative retinopathy generally remains stable during pregnancy but should be monitored carefully throughout gestation because of the potential for progression.

25. What is the White classification of diabetes in pregnancy?

In 1949, at the Joslin Clinic, Priscilla White developed a classification scheme for fetal and maternal pregnancy risk based on the prepregnancy state of women with T1D. She observed that patient age at diabetes onset, duration of diabetes, and severity of complications (vascular disease, nephropathy, retinopathy) significantly influenced maternal and perinatal outcomes. Since the new diabetes terminology was adopted in the late 1990s to define T1D and T2D by cause rather than by treatment, the White classification has been less commonly used by obstetricians to classify the duration and complications of women with diabetes, although it is still used by some institutions. Classes A1 and A2 were later added to classify women with GDM that is controlled with diet alone or with medications and continue to be used in practice (Table 8.1).

26. What are the glycemic goals in pregnancy?

The goals of glucose control during pregnancy are to reduce adverse perinatal outcomes. The optimal glycemic levels in pregnancy to prevent adverse outcomes are not known with certainty. The current American Diabetes Association (ADA) and ACOG recommendations for glycemic targets are as follows: fasting glucose < 95 mg/dL; 1-hour postprandial glucose < 140 mg/dL; and 2-hour postprandial glucose < 120 mg/dL. The results from the multicenter HAPO (Hyperglycemia and Adverse Pregnancy Outcomes) trial, which studied 25,000 pregnant women in nine countries, suggested that abnormal fetal growth occurs along a continuum and at lower glucose values than previously recognized. However, more intensive goals have not been tested in an adequately powered randomized controlled trial (RCT) to determine whether they can achieve a reduction in macrosomia without increasing the risk of SGA or other adverse perinatal outcomes, especially in women with T1DM who may have hypoglycemia unawareness. Pregnant women with T1DM and severe hypoglycemia unawareness should consider CGM to improve their diabetes management. More liberal goals for fasting (e.g., 80–110 mg/dL) and 2-hour postprandial (e.g., 120-150 mg/dL) glucose levels may be considered because of the risk of severe protracted hypoglycemia, which is a significant hazard to the mother and the fetus. Because macrosomia is related to both fasting glucose and postprandial glucose excursions, it is recommended that pregnant women with diabetes monitor premeal and postprandial glucose values regularly.

27. What is the role of CGM in pregnancy?

CGM is a useful tool, especially among women with T1D or T2D who are having difficulty with glycemic control, have frequent hypoglycemic episodes or hypoglycemia unawareness, or have unclear compliance patterns that may hinder better delineation of glucose patterns and directed insulin adjustments. CGM provides glucose data

Table 8.1. Modified White Classification of Pregnant Women With Diabetes.

CLASS	AGE AT ONSET (YEARS)	DURATION (YEARS)	VASCULAR DISEASE	MEDICATION
Gestational Diabetes				
A1	Any	Pregnancy	None	None
A2	Any	Pregnancy	None	Yes
Pregestational Diabetes				
B	Age > 20	< 10	None	Yes
C	Age 10–19	10–19	None	Yes
D	Age < 10	> 20	Benign retinopathy	Yes
F	Any	Any	Nephropathy	Yes
R	Any	Any	Proliferative retinopathy	Yes
T	Any	Any	Renal transplant	Yes
H	Any	Any	Coronary artery disease	Yes

that can be used to manage insulin therapy in real time. The CONCEPTT (Continuous Glucose Monitoring in Pregnant Women with Type 1 Diabetes) trial demonstrated more time in glycemic target range, less hyperglycemic episodes, lower rates of LGA infants, and lower neonatal intensive care unit (NICU) admissions among women with T1D using continuous glucose monitors during the pregnancy.

28. Discuss the role of the insulin pump in pregnancy.
    Pregnancy involves frequent physiologic changes in insulin resistance, glucose uptake, and responses to exercise, as well as the stresses of labor and delivery. Insulin pumps are advantageous in this setting and allow for more subtle, time-specific insulin dose changes. Experience in the use of insulin pumps in the treatment of T1D during pregnancy continues to increase. Insulin pump therapy may be especially helpful for women with T1D who have insulin sensitivity and variable insulin requirements throughout the night. Most trials have found that insulin pump therapy is equivalent to multiple daily injections (MDIs) using basal-bolus insulin; a few studies have reported improved HbA$_{1c}$ without an increase in hypoglycemic episodes. However, DKA can occur more rapidly with pump failure because only rapid-acting insulin is used in pumps. Because pump failures place pregnant women at significant risk for DKA, hyperglycemia and hypoglycemia, and consequent adverse pregnancy outcomes, insulin pump therapy is not ideal for all patients. Pump therapy is more likely to be successful if it is initiated before pregnancy, the women have reliable glycemic control with use of MDIs with basal-bolus insulin, they can accurately count carbohydrates, and effectively use carbohydrate-to-insulin ratios.

    Sensor-integrated insulin delivery systems (hybrid closed-loop pumps) have not yet been widely studied in pregnancy. However, a recent RCT demonstrated that hybrid closed-loop therapy in pregnant women with T1D, including a subset of women who continued to use the system through labor and delivery, achieved a higher percentage of glucose time in range compared with patients using a pump with a nonintegrated continuous glucose monitor. Hybrid closed-loop systems that currently use algorithms that target a glucose level of 120 mg/dL may not be ideal in pregnancy because nocturnal glucose targets during pregnancy are 80 to 100 mg/dL.

29. Discuss the role of glargine and detemir in pregnancy.
    Detemir (Levemir) is approved by the FDA for use in pregnancy and may result in less nocturnal hypoglycemia compared with neutral protamine Hagedorn (NPH) insulin, although the peaks of both detemir and NPH can be variable during pregnancy. For women with severe hepatic insulin resistance, NPH or detemir before bedtime may be needed to achieve sufficient fasting glucose control. Experience with insulin glargine (Lantus) in pregnancy is fairly extensive. Glargine does not cross the placenta. Similar pregnancy outcomes have been reported in women taking glargine and those taking NPH. Either glargine or detemir may be useful in women experiencing recurrent hypoglycemia on NPH or women who have unpredictable eating patterns and meal timing.

30. What is the role of rapid-acting insulin analogues in pregnancy?
    Lispro (Humalog) and aspart (Novolog) have been used in pregnancy and shown to be safe and effective. Immediate perinatal outcomes are similar between regular insulin and lispro; however, compared with regular insulin, lispro has been reported to improve overall glycemic control during pregnancy, with lower total insulin requirements. These rapid-acting analogues better reduce postprandial hyperglycemia and the risk of hypoglycemia compared with regular insulin. Considering the pharmacokinetic challenges with regular insulin, meal timing is critical to ensure that regular insulin is administered at least 30 minutes before the first bite of food. Using rapid-acting insulin before each meal according to carbohydrate intake can help achieve optimal postprandial control, especially in women with T1D or in women with T2D who have marked variation in the timing and the amount of their carbohydrate intake.

31. How common is hypoglycemia in women with T1D during pregnancy and in the postpartum period?
    Pregnant women with T1D have higher risks for hypoglycemia during the first and early second trimester because of the relative insulin sensitivity during this time and the diminished counterregulatory hormonal responses to hypoglycemia that occur in pregnancy. Maternal hypoglycemia has declined recently with the more available use of continuous glucose monitors. In women with T1D not using continuous glucose monitors, occasional monitoring in the middle of the night is recommended because of the increased risk of nocturnal hypoglycemia, especially if the woman has hypoglycemia unawareness. The hormone-driven insulin resistance of the second and third trimesters declines rapidly after delivery of the placenta, and therefore, women need to decrease their insulin doses to one third to one half of their pregnancy insulin requirements after delivery, particularly if they are breastfeeding. Insulin doses then typically increase over several weeks closer to pre-pregnancy doses unless breastfeeding is continued.

32. Discuss fetal measures of well-being and surveillance required in pregnant women with diabetes.
    The pregnancy risks for women with T2D are similar to women with T1D, but patients with T2D often have coexisting obesity and other comorbidities. In addition to poor glycemic control, factors that increase the risk for poor outcomes include obesity, hypertension, undiagnosed sleep breathing disorders, and occult cardiopulmonary disease. Failure to achieve optimal glycemic control in early pregnancy in women with any type

of preexisting diabetes may have teratogenic effects or lead to early fetal loss. Poor control later in pregnancy increases the risk of intrauterine fetal demise, LGA infants, and long-term metabolic and cardiovascular complications in the newborn.

The rates of stillbirth among women with T1D or T2D is five-fold higher than women without diabetes and ~ 50% of cases are unexplained. Fetal hypoxia and cardiac dysfunction associated with cardiac enlargement and asymmetric septal hypertrophy result from poor glycemic control and are probably the most important pathogenic factors. Fetal hyperglycemia and hyperinsulinemia result in excess fetal growth, increased fetal oxygen consumption, and relative tissue hypoxia. It is recommended that all women with pregnancies complicated by diabetes undergo early ultrasonography examination to confirm the viability and dating of the pregnancy and a formal anatomy scan at 18 to 20 weeks to evaluate for fetal anomalies. Fetal echocardiogram should be performed at 20 to 24 weeks' gestation for a more detailed fetal cardiac evaluation if the HbA_{1c} level was significantly elevated or cardiac anatomy was suboptimally viewed on a formal anatomy scan. Daily fetal movement monitoring should start at ≈ 28 weeks' gestation, and fetal surveillance should begin at ≈ 32 weeks' gestation. The optimal frequency or mode of antenatal monitoring is unknown. Fetal ultrasonography for evaluating growth should be considered at 28 to 32 weeks' gestation and before delivery to aid in delivery planning. Delivery timing should be individualized for each patient, considering glycemic control, maternal comorbidities, and fetal well-being. Generally, women with well-controlled GDM class A1 deliver between 39 to 41 weeks, those with GDM class A2 deliver at 39 to 40 weeks, and those with poorly controlled diabetes (whether preexisting or GDM) deliver between 37 to 38 weeks.

33. What is the risk of DKA in pregnancy?

DKA may occur with lower blood glucose levels (often referred to as "euglycemic DKA") because of the decreased buffering capacity in pregnancy (i.e., respiratory alkalosis with compensatory metabolic acidosis), increased glomerular glucose filtration, continuous glucose utilization by the fetal–placental unit, and increased plasma volume. In addition, an early switch from carbohydrate metabolism to lipolysis occurs in pregnant women who have depleted their glycogen stores after a 12-hour fast, resulting in relative starvation ketosis.

Any pregnant woman with T1D who is unable to keep down food or fluids or who has persistent severe hyperglycemia should check urine ketones at home. If ketones cannot be cleared quickly from urine, a chemistry panel should be ordered to rule out an increased anion gap, regardless of the woman's glycemic status. Often, the only precipitating factor for DKA in pregnancy is nausea and vomiting, but other causes, such as urinary tract infections, should be aggressively investigated. Women with T2D and even women with GDM can also develop DKA, especially in the context of prolonged fasting, infections, use of beta-agonists for preterm labor, or steroids to promote fetal lung maturity. All pregnant women with diabetes during pregnancy should be counseled on the signs and symptoms of DKA.

34. How does maternal DKA affect the fetus?

Although rates of fetal demise after DKA have declined (15%), the rates remain significantly higher than baseline (2%–3%) among women with T1D. Women with DKA are more likely to have preterm birth, fetal demise, and NICU admissions. Risk factors for fetal loss include maternal intensive care unit (ICU) admission, later gestation, delayed treatment, and higher serum osmolality in the presence of DKA. Identifying and treating any maternal inciting conditions, abnormal glycemia, acid/base abnormalities, and volume deficits are necessary to improve fetal status.

35. What must the physician remember about DKA in pregnancy?

Pregnant women unable to take oral nutrients require an additional 100 to 150 g/day of intravenous glucose to meet the metabolic demands of the fetal–placental unit. Without adequate carbohydrate (often a D10W glucose solution is necessary), fat will be burned for fuel, and the patient with DKA will remain ketotic.

KEY POINTS: DIABETES IN PREGNANCY

- Although hyperglycemia is a major teratogen, the risk for congenital anomalies can be decreased to the baseline population risk with optimal glycemic control before conception and during the first 10 weeks of gestation.
- Diabetic ketoacidosis may occur at glucose levels < 200 mg/dL in pregnant women with T1D or T2D and may also occur in women with GDM.
- Inadequately controlled diabetes may place the fetus at risk for developing childhood obesity, metabolic syndrome, nonalcoholic fatty liver, and glucose intolerance.
- Women who develop gestational diabetes have a 30% to 74% risk of developing T2D within 5 to 10 years.
- Pregnancy does not usually accelerate the progression of diabetic nephropathy unless kidney disease is severe; however, proteinuria, diabetic retinopathy, and autonomic neuropathy may worsen.
- Insulin requirements often decrease in the first trimester, placing the mother at high risk of severe hypoglycemia, especially at night, but insulin requirements may double or triple in the late second and third trimesters as a result of the insulin resistance of pregnancy.

Continued

36. What is GDM, and how is it diagnosed?

The ACOG defines GDM as a "condition in which carbohydrate intolerance develops during pregnancy." GDM is associated with increased adverse perinatal outcomes, maternal progression to T2D and CVD, and long-term risks for cardiometabolic disease in the offspring. It is recommended that all pregnant women undergo glucose testing between 24 to 28 weeks to screen for GDM.

TWO-STEP APPROACH

Before 2010, the two-step approach to testing for GDM was universally advocated in the United States. According to the glucose test thresholds set by the institution, GDM is diagnosed after a failed 50 g oral glucose challenge test (OGCT) and if *two* of four values are abnormal on the 3-hour oral glucose tolerance test (OGTT). The 50-g, 1-hour OGCT is the accepted *screening* method by the ACOG and the National Institutes of Health (NIH) for the presence of GDM. A positive result on screening is in the range of $\geq$ 130 to 140 mg/dL. The sensitivity and specificity of the test depend on what threshold value is chosen by an institution, commonly selected according to the prevalence of GDM in the population being screened. The test does not have to be performed during a fasting state, and a serum sample must be drawn exactly 1 hour after administering the oral glucose.

The 100-g, 3-hour OGTT thresholds to diagnose GDM are predictive of the risk of diabetes developing after pregnancy. The most commonly used 3-hour OGTT thresholds are the Carpenter and Coustan criteria (Table 8.2). The test should be performed after 3 days of an unrestricted carbohydrate diet and while the patient is fasting for at least 8 hours. Using the Carpenter and Coustan glucose criteria, at least two abnormal values are needed for the diagnosis of GDM. Recently, the ACOG acknowledged that increased adverse outcomes similar to those in pregnancies complicated by GDM may occur in women with only one abnormal value on the 3-hour OGTT, but further studies are necessary to determine whether this population would benefit from treatment. If the 100-g, 3-hr OGTT test is performed and only one value is abnormal, a repeat 100-g, 3-hour test should be performed 1 month later because a single elevated glucose value increases the risk of LGA infants, and one third of these patients will ultimately meet the diagnostic criteria for GDM (see Table 8.2). Unfortunately, this two-step approach can delay diagnostic testing and treatment.

ONE-STEP APPROACH

The HAPO trial demonstrated a strong, continuous association between maternal glucose levels and adverse pregnancy outcomes (i.e., LGA infants, elevated cord C-peptide indicative of fetal hyperinsulinemia, primary cesarean deliveries, and neonatal hypoglycemia) from glucose values that were below those diagnostic of GDM. On the basis of these perinatal findings, the IADPSG recognized an increased risk of LGA infants by using a *single* abnormal threshold glucose value and developed diagnostic glucose thresholds that were lower than the existing recommended diagnostic cut-off values (see Table 8.2) and that predicted a 1.75-fold increased risk for LGA infants by using a 75-g, 2-hour OGTT. If a twofold increased risk had been used, higher glucose thresholds would have been defined. The test similarly is performed after 3 days of an unrestricted carbohydrate diet and while the patient is fasting for at least 8 hours. One abnormal value is needed for the diagnosis of GDM.

An NIH Consensus Development Conference on diagnosing GDM in 2013 reviewed the existing literature and concluded that adopting the IADPSG (one-step approach) would "increase the prevalence of GDM, and the corresponding costs and interventions, without clear demonstration of improvements in the most clinically important health and patient-centered outcomes." Additionally, obesity alone is a strong risk factor for LGA, and the effectiveness of only targeting and treating mild hyperglycemia in the context of obesity is not yet clear. Unfortunately, lack of a consensus for the diagnosis of GDM in the United States between the ACOG/NIH and the IADPSG (adopted by the Endocrine Society and the WHO), with the ADA considering either option, has resulted in dividing practitioners, forcing them to choose one set of criteria over the other and resulting in complete lack of standardization. There are no RCTs comparing the

Table 8.2. Criteria for a Positive 100-g Oral Glucose Tolerance Test[a] (Carpenter and Coustan).

Fasting glucose	$\geq$ 95 mg/dL
1-hour glucose	$\geq$ 180 mg/dL
2-hour glucose	$\geq$ 155 mg/dL
3-hour glucose	$\geq$ 140 mg/dL

Criteria for a Positive 75-g Oral Glucose Tolerance Test[b] (IADPSG)

Fasting glucose	$\geq$ 92 mg/dL
1-hour glucose	$\geq$ 180 mg/dL
2-hour glucose	$\geq$ 153 mg/dL

Overt Diabetes[c]

Fasting glucose	$\geq$ 125 mg/dL
HbA_{1c}	$\geq$ 6.5%
2-hour (75-g)	$\geq$ 200 mg/dL
Random glucose	$\geq$ 200 mg/dL

HbA_{1c}, Glycosylated hemoglobin; *IADPSG,* International Association of the Diabetes and Pregnancy Study Groups.
[a]Two abnormal values needed.
[b]One abnormal value needed.
[c]Any of above.

diagnostic criteria or demonstrating that implementation and treatment based on the IADPSG criteria will result in lower rates of LGA infants or other adverse pregnancy outcomes compared with the two-step, ACOG/NIH–endorsed approach.

37. Discuss the controversy regarding early screening for diabetes and its limitations in pregnancy.
    The ACOG, the ADA, the Endocrine Society, and the United States Preventive Services Task Force (USPTF) support universal GDM testing at 24 to 28 weeks' gestation. With the increasing prevalence of obesity in women, delayed childbearing, the high number of pregnant women who present without pregestational diabetes testing, and the observed degree of hyperglycemia at diagnosis or its manifestation early in pregnancy (before 24 weeks), there is concern that women are entering pregnancy with undiagnosed preexisting (overt) diabetes. Regardless of age, women with T2D or an early diagnosis of diabetes in pregnancy (who often have prediabetes) have a much higher risk of maternal and fetal complications, including major malformations, particularly if their HbA_{1c} is $\geq$ 6.5%. Therefore the ADA, the ACOG, and the IADPSG recommend early testing during the initiation of prenatal care among women at high risk for diabetes (Table 8.3). Because the optimal test to diagnose GDM early in gestation has not been well studied, nor has the efficacy of early treatment been demonstrated, there is lack of consensus over the best way to screen for "early GDM." The ACOG recommends early diabetes screening with use of the *nonpregnant* 75-g, 2-hour OGTT method (HbA_{1c}, fasting, and 2-hour glucose levels) to identify women with potentially undiagnosed T2D or the two-step screening process for GDM (see Table 8.2).
    The ADA recommends that the diagnosis of overt diabetes be considered among women diagnosed for the first time in pregnancy with any of the following criteria: HbA_{1c} $\geq$ 6.5%, fasting blood glucose (FBG) $\geq$ 126 mg/dL, 2-hour glucose $\geq$ 200 mg/dL after a 75-g oral glucose load, or symptoms of hyperglycemia with a random glucose $\geq$ 200 mg/dL; these are the same criteria for diagnosing diabetes outside of pregnancy (see Table 8.2). GDM is diagnosed if glucose intolerance was identified during pregnancy *and* the women did not meet the criteria for overt diabetes. Unfortunately, according to the one-step and two-step diagnostic approaches, there are no specific criteria to diagnose early GDM because both diagnostic criteria were developed for women at 24 to 28 weeks' pregnancy. Because there is evidence that women who already demonstrate glucose intolerance early in pregnancy may have similar outcomes as women with preexisting diabetes, there are studies underway attempting to develop outcome-based criteria for the diagnosis of "early" GDM.
    The recommendations given by the IADPSG to diagnose overt diabetes in early pregnancy have resulted in opponents emphasizing that some high-risk women with only impaired glucose tolerance (by OGTT) will be missed if the new criteria are used because a practitioner can choose whether or not to obtain HbA_{1c}, FBG, or 75-g, 2-hour OGTT early in pregnancy. Profound differences for the sensitivity of FBG versus a 1- or 2-hour, 75-g glucose value in diagnosing GDM have been demonstrated among different ethnic populations. In the Asian

Table 8.3. ADA and ACOG Risk Factors.

1. Early testing should be considered in overweight or obese (BMI $\geq$ 25 kg/m^2 or $\geq$ 23 kg/m^2 in Asian Americans) adults who have one or more of the following risk factors:
   - First-degree relative with diabetes
   - High-risk race/ethnicity (e.g., African American, Hispanic American, Native American, Asian American, Pacific Islander)
   - History of cardiovascular disease
   - Hypertension ($\geq$ 140/90 mm Hg or on therapy for hypertension)
   - HDL cholesterol level $\leq$ 35 mg/dL (0.90 mmol/L) and/or a triglyceride level $\geq$ 250 mg/dL (2.82 mmol/L)
   - Women with polycystic ovary syndrome
   - Physical inactivity
   - Other clinical conditions associated with insulin resistance (e.g., severe obesity, acanthosis nigricans)
2. Patients with prediabetes (HbA$_{1c}$ $\geq$ 5.7%, impaired glucose tolerance, or impaired fasting glucose) should be tested yearly.
3. Women who were diagnosed with GDM should have lifelong testing at least every 3 years.

ACOG, American College of Obstetrics and Gynecology; *ADA,* American Diabetes Association; *BMI,* body mass index; *GDM,* gestational diabetes mellitus; *HbA$_{1c}$,* glycosylated hemoglobin; *HDL,* high-density lipoprotein.

population, for example, women will commonly have impaired glucose tolerance (IGT) after a glucose load but have FBG within the normal range. Hispanic women, in contrast, primarily fail their glucose test by having an elevated FBG caused by hepatic insulin resistance and increased gluconeogenesis.

HbA$_{1c}$ evaluation is the least sensitive test to diagnose either prediabetes or diabetes, especially during pregnancy with the increase in plasma volume, erythrocyte turnover, and altered degrees of glycosylation. A HbA$_{1c}$ level $\geq$ 5.7% has been advocated to diagnose glucose intolerance early in pregnancy. However, it does not have the sensitivity or the specificity to be used to diagnose GDM, and therefore, women having or exceeding this value should be advised to follow this up with an OGTT. The FBG is less sensitive than the post–glucose load value on a 75-g, 2-hour OGTT for diagnosing prediabetes or diabetes. Furthermore, there are some data indicating that fasting glucose values are higher in the first trimester before they decline throughout gestation, suggesting that a glucose of 92 mg/dL may not be the optimal fasting value to diagnose GDM early in pregnancy. Currently, there is no consensus regarding a preferred early testing strategy to diagnose GDM, although the ACOG endorses use of the same diagnostic criteria in early pregnancy as well as in late pregnancy. Clearly, the identification and treatment of early GDM based on adverse pregnancy outcomes is a major priority, given that the fetus can begin secreting insulin by 12–14 weeks. Increasing data suggest that early metabolic changes are important in the developing fetus with short-term and long-term risks. If diagnosis and treatment are not initiated early in gestation, testing should be done at 24 to 28 weeks' gestation by using either the 100-g, 3-hour OGTT (ACOG) or the 75-g, 2-hour OGTT (IADPSG).

38. **What causes GDM?**
GDM is caused by abnormalities in at least three aspects of fuel metabolism: (1) insulin resistance in fat and muscle, (2) increased hepatic glucose production, and (3) impaired insulin secretion. Although insulin levels may be high, the increased insulin resistance of pregnancy still results in inadequate compensation because impaired beta cell function leads to insufficient insulin secretion to maintain euglycemia in the presence of insulin resistance. The insulin resistance is thought to result from increased production of human placental lactogen, placental growth hormone, tumor necrosis factor-alpha (TNF-α), and inflammatory cytokines. Women who develop GDM have lower pregravid insulin sensitivity compared with matched control groups, and some abnormalities may persist after delivery. The majority of women with GDM are overweight, and many have characteristics of metabolic syndrome before pregnancy. Thin or normal-weight women who develop GDM are in the minority, but more "normal weight" phenotypes are being recognized during pregnancy, and they likely represent a higher risk group for future cardio-metabolic disease, or they are misdiagnosed and have autoimmune diabetes or monogenic types of diabetes.

A small percentage of women diagnosed with GDM have maturity-onset diabetes of the young (MODY), most commonly MODY-2. Thus, a strong family history is important information, especially if diabetes occurred in family members who were not overweight. Genetic testing for MODY can be offered because the fetus has a 50% risk of inheritance. More commonly, women who are underweight or normal weight may have latent autoimmune diabetes of adulthood (LADA), in which the increased insulin requirements of pregnancy result in hyperglycemia in the presence of ongoing autoimmune beta cell destruction. They may be diagnosed for the first time in pregnancy or in the postpartum period. These women should be tested for glutamic acid decarboxylase (GAD) and antiislet antibodies.

39. **Summarize the role of impaired insulin secretion in GDM.**
Although women with GDM have hyperinsulinemia, most have an impaired insulin response compared with BMI-matched women without GDM. Impaired insulin secretion renders the woman unable to meet the requirement for

greater insulin production necessitated by the rising insulin resistance and increased hepatic glucose production as gestation advances. Pregnancy is a 9-month "stress test" and illustrates the potential for the later development of T2DM, because the marked insulin resistance of pregnancy necessitates a two- to three-fold increase in insulin secretion. If the beta cells are unable to secrete the necessary insulin, a clinically evident abnormality in glucose metabolism results. Beta cell defects persist postpartum and the severity of the defect is predictive of the risk of later developing T2DM.

40. **Summarize the risks to the mother with GDM**
    The immediate risks to the mother with GDM are an increased incidence of cesarean delivery ($\approx$ 30%), preeclampsia ($\approx$ 10%–30%), and polyhydramnios ($\approx$ 10%–20%), which can result in preterm labor. The long-term risks to the mother are related to recurrent GDM in future pregnancies (30%–50% recurrence) and the substantial risk of developing T2D and CVD.
    Women with GDM have an extremely high risk (33%–74%) of developing T2D in the subsequent 5 to 10 years. Risk factors include fasting hyperglycemia, pharmacotherapy requirement for managing glycemia, GDM diagnosed before 24 weeks of gestation (preexisting glucose intolerance), obesity, ethnicity associated with a high prevalence of T2D, multiple subsequent pregnancies, postpartum weight retention, and IGT or impaired fasting glucose (prediabetes) at postpartum week 6. The offspring of women with diabetes are at higher risk for obesity, T2D, and metabolic syndrome.

41. **What are the complications in an infant born to a mother with GDM?**
    Infants born to mothers with GDM are at increased risk for macrosomia, LGA, small-for-gestational age (SGA), shoulder dystocia, neonatal hypoglycemia, consequences of prematurity, hyperbilirubinemia, polycythemia, cardiac septal hypertrophy, and long-term programming effects, including T2D, CVD, and obesity. Even with the advent of screening and aggressive GDM management, the incidence of individual neonatal complications ranges from 12% to 28%. The influence of maternal obesity on these adverse outcomes among women with GDM and the true incidence of long-term metabolic consequences of these infants remain unknown.

42. **Summarize the mechanism behind abnormal fetal growth in GDM and preexisting diabetes.**
    The uptake and relationship of fetal nutrients is not well characterized. Increased maternal availability of substrates, such as glucose, amino acids, FFA, and triglycerides allows for greater placental transport to the fetus, resulting in fetal overgrowth and fat accretion. The glucose concentration difference between the maternal and fetal compartments drives the flux of glucose to the fetus. Glucose strongly influences the maintenance of beta cell mass. Hyperglycemia results in fetal pancreatic islet hypertrophy and beta cell hyperplasia with consequent fetal production of high levels of insulin, which is a potent growth hormone. Fetal hyperinsulinemia increases glucose uptake and clearance in fetal tissues, causing an exaggerated glucose gradient from mother to fetus and potentially lowering maternal postprandial glucose, resulting in what can appear to be optimal glycemic control in the mother (fetal–placental steal syndrome).

43. **Describe the role of lipids in GDM.**
    Among women with GDM and obesity, some studies support that maternal lipids (triacylglycerols and nonesterified fatty acids) are more highly correlated with birth weight compared with glucose and obesity; maternal triglycerides also appear to contribute significantly to infant adiposity. The placenta expresses lipoprotein lipase (LPL), which hydrolyzes maternal triglycerides to FFA, which can be transported across the placenta. Upregulation of many genes involved with lipid transport and storage, inflammation, and oxidative processes characterize GDM placentas and may affect nutrient transport and fetal fat accretion.
    The placenta plays a key role in the regulation of nutrient transport in GDM, contributing to macrosomia or LGA infants (Fig. 8.1). Glucose and amino acids are critical for the development of the fetus, but the transfer of lipids to the fetal compartment is important for cellular and brain development, fat accretion, and overall fetal growth. The placental transport mechanism for lipids is complex and remains poorly understood. GDM is associated with dysregulated maternal lipid metabolism, decreased placental fatty acid oxidation, increased inflammatory cytokines, and differentially methylated genes being involved in energy and lipid metabolism, all of which can influence fetal fat accretion and growth. Increased fat availability to the fetus leads to adiposity and visceromegaly (especially heart, liver, and pancreas), which can increase fetal abdominal girth disproportionate to other body measurements (body-to-head disproportion) and lead to increased shoulder dystocia, birth trauma, and cesarean deliveries. These early metabolic changes in the offspring place it at risk for future metabolic disease and obesity.

44. **What other fetal complications may result from GDM or preexisting diabetes?**
    - Fetal malformations are more common among women with preexisting diabetes compared with women without diabetes. Multiple organ systems are susceptible to a hyperglycemic environment. Malformations reported to be associated with diabetes include, but are not limited to, cardiac, skeletal, genitourinary, renal, and gastrointestinal malformations. Anomalies associated with diabetes occur before week 8 of gestation. Although there is no single syndrome specific to diabetes, caudal regression syndrome is a condition strongly associated with diabetes and characterized by agenesis or hypoplasia of the femur and lower vertebrae.

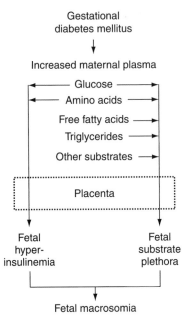

**Gestational
diabetes mellitus**

↓

Increased maternal plasma

Glucose

Amino acids

Free fatty acids

Triglycerides

Other substrates

Placenta

Fetal
hyper-
insulinemia

Fetal
substrate
plethora

↓

Fetal macrosomia

Fig. 8.1 The mechanism by which gestational diabetes mellitus leads to fetal macrosomia.

- With poor glucose control, there is also an increased risk of spontaneous abortions and intrauterine fetal demise because of fetal acidemia and hypoxia.
- Cardiac septal hypertrophy is demonstrated in 35% to 40% of pregnancies with diabetes.
- Shoulder dystocia with subsequent brachial plexus injury (Erb's or Klumpke's palsy, Horner's syndrome), facial nerve palsy, cephalohematoma, and clavicular fractures; fetal distress; low Apgar scores; and birth asphyxia, when unrecognized.
- Respiratory distress syndrome may occur in up to 30% of infants because of decreased lung surfactant synthesis with poor glycemic control.
- Common metabolic abnormalities in the infant of a mother with diabetes include neonatal hypoglycemia from sustained hyperinsulinemia, hypocalcemia, polycythemia, and hyperbilirubinemia.
- Excess FFA and triglycerides delivered to the fetus may also contribute to excess fetal growth and continues to be a subject of increased research to discern whether these substrates may need to be targeted for lowering.

45. Describe the fetal-based management strategy and fetal surveillance in GDM

    Amniotic fetal insulin levels, a marker of fetal hyperinsulinemia, correlates strongly with the fetal abdominal circumference at 28 to 32 weeks' gestation. A number of RCTs have demonstrated that using fetal overgrowth as a guide to metabolic intervention among women with mild GDM is beneficial. Insulin treatment, compared with diet-only interventions, has been shown to decrease both mild maternal hyperglycemia and FFAs and to reduce the rates of LGA infants.

    The optimal method or frequency of fetal surveillance to prevent adverse outcomes among women with GDM has not been established. Current recommendations are for women who require pharmacotherapy or have suboptimal glycemic control to have a fetal nonstress test (NST), a modified biophysical profile (amniotic fluid index plus fetal NST), or a biophysical profile (ultrasonographic evaluation of fetal well-being) once or twice a week beginning at 32 to 34 weeks' gestation. Delivery timing should be individualized, considering other maternal comorbidities, glycemic control, pharmacotherapy, and fetal well-being. Shoulder dystocia is more likely to occur at any given birth weight to infants born to women with diabetes compared with those born to women without diabetes. Because macrosomia and LGA size are the most common fetal complications among women with GDM and pregestational diabetes, it is recommended that a scheduled cesarean delivery be offered for an estimated fetal weight of ≥ 4500 g.

46. Discuss the long-term sequelae of GDM or preexisting diabetes in the offspring of affected mothers.

    The offspring of women with diabetes are at higher risk for obesity, T2D, and metabolic syndrome. The incidence of childhood T2D was approximately 10-fold higher in the offspring of Pima Indian mothers with diabetes compared with the offspring of mothers who did not develop diabetes until after pregnancy. Proliferation of fetal adipocytes and pancreatic beta cells may be responsible for "fetal programming" the later development of obesity and metabolic syndrome, in addition to changes in appetite regulation, mitochondrial capacity, and adipogenic potential of stem cells. Interestingly, newborns of obese mothers with GDM already have 68% more intrahepatic fat, as demonstrated by magnetic resonance imaging/magnetic resonance spectroscopy (MRI/MRS) compared with newborns of normal-weight mothers; this might serve as the "first hit," increasing their risk for developing nonalcoholic fatty liver disease. Growing evidence supports an association between a metabolically abnormal in utero environment and epigenetic modifications in newborns. Further studies are needed to determine the contributions of epigenetic disturbances to metabolic function and long-term developmental programming consequences.

47. **What is the role of exercise in patients with GDM or preexisting diabetes?**
Both the ACOG and the ADA advise that pregnant women adopt the national guidelines with regard to engaging in cardiovascular exercise 20 minutes daily and resistance activity 2 to 3 days per week, provided there is no obstetric contraindication. Moderate exercise is well tolerated and safe in pregnancy. Exercise introduced early in pregnancy decreases gestational weight gain and the risk of developing GDM, without increasing the rates of SGA. However, exercise initiated in the second half of pregnancy has not been shown to decrease the rates of GDM. In women with GDM, exercise improves fasting glucose levels and postprandial glucose excursions, decreases excessive weight gain, and reduces adverse perinatal outcomes, such as cesarean delivery and macrosomia. Some women may be able to avoid insulin therapy by walking for 20 minutes after each meal. Women should be encouraged to engage in physical activity before pregnancy and to continue through the postpartum period because exercise has long-lasting benefits for the GDM mother, who is at risk of developing T2D in the future.

48. **When is an exercise program contraindicated?**
Women who do not have absolute contraindications for exercise should be encouraged to continue or begin both cardiovascular and resistance activity during pregnancy. Absolute contraindications include hemodynamically significant heart disease, restrictive lung disease, incompetent cervix, persistent second or third trimester bleeding, active premature labor, severe preeclampsia, and severe anemia. Women with medical or obstetric comorbidities should speak with their providers to individualize exercise recommendations.

49. **What is the best diet therapy for women with GDM, and how much weight should they gain?**
After GDM is diagnosed, women should have formal dietary guidance and support, set exercise goals with their provider, and receive education on capillary SMBG to have objective information to determine whether glycemic goals are being met throughout the pregnancy. All pregnant women should have a foundation of healthy nutrient-dense food choices and physical exercise, which includes cardiovascular and resistance activity. Both fasting and postprandial glucose levels have been associated with the risk of LGA infants. Most women diagnosed with GDM can maintain their target postprandial blood glucose levels through nutritional and lifestyle modifications (reduced carbohydrate meals and walking after meals), but fasting glucose targets are more difficult to achieve in those who have fasting hyperglycemia. Distributing consumption of complex carbohydrates throughout the day, adding good-quality protein and fat sources, and minimizing prolonged periods of fasting can improve glycemic control. Saturated fats should also be limited because of their effect to increase insulin resistance and their independent contribution to excess triglycerides and FFAs for fetal fat accretion.

Excessive weight gain in pregnancy is associated with increased adverse perinatal outcomes, such as LGA infants. Some data support that in overweight or obese women with GDM, not gaining any weight is safe, and it may, in fact, reduce the need for medical therapy. Weight loss during pregnancy is not advocated. Although the optimal weight gain parameters for women with diabetes in pregnancy to promote the most favorable pregnancy outcomes are unknown and should, therefore, be individualized, the Institute of Medicine (IOM) recommends weight gain goals for each BMI category in pregnancy: BMI < 18.5 kg/m^2, 28 to 40 lb; BMI 18.5 to 24.9 kg/m^2, 25 to 35 lb; BMI 25 to 29.9 kg/m^2, 15 to 25 lb; BMI ≥ 30 kg/m^2, 11 to 20 lb.

50. **When should medical therapy be used to treat GDM?**
Women who receive nutritional education, counseling regarding the benefits of exercise, undertake other lifestyle behavioral modifications and continue to have fasting blood glucose levels > 95 mg/dL, 1-hour postprandial glucose levels > 140 mg/dL, or 2-hour postprandial glucose levels > 120 mg/dL should be started on medical therapy. Women with GDM and ultrasonographic findings consistent with LGA size are also candidates for medical management. Insulin is the preferred pharmacologic agent. GDM is often managed with twice-daily injections of NPH insulin and rapid-acting insulin analogues (lispro or aspart) at meal times or regular insulin with breakfast and dinner. Detemir and glargine can also be used as basal insulins instead of NPH. In women who are adversed to administration of insulin injections more than once per day, the combination of basal insulin (NPH, detemir, glargine) at night for fasting hyperglycemia and glyburide 1 hour before breakfast and dinner for postprandial hyperglycemia may be effective, but this requires further validation through prospective studies. Serious hypoglycemia is uncommon among women with GDM who receive insulin teaching because of their underlying insulin resistance and symptomatic hypoglycemia awareness.

Although insulin is the preferred agent for GDM, there are some convenience benefits, but long-term safety data with oral agents are limited. Caution should be exercised because glyburide and metformin cross the placenta and the resultant potential risks of fetal exposure for intrauterine programming and long-term health consequences. Mothers who are unable to safely self-administer insulin or have a strong preference for oral agents may be candidates for metformin or glyburide, with individualized counseling and care.

Glyburide: Glyburide crosses the placenta less compared with all other sulfonylureas but still may affect fetal insulin levels. It may also increase placental glucose transporter 1 (GLUT-1) expression in a dose-dependent fashion, increasing the potential for greater glucose transport to the fetus, in addition to its potential influence on the fetal pancreas. If given at all during pregnancy, its use should be restricted to women with GDM. In two multicenter trials comparing insulin and glyburide in the treatment of GDM, neonatal outcomes were not different between the groups, but there were higher frequencies of maternal hypoglycemia with glyburide. Meta-analyses have also demonstrated increased rates of macrosomia and neonatal hypoglycemia with sulfonylurea use compared with insulin use in GDM. However, suboptimal dosing of glyburide and poor study designs may explain the less favorable outcomes in prior studies. Glyburide should be dosed at least 30 to 60 minutes before meal times because insulin secretion stimulated by glyburide does not peak until 3 to 4 hours after a dose; its pharmacokinetic properties suggest that it should not be used before bedtime to control fasting hyperglycemia. Approximately 20% to 35% of women with GDM will fail glyburide therapy and require insulin treatment to achieve adequate glycemic control. Risk factors associated with glyburide treatment failure include diagnosis of GDM at < 24 weeks' gestation, fasting hyperglycemia, recurrent pregnancies, inappropriate administration, and more severe hyperglycemia.

Metformin: It is recommended that metformin use in GDM be limited to prospective trials, but many practitioners currently use it because of its lower risk of hypoglycemia, ease of use, and the challenges of treating a rapidly growing GDM population. The MiG (Metformin in Gestation) RCT of 751 women with GDM randomized to metformin or insulin at ≈ 24 to 28 weeks demonstrated no immediate adverse neonatal outcomes and reported decreased maternal weight gain and preeclampsia in the insulin group and increased rates of maternal hypertriglyceridemia and preterm birth in the metformin group. In the metformin group, 46% of women with GDM required supplemental insulin to meet glycemic pregnancy targets. A recent Cochrane analysis showed that metformin does not appear to improve pregnancy outcomes or prevent GDM.

Metformin has several intracellular effects that can inhibit growth, suppress mitochondrial respiration, have epigenetic modifications on gene expression, mimic fetal nutrient restriction, and alter postnatal gluconeogenic responses. These findings raise concerns about its potential effects on the developmental programming of metabolic disease in the offspring of women with GDM. Childhood follow-up studies from trials using metformin among women with GDM or polycystic ovary syndrome (PCOS) demonstrated increased child weights and fat mass among the offspring of some mothers who were randomized to metformin therapy. Follow-up from the MiG trial did not show differences in glucose, lipids, insulin resistance, or liver function test measures in either subgroup of the offspring exposed to metformin compared with insulin. These findings are consistent with animal studies, in which normally grown fetuses exposed to metformin exhibit postnatal overgrowth, particularly after consuming high-fat Western-style diets, underscoring the importance of high-quality nutrition postnatally for long-term health prevention. Although the Society of Maternal-Fetal Medicine supports metformin as an alternative to insulin in GDM, these recommendations do not address long-term outcomes in the offspring but were released before the MiG and PCOS trials released their longer-term childhood data.

51. What are the important postpartum management issues for women with pregestational or gestational diabetes? New life adjustments, sleep deprivation, fatigue, erratic meal timing, metabolic changes and improved insulin sensitivity, and breastfeeding all challenge women in the postpartum period. Issues that require attention to optimize maternal health include maintaining appropriate glycemic control, sustaining high-quality nutrition practices, exercising, weight loss, breastfeeding, blood pressure and renal protection management, and contraception. The majority of women with pregestational diabetes have dramatic decreases in their insulin requirements in the immediate postpartum period. Women who are breastfeeding likely require lower insulin doses than their prepregnancy doses. Glycemic goals are not as strict as those for the pregnancy period. Women with T1D should be checked for TPO antibodies and have TSH measured to check for postpartum thyroiditis. If antibodies are positive, there is a 50% risk of postpartum thyroiditis.

Women with diabetes should be encouraged to breastfeed unless other contraindicating conditions are present. Because women with GDM and pregestational diabetes are at risk for delayed onset of lactogenesis and breast-milk production, referral to a lactation specialist is valuable in this population. Women with T1D who breastfeed have overall lower insulin requirements compared with those who do not, necessitating a variable reduction in insulin of at least 10% less than prepregnancy requirements. Because of fluctuating glucose levels and the high risk for maternal hypoglycemia during breastfeeding, glucose goals should be relaxed after delivery. Both metformin and glyburide appear to be compatible with breastfeeding, but women requiring high doses of glyburide should notify their pediatrician. Breastfeeding duration and intensity is associated with less atherogenic maternal lipid profiles and lower incidences of T2D and metabolic syndrome among women with a history of GDM.

Inability to lose pregnancy weight is one of the strongest risk factors for progression to T2D. The postpartum period offers a unique opportunity to continue healthy habits learned during the pregnancy; these can improve the long-term health of the woman, the child, and the entire family unit. However, women with preexisting diabetes are often lost to follow-up, their glycemic control deteriorates, and they do not address or obtain effective contraception, placing them at risk for adverse outcomes in subsequent pregnancies. Women with GDM have an increased risk for T2D in the future. They also often go without appropriate follow-up, running the risk of becoming pregnant with undiagnosed T2D and major malformations in their offspring. The importance of diagnosing impaired glucose intolerance or prediabetes lies in its value to determine the degree of abnormal glucose homeostasis and predict the progression to T2D. Up to 70% of individuals with prediabetes of will progress to T2D at a rate of approximately 5% to 10% per year. Because decreased beta cell function is already present in the prediabetes stage, weight loss and goals involving healthy lifestyle, healthy eating behaviors, and exercise should be instituted in this high-risk group of women. Metformin can be considered if lifestyle changes fail or if the women have difficulty sustaining these behavior modifications.

52. What interventions may reduce the risk of developing T2D?

Counseling with regard to sustaining the diet modifications encouraged during pregnancy, continuing regular exercise, and losing pregnancy weight are essential to improve insulin sensitivity, long-term health, and prevent progression to T2D and other weight-related diseases. Moreover, compared with women who gain weight within the recommended parameters, those who gain more weight during pregnancy than that recommended by the IOM have higher postpartum weight retention, placing them at higher risks in subsequent pregnancies. Among Hispanic women with a history of GDM, postpartum weight gain was most strongly associated with declining beta cell compensation. Women with GDM who have interpregnancy weight gain have a higher recurrence of GDM in subsequent pregnancies compared with women who lose weight between pregnancies. Breastfeeding decreases the risk for mothers with GDM from developing T2D within the following 2 years by 53% and by 40% over 19 years. Lactation duration is independently associated with a lower incidence of diabetes, but any amount or duration has been found to be beneficial.

Adhering to high-quality dietary patterns, such as the Mediterranean and DASH diets, reduces the risk of the progression to T2D among women with GDM. A subgroup analysis of the Diabetes Prevention Program (DPP) trial examined women with prediabetes with a history of GDM and showed that they had a much higher risk of developing T2D (11.4% per year) compared with women with prediabetes but without a history of GDM (6.9% per year) over a 10-year follow-up period. This risk was reduced with diet, exercise of 150 minutes per week, and a 7% weight-loss goal (35% risk reduction) or metformin (40% risk reduction).

Women should be advised to return to their prepregnancy weight by 6 to 12 months after delivery through healthy eating behaviors and exercise. Overweight and obese women should continue to work toward additional weight loss to improve their overall health. If diet and exercise are unsuccessful or do not normalize glucose tolerance, metformin should be considered, especially in women with both impaired fasting glucose (IFG) and IGT. Women with GDM should have cardiovascular and diabetic screening every 1 to 3 years after delivery in addition to discussing health goals with their primary care physician.

Because parents highly influence their children's eating habits, sustaining healthy nutrition and lifestyle modifications learned during the pregnancy is important to improve the overall health of the family unit. Children whose mothers emphasize health goals consume more healthy food and less unhealthy food.

53. Discuss the importance of glucose monitoring and subsequent testing during the postpartum period.

Women with pregestational diabetes should continue vigilant home glucose monitoring in the postpartum period because insulin requirements drop almost immediately and often dramatically at this time, increasing the risk of hypoglycemia. Although glycemic targets are relaxed after delivery, glucose monitoring remains important to keep glycemia within range to promote appropriate wound healing from cesarean section incisions and perineal or vulvar lacerations.

Women with GDM are generally followed up in the immediate postpartum period with fasting glucose assessments to determine their metabolic status. If testing falls within normal glycemic ranges, they are not required to continue glucose monitoring during the postpartum period. Because approximately 1 in 20 women with GDM will meet the criteria for diabetes on postpartum testing, it is recommended that all women with a history of GDM be reassessed at postpartum weeks 6 to 12 with a 75-g, 2-hour OGTT. The following criteria are used for diagnosis: diabetes FBG $\geq$ 126 mg/dL and/or 2-hour glucose $\geq$ 200 mg/dL; IFG–FBG 100 to 125 mg/dL; and IGT 2-hour glucose 140 to 199 mg/dL. If only FBG is measured, women with persistent IGT will be missed. HbA_{1c} measurement is not sensitive in diagnosing prediabetes at postpartum week 6 because it is often confounded by iron-deficiency anemia, postpartum blood loss, postpartum fluid shifts, and reflects glycemia over a 3-month period, which would include the last 6 weeks of pregnancy.

The ADA and the ACOG recommend retesting every 1 to 3 years by using FBG, HbA_{1c}, or 75-g, 2-hour OGTT; cardiovascular screening should also be performed with similar frequency. The 75-g, 2-hour OGTT remains the most sensitive method for detecting any glucose intolerance. Women who fulfill the criteria for prediabetes on their 75-g OGTT may have up to a 70% to 80% chance of developing T2D in 5 to 10 years and are, thus, considered an extremely high-risk group. At a minimum, HbA_{1c} levels should be checked every 1 to 3 years; however, $HbA_{1c} \geq$ 5.7% has poor sensitivity compared with FBG or 75-g, 2-hour OGTT at 6 weeks to 1 year. To improve the pregnancy outcomes in subsequent pregnancies and the long-term health for women who have completed childbearing, routine diabetes and cardiovascular testing should be performed, in addition to setting health goals.

54. Discuss using the postpartum period as a window of opportunity for preconception counseling and ensuring adequate contraception.

The postpartum period is the preconception period for subsequent pregnancies. Reliable LARC is strongly encouraged in all women with pregestational diabetes or GDM because at least 50% of pregnancies are unplanned. Contraception provides the opportunity to improve a woman's health between pregnancies, prevent short-interval pregnancies, ensure that appropriate prenatal supplements are consumed, and reduce the risk for adverse perinatal outcomes in future pregnancies. It is well established that women with diabetes can have better perinatal outcomes with preconception care and well-controlled glycemia. Women should aim for an HbA_{1c} level $< 6.5\%$ before conception to reduce the risk of congenital anomalies, miscarriage, and developmental fetal programming. It is recommended that women with diabetes regularly see their primary care provider and/or endocrine care provider to individualize reliable contraception, strongly consider LARC options, optimize glycemic and cardiovascular profiles, assess for and manage any microvascular and macrovascular diseases, review medications, and improve preconception weight, nutrition, and lifestyle behaviors.

55. Which contraceptive agents can be used by women with diabetes or a history of GDM?

All contraceptive methods have good safety profiles and overall efficacy among women with diabetes. Barrier and oral contraceptive methods are available, but inconsistent use can lead to decreased efficacy. Hormonal contraception does not appear to cause microvascular disease or alter carbohydrate metabolism according to currently available data, but a woman with multiple cardiovascular risk factors should avoid combined oral contraceptive (COC) agents. Women with poorly controlled hypertension or hypertriglyceridemia and those who are at risk for thromboembolic disease in addition to their diabetes are not good candidates for estrogen-containing oral contraceptives. Triglycerides should be measured after the initiation of oral contraceptives in women with diabetes or known hyperlipidemia, given the higher incidence of hypertriglyceridemia and the associated risk of pancreatitis with oral estrogen use.

LARC methods, such as the intrauterine device (IUD) and implant devices, are reliable, low-risk, and preferred methods for contraception among women with diabetes. There is no increase in pelvic inflammatory disease with the use of an IUD in women with well-controlled T1D or T2D in the postinsertion period. Therefore, an IUD (containing either copper or progestin) is a very attractive option in women who do not desire pregnancies in the near future. The etonogestrel implant (Nexplanon) does not worsen carbohydrate intolerance and is also a good choice for women for up to 3 years.

Progesterone agents, such as Depo-Provera (medroxyprogesterone acetate) and norethindrone, are less favorable alternatives because Depo-Provera may affect carbohydrate tolerance and norethindrone alone ("Minipill") is less efficacious. Depo-Provera has been associated with an increased risk of T2D in nursing mothers with a history of GDM, primarily because of excess weight gain associated with its use. Bilateral tubal ligation is a permanent form of birth control that requires surgical intervention. It can be performed safely among women with diabetes and offers the best perioperative results if the woman has good glycemic control. The significant benefits and potential side effects of hormonal contraceptives need to be individualized, taking into consideration the high maternal and fetal risks of an unplanned or unwanted pregnancy, especially in mothers with diabetes.

56. How common is postpartum thyroiditis in women with T1D, and when does it appear?

Women with T1D have a three- to fourfold higher risk ($\approx 20\%$) of developing postpartum thyroiditis compared with the general population, particularly if they are TPO antibody positive. The classic presentation for postpartum thyroiditis is a hyperthyroid phase that occurs 2 to 4 months after delivery, followed by a hypothyroid phase in the subsequent 4- to 8-month period, and then a return to the euthyroid state by the end of the first year in 75% to 80% of patients. It can also present with isolated hypothyroidism or isolated thyrotoxicosis. Given the significance of this disorder, measurement of TSH is recommended in patients with T1D with positive TPO antibodies at 3 months and at 6 months after delivery or with any suggestive symptoms.

BIBLIOGRAPHY

ACOG Committee Opinion No. 650: Physical activity and exercise during pregnancy and the postpartum period. (2015). *Obstetrics and Gynecology, 126*(6), e135–e142.

Alexander, E. K., Pearce, E. N., Brent, G. A., Brown, R. S., Chen, H., Dosiou, C., . . . Sullivan, S. (2017). 2017 Guidelines of the American Thyroid Association for the diagnosis and management of thyroid disease during pregnancy and the postpartum. *Thyroid, 27*(3), 315–389.

American College of Obstetricians and Gynecologists. (2015). Practice Bulletin No. 148: thyroid disease in pregnancy. *Obstetrics and Gynecology, 125*(4), 996–1005.

American College of Obstetricians and Gynecologists' Committee on Practice Bulletins—Obstetrics. (2016). Practice Bulletin No. 173: Fetal macrosomia. *Obstetrics and Gynecology, 128*(5), e195–e209.

American Diabetes Association. (2018). Classification and diagnosis of diabetes: standards of medical care in diabetes—2018. *Diabetes Care, 41*(Suppl. 1), S13–S27.

Aroda, V. R., Christophi, C. A., Edelstein, S. L., Zhang, P., Herman, W. H., Barrett-Connor, E., . . . Ratner, R. E. (2015). The effect of lifestyle intervention and metformin on preventing or delaying diabetes among women with and without gestational diabetes: the Diabetes Prevention Program outcomes study 10-year follow-up. *Journal of Clinical Endocrinology and Metabolism, 100*(4), 1646–1653.

Balsells, M., Garcia-Patterson, A., Sola, I., Roque, M., Gich, I., & Corcoy, R. (2015). Glibenclamide, metformin, and insulin for the treatment of gestational diabetes: a systematic review and meta-analysis. *BMJ, 350*, h102.

Barbour, L. A., & Hernandez, T. L. (2018). Maternal non-glycemic contributors to fetal growth in obesity and gestational diabetes: spotlight on lipids. *Current Diabetes Reports, 18*(6), 37.

Barbour, L. A., Farabi, S. S., Friedman, J. E., Hirsch, N. M., Reece, M. S., Van Pelt, R. E., & Hernandez, T. L. (2018). Postprandial triglycerides predict newborn fat more strongly than glucose in women with obesity in early pregnancy. *Obesity (Silver Spring), 26*(8), 1347–1356.

Barbour, L. A., Scifres, C., Valent, A. M., Friedman, J. E., Buchanan, T. A., Coustan, D., ... Loeken, M. R. (2018). A cautionary response to SMFM statement: pharmacological treatment of gestational diabetes. *American Journal of Obstetrics and Gynecology, 219*(4), 367.e1–367.e7.

Barrett, H. L., Dekker Nitert, M., McIntyre, H. D., & Callaway, L. K. (2014). Normalizing metabolism in diabetic pregnancy: is it time to target lipids? *Diabetes Care, 37*(5), 1484–1493.

Bateman, B. T., Patorno, E., Desai, R. J., Seely, E. W., Mogun, H., Dejene, S. Z., ... Huybrechts, K. F. (2017). Angiotensin-converting enzyme inhibitors and the risk of congenital malformations. *Obstetrics and Gynecology, 129*(1), 174–184.

Bourjeily, G., Danilack, V. A., Bublitz, M. H., Lipkind, H., Muri, J., Caldwell, D., ... Rosene-Montella, K. (2017). Obstructive sleep apnea in pregnancy is associated with adverse maternal outcomes: a national cohort. *Sleep Medicine, 38*, 50–57.

Buschur, E., Stetson, B., & Barbour, L. A. (2018). Diabetes in pregnancy. In K. R. Feingold, B. Anawalt, & A. Boyce (Eds.), *Endotext* [Internet]. South Dartmouth, MA: MDText.com.

Casey, B. M., Thom, E. A., Peaceman, A. M., Varner, M. W., Sorokin, Y., Hirtz, D. G., ... Rouse, D. J. (2017). Treatment of subclinical hypothyroidism or hypothyroxinemia in pregnancy. *New England Journal of Medicine, 376*(9), 815–825.

Catalano, P. M., & Shankar, K. (2017). Obesity and pregnancy: mechanisms of short term and long term adverse consequences for mother and child. *BMJ, 356*, j1.

Catalano, P. M., Tyzbir, E .D., Wolfe, R. R., Roman, N. M., Amini, S. B., & Sims, E. A. (1992). Longitudinal changes in basal hepatic glucose production and suppression during insulin infusion in normal pregnant women. *American Journal of Obstetrics and Gynecology, 167*(4 Pt 1), 913–919.

Caughey, A. B., & Valent, A. M. (2016). When to deliver women with diabetes in pregnancy? *American Journal of Perinatology, 33*(13), 1250–1254.

Committee on Practice Bulletins—Obstetrics. (2018). ACOG Practice Bulletin No. 190: Gestational diabetes mellitus. *Obstetrics and Gynecology, 131*(2), e49–e64.

Crowther, C. A., Hiller, J. E., Moss, J. R., McPhee, A. J., Jeffries, W. S., & Robinson, J. S. (2005). Effect of treatment of gestational diabetes mellitus on pregnancy outcomes. *New England Journal of Medicine, 352*(24), 2477–2486.

Crume, T. L., Ogden, L., Daniels, S., Hamman, R. F., Norris, J. M., & Dabelea, D. (2011). The impact of in utero exposure to diabetes on childhood body mass index growth trajectories: the EPOCH study. *Journal of Pediatrics, 158*(6), 941–946.

Deshpande, N. A., James, N. T., Kucirka, L. M., Boyarsky, B. J., Garonzik-Wang, J. M., Montgomery, R. A., & Segev, D. L. (2011). Pregnancy outcomes in kidney transplant recipients: a systematic review and meta-analysis. *American Journal of Transplantation, 11*(11), 2388–2404.

Desoye, G., & Nolan, C. J. (2016). The fetal glucose steal: an underappreciated phenomenon in diabetic pregnancy. *Diabetologia, 59*(6), 1089–1094.

Dodd, J. M., Grivell, R. M., Deussen, A. R., & Hague, W. M. (2018). Metformin for women who are overweight or obese during pregnancy for improving maternal and infant outcomes. *Cochrane Database of Systematic Reviews, 7*, CD010564.

Dong, D., Reece, E. A., Lin, X., Wu, Y., Arias Villela, N., & Yang, P. (2016). New development of the yolk sac theory in diabetic embryopathy: molecular mechanism and link to structural birth defects. *American Journal of Obstetrics and Gynecology, 214*(2), 192–202.

Dudley, D. J. (2007). Diabetic-associated stillbirth: incidence, pathophysiology, and prevention. *Obstetrics and Gynecology Clinics of North America, 34*(2), 293–307, ix.

Dutton, H., Borengasser, S. J., Gaudet, L. M., Barbour, L. A., & Keely, E. J. (2018). Obesity in pregnancy: optimizing outcomes for mom and baby. *Medical Clinics of North America, 102*(1), 87–106.

Eyal, S., Easterling, T. R., Carr, D., Umans, J. G., Miodovnik, M., Hankins, G. D., ... Hebert, M. F. (2010). Pharmacokinetics of metformin during pregnancy. *Drug Metabolism and Disposition, 38*(5), 833–840.

Feig, D. S., Donovan, L. E., Corcoy, R., Murphy, K. E., Amiel, S. A., Hunt, K. F., ... Murphy, H. R. (2017). Continuous glucose monitoring in pregnant women with type 1 diabetes (CONCEPTT): a multicentre international randomised controlled trial. *Lancet, 390*(10110), 2347–2359.

Friedman, J. E. (2015). Obesity and gestational diabetes mellitus pathways for programming in mouse, monkey, and man—where do we go next? The 2014 Norbert Freinkel Award Lecture. *Diabetes Care, 38*, 1402–1411.

Gunderson, E. P. (2014). Impact of breastfeeding on maternal metabolism: Implications for women with gestational diabetes. *Current Diabetes Reports, 14*(2), 460.

Gunderson, E. P., Hurston, S. R., Ning, X., Lo, J. C., Crites, Y., Walton, D., ... Quesenberry, C. P., Jr. (2015). Lactation and progression to type 2 diabetes mellitus after gestational diabetes mellitus: a prospective cohort study. *Annals of Internal Medicine, 163*(12), 889–898.

Gunderson, E. P., Lewis, C. E., Lin, Y., Sorel, M., Gross, M., Sidney, S., ... Quesenberry, C. P., Jr. (2018). Lactation duration and progression to diabetes in women across the childbearing years: the 30-year CARDIA study. *JAMA Internal Medicine, 178*(3), 328–337.

Hanem, L. G. E., Stridsklev, S., Júlíusson, P. B., Salvesen, Ø., Roelants, M., Carlsen, S. M., ... Vanky, E. (2018). Metformin use in PCOS pregnancies increases the risk of offspring overweight at 4 years of age: follow-up of two RCTs. *Journal of Clinical Endocrinology and Metabolism, 103*(4), 1612–1621.

HAPO Study Cooperative Research Group, Metzger, B. E., Lowe, L. P., Dyer, A. R., Trimble, E. R., Chaovarindr, U., ... Sacks, D. A. (2008). Hyperglycemia and adverse pregnancy outcomes. *New England Journal of Medicine, 358*(19), 1991–2002.

Harmon, K. A., Gerard, L., Jensen, D. R., Kealey, E. H., Hernandez, T. L., Reece, M. S., ... Bessesen, D. H. (2011). Continuous glucose profiles in obese and normal-weight pregnant women on a controlled diet: metabolic determinants of fetal growth. *Diabetes Care, 34*(10), 2198–2204.

Hay, W. W., Jr. (2006). Placental-fetal glucose exchange and fetal glucose metabolism. *Transactions of the American Clinical and Climatological Association, 117*, 321–339, discussion 339–340.

Hernandez, T. L., Friedman, J. E., Van Pelt, R. E., & Barbour, L. A. (2011). Patterns of glycemia in normal pregnancy: should the current therapeutic targets be challenged? *Diabetes Care, 34*(7), 1660–1668.

Hernandez, T. L., Mande, A., & Barbour, L. A. (2018). Nutrition therapy within and beyond gestational diabetes. *Diabetes Research and Clinical Practice, 145*, 39–50. doi:10.1016/j.diabres.2018.04.004.

Koyanagi, A., Zhang, J., Dagvadorj, A., Hirayama, F., Shibuya, K., Souza, J. P., & Gülmezoglu, A. M. (2013). Macrosomia in 23 developing countries: an analysis of a multicountry, facility-based, cross-sectional survey. *Lancet, 381*(9865), 476–483.

Kozhimannil, K. B., Pereira, M. A., & Harlow, B. L. (2009). Association between diabetes and perinatal depression among low-income mothers. *JAMA, 301*(8), 842–847.

Lain, K. Y., & Catalano, P. M. (2007). Metabolic changes in pregnancy. *Clinical Obstetrics and Gynecology, 50*(4), 938–948.

Landon, M. B., Spong, C. Y., Thom, E., Carpenter, M. W., Ramin, S. M., Casey, B., . . . Anderson, G. B. (2009). A multicenter, randomized trial of treatment for mild gestational diabetes. *New England Journal of Medicine, 361*(14), 1339–1348.

Morrison, F. J. R., Movassaghian, M., Seely, E. W., Curran, A., Shubina, M., Morton-Eggleston, E., . . . Turchin, A. (2017). Fetal outcomes after diabetic ketoacidosis during pregnancy. *Diabetes Care, 40*(7), e77–e79.

Nicklas, J. M., & Barbour, L. A. (2015). Optimizing weight for maternal and infant health - tenable, or too late? *Expert Review of Endocrinology & Metabolism, 10*(2), 227–242.

Reutrakul, S., Zaidi, N., Wroblewski, K., Kay, H. H., Ismail, M., Ehrmann, D. A., & Van Cauter, E. (2013). Interactions between pregnancy, obstructive sleep apnea, and gestational diabetes mellitus. *Journal of Clinical Endocrinology and Metabolism, 98*(10), 4195–4202.

Rowan, J. A., Hague, W. M., Gao, W., Battin, M. R., Moore, M. P., & MiG Trial Investigators. (2008). Metformin versus insulin for the treatment of gestational diabetes. *New England Journal of Medicine, 358*(19), 2003–2015.

Rowan, J. A., Rush, E. C., Plank, L. D., Lu, J., Obolonkin, V., Coat, S., & Hague, W. M. (2018). Metformin in gestational diabetes: the offspring follow-up (MiG TOFU): body composition and metabolic outcomes at 7-9 years of age. *BMJ Open Diabetes Research & Care, 6*(1), e000456.

Sacks, D. A., Hadden, D. R., Maresh, M., Deerochanawong, C., Dyer, A. R., Metzger, B. E., . . . Trimble, E. R. (2012). Frequency of gestational diabetes mellitus at collaborating centers based on IADPSG consensus panel-recommended criteria: the Hyperglycemia and Adverse Pregnancy Outcome (HAPO) study. *Diabetes Care, 35*, 526–528.

Schwartz, R. A., Rosenn, B., Aleksa, K., & Koren, G. (2015). Glyburide transport across the human placenta. *Obstetrics and Gynecology, 125*(3), 583–588.

Sénat, M. V., Affres, H., Letourneau, A., Coustols-Valat, M., Cazaubiel, M., Legardeur, H., . . . Bouyer, J. (2018). Effect of glyburide vs subcutaneous insulin on perinatal complications among women with gestational diabetes: a randomized clinical trial. *JAMA, 319*(17), 1773–1780.

Stewart, Z. A., Wilinska, M. E., Hartnell, S., Temple, R. C., Rayman, G., Stanley, K. P., . . . Murphy, H. R. (2016). Closed-loop insulin delivery during pregnancy in women with type 1 diabetes. *New England Journal of Medicine, 375*(7), 644–654.

Tobias, D. K., Stuart, J. J., Li, S., Chavarro, J., Rimm, E. B., Rich-Edwards, J., . . . Zhang, C. (2017). Association of history of gestational diabetes with long-term cardiovascular disease risk in a large prospective cohort of US women. *JAMA Internal Medicine, 177*(12), 1735–1742.

Valent, A. M., Newman, T., Kritzer, S., Magner, K., & Warshak, C. R. (2017). Accuracy of sonographically estimated fetal weight near delivery in pregnancies complicated with diabetes mellitus. *Journal of Ultrasound in Medicine, 36*(3), 593–599.

Visser, J., Snel, M., & Van Vliet, H. A. (2013). Hormonal versus non-hormonal contraceptives in women with diabetes mellitus type 1 and 2. *Cochrane Database of Systematic Reviews*, (3), CD003990.

Wahabi, H. A., Alzeidan, R. A., Bawazeer, G. A., Alansari, L. A., & Esmaeil, S. A. (2010). Preconception care for diabetic women for improving maternal and fetal outcomes: a systematic review and meta-analysis. *BMC Pregnancy and Childbirth, 10*, 63.

Wexler, D. J., Powe, C. E., Barbour, L. A., Buchanan, T., Coustan, D. R., Corcoy, R., . . . Catalano, P. M. (2018). Research gaps in gestational diabetes mellitus: executive summary of a National Institute of Diabetes and Digestive and Kidney Diseases Workshop. *Obstetrics and Gynecology, 132*(2), 496–505.

White, P. (1949). Pregnancy complicating diabetes. *American Journal of Medicine, 7*(5), 609–616.

HYPOGLYCEMIC DISORDERS

Helen M. Lawler

CHAPTER 9

1. **What is the definition of hypoglycemia in people without diabetes?**
   In an individual without diabetes, hypoglycemia is defined by the presence of Whipple's triad:
   1. Hypoglycemic symptoms
   2. Low blood glucose (BG) level < 55 mg/dL (3 mmol/L) while symptoms are occurring
   3. Resolution of hypoglycemic symptoms with correction of the low BG level

2. **What are the clinical symptoms of hypoglycemia?**
   The symptoms of hypoglycemia can be divided into *neurogenic symptoms* and *neuroglycopenic symptoms*. Neurogenic symptoms are catecholamine mediated (palpitations, tremulousness, and anxiety) and cholinergic mediated (hunger, diaphoresis, and paresthesias). Neuroglycopenic symptoms include mental fogginess, confusion, irritability, behavioral changes, seizures, loss of consciousness, and coma.

3. **What is the importance of the timing of these symptoms in relation to food intake?**
   Fasting hypoglycemia refers to low BG levels that occur more than 4 hours after the last meal, especially after missed meals or an overnight fast. *Postprandial* or *reactive hypoglycemia* occurs within 4 hours after food intake. Postprandial hypoglycemia is typically seen with postgastric bypass hypoglycemia and the noninsulinoma pancreatogenous hypoglycemia syndrome. Patients with insulinomas typically have fasting hypoglycemia, but postprandial hypoglycemia can also occur. Because many conditions can cause fasting and/or postprandial hypoglycemia, the timing of the hypoglycemia in relation to meals is not always a reliable indicator of the etiology.

4. **What are the causes of hypoglycemia in adults?**
   The causes of hypoglycemia are usually divided into those that are insulin mediated (hyperinsulinemic hypoglycemia) and non–insulin mediated (hypoinsulinemic hypoglycemia).

Hyperinsulinemic Hypoglycemia	Non–Insulin-Mediated Hypoglycemia
Insulinoma	Critical illness (sepsis; hepatic, renal, or heart failure)
Postgastric bypass hypoglycemia (PGBH)	Starvation
Noninsulinoma pancreatogenous hypoglycemia syndrome (NIPHS)	Alcohol
Exogenous insulin therapy for diabetes	Glycogen storage diseases or other hepatic enzyme defects
Insulin secretagogue therapy for diabetes (sulfonylureas, meglitinides)	Adrenal insufficiency
Factitious hypoglycemia (surreptitious insulin or insulin secretagogue use)	Non–islet cell tumors (insulin-like growth factor [IGF] mediated)
Insulin autoimmune syndrome (antibody to insulin or insulin receptor)	Consumption of unripe ackee fruit ("Jamaican vomiting sickness")
Nondiabetes drugs	Nondiabetes drugs

5. **What is idiopathic postprandial syndrome?**
   Idiopathic postprandial syndrome refers to symptoms suggestive of hypoglycemia that occur after eating but without biochemical evidence of hypoglycemia. Once other etiologies for hypoglycemia-like symptoms (hyperthyroidism, pheochromocytoma, and migraines) have been excluded, it is then more appropriate to identify those symptoms without biochemical hypoglycemia (and, thus, absent Whipple's triad) as idiopathic postprandial syndrome. Frequently, underlying anxiety, neuropsychiatric disease, or situational stress reactions are the real culprits of idiopathic postprandial syndrome, which the patient characterizes or self-diagnoses as reactive hypoglycemia.

6. What are the artifactual causes of hypoglycemia?

Pseudohypoglycemia occurs in some chronic leukemias when the leukocyte counts are markedly elevated. This artifactual hypoglycemia results from utilization of glucose by leukocytes after the blood sample has been drawn. Pseudohypoglycemia may also occur with hemolytic anemia or polycythemia vera through similar mechanisms. In addition, a discordance between capillary and venous glucose levels can cause pseudohypoglycemia. This has been reported in patients with Raynaud's phenomenon, peripheral vascular disease, and shock resulting from low capillary blood flow. Artifactual hypoglycemia may also be seen with improper sample collection or storage, errors in analytic methodology, or confusion between whole blood and plasma glucose values. Plasma glucose is about 15% higher than the corresponding whole BG values.

7. When hypoglycemia occurs, what counterregulatory events occur to preserve glucose for brain metabolism?

A normal initial physiologic response to declining BG levels is suppression of insulin secretion and stimulation of glucagon and epinephrine secretion. Glucagon and epinephrine are the dominant counterregulatory hormones. Their metabolic effects are immediate: stimulation of hepatic glycogenolysis and later gluconeogenesis, resulting in increased hepatic glucose production to restore BG levels to the physiologic range. Glucagon is the more important counterregulatory hormone present during acute hypoglycemia because epinephrine does not appear to be essential if glucagon is present. If glucagon secretion is decreased or absent, epinephrine serves as the principal counterregulatory hormone. Other hormones that respond to hypoglycemic stress are cortisol and growth hormone, but their effects are delayed.

8. What is hyperinsulinemic hypoglycemia, and which conditions cause islet beta cell hyperfunction?

Hyperinsulinemic hypoglycemia refers to hypoglycemia [plasma glucose < 55 mg/dL (< 3 mmol/L)] associated with a serum insulin level ≥ 3 μU/mL, C-peptide ≥ 0.2 nmol/L, proinsulin ≥ 5 pmol/L, and beta-hydroxybutyrate ≤ 2.7 mmol/L. If hyperinsulinemic hypoglycemia is present, a glucose rise of > 25 mg/dL (1.4 mmol/L) is also anticipated in response to administration of intravenous glucagon. This is because elevated insulin levels inhibit hepatic glycogenolysis and preserve hepatic glycogen stores. Glucagon administration causes the release of glucose from the preserved hepatic glycogen stores. Hyperinsulinemic hypoglycemia suggests the presence of islet beta cell hyperfunction (insulinoma, NIPHS, or PGBH), therapeutic or surreptitious use of insulin or oral hypoglycemic agents, or insulin autoimmune syndrome. Of note, approximately 85% of insulinomas are single benign tumors, 7% are multiple benign tumors, and 6% are malignant tumors.

9. Which laboratory tests are useful in evaluating Whipple's triad?

Once Whipple's triad is confirmed, a complete blood count, comprehensive metabolic panel, 8 AM serum cortisol level, and serum insulin antibody levels should be obtained at the clinic visit. Obtaining values for serum insulin, proinsulin, C-peptide, and beta-hydroxybutyrate, along with a sulfonylurea screen, while hypoglycemia is occurring is the critical step. If these data are not available from an episode of spontaneous hypoglycemia, a prolonged (72-hour) supervised fast is recommended to determine the cause of Whipple's triad. During a prolonged fast, ~ 100% of patients with an insulinoma will have Whipple's triad within 72 hours, 95% within 48 hours, and 67% within 24 hours.

Patients with NIPHS and PGBH usually experience only postprandial hypoglycemia and do not generally have fasting hypoglycemia. An oral glucose tolerance test (OGTT) is not recommended to evaluate postprandial hypoglycemia because hypoglycemia occurs with similar frequencies in patients with hypoglycemic symptoms and in asymptomatic control patients. Instead, a mixed meal tolerance test (MMTT) is recommended. During the MMTT, the patient consumes a solid or liquid meal similar in content, if possible, to meals that usually provoke symptoms and is then observed for up to 5 hours. Plasma glucose, insulin, proinsulin, and C-peptide levels are obtained at baseline and every 30 minutes for 5 hours.

10. Describe PGBH.

Hypoglycemia can sometimes occur after Roux-en-Y gastric bypass (RYGB) surgery and other procedures that alter the anatomy of the upper gastrointestinal tract. The prevalence is reported to be 0.2% to 1.0%, although one third of bariatric surgery patients responding to a mail survey reported hypoglycemic symptoms, with 11.6% reporting more serious symptoms, including needing third-party assistance. PGBH is defined as postprandial hypoglycemia, often with neuroglycopenic symptoms that occur at least 6 months after bariatric surgery despite adherence to an acceptable bariatric diet. The MMTT or provocation meal test reveals a rapid rise in BG often with glucose values > 200 mg/dL accompanied by a robust insulin and GLP-1 response, followed by the development of hypoglycemia. The pathogenesis of PGBH is currently unknown, but pathologic findings of nesidioblastosis are often seen.

11. How do you treat PGBH?

Treatment involves advising patients to eat a diet high in protein, to limit carbohydrates to under 30 g per meal, and to limit added sugar to under 4 g per meal. If hypoglycemia persists after dietary modification, an alpha-glucosidase inhibitor, such as acarbose or miglitol, is often used. Alpha-glucosidase inhibitors impair carbohydrate absorption and thereby reduce the postprandial rise in glucose and insulin. Although data are limited, diazoxide, somatostatin analogues, and calcium channel blockers have all been used with varying degrees of success. In severe cases refractory to dietary modification and pharmacotherapy, options include reversal of the RYGB, surgical restoration of gastric restriction, and continuous tube feeds through a gastrostomy tube inserted into the remnant stomach. However, the success rate of ~ 70% with reversal of the RYGB is not ideal. Of note, treatment with pancreatectomy has fallen out of favor due to high morbidity and incomplete resolution or recurrence of hypoglycemia.

12. **What is NIPHS?**

NIPHS is a very rare cause of endogenous hyperinsulinemic hypoglycemia presenting in adulthood. Affected patients have primarily postprandial hypoglycemia caused by islet cell hypertrophy. Pathologic findings (nesidioblastosis) are similar to those seen in neonates and infants with persistent hyperinsulinemic hypoglycemia and in adults with PGBH. PGBH and NIPHS have similar clinical presentations and pathologic findings, but NIPHS occurs in the absence of prior bariatric surgery and is classified as a separate entity.

13. **How do you treat NIPHS?**

The treatment for NIPHS and PGBH are the same. Mild cases may respond to dietary modification alone. Simple carbohydrate consumption should be limited, and higher protein and fiber diets are encouraged to blunt postprandial glucose and insulin excursions. Acarbose can also be added, if needed. Diazoxide, somatostatin analogues, and calcium channel blockers have also been used with varying degrees of success. In severe cases, a partial or rarely complete pancreatectomy may be necessary.

14. **How do you distinguish an insulinoma from factitious hypoglycemia?**

Insulinomas are characterized by hypoglycemia with elevated or inappropriately normal serum insulin, C-peptide, and proinsulin levels. Surreptitious insulin administration is identified by finding elevated serum insulin but low levels of C-peptide and proinsulin, because endogenous insulin secretion is suppressed in this situation. Circulating insulin antibodies may be positive with surreptitious insulin administration and with the insulin autoimmune syndrome. However, patients with insulin autoimmune syndrome have elevated C-peptide and proinsulin levels. Surreptitious sulfonylurea or meglitinide ingestion is suggested by finding elevated serum insulin, C-peptide, and proinsulin levels with a positive drug screen for oral hypoglycemic agents.

15. **What procedures are helpful to localize the cause of pancreatic islet cell hyperinsulinemia?**

Once biochemical evidence of an insulinoma is confirmed, abdominal imagining should be the next step. Noninvasive imaging options include transabdominal ultrasonography, abdominal computed tomography (CT), and magnetic resonance imaging (MRI). A positron emission tomography (PET)/CT with ^{68}Ga-DOTA-exendin-4 has also recently been used to localize insulinomas. Some insulinomas are extremely small (less than a few millimeters) and easily escape detection on noninvasive imaging. Endoscopic ultrasonography may be useful in these cases. Selective arterial calcium infusions can also localize occult tumors and help distinguish between an isolated insulinoma and diffuse disease. Intraoperative ultrasonography is also useful for localizing pancreatic tumors.

16. **If surgical resection of an insulinoma is not possible or the patient has metastatic or inoperable carcinoma, adenomatosis, or hyperplasia, what management options may control the hypoglycemia?**

Dietary changes, such as frequent feedings and snacks, can be helpful. The most commonly used medication is diazoxide, which inhibits insulin secretion. Somatostatin analogues (octreotide, lanreotide), verapamil, and phenytoin can also be effective. Endoscopic ethanol ablation has been used successfully in nonsurgical candidates and, therefore, is another option if there is sufficient expertise in this procedure available. For islet cell carcinoma, various chemotherapeutic agents can be used (see Chapter 61).

17. **If other family members have pancreatic tumors, what condition is suggested?**

Multiple endocrine neoplasia type 1 (MEN-1) occurs as an autosomal dominant condition characterized by functioning and nonfunctioning pituitary tumors, parathyroid hyperplasia, and islet cell tumors, most commonly gastrinomas (Zollinger-Ellison syndrome) and insulinomas. When this condition is suspected, family members should be screened genetically or tested for the components of MEN-1. However, only about 5% to 10% of insulinomas are associated with MEN-1 (see Chapter 60).

18. **What are the causes of childhood hypoglycemia?**

Hyperinsulinemic hypoglycemia in children can result from the same etiologies that cause this condition in adults but persistent hyperinsulinemic hypoglycemia of infancy (PHHI) is the most common cause of persistent hypoglycemia in infants. PHHI has also been referred to as *congenital hyperinsulinism, primary islet cell hypertrophy,* and *familial hyperinsulinemic hypoglycemia.* Nesidioblastosis, characterized by abnormal hypertrophied beta cells, is seen on pathologic examination of surgical specimens. Non–insulin-mediated hypoglycemia in infants and young children suggests an inborn error of metabolism, such as defective gluconeogenesis and/or glycogen metabolism (i.e., glycogen storage disease type 1: glucose-6-phosphatase-deficiency) or a fatty acid oxidation disorder. Adrenal insufficiency also causes non–insulin-mediated hypoglycemia in childhood.

19. **What are the most common drugs that cause hypoglycemia in adults?**
It is important to rule out insulin and oral insulin secretagogues (sulfonylureas, meglitinides) as the cause of hypoglycemia. Other drugs that have at least moderate quality of evidence supporting an association with hypoglycemia include indomethacin, quinine, pentamidine, quinolones, tramadol, and cibenzoline.

20. **How does alcohol cause hypoglycemia?**
Ethanol acutely inhibits hepatic gluconeogenesis. Hypoglycemia from alcohol ingestion generally occurs only in patients who also have impaired glycogenolysis caused by depletion of hepatic glycogen stores from fasting or chronic malnutrition. It is, therefore, the combination of acutely impaired gluconeogenesis and ineffective glycogenolysis that results in alcohol-induced hypoglycemia.

21. **What is the mechanism of non–islet cell tumor hypoglycemia (NICTH)?**
Hypoglycemia can occur most commonly with large mesenchymal or epithelial cell tumors, myelomas, fibromas, carcinoid tumors, colorectal carcinomas, and hepatocellular carcinomas. NICTH is an infrequent complication of malignancy and can be caused by various mechanisms. Most commonly, these tumors secrete incompletely processed IGF-2 and rarely IGF-1, which bind to insulin receptors to cause hypoglycemia. In addition, IGF-2 also suppresses growth hormone and glucagon. Thus, IGF-2 promotes continued glucose utilization and inhibits glycogenolysis and gluconeogenesis. Less commonly, non–islet cell tumors can produce insulin or insulin receptor antibodies. Hypoglycemia can also occur as a result of bilateral adrenal gland or liver destruction from widespread tumor invasion or metastases.

22. **What autoimmune syndromes are associated with hypoglycemia?**
Autoantibodies directed against insulin receptors or insulin itself may provoke hypoglycemia. Antiinsulin receptor antibodies bind directly to and stimulate insulin receptors and thereby mimic insulin action in tissues. Antiinsulin antibodies bind circulating insulin and randomly dissociate from insulin at inappropriate times, causing a sudden rise in free insulin levels and subsequent hypoglycemia. This disorder is observed most often in patients from Japan, usually in association with other autoimmune diseases.

23. **When is hypoglycemia attributed to underlying medical illness?**
Patients with critical illness have multiple reasons for developing hypoglycemia, including hepatic dysfunction, renal insufficiency, medications, and poor dietary intake. Hepatic failure leads to hypoglycemia because of the liver's role in gluconeogenesis and glycogenolysis. Renal failure likely causes hypoglycemia as a result of reduced renal clearance of insulin and decreased renal glucose production caused by impaired renal gluconeogenesis. During sepsis, elevated cytokines may increase glucose utilization and inhibit gluconeogenesis, causing hypoglycemia when glycogen stores are not sufficient. Starvation states, such as anorexia nervosa, also cause hypoglycemia as a result of depletion of glycogen stores and lack of substrate for gluconeogenesis.

KEY POINTS

- Hypoglycemia in a person without diabetes is defined by the presence of Whipple's triad.
- Obtaining fasting values for insulin, proinsulin, C-peptide, and beta-hydroxybutyrate along with a sulfonylurea screen while hypoglycemia is occurring is critical. If these data have not been acquired, a 72-hour supervised fast is recommended to determine the cause of Whipple's triad.
- If hyperinsulinemic hypoglycemia is present, a glucose rise of > 25 mg/dL (1.4 mmol/L) is anticipated in response to the administration of intravenous glucagon, which acutely stimulates hepatic glycogenolysis.
- Hyperinsulinemic hypoglycemia suggests islet beta cell hyperfunction (insulinoma, noninsulinoma pancreatogenous hypoglycemia syndrome [NIPHS], or postgastric bypass hypoglycemia [PGBH]), the surreptitious use of insulin or oral hypoglycemic agents, or insulin autoimmune hypoglycemia.
- Non–insulin-mediated hypoglycemia may be secondary to critical illness, starvation, alcohol abuse, adrenal insufficiency, non–islet cell tumors, glycogen storage diseases, or consumption of an unripe ackee fruit.

BIBLIOGRAPHY

Charles, M. A., Hofeldt, F., Shackelford, A., Waldeck, N., Dodson, L. E., Jr., Bunker, D., . . . Eichner, H. (1981). Comparison of oral glucose tolerance tests and mixed meals in patients with apparent idiopathic postabsorptive hypoglycemia: absence of hypoglycemia after meals. *Diabetes, 30*(6), 465–470.

Cryer, P. E. (2015). Minimizing hypoglycemia in diabetes. *Diabetes Care, 38*(3), 1583–1591.

Cryer, P. E., Axelrod, L., Grossman, A. B., Heller, S. R., Montori, V. M., Seaquist, E. R., & Service, F. J. (2009). Evaluation and management of adult hypoglycemic disorders: an Endocrine Society clinical practice guideline. *Journal of Clinical Endocrinology and Metabolism, 94*(3), 709–728.

Cryer, P. E., & Gerich, J. E. (1985). Glucose counterregulation, hypoglycemia, and intensive insulin therapy in diabetes mellitus. *New England Journal of Medicine, 313*, 232–241.

Cuthbertson, D.J., Banks, M., Khoo, B., Antwi, K., Christ, E., Campbell, F., . . . Wild, D. (2016). Application of Ga(68)-DOTA-exendin-4 PET/ CT to localize an occult insulinoma. *Clinical Endocrinology, 84*, 789–791.

Dynkevich, Y., Rother, K. I., Whitford, I., Qureshi, S., Galiveeti, S., Szulc, A. L., ... Roth, J. (2013). Tumors, IGF-2, and hypoglycemia: insights from the clinic, the laboratory, and the historical archive. *Endocrinology Review, 34*, 798–826.

El Khoury, M., Yousuf, F., Martin, V., & Cohen, R. M. (2008). Pseudohypoglycemia: a cause for unreliable finger-stick glucose measurements. *Endocrine Practice, 14*(3), 337–339.

Golightly, L. K., Simendinger, B. A., Barber, G. R., Stolpman, N. M., Kick, S. D., & McDermott, M. T. (2017). Hypoglycemic effects of tramadol analgesia in hospitalized patients: a case-control study. *Journal of Diabetes and Metabolic Disorders, 16*, 30.

Hirshberg, B., Livi, A., Bartlett, D. L., Libutti, S. K., Alexander, H. R., Doppman, J. L., ... Gorden, P. (2000). Forty-eight-hour fast: the diagnostic test for insulinoma. *Journal of Clinical Endocrinology and Metabolism, 85*, 3222–3226.

Lee, C. J., Clark, J. M, Schweitzer, M., Magnuson, T., Steele, K., Koerner, O., & Brown, T. T. (2015). Prevalence of and risk factors for hypoglycemic symptoms after gastric bypass and sleeve gastrectomy. *Obesity (Silver Spring), 23*, 1079–1084.

Maitra, S. R., Wojnar, M. M., & Lang, C. H. (2000). Alterations in tissue glucose uptake during the hyperglycemic and hypoglycemic phases of sepsis. *Shock, 13*, 379–385.

Metzger, S., Nusair, S., Planer, D., Barash, V., Pappo, O., Shilyansky, J., & Chajek-Shaul, T. (2004). Inhibition of hepatic gluconeogenesis and enhanced glucose uptake contribute to the development of hypoglycemia in mice bearing interleukin-1beta-secreting tumor. *Endocrinology, 145*, 5150–5160.

Millstein, R., & Lawler, H. M. (2017). Hypoglycemia after gastric bypass: an emerging complication. *Cleveland Clinic Journal of Medicine, 84*(4), 319–328.

Murad, M. H., Coto-Yglesias, F., Wang, A. T., Sheidaee, N., Mullan, R. J., Elamin, M. B., . . . Montori, V. M. (2009). Drug-induced hypoglycemia: a systematic review. *Journal of Clinical Endocrinology and Metabolism, 94*, 741–745.

Noone, T. C., Hosey, J., Firat, Z., & Semelka, R. C. (2005). Imaging and localization of islet-cell tumours of the pancreas on CT and MRI. *Best Practice & Research: Clinical Endocrinology & Metabolism, 19*, 195–211.

Sarwar, H., Chapman, W. H., III, Pender, J. R., Ivanescu, A., Drake, A. J., III, Pories, W. J., & Dar, M. S. (2014). Hypoglycemia after Roux-en-Y gastric bypass: the BOLD experience. *Obesity Surgery, 24*, 1120–1124.

Saxon, D. R., McDermott, M. T., & Michels, A. W. (2016). Novel management of insulin autoimmune syndrome with rituximab and continuous glucose monitoring. *Journal of Clinical Endocrinology and Metabolism, 101*, 1931–1934.

Service, F. J., McMahon, M. M., O'Brien, P. C., & Ballard, D. J. (1991). Functioning insulinoma—incidence, recurrence, and long-term survival of patients: a 60-year study. *Mayo Clinic Proceedings, 66*, 711–719.

Whipple, A. O. (1938). The surgical therapy of hyperinsulinism. *Journal of International Chirurgie, 3*, 237.

CHAPTER 10

LIPID DISORDERS

Emily B. Schroeder and Michael T. McDermott

1. What are the major lipids in the bloodstream?

   Cholesterol and triglycerides (TGs) are the major circulating lipids. Cholesterol is used by all cells for the synthesis and repair of membranes and intracellular organelles and by the adrenal glands and gonads as a substrate to synthesize adrenal and gonadal steroid hormones. TGs are an energy source and can be stored as fat in adipose tissue or used as fuel by muscle and other tissues.

2. What are lipoproteins?

   Cholesterol and TGs are not water soluble and, thus, cannot be transported through the circulation as individual molecules. Lipoproteins are large, spherical particles that package these lipids into a core surrounded by a shell of water-soluble proteins and phospholipids. Lipoproteins serve as vehicles that transport cholesterol and TGs from one part of the body to another.

3. What are the major lipoproteins in the bloodstream?

   Chylomicrons, very-low-density lipoproteins (VLDLs), low-density lipoproteins (LDLs), and high-density lipoproteins (HDLs) are the major circulating lipoproteins. Their functions are as follows:

   Lipoprotein Function

Lipoprotein	Function
Chylomicron	Transport exogenous TGs from the gut to adipose tissue and muscle
VLDL	Transport endogenous TGs from the liver to adipose tissue and muscle
LDL	Transport cholesterol from the liver to peripheral tissues
HDL	Transport cholesterol from peripheral tissues to the liver

   HDL, High-density lipoprotein; *LDL*, low-density lipoprotein; *TG*, triglycerides; *VLDL*, very-low-density lipoprotein.

4. What are apoproteins?

   Apoproteins are located on the surface of lipoproteins. They function as ligands for binding to lipoprotein receptors and as cofactors for metabolic enzymes. Their functions are as follows:

   Apoprotein Function

Apoprotein	Function
Apoprotein A	Ligand for peripheral HDL receptors
Apoprotein B	Ligand for peripheral LDL receptors
Apoprotein E	Ligand for hepatic receptors for remnant particles
Apoprotein C-II	Cofactor for LPL

   HDL, High-density lipoprotein; *LDL*, low-density lipoprotein; *LPL*, lipoprotein lipase.

5. Name other enzymes and transport proteins that are important in lipoprotein metabolism.

   See Table 10.1 and Fig. 10.1.

6. Describe the function and metabolism of LDL.

   LDL transports cholesterol from the liver to peripheral tissues, where surface apoprotein B-100 binds to cellular LDL receptors (LDLRs). LDLR clustering in clathrin-coated pits on the cell membrane, promoted by LDLR adaptor protein-1 (LDLRAP-1), is necessary for efficient LDL uptake. After LDL is internalized, it is degraded to free cholesterol (FC) for intracellular use. Excess LDL is cleared from the circulation by scavenger macrophages.

7. What is proprotein convertase subtilisin/kexin type 9 (PCSK9)?

   PCSK9 is a cellular protein that promotes the degradation of LDLR within lysosomes, thereby preventing recycling of the LDLR to the cell surface to internalize more LDL. Activating mutations of the gene for PCSK9 cause a rare form of familial hypercholesterolemia, and inactivating mutations result in low serum LDL cholesterol (LDL-C) levels. This makes PCSK9 an interesting target for pharmacotherapy (see Question 31).

Table 10.1. Enzymes and Transport Proteins Important in Lipoprotein Metabolism.

ENZYME/TRANSPORT PROTEIN	FUNCTION
3-hydroxy-3-methyl-glutaryl-coenzyme A (HMG CoA) reductase	The rate-limiting enzyme in hepatic cholesterol synthesis
Lipoprotein lipase (LPL)	Removes TG from chylomicrons and VLDL in adipose tissue, leaving remnant particles
Hepatic lipase (HL)	Removes additional TG from remnant particles in the liver, converting them into LDL
Lecithin cholesterol acyl transferase (LCAT)	Esterifies cholesterol molecules on the surface of HDL, drawing them into the HDL core
Cholesterol ester transfer protein (CETP)	Shuttles esterified cholesterol back and forth between HDL and LDL

HDL, High-density lipoprotein; LDL, low-density lipoprotein; TG, triglycerides; VLDL, very low-density lipoprotein.

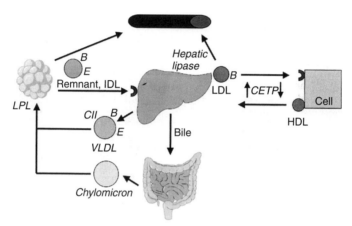

Fig. 10.1. Lipoprotein metabolism. B, Apolipoprotein B; CETP, cholesterol ester transfer protein; CII, apolipoprotein C-II; E, apolipoprotein E; HDL, high-density lipoprotein; IDL, intermediate-density lipoprotein; LDL, low-density lipoprotein; LPL, lipoprotein lipase; VLDL, very-low-density lipoprotein.

8. What is the function of HDL?

   HDL removes excess cholesterol from cells by two mechanisms. Nascent pre–beta HDL is made in the liver and intestine. Surface Apo A1 on pre–beta HDL acquires FC through the adenosine triphosphate (ATP)–binding cassette transporter A1 (ABCA1) on arterial wall macrophages. Plasma lecithin cholesterol acyl transferase (LCAT) then esterifies FC to cholesterol ester (CE), forming a mature beta HDL particle. Mature beta HDL accepts additional FC from arterial macrophages through the ABCA1 transporter and the scavenger receptor, class B, type 1 (SR-B1) receptor. Cholesterol ester transfer protein (CETP) transfers some CE back to the LDL particles, and the mature HDL transports the remaining CE to the liver, where transfer occurs through hepatic SR-B1 receptors. In addition to reverse cholesterol transport, HDL also reduces LDL oxidation, inhibits vascular inflammation, and improves endothelial function. All of these functions make HDL a potent antiatherogenic lipoprotein.

9. Describe the pathogenesis of the atherosclerotic plaque and arterial thrombosis.

   LDL can be modified by oxidation. Scavenger macrophages located beneath the intimal surface of arteries engulf oxidized LDL, becoming lipid-laden foam cells, which secrete growth factors that stimulate smooth muscle cell proliferation. These developing plaques also secrete cytokines that attract inflammatory cells, which secrete proteolytic enzymes; these enzymes erode the fibromuscular plaque cap, making it prone to rupture. When rupture occurs, platelets aggregate and release chemicals that promote vasoconstriction and initiate thrombus formation, which may ultimately occlude the artery.

10. Explain the function and metabolism of TGs.

    Food and hepatic synthesis are the major sources of TGs. They are transported by chylomicrons (dietary TGs) and VLDL (endogenous TGs) to adipose tissue and muscle, where LPL and cofactor apoprotein C-II break down TGs into fatty acids (FAs) and monoglycerides. FAs enter adipose cells to be stored as fat or muscle cells to be used as fuel. The chylomicron and VLDL remnant particles return to the liver, where HDL converts VLDL remnants into LDL.

11. Are elevated serum TG levels harmful?

Increased serum TG levels are associated with atherosclerosis and increased rates of coronary disease. The American Heart Association states that TGs are not directly atherogenic but represent an important biomarker of cardiovascular risk because of their association with an atherogenic lipid profile (low HDL cholesterol levels and small, dense LDL particles), as well as obesity, insulin resistance, and metabolic syndrome (MS). It has not yet been shown that decreasing TG levels will decrease coronary disease risk. TG values > 1000 mg/dL significantly increase the risk of acute pancreatitis.

12. What is metabolic syndrome (MS)?

MS is a condition that is diagnosed when a patient has any three of the following: elevated fasting glucose ($\geq$ 110 mg/dL), high TGs ($\geq$ 150 mg/dL), low HDL (< 40 mg/dL for men, < 50 mg/dL for women), hypertension ($\geq$ 130/85 mm Hg), and abdominal obesity (waist > 40 inches in men, > 35 inches in women). The common thread among the disorders that comprise MS appears to be insulin resistance. MS carries a high risk for atherosclerotic vascular disease.

13. What is lipoprotein(a)?

Apoprotein(a) has approximately 85% amino-acid sequence homology with plasminogen. When an apoprotein(a) molecule attaches to apoprotein B on the surface of an LDL particle, the new particle is referred to as *lipoprotein(a)*. Excessive lipoprotein(a) promotes atherosclerosis, possibly because it is easily oxidized and engulfed by macrophages, because it inhibits thrombolysis, or both.

14. What are primary dyslipidemias?

Primary dyslipidemias are inherited disorders of lipoprotein metabolism. The major primary dyslipidemias and their lipid phenotypes are as follows:

Primary Dyslipidemias

Primary Dyslipidemia	Phenotype
Familial hypercholesterolemia (FH)	↑↑ Cholesterol
Polygenic hypercholesterolemia	↑ Cholesterol
Familial combined hyperlipidemia (FCH)	↑ Cholesterol and ↑ triglycerides (TGs)
Familial dysbetalipoproteinemia (FDL)	↑ Cholesterol and ↑ TGs
Familial hypertriglyceridemia (FHT)	↑ TGs
Familial hyperchylomicronemia (FHC)	↑↑ TGs

15. What is familial hypercholesterolemia (FH)?

FH is an inherited disease characterized by extreme elevations of serum cholesterol but normal serum TG levels. The population frequency is 1:500 for heterozygous familial hypercholesterolemia (HeFH), which generally presents with serum cholesterol levels of 300 to 800 mg/dL, and 1:1,000,000 for homozygous familial hypercholesterolemia (HoFH), which results in serum cholesterol levels of 600 to > 1000 mg/dL. Most patients have genetic mutations resulting in deficient or dysfunctional LDLRs. Other less common monogenic hypercholesterolemic disorders include apoprotein B mutations that produce a defective apoprotein B that cannot bind to LDLR, PCSK9 mutations that cause accelerated LDLR degradation, LDLRAP-1 mutations that prevent normal clustering of LDLR in cell surface clathrin-coated pits, and ATP-binding cassette G5 or G8 (ABCG5/8) mutations that cause abnormal cellular transport of cholesterol and plant sterols (sitosterolemia). These disorders are characterized by premature coronary artery disease (CAD), often before 20 years of age in HoFH, and tendon xanthomas.

16. What is familial combined hyperlipidemia (FCH)?

FCH is an inherited disorder characterized by variable elevations of both serum cholesterol and TG levels. Affected individuals have excessive hepatic apoprotein B synthesis, with increased numbers of apoprotein B–containing VLDL and LDL particles. These patients are prone to premature CAD. It most likely has a genetically complex basis, with the phenotype resulting from the interaction of the environment and multiple susceptibility genes.

17. What is familial dysbetalipoproteinemia (FDL)?

FDL is also known as *broad beta disease, remnant removal disease,* or *type III hyperlipoproteinemia.* It is an inherited condition characterized by increased serum total cholesterol, moderate hypertriglyceridemia (300–400 mg/dL), and normal high-density lipoprotein cholesterol (HDL-C) levels. This disorder results from an abnormal apoprotein E phenotype (E2/E2), which binds poorly to hepatic receptors, resulting in impaired clearance of circulating VLDL remnants by the liver. Affected individuals often have premature CAD. Planar xanthomas in the creases of the palms and soles of the feet are a characteristic finding in patients with FDL.

18. **What is polygenic hypercholesterolemia?**

Polygenic hypercholesterolemia, which is characterized by mild-to-moderate elevations of serum cholesterol alone, is the most common type of inherited hypercholesterolemia. This condition generally occurs when one or more mild defects of cholesterol metabolism combine to elevate the serum cholesterol level. Affected individuals have an increased risk of CAD.

19. **What are familial hypertriglyceridemia (FHT) and familial hyperchylomicronemia (FHC)?**

FHT is characterized by moderate-to-severe elevations of serum TGs with normal serum cholesterol levels. It has a complex polygenic etiology. FHC is characterized by extremely high serum TG and chylomicron levels. FHC is caused by inactivating mutations in the gene for lipoprotein lipase (LPL) or apoprotein CII and mutations of the apolipoprotein AV (*APOAV*) gene. Severe hypertriglyceridemia with chylomicronemia may predispose to the development of eruptive xanthomas, lipemia retinalis, hepatosplenomegaly, and acute pancreatitis.

20. **How do you distinguish between FCH and FDL?**

Because FCH and FDL are characterized by combined elevations of both cholesterol and TGs, additional tests may be necessary to make the distinction. Patients with FCH have increased serum apoprotein B levels, whereas patients with FDL have an E2/E2 apoprotein E phenotype and a broad beta-band on lipoprotein electrophoresis. Family studies are also helpful.

21. **What causes familial low HDL?**

Familial hypoalphalipoproteinemia (familial low HDL) is characterized by extremely low serum HDL levels and premature CAD. Inactivating mutations in the genes that encode apolipoprotein A1 (APOA1), ABCA1, or LCAT result in HDL-C levels of < 5 to 10 mg/dL. LPL mutations reduce HDL-C to a lesser degree.

22. **What are secondary dyslipidemias?**

Secondary dyslipidemias are serum lipid elevations that result from systemic diseases, such as diabetes mellitus, hypothyroidism, nephrotic syndrome, renal disease, obstructive liver disease, dysproteinemias, and lipodystrophies. Lipids may also be increased by medications, such as beta-blockers, thiazide diuretics, estrogens, progestins, androgens, retinoids, corticosteroids, cyclosporin A, antipsychotics, and protease inhibitors. These disorders usually improve when the primary condition is treated or the offending drugs are discontinued.

23. **What are the causes of acquired hypertriglyceridemia?**

Hypertriglyceridemia can be caused by insulin resistance or obesity, other medical conditions (diabetes, human immunodeficiency virus [HIV] infection, nephrotic syndrome, hypothyroidism, connective tissue disease), alcohol abuse, and medications (estrogens, glucocorticoids, antiretroviral medications, retinoids, some antihypertensive medications).

KEY POINTS: CAUSES OF LIPID DISORDERS

- Elevated low-density lipoprotein (LDL) cholesterol is a major risk factor for coronary artery disease (CAD).
- Low high-density lipoprotein (HDL) cholesterol is also a significant risk factor for CAD.
- High serum triglycerides (TGs) are associated with increased risk of CAD, but it is unclear whether lowering TG levels decreases CAD risk.
- Serum TG levels > 1000 mg/dL significantly increase the risk of acute pancreatitis.
- Inflammation within the atherosclerotic plaque plays a major role in plaque rupture and the occurrence of acute coronary events.

24. **Describe the general approach to the treatment of dyslipidemia.**

Management of dyslipidemias usually requires a multifaceted approach and may include treatment of secondary causes, lifestyle changes, medical therapy, and rarely apheresis.

25. **What are the American College of Cardiology/American Heart Association (ACC/AHA) recommendations for lifestyle changes to improve atherosclerotic cardiovascular disease (ASCVD) risk?**

For individuals who would benefit from LDL-C cholesterol lowering, the ACC/AHA guidelines recommend:
- Consuming a dietary pattern that emphasizes vegetables, fruits, and whole grains; includes low-fat dairy products, poultry, fish, legumes, nontropical vegetable oils, and nuts; and limits intake of sweets, sugar-sweetened beverages, and red meats. This can be achieved by following diet plans, such as the DASH (Dietary Approaches to Stop Hypertension) diet.
- Aiming for 5% to 6% of calories from saturated fats.
- Reducing the percent of calories from saturated fats and *trans* fats.

26. **What medications are currently available for the treatment of dyslipidemias?**

See Tables 10.2 and 10.3.

Table 10.2. Medications for the Treatment of Dyslipidemia.

	AVAILABLE AGENTS	LDL EFFECT (%)	TG EFFECT (%)	HDL EFFECT (%)
Statins	Rosuvastatin Atorvastatin Pitavastatin Simvastatin Pravastatin Lovastatin Fluvastatin	↓ 20%–60%	↓ 0%–30%	↑ 0%–15%
PCSK9 inhibitors	Alirocumab Evolocumab	↓ 30%–70%	↓ 0%–25%	↑ 5%–10%
Cholesterol absorption inhibitors	Ezetimibe	↓ 18%–25%	None	↓ 5%–10%
Bile acid sequestrants	Cholestyramine Colestipol Colesevelam	↓ 15%–30%	None or slight increase	None or slight increase
Nicotinic acid	Niacin Niacin ER	↓ 10%–25%	↓ 25%–30%	↑ 15%–35%
Fibrates	Fenofibrate Gemfibrozil	↓ 0%–20%; can increase	↓ 30%–45%	↑ 5%–10%
Omega-3 fatty acids	EPA DHA	↑ 0%–10%	↓20%–50%	↑5%–10%

EPA, Eicosapentaenoic acid; *DHA*, docosahexaenoic acid; *HDL*, high-density lipoprotein; *LDL*, low-density lipoprotein; *TG*, triglycerides; *VLDL*, very-low-density lipoprotein.

Table 10.3. Statins by Degree of Intensity.

HIGH-INTENSITY STATIN THERAPY	MODERATE-INTENSITY STATIN THERAPY	LOW-INTENSITY STATIN THERAPY
Atorvastatin 40–80 mg Rosuvastatin 20–40 mg	Atorvastatin 10–20 mg Rosuvastatin 5–10 mg Simvastatin 20–40 mg Pravastatin 40–80 mg Lovastatin 40 mg Fluvastatin XL 80 mg Fluvastatin 40 mg twice a day Pitavastatin 2–4 mg	Simvastatin 10–20 mg Pravastatin 10–20 mg Lovastatin 20 mg Fluvastatin 20–40 mg Pitavastatin 1 mg

Doses are once a day unless otherwise specified.

27. When treatment is recommended by the ACC/AHA for hypercholesterolemia?

The 2013 ACC/AHA guidelines moved away from a treat-to-target approach and, instead, recommended treating specific groups of individuals with high ASCVD risk (Table 10.4). These groups include people with:
1. Clinical ASCVD.
2. LDL ≧ 190 mg/dL.
3. LDL = 70 to 189 mg/dL, diabetes, age 40 to 75 years.
4. LDL = 70 to 189 mg/dL, no diabetes, age 40 to 75 years, 10-year ASCVD risk ≧ 7.5%.

For individuals over age 75 years, risks and benefits should be discussed with the patient to allow for shared decision making. In addition, risks and benefits should be discussed with individuals ages < 40 years with high ASCVD risk.

28. Describe the mechanism of action of statin medications.

Statins inhibit 3-hydroxy-3-methyl-glutaryl-coenzyme A reductase (HMG CoA reductase), the rate-limiting enzyme in cholesterol synthesis. This leads to a decrease in cholesterol synthesis and an increase in hepatic LDL receptor-mediated LDL removal from the circulation. The most commonly used statins, in increasing order of relative LDL-lowering potencies, are: fluvastatin < pravastatin < lovastatin < simvastatin < atorvastatin < rosuvastatin < pitavastatin (Table 10.3). The initial statin dose will produce the greatest LDL cholesterol reduction. Each subsequent doubling of the statin dose will, on average, result only in an additional 6% decrease in serum LDL cholesterol.

Table 10.4. ACC/AHA Recommendations for Treatment of Specific ASCVD Risk Groups.

POPULATION	STATIN INTENSITY
Clinical ASCVD Age 21–75 years	High
Clinical ASCVD Age > 75 years	Moderate (shared decision-making)
LDL ≧ 190 mg/dL Age 21–75 years	High
LDL ≡ 70–189 mg/dL Diabetes Age 40–75 years 10-year ASCVD risk ≧ 7.5%	High
LDL ≡ 70–189 mg/dL Diabetes Age 40–75 years 10-year ASCVD risk < 7.5%	Moderate
LDL ≡ 70–189 mg/dL No diabetes Age 40–75 years 10-year ASCVD risk ≧ 7.5%	Moderate/high
LDL ≡ 70–189 mg/dL No diabetes Age 40–75 years 10-year ASCVD risk 5.0%–7.5%	Moderate

29. **What are the potential side effects of statins?**

Myalgias occur in 5% to 15% of patients. True myositis is much less common, and rhabdomyolysis is very rare (≈ 1:10,000). For creatinine kinase (CK) elevations > 5 times the upper limit of normal or if the patient has moderate to severe symptoms, the statin should be stopped. Once the patient is asymptomatic and the CK is reduced, then reasonable approaches include: a trial of low-dose fluvastatin or pravastatin; alternate daily or weekly dosage of a more potent statin, such as rosuvastatin or pitavastatin; or a combination of a low-dose statin with a nonstatin cholesterol agent (ezetimibe or bile acid sequestrant). Over-the-counter preparations containing natural statin-like agents, such as red yeast rice, can also be tried, although such products undergo limited quality control and have low efficacy. For patients with mild symptoms and CK elevations < 5 times the upper limit of normal, the statin may be continued. If symptoms worsen, then the CK should be rechecked.

There have also been concerns about increased rates of memory loss with use of statins. However, blinded studies do not show higher rates of myalgias or memory loss. Statins do increase the risk of metabolic syndrome, prediabetes, and diabetes, as was shown in the JUPITER (Justification for the Use of Statins in Prevention: an Intervention Trial Evaluating Rosuvastatin) trial.

30. **Does aggressive cholesterol-lowering therapy effectively and safely reduce the risk of CAD?**

Clinical trials have repeatedly demonstrated the efficacy of aggressive cholesterol lowering with statins in reducing myocardial infarction, strokes, and cardiovascular mortality in patients with a previous history of CAD (secondary prevention). A meta-analysis from the Cholesterol Treatment Trialists' Collaboration suggests that each 1 mmol/L (38.7 mg/dL) reduction in LDL-C results in an approximately 20% reduction in the annual rate of cardiovascular disease (CVD) events.

The role of statins in the setting of primary prevention is less clear. Although some trials have shown that LDL-C reduction with medical therapy decreases the rate of CVD events and CVD mortality, their effects on all-cause mortality remain uncertain. In addition, the cost effectiveness of statins and the overall effect on quality of life in the setting of primary prevention is unclear. Therefore, a risk-stratification approach, as advocated by the ACC/AHA 2013 guidelines, is most prudent.

31. **Describe the role of PCSK9 inhibitors.**

PCSK9 inhibitors are the newest class of cholesterol-lowering medications. The PCSK9 inhibitors currently approved in the United States are evolocumab and alirocumab. These monoclonal antibodies to PCSK9 prevent the binding of PCKS9 to the LDL–LDLR complex. This causes increased recycling of LDLR to the cell membrane and enhanced LDL clearance with reductions in LDL-C levels of 50% to 70%. Cardiovascular event reduction has also been demonstrated in several large randomized controlled trials (RCTs). Use of this class has been restricted mainly because of the high cost of these medications

32. What is the appropriate role for niacin?
Niacin reduces LDL-C, lipoprotein(a), and TGs and increases HDL-C. Although older RCTs showed modest benefits of niacin in ASCVD events, newer RCTs and a recent meta-analysis did not show any benefit of niacin as mono-therapy or when added to a statin. The use of niacin is currently very limited as a result of the findings of these newer studies, the many side effects of niacin (particularly flushing), and the new medication options. Niacin is still an option for patients who do not tolerate other medications or who have elevated lipoprotein(a) levels.

33. What is the appropriate role for ezetimibe?
Ezetimibe, which inhibits intestinal cholesterol absorption, lowers LDL-C by 17% to 20% when used as monother-apy. It is somewhat more effective when used in combination with statins, lowering LDL-C by 25%. Ezetimibe added to statin therapy in high-risk individuals has modest effects on ASCVD events.

34. What is the appropriate role for fibrates?
Fibrates, which decrease VLDL production, are the most effective TG-lowering agents. They also increase HDL-C and modestly decrease LDL-C. Although they can reduce LDL-C to a modest degree in some patients without hypertriglyceridemia and in those with FDL, they are not a first-line therapy for treating isolated elevations in LDL-C and should be thought of primarily as a treatment for hypertriglyceridemia.

KEY POINTS: TREATMENT OF LIPID DISORDERS

- Statins are the most effective low-density lipoprotein cholesterol (LDL-C)–lowering agents and have the strongest evidence base for reducing cardiovascular events.
- Proprotein convertase subtilisin/kexin type 9 (PCSK9) inhibitors are also potent reducers of LDL-C levels, and there is evidence for cardiovascular event reduction, but their use is currently limited by their high cost.
- Additional LDL reduction can be achieved by adding ezetimibe, niacin, and bile acid resins.
- Fibrates are the most effective triglyceride (TG)-lowering agents, but additional reductions can be achieved by adding niacin, fish oils, and high-dose statins.
- Management of dyslipidemias usually requires a multifaceted approach, which may include treatment of secondary causes, lifestyle changes, medical therapy, and rarely apheresis.
- The 2013 American College of Cardiology/American Heart Association (ACC/AHA) guidelines moved away from a treat-to-target approach and, instead, recommended treating certain groups of individuals with high risk for ASCVD.

35. What other aggressive therapies are available for FH?
Mipomersen is an antisense oligonucleotide apoprotein B inhibitor; it lowers LDL-C by ≈ 25% to 38%. Lomitapide is a microsomal TG transfer protein inhibitor; it lowers LDL-C by ≈ 40% to 50%. These two medications can have significant hepatotoxicity and are very expensive; furthermore, neither medication has been shown to reduce cardiovascular events. As a result they are seldom used but are available in limited circumstances. LDL apheresis lowers LDL by 70% to 80% and has been shown to reduce cardiovascular events and improve quality of life. This modality is available mainly in specialty centers and is used when combination therapy with statins and PCSK9 inhibitors are insufficiently effective or cannot be used.

36. What is the role of assessment of lipoprotein(a)?
Elevations of lipoprotein(a) are primarily caused by inheritance of apoprotein(a) alleles and are associated with an increased risk of ASCVD events. However, convincing evidence that lowering lipoprotein(a) reduces ASCVD events is lacking. Therefore, the main reason to assess lipoprotein(a) levels is for risk stratification, which may motivate more aggressive treatment other ASCVD risk factors.

37. How should the patient with severe hypertriglyceridemia be managed?
Serum TG levels above 1000 mg/dL must be lowered quickly because of the high risk of precipitating acute pan-creatitis. Medications alone are not effective when TG levels are this high. Patients must immediately be placed on a very low fat (< 5% fat) diet until the TG level is < 1000 mg/dL. Such a diet lowers serum TGs by ≈ 20% each day. Contributing factors, most commonly uncontrolled diabetes mellitus, alcohol abuse, estrogen use, and use of HIV medications, must simultaneously be addressed. After serum TG levels are < 1000 mg/dL, the most effective medications to reduce serum TGs further are fibrates. If these medications do not lower serum TG sufficiently, niacin, fish oils, or a statin may be added to the regimen.

BIBLIOGRAPHY

AIM-HIGH Investigators; Boden, W. E., Probstfield, J. L., Anderson, T., Chaitman, B. R., Desvignes-Nickens, P., . . . Weintraub, W. (2011). Niacin in patients with low HDL cholesterol levels receiving intensive statin therapy. *New England Journal of Medicine, 365*(24), 2255–2267.

Brahm, A. J., & Hegele, R. A. (2016). Combined hyperlipidemia: familial but not (usually) monogenic. *Current Opinion in Lipidology, 27*(2), 131–140.

Canner, P. L., Berge, K. G., Wenger, N. K., Stamler, J., Friedman, L., Prineas, R. J., & Friedewald, W. (1986). Fifteen year mortality in Coronary Drug Project patients: long-term benefit with niacin. *Journal of the American College of Cardiology, 8*(6), 1245–1255.

Cannon, C. P., Blazing, M. A., Giugliano, R. P., McCagg, A., White, J. A., Theroux, P., . . . Califf, R. M. (2015). Ezetimibe added to statin therapy after acute coronary syndromes. *New England Journal of Medicine, 372*(25), 2387–2397.

Cannon, C. P., Giugliano, R. P., Blazing, M. A., Harrington, R. A., Peterson, J. L., Sisk, C. M., . . . Califf, R. M. (2008). Rationale and design of IMPROVE-IT (IMProved Reduction of Outcomes: Vytorin Efficacy International Trial): comparison of ezetimibe/simvastatin versus simvastatin monotherapy on cardiovascular outcomes in patients with acute coronary syndromes. *American Heart Journal, 156*, 826–832.

Cholesterol Treatment Trialists' (CTT) Collaboration. (2010). Efficacy and safety of more intensive lowering of LDL cholesterol: a meta-analysis of data from 170,000 participants in 26 randomised trials. *Lancet, 376*, 1670–1681.

Cholesterol Treatment Trialists' (CTT) Collaborators; Mihaylova, B., Emberson, J., Blackwell, L., Keech, A., Simes, J., . . . Baigent, C. (2012). The effects of lowering LDL cholesterol with statin therapy in people at low risk of vascular disease: meta-analysis of individual data from 27 randomised trials. *Lancet, 380*(9841), 581–590.

Chou, R., Dana, T., Blazina, I., Daeges, M., & Jeanne, T. L. (2016). Statins for prevention of cardiovascular disease in adults: evidence report and systematic review for the US Preventive Services Task Force. *JAMA, 316*(19), 2008–2024.

Chroni, A., & Kardassis, D. (2018). HDL dysfunction caused by mutations in apoA-I and other genes that are critical for HDL biogenesis and remodeling. *Current Medicinal Chemistry*. doi:10.2174/0929867325666180313114950. [Epub ahead of print]

Cornier, M. A., & Eckel, R. H. (2015). Non-traditional dosing of statins in statin-intolerant patients-is it worth a try? *Current Atherosclerosis Reports, 17*(2), 475.

Davidson, M. H., Ballantyne, C. M., Jacobson, T. A., Bittner, V. A., Braun, L. T., Brown, A. S., . . . Dicklin, M. R. (2011). Clinical utility of inflammatory markers and advanced lipoprotein testing: Advice from an expert panel of lipid specialists. *Journal of Clinical Lipidology, 5*, 338–367.

Davidson, M. H. (2013). Emerging low-density lipoprotein therapies: Targeting PCSK9 for low-density lipoprotein reduction. *Journal of Clinical Lipidology, 7*(Suppl. 3), S11–S15.

Eckel, R. H., Jakicic, J. M., Ard, J. D., de Jesus, J. M., Houston Miller, N., Hubbard, V. S., . . . Tomaselli, G. F. (2014). 2013 AHA/ACC guideline on lifestyle management to reduce cardiovascular risk: a report of the American College of Cardiology/American Heart Association Task Force on Practice Guidelines. *Circulation, 129*(25 Suppl. 2), S76–S99.

Emerging Risk Factors Collaboration. (2012). Lipid-related markers and cardiovascular disease prediction. *JAMA, 307*, 2499–2506.

Frick, M. H., Elo, O., Haapa, K., Heinonen, O. P., Heinsalmi, P., Helo, P., . . . Manninen, V. (1987). Helsinki Heart Study: primary-prevention trial with gemfibrozil in middle-aged men with dyslipidemia. Safety of treatment, changes in risk factors, and incidence of coronary heart disease. *New England Journal of Medicine, 317*(20), 1237–1245.

Gupta, A., Thompson, D., Whitehouse, A., Collier, T., Dahlof, B., Poulter, N., . . . Sever, P. (2017). Adverse events associated with unblinded, but not with blinded, statin therapy in the Anglo-Scandinavian Cardiac Outcomes Trial-Lipid-Lowering Arm (ASCOT-LLA): a randomised double-blind placebo-controlled trial and its non-randomised non-blind extension phase. *Lancet, 389*(10088), 2473–2481.

Hou, R., & Goldberg, A. C. (2009). Lowering low-density lipoprotein cholesterol: statins, ezetimibe, bile acid sequestrants, and combinations: comparative efficacy and safety. *Endocrinology and Metabolism Clinics of North America, 38*, 79–97.

HPS2-THRIVE Collaborative Group, Landray, M. J., Haynes, R., Hopewell, J. C., Parish, S., Aung, T., . . . Armitage, J. (2014). Effects of extended-release niacin with laropiprant in high-risk patients. *New England Journal of Medicine, 371*(3), 203–212.

Jun, M., Foote, C., Lv, J., Neal, B., Patel, A., Nicholls, S. J., . . . Perkovic, V. (2010). Effects of fibrates on cardiovascular outcomes: a systematic review and meta-analysis. *Lancet, 375*, 1875–1884.

Keech, A., Simes, R. J., Barter, P., Best, J., Scott, R., Taskinen, M. R., . . . Laakso, M. (2005). Effects of long-term fenofibrate therapy on cardiovascular events in 9795 people with type 2 diabetes mellitus (the Field Study): randomised controlled trial. *Lancet, 366*, 1849–1861.

Larsen, M. L., Illingworth, D. R., & O'Malley, J. P. (1994). Comparative effects of gemfibrozil and clofibrate in type III hyperlipoproteinemia. *Atherosclerosis, 106*(2), 235–240.

Miller, M., Stone, N. J., Ballantyne, C., Bittner, V., Criqui, M. H., Ginsberg, H. N., . . . Pennathur, S. (2011). Triglycerides and cardiovascular disease: a scientific statement from the American Heart Association. *Circulation, 123*, 2292–2333.

Ridker, P. M., Pradhan, A., MacFadyen, J. G., Libby, P., & Glynn, R. J. (2012). Cardiovascular benefits and diabetes risks of statin therapy in primary prevention: an analysis from the JUPITER trial. *Lancet, 380*(9841), 565–571.

Sattar, N., Preiss, D., Murray, H. M., Welsh, P., Buckley, B. M., de Craen, A. J., . . . Ford, I. (2010). Statins and risk of incident diabetes: a collaborative meta-analysis of randomised statin trials. *Lancet, 375*(9716), 735–742.

Saxon, D. R., & Eckel, R. H. (2016). Statin intolerance: a literature review and management strategies. *Progress in Cardiovascular Diseases, 59*(2), 153–164.

Schandelmaier, S., Briel, M., Saccilotto, R., Olu, K. K., Arpagaus, A., Hemkens, L. G., & Nordmann, A. J. (2017). Niacin for primary and secondary prevention of cardiovascular events. *Cochrane Database of Systematic Reviews, 6*, CD009744.

Semenkovich, C. F., Goldberg, A. C., & Goldberg, I. J. (2011). Disorders of lipid metabolism. In S. Melmed, K. S. Polonsky, P. R. Larsen, & H. M. Kronenberg (Eds.), *Williams textbook of endocrinology* (12th ed.). Philadelphia, PA: Elsevier Saunders.

Silverman, M. G., Ference, B. A., Im, K., Wiviott, S. D., Giugliano, R. P., Grundy, S. M., . . . Sabatine, M. S. (2016). Association between lowering LDL-C and cardiovascular risk reduction among different therapeutic interventions: a systematic review and meta-analysis. *JAMA, 316*(12), 1289–1297.

Stone, N. J., Robinson, J. G., Lichtenstein, A. H., Bairey Merz, C. N., Blum, C. B., Eckel, R. H., . . . Tomaselli, G. F. (2014). 2013 ACC/AHA guideline on the treatment of blood cholesterol to reduce atherosclerotic cardiovascular risk in adults: a report of the American College of Cardiology/American Heart Association Task Force on Practice Guidelines. *Circulation, 129*(25 Suppl. 2), S1–S45.

Vale, N., Nordmann, A. J., Schwartz, G. G., de Lemos, J., Colivicchi, F., den Hartog, F., . . . Briel, M. (2014). Statins for acute coronary syndrome. *Cochrane Database of Systematic Reviews*, (9), CD006870.

CHAPTER 11

OBESITY

Elizabeth A. Thomas and David Saxon

1. **Define the terms "overweight" and "obesity."**
   Overweight and obesity are defined as degrees of excess weight that are associated with increases in morbidity and mortality. In 1998, the National Heart, Lung, and Blood Institute of the National Institutes of Health (NIH) published guidelines on the diagnosis and treatment of overweight and obesity. The expert panel advocated using specific body mass index (BMI) cut-off points to diagnose both conditions. BMI is calculated by dividing a person's weight in kilograms by his or her height in meters squared. A BMI (kg/m^2) of ≤ 25 is considered normal; 25 to 29.9 is considered overweight; 30 to 34.9 is considered mild obesity; 35 to 39.9 is considered moderate obesity; and ≥ 40 is considered severe or morbid obesity.

2. **Does fat distribution affect the assessment of risk in the patient with overweight or obesity?**
   Yes. Accumulation of excessive adipose tissue in a central- or upper-body distribution (android or male pattern) is associated with a greater risk of adverse metabolic health consequences compared with lower-body obesity (gynecoid or female pattern). Abdominal adiposity is an independent predictor of risk for diabetes, hypertension, dyslipidemia, and coronary artery disease. The absolute amount of intraabdominal or visceral fat is most closely linked to these adverse health risks.

3. **Explain the role of waist circumference in risk stratification.**
   Waist circumference is the favored measurement for risk stratification on the basis of fat distribution. Men with a waist circumference > 40 inches (> 102 cm) and women whose waist circumference is > 35 inches (> 88 cm) have increased risk. Waist circumference is most useful for risk stratification in people with BMI between 25 and 30 kg/m^2. In this intermediate-risk group, those with increased waist circumference should undertake greater efforts directed at preventing further weight gain, whereas those with a smaller waist circumference can be reassured that their weight likely does not pose major health hazards.

4. **How is waist circumference measured?**
   Waist circumference should be measured with a tape placed parallel to the floor, at the level of the iliac crest, at the end of a relaxed expiration.

5. **What adverse health consequences are associated with obesity?**
   Obesity is clearly associated with diabetes, hypertension, hyperlipidemia, coronary artery disease (CAD), degenerative arthritis, gallbladder disease, and cancers of the endometrium, breast, prostate, and colon. It has also been associated with urinary incontinence, gastroesophageal reflux, infertility, sleep apnea, and congestive heart failure (CHF). The incidence of these conditions rises steadily as body weight increases (Figs. 11.1 and 11.2). Risks increase with even modest weight gain. Health risks are magnified with advancing age and a positive family history of obesity-related diseases.

6. **Summarize the economic consequences of obesity.**
   The annual total direct and indirect U.S. health care costs associated with obesity were estimated to exceed $275 billion in 2016. Much of the direct cost of obesity results from the high cost of treating obesity-related comorbidities, such as cardiovascular disease and type 2 diabetes (T2D).

7. **What are the psychological complications of obesity?**
   Situational depression and anxiety related to obesity are common. The person with obesity may suffer from discrimination that contributes further to difficulty with poor self-image and social isolation. It may be difficult in some patients to determine whether depression is accelerating weight gain or whether weight gain is exacerbating an underlying depression, but treating both conditions may improve quality of life. Work by the Rudd Center and other groups has highlighted the bias that patients with obesity experience, even in doctors who care for them. It is important for treating physicians to at least be aware of a tendency to blame patients with obesity for their condition and to overcome this common bias, if present, as much they can.

8. **How common is obesity?**
   Obesity has reached epidemic proportions in the United States. The National Health and Nutrition Examination Survey (NHANES) conducted by the federal government uses direct measures of height and weight in a representative

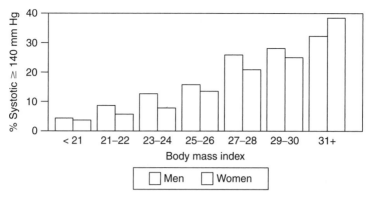

Fig. 11.1. Body mass index and the risk of hypertension. (From Health Canada. (1989). *Canadian Guidelines for Healthy Weights* (p. 69). Catalogue No. H39-134 1989e.)

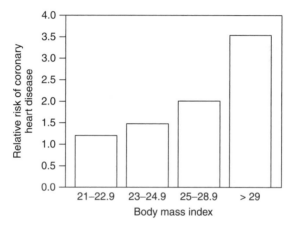

Fig. 11.2. Body mass index and the risk of coronary artery disease.

sample of Americans to estimate the prevalence of obesity. The latest data from the NHANES showed that in 2015 to 2016, the prevalence of obesity was 39.8% in adults and 18.5% in the young. The overall prevalence of obesity is higher among non-Hispanic black and Hispanic adults than among non-Hispanic white and non-Hispanic Asian adults. The same pattern is seen among the young.

9. What caused the dramatic rise in the prevalence of obesity in the 1980s and 1990s?
   The prevalence of obesity, indeed, rose significantly over this short period; it seems that the primary culprit is a changing environment that promotes increased food intake and reduced physical activity. This statement should not be taken to mean, however, that body weight is not subject to physiologic regulation. The control of body weight is complex, with multiple interrelated systems controlling caloric intake, the macronutrient content of the diet, energy expenditure, and fuel metabolism.

10. Describe the current model for obesity as a chronic disease.
    Obesity is now viewed as a chronic, often progressive, metabolic disease, much like diabetes or hypertension. This view requires a conceptual shift from the previous widely held belief that obesity is simply a cosmetic or behavioral problem. Development of obesity requires a period of positive energy balance during which energy intake exceeds energy expenditure. Maintaining energy balance is one of the most important survival mechanisms of any organism. A sustained negative imbalance between energy intake and expenditure can become potentially life threatening within a relatively short time. To maintain energy balance, the organism must assess energy stores within the body; assess the nutrient content of the diet; determine whether the body is in negative energy or nutrient balance; and adjust hormone levels, energy expenditure, nutrient movement, and eating behavior in response to these assessments.

11. Do abnormal genes cause obesity?

Obesity is clearly more common in people who have family members who are also obese. Genetics appear to be responsible for 30% to 60% of the variance in weight in most populations. The problem of human obesity, however, involves an interaction between genetic susceptibility and environmental triggers. The genes that we possess to regulate body weight evolved somewhere between 200,000 and 1 million years ago, at which time the environmental factors controlling nutrient acquisition and habitual physical activity were dramatically different. A number of single gene defects have been identified that cause severe childhood obesity. These include mutations in the leptin gene, leptin receptor, the melanocortin 4 receptor (*MC4-R*) gene, brain-derived neurotrophic factor (BDNF), single-minded homologue 1 (SIM-1), and others. However, these mutations are quite rare, explaining < 8% of severe early-onset obesity. Genome-wide association studies (GWAS) have identified > 20 genes that are associated with common forms of human obesity. The most common of these is the *FTO* gene. The allele of this gene that is associated with weight gain is present in 15% of humans. However, the weight gain associated with this high-risk allele is only 3 kg. Thus, common human obesity appears to be the result of alterations in a large number of genes each having relatively small effects (polygenic).

12. What is leptin?

Leptin is a hormone secreted exclusively by adipose tissue in direct proportion to fat mass. It was discovered in 1994. Leptin acts through receptors located on neurons in the arcuate nucleus of the hypothalamus and other brain regions to regulate both food intake and energy expenditure. Changes in leptin levels in the hypothalamus alter the production of a number of neuropeptides, including proopiomelanocortin (POMC) and agouti-related peptide (AGRP).

13. Does leptin deficiency cause human obesity?

In a handful of cases, genetic deficiency of either leptin or its receptor has been found to cause severe early-onset obesity. Treating individuals with leptin deficiency with leptin results in dramatic weight loss. However, leptin levels are typically increased in obese compared with lean persons in proportion to their increased fat mass. Studies in which recombinant human leptin was administered to those typically obese produced minimal weight loss. These findings suggest that common forms of human obesity are associated with leptin resistance, not leptin deficiency.

14. Explain how the melanocortin system is involved in weight regulation.

Alpha-melanocortin (alpha-MSH) is one of the hormone products of the *POMC* gene. This neuropeptide acts in the hypothalamus on melanocortin receptors, particularly the MC4-R subtype to regulate body weight. By stimulating the MC4-R, alpha-MSH inhibits food intake, whereas the natural antagonist AGRP, also made in the hypothalamus, stimulates food intake. MC4-R agonists have been developed. Although these drugs decrease food intake and reduce body weight in obese rodents, they have not been found to be useful as single agents in humans with obesity. The failure of these drugs and others that work through hypothalamic regulatory pathways to produce significant weight loss in such individuals has raised questions as to the role of these systems in common forms of human obesity.

15. What is ghrelin?

Ghrelin is a hormone originally identified as a growth hormone–releasing hormone (GHRH) produced by the stomach and proximal small intestine that appears to regulate appetite. Ghrelin levels rise before meals and promptly fall following food intake. Self-reported hunger mirrors serum ghrelin levels. Twenty four-hour ghrelin levels rise when people go on an energy-restricted diet and are dramatically reduced after gastric bypass surgery. Ghrelin has been described as a "hunger hormone" and is another possible target for weight loss drugs. The bioactive form of the hormone, acylated ghrelin, has a fatty acid attached to the parent hormone. Drugs that alter the production of acylated ghrelin are also being investigated.

16. Does a decrease in energy expenditure play a role in the development of obesity?

The development of obesity requires an imbalance between caloric intake and caloric expenditure. For fat mass to increase, there must be an imbalance between the amount of fat deposited compared with the amount of fat oxidized. One possibility is that some individuals become obese because of a reduction in their energy expenditure. Despite the common idea that a "low metabolic rate" predisposes to obesity, there is little evidence that this is true.

17. What are the components of energy expenditure?

1. *Basal metabolic rate (BMR):* The amount of energy needed to maintain body homeostasis by maintaining body temperature, maintaining cardiopulmonary integrity, and maintaining electrolyte stability.
2. *Thermic effect of food:* A relatively small component (5%–10%) that represents the energy cost associated with the assimilation of a meal.
3. *Physical activity energy expenditure (PAEE):* This is the most variable component. It can account for as little as 10% to 20% of total energy expenditure in those who are sedentary or as much as 60% to 80% of total energy expenditure in training athletes. PAEE increases with planned physical activity or with activities of daily living (ADLs), such as stair climbing or even fidgeting. The unconscious component of physical activity has been termed *nonexercise activity thermogenesis* (NEAT) and may be a regulated parameter.

18. Explain the concept of energy balance.

When an individual is weight stable, total daily energy expenditure equals total daily energy intake. Total energy expenditure is linearly related to lean body mass. Studies that have used sophisticated methods for measuring energy expenditure have clearly shown that individuals with obesity consume more calories compared with lean individuals. The person with obesity who says that he or she eats only a small amount but is gaining weight may be telling the truth in the short term, but over longer periods, high caloric intakes are required to maintain the obese state. Although reduced levels of PAEE may predispose to obesity, BMR is not reduced in individuals with obesity. The central cause of obesity is the failure to couple energy intake to energy expenditure accurately over time.

19. Are there other factors involved in the increase in the prevalence of obesity?

Investigators have identified a range of novel environmental factors that may be related to the increase in obesity seen over the last 40 years. One area that has received a good deal of attention is reduced sleep time. It is clear that on average Americans are sleeping less than they did 50 years ago. Epidemiologic studies have shown that shortened sleep time is associated with obesity, and experimental studies have shown that sleep restriction is associated with insulin resistance, increased appetite, and a change in fat oxidation. Medication use is another factor that may be involved in promoting obesity. Widely used medications that promote weight gain include antipsychotic medications, sulfonylureas, insulin, thiazolidinediones, and progesterone-containing birth control medications. Other novel factors that are potentially involved include the aging of the population, increasing number of ethnic minorities in the United States, increases in the use of climate control systems in houses and public buildings (mice housed in thermoneutral environments weigh more than mice housed at lower temperatures), and increases in environmental toxins (some studies suggest that adipose tissue increases in response to environmental toxins in an effort to sequester them).

20. What options are available for treating the patient with obesity?

Treatment options for individuals who are overweight or obese include diet, exercise, pharmacotherapy, surgery, and combinations of these modalities. The specific modality should be based on the individual's BMI and associated health problems. A more aggressive treatment approach is warranted in those whose BMI is higher and those with weight-related health problems. Behavioral approaches can be advocated for all individuals who are overweight or obese. Pharmacologic treatment should be considered in those with BMI > 27 kg/m^2 in the presence of medical complications or > 30 kg/m^2 in the absence of medical complications. Surgical treatment is currently reserved for those with BMI > 40 kg/m^2, or BMI > 35 kg/m^2 with comorbidities. Recent evidence suggests that bariatric surgery is also helpful for patients with diabetes whose BMI is < 35 kg/m^2.

21. What is the goal of a weight loss program?

Before discussing the treatment options with a patient, it is important to determine the goal of the treatment program. Many patients with obesity have unrealistic expectations about the amount of weight that they could lose through a weight loss program. Most would like to achieve ideal body weight and are disappointed if they lose only 5% to 10% of their initial weight. These desires stand in stark contrast to the magnitude of weight loss that has been seen with all treatment modalities short of bariatric surgery. The most effective diet, exercise, or drug treatment programs available result in roughly a 5% to 10% weight loss in most people.

22. Is a 5% to 10% reduction helpful in terms of health improvement?

This degree of weight reduction has been associated with improvements in health-related measures, such as lower blood pressure, reductions in low-density lipoprotein cholesterol (LDL-C) levels, improved functional capacity, and a markedly reduced risk of diabetes. Most experts now believe that a sustained 5% to 10% weight loss (e.g., a weight loss of 11–12 lb for someone who initially weighed 220 lb) is a realistic goal with measurable health benefits. Alternatively, prevention of further weight gain may be a reasonable and attainable goal, or the health care provider may simply encourage the patient to focus on eating and activity habits and not on a weight goal at all.

23. How can a patient's readiness to change his or her diet or physical activity be assessed?

Stages of change theory can help the clinician focus counseling activities within the context of a brief office visit. Prochazka has hypothesized that a person passes through six predictable stages before he or she is able to change long-standing behaviors, such as unhealthy diet, poor physical activity patterns, or smoking: (1) precontemplative, (2) contemplative, (3) planning, (4) action, (5) maintenance, and (6) relapse. Identifying the stage that the patient is in and targeting counseling efforts to that stage may improve the effectiveness of the counseling activities.

24. What is "motivational interviewing," and how is it used in counseling a patient with obesity?

Motivational interviewing is a counseling style that was developed for use in those with alcoholism. The method is useful when interacting with patients who are ambivalent about changing their diet or physical activity behaviors. The strategies used focus on resolving this ambivalence by having patients explore their reasons for wanting to change and the reasons for finding their current behavior more comfortable. The method grows out of the idea that motivation cannot be created, but for many patients, the motivation is already there; it simply needs to be identified and redirected.

25. Discuss the role of diet in the treatment of the patient with obesity.

The mainstays of dietary modification in weight loss therapy have been diets low in fat and reduced in calories; however, studies have shown that no one specific diet is superior to all others. Compelling evidence in favor of this approach comes from the Diabetes Prevention Project (DPP) and other related trials in individuals at high risk of diabetes. Whatever changes the person makes must be sustained to be beneficial. The clinician should assess the current diet by taking a thorough nutritional history, which may involve a verbal 24- or 72-hour diet recall. Alternatively, the patient may keep a written 3- to 7-day food diary. Assessing meal patterns is important because many people skip breakfast and eat lunch erratically. Attention should be paid to how often the person eats out, especially fast food. Many patients are able to identify key foods that are a problem for their weight loss efforts. Small, gradual changes may be more successful than drastic ones.

26. Should patients be encouraged to attend a commercial weight loss program?

Yes. Current guidelines suggest the most effective behavioral treatment for obesity is a high-intensity, comprehensive weight loss intervention provided in individual or group sessions by a trained interventionist, along with the principal components of the program—a moderately reduced calorie diet, increased physical activity, and behavioral support to facilitate adherence. Most people know what they should eat. The problem is that they either do not pay attention to what they eat or do not find a "healthy diet" palatable. The use of commercial programs, such as Weight Watchers or TOPS (Taking Off Pounds Sensibly), can provide reasonable nutritional counseling, along with social support, which often cannot be provided in the context of a busy office practice. Many patients are surprised at the cost of these programs, which may be a deterrent to their continued use. However, this kind of program involves no risk and may be cheaper in the long term compared with pharmacologic treatment. The scientific literature supports the notion that for many people, commercial weight loss programs are a reasonable option.

27. Are meal replacements useful in a weight loss program?

For some people, it is difficult to control calories through self-selected meals. Time may not be available for food preparation, and convenience may override health concerns. For such people, meal replacements, which are reduced-calorie, nutritionally complete meals, are a reasonable option with scientifically proven effectiveness if used as a long-term strategy. In fact, this approach was used in the NIH-funded Look Ahead Trial, and participants who were in the highest quartile of meal replacement use were four times more likely to meet their weight loss goals.

28. What are low-calorie diet (LCD) and very-low-calorie diet (VLCD)? When should their use be considered?

A VLCD is a nutritionally complete diet of 800 kcal/day that produces rapid weight loss. An LCD contains between 800 to 1000 kcal/day. Commercially available products typically consist of liquid meals that have been supplemented with essential amino acids, essential fatty acids, vitamins, and micronutrients taken four to five times per day. Supplementing the commercial product with fruits and vegetables converts a VLCD to an LCD and may make the diet more tolerable for patients. Recent data suggest that VLCDs and LCDs may produce a degree of weight loss that is better than traditional dietary approaches and closer to what is seen with bariatric surgery. These diets may also be useful for the patient who needs short-term weight loss for a diagnostic or surgical procedure. Gallstone formation is a recognized complication of these diets.

29. What is alternate-day fasting? What is time-restricted feeding?

There are a multitude of dietary strategies that may lead to weight loss success for some individuals. Two strategies that have recently become more popular and are starting to have a stronger evidence base are alternate-day fasting and time-restricted feeding. There are several forms of alternate-day fasting, but probably the most commonly used version involves "modified" fasting, where 500 calories are an allowable intake on fasting days. Time-restricted feeding is a form of intermittent fasting, where eating is reserved for a certain period of the day only, such as from 8 AM until 4 PM. The remainder of the day is the fasting period, and this schedule is repeated on a daily basis.

KEY POINTS: OBESITY

- Obesity is defined as a body mass index (BMI) > 30 kg/m^2.
- A 5% to 10% weight loss is a good goal with known health benefits.
- Current guidelines suggest the most effective behavioral treatment for obesity is a comprehensive weight loss intervention addressing the three components of diet, exercise, and support for behavioral change.
- The U.S. Food and Drug Administration (FDA)–approved medications to help overweight and patients with obesity lose weight are phentermine, orlistat, lorcaserin, phentermine/topiramate ER, naltrexone/bupropion SR, and liraglutide 3 mg.

30. What medications are available to treat obesity?
- Phentermine (Adipex-P, Fastin, Ionamin, Lomaira)
- Orlistat (Xenical, Alli)

- Lorcaserin (Belviq)
- Phentermine plus topiramate extended release (ER) (Qsymia)
- Naltrexone plus bupropion sustained release (SR) (Contrave)
- Liraglutide (Saxenda)
  (See Table 11.1.)

31. Discuss the role of exercise in a weight loss program.

Increased physical activity appears to be a central part of a successful weight loss program. Although exercise does not produce much added weight loss over diet alone in the short term, it appears to be extremely important in maintaining the reduced state. The National Weight Control Registry is a group of 3000 people who were included for having successfully lost 30 lb and keeping it off for a least 1 year. They self-reported 2000 kcal/wk of planned physical activity (60-80 min/day on most days of the week). A discussion of physical activity should begin with a physical activity history. Ask about the frequency of engaging in planned physical activity and any physical limitations that make it difficult to exercise. Then, ask about hours per day of sedentary behavior, including television viewing and computer time. Finally, discuss ADLs, including work-related activities. Assess the individual's readiness to change his or her physical activity.

32. How much physical activity is necessary to prevent weight gain as opposed to maintaining a reduced weight?

In 2008, the federal government published physical activity guidelines for Americans. These guidelines recommend that all adults do 150 min/wk of moderate-intensity aerobic physical activity or 75 min/wk of vigorous-intensity aerobic physical activity. In addition, the guidelines recommend that muscle-strengthening activities that involve all major muscle groups be performed on $\geq$ 2 days/wk. This level of activity is designed to prevent weight gain. It appears that 60 to 90 min/day of moderate physical activity may be needed for maintenance of weight loss. Individuals included in the National Weight Control Registry perform physical activity of, on average, 12,000 steps/day, to maintain a reduced obese state.

33. What major medical organizations and societies support the use of antiobesity pharmacotherapy for the treatment of obesity?

In recent years, numerous medical organizations and societies have published guidelines that support the use of antiobesity medications in certain individuals. Some of the organizations include the Endocrine Society, the American Association of Clinical Endocrinology, the American Heart Association, the American College of Cardiology, The Obesity Society, and Veterans Health Administration.

34. When are antiobesity medications indicated?

Weight loss medications (see Table 11.1) are indicated as an adjunct to a reduced-calorie diet and increased physical activity for chronic weight management in adults with an initial BMI of $\geq$ 30 kg/m^2, or $\geq$ 27 kg/m^2 in the presence of at least one weight-related comorbid condition.

35. What barriers exist to the more widespread use of antiobesity medications?

Medications for weight loss have a checkered history, and concerns about drug safety deter many providers from prescribing any weight loss medications. Fenfluramine (part of "fen-phen") and sibutramine were removed from the market in several countries because of their association with an increased rate of cardiac valvulopathy and cardiovascular events, respectively. Rimonabant was a promising cannabinoid receptor-1 blocker that was briefly approved in Europe but never reached the market in the United States because of serious psychiatric side effects. Other well-recognized barriers to the use of weight loss medications include the perception by some that obesity is not a disease that warrants pharmacologic therapy, lack of provider training regarding the proper use of the medications, and general absence of insurance coverage for weight loss medications.

36. Are phentermine and amphetamine related?

Yes, phentermine is chemically related to amphetamine and works predominantly on the neurotransmitter norepinephrine to reduce appetite. The addictive effects of amphetamine are thought to result from its actions on the neurotransmitter dopamine. Phentermine has substantially fewer dopaminergic effects compared with amphetamine and, thus, has minimal potential for addiction.

37. Is phentermine effective? What is the usual dose?

Phentermine is the most commonly prescribed weight loss medication in the United States. Compared with placebo, phentermine produces roughly a 5% weight loss in 50% to 60% of those who take it. The dose used ranges from 15 to 37.5 mg/day. A newer formulation of 8 mg that can be taken up to three times daily before meals has recently become available.

38. Discuss the side effects of phentermine.

Phentermine is a central stimulant and can cause hypertension, tachycardia, nervousness, headache, difficulty sleeping, and tremor in some individuals. It should not be used in those with uncontrolled hypertension. Blood

Table 11.1. FDA-Approved Weight Loss Medications.[a]

	PHENTERMINE	ORLISTAT (XENICAL, ALLI)	PHENTERMINE/ TOPIRAMATE (QSYMIA)	LORCASERIN (BELVIQ)	NALTREXONE/ BUPROPION (CONTRAVE)	LIRAGLUTIDE 3.0 MG (SAXENDA)
Mechanism of action	Appetite suppressant/ sympathomimetic	Gastrointestinal lipase inhibitor	Phentermine: sympathomimetic Topiramate: mechanism unknown	Appetite suppressant: selective serotonin 2C receptor agonist	Naltrexone: opioid antagonist Bupropion: reuptake inhibitor of dopamine and norepinephrine Suppresses appetite and reward	GLP-1 agonist Enhances satiety, slows gastric emptying
Dose	15–37.5 mg daily (dose in AM)	60–120 mg before meals	3.75/23 mg, 7.5/46 mg, 11.25/69 mg, 15/92 mg	10 mg twice daily or 20 mg extended release (ER)	8/90 mg (titrate up to 32/360 mg daily)	3.0 mg daily (titrate up by 0.6 mg weekly)
Side effects	Increased heart rate and blood pressure, insomnia, dry mouth, headache, tremor	Diarrhea, oily stools, malabsorption of fat-soluble vitamins, possible liver toxicity	Increased heart rate and blood pressure, insomnia, agitation, dry mouth, headache, tremor, suicidal thoughts, acute glaucoma, mood/sleep disorders, cognitive impairment, metabolic acidosis, increased creatinine	Minimal: headache, dizziness, and nausea (rare priapism, monitor for depression)	Increased heart rate and blood pressure, nausea, constipation, headache Precautions: suicidal thoughts/behaviors, opiates	Nausea, vomiting, diarrhea, constipation, dyspepsia, abdominal distention/flatulence
Effectiveness (weight loss compared with placebo)	≈ 5%	≈ 4–5%	7.5/46: ≈ 8% 15/92: ≈ 10%	≈ 4–5%	≈ 5%	≈ 5–7%
Contraindications[b]	Uncontrolled hypertension, coronary artery disease, congestive heart failure	Malabsorption, chronic diarrhea, cholestasis, history of hyperoxaluria or calcium oxalate nephrolithiasis	Recent cardiovascular event, ESRD, hepatic impairment, cholelithiasis, nephrolithiasis, uncontrolled depression, MAOIs or carbonic anhydrase inhibitors	SSRIs, SNRIs, TCAs, bupropion, triptans, MAOIs, lithium, tramadol, antipsychotics, valvular heart disease	Uncontrolled hypertension, seizures, bupropion, eating disorders, opioid use, MAOIs, alcohol use	Personal or family history of medullary thyroid cancer, severe gastrointestinal disease, gastroparesis, history of pancreatitis, history of suicide attempts

[a]All listed medications are FDA approved for long-term use, except for phentermine, which is approved for 3-months' use.
[b]All weight loss medications are contraindicated during pregnancy.
ESRD, End-stage renal disease; FDA, U.S. Food and Drug Administration; GLP-1, glucagon-like peptide 1; MAOI, monoamine oxidase inhibitor; SMRI, serotonin and norepinephrine reuptake inhibitor; SSRI, selective serotonin reuptake inhibitor; TCA, tricyclic antidepressant.

pressure should be monitored closely after initiation of this medicine. There is no evidence that when used alone (in contrast to the combination of phentermine with fenfluramine), it is associated with cardiac valvular or pulmonary vascular toxicity. Phentermine is only approved by the FDA for 3-month use. However, it has been widely prescribed longer than any other weight loss agent, and there has been no evidence of serious long-term side effects.

39. **How does orlistat work? What is the usual dose?**

Orlistat is a pancreatic lipase inhibitor. At the prescription strength of 120 mg three times a day with meals (trade name Xenical), it reduces the absorption of dietary fat by roughly 30% by inhibiting the enzyme responsible for fat digestion. The average weight loss seen is about 5%. This medication may be preferred in those with mood disorders, heart disease, or poorly controlled hypertension. A 60-mg form (trade name Alli) has been approved by the FDA and is available over the counter. This strength is less effective than the prescription strength, giving roughly a 2% to 4% weight loss.

40. **What are the side effects of orlistat?**

The main side effects result from the malabsorption of fat. Patients who eat a high-fat meal experience greasy stools and may even have problems with incontinence of stool. If the patient chooses to skip the medication, he or she can eat a high-fat meal without side effects and without the benefit that the medication would otherwise provide. The FDA has approved orlistat for long-term use, and there is no specific mention in the package insert of when it should be stopped. Because of the potential to cause fat-soluble vitamin deficiencies, patients should be instructed to take a multivitamin daily. Orlistat should be used with caution in those taking warfarin (Coumadin) and is contraindicated in those on cyclosporine.

41. **Discuss the use of lorcaserin.**

Lorcaserin is a selective 5-hydroxytryptamine (HT) 2C (5-HT2C) receptor agonist that modifies serotonin signaling to reduce food intake. Specifically, the activation of the 5-HT2C receptor leads to the activation of POMC production, which causes satiety. The 5-HT2C receptor is located almost exclusively in the brain. Average weight loss with lorcaserin was approximately 4% to 5% in clinical trials. The medication is sold under the trade name Belviq and is available in twice-daily dosing and also in a once-daily ER form.

42. **Discuss the use of phentermine plus topiramate ER in obesity treatment.**

Topiramate is indicated for the treatment of seizure disorder and migraine. In clinical trials, individuals taking phentermine plus topiramate experienced a mean weight loss of 8% to 10%. The recommended dose is phentermine 7.5 mg plus topiramate ER 46 mg. The higher dosage of phentermine 15 mg plus topiramate 92 mg can also be prescribed. The combination medication (trade name Qsymia) cannot be used during pregnancy because data have shown that fetuses exposed to topiramate during the first trimester are at increased risk of oral clefts (cleft lip with or without cleft palate). Females of reproductive age should have a negative pregnancy test result before starting the medication, should use effective contraception and should have pregnancy tests every month while on the medication. Additionally, the medication cannot be used in patients with glaucoma or hyperthyroidism.

43. **Discuss the use of naltrexone plus bupropion SR in obesity treatment.**

Bupropion is a dopamine and norepinephrine reuptake inhibitor that stimulates POMC neurons. When combined with naltrexone (an opioid antagonist), bupropion enhances efficacy by releasing feedback inhibition of POMC neurons that naltrexone potentiates. The combination of the two medications was approved by the FDA in 2014 for chronic weight management (trade name Contrave). The average weight loss with the combined medication was approximately 5% in clinical trials. Common side effects include nausea, constipation, headache, and dizziness. The medication should not be used in patients with uncontrolled hypertension, seizure disorders, or anorexia or bulimia; in those with drug or alcohol withdrawal; and in patients concurrently taking monoamine oxidase inhibitors.

44. **Discuss the use of liraglutide in obesity treatment.**

Liraglutide is a glucagon-like peptide-1 (GLP-1) inhibitor that was initially approved at lower doses for diabetes (trade name Victoza). Studies indicated that more weight loss was achieved with the medication when given at higher doses. In 2014, the FDA approved liraglutide specifically for the chronic management of obesity at a dose of 3 mg (trade name Saxenda). The average weight loss in the major clinical trial of the medication was 7.2kg. Common side effects are nausea and vomiting, and there is concern about an increased risk of pancreatitis with the medication. Patients with a personal or family history of medullary thyroid cancer and/or multiple endocrine neoplasia type 2 (MEN-2) should avoid the medication. There is some clinical trial evidence that liraglutide delays the progression from prediabetes to diabetes.

45. **How long will a weight loss medication need to be taken?**

Medications used to promote weight loss will work only as long as they are taken and most weight loss is achieved in the first 3 to 6 months of therapy. If a patient loses weight while taking a medication and then stops using it, he or she is likely to regain the lost weight. If a physician and a patient decide to try a weight loss medication, it should be taken for a minimum of 3 months to determine whether the patient will experience a weight loss benefit. Then, some form of chronic use should be considered, given the available information about the risks and potential benefits of the medication. There are also data supporting the intermittent use of weight loss medications.

WEBSITES

http://www.win.niddk.nih.gov/statistics/index.htm
http://www.acsm.org
http://www.motivationalinterview.org
http://www.niddk.nih.gov/health/nutrit/nutrit.htm
http://www.health.gov/paguidelines/factsheetprof.aspx

BIBLIOGRAPHY

Apovian, C. M., Aronne, L. J., Bessesen, D. H., McDonnell, M. E., Murad, M. H., Pagotto, U., ... Still, C. D. (2015). Pharmacological management of obesity: an Endocrine Society clinical practice guideline. *Journal of Clinical Endocrinology and Metabolism, 2*, 342–362.

Bessesen, D. H., & Van Gaal, L. F. (2018). Progress and challenges in anti-obesity pharmacotherapy. *Lancet Diabetes & Endocrinology, 3*, 237–248.

Dansinger, M. L., Gleason, J. A., Griffith, J. L., Selker, H. P., & Schaefer, E. J. (2005). Comparison of the Atkins, Ornish, Weight Watchers, and Zone diets for weight loss and heart disease risk reduction: a randomized trial. *JAMA, 293*, 43–53.

Fidler, M. C., Sanchez, M., Raether, B., Weissman, N. J., Smith, S. R., Shanahan, W. R., ... & BLOSSOM Clinical Trial Group. (2011). A one-year randomized trial of lorcaserin for weight loss in obese and overweight adults: the BLOSSOM trial. *Journal of Clinical Endocrinology and Metabolism, 96*, 3067–3077.

Finkelstein, E. A., Trogdon, J. G., Cohen, J. W., & Dietz, W. (2009). Annual medical spending attributable to obesity: payer-and service-specific estimates. *Health Affairs, 28*, w822–w831.

Flegal, K. M., Kruszon-Moran, D., Carroll, M. D., Fryar, C. D., & Ogden, C. L. (2016). Trends in obesity among adults in the United States, 2005 to 2014. *JAMA, 21*, 2284–2291.

Foster, G. D., Wyatt, H. R., Hill, J. O., McGuckin, B. G., Brill, C., Mohammed, B. S., ... Klein, S. (2003). A randomized trial of a low-carbohydrate diet for obesity. *New England Journal of Medicine, 348*, 2082–2090.

Gadde, K. M., Allison, D. B., Ryan, D. H., Peterson, C. A., Troupin, B., Schwiers, M. L., & Day, W. W. (2011). Effects of low-dose, controlled-release, phentermine plus topiramate combination on weight and associated comorbidities in overweight and obese adults (CONQUER): a randomised, placebo-controlled, phase 3 trial. *Lancet, 377*(9774), 1341–1352.

Hales, C. M., Carroll, M. D., Fryar, C. D., & Ogden, C. L. (2017). Prevalence of obesity among adults and youth: United States, 2015–2016. *NCHS Data Brief, (288)*, 1–8.

Hession, M., Rolland, C., Kulkarni, U., Wise, A., & Broom, J. (2009). Systematic review of randomized controlled trials of low-carbohydrate vs. low-fat/low-calorie diets in the management of obesity and its comorbidities. *Obesity Reviews, 10*(1), 36–50.

Heymsfield, S. B., van Mierlo, C. A., van der Knaap, H. C., Heo, M., & Frier, H. I. (2003). Weight management using a meal replacement strategy: meta and pooling analysis. *International Journal of Obesity and Related Metabolic Disorders, 27*, 537–549.

Heymsfield, S. B., & Wadden, T. A. (2017). Mechanisms, pathophysiology, and management of obesity. *New England Journal of Medicine, 376*(3), 254–266.

Jensen, M. D., Ryan, D. H., Apovian, C. M., Ard, J. D., Comuzzie, A. G., Donato, K. A., ... Tomaselli, G. F. (2014). 2013 AHA/ACC/TOS guideline for the management of overweight and obesity in adults: a report of the American College of Cardiology/American Heart Association Task Force on Practice Guidelines and The Obesity Society. *Circulation, 129*, S102-S138.

Knowler, W. C., Barrett-Connor, E., Fowler, S. E., Hamman, R. F., Lachin, J. M., Walker, E. A., & Nathan, D. M. (2002). Reduction in the incidence of type 2 diabetes with lifestyle intervention or metformin. *New England Journal of Medicine, 346*, 393–403.

Lauderdale, D. S., Knutson, K. L., Rathouz, P. J., Yan, L. L., Hulley, S. B., & Liu, K. (2009). Cross-sectional and longitudinal associations between objectively measured sleep duration and body mass index: the CARDIA Sleep Study. *American Journal of Epidemiology, 170*, 805–813.

Moyer, V. A., & U.S. Preventive Services Task Force. (2012). Screening for and management of obesity in adults: U.S. Preventive Services Task Force recommendation statement. *Annals of Internal Medicine, 157*(5), 373–378.

Nissen, S. E., Wolski, K. E., Prcela, L., Wadden, T., Buse, J. B., Bakris, G., ... Smith, S. R. (2016). Effect of naltrexone-bupropion on major adverse cardiovascular events in overweight and obese patients with cardiovascular risk factors: a randomized clinical trial. *JAMA, 315*(10), 990–1004.

Pi-Sunyer, X., Astrup, A., Fujioka, K., Greenway, F., Halpern, A., Krempf, M., ... Wilding, J. P. (2015). A randomized, controlled trial of 3.0 mg of liraglutide in weight management. *New England Journal of Medicine, 373*(1), 11–22.

Ramachandrappa, S., & Farooqi, I. S. (2011). Genetic approaches to understanding human obesity. *Journal of Clinical Investigation, 121*(6), 2080–2086.

Samaha, F. F., Iqbal, N., Seshadri, P., Chicano, K. L., Daily, D. A., McGrory, J., ... Stern, L. (2003). A low-carbohydrate as compared with a low-fat diet in severe obesity. *New England Journal of Medicine, 348*, 2074–2081.

Tuomilehto, J., Lindström, J., Eriksson, J. G., Valle, T. T., Hämäläinen, H., Ilanne-Parikka, P., ... Uusitupa, M. (2001). Prevention of type 2 diabetes mellitus by changes in lifestyle among subjects with impaired glucose tolerance. *New England Journal of Medicine, 344*, 1343–1350.

Wadden, T. A., Neiberg, R. H., Wing, R. R., Clark, J. M., Delahanty, L. M., Hill, J. O., ... Vitolins, M. Z. (2008). One-year weight losses in the Look AHEAD study: factors associated with success. *Obesity (Silver Spring), 17*(4), 713–722.

Wadden, T. A., Butryn, M. L., Hong, P. S., & Tsai, A. G. (2014). Behavioral treatment of obesity in patients encountered in primary care settings: A systematic review. *JAMA, 312*(17), 1779-1791.

II

BONE AND MINERAL DISORDERS

CHAPTER 12

OSTEOPOROSIS AND OTHER METABOLIC BONE DISEASES: EVALUATION

Michael T. McDermott

1. **What is osteoporosis?**
   Osteoporosis is a skeletal disorder characterized by compromised bone strength, which predisposes to the development of fragility fractures. Bone strength is determined by both *bone mass* and *bone quality*. The diagnosis of osteoporosis is established by the presence of a true fragility fracture or, in patients who have never sustained a fragility fracture, by measuring bone mineral density (BMD) or using the Fracture Risk Assessment Tool (FRAX).

2. **What does fragility fracture mean?**
   Fragility fractures are those that occur spontaneously or following minimal trauma, defined as falling from a standing height or less. Fractures of the vertebrae, hips, and distal radius (Colles' fracture) are the most characteristic fragility fractures, but patients with osteoporosis are prone to all types of fractures. Up to 40% of women and 13% of men develop one or more osteoporotic fractures during their lifetime. Osteoporosis accounts for approximately 1.5 million fractures in the United States each year.

3. **Describe the complications of osteoporotic fragility fractures.**
   Vertebral fractures cause loss of height, anterior kyphosis (dowager's hump), reduced pulmonary function (forced vital capacity [FVC] decreases by 9% per fracture), and an increased mortality rate. Approximately one third of all vertebral fractures are painful but two thirds are asymptomatic. Hip fractures are associated with permanent disability in nearly 50% of patients and with a 20% excess mortality rate compared with the age-matched population without fractures.

4. **What factors contribute most to the risk of developing an osteoporotic fracture?**
   - Low bone mineral density (BMD) [twofold increased risk for every one standard deviation (T-score) decrease of BMD]
   - Age (twofold increased risk for every decade of age above 60 years)
   - Previous fragility fracture (fivefold increased risk for a previous fracture)
   - Frequent falls
   - Corticosteroid use

5. **How is the diagnosis of osteoporosis made?**
   Osteoporosis can be diagnosed by any one of three criteria: fragility fracture, low BMD, high FRAX risk score.

FRAGILITY FRACTURE CRITERIA

- The presence or history of a fragility fracture establishes a diagnosis of osteoporosis, regardless of the BMD T-score.

BONE DENSITOMETRY CRITERIA

- BMD T-score below -2.5 at any site indicates the presence of osteoporosis in a patient aged > 50 years without fractures; the diagnostic T-score ranges are as follows:

T-score ≥ -1	Normal
T-score between -1 and -2.5	Osteopenia
T-score ≤ -2.5	Osteoporosis

- In a premenopausal woman or man aged < 50 years, the diagnosis can be made based on a BMD Z-score of ≤ -2.0 at the lowest skeletal site.

FRAX RISK ASSESSMENT CRITERIA

- A FRAX risk score (10 years) $\geq$ 3% for hip fracture or $\geq$ 20% for major osteoporosis fractures can also be used to diagnose osteoporosis.

6. How do you determine whether a patient has had a previous vertebral fracture?

Back pain or tenderness are helpful clues but may be absent because two thirds of vertebral fractures are asymptomatic. Height loss of $\geq$ 2 inches or dorsal kyphosis are highly suggestive clinical findings. Vertebral imaging with lateral spine films or vertebral fracture assessment (VFA) on dual energy x-ray absorptiometry (DXA) images are the most accurate ways to detect existing vertebral fractures.

7. How is BMD currently measured?

DXA is the most widely used method in current practice. Radiation exposure is minimal, with only 1 to 3 μSv/site compared with 50 to 100 μSv for one chest radiograph. BMD can also be measured by computed tomography (CT) (50 μSv) and ultrasonography (no radiation). Central measurements (spine and hip) are the best predictors of fracture risk and have the best precision for longitudinal monitoring. Peripheral measurements (heel, radius, hands) are widely available and less expensive but are less accurate. Bone densitometry testing is covered in more detail in Chapter 13.

8. What are the currently accepted indications for BMD measurement?

- Age $\geq$ 65 years (women); age $\geq$ 70 years (men)
- Estrogen deficiency plus one risk factor for osteoporosis
- Vertebral deformity, fracture, or osteopenia by x-ray
- Primary hyperparathyroidism
- Glucocorticoid therapy, $\geq$ 5 mg/day of prednisone for $\geq$ 3 months
- Monitoring the response to an osteoporosis medication approved by the U.S. Food and Drug Administration (FDA)

9. How do you read a bone densitometry report?

T-score: Number of standard deviations (SDs) the patient is below or above the mean value for young (20–30 years old) normal subjects (peak bone mass). The T-score is the best overall predictor of fracture risk.

Z-score: Number of SDs the patient is below or above the mean value for age-matched normal subjects. The Z-score indicates whether or not the BMD is appropriate for age. A low Z-score is predictive of an underlying secondary cause other than age or menopause.

Absolute BMD: The actual BMD expressed in g/cm^2. This is the value that should be used to calculate changes in BMD during longitudinal follow-up.

10. What estimates of bone loss and fracture risk can be made from a patient's bone mineral density measurement with DXA?

T-Score	Bone Loss (%)	Increase in Fracture Risk
−1	12%	2 times
−2	24%	4 times
−3	36%	8 times
−4	48%	16 times

Note: Thirty percent of BMD loss must occur before osteopenia is detected on a routine radiograph; this degree of loss suggests a T score of −2.5.

11. How do you use FRAX?

FRAX (www.shef.ac.uk/FRAX/) is a free computer-based program developed by the World Health Organization (WHO). This tool uses clinical risk factors, with or without femoral neck BMD, to provide a 10-year absolute risk estimate for developing a hip or another major osteoporotic fracture (wrist, proximal humerus, etc.). It is recommended for use in making treatment decisions in drug-naïve patients age > 40 years with *osteopenia* on BMD testing and without fragility fractures. Treatment is advised for those who have a 10-year risk $\geq$ 3% for hip fracture or $\geq$ 20% for major osteoporosis fractures.

12. What is a trabecular bone score, and how is it used?

Trabecular bone score (TBS) is a newer technique developed to evaluate bone quality. TBS uses data from existing DXA lumbar spine images to produce a gray-level textural index that correlates well with fracture risk in postmenopausal women and in men age $\geq$ 50 years. It can be used in conjunction with DXA to assist with decisions about initiation of osteoporosis therapy. TBS can also be entered into FRAX. It should not be used alone and is not validated as a tool for monitoring therapy. TBS is particularly useful in disorders for which DXA alone significantly underestimates fracture risk, such as glucocorticoid-induced osteoporosis and diabetes mellitus.

13. What are the major risk factors for the development of osteoporosis?

Nonmodifiable	Modifiable
Advanced age	Low calcium intake
Race (Caucasian, Asian)	Low vitamin D intake
Female gender	Estrogen deficiency
Early menopause	Sedentary lifestyle
Slender build (< 127 lb)	Cigarette smoking
Positive family history (hip fracture)	Alcohol excess (> 2 drinks/day)
	Caffeine excess (> 2 servings/day)

Note: Mental disorders, use of antipsychotic medications, and hyponatremia are newly identified conditions that result in an increased fracture risk.

14. What other conditions must be considered as causes of low BMD?

Osteomalacia[a]	Celiac disease
Osteogenesis imperfecta	Inflammatory bowel disease
Ehlers-Danlos syndrome	Gastrectomy/bowel bypass surgery
Hyperparathyroidism	Primary biliary cirrhosis
Hyperthyroidism	Multiple myeloma
Hyperprolactinemia	Rheumatoid arthritis/Systemic lupus erythematosus
Alcoholism	Ankylosing spondylitis
Hypogonadism	Renal failure
Cushing's syndrome	Renal tubular acidosis
Eating/Exercise disorders	Idiopathic hypercalciuria
High-risk medications[b]	Systemic mastocytosis

[a]Osteomalacia will be covered in more detail in Chapter 15.
[b]Glucocorticoids, excess thyroid hormone, anticonvulsants, heparin, lithium, selective serotonin reuptake inhibitors (SSRIs), aromatase inhibitors, premenopausal tamoxifen, leuprolide, cyclosporine. Probable/Possible: Thiazolidinediones, proton pump inhibitors, excess vitamin A.

15. Outline a cost-effective evaluation to rule out other causes of low bone mass.
Calcium, albumin, phosphorous, creatinine, carbon dioxide (CO_2)
Alkaline phosphatase
25-hydroxy vitamin D (25 OH vitamin D)
Testosterone (men)
Thyroid-stimulating hormone (TSH) (if hyperthyroidism suspected clinically)
Celiac disease testing (Caucasians with symptoms or low 25 OH vitamin D)
Urine (24 hour) calcium, sodium, creatinine
Serum protein electrophoresis (SPEP) (if age > 50 years and abnormal complete blood cell count [CBC])
    Note: Approximately one third of women and two thirds of men will have an abnormality detected with this evaluation. Therefore, this cost-effective evaluation is recommended in all patients with osteoporosis. A low Z-score suggests that an underlying secondary cause is even more likely to be present.

16. What are the most significant risk factors for frequent falls?
Frailty
Use of sedatives
Visual impairment
Cognitive impairment
Lower extremity disability
Obstacles to ambulation in the home
    Note: The most predictive factor for a future fall is a previous fall within the past 6 months. Almost all hip fractures occur as a result of falls. Falls have been shown to predict fractures independently of the FRAX score.

17. How does osteoporosis differ in men?
Approximately 1 to 2 million men in the United States have osteoporosis. The diagnostic criteria are the same in men as in women (fragility fracture, T-score ≤ −2.5, FRAX scores). Nearly two thirds of men with osteoporosis have an identifiable secondary cause of bone loss, most often alcohol abuse, glucocorticoid use, and hypogonadism, including gonadotropin-releasing hormone (GnRH) analogue use for prostate cancer. Treatment is the same in men as in women, although testosterone replacement in men with hypogonadism is an effective adjunctive strategy.

18. How do glucocorticoids cause osteoporosis?

Glucocorticoids adversely affect both phases of bone remodeling, leading to rapid loss of bone. They impair bone formation by promoting apoptosis of existing osteoblasts and reducing the development of new osteoblasts. They increase bone resorption by decreasing the production of sex steroids and osteoprotegerin, an endogenous inhibitor of bone resorption. Osteocytes are also affected and undergo apoptosis.

Note: Patients on glucocorticoids fracture at higher or better BMD values (T-scores) compared with patients with other types of osteoporosis.

19. How should patients on glucocorticoids be monitored?

Patients starting glucocorticoid therapy (prednisone dose ≥ 5 mg/day or equivalent) with a planned duration of treatment of ≥ 3 months or on existing treatment for ≥ 3 months should have their BMD tested and FRAX score calculated at the start of therapy and preferably every 12 months as long as glucocorticoid therapy is continued.

20. Discuss the causes and treatment of osteogenesis imperfecta.

Osteogenesis imperfecta (OI) results from defective osteoblast function, most commonly caused by mutations in genes that encode the alpha-1 and alpha-2 chains of type I collagen (*COL1A1* and *COL1A2*). Autosomal recessive OI is caused by mutations in genes that encode proteins involved in type I collagen posttranslational modification (*FKBP10*, *CRTAP*, *LEPRE1*, and *PPIB*) or other regulators of bone formation and homeostasis (*SERPINH1*, *SERPINF1*, *SP7/OSX*, and *IFITM5*). OI varies in clinical and radiographic features and severity.

Therapy goals are to reduce fractures and pain, and to prevent bone deformities and functional impairment. Data on the risks and benefits of pharmacologic therapy are sparse. Bisphosphonates are used for most forms of OI, but not in type VI, in which bone mineralization is defective and bisphosphonates may cause harm. Anabolic therapy has been used in other patients, but its effects are dependent on the underlying mutation. Patients with OI are best managed in centers with experience in treating this condition.

21. What is hypophosphatasia?

Hypophosphatasia results from inherited inactivating mutations of the gene that encodes the tissue-nonspecific alkaline phosphatase isoenzyme (*ALPL*). The severity of the enzyme defect determines the clinical features, which vary from fetal demise to disabling pediatric forms to milder adult forms manifested by rickets or osteomalacia, dental abnormalities, multiple fractures, or just osteoporosis. Low serum alkaline phosphatase, elevated vitamin B_6 or pyridoxal phosphate, and high urine phosphoethanolamine levels suggest the diagnosis, which can be confirmed with genetic testing. Recently, enzyme replacement with asfotase alfa has become available for treatment.

22. Define osteopetrosis.

Osteopetrosis (marble bone disease) results from defective osteoclast function. Mutations have been identified in the following genes: *TCIRG1* (proton pump), *CLCN7* (chloride channel), *CAII* (carbonic anhydrase II) and *gl/gl* (unknown function). Each of these gene abnormalities leads to the inability of osteoclasts to create an acidic environment in the resorption pit under its ruffled border needed for the dissociation of calcium hydroxyapatite from bone matrix. The impaired bone resorption produces dense, chalky, fragile bones and bone marrow replacement. Skeletal radiography shows generalized osteosclerosis. The diagnosis is made via genetic testing. Bone marrow transplantation to provide normal osteoclasts may be needed in severe cases, whereas high-dose calcitriol to stimulate osteoclasts can be effective in the milder forms.

23. What is familial hyperphosphatemic tumoral calcinosis?

Familial hyperphosphatemic tumoral calcinosis results from inactivating mutations of the gene that encodes fibroblast growth factor 23 (FGF 23). FGF 23 normally acts through the FGF 23 receptor and coreceptor Klotho, to regulate (lower) serum phosphorus by enhancing renal phosphate loss and reducing intestinal phosphate absorption by lowering serum 1,25 (OH)2 vitamin D levels through inhibition of renal 1 alpha hydroxylase. Patients with this condition make insufficient amounts of functional FGF 23 and, as a result, develop painful ectopic calcifications and elevated serum phosphorus levels.

KEY POINTS

- The major risk factors for fragility fractures are low bone mass, advancing age, previous fragility fractures, corticosteroid use, and the propensity to fall.
- Disorders causing secondary bone loss are present in approximately one third of women and two thirds of men who have osteoporosis.
- Patients with osteoporosis should have a complete history and physical examination, and key, cost-effective laboratory tests should be performed to identify any underlying responsible disorders.
- High doses and prolonged use of glucocorticoids produce greater risk, but all doses of oral glucocorticoids and even inhaled steroids increase the risk of osteoporotic fractures.
- Glucocorticoid-induced osteoporosis results from a combination of suppressed bone formation and enhanced bone resorption, accounting for the rapid bone loss often seen in glucocorticoid-treated patients.

TOP SECRETS

The presence of a fragility fracture helps make the diagnosis of osteoporosis, regardless of the patient's bone mineral density or FRAX score.

Each vertebral fracture reduces pulmonary FVC by about 9%. FRAX is designed to assess fracture risk for therapeutic decision making only in osteoporosis drug-naïve patients who have osteopenia on bone mineral density testing. Glucocorticoids cause rapid bone loss because they adversely affect both major areas of bone remodeling, simultaneously inhibiting bone formation and promoting bone resorption.

 WEBSITES

The National Osteoporosis Foundation: www.nof.org
NIH Osteoporosis and Related Bone Diseases—National Resource Center: www.osteo.org
American Society for Bone and Mineral Research: www.asbmr.org
Bones and Osteoporosis: www.bones-and-osteoporosis.com
International Society for Clinical Densitometry: www.iscd.org

BIBLIOGRAPHY

Black, D. M., & Rosen, C. J. (2016). Postmenopausal osteoporosis. *New England Journal of Medicine, 374*, 254–262.
Bolton, J. M., Morin, S. N., Majumdar, S. R., Sareen, J., Lix, L. M., Johansson, H., . . . Leslie, W. D. (2017). Association of mental disorders and related medication use with risk for major osteoporotic fractures. *JAMA Psychiatry, 74*, 641–648.
Buckley, L., Guyatt, G., Fink, H. A., Cannon, M., Grossman, J., Hansen, K. E., . . . McAlindon, T. (2017). 2017 American College of Rheumatology guideline for the prevention and treatment of glucocorticoid-induced osteoporosis. *Arthritis & Rheumatology, 69*, 1521–1537.
Camacho, P. M., Petak, S. M., Binkley, N., Clarke, B. L., Harris, S. T., Hurley, D. L., . . . Watts, N. B. (2016). American Association of Clinical Endocrinologists and American College of Endocrinology clinical practice guidelines for the diagnosis and treatment of postmeno-pausal osteoporosis – 2016. *Endocrine Practice, 22*(Suppl. 4), 1–42.
Carpenter, T. O. (2011). The expanding family of hypophosphatemic syndromes. *Journal of Bone and Mineral Research, 30*, 1–9.
Carpenter, T. O., Imel, E. A., Holm, I. A., Jan de Beur, S. M., & Insogna, K. L. (2011). A clinician's guide to X-linked hypophosphatemia. *Journal of Bone and Mineral Research, 26*, 1381–1388.
Damilakis, J., Adams, J. E., Guglielmi, G., & Link, T. M. (2010). Radiation exposure in x-ray-based imaging techniques used in osteopo-rosis. *European Radiology, 20*, 2707–2714.
Drake, M. T., Murad, M. H., Mauck, K. F., Lane, M. A., Undavalli, C., Elraiyah, T., . . . Montori, V. M. (2012). Clinical Review. Risk factors for low bone mass-related fractures in men: a systematic review and meta-analysis. *Journal of Clinical Endocrinology and Metabolism, 97*, 1861–1870.
Eastell, R., & Szulc, P. (2017). Use of bone turnover markers in postmenopausal osteoporosis. *Lancet Diabetes & Endocrinology, 5*, 908–923.
Gattineni, J. (2014). Inherited disorders of calcium and phosphate metabolism. *Current Opinion in Pediatrics, 26*, 215–222.
Harvey, N. C., Odén, A., Orwoll, E., Lapidus, J., Kwok, T., Karlsson, M. K., . . . Johansson, H. (2018). Falls predict fractures independently of FRAX probability: a meta-analysis of the osteoporotic fractures in men (MrOS) study. *Journal of Bone and Mineral Research, 33*, 510–516.
Imel, E. A., & Econs, M. J. (2012). Approach to the hypophosphatemic patient. *Journal of Clinical Endocrinology and Metabolism, 97*, 696–706.
Kinoshita, Y., & Fukumoto, S. (2018). X-linked hypophosphatemia and FGF23-related hypophosphatemic diseases: prospect for new treatment. *Endocrine Reviews, 39*, 274–291. doi:10.1210/er.2017-00220.
Licata, A. A., Binkley, N., Petak, S. M., & Camacho, P. M. (2018). Consensus statement by the American Association of Clinical Endocri-nologists and American College of Endocrinology on the quality of DXA scans and reports. *Endocrine Practice, 24*, 220–229.
Lindsay, R., Silverman, S. L., Cooper, C., Hanley, D. A., Barton, I., Broy, S. B. .... Seeman, E. (2001). Risk of new vertebral fracture in the year following a fracture. *JAMA, 285*, 320–323.
Long, F. (2011). Building strong bones: molecular regulation of the osteoblast lineage. *Nature Reviews Molecular Cell Biology, 13*, 27–38.
Marie, P. J., & Cohen-Solal, M. (2018). The expanding life and functions of osteogenic cells: from simple bone-making cells to multifunctional cells and beyond. *Journal of Bone and Mineral Research, 33*, 199–210.
Martineau, P., & Leslie, W. D. (2017). Trabecular bone score (TBS): method and applications. *Bone, 104*, 66–72.
Mittan, D., Lee, S., Miller, E., Perez, R. C., Basler, J. W., & Bruder, J. M. (2002). Bone loss following hypogonadism in men with prostate cancer treated with GnRH analogs. *Journal of Clinical Endocrinology and Metabolism, 87*, 3656–3661.
Painter, S. E., Kleerekoper, M., & Camacho, P. M. (2006). Secondary osteoporosis: a review of the recent evidence. *Endocrine Practice, 12*, 436–445.
Palomo, T., Vilaç/Ba, T., & Lazaretti-Castro, M. (2017). Osteogenesis imperfecta: Diagnosis and treatment. *Current Opinion in Endocrinology Diabetes and Obesity, 24*, 381–388.
Rothman, M. S., Lewiecki, E. M., & Miller, P. D. (2017). Bone density testing is the best way to monitor osteoporosis treatment. *American Journal of Medicine, 130*, 1133–1134.
Ryan, C. S., Petkov, V. I., & Adler, R. A. (2011). Osteoporosis in men: the value of laboratory testing. *Osteoporosis International, 22*, 1845–1853.
Shapiro, J. R., & Lewiecki, E. M. (2017). Hypophosphatasia in adults: clinical assessment and treatment considerations. *Journal of Bone and Mineral Research, 32*, 1977–1980.

Silva, B. C., Broy, S. B., Boutroy, S., Schousboe, J. T., Shepherd, J. A., & Leslie, W. D. (2015). Fracture risk prediction by non-BMD DXA measures: the 2015 ISCD Official Positions Part 2: Trabecular Bone Score. *Journal of Clinical Densitometry, 18*, 309–330.

Silva, B. C., Leslie, W. D., Resch, H., Lamy, O., Lesnyak, O., Binkley, N. . . . Bilezikian, J. P. (2014). Trabecular bone score: a noninvasive analytical method based upon the DXA image. *Journal of Bone and Mineral Research, 29*, 518–530.

Targownik, L. E., Lix, L. M., Metge, C. J., Prior, H. J., Leung, S., & Leslie, W. D. (2008). Use of proton pump inhibitors and risk of osteoporosis-related fractures. *CMAJ, 179*, 319–326.

Tolar, J., Teitelbaum, S. L., & Orchard, P. J. (2004). Osteopetrosis. *New England Journal of Medicine, 351*, 2839–2849.

Usala, R. L., Fernandez, S. J., Mete, M., Cowen, L., Shara, N. M., Barsony, J., & Verbalis, J. G. (2015). Hyponatremia is associated with increased osteoporosis and bone fractures in a large US health system population. *Journal of Clinical Endocrinology and Metabolism, 100*, 3021–3031.

Whyte, M. P., Greenberg, C. R., Salman, N. J., Bober, M. B., McAlister, W. H., Wenkert, D., . . . Landy, H. (2012). Enzyme-replacement therapy in life-threatening hypophosphatasia. *New England Journal of Medicine, 366*, 904–913.

Whyte, M. P., Rockman-Greenberg, C., Ozono, K., Riese, R., Moseley, S., Melian, A., . . . Hofmann, C. (2016). Asfotase alfa treatment improves survival for perinatal and infantile hypophosphatasia. *Journal of Clinical Endocrinology and Metabolism, 101*, 334–342.

Wu, C. C., Econs, M. J., DiMeglio, L. A., Insogna, K. L., Levine, M. A., Orchard, P. J., . . . Polgreen, L. E. (2017). Diagnosis and management of osteopetrosis: consensus guidelines from the osteopetrosis working group. *Journal of Clinical Endocrinology and Metabolism, 102*, 3111–3123.

CHAPTER 13

MEASUREMENT OF BONE MASS

Christine M. Swanson

1. What is bone mineral density (BMD)?

   BMD usually refers to areal bone mineral density (aBMD), a two-dimensional (2D) approximation of bone mass, estimated as grams per centimeter squared (g/cm^2). aBMD is dependent on bone size (smaller bones appear less dense). It is obtained from a dual energy x-ray absorptiometry (DXA) scan and derived by dividing the bone mineral content (BMC) in grams by the bone area in centimeters squared. BMC is a measure of the mineral (primarily calcium) found in bone. The amount of x-ray energy absorbed by calcium reflects the BMC. Although less commonly used clinically, volumetric BMD (vBMD) can be measured at the lumbar spine (L-spine) and hip with three-dimensional (3D) quantitative computed tomography (QCT). vBMD is expressed in g/cm^3 and is not dependent on bone size. "BMD" in this chapter will refer to aBMD, unless otherwise noted.

2. What techniques are used to measure bone mass, and what is the preferred method?

   The most commonly used and accepted technique for measuring bone mass is central DXA. Central DXA is preferred because it is noninvasive, is of low cost, has relatively minimal radiation exposure (1–10 μSv) with short scanning times, good precision, and extensive data supporting its relationship to fracture risk and response to treatment. Central DXA estimates aBMD at the L-spine, hip (including femoral neck), and sometimes forearm. The most commonly used DXA machines are made by Hologic, General Electric Healthcare (GE Lunar), and Norland. Portable peripheral DXA (pDXA) can assess BMD at peripheral sites (e.g., radius). DXA-generated BMD from central sites have superior fracture risk prediction, but pDXA can be used to assess fracture risk. pDXA should not be used to diagnose osteoporosis or to monitor BMD. The term "DXA" in this chapter will refer to central DXA, unless otherwise noted. Quantitative ultrasonography (QUS) uses the velocity of ultrasound passing through bone to assess calcaneal BMD. QUS is often discordant from central DXA. Central DXA is preferred, but if unavailable, QUS can be used for fracture risk assessment and initiating treatment but not for monitoring. QCT assesses vBMD but requires more time and radiation exposure than DXA. Some software applications can provide DXA-equivalent aBMD values from QCT at the proximal femur. Peripheral QCT (pQCT) devices assess vBMD at the tibia and forearm. High-resolution peripheral QCT (HRpQCT) measures vBMD at the distal radius or tibia, can differentiate cortical and trabecular bone compartments, can be used to estimate bone strength with finite element analysis (FEA), and is primarily used for research. Routine x-rays are not sensitive enough to assess BMD because demineralization is not visually apparent on radiography until $\geq$ 40% of bone density is lost.

3. Why is BMD important?

   BMD is one of the most important determinants of bone strength and fracture risk. Fracture risk increases as BMD decreases and fracture risk doubles for every standard deviation decrease below the young adult mean (i.e., T-score). Hip BMD predicts hip fracture risk, and BMD at the hip and L-spine predict vertebral fracture risk. BMD from DXA is used to assess fracture risk, diagnose low bone mass/osteoporosis, and monitor changes in bone density over time while on or off osteoporosis medications. Serial DXA examinations must be performed on the same machine at the same facility for accurate BMD trends over time (see Question 13).

4. Who should get a bone density screening test?

   The National Osteoporosis Foundation (NOF) recommends screening DXA be performed in certain groups (Table 13.1). Baseline and serial bone density examinations should be considered in those who are initiating or have been on bone-harming medications (e.g., glucocorticoids, aromatase inhibitors, antiepileptic medications, etc.), those initiating or already on pharmacologic therapy for osteoporosis, and/or those at risk for bone loss. Insurance coverage of DXA in certain groups may vary (e.g., screening DXA in men).

5. What anatomic sites are routinely measured?

   A minimum of two anatomic sites are recommended for BMD assessment. Central DXA typically measures BMD at the L-spine (L1–4) in the anteroposterior (not lateral) orientation, and one or both proximal femurs. The two most important regions of interest (ROIs) at the proximal femur are the femoral neck and the total hip (which includes the femoral neck). Other proximal femur sites reported (e.g., Ward's triangle, trochanteric) are not commonly used in clinical practice. If both hips are measured, BMD and T-score from each side should be used individually because there are insufficient data to determine whether mean T-scores for bilateral hip BMD can be used for diagnosis. Forearm BMD can also be obtained in certain circumstances.

Table 13.1. NOF Recommends Performing Screening DXA in the Following Groups:

Women aged ≥ 65 years and men aged ≥ 70 years

Postmenopausal women and men who are ≥ 50 years of age with an adult fracture or risk factor for osteoporosis/fracture
Risk factors include (but are not limited to):
- Low body weight/BMI
- Use of bone-harming medications (e.g., glucocorticoids, antiepileptic drugs, aromatase inhibitors, etc.)
- Disease or condition associated with bone loss (e.g., hypogonadism, hyperparathyroidism, premature menopause, etc.)
- Rheumatoid arthritis
- Family history of osteoporosis and hip fracture
- Tobacco use
- Excessive alcohol use

Individuals within 6 months of initiation of long-term glucocorticoid therapy

Anyone with "low bone mass" on radiography

BMI, Body mass index; *DXA,* dual energy x-ray absorptiometry; *NOF,* National Osteoporosis Foundation.

6. When should forearm BMD be obtained, and which forearm site is clinically relevant?
   The forearm is an anatomic site with a high amount of cortical bone. BMD at the distal 33% radius of the *non-dominant* forearm should be obtained if the patient has a disease or condition associated with greater bone loss at primarily cortical sites (e.g., primary hyperparathyroidism), if the patient's weight exceeds the weight limit of the DXA machine, or if other anatomic sites cannot be used or accurately assessed (e.g., hardware). The forearm typically does not respond well to pharmacologic therapy (and may even decline with anabolic agents) and is not a preferred site for serial BMD monitoring.

7. When should a vertebra or the entire L-spine be excluded?
   A vertebra should be excluded if:
   - It is clearly anatomically abnormal (e.g., known compression fracture, hardware, etc.).
   - There is > 1.0 T-score difference between adjacent vertebrae.
     A minimum of two vertebrae are required for accurate L-spine BMD assessment. Therefore, the entire L-spine should be excluded if there are not a minimum of two vertebrae that can be adequately evaluated.

8. What is a T-score, and when should it be used?
   A T-score represents the number of standard deviations a person's BMD is above/below the average for young, Caucasian, healthy individuals at peak bone mass. It should be used for postmenopausal women and men aged ≥ 50 years. The International Society for Clinical Densitometry (ISCD) recommends that a normative female database be used for women and men, but some institutions may use a male database for male patients.

9. What is a Z-score, and when should it be used?
   A Z-score represents the number of standard deviations a person's BMD is above/below the average of age-, gender-, and often race-matched persons. A Z-score should be used instead of the T-score for premenopausal women and men aged < 50 years. Z-scores are also informative for postmenopausal women and men aged ≥ 50 years because a low Z-score (at any age) may indicate an underlying, secondary cause of low bone mass that should be evaluated with history, physical examination, and appropriate laboratory workup.

10. What are the cut-off values for an abnormal Z-score?
    A Z-score ≤ −2.0 in premenopausal women and men aged < 50 years is considered abnormal for age and gender. Although pharmacologic therapy is sometimes indicated for patients with Z-scores in this range, there is little information available. A decision to treat should be based on a thorough consideration of risks and benefits.

11. What are the cut-off values for an abnormal T-score?
    WHO classifications are based on central DXA aBMD measurements and apply to postmenopausal women and men aged ≥ 50 years (Table 13.2). The diagnosis is based on the lowest T-score at any site. For example, if the left total hip T-score is −2.1 and the L1–L4 T-score is −2.5, the patient's diagnosis is osteoporosis, not osteopenia, at the total hip and osteoporosis at the L-spine. The T-score cut-off value of −2.5 was chosen because it identified approximately 30% of postmenopausal women as having osteoporosis, which is approximately equivalent to the lifetime risk of fracture at the sites measured. It is important to remember that a person can also meet NOF criteria for osteoporosis, regardless of BMD, if they had a fragility fracture, and/or have an elevated fracture risk. Ten-year fracture risk can be estimated using FRAX (www.sheffield.ac.uk/FRAX/). FRAX can be applied to individuals aged

Table 13.2. WHO Classification of BMD (From Central DXA).

T-SCORE	DIAGNOSIS
−1.0 or higher	Normal BMD
−1.1 to −2.4	Low bone mass (also called "osteopenia")
−2.5 or lower	Osteoporosis

BMD, Bone mineral density; *DXA,* dual energy x-ray absorptiometry; *WHO,* World Health Organization.

40 to 90 years. United States FRAX treatment thresholds are ≥ 20% risk for major osteoporotic fracture and ≥ 3% risk for hip fracture over the next 10 years. DXA can only generate BMD and T-scores, it cannot discern why BMD is low. For example, it cannot differentiate osteoporosis and osteomalacia (e.g., vitamin D deficiency). When low BMD is identified by DXA, an appropriate evaluation should be performed to exclude underlying, secondary causes of low bone mass, including history, physical examination, and laboratory workup.

12. How should BMD measurements be used to assess the need for pharmacologic treatment in postmenopausal women and men aged ≥ 50 years?
   Clinical judgment should be used to determine the need for pharmacologic treatment in each individual based on all available data, not just BMD. After appropriate medical evaluation to exclude underlying, secondary causes of low BMD, the NOF and the American Association of Clinical Endocrinologists (AACE) suggest pharmacologic treatment be considered in postmenopausal women and men ≥ 50 years of age with:
   • A T-score ≤ −2.5 at any site
   • A fragility fracture—defined as a nontraumatic fracture or fracture sustained after a fall from standing height or less that would not otherwise be expected to cause a fracture. Typically applies to a fracture at an osteoporotic site such as the hip, spine, humerus, forearm, and pelvis, not fractures in the face, hands, or feet.
   • Low bone mass (T-score of −1.1 through −2.4) and a 10-year risk of major osteoporotic fracture ≥ 20% or hip fracture ≥ 3% based on FRAX (cutoffs for United States. May differ by country.).
   　　Nonpharmacologic management should also be considered, including fall prevention, smoking cessation, getting adequate calcium, vitamin D, and protein, and avoiding excess alcohol.

13. How do you trend bone density over time? What is a significant change in BMD?
   BMD (g/cm^2), not T-scores, should be trended over time. There are differences in BMD assessment in the various commercially available DXA machines (e.g., Hologic, GE Lunar, Norland). In addition, inherent machine error and differences in patient positioning contribute to measurement error. Therefore, only BMD obtained on the same machine at the same facility (ideally performed by the same DXA technician) can be accurately trended over time. A statistically significant change in BMD is one that meets or exceeds the error of the machine (also known as the least significant change [LSC]). Each DXA facility should report the LSC for their facility/machine/DXA technician for each anatomic site. If not reported, a change > 3% is generally considered significant. DXA should be repeated when the change in BMD is expected to exceed the LSC.

14. What anatomic sites are most important for BMD monitoring?
   Anatomic sites with a high percentage of trabecular bone (e.g., L-spine) will change the fastest. In addition, sites with the best precision of measurement are preferred. Therefore, the preferred sites for monitoring (in descending order) are L-spine, total hip, and femoral neck.

15. What are common reasons for inaccurate BMD assessment or BMD trend at the L-spine?
   Laminectomy and lytic bone lesions can falsely lower BMD at the L-spine. More commonly, L-spine BMD is artificially increased, particularly in individuals aged ≥ 65 years. Arthritis, scoliosis, osteophytes, compression fractures, vertebral hemangiomas, internal artifacts overlying lumbar vertebra (e.g., abdominal aortic calcifications, pill bezoars), hardware or prior spine procedure (e.g., kyphoplasty, vertebroplasty), external artifacts (e.g., naval rings, clothing buttons), and osteoblastic bone metastases will falsely increase L-spine BMD and will inflate apparent BMD gains over time at this site. L-spine BMD may not be accurate if a nuclear medicine study or other imaging study that requires oral contrast has been performed recently. Vertebral fractures cannot be diagnosed by DXA unless vertebral fracture assessment (VFA) software is used; therefore, spine x-rays and/or magnetic resonance imaging (MRI) must be performed if vertebral compression fractures are suspected. Spine imaging is important for diagnosis because ≈ 50% of vertebral fractures are clinically silent. DXA images should be evaluated to ensure L1–L4 are accurately labeled and that the same vertebral levels are assessed over time (Fig. 13.1).

16. What are common reasons for inaccurate BMD assessment or BMD trend at the total hip?
   Overlying clothing artifact and differences in hip rotation, femur angle (excessive femur abduction/adduction), and ROI placement can alter accurate BMD assessment and trend over time (Fig. 13.2). The femur should be internally rotated 15 to 20 degrees so that the lesser trochanter is barely seen, if at all. If the lesser trochanter is seen, subsequent examinations should match the degree of rotation on previous examinations to avoid artifactual

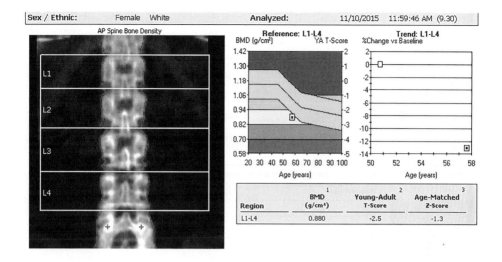

| Sex / Ethnic: | Female White | | Analyzed: | | 11/10/2015 11:59:46 AM (9.30) |

Fig. 13.1. Erroneous lumbar spine (L-spine) bone mineral density (BMD) loss. BMD in a 57-year-old Caucasian female showing 13.1% BMD loss at the L-spine *(top)* compared with prior examination performed 7 years earlier *(bottom)*. Bone loss is erroneous because different vertebral levels were assessed (compare ROI box placement in 2008 versus 2015 images).

changes in BMD. Unlike the spine, osteoarthritis at the hip joint does not affect BMD assessment at the total hip. The hip should be excluded if hardware is present.

17. What is a trabecular bone score (TBS), and when should it be used?
   The trabecular bone score (TBS) software analyzes pixel gray-level variations in L-spine DXA images (in real time or on previously obtained scans) to assess trabecular microarchitecture, an important determinant of bone strength (Fig. 13.3). TBS is a rough estimate of bone quality and predicts fracture risk independent of BMD. TBS is

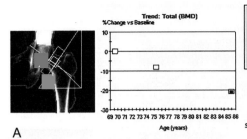

A

Image not for diagnosis

Trend: Total (BMD)
%Change vs Baseline

	Trend: Total			
Measured Date	Age (years)	BMD (g/cm²)	Change vs Previous (%)	Previous (g/cm²)
06/19/2017	85.4	0.553	-13.9	-0.089
04/10/2007	75.2	0.642	-8.3	-0.058
09/25/2001	69.7	0.700	-	-

Statistically 68% of repeat scans fall within 1SD (± 0.026 g/cm² for Left Femur Total)

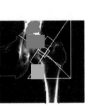

B

Trend: Total (BMD)
%Change vs Baseline

	Trend: Total			
Measured Date	Age (years)	BMD (g/cm²)	Change vs Previous (%)	Previous (g/cm²)
06/19/2017	85.4	0.591	-8.9	-0.058
04/10/2007	75.2	0.649	-10.5	-0.076
09/25/2001	69.7	0.725	-	-

Statistically 68% of repeat scans fall within 1SD (± 0.026 g/cm² for Right Femur Total)

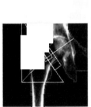

C

Image not for diagnosis

Trend: Total (BMD)
%Change vs Baseline

	Trend: Total			
Measured Date	Age (years)	BMD (g/cm²)	Change vs Previous (%)	Previous (g/cm²)
06/19/2017	85.4	0.578	-10.0	-0.064
04/10/2007	75.2	0.642	-8.3	-0.058
09/25/2001	69.7	0.700	-	-

Statistically 68% of repeat scans fall within 1SD (± 0.026 g/cm² for Left Femur Total)

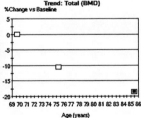

D

Trend: Total (BMD)
%Change vs Baseline

	Trend: Total			
Measured Date	Age (years)	BMD (g/cm²)	Change vs Previous (%)	Previous (g/cm²)
06/19/2017	85.4	0.591	-8.9	-0.058
04/10/2007	75.2	0.649	-10.5	-0.076
09/25/2001	69.7	0.725	-	-

Statistically 68% of repeat scans fall within 1SD (± 0.026 g/cm² for Right Femur Total)

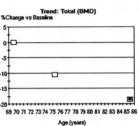
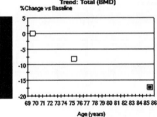

Fig. 13.2. Asymmetric bone mineral density (BMD) change at bilateral total femurs. Relatively greater BMD loss at the left compared with right total hip **(A, B)** from 2007 to 2017. When a red region of interest (ROI) line is correctly drawn on the left femur to more closely approximate the bone **(C)**, BMD loss is more symmetric at the right and left total hips **(C, D)**.

associated with vertebral, hip, and major osteoporotic fracture risk in postmenopausal women, major osteoporotic fracture risk in postmenopausal women with diabetes mellitus type 2, and risk of hip and major osteoporotic fractures in men age ≥ 50 years. Treatment decisions should not be based on TBS alone; however, FRAX assessments can be adjusted for TBS. Current data are insufficient to recommend the use of TBS to monitor pharmacologic therapy.

18. What additional considerations are needed for BMD assessment in children?

DXA assessment in children is typically performed at the L-spine and total body (minus head). T-scores should not be used in this population because aBMD is dependent on bone size and children have not reached peak bone

Bone Mineral Density images   TBS Images and associated reference curves

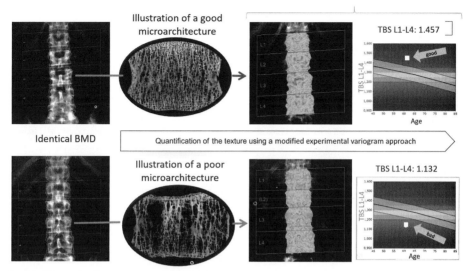

Fig. 13.3. Difference in trabecular bone score (TBS)/microarchitecture for two women with the same lumbar spine bone mineral density (BMD). The woman with lower TBS would have a higher fracture risk than the woman with a higher TBS. (Adapted from Ulivieri, F. M., Silva, B. C., Sardanelli, F., Hans, D., Bilezikian, J.P., & Caudarella, R. (2014). Utility of the trabecular bone score (TBS) in secondary osteoporosis. *Endocrine, 47*(2), 435–448.)

mass. Bone mineral apparent density (BMAD in g/cm³) can estimate vBMD at the L-spine and femoral neck to overcome the limitations of bone size in a 2D DXA image. Osteoporosis diagnosis should not be made based on BMD alone and requires clinical context in younger populations.

KEY POINTS

- aBMD from central DXA is the preferred method for assessing bone mass.
- T-scores are preferentially used to diagnose low bone mass and osteoporosis in postmenopausal women and men aged ≥ 50 years but Z-scores can still provide insight into the possible underlying causes of low bone mass and osteoporosis.
- DXA cannot establish why BMD is low—an appropriate medical evaluation to exclude secondary causes of osteoporosis (e.g., osteomalacia) should be performed.
- Review of DXA images is critical to ensure BMD assessment and trend are accurate.
- TBS is an assessment of trabecular microarchitecture using L-spine DXA images and can be used to augment fracture risk assessment and treatment decisions.

BIBLIOGRAPHY

Bates, D. W., Black, D. M., & Cummings, S. R. (2002). Clinical use of bone densitometry: clinical applications. *Journal of the American Medical Association, 288*(15), 1898–1900.

Blake, G., Adams, J. E., & Bishop, N. (2013). DXA in adults and children. In C. J. Rosen & R. Bouillon (Eds.), *Primer on the metabolic bone diseases and disorders of mineral metabolism* (8th ed., pp. 251–263). Ames, IA: John Wiley & Sons.

Bonnick, S. L. (2010). *Bone densitometry in clinical practice: application and interpretation* (3rd ed.). New York, NY: Humana Press.

Bousson, V., Bergot, C., Sutter, B. Levitz, P., Cortet, B., & Scientific Committee of the Groupe de Recherche et d'Information sur les Ostéoporoses. (2012). Trabecular bone score (TBS): available knowledge, clinical relevance, and future prospects. *Osteoporosis International, 23*(5), 1489–1501.

Camacho, P. M., Petak, S. M., Binkley, N., Clarke, B. L., Harris, S. T., Hurley, D. L., . . . & Watts, N. B. (2016). American Association of Clinical Endocrinologists and American College of Endocrinology clinical practice guidelines for the diagnosis and treatment of postmenopausal osteoporosis. *Endocrine Practice, 22*(Suppl. 4), 1–42.

Cosman, F., de Beur, S. J., LeBoff, M. S., Lewiecki, E. M., Tanner, B., Randall, S., & Lindsay, R. (2015). Clinician's guide to prevention and treatment of osteoporosis. *Osteoporosis International, 26*(7), 2045–2047.

Cummings, S. R., Bates, D., & Black, D. M. (2002). Clinical use of bone densitometry: scientific review. *Journal of the American Medical Association, 288*(15), 1889–1897.

Gourlay, M. L., Fine, J. P., Preisser, J. S., May, R. C., Li, C., Lui, L.Y., . . . Ensrud, K. E. (2012). Bone-density testing interval and transition to osteoporosis in older women. *New England Journal of Medicine, 366*(3), 225–233.

Hans, D., Šteňová, E., & Lamy, O. (2017). The trabecular bone score (TBS) complements DXA and the FRAX as a fracture risk assessment tool in routine clinical practice. *Current Osteoporosis Reports, 15*(6), 521–531.

International Society for Clinical Densitometry. (2015). *Official Positions Brochure.* Middletown, CT: ISCD.

Kanis, J. A., Hans, D., Cooper, C, Baim, S., Bilezikian, J. P., Binkley, N., . . . McCloskey, E. V. (2011). Interpretation and use of FRAX in clinical practice. *Osteoporosis International, 22*(9), 2395–2411.

Lewiecki, E. M., Binkley, N., Morgan, S. L., Shuhart, C. R., Camargos, B. M., Carey, J. J., . . . Leslie, W. D. (2016). Best practices for dual-energy x-ray absorptiometry measurement and reporting: international society for clinical densitometry guidance. *Journal of Clinical Densitometry, 19*(2), 127–140.

Licata, A. A., & Williams, S. E. (2014). A DXA primer for the practicing clinician: a case-based manual for understanding and interpreting bone densitometry. New York, NY: Springer.

Miller, P. D., Zapalowski, C., Kulak, C. A., & Bilezikian, J. P. (1999). Bone densitometry: the best way to detect osteoporosis and to monitor therapy. *Journal of Clinical Endocrinology and Metabolism, 84*(6), 1867.

WHO Study Group. (1994). *Assessment of fracture risk and its application to screening for postmenopausal osteoporosis, WHO Technical Report Series 843.* Geneva, Switzerland: World Health Organization.

CHAPTER 14

OSTEOPOROSIS MANAGEMENT

Michael T. McDermott

1. **What nonpharmacologic measures help prevent and treat osteoporosis?**
   Adequate calcium intake (diet plus supplements):
   > 1000 to 1200 mg/day, premenopausal women and men
   > 1200 to 1500 mg/day, postmenopausal women and men age $\geq$ 65 years
   Adequate vitamin D intake: 800 to 1200 IU/day.
   Regular exercise: aerobic and resistance
   Limitation of alcohol consumption to $\leq$ 2 drinks/day
   Limitation of caffeine consumption to $\leq$ 2 servings/day
   Smoking cessation
   Fall prevention
   Note: Taking more than the stated amounts of calcium and vitamin D is not recommended. Higher intakes may be associated with kidney stones as well as more vascular calcifications, particularly in patients with renal insufficiency.

2. **How can dietary calcium intake be accurately assessed?**
   The major bioavailable sources are dairy products and calcium-fortified fruit drinks. When taking a diet history, the following approximate calcium contents should be assigned for dairy product intake:

Milk/Yogurt	300 mg/cup
Cheese	300 mg/oz
Fruit juice with calcium	300 mg/cup

   In addition to calcium from dairy, add another 300 mg for the general nondairy diet to give an overall reasonable estimate of total daily calcium intake.

3. **How do you ensure adequate intake of calcium?**
   Low-fat dairy products are the *best* sources of calcium. Calcium supplements should be added when the desired goals cannot be reached with dietary sources. Calcium carbonate and calcium citrate are both well absorbed when taken with meals. Gastric acid is needed for normal calcium absorption; calcium carbonate absorption may be significantly reduced in patients who have achlorhydria or who use proton pump inhibitors (PPIs). Calcium citrate absorption is less affected by PPI use. Calcium citrate is also a better choice in patients with a history of kidney stones because citric acid is often low in the urine of stone formers.

4. **What are the best ways to achieve adequate vitamin D intake?**
   There are two natural forms of vitamin D: cholecalciferol (D_3) and ergocalciferol (D_2). Fatty fish (salmon, tuna, mackerel; D3 = 400 IU/3.5 oz), fortified milk (400 IU/quart), and cereal products (50 IU/cup) are good dietary sources. Vitamin D_2 and D_3 supplements are available over the counter in multiple doses, and 50,000 IU vitamin D_2 supplements can be given by prescription. Ten minutes of midday summer sunlight exposure to a fair-skinned person in a tank-top and shorts not wearing sunscreen produces 10,000 IU of vitamin D_3. Dark-skinned individuals and the elderly get less production. However, many individuals wear sunscreen (sun protection factor [SPF] > 8), which prevents vitamin D synthesis in the skin. Therefore, oral vitamin D is necessary for most people. The optimal vitamin D intake is 800 to 1200 IU daily and should not exceed 4000 IU/day with long-term use.

5. **How do you treat patients with vitamin D deficiency?**
   The goal serum 25-hydroxy (25-OH) vitamin D level is 30 to 100 ng/mL. In general, 1000 units (U) daily of vitamin D will raise the serum level by 6 to 10 ng/mL. The following is recommended:

25-OH Vitamin D Level	Management
20–30 ng/mL	2000 U vitamin D_3 daily
10–20 ng/mL	50,000 U vitamin D_2 weekly for 3 months; then 2000 U vitamin D_3 daily
< 10 ng/mL	50,000 U vitamin D_2 twice weekly for 3 months; then, 2000 U vitamin D_3

   Patients with malabsorption syndromes, bowel bypass surgery, and severe liver disease and those who take antiepileptic drugs may require higher doses. Some may need to be treated with calcitriol. Patients who are

Bone remodeling

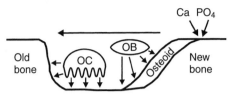

Fig. 14.1. Bone remodeling. *OB*, Osteoblast; *OC*, osteoclast. i

obese, because of their larger volume of distribution of this fat-soluble vitamin, may require higher doses or longer durations of treatment. However, noncompliance is the most common reason that patients with persistently low vitamin D levels on therapy do not increase their levels.

6. Does calcium or vitamin D supplementation promote vascular calcification or coronary artery disease (CAD)?
   The suggestion that calcium and/or vitamin D supplementation promotes calcification of coronary arteries arose from several early, small studies that gained significant attention from the popular press. However, subsequent large reviews and meta-analyses demonstrated that the existing published evidence does not support the hypothesis that calcium and/or vitamin D supplementation, in recommended doses, increases the risk of CAD or CAD mortality. As stated above, however, excessive doses should be avoided.

7. When should pharmacologic therapy be initiated for osteoporosis?
   Pharmacologic therapy should be advised for patients who have any *one* of the following:
   • History of a fragility fracture (vertebral, hip, wrist, humerus)
   • T-score ≤ −2.5 (at any site)
   • Fracture Risk Assessment Tool (FRAX) 10-year risk score ≥ 3% for hip fracture or ≥ 20% for major osteoporosis fractures
      FRAX (Search Engine: FRAX), developed by the World Health Organization (WHO), is recommended for making treatment decisions in drug-naïve patients with osteopenia on bone mineral density (BMD) testing.

8. Describe bone remodeling.
   Bone remodeling is the process that removes old bone and replaces it with new bone. Osteoclasts attach to bone surfaces and secrete acid and enzymes that dissolve away underlying bone. Osteoblasts then migrate into these resorption pits and secrete osteoid, which becomes mineralized with calcium phosphate crystals (hydroxyapatite). Osteocytes serve as the mechanoreceptors that sense skeletal stress and send signals, such as sclerostin, to orchestrate bone remodeling in areas of bone that need renewal. See Fig. 14.1.

9. What are RANK, RANK-L, and osteoprotegerin?
   RANK (receptor activator of nuclear factor κ) is a specific receptor on osteoclasts for RANK-L (RANK ligand). RANK-L, which is expressed on the surface of osteoblasts and other cells, binds to RANK to stimulate osteoclastic bone resorption. Osteoprotegerin (OPG) is a soluble decoy receptor produced by osteoblasts and bone marrow stromal cells that binds to RANK-L, preventing it from interacting with RANK. Bone resorption is driven by RANK-L and inhibited by OPG.

10. How do the pharmacologic agents for osteoporosis work?
    Osteoporosis medications are classified into two main categories: antiresorptive agents and anabolic agents. Antiresorptive medications include the bisphosphonates, denosumab, estrogens, raloxifene, and calcitonin; these agents work by inhibiting osteoclastic bone resorption. Teriparatide and abaloparatide are the currently available anabolic agents; they work by stimulating osteoblastic bone formation.

11. What pharmacologic agents are approved by the U.S. Food and Drug Administration (FDA), and how are they used?

Mechanism	Route	Dose	Frequency
Antiresorptive Agents			
Bisphosphonates			
Alendronate (Fosamax)	Oral	10 mg	Daily
		70 mg	Weekly
Risedronate (Actonel)	Oral	5 mg	Daily
		35 mg	Weekly
		150 mg	Monthly

Mechanism	Route	Dose	Frequency
Risedronate SR (Atelvia)	Oral	35 mg	Weekly
Ibandronate (Boniva)	Oral	150 mg	Monthly
	IV[a]	3 mg	Every 3 months
Zoledronic acid (Reclast)	IV[a]	5 mg	Yearly
Non-Bisphosphonates			
Denosumab (Prolia)	SQ	60 mg	Every 6 months
Raloxifene (Evista)	Oral	60 mg	Daily
Calcitonin (Miacalcin)	Nasal	200 U	Daily
	SQ +	100 U	Daily
Estrogen Therapy (multiple preparations and regimens)			
Anabolic Agents			
Teriparatide (Forteo)	SQ +	20 mcg	Daily
Abaloparatide (Tymlos)	SQ	80 mcg	Daily

[a]Infusion times: IV ibandronate 1 to 3 minutes; IV zoledronic acid 15 to 30 minutes.

IV, Intravenous; *SQ,* subcutaneous; *SR,* sustained release.

12. Explain how bisphosphonates work.

Bisphosphonates are pyrophosphate analogues that avidly bind to bone and are subsequently ingested by osteoclasts during bone remodeling. They inhibit osteoclast function by blocking the enzyme farnesyl diphosphate synthase (FPPS) in the 3-hydroxy-3-methyl-glutaryl-coenzyme A (HMG CoA) reductase (mevalonate) pathway. FPPS inhibition prevents the formation of essential metabolites (Ras, Rho, Rac) that normally connect small proteins to the cell membrane, a process known as *prenylation,* which is critical for subcellular protein trafficking. This interferes with the lipid modification of the osteoclast cell membrane and cytoskeleton that is required for maintenance of the "ruffled border", resulting in impaired osteoclast activity and accelerated osteoclast apoptosis. Because bone formation is not initially affected, bone formation temporarily exceeds resorption and bone mass increases. After about 24 months, bone formation declines to the level of resorption, and bone mass stabilizes. Over this time, bone mass increases 4% to 8% in the spine and 3% to 6% in the hip. This is accompanied by a 33% to 68% relative risk reduction for incident vertebral fractures (all agents) and a 40% to 50% reduction in hip fractures (alendronate, risedronate, and zoledronic acid only).

13. Describe how bisphosphonates should be taken.

Bisphosphonates have very poor intestinal absorption (< 1%), which is further inhibited by the presence of food or medications in the gastrointestinal tract. The major side effect of the oral bisphosphonates is esophageal and gastrointestinal pain. To maximize intestinal absorption and to minimize gastrointestinal toxicity, they should be taken first thing each morning on an empty stomach with a full glass of water. The patient should then remain upright and take nothing by mouth for at least 30 to 60 minutes after medication ingestion. Gastrointestinal side effects can be avoided and adherence improved with use of the intravenous (IV) bisphosphonates (zoledronic acid, ibandronate).

Because of the risk of osteonecrosis of the jaw (ONJ) with antiresorptive therapies, it is recommended that providers perform an oral examination before starting bisphosphonate therapy and any planned invasive dental work (extractions, implants) should be done before starting a bisphosphonate.

14. What is denosumab, and how does it work in osteoporosis?

Denosumab (Prolia) is a monoclonal antibody directed against RANK-L, which is expressed on the surface of osteoblasts. Denosumab prevents RANK-L from binding to RANK to stimulate osteoclastic bone resorption. In trials, denosumab increased lumbar spine bone mass by 6.5% and hip mass by 3.5%. This was accompanied by a 68% reduction in vertebral and 40% reduction in hip fractures over 3 years. Denosumab is cleared by the reticuloendothelial system and can, therefore, be used in patients with osteoporosis and stage 4 chronic kidney disease (creatinine clearance [CrCl] 15–30 cc/min). It is given as 60 mg subcutaneously (SQ) every 6 months in a clinic or an infusion center. This medication is well tolerated, but there is concern that the rate of infections could increase because RANK-L is also expressed on T-helper cells and involved in dendritic cell activation.

Because of the risk of ONJ with antiresorptive therapies, any planned invasive dental work (extractions, implants) should be done before starting denosumab, if possible. It is also recommended that providers carry out an oral examination before starting denosumab therapy.

15. What happens when denosumab is stopped, and what precautions are recommended?

Discontinuation of denosumab has been reported to result in rapid bone loss, and some patients have developed multiple vertebral fractures. For this reason, if denosumab therapy is stopped after at least two doses, it is recommended that bisphosphonate therapy be started; if an oral bisphosphonate is used, it should be started 6 months after the last denosumab injection, whereas if IV zoledronic acid is chosen, it is recommended that it be given 9 months after the last denosumab injection. An alternative to bisphosphonate therapy would be anabolic therapy with teriparatide or abaloparatide.

16. What is ONJ, and which medications may cause it?

ONJ presents as persistently exposed bone following an invasive dental procedure (extractions and implants); it does not occur after root canal procedures or fillings. It has been reported mainly in patients on antiresorptive medications (bisphosphonates or denosumab) and does not occur with the anabolic bone agents. ONJ develops most often during high-dose, frequent administration of antiresorptive agents for the treatment of multiple myeloma or bone metastases; however, it has also been reported in patients taking antiresorptive agents for osteoporosis. Good oral hygiene and regular dental care are the best preventive measures. As discussed above, an oral examination should be done by the prescribing provider before starting bisphosphonates or denosumab and initiating antiresorptive therapy should be delayed if invasive dental work is being planned. For patients already on these agents, temporarily stopping antiresorptive therapy for invasive dental procedures (3 months before the procedure) is a common and reasonable practice but has not been shown to prevent ONJ. Some oral surgeons require that a serum C-telopeptide be in the normal range before they will perform surgery.

17. What about atypical femoral fractures (AFFs) with antiresorptive medication use?

AFFs have also been reported in patients being treated with antiresorptive agents; anabolic agents have not been implicated as causative agents. This complication has occurred almost exclusively in those on long-term antiresorptive therapy (> 5 years). Any such patient with unexplained thigh pain should be evaluated with radiography looking for a "bird beak" on the lateral aspect of the femoral shaft, indicating a stress fracture (Fig. 14.2). These fractures are frequently bilateral and require femoral rods to stabilize. The risk is low (1 in 2000 patients) but appears increased in active patients, those on corticosteroids, and those with very low bone-turnover markers.

Periodic drug holidays for patients on bisphosphonates are recommended by many providers to reduce the risk of AFFs. The optimal durations of bisphosphonate therapy before considering a drug holiday are shown in Questions 27 and 28. A drug holiday decreases the risk of AFFs by 70%. Drug holidays are not currently recommended for denosumab because of the rapid bone loss and vertebral fractures that have been reported in some patients after discontinuation of this medication.

18. Briefly discuss the issues regarding hormone replacement therapy (HRT).

The Women's Health Initiative (WHI) study report in 2002 confirmed the efficacy of estrogen replacement therapy (ERT) and HRT for prevention of fractures but also confirmed a previously reported increased risk of breast cancer and cardiovascular events; following this report, the use of ERT and HRT significantly decreased. Currently, ERT (women without an intact uterus) and HRT (women with an intact uterus) are recommended mainly for limited use for up to 3 years to treat postmenopausal hot flashes, but more prolonged use is appropriate at the discretion of the provider after a thorough discussion with the patient. For a more complete discussion of ERT and HRT, see Chapter 56.

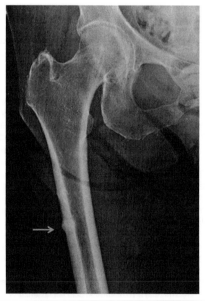

Fig. 14.2. Characteristic radiographic features of an atypical femur fracture.

19. Discuss the use of selective estrogen receptor modulators (SERMs) in the management of osteoporosis.

SERMs are agents that function as estrogen agonists in some tissues (bone) and estrogen antagonists in other tissues (breast). *Raloxifene (Evista)* is FDA approved for the treatment of postmenopausal osteoporosis. In clinical trials, it increased bone mineral density by 2% to 3% in both the spine and hip, and reduced the relative risk of vertebral fractures by 31% to 49% without an effect on hip fractures. Raloxifene has also been shown to reduce the risk (76%) of developing invasive breast cancer. The dose is 60 mg daily. Side effects include hot flashes, leg cramps, and an increased risk of thromboembolic disease (especially in smokers) similar to that seen with HRT. An ideal patient to receive raloxifene is a patient with osteoporosis and a personal or family history of breast cancer.

20. How can parathyroid hormone (PTH) and parathyroid hormone–related peptide (PTHrP) be anabolic agents for treating osteoporosis?

Persistently elevated serum levels of PTH) (hyperparathyroidism) or PTHrP promote osteoclastic bone resorption, hypercalcemia and bone loss. In contrast, intermittent daily pulses of exogenous PTH or PTHrP actually stimulate osteoblast differentiation, proliferation, and survival, resulting in osteoid formation and increased bone mass. They also decrease the production of the bone-inhibiting protein, sclerostin, from osteocytes.

21. Describe the currently available osteoanabolic agents.

Teriparatide (Forteo) is a 34–amino acid fragment of intact PTH that retains the ability to bind to and activate PTH receptors on osteoblasts and osteoblast precursors. It is self-administered daily at a 20 mcg/day dose SQ for 18 to 24 months. In trials, teriparatide increased lumbar spine BMD by 9% to 13% and hip BMD by 2.5% to 5%, while decreasing the relative risk of new vertebral fractures by 65% and nonvertebral fractures by 50%. The most common side effects are similar to those of placebo and include headache, arthralgias, nausea, orthostasis, and flushing. Teriparatide must be refrigerated for the duration of its use; it becomes inactivated if left unrefrigerated for over 24 hours.

Abaloparatide (Tymlos) is a 34 amino acid fragment of PTHrP that also activates osteoblast recruitment and activity. It is self-injected at an 80 mcg daily dose, and its use is limited to 24 months. Spine BMD has been shown to increase by 10.4% and hip BMD by 4% compared with placebo. In a head-to-head trial against teriparatide, abaloparatide reduced new vertebral fractures by 86%, nonvertebral fractures by 43%, and major osteoporosis fractures by 70% (the reduction in major osteoporosis fractures was statistically significantly better than with teriparatide). Side effects are similar to those reported with teriparatide. Abaloparatide does not require refrigeration.

Romosozumab is a monoclonal antibody developed to bind to and inactivate sclerostin, which is an endogenous inhibitor of the Wnt pathway. Wnt is the primary intracellular signaling pathway that stimulates osteoblast activity and new bone formation. Sclerostin acts as a brake to prevent excessive bone formation. Romosozumab inhibits sclerostin, and thereby stimulates bone formation. In clinical trials, romosozumab significantly increased BMD and prevented fragility fractures in patients with osteoporosis. At the time of writing, romosozumab is under review by the FDA and is not yet available.

22. Discuss the role of testosterone for the treatment of osteoporosis.

Men with osteoporosis and symptoms of hypogonadism may benefit from testosterone replacement therapy, especially if the serum testosterone level is less than 150 ng/dL. Testosterone replacement increases BMD in men with baseline low testosterone levels, but fracture reduction data have not been reported; for this reason, it is not an FDA-approved treatment for osteoporosis. Testosterone can be given intramuscularly (100–400 mg every 1–4 weeks; lower doses at more frequent intervals are preferred), as a transdermal patch (Androderm) or cream (Testim, AndroGel, Fortesta, Axiron), or as a buccal patch (Striant). Injectable testosterone pellets are not recommended because of the supraphysiologic testosterone levels that result from their use.

Testosterone therapy does not appear to cause prostate cancer but clearly increases the risk of exacerbation of existing prostate cancer. Testosterone therapy can precipitate or worsen sleep apnea. Evidence regarding cardiovascular (CV) safety of testosterone is currently controversial; however, the CV risk does appear to be increased in men who have on-treatment serum testosterone levels in the supraphysiologic range. Patients without improvement in hypogonadal symptoms should not continue these medications because other approved therapies for osteoporosis have demonstrated efficacy and safety data.

23. Have all these medications been shown to prevent fractures?

FDA-approved medications have all been demonstrated in randomized controlled trials (RCTs) to significantly reduce vertebral fractures in women with postmenopausal osteoporosis. Hip fractures have also been reduced by alendronate, risedronate, zoledronic acid, and denosumab. Nonvertebral fracture reduction has been reported with alendronate, risedronate, zoledronic acid, denosumab, teriparatide, and abaloparatide.

24. Should osteoporosis medications be used in combination?

No, not yet. Combining two antiresorptive medications should be avoided because of concern about excessive suppression of bone remodeling. Combining anabolic and antiresorptive medications is an appealing notion with emerging clinical trial data. The combination of teriparatide and alendronate had no synergy and resulted in inferior bone mass increases compared with teriparatide alone. In contrast, teriparatide combined with zoledronic acid or with denosumab did show synergy with regard to BMD improvements. Despite these promising results, combination therapy is not currently recommended because there are no data showing superior fracture reduction compared with monotherapy. Furthermore, the cost of using combinations is certainly additive and may cause significant problems with insurance coverage. Combination therapy is not recommended, but sequential therapy is clearly beneficial in many patients and is supported by a strong evidence base. Leaders in the field suggest that patients with severe osteoporosis may have maximal benefit by receiving anabolic therapy first, followed by an antiresorptive agent.

25. Summarize the benefits and risks of pharmacologic osteoporosis medications.

BENEFITS

Fracture reduction (significant for all FDA-approved agents)

RISKS

Common side effects
Upper gastrointestinal symptoms—oral bisphosphonates
Acute-phase reactions—IV bisphosphonates (first dose)
Transient decrease in serum calcium—zoledronic acid, denosumab
Transient increase in serum and urine calcium—teriparatide, abaloparatide
Uncommon/rare side effects
Osteonecrosis of the jaw—antiresorptive agents
Atypical femoral fractures—antiresorptive agents
Uveitis, keratitis, optic neuritis, orbital swelling—bisphosphonates
Hypercalcemia—teriparatide, abaloparatide

26. Describe a recommended risk-stratification strategy for osteoporosis therapy.

LOW-/MODERATE-RISK PATIENTS

Oral bisphosphonates (alendronate, risedronate, ibandronate)
Zoledronic acid
Denosumab

HIGH-RISK PATIENTS[a]

Zoledronic acid
Denosumab
Teriparatide
Abaloparatide

27. What is the optimal duration of treatment with osteoporosis medications?
    Oral bisphosphonates:
    • 5 years (low-/moderate-risk patients)
    • 6 to 10 years (high-risk patients[a])
    Zoledronic acid:
    • 3 years (low-/moderate-risk patients)
    • 6 years (high-risk patients[a])
    Denosumab—stopping not recommended without substituting another agent
    Teriparatide/Abaloparatide—24 months

28. Should patients on osteoporosis medications be given a drug holiday? If so, how long should the drug holiday last?
    Bisphosphonates are the only osteoporosis medication class for which a drug holiday should currently be considered. Drug holidays are not recommended with denosumab, teriparatide, or abaloparatide because of rapid bone loss after their discontinuation; if, and when, these medications are stopped, another agent should be substituted.

---

[a]High-risk patients—old age, prior fracture, very low BMD, high fall risk, glucocorticoid use.

Bisphosphonate drug holidays may be considered after a patient has had the optimal duration of treatment (see previous question). Bisphosphonate drug holidays should end under the following circumstances:
- A fragility fracture (spine, hip, wrist, humerus) occurs.
- Bone density decreases more than the least significant change (LSC) established for that specific instrument (see discussion on LSC below)
- Bone turnover markers (urine N-telopeptide, serum C-telopeptide, serum bone-specific alkaline phosphatase) increase by $\geq$ 30% or rise into the upper 50% of the reference range

29. How should BMD testing be used to monitor the response to osteoporosis therapy?
BMD testing to monitor osteoporosis therapy responses is most often repeated after 2 years of treatment. To accurately interpret serial changes, the LSC for the specific instrument must be known. The LSC is a precision estimate that informs the user about the minimum BMD change that should be considered significant. Standard procedures for performing the LSC assessment are available on the International Society for Clinical Densitometry website (www.iscd.org).

30. How do you interpret BMD changes in patients on osteoporosis medications?

BMD Change	Interpretation	Recommended Action
Increase $\geq$ LSC	Good response	Continue therapy
No Change or $<$ LSC	Adequate response	Continue therapy
Decrease $\geq$ LSC	Treatment failure	Evaluate; consider therapy change

BMD, Bone mineral density; *LSC*, least significant change.

31. What markers are available to assess bone remodeling, and how are they used?

Bone Formation	Bone Resorption
Serum alkaline phosphatase	Urine or serum N-telopeptides
Serum osteocalcin	Serum C-telopeptides
Serum P1NP	

P1NP, Total procollagen type 1 N-terminal propeptide.

Elevation of biomarkers predicts future bone loss. A 30% reduction of biomarkers after therapy is initiated verifies compliance and predicts an increase in bone mass. However, marked variability in biomarker measurement limits the utility of this tool.

32. What constitutes a treatment failure to osteoporosis therapy?
This is a controversial issue because all FDA-approved treatments, if taken as directed, significantly reduce the risk of fractures. However, no treatment completely eliminates the risk of fractures because treated patients are already at high risk. The current suggested criteria to define failure to respond to therapy are (any one of these): the development of $\geq$ 2 fragility fractures, decrease in BMD by more than the LSC of the specific DXA instrument, or increase in bone remodeling biomarkers by 30% or into the upper half of the reference range.

33. What do you do when BMD falls significantly during osteoporosis therapy?
The common causes of BMD loss on treatment and their management are listed below.

Cause	Management
Nonadherence $\longrightarrow$	Encourage adherence
Calcium deficiency $\longrightarrow$	Ensure adequate calcium intake
Vitamin D deficiency $\longrightarrow$	Ensure adequate vitamin D intake
Secondary bone loss $\longrightarrow$	Treat the cause
Treatment failure $\longrightarrow$	Change medication

34. Which medications are effective in preventing and treating glucocorticoid-induced osteoporosis (GIOP)?
Bisphosphonates (alendronate, risedronate, zoledronic acid) and teriparatide have been shown in RCTs to significantly improve BMD and reduce fractures in glucocorticoid-treated patients.

35. When should osteoporosis medications be considered in patients age $>$ 50 years who are taking glucocorticoid therapy?
The decision to initiate a bone-active agent is based on risk stratification using FRAX, lowest T-score value, and history of fragility fracture:
- *Low risk:* FRAX 10-year risk for a major osteoporotic fracture of $<$ 10%

- *Medium risk:* FRAX 10-year risk of 10% to 20%
- *High risk:* FRAX 10-year risk > 20%, *or* T-score ≤ −2.5 at any site, *or* a history of a previous fragility fracture
  Pharmacologic recommendations for postmenopausal women and men age > 50 years either starting or currently on glucocorticoids with an anticipated duration of therapy of ≥ 3 months are as follows:
- Low-risk patients on prednisone (or equivalent) ≥ 7.5 mg/day should start one of the following bisphosphonates: alendronate, risedronate, or zoledronic acid.
- Medium-risk patients on any dose (including prednisone < 7.5 mg/day) of glucocorticoids should start one of these same bisphosphonates.
- High-risk patients on any dose or duration (including < 3 months) of glucocorticoids should start one of these bisphosphonates. Teriparatide is another option for high-risk patients who have the lowest T-scores (below −2.5) and/or history of fragility fracture.
- In clinical practice, any patient not on a bone-active agent with a T-score below −1.5 and a loss of ≥ 4% of their BMD after a year on glucocorticoids should be evaluated for more aggressive therapy.

36. How should patients aged < 50 years be treated for GIOP?
    Premenopausal women and men aged < 50 years who have had a previous fragility fracture and are on prednisone ≥ 5 mg/day should receive a bisphosphonate regardless of their FRAX score or T-score. Zoledronic acid or teriparatide are the best options for the patients who are on higher doses (≥ 7.5 mg/day), longer duration (≥ 3 months), and have the worst T-scores (< −2.5). Therapeutic guidelines for premenopausal women with childbearing potential who have had a previous fragility fracture recommend a bisphosphonate only if they are taking ≥ 7.5 mg/day. Oral risedronate theoretically may be the safest in this circumstance because of the potential of less fetal toxicity should the patient become pregnant. Teriparatide is an alternative option.

27. Are there any guidelines for patients on intermittent pulses of IV glucocorticoids or inhaled steroids?
    Therapeutic guidelines for prevention and treatment of GIOP in patients receiving intermittent pulse glucocorticoids without daily therapy are lacking. Patients receiving ≥ 4 monthly IV pulses (1 g methylprednisolone equivalent) or high-dose oral pulses (prednisone ≥ 60 mg/day with taper over 2–4 weeks) within a 12-month period are at risk and should be treated based on the risk stratification outlined above. Patients on daily inhaled steroids (equivalent or higher dose than Advair 200 mcg/day) for a prolonged period (20 years) can lose bone (T-score 1 = 12%) and should be periodically monitored.

28. Develop an algorithm for the diagnosis and management of osteoporosis.
    See Fig. 14.3.

Osteoporosis Diagnosis and Management

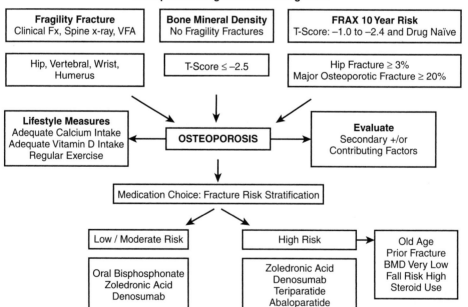

Fig. 14.3. Suggested osteoporosis diagnosis and management algorithm. High-risk patients: old age, prior fracture, very low BMD, high fall risk, glucocorticoid use. *FRAX,* Fracture Risk Assessment Tool; *VFA,* vertebral fracture assessment.]

KEY POINTS

- Nonpharmacologic measures that are effective for prevention and treatment of osteoporosis include adequate calcium and vitamin D nutrition, regular exercise, fall prevention, smoking cessation, and limitation of alcohol and caffeine intake.
- Pharmacologic therapy should be initiated in patients who have had a fragility fracture, a bone mineral density (BMD) T-score ≤ -2.5, or a Fracture Risk Assessment Tool (FRAX)–derived 10-year risk of $\geq 3\%$ for hip fractures and $\geq 20\%$ for other major osteoporosis fractures.
- There are two primary categories of effective medications for treating osteoporosis: antiresorptive agents and anabolic agents.
- Osteonecrosis of the jaw and atypical femoral fractures have been reported in some patients using antiresorptive medications but not anabolic medications.
- BMD loss during osteoporosis therapy is most often because of therapy nonadherence, but affected individuals should also be investigated for other causes of bone loss.
- Bisphosphonates and teriparatide improve BMD and reduce fractures in patients with glucocorticoid-induced osteoporosis.

TOP SECRETS

Medical therapy for osteoporosis should be offered to any patient who has had a fragility fracture, who has a bone mineral density T-score ≤ -2.5, or a FRAX 10-year risk of $\geq 3\%$ for a hip fracture or $\geq 20\%$ for any major osteoporosis fracture.

The greatest bone mineral density gains result from sequential therapy starting first with an osteoanabolic agent followed by treatment with an antiresorptive medication.

Rapid bone loss and multiple vertebral fractures associated with accelerated bone resorption have been reported after discontinuation of denosumab (Prolia).

ONJ and AFFs are uncommon complications that can result from the use of antiresorptive agents, but these complications do not occur with osteoanabolic agents.

BIBLIOGRAPHY

Adler, R. A. (2018). Management of endocrine disease: atypical femoral fractures: risks and benefits of long-term treatment of osteoporosis with anti-resorptive therapy. *European Journal of Endocrinology, 178*, R81–R87.

Adler, R. A., El-Hajj Fuleihan, G., Bauer, D. C., Camacho, P. M., Clarke, B. L., Clines, G. A., … Sellmeyer, D. E. (2016). Managing osteoporosis in patients on long-term bisphosphonate treatment: report of a task force of the American Society for Bone and Mineral Research. *Journal of Bone and Mineral Research, 31*, 16–35.

Anastasilakis, A. D., Polyzos, S. A., Makras, P., Aubry-Rozier, B., Kaouri, S., & Lamy, O. (2017). Clinical features of 24 patients with rebound-associated vertebral fractures after denosumab discontinuation: systematic review and additional cases. *Journal of Bone and Mineral Research, 32*, 1291–1296.

Axelsson, K. F., Nilsson, A. G., Wedel, H., Lundh, D., & Lorentzon, M. (2017). Association between alendronate use and hip fracture risk in older patients using oral prednisolone. *JAMA, 318*, 146–155.

Bindon, B., Adams, W., Balasubramanian, N., Sandhu, J., & Camacho, P. (2018). Osteoporotic fractures during bisphosphonate drug holiday. *Endocrine Practice, 24*, 163–169.

Black, D. M., & Rosen, C. J. (2016). Clinical practice. Postmenopausal osteoporosis. *New England Journal of Medicine, 374*, 254–262.

Bone, H. G., Wagman, R. B., Brandi, M. L., Brown, J. P., Chapurlat, R., Cummings, S. R., … Papapoulos, S. (2017). 10 years of denosumab treatment in postmenopausal women with osteoporosis: results from the phase 3 randomised FREEDOM trial and open-label extension. *Lancet Diabetes & Endocrinology, 5*, 513–523.

Bonnick, S., Johnston, C. C., Jr., Kleerekoper, M., Lindsay, R., Miller, P., Sherwood, L., & Siris, E. (2001). Importance of precision in bone density measurements. *Journal of Clinical Densitometry, 4*, 105–110.

Buckley, L., Guyatt, G., Fink, H. A., Cannon, M., Grossman, J., Hansen, K. E., … McAlindon, T. (2017). 2017 American College of Rheumatology guideline for the prevention and treatment of glucocorticoid-induced osteoporosis. *Arthritis & Rheumatology, 69*, 1521–1537.

Camacho, P. M., Petak, S. M., Binkley, N., Clarke, B. L., Harris, S. T., Hurley, D. L., … Watts N. B. (2016). American Association of Clinical Endocrinologists and American College of Endocrinology clinical practice guidelines for the diagnosis and treatment of postmenopausal osteoporosis – 2016. *Endocrine Practice, 22*(Suppl. 4), 1–42.

Chapurlat, R. (2018). Effects and management of denosumab discontinuation. *Joint Bone Spine, 85*, 515–517. doi:10.1016/j.jbspin.2017.12.013.

Chung, M., Tang, A. M., Fu, Z., Wang, D. D., & Newberry, S. J. (2016). Calcium intake and cardiovascular disease risk: an updated systematic review and meta-analysis. *Annals of Internal Medicine, 165*, 856–866.

Cosman, F., Crittenden, D. B., Adachi, J. D., Binkley, N., Czerwinski, E., Ferrari, S., … Grauer A. (2016). Romosozumab treatment in postmenopausal women with osteoporosis. *New England Journal of Medicine. 375*, 1532–1543.

Cosman, F., Miller, P. D., Williams, C. G., Hattersley, G., Hu, M. Y., Valter, I., … Black, D. (2017). Eighteen months of treatment with subcutaneous abaloparatide followed by 6 months of treatment with alendronate in postmenopausal women with osteoporosis: results of the ACTIVExtend trial. *Mayo Clinic Proceedings, 92*, 200–210.

Cosman, F., Nieves, J. W., & Dempster, D. W. (2017). Treatment sequence matters: anabolic and antiresorptive therapy for osteoporosis. *Journal of Bone and Mineral Research, 32*, 198–202.

Crandall, C. J., Newberry, S. J., Diamant, A., Lim YW, Gellad, W. F., Booth, M. J., … Shekelle, P. G. (2014). Comparative effectiveness of pharmacologic treatments to prevent fractures: an updated systematic review. *Annals of Internal Medicine, 161*, 711–723.

Cummings, S. R., Cosman, F., Lewiecki, E. M., Schousboe, J. T., Bauer, D. C., Black, D. M., … Randall, S. (2017). Goal-directed treatment for osteoporosis: a progress report from the ASBMR-NOF Working Group on Goal-Directed Treatment for Osteoporosis. *Journal of Bone and Mineral Research, 32*, 3–10.

Cummings, S. R., Ferrari, S., Eastell, R., Gilchrist, N., Jensen, J. B., McClung, M., … Brown, J. P. (2018). Vertebral fractures after discontinuation of denosumab: a post hoc analysis of the randomized placebo-controlled FREEDOM trial and its extension. *Journal of Bone and Mineral Research, 33*, 190–198.

Eastell, R., & Szulc, P. (2017). Use of bone turnover markers in postmenopausal osteoporosis. Osteoporosis treatment: recent developments and ongoing challenges. *Lancet Diabetes & Endocrinology, 5*, 908–923.

Holick, M. F. (2007). Vitamin D deficiency. *New England Journal of Medicine, 357*, 266–281.

Kendler, D. L., Marin, F., Zerbini, C. A. F., Russo, L. A., Greenspan, S. L., Zikan, V., … López-Romero, P. (2018). Effects of teriparatide and risedronate on new fractures in post-menopausal women with severe osteoporosis (VERO): a multicentre, double-blind, double-dummy, randomised controlled trial. *Lancet, 391*, 230–240. doi:10.1016/S0140-6736(17)32137-2.

Khan, A. A., Morrison, A., Hanley, D. A., Felsenberg, D., McCauley, L. K., O'Ryan, F., … Compston, J. (2015). Diagnosis and management of osteonecrosis of the jaw: a systematic review and international consensus. *Journal of Bone and Mineral Research, 30*, 3–23.

Khosla, S., & Hofbauer, L. C. (2017). Osteoporosis treatment: recent developments and ongoing challenges. *Lancet Diabetes & Endocrinology, 5*, 898–907.

Lamy, O., Gonzalez-Rodriguez, E., Stoll, D., Hans, D., & Aubry-Rozier, B. (2017). Severe rebound-associated vertebral fractures after denosumab discontinuation: 9 clinical cases report. *Journal of Clinical Endocrinology and Metabolism, 102*, 354–358.

Langdahl, B. L., Libanati, C., Crittenden, D. B., Bolognese, M. A., Brown, J. P., Daizadeh, N. S., … Grauer, A. (2017). Romosozumab (sclerostin monoclonal antibody) versus teriparatide in postmenopausal women with osteoporosis transitioning from oral bisphosphonate therapy: a randomised, open-label, phase 3 trial. *Lancet, 390*, 1585–1594.

Leder, B. Z., O'Dea, L. S., Zanchetta, J. R., Kumar, P., Banks, K., McKay, K., … Hattersley, G. (2015). Effects of abaloparatide, a human parathyroid hormone-related peptide analog, on bone mineral density in postmenopausal women with osteoporosis. *Journal of Clinical Endocrinology and Metabolism, 100*, 897–706.

Leder, B. Z., Tsai, J. N., Uihlein, A. V., Burnett-Bowie, S. A., Zhu, Y., Foley, K, … Neer, R. M. (2014). Two years of denosumab and teriparatide administration in postmenopausal women with osteoporosis (the DATA Extension study): a randomized controlled trial. *Journal of Clinical Endocrinology and Metabolism, 99*, 1694–1700.

Leder, B. Z., Tsai, J. N., Uihlein, A. V., Wallace, P. M., Lee, H., Neer, R. M., & Burnett-Bowie, S. A. (2015). Denosumab and teriparatide transitions in postmenopausal osteoporosis (the DATA-Switch study): extension of a randomised controlled trial. *Lancet, 386*, 1147–1155.

Lewiecki, E. M. (2003). Nonresponders to osteoporosis therapy. *Journal of Clinical Densitometry, 6*, 307–314.

Lewiecki, M., Cummings, S. R., & Cosman, F. (2013). Treat-to-target for osteoporosis: is now the time? *Journal of Clinical Endocrinology and Metabolism, 98*, 946–953.

Lewis, J. R., Radavelli-Bagatini, S., Rejnmark, L., Chen, J. S., Simpson, J. M., Lappe, J. M., … Prince, R. L. (2015). The effects of calcium supplementation on verified coronary heart disease hospitalization and death in postmenopausal women: a collaborative meta-analysis of randomized controlled trials. *Journal of Bone and Mineral Research, 30*, 165–175.

Lloyd, A. A., Gludovatz, B, Riedel, C., Luengo, E. A., Saiyed, R., Marty, E., … Donnelly, E. (2017). Atypical fracture with long-term bisphosphonate therapy is associated with altered cortical composition and reduced fracture resistance. *Proceedings of the National Academy of Sciences of the United States of America, 114*, 8722–8727.

Long, F. (2011). Building strong bones: molecular regulation of the osteoblast lineage. *Nature Reviews Molecular Cell Biology, 13*, 27–38.

Malouf-Sierra, J., Tarantino, U., García-Hernández, P. A., Corradini, C., Overgaard, S., Stepan, J. J., … Marin, F. (2017). Effect of teriparatide or risedronate in elderly patients with a recent pertrochanteric hip fracture: final results of a 78-week randomized clinical trial. *Journal of Bone and Mineral Research, 32*, 1040–1051.

Marie, P. J., & Cohen-Solal, M. (2018). The expanding life and functions of osteogenic cells: from simple bone-making cells to multifunctional cells and beyond. *Journal of Bone and Mineral Research, 33*, 199–210.

McClung, M. R. (2016). Cancel the denosumab holiday. *Osteoporosis International, 27*, 1677–1682.

McClung, M. R. (2017). Clinical utility of anti-sclerostin antibodies. *Bone, 96*, 3–7.

McClung, M. R. (2017). Using osteoporosis therapies in combination. *Current Osteoporosis Reports, 15*, 343–352.

McClung, M. R., Lewiecki, E. M., Geller, M. L., Bolognese, M. A., Peacock, M., Weinstein, R. L., … Miller, P. D. (2013). Effect of denosumab on bone mineral density and biochemical markers of bone turnover: 8-year results of a phase 2 clinical trial. *Osteoporosis International, 24*, 227–235.

McClung, M. R., Wagman, R. B., Miller, P. D., Wang, A., & Lewiecki, E. M. (2017). Observations following discontinuation of long-term denosumab therapy. *Osteoporosis International, 28*, 1723–1732.

Miller, P. D., Hattersley, G., Riis, B. J., Williams, G. C., Lau, E., Russo, L. A., … Christiansen, C. (2016). Effect of abaloparatide vs placebo on new vertebral fractures in postmenopausal women with osteoporosis: a randomized clinical trial. *JAMA, 316*, 722–733.

Miller, P. D., Pannacciulli, N., Brown, J. P., Czerwinski, E., Nedergaard, B. S., Bolognese, M. A., … Cummings, S. R. (2016). Denosumab or zoledronic acid in postmenopausal women with osteoporosis previously treated with oral bisphosphonates. *Journal of Clinical Endocrinology and Metabolism, 101*, 3163–3170.

Park-Wyllie, L. Y., Mamdani, M. M., Juurlink, D. N., Hawker, G. A., Gunraj, N., Austin, P. C., … Laupacis, A. (2011). Bisphosphonate use and the risk of subtrochanteric or femoral shaft fractures in older women. *JAMA, 305*, 783–789.

Qaseem, A., Forciea, M. A., McLean, R. M., & Denberg, T. D. (2017). Treatment of low bone density or osteoporosis to prevent fractures in men and women: a clinical practice guideline update from the American College of Physicians. *Annals of Internal Medicine, 166*, 818–839.

Rothman, M. S., Lewiecki, E. M., & Miller, P. D. (2017). Bone density testing is the best way to monitor osteoporosis treatment. *American Journal of Medicine, 130*, 1133–1134.

Ruggiero, S. L., Dodson, T. B., Fantasia, L., Goodday, R., Aghaloo, T., Mehrotra, B., & O'Ryan, F. (2014). American Association of Oral and Maxillofacial Surgeons position paper on medication-related osteonecrosis of the jaw – 2014 update. *Journal of Oral and Maxillofacial Surgery, 72*, 1938–1956.

Saag, K. G., Petersen, J., Brandi, M. L., Karaplis, A. C., Lorentzon, M., Thomas, T., ... Grauer, A. (2017). Romosozumab or alendronate for fracture prevention in women with osteoporosis. *New England Journal of Medicine, 377*, 1417–1427.

Shane, E., Burr, D., Abrahamsen, B., Adler, R. A., Brown, T. D., Cheung, A. M., ... Whyte, M. P. (2014). Atypical subtrochanteric and diaphyseal femoral fractures: second report of a task force of the American Society for Bone and Mineral Research. *Journal of Bone and Mineral Research, 29*, 1–23.

CHAPTER 15

OSTEOMALACIA, RICKETS, AND VITAMIN D INSUFFICIENCY

William E. Duncan

1. **What are osteomalacia and rickets?**

   Osteomalacia and *rickets* are terms that describe the clinical, histologic, and radiologic abnormalities of bone that are associated with more than 50 diseases and conditions. Osteomalacia is a disorder of mature (adult) bone, whereas rickets occurs in growing bone. Although rickets and osteomalacia were initially viewed as distinct clinical entities, the same pathologic processes may result in either disorder. In both conditions, mineralization of newly formed osteoid (the bone protein matrix) is inadequate or delayed. In rickets, there is defective chondrocyte differentiation as well as defective mineralization in both the bones and cartilage of the epiphyseal growth plates, resulting in growth retardation and skeletal deformities that are not typically seen in adults with osteomalacia.

2. **Why is it important to know about osteomalacia and rickets?**

   In the United States, at the beginning of the twentieth century, rickets caused by a deficiency of vitamin D was common in urban areas. In the 1920s, rickets was virtually eliminated by an appreciation of the antirachitic properties of sunlight and the use of cod liver oil (which contains significant concentrations of vitamin D). However, with the development of effective treatments for previously fatal diseases that affect vitamin D metabolism (e.g., chronic renal failure) and with an improved understanding of both vitamin D and mineral metabolism, many additional syndromes with osteomalacia or rickets as a feature have emerged. Many recent studies have demonstrated that undiagnosed vitamin D deficiency or insufficiency is common in the United States, and for a significant number of adult women with osteoporosis, vitamin D insufficiency may be an unsuspected component of their bone loss.

3. **Describe how vitamin D is synthesized and metabolized.**

   Serum vitamin D comes from two sources: dietary intake and conversion by ultraviolet (UV) irradiation of 7-dehydrocholesterol or ergosterol in the skin. Vitamin D is then transported through blood to the liver, where it is converted to 25-hydroxy (25-OH) vitamin D by the hepatic 25-hydroxylase enzyme. The 25-OH vitamin D is then converted in the kidney to the active hormone, 1,25-dihydroxy [(OH)$_2$] vitamin D, by the renal enzyme 1-alpha-hydroxylase. The active vitamin D metabolite has effects in many tissues, including the intestine (increases calcium absorption), the kidney (increases calcium reabsorption), the parathyroid glands (decreases PTH secretion), and bone (stimulates osteoblast maturation and bone matrix synthesis) (Fig. 15.1). Recent studies have suggested other possible roles for vitamin D in cardiovascular and neurologic diseases, insulin resistance and diabetes, malignancies, autoimmune conditions, and infections. From an understanding of how vitamin D is metabolized, it is apparent that even when dietary intake and UV-mediated vitamin D synthesis are normal, vitamin D deficiency may occur in association with severe malabsorptive, renal, or liver disease.

4. **List the causes of osteomalacia and rickets.**

   The primary abnormality of bone in patients with either osteomalacia or rickets is undermineralization of the bone matrix. The major mineral in bone is calcium hydroxyapatite $Ca_{10}(PO_4)_6(OH)_2$. Thus, any disease that results in decreased availability to bone of either calcium or phosphorus may result in osteomalacia or rickets (Table 15.1). Therefore, the causes of osteomalacia and rickets fall into three categories: (1) low calcium intake in children or disorders associated with abnormalities of vitamin D metabolism or action that limit the availability of calcium for mineralization of bone; (2) disorders associated with abnormalities of phosphorus metabolism; and (3) a small group of disorders in which there is normal vitamin D and mineral metabolism.

5. **Discuss the disease processes that interfere with the metabolism of vitamin D.**

   Clinically apparent vitamin D deficiency is rarely seen in the United States, except when there is limited exposure to sunlight and intake of vitamin D–fortified milk and other dairy products. However, many elderly Americans are at risk for occult vitamin D deficiency or insufficiency because of sun avoidance, the use of sunscreens, and an age-related decrease in the dermal synthesis of vitamin D, impaired hepatic and renal hydroxylation of vitamin D, and diminished intestinal responsiveness to 1,25-(OH)$_2$ vitamin D. Celiac disease or sprue, regional enteritis, intestinal bypass surgery, partial gastrectomy, chronic liver disease, primary biliary cirrhosis, pancreatic insufficiency, certain medications, and chronic renal failure have also been associated with the development of osteomalacia.

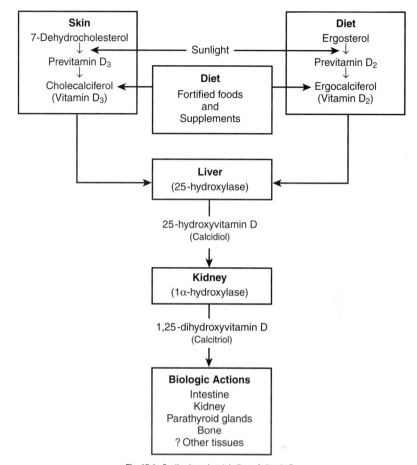

Fig. 15.1. Synthesis and metabolism of vitamin D.

6. List genetic disorders that interfere with vitamin D synthesis or action.
   Two extremely rare genetic syndromes are associated with rickets. Vitamin D–dependent rickets (VDDR) type I (also called *pseudo–vitamin D deficiency rickets*) is associated with an almost complete absence of renal 25-OH vitamin D-1alpha-hydroxylase activity. A second genetic syndrome, VDDR type II, results from a mutation of the vitamin D receptor gene which causes an end-organ resistance to $1,25(OH)_2$ vitamin D and a lack of vitamin D action.

7. Describe the regulation of serum phosphorus levels.
   Serum phosphorus is regulated by the coordinated action of $1,25(OH)_2$ vitamin D, parathyroid hormone (PTH), and fibroblast growth factor 23 (FGF 23). Phosphorus levels are increased by $1,25(OH)_2$ vitamin D, which enhances intestinal phosphate absorption. PTH lowers serum phosphorus by promoting renal phosphate excretion. FGF 23 lowers serum phosphate by forming a ternary complex with the FGF 23 receptor and the Klotho protein to enhance renal phosphate loss through renal sodium–phosphate transporters; FGF 23 also reduces intestinal phosphate absorption by lowering serum $1,25(OH)_2$ vitamin D levels through inhibition of renal 1alpha-hydroxylase and stimulation of renal 24 hydroxylase.

8. What conditions associated with abnormalities of phosphate metabolism result in osteomalacia or rickets?
   Nutritional phosphate deficiency, decreased intestinal absorption of phosphate resulting from ingestion of phosphate binders (e.g., aluminum hydroxide), and renal phosphate wasting can result in osteomalacia or rickets. Hereditary phosphate wasting is a genetically heterogeneous disease. X-linked hypophosphatemic rickets (XLHR) results from inherited loss-of-function mutations in the *PHEX* gene, leading to increased bone expression of FGF 23 as a result of decreased FGF 23 proteolysis. Autosomal dominant hypophosphatemic rickets (ADHR) results from

Table 15.1. Conditions Associated with Osteomalacia and Rickets.

CONDITION	PRIMARY MECHANISM[a]
Abnormal Vitamin D Metabolism or Action	
Nutritional deficiency	Vitamin D deficiency
Malabsorption	Vitamin D deficiency
Primary biliary cirrhosis	Malabsorption of vitamin D
Chronic renal disease	Impaired α-hydroxylation of 25-hydroxy vitamin D
Chronic liver disease	Impaired 25-hydroxylation of vitamin D
VDDR type I	1alpha-hydroxylase deficiency
VDDR type II	Mutation of the vitamin D receptor gene
Drugs (phenytoin, barbiturates, cholestyramine)	Increased catabolism and/or excretion of vitamin D
Phosphate Deficiency or Renal Phosphate Wasting	
Diminished phosphate intake	Phosphate deficiency
Excessive aluminum hydroxide intake	Increasing binding of intestinal phosphate
X-linked hypophosphatemic rickets	Genetic mutations causing phosphate wasting
Autosomal dominant hypophosphatemic rickets	Genetic mutations causing phosphate wasting
Tumor-induced osteomalacia	Urinary phosphate wasting caused by FGF 23
Miscellaneous renal tubular defects (RTA, FS)	Renal phosphate transport defect
Normal Vitamin D and Phosphate Metabolism	
Hypophophatasia	Alkaline phosphatase deficiency
Drugs (fluoride, aluminum, high-dose etidronate)	Inhibition of mineralization or stimulation of matrix synthesis
Osteogenesis imperfecta	Abnormal bone collagen
Fibrogenesis imperfecta ossium	Defective bone matrix

[a]Although only one mechanism for osteomalacia or rickets is given, other mechanisms also may contribute to the bone disease.
FGF 23, Fibroblast growth factor 23; *FS,* Fanconi's syndrome; *RTA,* renal tubular acidosis; *VDDR,* vitamin D–dependent rickets.

activating mutations in the gene that encodes FGF 23, resulting in increased FGF 23 levels. FGF 23 lowers serum phosphate by forming a ternary complex with the FGF 23 receptor and the Klotho protein to enhance renal phosphate loss through renal sodium–phosphate transporters; FGF 23 also reduces intestinal phosphate absorption by lowering serum $1,25(OH)_2$ vitamin D levels through inhibition of renal 1alpha-hydroxylase and stimulation of renal 24 hydroxylase. Tumor-induced osteomalacia (also called *oncogenic osteomalacia*) is a nonhereditary phosphate-wasting syndrome caused by neoplasms of mesenchymal origin which secret FGF 23 and produce osteomalacia.

9. Does chronic renal failure cause osteomalacia and rickets?

Chronic renal failure is associated with a number of bone diseases: osteoporosis, osteomalacia or rickets, osteitis fibrosa cystica (caused by longstanding secondary hyperparathyroidism), adynamic bone, and a combination of both osteomalacia and osteitis fibrosa cystica (termed *mixed renal osteodystrophy*). Rickets or osteomalacia is usually a late finding in the course of kidney disease and is rarely seen before patients begin dialysis. Rickets or osteomalacia associated with chronic renal failure is caused by decreased circulating concentrations of $1,25(OH)_2$ vitamin D, by aluminum intoxication from aluminum-containing antacids used as phosphate binders or an aluminum-contaminated dialysate, and possibly by the chronic metabolic acidosis associated with the renal failure.

10. What signs and symptoms are associated with osteomalacia?

In adults, osteomalacia may be asymptomatic. When symptomatic, osteomalacia may present with diffuse skeletal pain (often aggravated by physical activity or palpation of bone), muscle weakness, and sometimes muscle wasting. The muscle weakness often involves the proximal muscles of the lower extremities and may result in a waddling gait and difficulty rising from a chair or climbing stairs. The bone pain is described as dull and aching, and is usually located in the back, hips, knees, legs, and at sites of fractures. In patients with osteomalacia, fractures may result from even minor trauma.

11. Describe the clinical findings of rickets.

Because of the impaired calcification of cartilage at the growth plates in children with rickets, the clinical manifestations of rickets are significantly different from those of osteomalacia. Widening of the metaphyses (the growth zones between the epiphysis and diaphysis), slowed growth, and various skeletal deformities are prominent in this condition. The effects of rickets are greatest at sites where bone growth is most rapid. Because the rate and pattern of skeletal growth varies with age, the manifestations of rickets likewise will vary. One of the earliest signs of rickets in infants is *craniotabes* (an abnormal softness of the skull). In older infants and younger children, thickening of the forearm at the wrist and swelling of the costochondral junctions (also known as *rachitic rosary*), and Harrison's groove, a lateral indentation of the chest wall at the site of attachment of the diaphragm, may be present. In older children, bowing of the tibia and fibula may be observed. At any age, if rickets (or osteomalacia) is associated with hypocalcemia, paresthesias of the hands and around the mouth, muscle cramps, positive Chvostek's and Trousseau's signs, tetany, and seizures may be evident.

12. What are the biochemical abnormalities seen with osteomalacia and rickets caused by vitamin D deficiency?

The laboratory abnormalities associated with osteomalacia or rickets depend on the underlying defect or process causing the bone disease. To understand the biochemical abnormalities observed in conditions associated with the abnormal metabolism of vitamin D, an understanding of the body's response to hypocalcemia and knowledge of the vitamin D metabolic pathway is necessary. Thus, in patients with nutritional vitamin D deficiency or malabsorption, the low vitamin D concentrations result in a low or low normal serum calcium concentration, which serves as a stimulus for increased secretion of parathyroid hormone (causing secondary hyperparathyroidism). This secondary hyperparathyroidism, in turn, causes increased renal excretion of phosphate, decreased serum phosphate, elevated alkaline phosphatase concentrations, and reduced urinary calcium excretion.

13. What are the vitamin D metabolite concentrations associated with the diseases that interfere with vitamin D metabolism or action?

Depending on the abnormality of vitamin D metabolism, different vitamin D metabolite patterns may be observed. In nutritional vitamin D deficiency and malabsorption, serum 25-OH vitamin D levels are low. In VDDR type I, in which there is a deficiency of the renal 25-OH vitamin D-1alpha-hydroxylase enzyme, normal or increased serum 25-OH vitamin D and low or undetectable serum $1,25(OH)_2$ vitamin D concentrations are observed. In contrast, in VDDR type II, which causes a resistance of target organs to $1,25(OH)_2$ vitamin D, the levels of both $25(OH)_2$ vitamin D and $1,25(OH)_2$ vitamin D are elevated.

14. What radiographic findings are associated with osteomalacia and rickets?

The biochemical abnormalities associated with rickets and osteomalacia are usually evident before radiographic abnormalities are observed. The most common radiographic change in patients with osteomalacia is a reduction in bone mass. Pseudofractures (also called *Looser's zones* or *Milkman's fractures*) or complete fractures also may be observed. Pseudofractures are transverse radiolucent bands ranging from a few millimeters to several centimeters in length, usually perpendicular to the surface of the bones. They are most often bilateral and are particularly common in the femur, pelvis, and small bones of the hands and feet.

Certain radiographic abnormalities are primarily observed in children. These include fraying of the metaphyses of the long bones, widening of the unmineralized epiphyseal growth plates, and bowing of the legs. The skeletal deformities observed in children with rickets may persist into adulthood. Patients with osteomalacia may also have additional radiographic findings as a result of secondary hyperparathyroidism. Such findings include subperiosteal resorption of the phalanges, loss of the lamina dura of the teeth, widening of the spaces at the symphysis pubis and sacroiliac joints, and the presence of brown tumors or bone cysts.

15. Discuss the histologic features of osteomalacia.

The two diagnostic histologic findings of osteomalacia are the presence of widened osteoid seams and increased mineralization lag time (the time necessary for newly deposited matrix to mineralize). The mineralization lag time is assessed by administration of two short courses of oral tetracycline several weeks apart before a bone biopsy. Because tetracycline is deposited at the mineralization front in newly formed bone, the lag time may be determined by measuring the distance between the two fluorescent tetracycline bands in biopsy specimens of bone. Depending on the cause of the osteomalacia, hyperparathyroid bone changes may also be seen. Because of the many clinical signs and symptoms, radiographic findings, and biochemical abnormalities associated with osteomalacia or rickets, none of these tests or findings is diagnostic. The bone biopsy remains the gold standard in establishing the diagnosis of rickets and osteomalacia. The evaluation of a bone biopsy must be performed by personnel specially trained in the interpretation of bone histology.

16. Describe the therapy for osteomalacia and rickets caused by vitamin D deficiency.

The goal of therapy for patients with osteomalacia and rickets caused by an abnormality of vitamin D metabolism is to correct the hypocalcemia and the deficiency of active vitamin D metabolites by administration of calcium salts (as supplements or via diet) and vitamin D preparations. In the United States, vitamin D_2 (ergocalciferol), vitamin D_3 (cholecalciferol), $1,25(OH)_2$ vitamin D (calcitriol), and analogues of calcitriol are available. Each of these preparations has a different half-life and potency. The choice and dose of vitamin D preparation are determined by the underlying pathologic defect of vitamin D metabolism. For patients with nutritional vitamin D deficiency, treatment with vitamin D along with elemental calcium is often sufficient to heal the osteomalacia. Osteomalacia caused by hepatobiliary disease or chronic renal failure is managed with calcitriol or one of its analogues.

17. **What are the treatments for osteomalacia and rickets not caused by vitamin D deficiency?**
VDDR type I is treated with calcitriol in usual doses of 0.5 to 2.0 mcg daily because affected patients are unable to synthesize $1,25(OH)_2$ vitamin D but can respond to the physiologic levels of $1,25(OH)_2$ vitamin D if it is provided to them. In contrast, treatment of VDDR type II, which involves profound resistance to $1,25(OH)_2$ vitamin D, consists of administration of high doses of calcitriol, up to 60 mcg/day (an extraordinarily high dose), along with large doses of oral calcium. In severe cases, high-dose intravenous calcium infusions are required to heal the rickets in patients with VDDR type II. Hypophosphatemic rickets (XLHR and ADHR) must be treated with both phosphate replacement and calcitriol. Burosumab (Crysvita), a monoclonal antibody that binds to FGF 23, has also recently been approved by the U.S. Food and Drug Administration for the treatment of XLHR. Clinical trials showed that this drug normalizes phosphorus levels, improves bone mineralization, alleviates rickets in affected children, and promotes fracture healing in affected adults. Tumor removal or irradiation is required to treat tumor-induced osteomalacia. In chronic renal failure with aluminum-induced osteomalacia, aluminum is removed from the affected bone by treatment with the chelating agent deferoxamine. The bone disease can then be treated with calcium and calcitriol. Osteomalacia associated with renal tubular acidosis is treated with vitamin D and bicarbonate to correct the acidosis.

18. **How is vitamin D insufficiency diagnosed, and why is it important to diagnose it?**
The most stable and plentiful metabolite of vitamin D in human serum, 25-OH vitamin D, has a half-life of about 3 weeks, making it the most suitable indicator of vitamin D status. A global consensus conference has defined sufficient vitamin D status (based on serum 25-OH vitamin D levels) as > 50 nmol/L (20 ng/mL), insufficient vitamin D status as 30 to 50 nmol/L (12–20 ng/mL), and vitamin D deficiency as < 30 nmol/L (12 ng/mL). Insufficient vitamin D status is a common problem in the United States. Data from the National Health and Nutrition Examination Survey (2001–2004) population demonstrates that only 23% had circulating concentrations of 25-OH vitamin D > 30 ng/mL, and 6% had values < 10 ng/mL. As circulating 25-OH vitamin D concentrations decrease from sufficient vitamin D levels, there is an increasing negative impact on skeletal health. It therefore seems prudent to provide vitamin D supplementation to individuals with circulating 25-OH vitamin D levels < 50 nmol/L (20 ng/mL).

19. **What are the complications of treatment with vitamin D preparations?**
When high doses of vitamin D or one of the more potent vitamin preparations are used, it is important to carefully monitor for hypercalcemia. Mild hypercalcemia may be asymptomatic. However, severely hypercalcemic patients may complain of anorexia, nausea, vomiting, weight loss, headache, constipation, polyuria, polydipsia, and altered mental status. Impaired renal function, nephrocalcinosis, nephrolithiasis, and even death may eventually ensue. If vitamin D intoxication occurs, all calcium supplements and vitamin D preparations must be discontinued immediately and therapy for hypercalcemia instituted.

KEY POINTS: OSTEOMALACIA, RICKETS, AND VITAMIN D INSUFFICIENCY

- Osteomalacia and rickets are disorders resulting in inadequate or delayed mineralization of bone.
- Osteomalacia occurs in mature bone, whereas rickets occurs in growing bone. Thus, the clinical and radiographic findings of these two conditions differ.
- The causes of osteomalacia and rickets fall into three categories: (A) low calcium intake in children or disorders associated with abnormal vitamin D metabolism or action; (B) disorders associated with abnormal phosphate metabolism; and (C) a small group of disorders with normal vitamin D and mineral metabolism.
- Vitamin D insufficiency is common in the United States and has a negative impact on skeletal health.

BIBLIOGRAPHY

Adams, J. S., & Hewison, M. (2010). Update in vitamin D. *Journal of Clinical Endocrinology and Metabolism, 95*, 471.
Berry, J. L., Davies, M., & Mee, A. P. (2002). Vitamin D metabolism, rickets, and osteomalacia. *Seminars in Musculoskeletal Radiology, 6*, 173.
Carpenter, T. O. (2012). The expanding family of hypophosphatemic syndromes. *Journal of Bone and Mineral Metabolism, 30*, 1–9.
Carpenter, T. O., Imel, E. A., Holm, I. A., Jan de Beur, S. M., & Insogna, K. L. (2011). A clinician's guide to X-linked hypophosphatemia. *Journal of Bone and Mineral Research, 26*, 1381–1383.
Ginde, A. A., Liu, M. C., & Camargo, C. A., Jr. (2009). Demographic differences and trends of vitamin D insufficiency in the US population, 1988-2004. *Archives of Internal Medicine, 169*, 626.
Holick, M. F. (2006). Resurrection of vitamin D deficiency and rickets. *Journal of Clinical Investigation, 116*, 2062.
Holick, M. F. (2007). Vitamin D deficiency. *New England Journal of Medicine, 357*, 266.

Holick, M. F., Binkley, N. C., Bischoff-Ferrari, H. A., Gordon, C. M., Hanley, D. A., Heaney, R. P., . . . Weaver, C. M. (2011). Evaluation, treatment, and prevention of vitamin D deficiency: an endocrine society clinical practice guideline. *Journal of Clinical Endocrinology and Metabolism, 96,* 1911.

Imel, E. A., & Econs, M. J. (2012). Approach to the hypophosphatemic patient. *Journal of Clinical Endocrinology and Metabolism, 97,* 696–706.

Malloy, P. J., & Feldman, D. (2010). Genetic disorders and defects in vitamin D action. *Endocrinology and Metabolism Clinics of North America, 39,* 333.

Munns, C. F., Shaw, N., Kiely, M., Specker, B. L., Thacher, T. D., Ozono, K., . . . & Högler, W. (2016). Global consensus recommendations on prevention and management of nutritional rickets. *Journal of Clinical Endocrinology and Metabolism, 101,* 394.

Rosen, C. J. (2011). Vitamin D insufficiency. *New England Journal of Medicine, 364,* 248.

Rosen, C. J. (Ed.). (2013). *Primer on the metabolic bone diseases and disorders of mineral metabolism.* Ames, IA: Wiley-Blackwell.

Thacher, T. D., & Clarke, B. L. (2011). Vitamin D insufficiency. *Mayo Clinic Proceedings, 86,* 50.

Wolinsky-Friedland, M. (1995). Drug-induced metabolic bone disease. *Endocrinology and Metabolism Clinics of North America, 24,* 395.

CHAPTER 16

PAGET'S DISEASE OF BONE

Matthew P. Wahl and Christine M. Swanson

1. **What is Paget's disease of bone (PDB)?**
   PDB is a chronic disease characterized by abnormal bone remodeling in one or more bones. Pagetic osteoclasts (bone cells responsible for bone resorption) are abnormally large and overactive, causing focal areas of excessive bone resorption. Compensatory increases in bone formation (by osteoblasts) at pagetic sites result in disorganized, structurally weaker bone that is often increased in size. Sir James Paget first described this condition in 1876 and referred to it as *osteitis deformans*; however, there is evidence that the condition existed in Western Europe during the Roman period. PDB can lead to bone pain, skeletal deformities, pseudofractures, and osteoarthritis, although many patients with PDB are asymptomatic at diagnosis.

2. **What causes PDB?**
   The cause of PDB is unknown and may have genetic and environmental influences. Mutations in the *SQSTM1* gene, which encodes a protein that plays a role in osteoclast function, are seen in 40% to 50% of familial cases of PDB. Paramyxovirus infection has been proposed as a potential trigger for PDB as pagetic osteoclasts have been found to contain intranuclear structures resembling paramyxovirus nucleocapsids, although no virus has ever been cultured from pagetic osteoclasts. The incidence of PDB is decreasing worldwide, and this may reflect changes in environmental contributions to PDB.

3. **How does PDB typically present?**
   PDB is typically diagnosed when elevated serum alkaline phosphatase (ALP) or an abnormal radiograph (x-ray) is found incidentally in patients being evaluated for other reasons. Symptoms depend on the site and extent of involvement. At diagnosis, 30% to 40% of patients are symptomatic, with the most common symptom being bone pain. Frequently, bone pain develops later in the disease course—it is characterized as a deep and aching pain that occurs with rest or activity and is often worse at night.

4. **Who is typically affected by PDB?**
   PDB prevalence increases with age. It typically affects older adults and is uncommon before 40 years of age. Incidence of PDB also varies, depending on geography and gender. Men appear to be more commonly affected than women. PDB most commonly affects those of European descent and less commonly those of African and Asian descents. In the United States, PDB is estimated to affect 2% to 3% of the adult population age > 55 years.

5. **How is PDB diagnosed?**
   PDB can be diagnosed by using plain radiography. Typical findings of PDB on a radiograph include focal osteolysis with sclerotic changes, thickening of the cortex, coarse trabecular pattern, and bone enlargement (Fig. 16.1). ALP should be measured and is often, although not always, very elevated.

6. **What is the differential diagnosis of PDB?**
   The differential diagnosis for radiographic PDB may include chronic osteomyelitis, vertebral hemangioma, fibrous dysplasia, metastatic disease, metaphyseal dysplasia (Engelmann's disease), hyperostosis frontalis interna, familial expansile osteolysis, sternocostal clavicular hyperostosis, osteosarcoma and SAPHO (synovitis, acne, pustulosis, hyperostosis, osteitis) syndrome. Elevated ALP can be seen in liver or biliary disease, or any condition with increased bone turnover (e.g., osteomalacia, hyperparathyroidism, skeletal metastases).

7. **Which bones are involved in PDB?**
   PDB may be monostotic (involvement of one bone), or more commonly polyostotic (involvement of ≥ 2 bones). It has a predilection for the axial skeletal but can affect nearly any bone in the body. The most frequently involved bones are the pelvis (70%), femur (55%), lumbar spine (53%), skull (42%), and tibia (32%). Each individual pagetic site may progress or evolve over time; however, the number of skeletal sites involved is usually stable over time, and it is rare for new skeletal lesions to develop after diagnosis.

8. **What are the typical histologic and radiologic appearances and triphasic progression of pagetic bone lesions?**
   PDB progresses through three phases. First, there is a focal increase in bone resorption resulting from increased osteoclast activity by numerous enlarged, often multinucleated osteoclasts. Radiographic findings include bone loss, wedge-shaped areas of resorption in long bones, and circumscribed lytic lesions in the skull (osteoporosis circumscripta). Second, increased osteoblast activity and accelerated bone formation occur, resulting in disorganized collagen

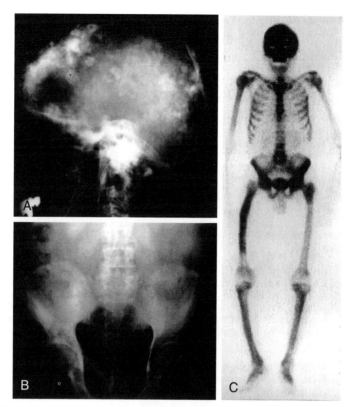

Fig. 16.1. The characteristic radiographic and scintigraphic findings seen in Paget's disease of bone. **(A)** A skull radiograph showing a thickened cranium with regions of dense sclerosis and osteopenia resulting in a "cotton wool" appearance. **(B)** A pelvic radiograph showing right hemipelvic loss of normal trabeculation, sclerosis, and cortical thickening, along with sclerosis of the iliopectineal line. **(C)** Full-body scintigraphy showing increased uptake in the skull, pelvis, lumbar spine, and bilateral femurs, with bowing of the right tibia, scapula, and bilateral proximal humerus.

architecture (mosaic or woven, instead of the normal lamellar pattern) and a mixed lytic/sclerotic phase. This abnormal bone has impaired strength and is at higher risk for fracture. On radiography, bones appear enlarged and sclerotic; bowing deformities, transverse linear radiolucencies ("pseudofractures"), and thickening of the calvarium may be seen. Finally, there is reduced bone cell activity and persistence of abnormal bone architecture, including enlarged, sclerotic bones.

9. Which laboratory tests should be obtained to evaluate and monitor PDB?
   ALP, calcium, albumin, liver function tests, and 25-hydroxy (25-OH) vitamin D levels should be obtained in patients with suspected or known PDB. ALP, a biomarker of osteoblastic activity, can be within normal limits in those with limited, monostotic disease or during the initial osteolytic phase of PDB, but rises during the osteoblastic phase and can correlate with disease activity. Measurement of ALP is the preferred assay in PDB. If liver disease is present or the ALP is normal, other markers of bone formation, such as bone-specific alkaline phosphatase (BSAP) or procollagen type I N-terminal propeptide (P1NP), can be checked. The elevated turnover marker can be monitored over time every 6 to 12 months to assess the patient's response to treatment and/or PDB activity.

10. What imaging is recommended to determine the extent of skeletal involvement in PDB and for monitoring?
    Plain radiography is used to diagnose PDB, but the extent of PDB involvement is best measured by using radionuclide bone scanning. Bone scan findings are nonspecific (e.g., false-positive findings may be seen at osteoarthritic sites); however, it is the most sensitive examination for identifying PDB lesions. Early symptomatic lesions may be apparent on bone scanning before radiography, whereas burned-out pagetic lesions that are easily seen on radiography may not have increased uptake on bone scanning. It is recommended that bone scanning be performed in newly diagnosed patients with PDB during their initial evaluation, followed by radiography of the involved sites. Computed tomography (CT), magnetic resonance imaging (MRI), and positron emission tomography (PET) are not routinely used in PDB.

Table 16.1. Bisphosphonates Used in the Treatment of Paget's Disease of Bone.

DRUG NAME	DOSAGE	DURATION
Zoledronate	5 mg IV (once, infused over 15 minutes)	N/A
Alendronate	40 mg per day by mouth	6 months
Risedronate	30 mg per day by mouth	2 months

IV, Intravenous; *N/A,* not applicable.

11. **What medications are available to treat PDB?**

   Adequate levels of calcium and vitamin D are essential in the treatment of PDB. Nitrogen-containing bisphospho-nates (Table 16.1) are considered first-line therapy in the treatment of PDB because they target the affected sites and effectively suppress bone resorption. These medications include intravenous (IV; zoledronic acid, also known as *zoledronate, pamidronate*) and oral formulations (alendronate, risedronate). Calcitonin is less effective and not commonly used. There are case reports of denosumab being used in the treatment of PDB; however, at this time, PDB is not an approved indication for denosumab use. Additionally, there are significant risks with stopping denosumab without subsequent antiresorptive therapy (declining bone mineral density, increased fracture risk) (see Anastasilakis, 2017).

12. **Which pharmacologic agent is the drug of choice for PDB?**

   Zoledronate, an IV infusion, is the drug of choice for PDB because it has the fastest, most dramatic, and sustained effect on ALP and on symptoms (pain, quality of life). After a single 5-mg IV dose, ALP levels normalize in 96% of patients or have at least a 75% reduction at 6 months. Zoledronate is effective even in patients with PDB who did not respond to previous treatment with other bisphosphonates. Sustained biochemical response to zoledronate may last for 6 years. Bisphosphonates are contraindicated in those with creatinine clearance (CrCl) < 35 mL/min.

13. **What are the indications for the treatment of PDB?**

   Bisphosphonate treatment should be considered for:
   - Symptoms, including bone pain that corresponds to a site of metabolically active PDB. Bisphosphonate therapy may help clarify if pain is due to bone or osteoarthritic pain.
   - Those at high risk of developing complications from PDB lesion (e.g., fracture in weight-bearing bones, headaches or nerve compression from involvement of the skull or spine, disease near major joints).
   - Before orthopedic or elective surgery at or near a pagetic site to reduce hypervascularity and perioperative blood loss.
   - Hypercalcemia in the setting of immobilization.

14. **What are the treatment goals in PDB?**

   Response to therapy is typically assessed with bone turnover markers. The preferred marker, ALP, normally decreases 1 to 2 weeks after zoledronate, reaching a nadir by 3 to 6 months. Bone resorption markers (e.g., serum C-telopeptides [CTx], urinary N-telopeptides [NTx]) fall more rapidly after treatment but are more expensive and cumbersome to obtain (i.e. must be drawn on morning, fasted serum or second void morning urine, respectively). Other bone formation markers (e.g., P1NP, BSAP) may be trended if ALP cannot be used (e.g., liver disease). Sustained remission may be indicated by bone turnover markers in the lower half of the reference range, and retreatment may be considered if pagetic symptoms recur or bone turnover markers become elevated. There are no data to support that ALP normalization decreases risk of long-term complications; however, trials have been limited in size and duration.

15. **What are the side effects of pharmacologic therapy?**

   Bisphosphonates have been associated with a small increased risk of osteonecrosis of the jaw (particularly with invasive dental procedures and in cancer patients) and atypical (subtrochanteric) femoral fractures. Bisphospho-nates can be nephrotoxic and are contraindicated in patients with impaired renal function (estimated glomerular filtration rate [eGFR] < 35 mL/min/1.73 m^2). Hypocalcemia can occur with bisphosphonate treatment, especially in those with vitamin D deficiency. Different formulations have specific side effects that should be considered, such as an acute-phase response (IV) and esophagitis/dyspepsia (oral). The acute-phase response may be more severe in patients with PDB than when used for osteoporosis because of greater osteoclast activity.

16. **What complications can arise in PDB?**

   Osteoarthritis, bone deformity, fracture, pseudofracture, and bone enlargement can be signs of longstanding PDB. Hearing loss can occur in patients with skull involvement and may be caused by cochlear damage from bony overgrowth. Other neurologic deficits resulting from impingement include spinal stenosis and radiculopathy. Obstructive hydrocephalus can occur if there is compression at the base of the skull. Pseudofractures are a characteristic finding in PDB and can progress to complete fractures. High-output cardiac failure (particularly in polyostotic disease) and hypercalcemia (when immobilized) are rarer complications of PDB. PDB lesions can rarely transform into a giant cell tumor (usually a benign condition) or osteosarcoma.

17. What is the risk of osteosarcoma in a patient with PDB?
Transformation of a pagetic site to osteosarcoma has a poor prognosis but is quite rare, occurring in < 1% of patients. Osteosarcoma should be suspected in patients with PDB who have increased bone pain and swelling, a new mass, or a new fracture at a pagetic site. MRI is useful in these instances to distinguish pagetic bone lesions from malignancies.

KEY POINTS

- Paget's disease of bone (PDB) is a chronic condition characterized by focal areas of abnormal osteoclasts that cause excessive bone resorption, followed by abnormal bone formation resulting in disorganized, weak bone.
- PDB commonly presents as an incidental discovery of elevated alkaline phosphatase or bone abnormality on a nonrelated imaging study.
- Radiography is used to diagnose PDB and nuclear medicine bone scans to evaluate extent of disease.
- The treatment of choice of PDB is intravenous zoledronate, and treatment is indicated in patients with PDB who have symptomatic bone pain, hypercalcemia, those at high risk of developing complications from PDB or those undergoing surgery at or near a pagetic site.

ACKNOWLEDGEMENTS

The authors would like to acknowledge the contributions of Dr. William E. Duncan, who was the author of this chapter in the previous edition. One of the authors (C.M.S.) is supported by K23 AR070275. Website: https://www.nof.org/pagets/

BIBLIOGRAPHY

Anastasilakis, A.D., Polyzos S.A., Makras, P., Aubry-Rozier, B., Kaouri, S., Lamy, O. (2017). Clinical Features of 24 Patients With Rebound-Associated Vertebral Fractures After Denosumab Discontinuation: Systematic Review and Additional Cases. *Journal of Bone and Mineral Research, 32*(6), 1291-1296.

Cundy, T. (2018). Paget's disease of bone. *Metabolism, 80*, 5–14.

Hosking, D., Lyles, K., Brown, J. P., Fraser, W. D., Miller, P., Curiel, M. D., . . . Reid, I. R. (2007). Long-term control of bone turnover in Paget's disease with zoledronic acid and risedronate. *Journal of Bone and Mineral Research, 22*(1), 142–148.

Langston, A. L., Campbell, M. K., Fraser, W. D., MacLennan, G. S., Selby, P. L., & Ralston, S. H. (2010). Randomized trial of intensive bisphosphonate treatment versus symptomatic management in Paget's disease of bone. *Journal of Bone and Mineral Research, 25*(1), 20–31.

Mangham, D. C., Davie, M. W., & Grimer, R. J. (2009). Sarcoma arising in Paget's disease of bone: declining incidence and increasing age at presentation. *Bone, 44*(3), 431–436.

Mays, S. (2010). Archaeological skeletons support a northwest European origin for Paget's disease of bone. *Journal of Bone and Mineral Research, 25*(8), 1839–1841.

Merlotti, D., Gennari, L., Martini, G., Valleggi, F., De Paola, V., Avanzati, A., & Nuti, R. (2007). Comparison of different intravenous bisphosphonate regimens for Paget's disease of bone. *Journal of Bone and Mineral Research, 22*(10), 1510–1517.

Paul Tuck, S., Layfield, R., Walker, J., Mekkayil, B., & Francis, R. (2017). Adult Paget's disease of bone: a review. *Rheumatology (Oxford, England), 56*(12), 2050–2059.

Ralston, S. H. (2008). Pathogenesis of Paget's disease of bone. *Bone, 43*(5), 819–825.

Ralston, S. H. (2013). Clinical practice. Paget's disease of bone. *New England Journal of Medicine, 368*(7), 644–650.

Reid, I. R., Lyles, K., Su, G., Brown, J. P., Walsh, J. P., del Pino-Montes, J., . . . Hosking, D. J. (2011). A single infusion of zoledronic acid produces sustained remissions in Paget disease: data to 6.5 years. *Journal of Bone and Mineral Research, 26*(9), 2261–2270.

Reid, I. R., Miller, P., Lyles, K., Fraser, W., Brown, J. P., Saidi, Y., . . . Hosking, D. (2005). Comparison of a single infusion of zoledronic acid with risedronate for Paget's disease. *New England Journal of Medicine, 353*(9), 898–908.

Seton, M., Moses, A. M., Bode, R. K., & Schwartz, C. (2011). Paget's disease of bone: the skeletal distribution, complications and quality of life as perceived by patients. *Bone, 48*(2), 281–285.

Shaker, J. L. (2009). Paget's disease of bone: a review of epidemiology, pathophysiology and management. *Therapeutic Advances in Musculoskeletal Disease, 1*(2), 107–125.

Singer, F. R., Bone, H. G., III, Hosking, D. J., Lyles, K. W., Murad, M. H., Reid, I. R., & Siris, E. S. (2014). Paget's disease of bone: An endocrine society clinical practice guideline. *Journal of Clinical Endocrinology and Metabolism, 99*(12), 4408–4422.

Siris, E. S., & Roodman, G. D. (2012). Paget's disease of bone. In C. Rosen (Ed.), *Primer on the metabolic bone diseases and disorders of mineral metabolism* (pp. 335–343). Hoboken, NJ: Wiley.

Tan, A., Goodman, K., Walker, A., Hudson, J., MacLennan, G. S., Selby, P. L., . . . Ralston, S. H. (2017). Long-term randomized trial of intensive versus symptomatic management in Paget's disease of bone: the PRISM-EZ study. *Journal of Bone and Mineral Research, 32*(6), 1165–1173.

Tan, A., & Ralston, S. H. (2014). Clinical presentation of Paget's disease: evaluation of a contemporary cohort and systematic review. *Calcified Tissue International, 95*(5), 385–392.

Wermers, R. A., Tiegs, R. D., Atkinson, E. J., Achenbach, S. J., & Melton, L. J., III. (2008). Morbidity and mortality associated with Paget's disease of bone: a population-based study. *Journal of Bone and Mineral Research, 23*(6), 819–825.

CHAPTER 17

HYPERCALCEMIA

Leonard R. Sanders

1. What is hypercalcemia, and how does protein binding affect the calcium level?

   Hypercalcemia is a corrected total serum calcium value above the upper limit of the normal range or an elevated ionized calcium value. Calcium is 50% free (ionized), 40% protein-bound, and 10% complexed to phosphate, citrate, bicarbonate, sulfate, and lactate. Only free calcium changes cause symptoms and signs. Of the protein-bound calcium, about 80% is bound to albumin and 20% to globulins. A decrease or increase in serum albumin of 1 g/dL from 4 g/dL decreases or increases the serum calcium by 0.8 mg/dL. An increase or decrease in serum globulin by 1 g/dL increases or decreases serum calcium by 0.16 mg/dL. Such protein changes do not affect free calcium and do not cause calcium-related symptoms.

2. How common are hypercalcemia and its main associated conditions?

   Hypercalcemia affects 0.5% to 1% of the general population. The incidence may increase to 3% among post-menopausal women. Primary hyperparathyroidism (PHPT) causes 70% of outpatient cases and 20% of inpatient cases of hypercalcemia. Cancer causes the majority of inpatient cases of hypercalcemia. About 10% to 30% of patients with malignancy experience hypercalcemia. Hyperparathyroidism and cancer cause 90% of all hypercal-cemia. About 10% to 20% of patients with hyperparathyroidism experience nephrolithiasis. Calcium oxalate stones are usually the most common stone type, but calcium phosphate stones are more characteristic.

3. How would you classify mild, moderate, and severe hypercalcemia?

   First, consider the patient's general health, hypercalcemic symptoms, and the normal upper limit for calcium in your laboratory. For example, a patient with renal failure and a serum phosphorus value of 8.5 mg/dL may have metastatic calcification with a serum calcium level of 10.5 mg/dL. Then the serum calcium (Ca) is corrected for the albumin concentration, as follows:

$$Ca_{corrected} = Ca_{observed} + [(4.0 - albumin) \times 0.8]$$

   With this in mind, a serum calcium value 1.5 to 3.5 mg/dL above the normal upper limit defines moderate hypercalcemia. Mild hypercalcemia occurs below this range and severe hypercalcemia above. Thus, if the normal upper limit for calcium is 10.5 mg/dL, a serum calcium value of 12 to 14 mg/dL indicates moderate hypercalce-mia. A serum calcium value < 12 mg/dL indicates mild hypercalcemia and a level greater than 14 mg/dL severe hypercalcemia.

4. Discuss the signs and symptoms of hypercalcemia.

   No symptoms are usually present with mild hypercalcemia (< 12 mg/dL). Moderate or severe hypercalcemia and rapidly developing mild hypercalcemia may cause symptoms and signs. Symptoms and signs involve (1) the central nervous system (lethargy, stupor, coma, mental changes, psychosis); (2) the gastrointestinal tract (anorexia, nausea, constipation, acid peptic disease, pancreatitis); (3) the kidneys (polyuria, nephrolithiasis); (4) the musculoskeletal system (arthralgias, myalgias, weakness); and (5) the vascular system (hypertension). The classic electrocardiography (ECG) change associated with hypercalcemia is a short QT interval. Occasionally, severe hypercalcemia also causes dysrhythmias, sinus arrest, disturbances in atrioventricular (AV) conduction, J waves (Osborn waves), and ST segment elevation mimicking myocardial infarction.

5. What are the sources of serum calcium?

   Bone calcium approximates 1 kg (99%) of body calcium. The body maintains normal serum calcium by integrated regulation of calcium absorption, resorption, and reabsorption. These processes occur, respectively, in the gut, bone, and kidney. Of 1000 mg/day of dietary calcium intake, the gut absorbs 300 mg/day, secretes 100 mg/day, and excretes 800 mg/day. Net absorption averages 200 mg/day. Calcium absorption is usually about 30% of dietary calcium; however, absorption may increase to > 50% when people take large doses of calcitriol. The kidney reabsorbs 98% of filtered calcium and excretes 200 mg/day. Bone exchanges about 500 mg of calcium per day with serum (Fig. 17.1).

6. What are the major anatomic and physiologic determinants of vitamin D?

   Diet, skin, liver, and kidney control the amount, synthesis, and secretion of vitamin D. Dietary sources of vitamin D include liver, fish oils, egg yolks, vitamin D–fortified foods, and vitamin D supplements. Skin exposure to ultraviolet sunlight activates 7-dehydrocholesterol to previtamin D, which subsequently rearranges to form vitamin D3

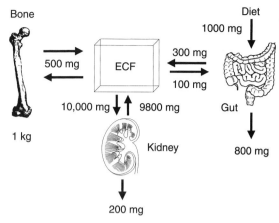

Fig. 17.1 Normal calcium balance. *ECF,* Extracellular fluid.

(cholecalciferol). Hepatic 25-hydroxylase then converts vitamin D to 25-hydroxy (25-OH) vitamin D. 25-OH vitamin D circulates and interacts with two renal mitochondrial hydroxylases. High parathyroid hormone (PTH), low phosphate, and low calcium levels stimulate 1-alpha-hydroxylase activity to increase conversion of 25-OH vitamin D to 1,25(OH)$_2$ vitamin D (calcitriol)—the most potent metabolite of vitamin D. Low PTH, high phosphate, and high calcium levels suppress 1-alpha-hydroxylase activity and stimulate 24-hydroxylase activity. This process inhibits calcitriol production and, through 24-hydroxylase, converts 25-OH vitamin D to 24,25-dihydroxy vitamin D [24,25(OH)$_2$ vitamin D], which promotes antiresorptive effects on bone and positive calcium balance. This same sequence occurs less intensely with normal levels of PTH, PO$_4$ (phosphate), and calcium. Calcitriol feeds back negatively on its own synthesis by suppressing 1-alpha-hydroxylase activity, stimulating 24-hydroxylase activity, decreasing PTH, and increasing calcium and phosphate. Calcitriol is also degraded primarily through the enzyme 24-hydroxylase. Renal 1-alpha-hydroxylase is most active, but this enzyme is also present in bone, brain, pancreas, heart, intestines, lymph nodes, adrenal gland, prostate, and other tissues (Fig. 17.2). Fibroblast growth factor 23 (FGF23) also has an important role in calcium and vitamin D metabolism.

7. What is FGF23, and what role does it play in calcium, phosphate, and vitamin D metabolism?
   FGF23 is a phosphaturic hormone produced by osteocytes in response to increases in serum levels of phosphate, 1,25(OH)$_2$ vitamin D, and PTH. FGF23 decreases serum phosphate, 1,25(OH)$_2$ vitamin D, and PTH by reducing proximal renal tubular phosphate reabsorption, stimulating 24-hydroxylase, inhibiting 1-alpha-hydroxylase, and variably inhibiting PTH synthesis and secretion by the parathyroid glands. FGF23 accumulates to very high levels in chronic kidney disease (CKD) and is associated with increased mortality in CKD.

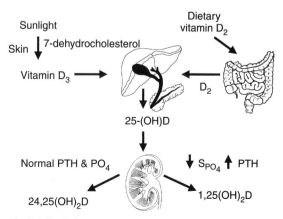

Fig. 17.2 Vitamin D metabolism. *PO$_4$,* Phosphate; *PTH,* parathyroid hormone.

8. **What are the classic and nonclassic effects of vitamin D, and what is the role of the vitamin D receptor?**

Calcitriol acts classically on intestine, bone, kidneys, and parathyroid glands to help regulate calcium and phosphate metabolism. When calcitriol activates the parathyroid vitamin D receptor (VDR), it decreases PTH messenger RNA (mRNA) synthesis by inhibiting the prepro-PTH gene at the vitamin D response element. This inhibition decreases PTH synthesis within the chief cell of the parathyroid gland and ultimately lowers PTH levels. Additionally, calcitriol increases intestinal calcium and phosphate absorption, increases bone calcium and phosphate resorption, enhances bone turnover, and enhances renal calcium and phosphate reabsorption. The VDR is a nuclear hormone receptor that is also regulated by calcium and PTH. Many proteins are downregulated and upregulated by the activated VDR. Downregulated proteins include PTH, 1-alpha-hydroxylase, bone matrix protein, bone sialoprotein, type I collagen, interferons, interleukins, tumor necrosis factor (TNF), epidermal growth factor receptors, renin, and peroxisome proliferator-activated receptor (PPAR) gamma-2. Upregulated proteins include osteopontin, matrix Gla protein, type IV collagen, interleukins, VDR, calcium-sensing receptor (CaSR), and 24-hydroxylase.

   Through activation of the VDR, calcitriol has many (nonclassic) effects other than those related to calcium and phosphorus metabolism. VDR activation may ameliorate arterial calcification, retard neuronal degeneration, enhance host defenses against bacterial infection and tumor growth, enhance Sertoli cell function and spermatogenesis, enhance insulin synthesis and secretion from pancreatic beta cells, and assist with glycogen and transferrin synthesis in liver parenchymal cells. Additionally, calcitriol has antiproliferative and prodifferentiating effects on myeloid cell precursors, cardiac and smooth muscle cells, and a variety of skin cells, including keratinocytes, fibroblasts, hair follicles, and melanocytes.

9. **What is the CaSR, and what role does it play in calcium metabolism?**

The CaSR is a membrane-bound calcium sensor–receptor. The most important locations of the CaSRs are the parathyroid glands and the renal tubular cells, but the receptors are located in many other tissues, including at low levels in pancreatic beta cells and thyroid C cells. The major function of the CaSR is to maintain extracellular calcium concentrations in the normal range and prevent hypercalcemia. In the parathyroid chief cells, the CaSR has a large extracellular domain of 700 amino acids (primary calcium binding site), a seven-segment transmembrane component, and a cytoplasmic carboxyl-terminal component of about 200 amino acids (primary effector site for metabolic changes). The CaSR belongs to subfamily C of the G protein–coupled receptor family. The CaSR senses the minutest change in ionized calcium (0.1 mg/dL) and regulates PTH secretion to maintain steady-state calcium levels within a narrow optimal range. These changes center on a set point for calcium-regulated PTH release that is unique for each individual. After activation by calcium, the CaSR activates phospholipase C, inhibits adenylate cyclase, and opens nonselective cation channels. This effect increases cytoplasmic calcium by mobilizing calcium from thapsigargin-sensitive intracellular stores and enhancing calcium influx through voltage-sensitive cation channels. These CaSR-induced changes in intracellular calcium act on the calcium response element of the prepro-PTH gene to decrease chief cell PTH mRNA synthesis, reduce PTH secretion, and decrease parathyroid gland hyperplasia. CaSR activation also activates the PAL cascade of phospholipase A2, arachidonic acid, and leukotrienes that degrades PTH stored in secretory granules. The parathyroid glands secrete both intact PTH (iPTH) and carboxy-terminal PTH (CPTH) fragments. Intact PTH acts directly on bone PTH receptors releasing calcium from bone. CPTH remains in the circulation much longer and at higher concentrations than iPTH and, although it was previously thought to be inactive, data now suggest that CPTH fragments can exert direct effects on bone cells through a novel class of CPTH receptors. CPTH fragments accumulate in renal failure. PTH functions to keep calcium in the normal range and helps prevent hypocalcemia. Cinacalcet and etelcalcetide are calcimimetic drugs that bind respectively to the transmembrane and extracellular domains of the CaSR and make it markedly more responsive to any level of ambient calcium.

10. **What is the function of the CaSR in the kidneys?**

In the kidney, as in the parathyroid glands, the CaSR functions to prevent hypercalcemia. Activation of the CaSR located on the basolateral membrane in the thick ascending limb of Henle's loop decreases tubular reabsorption of calcium and increases excretion. Activation of the renal CaSR generates an arachidonic acid metabolite that inhibits the luminal potassium channel and the sodium–potassium adenosine triphosphatase (ATPase) pump on the basolateral membrane. This diminishes the lumen-positive electrical gradient needed for passive calcium and magnesium reabsorption. Thus, there is less reabsorption and more excretion of calcium. Because PTH is decreased by the CaSR activated in the parathyroid gland, there is less PTH-mediated distal tubular reabsorption of calcium, net calcium loss, and lower plasma calcium.

11. **What are the overall effects of PTH, vitamin D, and FGF23 on calcium metabolism?**

Plasma calcium must be maintained within a narrow concentration range because of the key role it plays in a diverse array of physiologic processes, including intracellular signal transduction, muscle contraction, blood clotting, and neuronal transmission. Indeed, calcium in a given person is so tightly regulated that the average daily ionized calcium level does not deviate by > 0.3 mg/dL. Regulation of plasma calcium depends on normal amounts of PTH and calcitriol. Both hormones are also necessary for normal bone health. PTH and calcitriol provide the main control of serum calcium. Both PTH and calcitriol increase bone resorption by increasing osteoclast activity. At physiologic levels, PTH and calcitriol also increase bone formation. Because osteoclasts have no known receptors for either hormone, PTH and calcitriol stimulate osteoclast activity indirectly. Both hormones promote normal bone formation by direct action on the osteoblast line of cells. PTH enhances the activity of osteoblasts, which secrete such factors as interleukin-6 (IL-6) that stimulate osteoclastic bone resorption. PTH and calcitriol promote osteoclast differentiation from promonocytes to monocytes to macrophages to preosteoclasts, and finally to osteoclasts. This is accompanied by an increase in osteoclast number and activity, and decreased collagen synthesis. Calcitriol also increases calcium transport from bone to blood and maintains a favorable calcium–phosphate product necessary for normal bone mineralization. Both PTH and calcitriol stimulate osteoblast production of receptor activator of nuclear factor kappa B ligand (RANKL). RANKL binds to its membrane-bound receptor (RANK) on preosteoclasts and osteoclasts. This action stimulates osteoclast differentiation and osteoclast attachment to the bone via integrins and, ultimately, bone resorption. Both PTH and calcitriol also control osteoblast production and secretion of osteoprotegerin (OPG), which blocks the effects of excess RANKL and promotes normal bone metabolism. This process depends on the concentration of PTH and calcitriol. Higher PTH and calcitriol levels increase bone resorption abnormally and may cause hypercalcemia and loss of bone mass.

Bone resorption is the major mechanism of most occurrences of hypercalcemia (Table 17.1). However, PTH and calcitriol also act on the kidney to increase calcium reabsorption. PTH increases renal phosphate excretion, and calcitriol increases its reabsorption. PTH has no direct effect on the intestine, but calcitriol increases absorption of both calcium and phosphate. Higher calcium and calcitriol levels provide negative feedback on PTH secretion, whereas higher phosphate levels provide positive feedback. The net effect is normal bone function and plasma calcium at physiologic levels of PTH and calcitriol, and loss of bone mineral and hypercalcemia at high levels. FGF23 counters the effects of excess PTH and calcitriol by inhibiting synthesis of both hormones and increasing renal phosphate excretion.

12. How do calcium and phosphate interact with calcium-regulating hormones?
Table 17.2 summarizes the main factors controlling serum calcium. The arrows show direct actions of factors in the left column on factors in the top row, whereas the plus (+) and minus (−) signs show indirect actions. As a rule, the direct effects predominate as the net effect. Table 17.3 outlines the specific effects of each of these factors.

Table 17.1. Mechanisms and Causes of Hypercalcemia.

PRIMARY MECHANISM	CAUSE(S) OF HYPERCALCEMIA
Increased bone resorption	Hyperparathyroidism Local osteolytic hypercalcemia Humoral hypercalcemia of malignancy Thyrotoxicosis Pheochromocytoma Excessive vitamin A (usually > 25,000 IU/day) Lithium carbonate Immobilization Addison's disease
Increased renal reabsorption or decreased excretion	Milk-alkali syndrome Rhabdomyolysis Thiazide diuretics Familial hypocalciuric hypercalcemia Renal failure Lithium carbonate Addison's disease (volume contraction)
Increased gut absorption	Excessive vitamin D (usually > 10,000 IU/day) Berylliosis Candidiasis, coccidioidomycosis Eosinophilic granuloma Histoplasmosis Sarcoidosis Silicone implants Tuberculosis Inflammatory disorders Acquired immunodeficiency syndrome Lymphomas

Table 17.2. Interaction of Factors Controlling Serum Calcium.

	PTH	1,25(OH)₂D	CALCITONIN	CALCIUM	PO₄
Parathyroid hormone (PTH)	—	↑+	+	↑+	↓↑+
1,25(OH)₂D	↓−	↓−	+	↑	↑
Calcitonin	+	+	—	↓	↓
Calcium	↓	↓	↑	—	↓
Phosphate (PO₄)	↑+	↓	—	↓	—
Fibroblast growth factor-23 (FGF-23)	↓+	↓+	—	− +	↓−

Arrows (↑, increase; ↓, decrease) indicate direct effects; + and − indicate indirect effects; — indicates no effect.

Table 17.3. Summary of Calcium and Phosphate Control.

VARIABLE	DIRECT ACTION(S)
Parathyroid hormone (PTH)	Increased bone resorption of calcium and phosphate Increased distal renal tubular calcium reabsorption Decreased renal tubular phosphate reabsorption Increased renal production of 1,25(OH)₂ vitamin D Net effect: increased serum calcium and decreased phosphate
1,25(OH)₂ vitamin D	Increased bone resorption of calcium and phosphate Increased renal reabsorption of calcium and phosphate Increased gut absorption of calcium and phosphate Decreased parathyroid production of PTH Decreased renal production of 1,25(OH)₂ vitamin D Net effect: increased serum calcium and phosphate
Calcitonin	Decreased bone resorption of calcium and phosphate Decreased renal reabsorption of calcium and phosphate Decreased gut absorption of calcium and phosphate Net effect: decreased serum calcium and phosphate
Calcium	Decreased PTH synthesis and secretion Decreased 1,25(OH)₂ vitamin D production in the kidney Increased calcitonin release from the thyroid C cells Decreased phosphate
Phosphate	Decreased 1,25(OH)₂ vitamin D production in the kidney Decreased calcium Increased PTH synthesis in parathyroid chief cells
Fibroblast growth factor 23 (FGF23)	Decreased 1,25(OH)₂ vitamin D production in the kidney Decreased renal tubular phosphate reabsorption Decreased parathyroid production of PTH

13. List the main causes of hypercalcemia.
    The mnemonic VITAMINS TRAP (see Pont, 1989) includes most causes of hypercalcemia (Box 17.1).

14. How do various causes of hypercalcemia increase the serum calcium level?
    True hypercalcemia results from altered bone resorption, renal tubular reabsorption, and gut absorption of calcium. Although the bone (resorption and formation), kidney (reabsorption and excretion), and gut (absorption and secretion) each have two major processes involved with mineral metabolism, only resorption, reabsorption, and absorption play a significant role in hypercalcemia. An exception to this rule occurs when decreased renal function from renal or prerenal disease impairs calcium filtration and excretion. In Fig. 17.3, solid arrows represent potential causes of increased calcium, and dashed arrows represent potential causes of decreased calcium.

15. What are the mechanisms and causes of hypercalcemia?
    From the preceding discussions, one can appreciate that mechanisms of hypercalcemia are usually multifactorial. However, most hypercalcemic syndromes have a primary or predominant mechanism, as outlined in Table 17.1.

Box 17.1. Mnemonic for Causes of Hypercalcemia.

V = Vitamins
I = Immobilization
T = Thyrotoxicosis
A = Addison's disease
M = Milk-alkali syndrome
I = Inflammatory disorders
N = Neoplasm-related disease

S = Sarcoidosis
T = Thiazide diuretics (drugs)
R = Rhabdomyolysis
A = Acquired immunodeficiency syndrome
P = Paget's disease, parenteral nutrition, pheochromocytoma, parathyroid disease

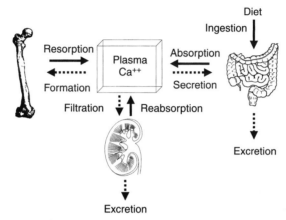

Fig. 17.3 Calcium (Ca^{++}) metabolism. Solid arrows represent potential causes of increased calcium, and dashed arrows represent potential causes of decreased calcium.

Most resorptive hypercalcemia is humoral (PTH, PTH-related peptide [PTHrP], transforming growth factor-alpha [TGF-alpha], TNF) or local osteolytic hypercalcemia (PTHrP, interleukins, prostaglandins). Increased calcium absorption usually occurs because of high $1,25(OH)_2$ vitamin D levels either from excess vitamin D ingestion or produced by tumors or granulomas. Ninety percent of hypercalcemia cases result from hyperparathyroidism or cancer.

KEY POINTS: HYPERCALCEMIA

- Therapy for hypercalcemia should be directed at the underlying etiology, including excess bone resorption, renal tubular reabsorption, and gut absorption.
- Although there are > 30 different causes of hypercalcemia, hyperparathyroidism and hypercalcemia of malignancy account for > 90% of cases.
- Most patients with severe hypercalcemia require normal saline hydration and multiple-drug therapy, but most therapies for hypercalcemia inhibit bone resorption.
- Zoledronic acid is the most potent bisphosphonate approved for the treatment of hypercalcemia and has the advantage over pamidronate of shorter infusion time and a longer duration of action.
- Cinacalcet is a calcimimetic that lowers serum parathyroid hormone (PTH), calcium, and phosphorus levels. It is approved for treatment of secondary hyperparathyroidism (HPT), parathyroid carcinoma, and primary HPT in patients with significant hypercalcemia when parathyroidectomy is not clinically appropriate. Although not approved for such situations, cinacalcet also lowers PTH and calcium in kidney transplant recipients who have persistently elevated PTH.

16. What is the relative frequency of skeletal lesions in patients with advanced cancer?
The relative frequency is as follows: myeloma 95% to 100%, breast and prostate 70%, thyroid 60%, bladder 40%, lung 35%, renal 25%, and melanoma 14% to 45%. Common sites of bone metastases are ribs, spine, pelvis, and proximal extremities.

17. What is the incidence of hypercalcemia in patients with cancer?
Hypercalcemia affects 15% to 30% of patients with cancer. It is most common in squamous cell carcinoma of the lung, head and neck; renal cell carcinoma; breast cancer; multiple myeloma; and lymphoma. About 80% of cancer-related hypercalcemia results from humoral causes and 20% from metastases to bone.

18. What are multiple endocrine neoplasia syndromes?

Multiple endocrine neoplasia (MEN) syndrome is associated with three familial syndromes, two of which manifest as hypercalcemia caused by hyperparathyroidism. MEN 1, or Wermer's syndrome, includes the three Ps: pituitary, parathyroid, and pancreatic tumors. Hypercalcemia caused by hyperparathyroidism is usually the first feature of this syndrome to appear. MEN 2 has two variants. Patients with MEN 2A, or Sipple's syndrome, have medullary carcinoma of the thyroid (MCT), pheochromocytoma, and hyperparathyroidism. Patients with MEN 2B have MCT, pheochromocytoma, multiple mucosal neuromas, and marfanoid habitus; they usually do not have hyperparathyroidism. In comparison with sporadic hyperparathyroidism, parathyroid tumors in MEN syndromes are more often bilateral, hyperplastic, and malignant.

19. How would you diagnose familial hypocalciuric hypercalcemia?

Familial hypocalciuric hypercalcemia (FHH), also called *familial benign hypercalcemia,* is caused by autosomal dominant *CaSR* gene mutations encoding inactive forms of the CaSR on parathyroid and renal tubular cell membranes. Important diagnostic features of FHH include the combination of no symptoms, a family history of benign hypercalcemia, mild hypercalcemia, normal-to-high serum PTH levels, and decreased renal calcium clearance with calcium/creatinine (Ca/Cr) clearance ratio < 0.01 or fractional excretion of calcium (FECa) $< 1\%$. The clinical importance of FHH is to distinguish it from PHPT to avoid needless and ineffective parathyroidectomy. Patients with PHPT usually have a FECa value $> 2\%$. Also, patients with FHH usually have a 24-hour urinary calcium level < 50 mg/24 hr, and those with HPT have values > 200 mg/24 hr.

20. What is the likely cause of hypercalcemia in the following patient?

An 18-year-old man has had serum calcium values of 10.5 to 11.8 mg/dL for 2 years. His physical examination results are normal, and he has a family history of hypercalcemia. Current laboratory values are as follows: calcium 11.5 mg/dL, intact PTH 70 pg/mL (normal NL < 65), plasma creatinine (PCr) 1.0 mg/dL, random urine calcium (UCa) 5 mg/dL, and urine creatinine (UCr) 90 mg/dL.

$$Ca/Cr \text{ clearance ratio} = [UCa \div PCa] \times [PCr \div UCr]$$
$$Ca/Cr \text{ clearance ratio} = [5 \text{ mg/dL} \div 11.5 \text{ mg/dL}] \times [1 \text{ mg/dL}/90 \text{ mg/dL}] = 0.005$$
$$FECa = 0.005 \times 100\% = 0.5\%$$

The history, family history, physical findings, laboratory values, and FECa $< 1\%$ support the diagnosis of FHH. However, testing for mutations in the *CaSR* gene may be needed to confirm the diagnosis.

21. What therapy is useful for hypercalcemia?

Most patients with severe hypercalcemia require treatment with multiple drugs. The lowest amount and least frequent dose that will achieve and maintain acceptable serum calcium levels should be given. The usual order of therapy is normal saline, calcitonin, zoledronic acid, and glucocorticoids, if indicated. Furosemide should be given only after good hydration, primarily to avoid volume overload and improve urinary volume. Bisphosphonates are relatively contraindicated with GFR < 30 mL/min per 1.73 m². Denosumab is a monoclonal antibody to RANKL that was approved by the U.S. Food and Drug Administration (FDA) in December 2014 for treatment of hypercalcemia of malignancy refractory to bisphosphonate therapy. Denosumab is not cleared by the kidney and may be used when zoledronic acid is ineffective or contraindicated, as in renal failure. However, caution should be used when the glomerular filtration rate (GFR) is < 30 mL/min per 1.73 m² and patients should be monitored closely for hypocalcemia for several weeks after administration. Gallium nitrate was effective but was discontinued by the manufacturer in 2012. Consult with nephrology for dialysis treatment for patients with renal failure and those with severe and refractory hypercalcemia and hypercalcemic crisis. See Table 17.4.

22. Describe the mechanisms of action of drug therapies for hypercalcemia.

See Table 17.5.

23. How might calcimimetic drugs be useful in therapy for hypercalcemia?

There are two FDA-approved calcimimetics that bind to the extracellular CaSRs on parathyroid cells and increase chief cell sensitivity to extracellular calcium. This effect shifts the PTH–calcium curve to the left, increasing parathyroid cell sensitivity to the PTH-suppressive effects of high extracellular calcium and decreasing responsiveness to the PTH-stimulatory effects of low calcium (see questions 8 and 9). Cinacalcet (generic as of 2018) is an oral calcimimetic that binds to the transmembrane domain of the CaSR and is FDA approved to treat secondary HPT in patients with end-stage renal disease on dialysis (2004), parathyroid carcinoma (2011), and hypercalcemia in patients with primary HPT who are unable to undergo parathyroidectomy (2011).

Etelcalcetide is an intravenous calcimimetic that binds to the extracellular domain of the CaSR at a site different from that of calcium; it was FDA approved in February 2017 for treatment of secondary HPT in adults with CKD on hemodialysis. Both calcimimetics decrease serum levels of PTH and calcium. Etelcalcetide appears to be more effective. By increasing CaSR calcium sensitivity in Henle's loop, cinacalcet also increases renal calcium excretion. Although not approved for the following uses, cinacalcet has improved persistent HPT after kidney transplantation, hypercalcemia caused by FHH, and lithium-induced hypercalcemia (see question 24). The net

Table 17.4. Therapy for Hypercalcemia.

THERAPY	DOSE	ROUTE	MONITOR/COMMENT
Saline	250–1000 mL/hr	IV	Cardiopulmonary function with examination, central venous pressure and chest radiograph, daily weights and input/output.
Furosemide	20–80 mg every 2–4 hr or 40 mg/hr CI	IV	Serum and urine electrolytes. Replace K, Mg, and PO_4 based on serum levels and urinary losses.
Salmon calcitonin	4–8 IU/kg every 6–12 hours	IM, SC	Allergic reaction. Give a skin test of 1 IU intradermally before treatment. Effective only during first 48–72 hr.
Prednisone/ methylprednisolone	40–60 mg daily for 10 days	PO/IV	Possible adjunct to calcitonin. Effective in $1,25(OH)_2$ vitamin D-associated hypercalcemia.
Zoledronic acid	4 mg IV over 20–30 minutes, may repeat in 7 days then every 2–4 weeks PRN	IV	Drug of choice for malignancy-associated hyper-calcemia. Dosage is decreased in stage 3 CKD to 3–3.5 mg. Avoid use for GFR < 30 mL/min. Monitor GFR. Hold for > 0.5 mg/dL increase in creatinine.
Pamidronate	60–90 mg over 2–24 hours every 1–3 weeks PRN	IV	Infuse 60 mg over 6–8 hours for GFR < 30 mL/min as one-time dose only and monitor GFR. Hold for > 0.5 mg/dL increase in creatinine.
Cinacalcet	30–90 mg 2–4 times daily	PO	Take with meals. Titrate every 2–4 weeks based on calcium and PTH measured at least 12 hr after dose.
Denosumab	120 mg every 4 weeks and days 8 and 15 of the first month of therapy	SC	For treatment of hypercalcemia of malignancy re-fractory to bisphosphonates. Takes 4–7 days for effect. Consider decreased dosage and frequently monitor for hypocalcemia when patient has vitamin D deficiency and GFR < 30 mL/min.
Dialysis	Low or no calcium dialysate	Hemodialysis Peritoneal dialysis	Hypercalcemic crisis or refractory hypercalcemia. Useful in renal failure. Nephrology consultation.

b.i.d., Twice daily; *CI*, continuous infusion; *CKD*, chronic kidney disease; *GFR*, glomerular filtration rate; *IM*, intramuscularly; *IV*, intravenously; *K*, potassium; *Mg*, magnesium; *Na*, sodium; *PO*, orally; *PO₄*, phosphate; *PRN*, as needed; *q.i.d.*, four times daily; *SC*, subcutaneously.

Table 17.5. Mechanisms of Action of Hypercalcemic Therapy.

DRUG	MECHANISM(S) OF ACTION
Saline	Dilutes serum calcium by volume expansion and increases urinary flow and calcium excretion.
Furosemide	Impairs renal sodium and calcium reabsorption in Henle's loop, increasing urinary flow and calcium excretion.
Calcitonin	Binds to receptors on osteoclasts, inhibiting osteoclast activity and decreasing bone resorption; also decreases renal reabsorption.
Glucocorticoids	Antagonism of vitamin D, causing decreased calcium absorption and reabsorption; in tumoral states, may be tumor lytic and may decrease production of osteoclast-activating factors and vitamin D.
Bisphosphonates	Impair osteoclast differentiation, recruitment, motility, and attachment; incorporate into bone matrix, making the matrix resistant to hydrolysis; overall effect is decreased bone resorption.
Cinacalcet	Calcimimetic that binds to the calcium-sensing receptor, making it markedly more responsive to calcium activation decreasing parathyroid hormone (PTH) and calcium.
Denosumab	Monoclonal antibody that binds to receptor activator of nuclear factor kappa B ligand (RANKL), pre-venting activation of the osteoclast RANK receptor and decreasing osteoclast bone resorption.
Dialysis	Direct removal of calcium from blood.

Note: For long-term hypocalcemic effects, drug therapy for hypercalcemia must antagonize one of the three main causes of hypercalcemia: bone resorption, renal reabsorption, or gut absorption. All hypercalcemia results from some abnormality in one of the three. Thus, one of these etiologies should be considered in the choice of drug therapy. As noted, most drug therapies for hypercalcemia impair bone resorption.

effect of calcimimetics is a dose-dependent reduction in PTH secretion, increase in urinary calcium excretion, and a decrease in serum calcium.

24. How does lithium cause hypercalcemia?

Lithium decreases urinary calcium through competitive inhibition of the CaSR in the thick ascending limb of Henle's loop, causing increased calcium reabsorption, decreased calcium excretion, and hypercalcemia. Urinary calcium may be low in lithium-treated patients, as it is in patients with FHH. Lithium also decreases the sensitivity of the parathyroid CaSR to calcium and shifts the PTH–calcium curve in the parathyroids to the right. Thus, for any given calcium level, there is less suppression of PTH secretion and synthesis, and higher serum PTH levels. Unlike in PHPT, serum phosphate tends to be normal and magnesium higher in lithium-treated patients. Because hypercalcemia and elevated PTH may persist after lithium is discontinued, therapy other than just discontinuing lithium may be indicated if the hypercalcemia is symptomatic. Cinacalcet has successfully corrected or ameliorated PTH and serum calcium levels in such patients. This effect is expected because cinacalcet sensitizes the CaSR to calcium and shifts the PTH-calcium curve to the left.

⊕ WEBSITES

National Cancer Institute: http://www.meb.uni-bonn.de/cancer.gov/CDR0000062737.html

Denosumab: a new agent in the management of hypercalcemia of malignancy: https://www.ncbi.nlm.nih.gov/pmc/articles/PMC4976858/

NIH Genetic and Rare Diseases Information Center—FHH: https://rarediseases.info.nih.gov/diseases/10828/familial-hypocalciuric-hypercalcemia

BIBLIOGRAPHY

Bringhurst, F. R., Demay, M. B., & Kronenberg, H. M. (2016). Hormones and disorders of mineral metabolism. In S. Melmed, K. S. Polonsky, P. R. Larsen, & H. Kronenberg (Eds.), *Williams textbook of endocrinology* (13th ed., p. 1254). Philadelphia, PA: Elsevier Saunders.

Carroll, R., & Matfin, G. (2010). Review: endocrine and metabolic emergencies: hypercalcaemia. *Therapeutic Advances in Endocrinology and Metabolism, 1*(5), 225–234.

Festen-Spanjer, B., Haring, C. M., Koster, J. B., & Mudde, A. H. (2008). Correction of hypercalcaemia by cinacalcet in familial hypocalciuric hypercalcaemia. *Clinical Endocrinology, 68,* 324–325.

Foley, K. F., & Boccuzzi, L. (2010). Urine calcium: laboratory measurement and clinical utility. *Laboratory Medicine, 41*(11), 683–686.

Goldner, W. (2016). Cancer-related hypercalcemia. *Journal of Oncology Practice, 12,* 426–432.

Kallas, M., Green, F., Hewison, M., White, C., & Kline, G. (2010). Rare causes of calcitriol-mediated hypercalcemia: a case report and literature review. *Journal of Clinical Endocrinology and Metabolism, 95*(7), 3111–3117.

Maalouf, N. M. (2012). Calcium homeostasis. In W. J. Kovacs, & S. R. Ojeda (Eds.), *Textbook of endocrine physiology* (6th ed., p. 381). New York, NY: Oxford University Press.

Martin, A., David, V., & Quarles, L. D. (2012). Regulation and function of the FGF23/Klotho endocrine pathways. *Physiology Review, 92*(1), 131–155.

Meehan, A. D., Udumyan, R., Kardell, M., Landén, M., Järhult, J., & Wallin, G. (2018). Lithium-associated hypercalcemia: pathophysiology, prevalence, management. *World Journal of Surgery, 42,* 415–424.

Mirrakhimov, A. E. (2015). Hypercalcemia of malignancy: an update on pathogenesis and management. *North American Journal of Medical Science, 7,* 483–493.

Peacock, M., Bilezikian, J. P., Bolognese, M. A., Borofsky, M., Scumpia, S., Sterling, L. R., ... Shoback, D. (2011). Cinacalcet HCL reduces hypercalcemia in primary hyperparathyroidism across a wide spectrum of disease severity. *Journal of Clinical Endocrinology and Metabolism, 96*(1), E9–E18.

Pont, A. (1989). Unusual causes of hypercalcemia. *Endocrinology and Metabolism Clinics of North America, 18,* 753–764.

Popovtzer, M. M. (2018). Disorders of calcium, phosphorus, vitamin D, and parathyroid hormone activity. In R. W. Schrier (Ed.), *Renal and electrolytes disorders* (8th ed., p. 163). Philadelphia, PA: Wolters Kluwer.

Renaghan, A. D., & Rosner, M. H. (2018). Hypercalcemia: etiology and management. *Nephrology Dialysis Transplantation, 33,* 549–551.

Shoback, D. M., Schafer, A. L., & Bikle, D. D. (2018). Metabolic bone disease. In D. G. Gardner & D. Shoback (Eds.), *Greenspan's basic & clinical endocrinology* (10th ed., p. 239). New York, NY: McGraw-Hill Education.

Tebben, P. J., Singh, R. J., & Kumar, R. (2016). Vitamin D-mediated hypercalcemia: mechanisms, diagnosis, and treatment. *Endocrinology Review, 37,* 521–547.

Thakker, R. V., Newey, P. J., Walls, G. V., Bilezikian, J., Dralle, H., Ebeling, P. R., ... Brandi, M. L. (2012). Clinical practice guidelines for multiple endocrine neoplasia type 1 (MEN1). *Journal of Clinical Endocrinology and Metabolism, 97*(9), 2990–3011.

Thosani, S., & Hu, M. I. (2015). Denosumab: a new agent in the management of hypercalcemia of malignancy. *Future Oncology, 11,* 2865–2871.

von Moos, R., Costa, L., Ripamonti, C. I., Niepel, D., & Santini, D. (2017). Improving quality of life in patients with advanced cancer: targeting metastatic bone pain. *European Journal of Cancer, 71,* 80–94.

Varghese, J., Rich, T., & Jimenez, C. (2011). Benign familial hypocalciuric hypercalcemia. *Endocrinology Practice, 17*(Suppl. 1), 13–17.

CHAPTER 18

HYPERPARATHYROIDISM

Leonard R. Sanders

1. **What is hyperparathyroidism?**

   Hyperparathyroidism (HPT) is a clinical disorder of calcium metabolism associated with increased bone resorption and specific symptoms and signs that result from excessive parathyroid hormone (PTH), hypercalcemia, or altered vitamin D, phosphate, and fibroblast growth factor 23 (FGF23) metabolism. The three types of HPT are primary, secondary, and tertiary.

2. **How common is primary HPT (PHPT)?**

   The prevalence of primary HPT (PHPT) in the United States is about 42 in 100,000 in the general population. The female-to-male ratio is 3:1. The incidence increases with age and approximates 3 to 4 in 1000 among postmenopausal women.

3. **What causes PHPT?**

   PHPT is characterized by abnormal regulation of PTH secretion by calcium, resulting in excessive PTH secretion and hypercalcemia. Although the cause of all PHPT is not known, genetic mutations that cause changes in the parathyroid chief cells may occur. These changes increase PTH secretion, in part as a result of an elevation of the calcium-suppressible PTH secretion set point and a change in the slope of the calcium–PTH curve that causes relatively nonsuppressible PTH secretion. Expression of the calcium-sensing receptor (CaSR) is reduced in parathyroid adenomas and hyperplasia, and may be partly responsible for decreased PTH suppressibility.

4. **What anatomic alterations occur in PHPT?**

   Most patients with PHPT have a single parathyroid adenoma (85%), whereas four-gland hyperplasia (10%) and multiple adenomas (< 5%) are less common, and parathyroid carcinomas are rare (< 1%). Greater than 95% of those with parathyroid adenomas have a single adenoma, and < 5% have ≥ 2 adenomas. Normal parathyroid glands weigh about 30 to 40 mg each. The average weight of parathyroid adenomas is 500 mg, but this depends on the longevity of the adenoma; some can weigh as much as 5 to 25 g. The largest reported tumor weighed 120 g, and the largest number of glands reported in one patient was eight.

5. **How do you diagnose PHPT?**

   Persistent hypercalcemia with increased or high-normal serum PTH levels usually confirms the diagnosis of PHPT. Associated low or low-normal serum phosphate and normal-to-high urinary calcium make PHPT more likely. PHPT is the most common cause of hypercalcemia and should be suspected whenever a patient has documented hypercalcemia. Because symptoms of PHPT are nonspecific or absent (see question 12), one must base the diagnosis primarily on laboratory studies. PHPT may present in three ways. PTH and calcium are elevated in 80% to 90% of patients with PHPT, normal PTH (20–64 pg/mL) and elevated calcium occur in 10% to 20%, and elevated PTH and normal calcium (normocalcemic PHPT) occur in 1%. Most patients with mild PHPT have no specific symptoms or signs, and PHPT is suspected after serum calcium is found elevated with routine multichannel laboratory screening.

6. **How does age complicate the diagnosis of HPT?**

   The laboratory reference range for intact PTH (10–65 pg/mL) and calcium (8.5–10.5 mg/dL) may be different in older adults and young individuals. These ranges may be different at different laboratories. The PTH reference range is not age adjusted, but a lower reference range of 10 to 45 pg/mL may be more appropriate for individuals aged < 45 years. PTH increases and calcium decreases with age. Why PTH increases with age is unclear, but the changes may be associated with age-related declines in renal function, vitamin D synthesis, and vitamin D and calcium absorption. Thus, PTH levels in the normal upper range are more likely to represent PHPT in patients who are younger than in those age > 50 years. Although serum calcium levels decline with age, the decline is usually related to decreasing albumin and does not affect serum PTH levels.

7. **How might you confirm the diagnosis of PHPT before recommending parathyroidectomy?**

   Obtain at least three fasting serum calcium levels and two PTH measurements at least several weeks apart. Ensure that the patient has normal renal function. Discontinue any thiazide diuretics for at least 1 week before measurement and discontinue lithium if safe to do so. Measure serum total calcium and calculate the correction for albumin and total protein levels; order an ionized calcium measurement if there is any doubt (see Chapter 17). If the serum calcium level is elevated and the PTH is high or high-normal, PHPT is usually present. If calcium is normal and PTH is high, secondary HPT (renal insufficiency, vitamin D deficiency, or calcium malabsorption) is much more likely. The 25-hydroxy (OH) vitamin D level should be > 30 ng/mL to exclude vitamin D deficiency. The second-generation PTH assays are the immunoradiometric assay (IRMA) and the immunochemiluminometric assay (ICMA). Both assays measure the intact biologically active PTH, both have similar reliability sufficient for diagnosis, and both measure PTH fragments other than PTH (1–84), including non–(1–84) PTH that accumulates in chronic kidney disease (CKD). Third-generation PTH assays target the amino-terminal 1 to 6 amino acids of the PTH (1–84) and are designated whole, bioactive, or intact PTH assays, but these have not offered a clinical benefit over the second-generation assays.

8. **What laboratories or conditions help with the differential diagnosis of PHPT?**
   Increased serum chloride (Cl), decreased phosphate (PO_4), a Cl/PO_4 ratio > 33, elevated urinary pH (6.0), and increased serum alkaline phosphatase levels support the diagnosis of PHPT but are not specific. If PTH is lower than expected, make sure that the patient is not taking excess biotin (vitamin B_7) that is known to falsely lower PTH levels in standard assays. Repeat the PTH measurement with the patient off biotin for a week. If PTH is lower than expected for PHPT in patients with hypercalcemia (< 20 pg/mL), consider cancer and other causes of hypercalcemia (see Chapter 17).

9. **What differentiates familial hypocalciuric hypercalcemia from PHPT?**
   Familial hypocalciuric hypercalcemia (FHH), or autosomal dominant familial benign hypercalcemia, often results from a loss-of-function mutation in the CaSR. If there is a family history of hypercalcemia and serum calcium and PTH levels are mildly elevated chronically, consider FHH. There is a 50% chance that a first-degree relative has FHH. Calculate the fractional excretion of calcium (FECa) (see Chapter 17). Urinary calcium is usually < 50 mg/24 hr, and the FECa is $< 1\%$. If the FECa is low, test family members for elevated PTH, hypercalcemia, and hypocalciuria. If they test positive, FHH is likely; however, results may overlap with PHPT, and genetic testing may be needed to confirm the diagnosis. Avoid neck exploration, which will not correct the hypercalcemia. In PHPT, FECa is usually $> 2\%$.

10. **How does CKD complicate the diagnosis of PHPT?**
    Renal failure increases serum PO_4 and decreases serum 1,25-dihydroxy $(OH)_2$ vitamin D (calcitriol) levels. Because PO_4 directly stimulates and calcitriol directly inhibits PTH secretion, serum PTH levels increase in renal failure (secondary HPT). High PO_4 and low calcitriol levels also directly decrease serum calcium. The resulting absolute or relative hypocalcemia further increases PTH secretion. Symptoms and signs of renal insufficiency, such as lethargy, depression, anorexia, nausea, constipation, and weakness, may be identical to those of PHPT. Thus, diagnosis of PHPT may be more difficult in renal failure; before parathyroidectomy in patients with CKD, parathyroid gland localization may be appropriate (question 24).

11. **What changes occur in renal failure that may complicate the results of the PTH assay?**
    In renal failure, PTH rises above normal because of the stimulatory effects of high serum PO_4 and low calcitriol levels. In addition, a non-(1–84) PTH molecular fragment (PTH 7–84), which has antagonistic actions to those of intact PTH, accumulates in renal failure and cross-reacts with intact PTH in the intact two-site assays. For this reason, measured levels of intact PTH in patients with renal failure may be > 1.5 to three times those of normal subjects to maintain physiologic PTH concentrations.

12. **What are the symptoms and signs of PHPT?**
    Greater than 85% of patients with PHPT are asymptomatic. However, vascular, musculoskeletal, gastrointestinal, and neurologic symptoms may occur in PHPT. The classic descriptive phrase for many of these features is "kidney stones, painful bones, abdominal groans, psychic moans, and fatigue overtones." The incidence of PHPT-associated nephrolithiasis is about 10% to 20%, and 5% of calcium stone formers have PHPT. Proximal muscle weakness is also characteristic. See Table 18.1 for other characteristic symptoms and signs.

13. **What is band keratopathy?**
    Band keratopathy is a classic but unusual sign of PHPT characterized by an irregular region of calcium phosphate deposition at the medial and lateral limbic margins of the outer edges of the corneas. The location is believed to be a result of diffusion of carbon dioxide from the air-exposed areas of the cornea, leaving an alkaline environment that favors precipitation of calcium phosphate crystals. Band keratopathy occurs only with a high calcium phosphate product. Diagnosis is made by ophthalmologic slit lamp examination. The sign differs from arcus senilis, an age-related, linear, concentric gray crescent separated from the extreme periphery (limbus corneae) by a rim of clear cornea that with time completely encircles the cornea.

14. **What are the classic radiographic findings in HPT?**
    The classic radiographic findings are subperiosteal bone resorption along the radial aspect of the middle and distal phalanges and distal clavicles. Salt-and-pepper skull is another classic finding. However, because most

Table 18.1. Hyperparathyroidism: Symptoms and Signs and Their Probable Causes.

SYMPTOMS AND SIGNS	PROBABLE CAUSE(S)
Renal: hypercalciuria, nephrolithiasis, nephrocalcinosis, polyuria, polydipsia, renal insufficiency, and distal renal tubular acidosis	Parathyroid hormone (PTH) stimulates bone resorption, hypercalcemia, bicarbonaturia, and phosphaturia, causing decreased tubular responsiveness to antidiuretic hormone (ADH), polyuria, calcium oxalate and phosphate crystallization, nephrocalcinosis, and renal insufficiency.
Neuromuscular: weakness, myalgia	Prolonged excessive PTH arguably causes direct neuropathy with abnormal nerve conduction velocities (NCVs) and characteristic electromyographic changes and myopathic features on muscle biopsy.
Neurologic and psychiatric: memory loss, depression, psychoses, neuroses, confusion, lethargy, fatigue, paresthesias	PTH and calcium cause peripheral neuropathy with abnormal NCVs and central nervous system damage with abnormal electroencephalographic changes.
Skeletal: bone pain, osteitis fibrosa, osteoporosis, and subperiosteal skeletal resorption	PTH increases bone resorption and acidosis with subsequent bone buffering and bone loss of calcium and phosphate.
Gastrointestinal: abdominal pain, nausea, heartburn, peptic ulcer, constipation, and pancreatitis	Hypercalcemia stimulates gastrin secretion, decreases peristalsis, and increases the calcium–phosphate product with calcium–phosphate deposition in and obstruction of pancreatic ducts.
Hypertension	PTH and hypercalcemia are associated with increased vasoconstriction.
Arthralgia, synovitis, arthritis	HPT is associated with increased crystal deposition from calcium phosphate (paraarticular calcification), calcium pyrophosphate (pseudogout), and uric acid/urate (gout)
Band keratopathy	Calcium–phosphate precipitation occurs in the medial and limbic margins of the cornea.
Anemia	Unknown

patients are diagnosed early, there are usually no radiographic findings associated with HPT. If HPT is prolonged, osteopenia or osteoporosis develops. Because cortical bone loss is higher in HPT, bone densitometry of the distal radius and hip is a good way to monitor for bone loss in patients who do not undergo parathyroidectomy. However, long-term excess PTH can cause a diffuse decrease in bone mineral, and three-site bone mineral density (BMD) measurement with dual energy x-ray absorptiometry (DXA) is often recommended.

15. What is the differential diagnosis of PHPT?

Because the main abnormality in PHPT is hypercalcemia, the differential diagnosis initially is that of hypercalcemia (see Chapter 17). A history and physical examination focused on symptoms and signs (question 12) may suggest one of the causes of hypercalcemia. If hypercalcemia is mild and the history and physical findings are nonspecific, PHPT is likely. The two most common causes of hypercalcemia are PHPT and malignancy. About 15% to 30% of patients with cancer develop hypercalcemia but are usually symptomatic. In humoral hypercalcemia of malignancy (HHM), the tumor usually produces a PTH-like hormone called *PTH-related peptide.*

16. What laboratory tests help to distinguish the three types of HPT?

See Table 18.2.

17. What pathophysiologic changes occur in PHPT?

PHPT causes excessive PTH secretion from parathyroid adenomas, hyperplasia, or rarely carcinoma. The increased PTH increases bone resorption, renal tubular calcium reabsorption, and calcitriol production, which increases intestinal absorption of calcium. All three processes contribute to hypercalcemia.

18. What pathophysiologic changes occur in secondary HPT?

Secondary HPT is excessive PTH secretion that occurs as a compensatory response to absolute or relative hyperphosphatemia, hypocalcemia, low calcitriol levels, and excess FGF23. Renal failure is the most common cause of secondary HPT and often produces PTH hypersecretion from all four of these stimuli. In renal failure, phosphorus increases because of decreased renal excretion. The increased phosphorous stimulates PTH secretion, decreases ionized calcium, decreases the production of $1,25(OH)_2$ vitamin D levels, and increases FGF23 from bone osteocytes. The lower calcium and vitamin D levels further increase PTH synthesis and secretion. Thus, controlling

Table 18.2. Parathyroid Hormone (PTH) and Calcium Levels in Hyperparathyroidism.

TYPE OF HYPERPARATHYROIDISM	PTH	CALCIUM
Primary	↑ Normal	↑
Secondary	↑	↓ Normal
Tertiary	↑↑	↑

↑, High; ↑↑, very high.

phosphorus levels with diet and phosphate binders and appropriate calcitriol supplementation may delay the onset of the secondary HPT of renal failure. Stimulation of the parathyroid cell CaSR, vitamin D receptor (VDR), and FGF23 receptor (FGFR) all decrease secretion of PTH by negative feedback. Other causes of hypocalcemia are vitamin D deficiency, dietary calcium malabsorption, and renal calcium leak. Secondary HPT is accompanied by parathyroid hyperplasia as the parathyroid glands enlarge to enhance their PTH-secretory capacity.

19. What pathophysiologic changes occur in tertiary HPT?

Tertiary HPT progresses from secondary HPT when prolonged hyperphosphatemia and hypocalcemia cause autonomous parathyroid hyperplasia and hypercalcemia. The spontaneous change from hypocalcemia to normocalcemia to hypercalcemia marks the transition from secondary HPT to tertiary HPT. PTH levels are often > 15 times the normal upper limit; this most commonly occurs in advanced CKD. Other findings include decreased parathyroid CaSR, VDR, and FGFR function and numbers. In tertiary HPT, PTH levels remain elevated despite vitamin D therapy and correction of hyperphosphatemia, and hypercalcemia persists despite reduction or discontinuation of vitamin D and calcium supplements. Tertiary HPT usually requires resection of at least three and one-half parathyroid glands to correct the hypercalcemia. However, adjusting vitamin D analogues and phosphate binders and administration of the oral or intravenous (IV) calcimimetics, cinacalcet or etelcalcetide, may reduce PTH and calcium to acceptable ranges and delay or obviate surgery.

20. How is hypercalcemia in HHM distinguished from PHPT?

The main distinguishing features of HHM are the levels of intact PTH and PTHrP. Table 18.3 shows the classic and most common patterns of these hormones. Patients with PHPT usually have elevated PTH and, although not usually measured, low or low-normal PTHrP. In contrast, patients with malignancy-associated hypercalcemia have low PTH levels (< 20 pg/mL). About 80% have increased PTHrP levels (PTHrP malignancy), and 20% have low PTHrP levels (non-PTHrP malignancy). Thus, measuring the two hormones distinguishes all three disorders (see question 21).

21. How do PTHrP and PTH differ?

PTHrP consists of three protein forms with 139, 141, and 173 amino acids. The first 139 amino acids are the same among the three forms. Eight of the first 13 N-terminal amino acids are identical to those of intact PTH (1–84), allowing PTHrP to bind to and stimulate the same receptors as PTH and to have similar hypercalcemic effects. But the two hormones have different effects on levels of $1,25(OH)_2$ vitamin D, partly because of their different secretion patterns. Both PTH (in PHPT) and PTHrP (in HHM) stimulate receptors that activate renal 1-alpha-hydroxylase. However, PTH secretion in PHPT is intermittent, whereas PTHrP secretion by malignant tumors is continuous, which probably downregulates these receptors, inhibiting 1-alpha-hydroxylase activity and decreasing $1,25(OH)_2$ vitamin D production. A continuous infusion of PTH causes similar decreases in $1,25(OH)_2$ vitamin D. Other mechanisms may further decrease $1,25(OH)_2$ vitamin D in PTHrP-associated HHM. HHM may also be associated with a 5- to 10-fold increase in the phosphaturic factor FGF23, which inhibits 1-alpha-hydroxylase activity and decreases $1,25(OH)_2$ vitamin D levels. The higher calcium levels typically encountered in HHM may also decrease 1-alpha-hydroxylase activity and $1,25(OH)_2$ vitamin D levels.

22. What hormonal and laboratory changes occur in PHPT?

Secretion of PTH in PHPT is intermittent; intermittent secretion avoids receptor downregulation and results in increased $1,25(OH)_2$ vitamin D formation. Serum calcium levels are higher in HHM than in PHPT, and these higher

Table 18.3. Hypercalcemia: PHPT and Malignancy.

	Serum Levels			
	INTACT PTH	PTHRP	1,25(OH)₂D	CALCIUM
PHPT	↑ Normal	↓	↑	↑
PTHrP malignancy	↓	↑	↓ Normal	↑
Non-PTHrP malignancy	↓	↓	↓ Normal	↑

↑, Increased; ↓, decreased; *PHPT*, primary hyperparathyroidism; *PTHrP*, parathyroid hormone–related protein.

calcium levels also decrease 1,25(OH)$_2$ vitamin D production. Thus, 1,25(OH)$_2$ vitamin D levels tend to be high in PHPT and low in HHM (see Table 18.3). Traditional associations with PHPT include hypophosphatemia, hyperchloremia, an increased chloride/phosphate ratio, and mild renal tubular acidosis. Unfortunately, such associations are nonspecific and too insensitive to be of diagnostic use. However, the triad consisting of hypercalcemia, elevated or high-normal PTH, and hypophosphatemia make the diagnosis of PHPT likely.

23. What PTH assay is most useful in the workup of hypercalcemia?
Intact PTH has 84 amino acids, with 70% metabolized by the liver and 20% metabolized by the kidneys; it has a half-life of 2 to 4 minutes. Less than 1% of the secreted intact hormone remains to interact physiologically with PTH receptors. Although the first 34 amino acids of the N-terminus contain the full biologic activity of the hormone, intact PTH (1–84) is the active hormone in vivo. The usual PTH measured in most laboratories is a second-generation assay using two sets of capture antibodies to the carboxy-terminal (39–84 amino acids) and a signal antibody specific for the amino-terminal (1–34 amino acids). This detects the "intact" PTH hormone. A modification of this intact PTH assay is a quick or rapid assay used in the operating room. Rapid PTH ICMA measurements of intact PTH are performed preoperatively and intraoperatively (10 minutes and sometimes 20 minutes after parathyroidectomy). A reduction in PTH of at least 50% indicates a successful operation.
In renal failure non–(1–84) PTH fragments accumulate, with the main PTH-C fragment being PTH 7–84. PTH-C fragments cross-react with the intact PTH assays and increase the healthy reference range for PTH to 1.5 to three times the normal upper limit. A third-generation PTH assay was developed to account for these molecules with signal antibodies to the 1- to 4–amino-terminal amino acids proving to more accurately quantify PTH 1–84. However, second- and third-generation assays are comparable in clinical medicine.

24. What methods best localize the parathyroid tumor in HPT?
Parathyroid imaging techniques are expensive and are not usually used for diagnosis but are commonly used as an aid to surgery. Technetium Tc99m sestamibi single-proton emission computed tomography (SPECT) may be > 85% to 90% sensitive, specific, and accurate and is commonly used. Sestamibi scanning is most accurate for localizing parathyroid adenomas but is much less useful for parathyroid hyperplasia. Ultrasonography is usually complementary to sestamibi scanning and, when combined with it, increases localization sensitivity to 95%. Hybrid SPECT/CT couples a SPECT camera with CT in a single integrated unit that offers better anatomic localization of scintigraphic findings that are identified on SPECT images.
Four-dimensional computed tomography (4D-CT) of the parathyroid, introduced in 2006, helps identify abnormal parathyroid glands, and provides a fourth dimension with IV contrast enhancement of parathyroid adenomas on early-phase imaging and persistent hyperenhancement on delayed imaging after contrast administration. The degree of early enhancement and slow washout of contrast correlates with metabolic activity of the parathyroid adenoma. Thus, 4D-CT demonstrates both function of parathyroid adenomas and excellent anatomy of the adenomas and surrounding structures. Combined sestamibi uptake and intraoperative gamma-probe localization is used to assist localization for minimally invasive parathyroidectomy (see next question). Less commonly, localization studies include cervical CT, magnetic resonance imaging (MRI), positron emission tomography (PET), intravenous digital subtraction angiography (IVDSA), arteriography, and selective venous sampling.

KEY POINTS: HYPERPARATHYROIDISM

- Primary hyperparathyroidism (PHPT) is associated with elevated PTH, hypercalcemia, osteoporosis, nephrolithiasis, and symptoms associated with these conditions.
- Recommendations for surgery in patients with asymptomatic PHPT includes any one of the following: serum calcium > 1.0 mg/dL above the normal upper limit; decreased estimated glomerular filtration rate (GFR) < 60 mL/min, calcium nephrolithiasis or nephrocalcinosis; 24-hr urine calcium > 400 mg/day and increased stone risk by biochemical analysis; reduced bone density with T-score ≥ −2.5; fragility fracture; vertebral compression fracture or increased risk of vertebral fracture; and age < 50 years.
- It is never wrong to recommend surgery for treatment of asymptomatic PHPT if the patient has no contraindications to surgery and has access to a skilled parathyroid surgeon. Symptomatic patients with neurocognitive, neuropsychiatric, gastrointestinal, and musculoskeletal symptoms that are thought to be related to PHPT should also be considered for surgery.
- Advantages of parathyroid surgery include cure of PHPT and hypercalcemia in most cases with a single operation, no need for regular prolonged follow-up, increased bone density, decreased fracture rate, decreased kidney stone formation, and potentially improved neurocognitive function.
- Parathyroid imaging is expensive and not usually used to confirm or exclude the diagnosis of PHPT. However, preoperative parathyroid localization studies are the norm and thyroid ultrasonography to screen for thyroid disease is also usually done before parathyroid surgery. Cervical ultrasonography performed by an experienced parathyroid sonographer is the least costly imaging modality and when combined with Tc99m sestamibi or 4D-CT is the most cost-effective strategy.

25. When should you use preoperative localization of a parathyroid adenoma?

Imaging is performed after deciding to proceed with parathyroidectomy and is performed for operative planning, and is almost always indicated before parathyroid surgery. Cervical ultrasonography performed by an experienced parathyroid sonographer is the least costly imaging modality and when combined with a sestamibi scan or 4D CT is the most cost-effective strategy. Preoperative imaging of the parathyroid glands and thyroid will often determine the type and extent of surgery performed. The type of imaging will often depend on the surgeon's preference, and the surgeon may want to evaluate the patient and order the imaging studies according to preference. Patients undergoing parathyroidectomy should undergo preoperative thyroid ultrasonography because of the high rate of concomitant thyroid disease that may require resection. Minimally invasive parathyroidectomy (MIP) using a small incision localized to one side of the neck is becoming the state-of-the-art surgical approach to treating PHPT and always requires preoperative localization. Minimally invasive radio-guided parathyroidectomy (MIRP) uses radio-active sestamibi uptake with an intraoperative gamma probe and provides for the least invasive and most accurate tumor localization. With MIRP, the operative time is shorter, the procedure can be done on an outpatient basis with use of local anesthesia, accurate localization of multiple adenomas is possible, and the patient can be discharged within hours of the procedure. Standard neck exploration, MIP, and MIRP all require an experienced parathyroid surgeon. Most surgeons will require one or more of the imaging studies summarized in question 24 before the operation.

26. Do all asymptomatic patients with HPT require surgical treatment?

No. Many asymptomatic patients with mild PHPT do not require surgery (see question 27). However, the only definitive therapy for PHPT is parathyroidectomy, and it is usually appropriate to recommend parathyroidectomy for patients with asymptomatic PHPT if they have access to an experienced parathyroid surgeon and have no contraindications to surgery. Advantages of parathyroid surgery are cure of PHPT and hypercalcemia in most cases with a single operation, no need for regular prolonged follow-up, decreased fracture rate, increased bone density, decreased frequency of kidney stones, and possible improvements in some neurocognitive elements.

27. What are the indications for parathyroidectomy in patients with asymptomatic PHPT?
   1. Serum calcium > 1.0 mg/dL above the upper normal limit
   2. Reduced bone density, as shown by DXA (T-score ≤ −2.5) at the lumbar spine, femoral neck, total hip, or distal one third radius; history of previous fragility fracture; vertebral fracture by x-ray, CT, MRI, or vertebral fracture assessment (VFA)
   3. Decreased estimated glomerular filtration rate (eGFR) to < 60 mL/min
   4. Calcium nephrolithiasis or nephrocalcinosis by radiography, ultrasonography, or CT
   5. 24-hour urine calcium > 400 mg/day and increased stone risk by urinary stone risk profile
   6. Age < 50 years
   7. Patients for whom medical surveillance is neither desired nor possible

28. How should you monitor patients with asymptomatic HPT who have not had parathyroidectomy?

Initially, obtain serum calcium and PTH measurements, DXA bone densitometry, and eGFR. Perform serum PTH, calcium and eGFR annually. Obtain three-site DXA bone densitometry (lumbar spine, hip, and forearm) every 1 to 2 years. Schedule office visits every 6 months and as needed to evaluate for symptoms of PHPT. Encourage adequate hydration and exercise, follow recommended guidelines for calcium intake established for all individuals and replete 25-OH vitamin D to levels > 30 ng/mL. Cinacalcet can be used to lower serum calcium levels and bisphosphonates can stabilize BMD.

29. How would you estimate GFR without performing 24-hour urine collection?

There are multiple equations for estimating GFR when kidney function is stable. Many laboratories provide an estimate of GFR whenever creatinine is measured on a multichannel laboratory test. Phone apps to estimate GFR are also available on Apple, android, and Windows cell phones. A good website to access most estimates for GFR is http://mdrd.com. Currently the CKD-EPI estimate of GFR is believed to be the most accurate.

30. What therapeutic options are available for patients unable to undergo surgery for PHPT?

The U.S. Food and Drug Administration (FDA) has approved two calcimimetics that bind to the extracellular CaSRs on parathyroid cells and increase chief cell sensitivity to extracellular calcium. This effect shifts the calcium–PTH curve to the left. Cinacalcet is an oral calcimimetic that binds to the transmembrane domain of the CaSR and is approved to treat secondary HPT in patients with end-stage renal disease on dialysis, hypercalcemia in patients with parathyroid carcinoma, and PHPT in patients unable to undergo surgery. Etelcalcetide is an IV calcimimetic that binds to the extracellular domain of the CaSR at a site different from that of calcium and is approved for treatment of secondary HPT in adults with CKD on hemodialysis. Both calcimimetics decrease serum calcium, PTH, and phosphorus levels. Etelcalcetide appears to be more effective. Bisphosphonates inhibit osteoclast-mediated bone resorption and can increase bone mass in patients with osteopenia and osteoporosis, as well as PHPT. Raloxifene may also preserve bone mass in patients who cannot tolerate bisphosphonates. Estrogens preserve bone mass, but their use remains controversial because of the associated potential risk of breast cancer and cardiovascular disease. Denosumab is a monoclonal antibody to receptor activator of nuclear factor-kappa B ligand (RANK-L) that decreases osteoclastic bone resorption and is FDA approved for the treatment of osteoporosis and hypercalcemia of malignancy. Angiographic ablation or percutaneous alcohol injection of parathyroid adenoma tissue are rarely used.

31. How would you evaluate and treat a patient with normocalcemic PHPT?

Normocalcemic PHPT (NCHPT) manifests as elevated serum PTH levels with normal corrected calcium levels. Studies now suggest that NCHPT is more common than previously thought and may cause complications, such as those of hypercalcemic HPT. To diagnose NCHPT, all secondary causes of HPT, such as vitamin D deficiency, CKD, calcium malabsorption, and renal leak hypercalciuria, should be evaluated and treated. Ionized calcium should be measured to confirm the normocalcemia. Vitamin D deficiency should be corrected to a 25-OH vitamin D level $\geq$ 30 ng/mL. After secondary HPT has been ruled out, the patient can be monitored and treated as for hypercalcemic HPT. However, referral for parathyroid surgery should not be routine for the normocalcemic patient with HPT but instead should be based on symptoms and signs (see questions 27 and 28).

32. What should you consider in the patient described below 3 months after minimally invasive parathyroidectomy with persistently elevated PTH?

The patient is a 60-year-old Caucasian woman, who preoperatively had 2 years of elevated calcium values averaging 11.2 mg/dL and PTH averaging 95 pg/mL. She had successful removal of a localized parathyroid adenoma via minimal parathyroidectomy surgery. Intraoperative PTH decreased to 45 pg/mL, and calcium decreased transiently to 8.2 mg/dL. She now has persistently normal calcium 9.0 to 9.5 mg/dL, 25-OH vitamin D 29 ng/mL, and elevated PTH 80 to 90 pg/mL 3 months postoperatively.

Of the focused parathyroidectomy surgeries with preoperative localization of the parathyroid adenoma, 90% to 95% are cured without four-gland explorations (question 24). Interestingly, about 25% of patients who are cured and have normal calcium levels after initial parathyroid surgery will have persistently elevated PTH many months later. So, the first consideration in this patient with 3 months of normal postoperative calcium is surgical cure with delayed return of PTH to normal. Older patients and those with higher preoperative PTH, lower 25-OH vitamin D, and CKD are more likely to have prolonged PTH elevations after curative parathyroidectomy. The prolonged return of PTH to normal may reflect mild secondary hyperparathyroidism associated with bone remineralization. It is important to correct low 25-OH vitamin D to $\geq$ 30 ng/mL and recommend usual calcium supplementation appropriate for age and gender.

⊕ WEBSITES

Parathyroid.com (good review of all aspects of parathyroid disease): http://www.parathyroid.com.
Khan, A. A., Hanley, D. A., Rizzoli, R., Bollerslev, J., Young, J. E., Rejnmark, L., ... Bilezikian, J. P. (2017). Primary hyperparathyroidism: review and recommendations on evaluation, diagnosis, and management. A Canadian and international consensus. *Osteoporosis International, 28*(1), 1–19. https://www.ncbi.nlm.nih.gov/pmc/articles/PMC5206263/.

BIBLIOGRAPHY

Bilezikian, J. P., Bandeira, L., Khan, A., & Cusano, N. E. (2018). Hyperparathyroidism. *Lancet, 391,* 168–178.
Bilezikian, J. P., Brandi, M. L., Eastell, R., Silverberg, S. J., Udelsman, R., Marcocci, C., & Potts, J. T., Jr. (2014). Guidelines for the management of asymptomatic primary hyperparathyroidism: summary statement from the fourth international workshop. *Journal of Clinical Endocrinology and Metabolism, 99,* 3561–3569.
Block, G. A., Bushinsky, D. A., Cheng, S., Cunningham, J., Dehmel, B., Drueke, T. B., ... Chertow, G. M. (2017). Effect of etelcalcetide vs cinacalcet on serum parathyroid hormone in patients receiving hemodialysis with secondary hyperparathyroidism. A randomized clinical trial. *Journal of the American Medical Association, 317*(2), 156–164.
Bringhurst, F. R., Demay, M. B., & Kronenberg, H. M. (2016). Hormones and disorders of mineral metabolism. In S. Melmed, K. S. Polonsky, & P. R. Larsen (Eds.), *Williams Textbook of Endocrinology* (13th ed., p. 1254). Philadelphia, PA: Elsevier.
Castellano, E., Attanasio, R., Latina, A., Visconti, G. L., Cassibba, S., & Borretta, G. (2017). Nephrolithiasis in primary hyperparathyroidism: a comparison between silent and symptomatic patients. *Endocrine Practice, 23,* 157–162.
Duke, W. S., Kim, A. S., Waller, J. L., & Terris, D. J. (2017). Persistently elevated parathyroid hormone after successful parathyroid surgery. *Laryngoscope, 127,* 1720–1723.
Kannan, S., Milas, M., Neumann, D., Parikh, R. T., Siperstein, A., & Licata, A. (2014). Parathyroid nuclear scan. A focused review on the technical and biological factors affecting its outcome. *Clinical Cases in Mineral and Bone Metabolism, 11*(1), 25–30.
Khan, A. A., Hanley, D. A., Rizzoli, R., Bollerslev, J., Young, J. E., Rejnmark, L., ... Bilezikian, J. P. (2017). Primary hyperparathyroidism: Review and recommendations on evaluation, diagnosis, and management. A Canadian and international consensus. *Osteoporosis International, 28,* 1–19.
Lal, G., & Clark, O. H. (2018). Endocrine surgery. In D. G. Gardner & D. M. Shoback (Eds.), *Greenspan's Basic & Clinical Endocrinology* (10th ed., p. 825). New York, NY: McGraw-Hill Education.
Lew, J., & Solorzano, C. (2009). Surgical management of primary hyperparathyroidism: state of the art. *Surgical Clinics of North America, 89,* 1205–1225.
Li, D., Radulescu, A., Shrestha, R. T., Root, M., Karger, A. B., Killeen, A. A., ... Burmeister, L. A. (2017). Association of biotin ingestion with performance of hormone and nonhormone assays in healthy adults. *Journal of the American Medical Association, 318*(12), 1150–1160.

Marcocci, C., Bollerslev, J., Khan, A. A., & Shoback, D. M. (2014). Medical management of primary hyperparathyroidism: proceedings of the fourth International Workshop on the Management of Asymptomatic Primary Hyperparathyroidism. *Journal of Clinical Endocrinology and Metabolism, 99,* 3607–3618.

Noureldine, S. I., Gooi, Z., & Tufano, R. P. (2015). Minimally invasive parathyroid surgery. *Gland Surgery, 4*(5), 410–419.

Pathak, P. R., Holden, S. E., Schaefer, S. C., Leverson, G., Chen, H., & Sippel, R. S. (2014). Elevated parathyroid hormone after parathyroidectomy delays symptom improvement. *Journal of Surgical Research, 190*(1), 119–125.

Rejnmark, L., Vestergaard, P., & Mosekilde, L. (2011). Clinical review—nephrolithiasis and renal calcifications in primary hyperparathyroidism. *Journal of Clinical Endocrinology and Metabolism, 96*(8), 2377–2385.

Šiprová, H., Fryšák, A., & Souček, M. (2016). Primary hyperparathyroidism, with a focus on management of the normocalcemic form: to treat or not to treat? *Endocrine Practice, 22,* 294–301.

Tucci, T. R. (2017). Normocalcemic primary hyperparathyroidism associated with progressive cortical bone loss—a case report. *Bone Reports, 7,* 152–155.

Walker, M. D., & Silverberg, S. J. (2018). Primary hyperparathyroidism. *Nature Reviews Endocrinology, 14*(2), 115–125.

Wilhelm, S. M., Wang, T. S., Ruan, D. T., Lee, J. A., Asa, S. L., Duh, Q. Y., ... Carty, S. E. (2016). The American Association of Endocrine Surgeons guidelines for definitive management of primary hyperparathyroidism. *Journal of the American Medical Association Surgery, 151*(10), 959–968.

Yeh, M. W., Zhou, H., Adams, A. L., Ituarte, P. H., Li, N., Liu, I. L., & Haigh, P. I. (2016). The relationship of parathyroidectomy and bisphosphonates with fracture risk in primary hyperparathyroidism. *Annals of Internal Medicine, 164,* 715–723.

CHAPTER 19

HYPERCALCEMIA OF MALIGNANCY

Michael T. McDermott

1. What are the three major types of hypercalcemia of malignancy?

   Humoral hypercalcemia of malignancy (HHM): Parathyroid hormone–related peptide (PTHrP) production by the primary tumor. PTHrP promotes both osteoclastic bone resorption and calcium reabsorption in the distal renal tubules. Other humoral substances that occasionally cause HHM include transforming growth factor-alpha (TGF-alpha) and tumor necrosis factor (TNF). HHM accounts for about 80% of all hypercalcemia of malignancy.

   Local osteolytic hypercalcemia (LOH): Cytokine production within osteolytic bone metastases. Cytokines stimulate aggressive local bone resorption and calcium release at metastatic sites. LOH accounts for about 20% of all hypercalcemia of malignancy.

   Calcitriol-mediated hypercalcemia: 1,25-dihydroxy [(OH)$_2$] vitamin D (calcitriol) production by the tumor. Calcitriol stimulates both intestinal calcium absorption and osteoclastic bone resorption. This condition accounts for $\approx$ 1% of all hypercalcemia of malignancy.

2. What is PTHrP?

   PTHrP is a protein that has sequence homology with the first 13 amino acids of parathyroid hormone (PTH). Both PTH and PTHrP bind to a common receptor (PTH/PTHrP receptor), resulting in stimulation of bone resorption and inhibition of renal calcium excretion. PTHrP is found in high concentrations in breast milk and amniotic fluid, but it can be detected in almost every tissue in the body; it is increased in the circulation during pregnancy. Its physiologic endocrine function may be to govern the transfer of calcium from the maternal skeleton and the bloodstream into the developing fetus and into breast milk. PTHrP is, by far, the most common humoral mediator of HHM.

3. What types of cancer most commonly cause HHM?

   Carcinoma of the lung, particularly squamous cell carcinoma, is the most common malignancy causing HHM. Other tumors associated with this disorder include squamous cell carcinomas of the head and neck, and of the esophagus, and adenocarcinomas of the breast, kidney, bladder, pancreas, and ovary. Non-Hodgkin's lymphoma and chronic myelogenous leukemia can also cause HHM.

4. What types of cancer are associated with LOH?

   Breast cancer with skeletal metastases, multiple myeloma, and lymphoma are the major cancers associated with LOH. These metastatic and primary bone tumors secrete cytokines directly into bone, where they stimulate aggressive local bone resorption. Cytokines that have been identified or proposed in LOH include PTHrP, DKK1 (Dickkopf WNT Signaling Pathway Inhibitor 1), lymphotoxin, interleukins, transforming growth factors, prostaglandins, and procathepsin D.

5. What types of cancer cause calcitriol-mediated hypercalcemia, and how does this happen?

   Hodgkin's and non-Hodgkin's lymphomas are the most common malignancies that cause hypercalcemia as a result of excess production of 1,25(OH)$_2$ vitamin D (calcitriol). However, the most common overall causes of this are granulomatous diseases, particularly sarcoidosis. In these conditions, lymphomas or granulomatous tissues express high levels of 1alpha hydroxylase, the enzyme that converts 25(OH) vitamin D into 1,25(OH)$_2$ vitamin D, the active form of the vitamin that stimulates intestinal absorption of calcium and phosphorus.

6. What are the key diagnostic features of the three types of hypercalcemia of malignancy?

   Table 19.1 shows how PTH, PTHrP, and 1,25(OH)$_2$ vitamin D testing can be used in the differential diagnosis of hypercalcemia of malignancy.

7. What is a good general diagnostic approach for a patient with hypercalcemia of unknown cause?

   Evaluation of hypercalcemia should always start with a good history and physical examination and measurement of PTH, creatinine, carbon dioxide (CO$_2$), and phosphorus. When the serum PTH is low, one must have a high degree of suspicion for hypercalcemia of malignancy. A good diagnostic approach to hypercalcemia is shown in Fig. 19.1.

8. What is the definition of a hypercalcemic crisis?

   A hypercalcemic crisis is defined as a serum calcium level > 14 mg/dL with associated symptoms. The symptoms and features most commonly seen with serum calcium levels this high include nausea, vomiting, dehydration, mental status changes, acute kidney injury, electrocardiography (ECG) changes, and cardiac dysrhythmias.

Table 19.1. Differential Diagnosis of Hypercalcemia of Malignancy.

PTH		PTHrP	1,25(OH)$_2$ VITAMIN D	VITAMIN D
Humoral hypercalcemia of malignancy	↓	↑		↓ or normal
Local osteolytic hypercalcemia	↓	↓		↓ or normal
Calcitriol-mediated hypercalcemia[a]	↓	↓		↑

[a]The most common overall causes of 1,25(OH)$_2$ vitamin D-mediated hypercalcemia, however, are granulomatous disorders, especially sarcoidosis, and not lymphomas. *PTH*, Parathyroid hormone; *PHTrP*, parathyroid hormone–related peptide.

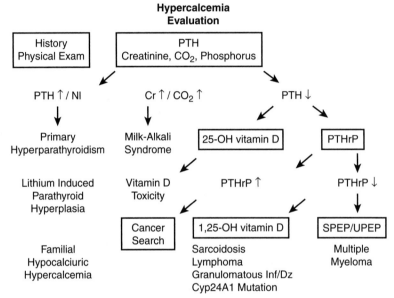

Fig. 19.1. Diagnostic approach to the patient with hypercalcemia. *CO$_2$,* Carbon dioxide; *Cr,* creatinine; *N1,* xxxxx; *OH,* hydroxy; *PTH,* parathyroid hormone; *PHTrP,* parathyroid hormone–related peptide; *SPEP,* xxxxx; *UPEP,* xxxxx.

9. What ECG changes are characteristic of severe hypercalcemia?
The classic ECG finding of severe hypercalcemia is a shortened QTC interval (hypocalcemia causes prolonged QCT interval, hypercalcemia causes shortened QCT interval). Other changes that can also be seen with severe hypercalcemia include first-degree heart block, scooped ST elevations in leads V1–V5, and scooped ST depressions in the inferior leads.

10. Describe the appropriate treatment approaches for the different types of hypercalcemia of malignancy.
Treatment of the primary malignancy is the most important long-term measure. To quickly and effectively lower serum calcium levels to a safe range, one must first attempt to determine the underlying mechanism and malignancy causing the hypercalcemia. Table 19.2 lists the measures that can be used selectively for treatment of the specific type of hypercalcemia.

Table 19.2. Treatment of Specific Types of Hypercalcemia of Malignancy.

PTHrP/Cytokine-Mediated Hypercalcemia of Malignancy (HHM, LOC, Myeloma)
Saline Infusion: 200–300 mL/hr to keep urine output at 100–150 mL/hr
Calcitonin: 4 IU/kg SQ or IM; repeat 4–8 IU/kg every 6–12 hours for 48 hours
Zoledronic acid (Zometa): 4 mg IV over 15 minutes (30 minutes in CKD)
Denosumab (Xgeva): 120 mg SQ every 4 weeks, if refractory to zoledronic acid
Dialysis: If refractory to the above measures

Table 19.2. Treatment of Specific Types of Hypercalcemia of Malignancy. *(Continued)*

Calcitriol [1,25(OH)$_2$ Vitamin D]–Mediated Hypercalcemia of Malignancy
Glucocorticoids: Prednisone 60 mg daily for 10 days
Saline Infusion: 200–300 mL/hr to keep urine output at 100–150 mL/hr
Calcitonin: 4 IU/kg SQ or IM; repeat 4–8 IU/kg every 6–12 hours for 48 hours
Zoledronic Acid (Zometa): 4 mg IV over 15 minutes (30 minutes in CKD)
Denosumab (Xgeva): 120 mg SQ every 4 weeks, if refractory to zoledronic acid
Dialysis: If refractory to the above measures

CKD, Chronic kidney disease; *HHM,* humoral hypercalcemia of malignancy; *IM,* intramuscular; *IV,* intravenous; *LOC,* local osteolytic hypercalcemia; *PHTrP,* parathyroid hormone–related peptide; *SQ,* subcutaneous.

KEY POINTS: HYPERCALCEMIA OF MALIGNANCY

- Humoral hypercalcemia of malignancy (HMM) usually results from solid tumor production of parathyroid hormone–related peptide (PTHrP), which binds to parathyroid hormone (PTH) and PTH/PTHrP receptors to stimulate bone resorption and renal tubular calcium reabsorption.
- Local osteolytic hypercalcemia (LOH) is caused by skeletal metastases that secrete cytokines directly into bone, stimulating aggressive localized bone resorption and calcium release.
- Calcitriol-mediated hypercalcemia occurs when marrow/hematologic malignancies express 1alpha hydroxylase, resulting in production of high levels of 1,25(OH)$_2$ vitamin D.
- The key initial diagnostic test in patients with hypercalcemia is measurement of serum PTH, which is elevated or high normal in primary hyperparathyroidism (most common cause of hypercalcemia) but is low or undetectable in hypercalcemia of malignancy and most other hypercalcemic disorders.
- Serum calcium levels can be lowered effectively in patients with hypercalcemia of malignancy with intravenous administration of saline and bisphosphonates.
- The development of hypercalcemia of malignancy portends a poor prognosis in most patients with cancer because it tends to occur in advanced tumor stages.

11. What is the prognosis for patients with hypercalcemia of malignancy?
    Because hypercalcemia often (but not always) correlates with advanced malignancy and metastatic disease, the overall prognosis is generally quite poor. In one study, the median survival of patients who developed hypercalcemia was only 30 days. However, this varies significantly, depending on the primary tumor/malignancy and response to antitumor therapy. Collaboration with the oncology providers and shared decision making with the patient and his or her family should guide further diagnostic and therapeutic considerations in a realistic manner. However, the patient's will to defeat the malignancy and to survive can never be underestimated.

BIBLIOGRAPHY

Adhikaree, J., Newby, Y., & Sundar, S. (2014). Denosumab should be the treatment of choice for bisphosphonate refractory hypercalcaemia of malignancy. *British Medical Journal Case Reports, 2014,* bcr2013202861.
Berenson, J. R. (2002). Treatment of hypercalcemia of malignancy with bisphosphonates. *Seminars in Oncology, 29,* 12–18.
Dietzek, A., Connelly, K., Cotugno, M., Bartel, S., & McDonnell, A. M. (2015). Denosumab in hypercalcemia of malignancy: a case series. *Journal of Oncology Pharmacy Practice, 21,* 143–147.
Edwards, B. J., Sun, M., West, D. P., Guindani, M., Lin, Y. H., Lu, H., . . . Murphy, W. A., Jr. (2016). Incidence of atypical femur fractures in cancer patients: the MD Anderson Cancer Center Experience. *Journal of Bone and Mineral Research, 31,* 1569–1576.
Hu, M. I., Glezerman, I. G., Leboulleux, S., Insogna, K., Gucalp, R., Misiorowski, W., . . . Jain, R. K. (2014). Denosumab for treatment of hypercalcemia of malignancy. *Journal of Clinical Endocrinology and Metabolism, 99,* 3144–3152.
Maier, J. D., & Levine, S. N. (2015). Hypercalcemia in the intensive care unit: a review of pathophysiology, diagnosis, and modern therapy. *Journal of Intensive Care Medicine, 30,* 235–252.
Major, P., Lortholary, A., Hon, J., Abdi, E., Mills, G., Menssen, H. D., . . . Seamen, J. (2001). Zoledronic acid is superior to pamidronate in the treatment of hypercalcemia of malignancy: a pooled analysis of two randomized, controlled clinical trials. *Journal of Clinical Oncology, 19,* 558–567.
Manne, J. (2016). Striking resemblance: Calcium-alkali syndrome. *American Journal of Medicine, 129,* 816–818.
Mirrakhimov, A. E. (2015). Hypercalcemia of malignancy: an update on pathogenesis and management. *North American Journal of Medical Science, 7,* 483–493.
Mundy, G. R., & Guise, T. A. (1997). Hypercalcemia of malignancy. *American Journal of Medicine, 103,* 134–145.
Ralston, S. H., Gallacher, S. J., Patel, U., Campbell, J., & Boyle, I. T. (1990). Cancer-associated hypercalcemia: morbidity and mortality. Clinical experience in 126 treated patients. *Annals of Internal Medicine, 112,* 499–504.
Rizzoli, R., Thiébaud, D., Bundred, N., Pecherstorfer, M., Herrmann, Z., Huss, H. J., . . . Body, J. J. (1999). Serum parathyroid hormone-related protein levels and response to bisphosphonate treatment in hypercalcemia of malignancy. *Journal of Clinical Endocrinology and Metabolism, 84,* 3545–3550.
Roodman, G. D. (2004). Mechanisms of bone metastasis. *New England Journal of Medicine, 350,* 1655–1664.
Stewart, A. F. (2005). Hypercalcemia associated with cancer. *New England Journal of Medicine, 352,* 373–379.

CHAPTER 20

HYPOCALCEMIA

Shari C. Fox

1. Define hypocalcemia.

   Hypocalcemia is the state in which the serum ionized calcium level drops below the normal range which, under normal conditions, corresponds to a serum total calcium level < 8.5 mg/dL (2.1 mmol/L).

2. How are serum calcium and serum albumin levels related?

   Approximately 50% of serum calcium is bound to albumin, to other plasma proteins, and to related anions, such as citrate, lactate, and sulfate. Of this, 40% is bound to protein, predominantly albumin, and 10% to 13% is attached to anions. The remaining 50% is unbound or ionized calcium. The total serum calcium level reflects both the bound and the unbound portions with a normal range of 8.5 to 10.5 mg/dL for most assays (2.1–2.5 mmol/L).

3. How is the serum total calcium corrected for a low serum albumin level?

   Serum total corrected calcium is calculated by the addition of 0.8 mg/dL (0.2 mmol/L) to the measured serum total calcium for every 1 g/dL that the serum albumin is below 4 g/dL. This is not a completely precise method, and therefore, serum ionized calcium measurements may be needed to confirm whether true hypocalcemia is present. The adjusted level of serum total calcium correlates with the ionized calcium level, which is the physiologically active form of serum calcium.

   $$\text{Corrected Ca (mg/dL)} = \text{Serum Ca (mg/dL)} + [0.8 \times (4.0 - \text{measured albumin g/dL})]$$

4. What is the most common cause of low total serum calcium?

   Hypoalbuminemia is the most common cause of low total serum calcium. In patients with chronic illness, malnutrition, cirrhosis, or volume overexpansion, serum albumin may be low, and this will reduce the total, but generally not the ionized, fraction of serum calcium. This could be thought of as "factitious" hypocalcemia.

5. What factors other than albumin influence the levels of serum ionized calcium?

   Serum pH influences the level of ionized calcium by causing decreased binding of calcium to albumin in acidosis and increased binding in alkalosis. As an example, respiratory alkalosis, seen in hyperventilation, causes a drop in the serum ionized calcium level. A shift of 0.1 pH units is associated with an ionized calcium change of 0.16 to 0.20 mg/dL (0.04–0.05 mmol/L). Increased levels of chelators, such as citrate, which may occur during large-volume transfusions of citrate-containing blood products, also may lower the levels of ionized calcium. Heparin may act similarly.

6. How is serum calcium regulated?

   Three hormones maintain calcium homeostasis: parathyroid hormone (PTH), vitamin D, and calcitonin. PTH acts in three ways to raise serum calcium levels: (1) PTH stimulates osteoclastic bone resorption; (2) PTH increases conversion of 25-hydroxy (OH) vitamin D to 1,25-dihydroxy (OH$_2$) vitamin D which then increases intestinal calcium and phosphorus absorption; and (3) PTH increases renal reabsorption of calcium. Calcitonin decreases the level of serum calcium by suppressing osteoclast activity in bone. The interplay of these hormones maintains calcium levels within a narrow range in a normal individual. In addition to those three hormones, calcium levels are also influenced by phosphate and magnesium levels.

7. What steps in vitamin D metabolism may influence serum calcium levels?

   Vitamin D is obtained through the diet or is formed in the skin in the presence of ultraviolet light. Vitamin D is converted to 25-OH vitamin D in the liver and finally to 1,25-dihydroxy(OH)$_2$ vitamin D, the most active form of vitamin D, in the kidney. 1,25(OH)$_2$ vitamin D acts directly on intestinal cells to increase calcium and phosphorus absorption. Deficiency in any of these steps may cause hypocalcemia.

8. What are the major causes of 'true' hypocalcemia?

   Among all the causes of hypocalcemia, postsurgical hypoparathyroidism, vitamin D deficiency, and autoimmune hypoparathyroidism are the most common. The multiple organ and hormonal regulatory systems involved in calcium homeostasis, however, create the potential for multiple causes of hypocalcemia. The etiology of hypocalcemia must be considered in relation to the level of serum albumin, the secretion of PTH, the level of vitamin D, and the presence or absence of hyperphosphatemia. Initially, hypocalcemia may be approached by a search for failure in

one or more of these systems. The systems primarily involved are the parathyroid glands, bone, kidney, and liver; the following list shows the clinical entities followed by their mechanisms:
- *Hypoparathyroidism:* decreased PTH production
- *Hypomagnesemia:* decreased PTH release, responsiveness, and action
- *Citrate toxicity from massive blood transfusions:* complexing of calcium with citrate
- *Pseudohypoparathyroidism:* PTH ineffective at target organs
- *Liver disease:* decreased albumin production, decreased 25-OH vitamin D production, drugs that stimulate 25-OH vitamin D metabolism
- *Renal disease:* renal calcium leak, decreased 1,25(OH)$_2$ vitamin D production, elevated serum phosphate (PO$_4$) from decreased PO$_4$ clearance; drugs that increase renal clearance of calcium
- *Bone disease:* drugs suppressing bone resorption; "hungry bone syndrome"—recovery from hyperparathyroidism or hyperthyroidism
- *Phosphate load:* endogenous—tumor lysis syndrome, hemolysis, and rhabdomyolysis; exogenous—phosphate-containing enemas, laxatives, and phosphorus burns
- *Pancreatitis:* sequestration/deposition of calcium in the pancreas; other
- *Toxic shock syndrome, other critical illnesses:* decreased PTH production or PTH resistance

9. What physical signs suggest hypocalcemia?
The hallmark of acute hypocalcemia is tetany, which is characterized by neuromuscular irritability. The tetany can be mild or more severe and is usually seen when the serum ionized calcium concentration is < 4.3 mg/dL (total serum calcium < 7.0–7.5 mg/dL). In addition to neuromuscular irritability, some patients have less specific symptoms, such as fatigue, anxiety, depression, and hyperirritability.
- *Mild tetany:* perioral numbness, paresthesia's of hands/feet, and muscle cramps
- *Severe tetany:* carpopedal spasms, laryngospasm, and focal or generalized seizures
- *Latent tetany:* Trousseau's and Chvostek's signs
    Chvostek's sign is an ipsilateral facial twitch elicited by tapping the skin over the facial nerve anterior to the external auditory meatus. Chvostek's sign is also present in 10% of normal individuals. Trousseau's sign is a forearm spasm induced by inflation of a blood pressure cuff to 20 mm Hg above the patient's systolic blood pressure for 3 to 5 minutes. Carpal spasm presents as flexion of the wrist and metacarpophalangeal joints, extension of the fingers, and adduction of the thumb.

10. What laboratory tests are clinically useful in distinguishing among the causes of hypocalcemia?
Table 20.1 summarizes the laboratory findings for common causes of hypocalcemia. Besides intact PTH and corrected (or ionized) calcium in serum, which are the most important initial tests, other tests that can be helpful depending on the clinical presentation and history include serum creatinine, phosphate, magnesium, vitamin D metabolites, alkaline phosphatase, amylase, and urinary calcium and magnesium.

11. Describe the symptoms of hypocalcemia.
- *Early symptoms:* numbness and tingling involving fingers, toes, and lips
- *Neuromuscular symptoms:* cramps, fasciculations, laryngospasm, and tetany
- *Cardiovascular symptoms:* arrhythmias, bradycardia, and hypotension
- *Central nervous system symptoms:* irritability, paranoia, depression, psychosis, organic brain syndrome, and seizures; "cerebral tetany", which is not a true seizure (see question 13), may also be seen in hypocalcemia; subnormal intelligence has also been reported
- *Chronic symptoms:* papilledema, basal ganglia calcifications, cataracts, dry skin, coarse hair, and brittle nails
    Symptoms reflect the absolute calcium concentration and the rate of fall in the calcium levels. Individuals may be unaware of symptoms because of gradual onset and may realize they have experienced an abnormality only when their sense of well-being improves with treatment.

12. What radiographic findings may be present with hypocalcemia?
Calcifications of basal ganglia may occur in the small blood vessels of that region. These occasionally may cause extrapyramidal signs but usually are asymptomatic. Of note, 0.7% of routine brain computed tomography (CT) scans show calcification of the basal ganglia.

13. What is cerebral tetany, and how does it differ from a true seizure?
Cerebral tetany manifests as generalized tetany without loss of consciousness, tongue biting, incontinence, or postictal confusion. Anticonvulsants may relieve the symptoms, but because they enhance 25-OH vitamin D catabolism, they also may worsen the hypocalcemia.

14. How does hypocalcemia affect cardiac function?
Calcium is involved in cardiac automaticity and is required for muscle contraction. Hypocalcemia can, therefore, result in arrhythmias and reduced myocardial contractility. This decrease in the force of contraction may be refractory to pressor agents, especially those that involve calcium in their mechanism of action. Through this

Table 20.1. Differential Diagnosis of Laboratory Evaluation of Most Common Causes of Hypocalcemia.

	CALCIUM (SERUM CORRECTED)	PTH	25-OH VITAMIN D	1,25-OH VITAMIN D	MAGNESIUM	PHOSPHORUS	CREATINE
Hypoparathyroidism	↓	↓	NI	↓	NI	↑	NI
Pseudohypoparathyroidism (PTH resistance)	↓	↑	NI	↓ or NI	NI	↑	NI
Liver disease	↓	↑	↓	↓ or NI		↓	NI
Hypomagnesemia	↓	↓ or NI	NI	NI	↓	NI	NI
Vitamin D deficiency	↓	↑	↓ or NI	↓ or NI or ↑	NI	↓ or NI	↓ or NI
Renal disease (secondary hyperparathyroidism)	↓	↑	NI	↓ or NI	↑ or NI	↑	↑

↑, Increased; ↓, decreased; NI, normal; PTH, parathyroid hormone.

process, beta-blockers and calcium channel blockers can exacerbate cardiac failure. With low serum calcium, the QT interval is prolonged, and ST changes may mimic those seen in ischemia. Although the relationship is variable, the calcium level inversely correlates moderately well with the interval from the Q-wave onset to the peak of the T wave.

15. **What are the potential ophthalmologic findings in hypocalcemia?**
Papilledema may occur with subacute and chronic hypocalcemia. Patients are most often asymptomatic, and the papilledema usually resolves with normalization of the serum calcium level. If symptoms develop or if papilledema does not resolve when the patient is normocalcemic, a cerebral tumor and benign intracranial hypertension must be excluded. Optic neuritis with unilateral loss of vision occasionally develops in patients with hypocalcemia. Lenticular cataracts may also occur with long-standing hypocalcemia but usually do not change in size after hypocalcemia is corrected.

16. **With which autoimmune disorders is hypocalcemia sometimes associated?**
Hypoparathyroidism may result from autoimmune destruction of the parathyroid glands. This disorder has been associated with adrenal, gonadal, and thyroid failure, as well as with alopecia areata, vitiligo, and chronic muco-cutaneous candidiasis. This combination of conditions, each associated with organ-specific autoantibodies, has been termed the autoimmune polyendocrinopathy syndrome, type 1 (see Chapter 59).

17. **Hypocalcemia is frequently encountered in intensive care settings. What are the potential causes?**
Low total serum calcium levels, which are found in 70% to 90% of patients receiving intensive care, result from multiple causes, including:
- Hypoalbuminemia
- Hypomagnesemia
- Hyperphosphatemia
- Anticoagulant therapy
- Rapid blood transfusions with citrate as a preservative
- Administration of anionic loads causing chelation (i.e., citrate, lactate, bicarbonate, phosphate, oxalate, ethylenediaminetetraacetic [EDTA] acid, and radiographic contrast media)
- Parathyroid failure and decreased vitamin D synthesis in severe illness
- Sepsis inducing some degree of resistance to the biologic effects of PTH
  Because of all the factors listed above, it is recommended that ionized serum calcium, rather than total serum calcium, be measured in patients with severe illness.

18. **Hypocalcemia is not unusual in patients with cancer. What conditions may lead to hypocalcemia in this patient group?**
- Tumor lysis syndrome causes hyperphosphatemia and associated formation of intravascular and tissue calcium-phosphate complexes.
- Multiple chemotherapeutic agents and antibiotics (amphotericin B and aminoglycosides) induce hypomagnese-mia, which, in turn, impairs secretion of PTH and causes resistance to PTH in skeletal tissue.
- Thyroid surgery and neck irradiation with transient or permanent hypoparathyroidism may cause hypocalcemia.
- Medullary carcinoma of the thyroid and pheochromocytoma may secrete calcitonin and, on rare occasions, this causes hypocalcemia.

19. **What drugs may cause hypocalcemia?**
Phenobarbital, phenytoin, primidone, rifampin, and glutethimide increase hepatic metabolism of 25-OH vitamin D and thereby may cause hypocalcemia. Aminoglycosides, diuretics (furosemide), and chemotherapeutic agents that induce renal magnesium wasting, and laxatives or enemas that create a large phosphate load, also may be asso-ciated with hypocalcemia. Heparin, ketoconazole, isoniazid, fluoride, foscarnet, and glucagon may also induce hypocalcemia by a variety of mechanisms. Osteoporosis treatments, such as bisphosphonates (especially the more potent ones, such as zoledronic acid) and denosumab, inhibit osteoclast function lower serum calcium levels, as does cinacalcet (a calcimimetic drug), which can acutely inhibit PTH release and lead to significant hypocalcemia in approximately 5% of patients treated.

20. **Which vitamin D metabolite is best for assessing total body vitamin D stores, 25-OH vitamin D or $1,25(OH)_2$ vitamin D?**
The serum 25-OH vitamin D level best reflects total body vitamin D stores. The conversion of 25-OH vitamin D to $1,25(OH)_2$ vitamin D is tightly controlled, and the level of serum $1,25(OH)_2$ vitamin D is usually maintained despite significant vitamin D depletion. Increases in PTH (secondary hyperparathyroidism) stimulate increased conversion of 25-OH vitamin D to $1,25(OH)_2$ vitamin D in this situation.

21. **How is hypocalcemia treated?**
Asymptomatic hypocalcemia requires supplementation with oral calcium and vitamin D derivatives to maintain the serum calcium level at least in the 7.5 to 8.5 mg/dL range. When the serum calcium falls acutely to a level at which the patient is symptomatic, intravenous administration is recommended. The dosage of calcium depends on

Table 20.2. Elemental Calcium Content of Commonly Used Preparations.

PREPARATION	ORAL DOSE	ELEMENTAL CALCIUM (mg)
Calcium Citrate		
Citracal	950 mg	200
Calcium acetate:		
PhosLo	667 mg	169
Calcium Carbonate		
Tums	500 mg	200
Tums Ex	750 mg	300
Oscal	625 mg	250
Oscal 500	1250 mg	500
Calcium 600	1500 mg	600
Titralac (suspension)	1000 mg/5 mL	400
INTRAVENOUS AGENTS	**VOLUME**	**ELEMENTAL CALCIUM (mg)**
Calcium chloride	2.5 mL of 10% solution	90
Calcium gluconate	10 mL of 10% solution	90
Calcium gluceptate	5 mL of 22% solution	90

the amount of elemental calcium present in each preparation (Table 20.2). For a hypocalcemic emergency, 90 or 180 mg of calcium gluconate in 50 mL of dextrose 5% (D5) or normal saline (NS) may be given as an intravenous bolus over 10 to 20 minutes. This dose will only temporarily raise the serum calcium (i.e., for 2–3 hours) and must, therefore, be followed by a slow infusion of 0.5 to 2.0 mg/kg/hr of either calcium gluconate or calcium chloride (calcium gluconate is preferred because it is less likely to lead to tissue necrosis if extravasated).

22. When is treatment with $1,25(OH)_2$ vitamin D (calcitriol) indicated?
    Under normal conditions, 25-OH vitamin D is converted to $1,25(OH)_2$ vitamin D (calcitriol) in the kidney through the stimulatory influence of PTH. Two conditions can, therefore, render the body unable to produce adequate amounts of calcitriol—hypoparathyroidism and renal failure. Because calcitriol is essential for normal intestinal calcium absorption, oral calcitriol (Rocaltrol) supplementation is indicated in patients who have either hypoparathyroidism or chronic renal failure. Of note, because vitamin D has weak biologic activity, these patients may be given large dosages of vitamin D (50,000–100,000 U/day) if calcitriol is unavailable.

23. What role can thiazide diuretics play in the treatment of hypocalcemia?
    Thiazide diuretics reduce urinary calcium excretion significantly, especially with 24-hour coverage (hydrochlorothiazide twice daily or chlorthalidone once daily). These medications can be used to reduce urinary calcium losses and increase serum calcium levels mildly in patients with hypocalcemia caused by conditions that are associated with increased urinary calcium excretion (hypoparathyroidism and idiopathic hypercalciuria).

24. Can recombinant human PTH (rhPTH) be used in the treatment of hypocalcemia?
    Subcutaneous injections of rhPTH 1 to 84 (Natpara) are indicated for patients with chronic hypoparathyroidism who cannot maintain stable serum and urinary calcium levels with calcium and vitamin D supplementation alone.

KEY POINTS: HYPOCALCEMIA

- Serum calcium levels must be corrected for serum albumin levels for accurate assessment.
- Tetany is the hallmark symptom of acute hypocalcemia.
- Multiple organ systems, minerals, anions, and drugs affect calcium levels and must be considered in the evaluation of hypocalcemia.
- Hypocalcemia is a frequent problem in trauma and intensive care settings, and is often a result of administration of intravenous agents.
- Hypocalcemia with severe symptoms requires rapid correction with IV calcium therapy.
- Asymptomatic hypocalcemia can initially be treated with oral calcium alone.
- Calcium plus active 1,25-dihydroxy vitamin D (e.g., calcitriol) is the initial treatment of hypocalcemia in patients with hypoparathyroidism and renal failure

BIBLIOGRAPHY

Ariyan, C. E., & Sosa, J. A. (2004). Assessment and management of patients with abnormal calcium. *Critical Care Medicine, 32,* S146–S154.

Bringhurst, F., Demay, M., Kronenberg, H. M. (2008). Hypocalcemic disorders. In S. Melmed, K. Polonsky, P. R. Larsen, & H. M. Kronenberg (Eds.), *Williams Textbook of Endocrinology* (11th ed., pp. 1241–1249). Philadelphia, PA: Saunders.

Dickerson, R. N. (2007). Treatment of hypocalcemia in critical illness—part 1. *Nutrition, 23,* 358–361.

Goltzman D. (2017, Dec. 28). Diagnostic approach to hypocalcemia. Retrieved from: https://www.uptodate.com.

Kastrup, E. K. (Ed.). (2003). *Drug facts and comparisons.* St. Louis, MO: Wolters Kluwer Health.

Lind, L., Carlstedt, F., Rastad, J., Stiernström, H., Stridsberg, M., Ljunggren, O., ... Ljunghall, S. (2000). Hypocalcemia and parathyroid hormone secretion in critically ill patients. *Critical Care Medicine, 28,* 93–99.

McEvoy, G. K. (Ed.). (2007). Calcium salts. In *AHFS Drug Information* (pp. 2655–2661). Bethesda, MD: American Society of Health-System Pharmacists.

Moe, S. M. (2008). Disorders involving calcium, phosphorus, and magnesium. *Primary Care, 35*(2), 215–237.

Orloff, L. A., Wiseman, S. M., Bernet, V. J., Fahey, T. J. 3rd., Shaha, A. R., Shindo, M. L., , ... Wang, M. B. (2018). American Thyroid Association statement on postoperative hypoparathyroidism: diagnosis, prevention, and management in adults. *Thyroid, 28*(7), 830–841.

Potts, J. T. (2005). Hypocalcemia. In D. L. Kasper (Ed.), *Principles of Internal Medicine* (16th ed., pp. 2263–2268). New York, NY: McGraw-Hill.

Sarko, J. (2005). Bone and mineral metabolism. *Emergency Medicine Clinics of North America, 23,* 703–721.

Schafer, A. L., & Shoback, D. M. (2016, January 3). Hypocalcemia: diagnosis and treatment. Retrieved from: https://www.endotext.org.

Shane, E. (1999). Hypocalcemia: pathogenesis, differential diagnosis and management. In M. J. Favus (Ed.), *Primer on the Metabolic Bone Diseases and Disorders of Mineral Metabolism* (4th ed., pp. 223–226). Philadelphia, PA: Lippincott Williams & Wilkins.

Winer, K. K., Ko, C. W., Reynolds, J. C., Dowdy, K., Keil, M., Peterson, D., , ... Cutler, G. B. Jr. (2003). Long-term treatment of hypoparathyroidism: a randomized controlled study comparing parathyroid hormone-(1-34) versus calcitriol and calcium. *Journal of Clinical Endocrinology and Metabolism, 88,* 4214–4220.

CHAPTER 21

NEPHROLITHIASIS

Leonard R. Sanders

1. How would you define hypercalciuria, kidney (renal) stones, renal calculi, nephrolithiasis, urolithiasis, renal lithiasis, and nephrocalcinosis?

   Hypercalciuria is urinary calcium excretion > 300 mg/day in men and > 250 mg/day in women. A more accurate definition is urinary calcium excretion > 4 mg/kg of ideal body weight per day in either gender. A 24-hour urine collection is needed to define hypercalciuria. However, a good estimate of the 24-hour urine calcium excretion is 1.1 times the calcium-to-creatinine (Ca/Cr) ratio on a random urine specimen. For example, if urine calcium is 20 mg/dL and urine creatinine is 70 mg/dL, then the Ca/Cr ratio would be 20:70 or 0.286 g (286 mg/day). The estimated 24-hour urinary calcium excretion would be 1.1 × 286 = 315 mg/day. *Kidney stones, renal calculi, nephrolithiasis, urolithiasis,* and *renal lithiasis* are synonymous terms that define the clinical syndrome of formation and movement of stones in the urinary collecting system. Renal calculi are abnormally hard, crystalline, insoluble substances that form specifically in the renal collecting system. Nephrocalcinosis is deposition of calcium salts in the renal parenchyma.

2. Who is at risk for the development of kidney stones?

   Kidney stones affect 12% of the world's population. The average prevalence of kidney stones in the United States has increased and is approximately 11% in men and 7% in women, with an overall prevalence of 9%. The lifetime risk for kidney stones is 19% in men and 9% in women. The yearly cost of kidney stone disease in the United States is $2.5 to $5.5 billion. Fifty percent of patients with kidney stones have a recurrence within 5 to 10 years. Stones occur most often between 30 and 60 years of age, and occur in Caucasians more than in other ethnicities. Women have had more stones in recent years, possibly related to increased age, fast food consumption (high in protein and salt), increased calories, decreased physical activity, and increased obesity. The Women's Health Initiative data suggest that estrogen hormone replacement therapy increases the risk of nephrolithiasis in healthy postmenopausal women. Risks for stones include a family history of stones, obesity, diabetes mellitus, metabolic syndrome, hypertension, autosomal dominant polycystic kidney disease, medullary sponge kidney, renal tubular acidosis, urine volume < 2 L/day, dietary calcium < 1000 mg/day, dietary sodium > 2 g/day, low water intake, high animal protein, and high intake of sugar-sweetened sodas (see question 4).

3. What are the composition and frequency of kidney stones in the United States?

   There are six major types of stones, as outlined in Fig. 21.1, which also shows the approximate frequency of occurrence of each type of stone.

4. What are the leading causes of nephrolithiasis?

   The most common causes of nephrolithiasis are the various types of polygenic idiopathic hypercalciuria (IH): absorptive hypercalciuria (AH) types AH-I to AH-III (renal phosphate leak) and renal hypercalciuria (RH). Other causes are primary hyperparathyroidism, hyperoxaluria, hyperuricosuria, hyperphosphaturia, hypocitraturia, hypomagnesuria, infection stones, gouty diathesis, renal tubular acidosis, cystinuria, calcifying nanoparticles, and alterations in the microbiome. Rarely, kidney stones may form from xanthine, triamterene, monosodium urate, ephedrine, guaifenesin, ciprofloxacin, and sulfonamides, and more commonly from protease inhibitors indinavir, atazanavir, and darunavir. Patients with idiopathic nephrolithiasis make up 10% to 20% of "stone formers" in whom routine workup yields no identifiable cause.

5. What conditions are associated with both renal stone disease and hypercalciuria?

   Calcium stones account for 80% of all kidney stones. Approximately 40% to 50% of calcium stone formers have hypercalciuria. Of those with hypercalciuria, 40% have IH, 5% have primary hyperparathyroidism, and 3% have renal tubular acidosis. Other causes of hypercalciuria include excessive dietary vitamin D, excessive calcium and alkali intake, sarcoidosis, Cushing's syndrome, hyperthyroidism, Paget's disease of bone, and immobilization. Nephrolithiasis is also associated with infection, acute and chronic kidney injury, coronary artery disease, obesity, type 2 diabetes mellitus, hypertension, and the metabolic syndrome.

6. What are the most important causes of normocalciuric calcium nephrolithiasis?

   The most important and most common causes of normocalciuric calcium nephrolithiasis are hypocitraturia (50%), hyperuricosuria (25%), hyperoxaluria (10%), and urinary stasis (5%).

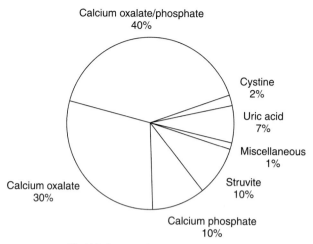

Fig. 21.1. Frequency of the types of kidney stones.

7. What is the process of renal stone formation?

Renal stone formation occurs in six steps: (1) Initially, urinary crystallization or precipitation of sparingly soluble salts and acids occurs. (2) Nucleation follows as crystals and urinary matrix ions form a stable framework for crystal enlargement through (3) growth and (4) aggregation. After the crystals sufficiently enlarge they become trapped and (5) retained in a narrow portion of the urinary collecting system at the end of the collecting ducts and near the renal papilla. Unless washed away by increased urinary flow, these aggregated crystals formed in the medullary interstitium are extruded and (6) adhere to the renal papillae to form a calcium-phosphate–based Randall's plaque nidus for further crystal accumulation and stone growth. Once stone growth occurs, the stone may detach from the renal papilla, move distally, and cause obstruction. Common sites for obstruction are the ureteropelvic junction (UPJ), mid-ureter (where it crosses over the iliac artery), and ureterovesical junction (UVJ).

8. What pathophysiologic factors influence the formation of renal stones?

Renal stones result from hereditary or acquired disorders causing supersaturation of stone precursors, deficiency of stone inhibitors, and possibly excess promoters. Supersaturation causes crystallization with mineral precursors, such as calcium and oxalate. Calcium oxalate crystals bind to anionic sialic acid–containing glycoproteins on the apical surfaces of renal tubular epithelial cells, allowing further growth. Other factors that increase stone formation include urinary stasis (medullary sponge kidney), decreased flow (obstruction), increased urine ammonium (infection), dehydration (concentrated urine), and increased urinary alkalinity (renal tubular acidosis [RTA]). Type I RTA promotes stone formation through the increased release of calcium and phosphorus from bone to buffer the chronic acidemia, with resulting hypercalciuria and hyperphosphaturia. The acidemia enhances proximal tubule reabsorption of citrate, with resulting hypocitraturia. The alkaline urine of RTA promotes precipitation of calcium phosphate stones. Acidemia with a positive urine anion gap ($UNa + UK - UCl$) is a clue to the presence of RTA.

9. What are the chemical precursors of renal stones?

Relatively high concentrations of salt and acid solutes determine crystalluria and stone formation. Calcium oxalate is most common and is supersaturated to four to five times its solubility in normal urine. Other precursors are calcium phosphate (hydroxyapatite) and calcium phosphate monohydrate (brushite). Uric acid, cystine, struvite (magnesium ammonium phosphate), and mucoprotein are undersaturated stone precursors. Drugs, such as ascorbic acid (conversion to oxalate) and triamterene (nidus for stone formation), also may promote renal stone formation.

10. What are the main inhibitors of renal stone formation, and how do they work?

Inhibitors include urinary citrate, pyrophosphate, magnesium, nephrocalcin, uropontin, glycosaminoglycans, and Tamm-Horsfall protein. Most inhibitors bind crystal precursors; for example, citrate binds calcium, making it less available to bind to oxalate. Inhibitors improve solubility and impair precipitation, nucleation, crystal growth, or aggregation. They also compete with stone precursor minerals, such as calcium oxalate, for binding to the apical surfaces of epithelial cells and inhibit epithelial cell adhesion and internalization of calcium oxalate crystals. Finally, inhibitors impair stone precursor transformation into a focus for crystallization and stone growth.

11. What is nephrocalcin, and what role does it play in the formation of renal stones?

Nephrocalcin is an anionic protein produced by the proximal renal tubule and Henle's loop. It usually inhibits the nucleation, crystal growth, and aggregation phases of stone formation. However, nephrocalcin isolated from some stone formers has defective structure and function and is found in the matrix of many calcium stones. Thus, nephrocalcin may have a dual role in stone formation. When normal, it acts as an inhibitor of stone formation. When abnormal, it may serve as a promoter by binding calcium and form a nidus for crystallization.

12. What are the promoters of renal stone formation?

Promoters of renal stone formation are poorly characterized but are believed to be primarily urinary mucoproteins and glycosaminoglycans. Under certain conditions, promoters enhance the formation of renal stones.

13. How does the kidney handle calcium?

Approximately 60% of the serum calcium is ionized or complexed and freely filtered by the glomerulus. The kidney reabsorbs 98% of the filtered calcium passively throughout the nephron. Sixty percent of the reabsorption occurs in the proximal convoluted tubule, 30% in Henle's loop, and 10% in the distal tubule. Furosemide impairs calcium reabsorption in Henle's loop and increases urinary calcium excretion. Thiazide diuretics impair distal tubule reabsorption of sodium, thereby increasing intracellular negativity and calcium reabsorption. Parathyroid hormone (PTH) increases distal tubular calcium reabsorption by enhancing calcium channel activity.

14. How would you calculate the normal filtered and excreted load of urinary calcium?

The serum calcium concentration is normally about 10 mg/dL. The kidney filters complexed and free calcium, which make up 60% of the total, or 6 mg/dL. The normal glomerular filtration rate (GFR) is 120 mL/min. Thus, the filtered load of calcium is 6 mg/100 mL $\times$ 120 mL/min $\times$ 1440 min/day = 10,368 mg/day. Because the kidney reabsorbs 98% of the filtered calcium, only 2% is excreted. Thus the kidney normally excretes about 200 mg of calcium/day (10,368 mg/day $\times$ 0.02 = 207 mg/day). If the excreted calcium level increases to 5%, the urinary calcium level increases to 500 mg/day.

KEY POINTS: PREVALENCE AND ETIOLOGY OF NEPHROLITHIASIS

- Kidney stone prevalence has increased in the United States and likely relates to dietary and lifestyle changes associated with increased obesity and metabolic syndrome; increased sodium and animal protein intake; and decreased fiber, fruits, vegetables, water, and dietary calcium intake.
- Approximately 14% of the U.S. population has a lifetime risk for at least one kidney stone.
- Stones form because of supersaturation of urinary stone precursors (e.g., calcium and oxalate), insufficient stone inhibitors (e.g., citrate), abnormal urine pH, or low urine volume.
- Stones are most commonly calcium based and result from hypercalciuria caused by excess absorption of dietary calcium, resorption of bone calcium, and decreased renal reabsorption of calcium.
- Low-calcium diets and restricting dietary calcium without limiting dietary oxalate increases oxalate absorption and the risk for calcium oxalate stones.

15. How do the serum calcium level and dietary sodium intake affect hypercalciuria?

To help prevent hypercalcemia, nonrenal elevation in serum calcium causes an increase in both filtered calcium and urinary calcium. Increased sodium delivery to Henle's loop and the distal tubule also raises urinary calcium. In non–stone formers, urinary calcium excretion increases about 40 mg for each 100 mEq of sodium excretion. In patients with hypercalciuric stones, calcium excretion increases up to 80 mg per each 100 mEq of sodium. Because urinary sodium excretion increases with higher dietary sodium intake, restricting dietary sodium reduces urinary calcium excretion. In patients with renal stones, the recommended daily dietary sodium is < 100 mEq (2300 mg) or about one teaspoon of salt (6000 mg).

16. What is the etiology and pathophysiology of IH?

IH affects 10% of the general population and 40% of stone formers. The four types of IH are AH-I, AH-II, AH-III, and RH. AH-I and AH-II result from increased intestinal sensitivity to calcitriol with intestinal calcium hyperabsorption and higher numbers of vitamin D receptors in osteoblasts, causing greater bone resorption and resorptive hypercalciuria. The latter accounts for decreased bone mass seen in many patients with AH-I and in some of those with AH-II. AH-III, an unusual disorder, is caused by a renal phosphate leak with urinary loss of phosphate, decreased serum phosphate, and increases in renal calcitriol production and intestinal calcium absorption. The level of the phosphaturic factor, fibroblast growth factor 23 (FGF23), is increased in some patients with calcium nephrolithiasis, hypophosphatemia, and renal phosphate leak. RH is characterized by impaired tubular reabsorption of calcium, which causes a decrease in serum calcium, elevations in PTH and calcitriol, and increases in bone resorption and intestinal calcium absorption.

Table 21.1. Forms of Idiopathic Hypercalciuria.

LABORATORY VALUE	AH-I	AH-II	AH-III	RH
Serum calcium	Normal	Normal	Normal	Normal
Serum phosphorus	Normal	Normal	↓	Normal
Serum intact PTH	Normal	Normal	Normal	↑
24-hour urinary calcium (1-g calcium diet)	↑	↑	↑	↑
Urine Ca/Cr ratio (1-g calcium load)	↑	↑	↑	↑
24-hour urinary calcium (400-mg calcium diet)	↑	Normal	↑	↑
Fasting urinary calcium (mg/dL GFR)	Normal	Normal	↑	↑

↑, Increased; ↓, decreased; *AH*, absorptive hypercalciuria; *Ca/Cr*, calcium/creatinine; *GFR*, glomerular filtration rate; *IH*, idiopathic hypercalciuria; *PTH*, parathyroid hormone; *RH*, renal hypercalciuria. See questions 17–20.

17. How would you distinguish among the various forms of IH?
    See Table 21.1.

18. When is it necessary to distinguish among the various forms of IH?
    Only complicated nephrolithiasis unresponsive to usual therapy requires differentiation (see the list of Websites on hypercalciuria review at the end of the chapter).

19. What explains the differences in serum levels of phosphorus and PTH in AH-III and RH?
    Serum phosphorus is low in AH-III because of a renal phosphate leak. The level of intact PTH is high in RH because the primary defect is decreased renal tubular calcium reabsorption, causing relative hypocalcemia that stimulates PTH.

20. How do changes in calcium intake help distinguish the different types of absorptive hypercalciuria and renal leak hypercalciuria? (See Table 21.1.)
    In AH-II, the 24-hour urine calcium normalizes with a restricted calcium diet (400 mg/day) because the absorptive excess is not as severe. However, the 24-hour urine calcium during calcium restriction remains high in AH-I because of marked calcium hyperabsorption, in AH-III because hypophosphatemia decreases renal tubular calcium reabsorption, and in RH because decreased renal tubular calcium reabsorption is the primary defect.
    High 24-hour urinary calcium is > 4 mg per kg ideal body weight. Normal 24-hour urinary calcium with a 400-mg/day calcium restriction is < 200 mg/day. For improved accuracy, urinary calcium measurements are at times expressed as GFR in milligrams per 100 milliliters to account for changes related to altered kidney function. The normal fasting urine calcium level is < 0.11 mg/100 mL GFR. The normal urine Ca/Cr ratio is < 0.20 after a 1-g oral load of calcium.

21. What defines low serum phosphorus on an 800-mg/day phosphorus-restricted diet?
    Low serum phosphorus is < 2.5 mg/dL on an 800-mg/day phosphorus diet.

22. What causes hyperoxaluria?
    Approximately 14% of urinary oxalate comes from dietary absorption and the remainder from metabolism of glyoxylate and ascorbic acid. Increased oxidation of glyoxylate to oxalate occurs in the rare autosomal recessive hereditary hyperoxaluria. The clinically more important enteric hyperoxaluria occurs with small bowel resection, bypass, or inflammation. Small bowel disease may cause bile salt and fat malabsorption, resulting in increased delivery of bile salts and fats to the colon. Bile salts damage colonic mucosa, increasing colonic permeability and oxalate absorption. Intestinal fatty acids are negatively charged and bind calcium and magnesium, decreasing the amounts of calcium and magnesium available for binding intestinal oxalate and leaving more oxalate free for intestinal absorption. Low-calcium diets do the same. Excess oxalate is primarily absorbed in the bile salt-damaged colon. Thus, patients with small bowel disease and an ileostomy do not hyperabsorb oxalate. Excessive dietary oxalate or ascorbic acid (> 2 g/day) also leads to hyperoxaluria. *Oxalobacter formigenes* metabolizes oxalate in the intestinal tract; reductions in these bacteria may also increase oxalate absorption. Recent evidence suggests that a healthy microbiome including the gram-negative bacteria *O. formigenes* may be important in reducing gut absorption of oxalate and urinary oxalate excretion.

23. Why is hyperoxaluria important in nephrolithiasis?
    Oxalate is a significant component of the most commonly formed stones (calcium oxalate) and contributes to urine supersaturation. Previously, it was believed to be a much stronger stimulus to calcium oxalate stone

formation compared with calcium. Newer data suggest that calcium may be just as potent; however, a high urinary concentration of either calcium or oxalate is a potent stimulus for calcium oxalate stone formation.

24. How does hyperuricosuria contribute to renal stones?

Uric acid stones develop in approximately 25% of patients with symptomatic tophaceous gout. Excessive urinary uric acid ($>$ 600 mg/day) supersaturates the urine, crystallizes, and forms uric acid stones. However, most uric acid stone formers do not have gout, hyperuricemia, or hyperuricosuria. But all have a urinary pH $<$ 5.5, which promotes uric acid stone formation. Approximately 25% of calcium stone formers have hyperuricosuria. Hyperuricosuria decreases the solubility of calcium oxalate. Monosodium urate may interfere with inhibitors, resulting in increased calcium oxalate stone formation. This disorder, called *hyperuricosuric calcium nephrolithiasis*, is characterized by normal serum calcium, urinary uric acid $>$ 600 mg/day, urine pH $>$ 5.5, and recurrent calcium stones.

25. How does urinary pH relate to renal stones?

Because uric acid has a pKa of 5.5, acid urine shifts the equilibrium so that the concentration of uric acid is higher than the concentration of sodium urate. At urine pH 6.5, only 10% is in the form of uric acid, and approximately 90% in the form of sodium urate. Because uric acid is 100 times less soluble than urate, uric acid stones are more likely to form in acid urine. This equilibrium is so important that uric acid stones virtually never develop unless the urinary pH is $<$ 5.5. Because of low urinary pH, uric acid stones occur more frequently in obesity and diabetes. Obesity and type 2 diabetes are associated with insulin resistance, renal steatosis, and renal lipotoxicity. This association results in decreased insulin-dependent renal production of ammonia, decreased urinary ammonium excretion, a lower urinary pH, and a propensity for uric acid stones. Additionally, obesity and type 2 diabetes are associated with hyperinsulinemia, which decreases distal nephron calcium reabsorption and increases net calcium excretion and the risk for calcium stones. Cystine stones are also more likely in acid urine, whereas calcium phosphate (brushite) stones usually form primarily in alkaline urine (pH $>$ 7.0). Calcium oxalate stones may develop in either acid or alkaline urine.

26. What conditions cause low levels of urinary citrate?

Patients with hypocitraturia excrete $<$ 320 mg/day while optimal levels are closer to 640 mg/day. Idiopathic hypocitraturia occurs in $<$ 5% of patients with calcium stones, and secondary hypocitraturia may occur in 30%. Citrate is freely filtered by the glomerulus, 75% is reabsorbed by the proximal renal tubule, and little citrate is secreted. Most secondary causes of hypocitraturia decrease urinary citrate by increasing proximal renal tubular reabsorption. Secondary causes of low citrate include dehydration, high animal protein and low fruit and vegetable intake, metabolic acidosis, hypokalemia, thiazide diuretics, carbonic anhydrase inhibitors, magnesium depletion, renal tubular acidosis, and diarrhea. Diarrhea also causes direct gastrointestinal loss of citrate and magnesium.

27. What is the role of diet in the formation of kidney stones?

The high animal protein (beef, poultry, pork, and fish) intake of many Americans ($>$ 1.5–2 g/kg/day) acidifies the urine with phosphoric, sulfuric, and uric acids; decreases urinary citrate; increases urinary calcium; and raises the risk for nephrolithiasis. Higher protein diets, such as the Atkins diet, worsen these effects. Increased sulfates and uric acid may act as cofactors in the formation of calcium oxalate and uric acid stones. High sodium intake increases urinary calcium excretion (see question 15). High calcium intake ($>$ 1500 mg) also contributes to hypercalciuria. However, low calcium intake ($<$ 600 mg) without low oxalate intake decreases oxalate binding in the gut, increases oxalate absorption, and increases urinary oxalate. A diet high in protein and salt (sodium chloride [NaCl]) impairs citrate excretion by inducing subclinical intracellular and extracellular acidosis and increased reabsorption of citrate. Fructose adversely affects the microbiome, increases uric acid production, and increases the risk of nephrolithiasis. Diets high in calories and low in fiber, fruits, and vegetables are associated with obesity and increased nephrolithiasis. High dietary oxalate (Table 21.2) increases calcium oxalate crystalluria. Orange juice may help prevent kidney stones by increasing urinary potassium and citrate. Potassium citrate as Urocit-K is commonly prescribed to increase urinary citrate; if from Micromedex, Urocit-K at 60 mEq/day raises urinary citrate by approximately 400 mg/day and increases urinary pH by approximately 0.7 units. However, an 8-oz glass of orange juice supplies 12 mEq potassium and 38 mEq citrate (which is more compared with that supplied by a 10-mEq/1080-mg tablet of Urocit-K). Cranberry juice has mixed reviews, but data now suggest that it should not be used in excess in stone disease because it may increase urinary oxalate. Citric acid juices (lemon and lime) supply little potassium and only one third as much citrate as orange juice. Although potassium citrate juices are more powerful at stone inhibition, nearly all citrus drinks are useful. An exception is grapefruit juice, which may increase stone formation by 30% to 50%. The clinician should be flexible with the patient's choice of fluid because the importance of the fluid intake may outweigh some of the theoretical negatives of the particular drink.

28. What are the presenting symptoms and signs of renal stones?

Approximately 30% of renal stones are asymptomatic and are found incidentally on radiographic studies. Seventy percent of renal stones are symptomatic. The patient may present with a dull ache in the posterior flank. However, the classic presenting symptom of renal stones is excruciating unilateral flank pain that waxes and wanes, and most patients have associated hematuria. The pain starts in the posterior lumbar area and then

Table 21.2. Selected High-Oxalate Foods.	
Fruits	Rhubarb
	Raspberries
	Blueberries
	Blackberries
	Gooseberries
	Strawberries
	Fruit cocktail
	Tangerines
	Purple grapes
	Citrus peel
Vegetables	Leafy dark greens
	Spinach
	Mustard greens
	Collard greens
	Cucumbers
	Green beans
	Beets
	Sweet potatoes
	Summer squash
	Celery
Others	Roasted coffee
	Ovaltine
	Tea
	Cocoa
	Chocolate
	Nuts
	Peanuts
	Wheat germ
	Baked beans
	Tofu

Adapted from Nelson, J. K., Moxness, K. E., Jensen, M. D., & Gastineau, C. F. (Eds.). (1994). *Mayo Clinic Diet Manual* (7th ed., pp. 315–362). St. Louis: Mosby.

radiates anteroinferiorly into the abdomen, groin, genital region, and medial thigh. Intense pain may last several hours and may be followed by dull flank pain. Nausea, vomiting, sweating, fever, and chills may occur. Patients with renal colic appear acutely ill and restless and move from side to side in an attempt to relieve the pain. Physical examination shows tenderness and guarding of the respective lumbar area. Deep abdominal palpation worsens discomfort, but rebound tenderness is absent. Urinary tract infection may be present. Obstruction, if present, is usually unilateral. Clinical evidence of renal failure is typically absent.

29. What is important in the history and physical examination of patients with kidney stones?
Obtain present, past, and family histories of stone disease, and ask about use of guaifenesin, ephedrine, indinavir, triamterene, sulfonamides, acyclovir, and vitamins A, C, and D. Determine fluid intake and sources of excess calcium, salt, oxalate, uric acid, and protein. Physical examination is generally not helpful except during acute disease (see question 28).

30. What tests are appropriate in the diagnosis of kidney stones?
Perform a complete urinalysis with focus on pH, hematuria, pyuria, bacteriuria, and crystalluria. If pH is high or there is bacteriuria, order a urine culture. Perform appropriate radiographic studies (see question 34). Have the patient strain all urine and save the stone, if passed, for stone analysis. If this is the patient's first stone, the pain subsides, and the stone is < 5 mm in diameter, conservative management with follow-up for several months is acceptable. Greater than 50% of stones in the proximal ureter and 75% of stones in the distal ureter < 5 mm in diameter pass spontaneously. Order vitamin D and a blood chemistry panel that includes serum sodium, potassium, chloride, carbon dioxide, creatinine, calcium, albumin, phosphorus, magnesium, and uric acid. Consider measurements of serum PTH and random urine for determination of the Ca/Cr ratio. If the patient has continued symptoms, if the stone is > 5 mm in diameter, or if obstruction is present, consult a urologist and plan for a more extensive evaluation. Include a 24-hour urine test for creatinine, sodium, calcium, phosphorus, magnesium, oxalate, citrate, uric acid, and urinary supersaturation. A 24-hour urine collection is adequate if creatinine is 15 to 20 mg/kg in men and 10 to 15 mg/kg in women. Consider repeating the 24-hour urine test to focus on

abnormalities 6 weeks after medical intervention. Discontinue multivitamins 5 days before collection to avoid antioxidant effects.

31. What is the therapeutic approach to patients with kidney stones?

Kidney stones do not require procedural intervention unless they are associated with or are likely to cause pain, obstruction, infection, or significant bleeding. Ureteral stones may also be treated conservatively (monitored) if there is no renal failure, fever, obstruction, infection, or pain. Pain can be controlled with nonsteroidal antiinflammatory drugs, but opioid analgesics may be necessary to treat acute pain exacerbations. Stones < 5 mm in diameter pass spontaneously within 4 to 6 weeks 75% of the time, but those > 10 mm in diameter usually do not. Passage of stones ranging from 5 mm to 10 mm in diameter is variable. Medical expulsive therapy (MET) with alpha-blockers, such as tamsulosin (0.4 mg daily), the calcium channel blocker nifedipine extended release (ER) (30 mg), and the phosphodiesterase type 5 inhibitor tadalafil (10 mg daily), may increase distal ureteral stone passage 65% by reducing ureteral spasm and improving peristalsis during acute colic episodes. MET therapy usually works within 4 weeks; tamsulosin is most effective, but combination MET therapy may be more successful. Corticosteroids may improve success by decreasing ureteral inflammation. Patients with symptomatic stones, stones > 5 mm in diameter, or multiple stones should be referred for urologic evaluation. Unless contraindicated, preventing stone recurrence requires: 2 to 3 L/day of fluid to increase urine output to > 2 L/day; intake of < 2 g/day of sodium; 0.8 to 1.0 g/kg ideal body weight of protein with more plant protein (two thirds of total) and less animal protein (one third); 1000 to 1200 mg/day of dietary calcium; and avoidance of grapefruit juice, excessive calcium supplements, oxalate, and vitamin C. If insufficient calcium is available in the diet and additional calcium supplements are needed for bone health, the calcium supplements should be taken with meals for a total daily calcium (meals + supplements) of 1000 to 1200 mg/day. Consider measuring 24-hour urine calcium, with and without the calcium supplement, to determine whether the supplement causes excessive urinary calcium that may require therapeutic changes.

KEY POINTS: TREATMENT OF NEPHROLITHIASIS

- Stones < 5 mm in diameter usually pass spontaneously and those > 10 mm in diameter usually do not. Stones 5 to 10 mm in diameter have variable outcomes. Distal ureteral stones are more likely to pass. If a ureteral stone is < 10 mm in diameter, alpha-1 blockers, calcium channel blockers, or tadalafil may help its passage.
- To prevent stone recurrence, encourage patients to drink 10 to 12 eight-ounce glasses of fluid (water and citrate-containing drinks). "Dilution is the solution." Dietary recommendations include 1000 to 1200 mg/day of dietary calcium, < 1.0 g/kg/day of protein with less animal protein (one third of total) and more plant protein (two thirds), and < 2000 mg/day of sodium.
- Addition of the Dietary Approaches to Stop Hypertension (DASH) as a basic diet with some modifications for sodium and oxalate, as necessary, decreases stone recurrence.
- Advise patients to avoid grapefruit juice, reduce dietary oxalate, and reduce ascorbic acid to 100 mg/day for calcium oxalate stone formers, and use calcium supplements with meals only if dietary calcium is insufficient to allow intake of 1000 to 1200 mg of calcium per day.
- Although potassium citrate is preferred for urinary alkalization and citrate replacement, citrus drinks, such as lemon, lime, and orange juice, may be substituted. Avoid grapefruit juice entirely and cranberry juice in excess.
- Refer patients to a urologist for continuing pain, obstruction, infection, severe bleeding, fever, or renal dysfunction.

32. What is the clinical significance of the urinalysis in patients with renal stones?

Most stone formers have macroscopic or microscopic hematuria and may have some crystalluria. The remainder of the urinalysis is usually normal. Crystals are normally absent in warm and freshly voided urine, and if present suggest a diagnosis. However, most urine specimens cool before examination, and crystals may form in normal urine with time and cooling. Thus, by the time urine is usually examined, the finding of crystalluria may have little clinical significance. An exception is the presence of cystine crystals, which are diagnostic of cystinuria. Persistently acidic urine (pH < 5.5) suggests uric acid or cystine stones. More alkaline urine (pH > 6.5–7.0) suggests calcium phosphate stones. Persistently alkaline urine (pH > 7.0–7.5) suggests the presence of urea-splitting organisms, such as *Proteus*, *Pseudomonas*, or *Klebsiella* species that cause recurrent urinary tract infections and strongly suggests struvite stones. Struvite stones never form unless the urine pH is alkaline.

33. What are the characteristics of urinary crystals in patients with renal stones?

Calcium oxalate monohydrate crystals may be dumbbell shaped, needle shaped, or oval, with the last resembling red blood cells. Calcium oxalate dihydrate crystals are pyramid shaped and have an envelope appearance. Calcium phosphate and uric acid crystals are too small for standard light microscopic resolution and look like amorphous debris. Uric acid crystals are characteristically yellow-brown in color. Less commonly, uric acid dihydrate crystals may be rhomboid shaped or resemble the four-sided diamonds on a deck of cards. If urine is fresh and warm, the crystals suggest a cause of the renal stone. However, all of these crystals may be found in normal cooled urine and are not necessarily diagnostic of disease. An exception is the presence of cystine crystals, which are flat, hexagonal plates resembling benzene rings—this always means cystinuria. Struvite (magnesium ammonium phosphate) crystals are rectangular prisms that resemble coffin lids.

34. How do radiographic tests help to evaluate patients with renal stones?
A plain radiograph of the abdomen (kidney–ureters–bladder [KUB]) should be obtained in all stone formers and shows stones with the following features: calcium (small, dense, and circumscribed); cystine (faint, soft, and waxy); and struvite (irregular and dense). Uric acid, xanthine, and indinavir stones are radiolucent and not seen. The progress of the stone can be easily monitored with the KUB. Phleboliths that can be confused with ureteral stones show a lucent center on KUB. Intravenous pyelography (IVP) localizes stones in the urinary tract and shows the degree of obstruction. A radiolucent obstruction on IVP suggests a uric acid stone. Ultrasonography reveals the size and location of larger stones, is sensitive for diagnosing obstruction, and may be best when radiation should be avoided, as in pregnancy. However, the initial radiographic procedure of choice for stone evaluation requires no patient preparation and is easy, sensitive, specific, and accurate. It should be ordered as follows: noncontrast helical (spiral) computed tomography (CT) with renal stone protocol using thin collimation of 2 to 3 mm. A newer technique that may replace noncontrast helical CT, but is not widely available, is dual-energy CT (DECT) with advanced postacquisition processing. DECT assesses stone attenuation at two different peak kilovolt (kVp) levels and can discriminate among several subtypes of urinary calculi without a formal stone analysis. Indinavir stones are not seen on KUB or CT scan and may be missed on IVP. Indinavir, atazanavir, and darunavir stones, which are diagnosed after suspicion is raised by history, physical examination, and signs of obstruction, may require contrast-enhanced CT scanning or IVP.

35. Which medications are used to treat various stone-forming conditions?
See Table 21.3.

Table 21.3. Oral Drug Therapy for Renal Stones.

DISORDER	DRUG	DOSAGE
Absorptive type I	Hydrochlorothiazide	12.5–25 mg twice daily
	Potassium citrate	10–30 mEq three times daily
	Cellulose sodium phosphate	5 g 1–3 times/day with meals
	Magnesium gluconate	1–1.5 g twice daily
	Magnesium oxide	400 mg twice daily
Absorptive type II	Hydrochlorothiazide	12.5–25 mg twice daily
Renal phosphate leak	Neutral sodium phosphate	500 mg three times daily
RH	Hydrochlorothiazide	12.5–25 mg twice daily
Hypocitraturia	Potassium citrate	10–30 mEq two to three times daily
Hyperuricosuria	Potassium citrate	10–30 mEq two to three times daily
	Allopurinol	100–300 mg/day
Enteric hyperoxaluria	Potassium citrate	10–30 mEq three times daily
	Magnesium gluconate	1–1.5 g twice daily
	Calcium citrate	950 mg four times daily
	Calcium carbonate	250–500 mg four times daily
	Cholestyramine	4 g three times daily
	Pyridoxine	100 mg/day
Cystinuria	Potassium citrate	10–30 mEq three times daily
	Tiopronin	100 mg 2–4 tablets three times daily
	Penicillamine	250–500 mg four times daily
	Pyridoxine	50 mg once daily
Struvite stones	Acetohydroxamic acid	250 mg 1–2 tablets three times daily
Antispasmodic therapy	Tamsulosin	0.4 mg once daily
	Nifedipine ER	30 mg once daily

Note: All medications are given orally. Dosages are estimated ranges and not absolute recommendations. Each drug must be adjusted according to the patient's tolerance. Use the lowest dosage necessary to attain the desired effect and avoid side effects. Always use drug therapy in addition to appropriate dietary changes and fluid input. Potassium citrate is better tolerated in lower dosages taken three times a day with meals. However, twice-daily dosing of extended-release potassium citrate may improve compliance. Potassium citrate is often required to correct thiazide-induced hypokalemia and hypocitraturia (see question 36). Chlorthalidone or indapamide may be substituted for hydrochlorothiazide for more convenient once-daily dosing (see question 37).

36. What are special considerations in the drug therapy of nephrolithiasis?

Potassium citrate, and not sodium citrate, for urine alkalinization to a pH > 7.0 is recommended for uric acid and cystine stones. Sodium citrate increases urinary sodium and calcium, and in alkaline urine, sodium urate may increase calcium stone formation. Cystine stone formers require higher fluid intake to reduce urinary cystine below its solubility limit of 200 to 250 mg/L and produce a urine output of 3 L/day. The cystine-binding thiol drugs tiopronin and penicillamine help reduce urinary cystine. Tiopronin has fewer side effects and should be tried first. Dietary purine and fructose restriction, adequate fluid intake, and potassium citrate often are the only therapy necessary for uric acid stones if uricosuria is < 800 mg/day. Use the xanthine oxidase inhibitor allopurinol with potassium citrate if uric acid stones continue or hyperuricemia is more severe. Use cellulose sodium phosphate (CSP) only for refractory stone disease in AH-I. CSP binds calcium and magnesium in the gut, decreases absorption of both, and may worsen osteopenia and increase urinary oxalate. Replace magnesium, as required. Monitor bone mass and treat osteopenia, as necessary.

37. Why are thiazide diuretics the first-line drug therapy for hypercalciuria-induced nephrolithiasis?

Thiazides are the first-line therapy because they increase proximal (indirectly) and distal (directly) tubular reabsorption of calcium. However, thiazides can cause depletion of potassium and citrate, which should be replaced with potassium citrate. Avoid triamterene, which can cause kidney stones. If potassium supplementation is added, use amiloride with caution to avoid hyperkalemia. The thiazide-like diuretics, chlorthalidone (12.5–50.0 mg daily) or indapamide (1.25–2.5 mg daily), may be preferred to hydrochlorothiazide for the convenience of once-daily dosing. Additionally, indapamide is less likely to cause lipid disturbances associated with the higher thiazide dosages needed to reduce urinary calcium.

38. How should you treat a symptomatic patient with a renal stone 1 to 2 cm in size?

Apply the therapeutic options in question 31. About 10% to 20% of all kidney stones require surgical removal because of size and symptoms. Many urologists treat symptomatic patients with 1 to 2 cm calcium stones in the renal pelvis or significant proximally obstructing stones (0.5–2.0 cm) with extracorporeal shock wave lithotripsy (ESWL). If the stone is too large or too hard, as estimated with CT, or is not in a good location for ESWL, percutaneous stone removal or a ureteroscopic approach may be indicated (see question 39). Additionally, because of the achievement of higher stone-free rates, many urologists choose percutaneous nephrolithotomy (PCNL) or mini-PCNL for 1- to 2-cm renal stones. Distal ureteral stones > 1 cm are best managed with ureteroscopic stone extraction.

39. How should you treat an asymptomatic patient with a renal stone 1 to 2 cm in size?

Treatment of the asymptomatic patient with a 1- to 2-cm renal stone is a toss-up. Each expert has an opinion based on the experience of the local medical community. Many asymptomatic stones can be monitored without intervention, other than that noted in question 31. Specifics of stone location, duration, obstruction, and overall patient health are important in the decision. Recurrent, enlarging, or multiple asymptomatic stones or stones with silent obstruction probably should be treated. Urology consultation is essential. Techniques considered by the urologist for stones that do not pass spontaneously include ureteroscopy (URS), percutaneous nephrostomy, ESWL, stent placement, PCNL, open nephrostomy, and robotic-assisted surgery. A combination of these techniques may be necessary for larger stones and depends on stone location. Flexible ureteroscopic lithotripsy with holmium:yttrium–aluminum–garnet (YAG) laser is less invasive and often as effective and safer than PCNL. Other techniques include percutaneous ultrasonic lithotripsy, endoscopic ultrasonic lithotripsy, percutaneous nephrolithotripsy, electrohydraulic lithotripsy, and URS with mechanical crushing, ultrasonography, or laser.

40. What treatment should be used if the stone is > 3 cm?

If the stone is > 3 cm, lithotripsy alone usually fails. The initial approach to patients with stones of this size includes endoscopic techniques, including PCNL and URS. In certain centers, robotic-assisted surgery is used to treat complex or large-volume renal stones. Open lithotomy is now unusual. Therapy for stones > 2 cm in size depends on the patient's overall status, wishes, and experiences, and the experiences of the patient's physician and urologist. A combination of techniques outlined in questions 38 and 39 is sometimes necessary.

⊕ WEBSITES

1. EMedicine: Nephrolithiasis: http://www.emedicine.com/med/topic1600.htm.
2. EMedicine: Hypercalciuria review: http://www.emedicine.com/med/topic1069.htm.
3. EMedicine: Hyperuricemia and gout review: http://www.emedicine.com/med/topic3028.htm.
4. EMedicine: Hypocitraturia review: http://www.emedicine.com/med/topic3030.htm.
5. EMedicine: Intracorporeal lithotripsy: http://www.emedicine.com/med/topic3034.htm.
6. American Urologic Association: Medical Management of Kidney Stones: http://www.auanet.org/guidelines/medical-management-of-kidney-stones-(2014)
7. American Urologic Association: Surgical Management of Stones: http://www.auanet.org/guidelines/surgical-management-of-stones
8. Favus MJ: Nephrolithiasis: https://www.ncbi.nlm.nih.gov/books/NBK279069/

BIBLIOGRAPHY

Aldoukhi, A. H., Roberts, W. W., Hall, T.L., & Ghani, K. R. (2017). Holmium laser lithotripsy in the new stone age: dust or bust? *Frontiers in Surgery, 4*(57), 1–6.

Alelign, T., & Petros, B. (2018). Kidney stone disease: an update on current concepts. *Advances in Urology, 2018*:3068365.

Brisbane, W., Bailey, M. R., & Sorensen, M. D. (2016). An overview of kidney stone imaging techniques. *Nature Reviews in Urology, 13*(11), 654–662.

Graham, A., Luber, S., & Wolfson, A. B. (2011). Urolithiasis in the emergency department. *Emergency Medical Clinics of North America, 29*, 519–538.

Han, H., Segal, A. M., Seifter, J. L., & Dwyer, J. T. (2015). Nutritional management of kidney stones (nephrolithiasis). *Clinical Nutrition Research, 4*(3), 137–152.

Kittanamongkolchai, W., Vaughan, L. E., Enders, F. T., Dhondup, T., Mehta, R. A., Krambeck, A. E., , … Rule, A. D. (2018). The changing incidence and presentation of urinary stones over 3 decades. *Mayo Clinic Proceedings, 93*(3), 291–299.

Maalouf, N. M., Sato, A. H., Welch, B. J., Howard B. V., Cochrane, B. B., Sakhaee, K., & Robbins, J. A. (2010). Postmenopausal hormone use and the risk of nephrolithiasis: results from the Women's Health Initiative hormone therapy trials. *Archives of Internal Medicine, 170*(18), 1678–1685.

Mehta, M., Goldfarb, D. S., & Nazzal, L. (2016). The role of the microbiome and kidney stone formation. *International Journal of Surgery, 36*, 607–612.

Meschi, T., Nouvenne, A., & Borghi, L. (2011). Lifestyle recommendations to reduce the risk of kidney stones. *Urology Clinics of North America, 38*, 313–320.

Bose, A., Monk, R. D., & Bushinsky, D. A. (2016). Kidney stones. In S. Melmed, K. S. Polonsky, P. R. Larsen, & H. M. Kronenberg. (Eds.), *Williams textbook of endocrinology* (13th ed., p. 1365). Philadelphia, PA: St. Louis, MO: Elsevier.

Popovtzer, M. M. (2018). Disorders of calcium, phosphorus, vitamin D, and parathyroid hormone activity. In R. W. Schrier (Ed.), *Renal and electrolytes disorders* (8th ed., p. 163). Philadelphia, PA: Wolters Kluwer.

Prochaska, M., & Curhan, G. C. (2018). Nephrolithiasis. In S. Gilbert & D. E. Weiner (Eds.), *Primer on kidney diseases* (7th ed., p. 420). Philadelphia, PA: Elsevier.

Sakhaee, K., Maalouf, N. M., & Sinnott, B. (2012). Clinical review—kidney stones 2011. Pathogenesis, diagnosis and management. *Journal of Clinical Endocrinology and Metabolism, 97*, 1847–1860.

Semins, M. J., & Matlaga, B. R. (2010). Medical evaluation and management of urolithiasis. *Therapeutic Advances in Urology, 2*(1), 3–9.

Siddiqui, K. M., & Albala, D. M. (2016). Robotic-assisted surgery and treatment of urolithiasis. *International Journal of Surgery, 36*, 673–675.

Siener, R., Seidler, A., Voss, S., & Hesse, A. (2016). The oxalate content of fruit and vegetable juices, nectars and drinks. *Journal of Food Composition and Analysis, 45*, 108–112.

Valovska, M. I., & Pais, Jr. V. (2018). Contemporary best practice urolithiasis and pregnancy. *Therapeutic Advances in Urology, 10*(4), 127–138.

Worcester, E. M., & Coe, F. L. (2010). Calcium kidney stones. *New England Journal of Medicine, 363*, 954–963.

Ziberman, D. E., Ferrandino, M. N., Preminger, G. M., Paulson, E. K., Lipkin, M. E., & Boll, D. T. (2010). In vivo determination of urinary stone composition using dual energy computerized tomography with advanced post-acquisition processing. *Journal of Urology, 184*, 2354–2359.

Ziemba, J. B., & Matlaga, B. R. (2017). Epidemiology and economics of nephrolithiasis. *Investigations in Clinical Urology, 58*, 299–306.

III

PITUITARY AND HYPOTHALAMIC DISORDERS

CHAPTER 22

PITUITARY INSUFFICIENCY

John J. Orrego

1. **What is pituitary insufficiency?**
   Pituitary insufficiency, also known as *hypopituitarism*, is a syndrome characterized by one or more anterior pituitary hormone deficiencies as a result of aplasia or hypoplasia, destruction, infiltration, or compression of the hypothalamus and/or pituitary gland. Pituitary insufficiency can be congenital or acquired; familial or sporadic; partial or complete; and transient (reversible) or permanent. Posterior pituitary failure, also known as central diabetes insipidus, characterized by decreased circulating antidiuretic hormone with polyuria and polydipsia, will be discussed in Chapter 29.

2. **Is central diabetes insipidus a manifestation of pituitary insufficiency?**
   Most patients with anterior pituitary insufficiency do not have concomitant posterior pituitary failure. However, in those in whom central diabetes insipidus is also present, craniopharyngioma, hypophysitis, metastatic cancer, and sarcoidosis should be suspected.

3. **How common is hypopituitarism in the general population?**
   A study conducted in northwestern Spain revealed that the incidence of hypopituitarism was 4.2 cases per 100,000 per year and that the prevalence was 45 cases per 100,000. There were no gender differences in this survey.

4. **What causes pituitary insufficiency?**
   Almost any disease that disturbs the normal interaction between the hypothalamus and the pituitary gland can produce anterior pituitary insufficiency. The most common cause of hypopituitarism is pituitary dysfunction associated with a pituitary adenoma and/or the effect of its treatment (surgery and/or radiation therapy). Among patients with pituitary macroadenomas, one third will present with one or more pituitary hormone deficiencies. Other frequent causes of hypopituitarism are shown in Table 22.1.

5. **How do patients with pituitary insufficiency first present?**
   The clinical manifestations of hypopituitarism depend on the extent and severity of the specific pituitary hormone deficiencies. If the onset is acute, the patient may be critically ill and present with hypotension and shock, obtundation, and even coma. However, if the onset is chronic and the pituitary deficiency is mild, the patient may only endorse fatigue and malaise.
   - *Adrenocorticotropic hormone (ACTH) deficiency (central adrenal insufficiency):* Fatigue, malaise, low-grade fever, diffuse myalgias and arthralgias, weakness, anorexia, weight loss, nausea, vomiting, abdominal pain, diarrhea, and postural lightheadedness.
   - *Thyroid-stimulating hormone (TSH) deficiency (central hypothyroidism):* Impaired mental activity, weight gain, fatigue, weakness, cold intolerance, dysphonia, somnolence, alopecia, facial puffiness, and constipation.
   - *Gonadotropin deficiency (central hypogonadism):* Men report decreased libido, erectile dysfunction, hot flashes, gynecomastia, and infertility. Women complain of oligo/amenorrhea, infertility, decreased libido, hot flashes, vaginal dryness, and dyspareunia.
   - *Growth hormone (GH) deficiency:* Fatigue, weakness, increased adiposity, decreased lean mass, exercise intolerance, and impaired sleep quality.
   - *Prolactin (PRL) deficiency:* Agalactia or hypolactia in the postpartum period.

6. **Are there any signs on physical examination that suggest pituitary insufficiency?**
   Other than delayed relaxation of deep tendon reflexes in patients with overt hypothyroidism (Woltman's sign), there are no specific or pathognomonic findings on physical examination in patients with hypopituitarism.
   - *ACTH deficiency:* Postural hypotension, tachycardia, pallor, alopecia, and areolar hypopigmentation. Women with longstanding ACTH deficiency often have loss of pubic and axillary hair.
   - *TSH deficiency:* Bradycardia, alopecia, facial/periorbital puffiness, madarosis (loss of the tail of the eyebrows), dysphonia, hypercarotenemia, and delayed relaxation of deep tendon reflexes (Woltman's sign).
   - *Gonadotropin deficiency:* If the onset of hypogonadism is prepubertal, both men and women will acquire eunuchoid features, including deficient secondary sex characteristics and excessive growth of the long bones. If the onset is postpubertal, men may have pallor, fine facial wrinkling, scarce body and facial hair, gynecomastia, increased adiposity and decreased muscle mass, and smaller and softer testicles. Women may have alopecia, hirsutism, reduced breast tissue mass, and vaginal atrophy.

Table 22.1. Etiology of Organic Hypopituitarism.

Neoplastic
Pituitary adenoma or carcinoma
Metastatic disease
Hematologic malignancies
Craniopharyngioma
Parasellar masses (meningioma, germinoma, glioma)

Traumatic
Surgery
Radiation
Traumatic brain injury

Vascular
Sheehan's syndrome
Apoplexy
Aneurysm

Infiltrative/Inflammatory
Hypophysitis
Sarcoidosis
Histiocytosis X
Hemochromatosis

Infectious
Bacterial abscess
Tuberculosis
Fungal infections
Parasitic infections

- *GH deficiency:* Fine facial wrinkling, increased adiposity, and decreased muscle mass. The onset of GH deficiency before growth plate closure will cause short stature.
- *PRL deficiency:* Postpartum agalactia.

7. How is hypopituitarism diagnosed?

In the setting of typical and overt manifestations of hypopituitarism, basal serum hormone measurements may suffice. However, in patients with more subtle manifestations, dynamic endocrine testing may be indicated.

- *ACTH deficiency:* Nonspecific laboratory findings include hyponatremia, normochromic, normocytic anemia, and eosinophilia. In the noncritical setting, morning (7–9 AM) serum cortisol levels < 3 mcg/dL and > 15 mcg/dL practically rule in and rule out adrenal insufficiency, respectively. When cortisol values are between 3 and 15 mcg/dL or if there is any doubt about the diagnosis, standard-dose corticotropin (ACTH) stimulation testing should be performed. An ampule of cosyntropin (250 mcg) is administered intramuscularly or intravenously, and serum cortisol is obtained at 0, 30, and 60 minutes. Adrenal insufficiency is excluded if either the 30-minute or the 60-minute cortisol level is > 18 mcg/dL. If it is not obvious that the etiology is central in origin, an inappropriately low or normal morning (7–9 AM) plasma ACTH level will confirm this suspicion.
- *TSH deficiency:* Hyponatremia, macrocytic anemia, hyperlipidemia, and elevated creatine phosphokinase (CPK), lactate dehydrogenase (LDH), and aspartate aminotransferase (AST) can be seen. However, central hypothyroidism is confirmed when the serum free thyroxine (T_4) level is below the laboratory reference range in conjunction with a low, normal, or slightly elevated TSH concentration in the setting of pituitary disease.
- *Gonadotropin deficiency:* Normochromic, normocytic anemia may be seen in men with hypogonadism. Decreased fasting morning (before 10 AM) testosterone levels in men and low estradiol concentrations in premenopausal normoprolactinemic women with oligomenorrhea or amenorrhea, in conjunction with inappropriately low or normal luteinizing hormone (LH) and follicle-stimulating hormone (FSH) levels, are indicative of central hypogonadism. In postmenopausal women, the absence of high serum FSH and LH is consistent with gonadotropin deficiency.
- *GH deficiency:* In patients with clear-cut features of GH deficiency, $\geq$ three pituitary hormone deficits, and insulin-like growth factor 1 (IGF-1) level below the lower limit of normal for age and gender is indicative of GH deficiency. Otherwise, GH stimulation testing, using appropriately controlled body mass index (BMI) cut-offs to assess peak GH values, is required to make this diagnosis. Because growth hormone–releasing hormone (GHRH) is presently unavailable in the United States and the insulin tolerance test is not commonly performed for fear of complications associated with hypoglycemia, the glucagon stimulation test has become increasingly utilized to rule out GH deficiency. Glucagon 1 mg (1.5 mg if weight > 90 kg) is administered intramuscularly and blood for GH and glucose is collected at 0, 30, 60, 90, 120, 150, 180, 210, and 240 minutes. A peak GH level < 3 mcg/L is indicative of GH deficiency.
- *PRL deficiency:* Low or undetectable serum PRL concentration.

8. What is the role of pituitary magnetic resonance imaging (MRI) scanning in hypopituitarism?

Any patient with unexplained hypopituitarism or hyperprolactinemia, or with symptoms of tumor mass effect should undergo pituitary MRI scanning with and without contrast. Patients with suspected functional hypopituitarism (i.e., after use/abuse of anabolic–androgenic steroids or glucocorticoids) do not usually need pituitary imaging. Men with unexplained and isolated central hypogonadism with confirmed serum testosterone levels < 150 ng/mL should be imaged.

9. How common is pituitary insufficiency after traumatic brain injury (TBI)?

The overall incidence of TBI in the United States has been estimated to be 538 cases per 100,000. The likelihood of pituitary insufficiency is directly related to the severity of the injury. Anterior pituitary deficiencies are more common acutely than 3 and 12 months afterward. In a study of patients with TBI, 76% had hormonal deficiencies in the acute phase; these persisted in only 13% and 11% of the patients after 3 and 12 months, respectively. GH and gonadotropin deficiencies are the two most common disturbances. The causative mechanism seems to be hemorrhagic infarction of the hypothalamus and/or the pituitary gland as a result of direct damage to these structures, increased intracranial pressure, hypoxia, or bleeding.

10. How soon after radiation therapy should pituitary insufficiency be expected?

Any radiation fields that include the hypothalamic–pituitary area can cause neuroendocrine dysfunction. Irradiation for sellar and parasellar tumors, primary brain tumors, nasopharyngeal carcinoma, acute lymphoid leukemia, and tumors of the skull base have been shown to compromise hypothalamic/pituitary function. Depending on the radiation dose and the presence of preexisting pituitary disease, it may take from several months to many years for pituitary insufficiency to develop. The 5-year cumulative incidence of GH deficiency, gonadotropin deficiency, ACTH deficiency, and TSH deficiency in patients with pituitary tumors (radiation dose: 30–50 Gy) and those with nasopharyngeal carcinoma (radiation dose: > 60 Gy) were 100%, 57%, 61%, and 27%, respectively, and 63%, 31%, 27%, and 15%, respectively. Regular testing is mandatory to ensure timely diagnosis and early treatment.

11. What is Sheehan's syndrome?

Sheehan's syndrome is a form of hypopituitarism that occurs in women after delivering a baby, as a result of infarction within the adenohypophysis caused by massive uterine hemorrhage and hypovolemia. Typically, these women are unable to lactate for their newborn and have persistent amenorrhea and symptoms of hypocortisolemia and hypothyroidism. Pituitary MRI imaging shows an atrophic or small pituitary gland and, sometimes, an empty sella. Pathologic studies have shown replacement of organizing necrotic areas by a fibrous scar. The pituitary gland cannot regenerate; new cells do not form to replace the necrotized cells. With modernization of medicine and improved obstetric care, the incidence of Sheehan's syndrome has plummeted in industrialized countries.

12. What is pituitary apoplexy?

Pituitary apoplexy is the abrupt destruction of the majority of the anterior pituitary cells, resulting from an infarction of and/or acute hemorrhage into the pituitary gland or a pituitary adenoma. Not infrequently, pituitary apoplexy is the first manifestation of a pituitary macroadenoma. Precipitating factors include anticoagulation therapy, bleeding disorders, head trauma, diabetes mellitus, and radiation therapy. Patients usually present with severe headaches, obtundation, ophthalmoplegia, visual loss, hypotension, and shock. Acute hemorrhage into a pituitary adenoma on pituitary MRI scanning and demonstration of biochemical hypopituitarism confirm the diagnosis. Rapid glucocorticoid and thyroid replacement therapies and surgical decompression, if needed, are life-saving measures. Of note, small hemorrhages within pituitary adenomas may be incidentally detected during annual MRI surveillance of these tumors.

13. Describe the different types of hypophysitis.

Hypophysitis is a general term used to describe chronic inflammation of the pituitary gland and can be classified according to the anatomic location of the pituitary involvement, the cause, and the histopathologic appearance. On the basis of clinical, radiologic, and pathologic findings, the condition is classified as adenohypophysitis, infundibuloneurohypophysitis, and panhypophysitis. Depending on the etiology, it can be considered primary or secondary, the latter having a clear cause. Histopathologically, it is classified as lymphocytic, granulomatous, plasmacytic (immunoglobulin G4 [IgG4]–associated), and xanthomatous. Lymphocytic hypophysitis, the most common form, is characterized by a marked infiltration of lymphocytes that populate the pituitary gland both diffusely and occasionally in focal clusters. The lymphocytes are accompanied by scattered plasma cells, eosinophils, and fibroblasts, and by fibrosis in later stages. It is three times more common in women than in men and uniquely presents in association with late pregnancy and the early postpartum period in about 40% of affected women. Hypophysitis may also occur as a complication of anti–cytotoxic T-lymphocyte-associated antigen 4 (CTLA-4) immunotherapy, mostly with ipilimumab (Yervoy), which is used to treat melanoma. Patients usually present with the triad of headaches, hypopituitarism, and pituitary enlargement within 8 to 10 weeks after beginning treatment. This complication affects 15% of patients treated with ipilimumab.

14. What is empty sella syndrome?

Empty sella turcica occurs as a result of intrasellar herniation of the suprasellar subarachnoid space with compression of the pituitary gland producing, in many cases, a remodeling of the sella; this results from a combination of an incomplete diaphragm sella and increased cerebrospinal fluid pressure. It is classified as primary or secondary. Primary empty sella is more common in multiparous, hypertensive women who are obese. A common complaint is headaches; pituitary function is usually normal. Secondary empty sella is caused by pituitary disease, surgery, or irradiation. The predominant clinical finding in these patients is visual abnormality, resulting from arachnoidal adhesions and traction on the optic apparatus. Some patients can also have mild hyperprolactinemia caused by stretching of the pituitary stalk.

15. Describe functional causes of pituitary insufficiency.
    It is important to exclude functional hypopituitarism when patients present with an isolated pituitary deficit. Patients receiving high doses of oral glucocorticoids for > 6 weeks or those having frequent articular or epidural glucocorticoid injections or using high doses of potent inhaled glucocorticoids have suppressed plasma ACTH levels and may develop transient adrenal atrophy. Depending on dosing and length of exposure to glucocorticoids, these patients may or may not exhibit cushingoid features. Body builders withdrawing from anabolic–androgenic steroids can exhibit undetectable LH and FSH and very low testosterone levels in conjunction with polycythemia. Hypothalamic amenorrhea, characterized by low serum levels of estradiol, LH, and FSH, can be caused by anorexia nervosa, strenuous exercise, and high levels of stress. Hyperprolactinemia also suppresses secretion of LH, FSH, and gonadal steroids; decreased testosterone or estrogen concentrations usually normalize after correcting hyperprolactinemia with dopamine agonists. Critical illness and high-dose opioids may suppress both the hypothalamic–pituitary–adrenal and the hypothalamic–pituitary–gonadal axes.

16. How is pituitary insufficiency treated?
    The goal of therapy is to replace hormone deficits as close to the physiologic pattern as possible.
    - *ACTH deficiency:* Hydrocortisone 15 to 20 mg per day, in two or three divided doses, or prednisone 5 mg per day, is commonly used to replace cortisol. Patients using divided doses of hydrocortisone should take 10 to 15 mg in the morning upon awakening and 5 to 10 mg in the afternoon (two-dose regimen), or 10 to 15 mg in the morning and 5 to 10 mg at lunch and again in the late afternoon (three-dose regimen). Because ACTH is not the main regulator of aldosterone secretion, patients with central adrenal insufficiency do not need fludrocortisone. Although it has been suggested that some women with decreased libido and muscle weakness may benefit from taking low doses of dehydroepiandrosterone (DHEA), recent guidelines recommend against its use because of limited data concerning its efficacy and safety. Patients should be educated about stress dosing and emergency glucocorticoid administration, and instructed about obtaining an emergency card/bracelet/necklace regarding adrenal insufficiency.
    - *TSH deficiency:* Levothyroxine (LT_4) in doses sufficient to achieve and maintain serum free T_4 levels in the mid- to upper half of the reference range should be used to treat central hypothyroidism. Treatment with liothyronine (LT_3) or desiccated thyroid extracts should be discouraged.
    - *Gonadotropin deficiency:*
      - If no contraindications are present, men should be treated with testosterone to alleviate hypogonadal symptoms, improve bone mineral density (BMD), and prevent anemia related to testosterone deficiency. The choice of testosterone formulations depends on patient preference, cost, and risk of specific adverse effects.
      - If no contraindications are present, premenopausal women should be treated with hormone replacement therapy until age 45 to 55 years to alleviate vasomotor symptoms of hypoestrogenism, improve vaginal atrophy and dysuria, prevent bone loss, and reduce the risk of cardiovascular disease and mortality. Unopposed estrogens are given to women who have undergone a hysterectomy and combined estrogen–progesterone preparations are used for those with an intact uterus to prevent endometrial hyperplasia.
    - *GH deficiency:* GH replacement therapy may be offered to adult patients with rigorously proven GH deficiency, no contraindications, and persistently reduced sense of well-being, energy, quality of life, muscle strength, and lean body mass, despite adequate replacement of other pituitary deficiencies. The starting dose for patients age < 60 years is 0.2 to 0.4 mg per day and that for patients age > 60 years is 0.1 to 0.2 mg per day. GH replacement results in improved body composition, BMD, muscle strength, and lipoprotein metabolism. Side effects associated with GH replacement include fluid retention, arthralgias and myalgias, carpal tunnel syndrome, paresthesias, and sleep apnea.

17. How are the different hormonal treatments monitored?
    Monitoring central adrenal insufficiency and central hypothyroidism is not as clear-cut as monitoring their primary counterparts.
    - *ACTH deficiency:* Because there is no reliable marker to determine exact glucocorticoid requirements, dose adjustments depend on clinical status, comorbid conditions, and the patient's sense of well-being.
    - *TSH deficiency:* Serum TSH levels cannot be used to adjust thyroid replacement dosing in patients with central hypothyroidism. Serum free T_4, obtained before the LT_4 dose, should be used instead. The target free T_4 level should be in the mid- to upper half of the reference range.
    - *Gonadotropin deficiency:*
      - Testosterone replacement therapy is monitored with serum testosterone levels. In patients on testosterone injections, the testosterone level should be obtained half-way between shots. In those on topical testosterone, it

should be obtained 4 to 12 hours after its application. Hematocrit and hemoglobin should be obtained twice a year to rule out polycythemia.

- In women on estrogen/progesterone replacement, follow-up includes assessing symptoms and monitoring for side effects. Measuring serum estradiol is not beneficial.
- *GH deficiency:* GH doses should be titrated by 0.1 to 0.2 mg per day at 6-week intervals, targeting age-adjusted IGF-1 levels in the midnormal range. Once this target is achieved, IGF-1 should be measured every 6 months. If side effects occur, the dose should be reduced. Younger patients, those who are morbidly obese, and women, mainly if taking oral estrogens, usually require higher starting and maintenance doses of GH.

18. What are the risks of hormonal overreplacement in hypopituitarism?

Excessive glucocorticoid doses in patients with central adrenal insufficiency can cause weight gain, metabolic syndrome, increased overall and cardiovascular mortality, bone loss, and, especially in men, increased vertebral fracture risk despite the restoration of gonadal status. Low-dose hydrocortisone replacement may actually increase bone formation and promote a positive bone-remodeling balance. LT_4 overreplacement in central hypothyroidism increases the risk of atrial fibrillation, increases overall and cardiovascular-specific mortality and morbidity, and promotes bone turnover, resulting in an increased fracture risk, mainly in postmenopausal women. Higher LT_4 doses have been associated with a higher prevalence of vertebral fractures. The overall impact of estrogen and testosterone replacement on cardiovascular disease in patients with central hypogonadism is unclear. Estrogen replacement therapy through age 50 years may reduce the risk of cardiovascular disease and mortality.

19. Management of hypopituitarism in pregnancy.

Because fertility is usually impaired in women with pituitary insufficiency, they rarely have spontaneous pregnancies.

- *ACTH deficiency:* Hydrocortisone, which does not cross the placenta, should be the drug of choice. Higher doses may be required (20%–40% more), particularly during the third trimester. Dexamethasone, which is not inactivated in the placenta, should be avoided. Pregnant patients should be closely monitored for clinical manifestations of glucocorticoid under- and overreplacement. Stress dosing is recommended during the active phase of labor.
- *TSH deficiency:* Serum TSH levels cannot be used to adjust thyroid replacement dosing in patients with central hypothyroidism. Serum free T_4, obtained before the LT_4 dose, should be used instead. The target free T_4 level should be in the mid to upper half of the reference range.
- *GH deficiency:* Because there are no prospective studies evaluating the efficacy and safety of GH therapy during pregnancy, and the fact that the placenta synthesizes GH, GH replacement therapy should be discontinued during pregnancy.

20. Do antiepileptic medications interact with hormone replacement therapy?

Some antiepileptic drugs (AEDs), including phenytoin, carbamazepine, oxcarbamazepine, and topiramate, enhance hepatic cytochrome P450 (CYP450) isoenzyme activity, increasing the catabolism of certain hormonal preparations and resulting in lower serum concentrations of these hormones. For example, patients with central adrenal insufficiency taking dexamethasone or prednisone, who are also on AEDs, may need to increase their glucocorticoid doses. This is less likely to be an issue with hydrocortisone. Because AEDs may speed up T_4 clearance and displace thyroid hormones from their binding proteins, free T_4 levels should be checked 6 weeks after starting, stopping, or switching AEDs, and LT_4 doses adjusted accordingly. Of note, phenytoin may also affect free T_4 measurements if methods other than equilibrium dialysis are used. Certain AEDs increase sex hormone–binding globulin concentrations, decreasing the bioavailability of estradiol and testosterone, potentially affecting the efficacy of gonadal hormone treatment.

21. Are there any interactions between replacement hormones?

Because GH therapy can decrease circulating free T_4 levels in adults with GH deficiency, free T_4 should be measured 6 weeks after initiation of GH replacement and after each dose escalation to rule out a mild case of central hypothyroidism. This also applies to those patients with central hypothyroidism already receiving LT_4 who are being started on GH therapy. Patients with GH deficiency have increased activity of 11-beta hydroxysteroid dehydrogenase type 1, resulting in increased conversion of cortisone to cortisol. Thus, GH replacement, by decreasing the conversion of cortisone to cortisol, may expose occult central adrenal insufficiency in patients with borderline ACTH reserve or those receiving subtherapeutic doses of glucocorticoids. Gonadal steroids influence GH-mediated hepatic IGF-1 generation. Because oral estrogens decrease IGF-1 levels, women on estrogen replacement therapy need higher doses of GH to reach their target IGF-1 concentrations. Commencement of glucocorticoid replacement therapy can unmask central diabetes insipidus. Finally, because thyroid hormone increases the metabolic clearance rate of cortisol, initiating LT_4 in patients with coexistent but unrecognized adrenal insufficiency can precipitate an adrenal crisis.

22. Is life expectancy altered by hypopituitarism?

All-cause mortality and vascular death are increased in patients with hypopituitarism compared with age- and gender-matched controls. A recent meta-analysis concluded that the standardized mortality ratio associated with

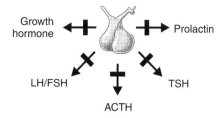

Fig. 22.1 Possible hormone deficiencies in hypopituitarism. *ACTH*, Adrenocorticotropic hormone; *FSH*, follicle-stimulating hormone; *LH*, luteinizing hormone; *TSH*, thyroid-stimulating hormone.

hypopituitarism in men is 2.06 (95% confidence interval [CI], 1.94–2.20] and in women is 2.80 (95% CI, 2.59–3.02). Pituitary irradiation seems to confer an increased risk of death from cerebrovascular disease.

KEY POINTS

- Hypopituitarism is characterized by one or more pituitary hormone deficiencies as a result of congenital or acquired hypothalamic and/or pituitary dysfunction.
- The most common cause of acquired hypopituitarism is pituitary dysfunction associated with pituitary macroadenomas and/or the effect of their treatment (surgery and radiation therapy).
- If pituitary insufficiency is suspected, basal and/or dynamic pituitary function testing should be performed.
- The best biochemical indicator of thyroid replacement therapy adequacy in patients with central hypothyroidism is a free thyroxine (T_4) concentration in the mid- to upper-half of the reference range.
- A dedicated pituitary magnetic resonance imaging (MRI; more slices through the sellar and parasellar regions) with and without contrast, rather than a brain MRI, should be ordered in patients with hypopituitarism, when indicated.
- Traumatic brain injury and subarachnoid hemorrhage are increasingly recognized as causes of hypopituitarism.

BIBLIOGRAPHY

Aimaretti, G., Ambrosio, M. R., Di Somma, C., Gasperi, M., Cannavò, S., Scaroni, C., … Ghigo, E. (2005). Residual pituitary function after brain injury-induced hypopituitarism: a prospective 12-month study. *Journal of Clinical Endocrinology and Metabolism, 90,* 6085–6092.

Appelman-Dijkstra, N. M., Kokshoorn, N. E., Dekkers, O. M., Neelis, K. J., Biermasz, N. R., Romijn, J. A., … Pereira, A. M. (2011). Pituitary dysfunction in adult patients after cranial radiotherapy: systematic review and meta-analysis. *Journal of Clinical Endocrinology and Metabolism, 96,* 2330–2340.

Crowley, R. K., Argese, N., Tomlinson, J. W., & Stewart, P. M. (2014). Central hypoadrenalism. *Journal of Clinical Endocrinology and Metabolism, 99,* 4027–4036.

Darzy, K. H., & Shalet, S. M. (2009). Hypopituitarism following radiotherapy. *Pituitary, 12,* 40–50.

De Marinis, L., Bonadonna, S., Bianchi, A., Maira, G., & Giustina, A. (2005). Primary empty sella. *Journal of Clinical Endocrinology and Metabolism, 90,* 5471–5477.

Faje, A. T., Sullivan, R., Lawrence, D., Tritos, N. A., Fadden, R., Klibanski, A., & Nachtigall, L. (2014). Ipilimumab-induced hypophysitis: a detailed longitudinal analysis in a large cohort of patients with metastatic melanoma. *Journal of Clinical Endocrinology and Metabolism, 99,* 4078–4085.

Fleseriu, M., Hashim, I. A., Karavitaki, N., Melmed, S., Murad, M. H., Salvatori, R., & Samuels, M. H. (2016). Hormonal replacement in hypopituitarism in adults: an Endocrine Society clinical practice guideline. *Journal of Clinical Endocrinology and Metabolism, 101,* 3888–3921.

Gutenberg, A., Hans, V., Puchner, M. J., Kreutzer, J., Brück, W., Caturegli, P., & Buchfelder, M. (2006). Primary hypophysitis: clinical-pathological correlations. *European Journal of Endocrinology, 155,* 101–107.

Kovacs, K. (2003). Sheehan syndrome. *Lancet, 361,* 520–522.

Nawar, R. N., AbdelMannan, D., Selman, W. R., & Arafah, B. M. (2008). Pituitary tumor apoplexy: a review. *Journal of Intensive Care Medicine, 23,* 75–90.

Nielsen, E. H., Lindholm, J., & Laurberg, P. (2007). Excess mortality in women with pituitary disease: a meta-analysis. *Clinical Endocrinology (Oxford), 67,* 693–697.

Persani, L. (2012). Central hypothyroidism: pathogenic, diagnostic, and therapeutic challenges. *Journal of Clinical Endocrinology and Metabolism, 97,* 3068–3078.

Regal, M., Paramo, C., Sierra, S. M., & Garcia-Mayor, R. V. (2001). Prevalence and incidence of hypopituitarism in an adult Caucasian population in northwestern Spain. *Clinical Endocrinology (Oxford), 55,* 735–740.

Schneider, H. J., Aimaretti, G., Kreitschmann-Andermahr, I., Stalla, G. K., & Ghigo, E. (2007). Hypopituitarism. *Lancet, 369,* 1461–1470.

Sherlock, M., Ayuk, J., Tomlinson, J. W., Toogood, A. A., Aragon-Alonso, A., Sheppard, M. C., … Stewart, P. M. (2010). Mortality in patients with pituitary disease. *Endocrine Reviews, 31,* 301–342.

Toogood, A. A, & Stewart, P. M. (2008). Hypopituitarism: clinical features, diagnosis, and management. *Endocrinology and Metabolism Clinics of North America, 37,* 235–261.

CHAPTER 23

NONFUNCTIONING PITUITARY TUMORS AND PITUITARY INCIDENTALOMAS

Janice M. Kerr and Michael T. McDermott

1. Describe the incidence of pituitary adenomas.

   Pituitary adenomas are benign, monoclonal neoplasms of anterior pituitary cells. A pituitary incidentaloma is a previously unsuspected pituitary lesion that is detected on radiography performed for an unrelated reason. The prevalence of adenomas varies by detection method, including: $\approx$ 10% by autopsy series and $\approx$ 20% in radiographic series. Most incidentalomas are microadenomas (> 90%). Despite the prevalence of pituitary adenomas, clinically-evident pituitary disease is less common, estimated at $\approx$ 80 to 100 cases per 100,000 persons.

   In most epidemiologic studies, nonfunctioning adenomas are the second most common adenoma type after prolactinomas.

2. How are pituitary adenomas classified?

   Pituitary adenomas are characterized as follows:
   - *Cell of origin:* Gonadotroph, lactotroph, somatotroph, corticotroph, or thyrotroph-derived as determined by immunohistochemical staining for the pituitary hormones and the transcription factors that determine pituitary cell lineages (e.g., T-Pit = corticotrophs; SF-1 = gonadotrophs; and Pit-1 = thyrotrophs, somatotrophs, and lactotroph cells).
   - *Size:* Microadenomas < 1 cm; macroadenomas $\geq$ 1 cm; and giant adenomas > 4 cm.
   - *Clinical evidence of hormone over-production:* As discussed in the other chapters, pituitary tumors may manifest with clinically distinct syndromes on the basis of their hormone production (e.g., growth hormone [GH] tumors = acromegaly; adrenocorticotropic hormone [ACTH] tumors = Cushing's disease; prolactinoma = galactorrhea [in females]. In contrast, a nonfunctional adenoma (NFA) is characterized by the clinical absence of pituitary hormone excess. Most NFAs are of gonadotroph origin but are not clinically apparent because of inefficient synthesis or secretion of intact follicle-stimulating hormone-beta (FSH-beta) or luteinizing hormone-beta (LH-beta) molecules with the alpha subunit glycoprotein.

3. What is the differential diagnosis of a sellar mass?

   The differential diagnosis of sellar masses is broad and includes (in relative order of frequency): pituitary adenomas, rest cell tumors (e.g., Rathke's cleft cysts, craniopharyngiomas), arachnoid cysts, mesenchymal/stromal tumors (e.g., meningiomas, chordomas), neuronal/paraneuronal tumors (e.g., gangliocytomas, neuroblastomas), primary and secondary hypophysitis, tumors of the posterior pituitary (e.g., pituicytomas, spindle cell oncocytomas), germ cell tumors, and metastatic diseases. Importantly, normal physiologic hypertrophy, or pseudotumor, of the pituitary gland can occur, such as during hypothyroidism, puberty, and pregnancy, and this can be misdiagnosed as a pituitary tumor (Fig. 23.2C).

4. Describe the common presentation for NFAs.

   Nonfunctional pituitary adenomas comprise an estimated $\approx$ 30% of pituitary tumors. NFAs typically occur in patients in the fifth to sixth decades of life and have a slight male predominance. The clinical spectrum of NFAs varies from being asymptomatic and detected incidentally (< 10% of adenomas), to presenting with large tumors with mass effects. Delayed diagnosis is common because NFAs lack a characteristic clinical syndrome of hormone overproduction; therefore, these tumors are often macroadenomas at the time of diagnosis (80%), and patients are often symptomatic from tumor-compressive effects on nearby neurologic or vascular structures (Fig. 23.1). Common symptoms may include:
   - *Headaches:* Via stretched dural membranes containing pain receptors, increased intrasellar pressure, and/or activation of trigeminal pain pathways in the cavernous sinuses.
   - *Vision defects:* Large tumors initially compress the inferior aspect of the optic chiasm and the superior nasal retinal fibers, resulting in superior temporal visual field defects. With further compression of the central portion of chiasm, inferior vision loss and classic bitemporal hemianopsia occur. Depending on the pattern of tumor compression, the vision defects may be asymmetric, unilateral, bilateral, or central.
   - *Pituitary hormone deficiencies:* From interruption of pituitary-specific releasing hormone delivery through the pituitary stalk, anterior pituitary gland compression, and/or hyperprolactinemia (from stalk effect). Gonadotropins (LH, FSH) and GH are the most common deficiencies, occurring in > 50% of patients. Thyroid and adrenal hormone deficiencies are less common, occurring in < 30% of patients.

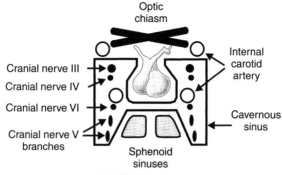

Fig. 23.1 Pituitary fossa.

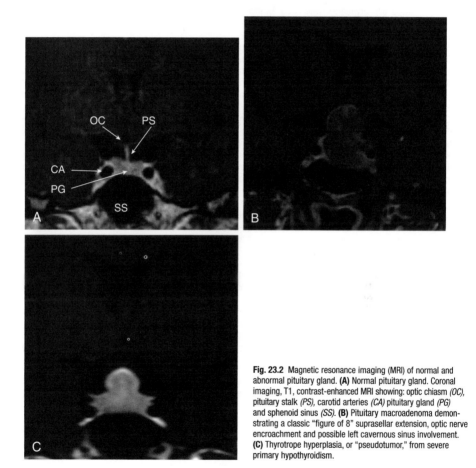

Fig. 23.2 Magnetic resonance imaging (MRI) of normal and abnormal pituitary gland. **(A)** Normal pituitary gland. Coronal imaging, T1, contrast-enhanced MRI showing: optic chiasm *(OC)*, pituitary stalk *(PS)*, carotid arteries *(CA)* pituitary gland *(PG)* and sphenoid sinus *(SS)*. **(B)** Pituitary macroadenoma demonstrating a classic "figure of 8" suprasellar extension, optic nerve encroachment and possible left cavernous sinus involvement. **(C)** Thyrotrope hyperplasia, or "pseudotumor," from severe primary hypothyroidism.

- *Ophthalmoplegia/Diplopia:* From cranial nerve (CN) III (oculomotor), IV (trochlear), VI (abducens), or V (trigeminal) compression. Palsy of CN III is most common (presents as ptosis and "down and out" eye position), followed by CN VI palsy (presents as convergent strabismus) and then CN IV palsy (presents as vertical diplopia).
- *Pituitary apoplexy:* A clinical syndrome of headache, visual deficits, ophthalmoplegia, and/or altered mental status caused by the sudden hemorrhage or infarction of the pituitary gland. It complicates an estimated 10 to 15% of pituitary adenomas, and importantly is associated with a high incidence of central adrenal insufficiency (75%) and central hypothyroidism (50%).

- *Cerebrospinal fluid leak/Rhinorrhea:* From inferior tumor extension through the sphenoid bone and into the sphenoid sinus.
- *Rare presentations:* Very rarely, patients may present with (1) stroke from internal carotid artery occlusion, (2) seizures from temporal lobe tumor involvement, and (3) giant tumors rarely obstruct the foramen of Monro, leading to intracranial hypertension and hydrocephalus.

5. What are the types of nonfunctioning adenomas?

Nonfunctional pituitary tumors are subtyped by immunohistochemical staining for the various pituitary hormones and the pituitary-specific transcription factors that delineate their pituitary cell lineages. NFAs constitute a heterogeneous group of tumors, including the following:
- Gonadotrophs the vast majority of cases [80%]—stain for LH-beta, FSH-beta, and/or alpha subunit and/or the transcription factor SF-1.
- Null cell tumors (negative immunoreactivity for both pituitary hormones and pituitary transcription factors).
- Silent adenomas (e.g., corticotroph adenomas—positive ACTH/T-Pit staining; somatotroph adenomas—positive GH/Pit-1 staining; or thyrotropinomas—positive thyroid-stimulating hormone [TSH]/ Pit-1 staining), but without clinical stigmata of hormone excess.
- Plurihormonal pituitary tumors (which stain for multiple pituitary hormones), although generally are not clinically evident.

6. What is the significance of silent and plurihormonal pituitary tumors?

The diagnosis of a silent or a plurihormonal adenoma is important because of their typical aggressive behavior, high degrees of invasiveness, and high rates of recurrence. Patients with these tumors are typically refractory to standard treatments and often require repeat surgical resections and/or radiation treatments. In addition, a subset of silent tumors, particularly the silent ACTH- or GH-secreting tumors, may later progress to functionally-apparent disease, usually in association with tumor growth.

7. Are nonfunctioning pituitary adenomas heritable?

Less than 5% of NFAs are associated with hereditary syndromes, or germline mutations, which include multiple endocrine neoplasia type 1 and type 4 (MEN-1, MEN-4), familial isolated pituitary adenomas (FIPA), or succinate dehydrogenase mutations. NFAs are an uncommon manifestation of FIPA (< 20%), but this should be considered in young patients (age < 30 years), particularly if associated with large or aggressive tumors and a positive family history of pituitary adenomas.

8. Is the pathogenesis for sporadic nonfunctioning pituitary tumors known?

Analyses of sporadic NFAs have revealed a number of interesting candidate mutations: loss of tumor suppressor genes, oncogenic drivers, and epigenetic mutations. However, these are identified in only a relatively small subset of tumors.

9. How should a pituitary adenoma, including a pituitary incidentaloma, initially be evaluated?

A thorough history and physical examination can detect symptoms and/or signs of pituitary hormone excess or hypopituitarism. Baseline pituitary hormone testing should include the following serum/plasma measurements: an a.m. cortisol, ACTH, prolactin (PRL), GH, insulin-like growth factor 1 (IGF-1), TSH, free thyroxine (free T_4), LH, FSH, testosterone (men), and estradiol (women). A dehydroepiandrosterone sulfate (DHEA-S) level is also helpful in assessing for possible central adrenal insufficiency because it is the earliest adrenal marker of deficiency. Additional screening tests for Cushing's disease are recommended *only* if clinically indicated. In assessing for preoperative hypopituitarism, emphasis should be placed on diagnosing and replacing thyroid hormone and glucocorticoid deficiencies, as needed.

10. Does an elevated serum PRL level indicate that a tumor is a functioning prolactinoma?

No. The secretion of PRL is negatively regulated by hypothalamic dopamine (DA) via the pituitary stalk. Stalk compression from a large nonfunctioning tumor can impair DA delivery and, thus, increase PRL levels. The serum PRL rarely exceeds 100 to 150 ng/mL in such cases, whereas it is usually much higher with PRL–secreting tumors (e.g., PRL levels > 500 ng/mL with macroprolactinomas). In rare cases when the distinction between a prolactinoma and a NFA is difficult, a brief empiric trial of a DA agonist can be considered. The hallmarks of a NFA with hyperprolactinemia from stalk effect are that the PRL level often becomes undetectable (< 1 ng/mL) on even low-dose cabergoline, and the tumor does not shrink appreciably even after several months of DA treatment.

11. What additional testing is needed to evaluate a pituitary adenoma?

Ideally, a high-resolution, gadolinium-enhanced, pituitary-dedicated magnetic resonance imaging (MRI) should be performed to characterize the pituitary lesion and its proximity to adjacent structures. Conversely, a contrast-enhanced computed tomography can be performed if a MRI is contraindicated (i.e., corporal metal, pacemakers). Compared with the normal pituitary gland (see Fig. 23.2A), pituitary macroadenomas are characteristically hypo-enhancing lesions on contrast-enhanced T1 MRI imaging (see Fig. 23.2B). It is also worth noting that normal pituitary hyperplasia, as from severe hypothyroidism or pregnancy, can present as a "pseudotumor," which is characteristically homogenously enhancing and uniformly isointense on T1 imaging (see Fig. 23.2C).

Visual field testing is recommended for pituitary tumors that abut or distort the optic chiasm. Ideally, these patients should be referred to a neuro-ophthalmologist for assessment of visual acuity and visual fields. In addition, optical coherence tomography evaluation may be used as a general tool to assess visual loss and predict recovery.

12. What are the treatment indications and options for incidentalomas and nonfunctioning pituitary tumors?
With the exception of prolactinomas, functional pituitary adenomas, including incidentalomas, should be managed first line with transsphenoidal surgery (TSS). In addition, TSS is first-line therapy for nonfunctioning adenomas with the following indications:
- Symptoms of visual field deficits, vision loss or ophthalmoplegia
- Compression of the optic apparatus on MRI
- Endocrine dysfunction, including hypopituitarism or stalk effect causing hyperprolactinemia
- Pituitary apoplexy
- Refractory headaches not attributable to other headache syndromes or etiologies
- Other neurologic deficits related to compression from the tumor

Importantly, TSS should be performed by an experienced neurosurgeon who routinely performs either microscopic or endoscopic transsphenoidal techniques, and ideally as part of an expert pituitary-dedicated team (e.g., endocrinologists, neuropathologists, radiation oncologists). Lastly, radiation therapy is usually second-line therapy for a NFA if surgery is contraindicated or not desired.

13. Are there any medical therapies for nonfunctioning adenomas?
No. There are currently no effective, or U.S. Food and Drug Administration–approved, medical therapies for NFAs. Despite the presence of DA receptors on NFAs, the efficacy of DA agonists (i.e., bromocriptine and cabergoline) on tumor growth control varies widely. In addition, there is insufficient evidence to recommend the use of somatostatin receptor agonists (e.g., octreotide, lanreotide, pasireotide) for NFAs. Lastly, temozolomide (TMZ) can be considered in rare cases of very aggressive and malignant pituitary tumors.

14. How should a pituitary nonfunctioning adenoma, including a pituitary incidentaloma, be followed?
For NFA/microadenomas, follow-up MRI imaging is recommended at 1-, 2-, and 5-year intervals. Pituitary hormone reevaluation should be considered if there has been significant interval tumor growth, or as clinically indicated. TSS is recommended for any significant interval tumor growth associated with vision defects, loss of pituitary gland function, intractable headaches, or evidence of hormone overproduction. For stable tumor size over a 5-year period, particularly with tumors < 5 mm, consideration can be given to foregoing additional imaging.

NFA/macroadenomas that are not treated surgically require closer MRI follow-up because of the risk of tumor growth. Specifically, follow-up MRI imaging at 6 months and then annually for 5 years is recommended. Transsphenoidal resection is recommend for any significant interval tumor growth associated with vision defects, loss of pituitary gland function, intractable headaches, or evidence of hormone overproduction (in cases of previous "silent" tumors). For asymptomatic tumors over a prolonged period, decreased imaging frequency (every 2–5 years) can be considered.

15. What is the natural history of nonfunctioning pituitary tumors?
The growth frequency of NFAs is estimated to be ≈ 10% to 13% for microadenomas and ≈ 34% to 40% for macroadenomas over 8 years. Progressive tumor growth usually proceeds at very slow rates (1–2 mm/year). Long term, microadenomas rarely grow to be > 1 cm in size. Lastly, the incidence of pituitary apoplexy is approximately 1.1 per 100 patient-years for macroadenomas and 0.4 per 100 patient-years for microadenomas.

16. How successful is transsphenoidal surgery for nonfunctioning adenomas?
- *Transsphenoidal resection:* The rates of successful NFA resection are a function of the tumor size and degree of invasiveness. Gross total resection rates are highest for tumors localized exclusively in the sella, but decreases to < 50% when there is cavernous sinus invasion or bony involvement.
- *Pituitary hormone function:* Transsphenoidal surgery, when performed in experienced neurosurgical centers, maintains normal pituitary gland function in the vast majority of NFA cases when function is normal preoperatively (> 85–90%) and usually improves or normalizes (15%–30%) any preoperative hormone deficiencies. In addition, new-onset pituitary hormone deficiencies, after an uncomplicated TSS, are uncommon at experienced neurosurgical centers (~ 5 to 7%). Patients with pituitary apoplexy, or who underwent repeat aggressive surgical resections, are unlikely to recovery anterior pituitary gland function. Recovery of pituitary hormone production is best assessed at 6 to 12 weeks after surgery. The recommended evaluation includes basal pituitary hormone testing (as stated above) and stimulation testing (e.g., cosyntropin or GH deficiency testing) only as indicated.
- *Headaches:* Headaches, particularly those associated with a retroorbital tumor location and large tumors (> 1 cm), are relieved in an estimated ≈ 70% of NFA patients postoperatively.
- *Vision:* Most patients with preoperative vision deficits improve, although many do not normalize entirely (≈ 30% of cases). The time course of visual field recovery includes an immediate improvement in the first week postoperatively (≈ 50%), followed by a slower recovery phase over the next 6 to 12 months. A worse prognosis for visual recovery is associated with a longer duration of preoperative vision loss.

17. What are the risks of regrowth and treatment options for persistent/recurrent NFAs?

The long-term risk of NFA recurrence, after TSS, is estimated to be 33% to 47% and 6% to 16% for patients with, and without, radiographic evidence of residual tumors, respectively, on 3-month post-TSS imaging. Risk factors for regrowth include large/invasive tumors, cavernous sinus/bony/dural involvement, and silent or plurihormonal NFAs. The role of proliferation markers on pathology analyses (e.g., Ki-67, pituitary tumor-transforming gene) for predicting adenoma recurrence is not currently well defined.

For recurrent/persistent tumors, repeat TSS can be considered in select cases where there is radiologic evidence for a surgically-accessible sellar tumor, particularly if associated with mass effects. In general, with each subsequent neurosurgery, the likelihood for gross total resection decreases, and the risk of postsurgical complications increases. Lastly, in nonsurgical cases, radiation therapy is advised when the pituitary tumor remnants are growing significantly or are symptomatic.

18. How effective is radiation therapy for NFAs?

External beam radiation therapy is excellent for controlling NFA growth; > 90% progression-free survival rates have been reported at 10 years in most series. Tumor control occurs regardless of the radiation technique or NFA subtype. Two general radiation modalities are used for pituitary adenomas: (1) conventional/conformal radiation, which is delivered in daily small fractions (1.8–2.0 Gy/day) over 5 to 6 weeks (45–54 Gy total); or (2) stereotactic radiosurgery (SRS), which is high-dose focused radiation, delivered as photons (e.g., Gamma knife, Cyberknife, LINAC) or protons (proton beam radiation). SRS treatment typically occurs as a single treatment or during a few (2–5) sessions (fractionated stereotactic radiotherapy), with a lower total radiation dose (15–20 Gy), but relatively high tumor dose. When feasible, SRS is generally preferred over conventional radiation because of its comparable treatment efficacy, patient convenience and possible lower rates of hypopituitarism. The choice of radiation is ultimately based on the tumor size and its proximity to the optic chiasm. Specifically, only smaller pituitary adenomas (< 3 cm) that are at least 5 mm from the optic chiasm (because of nerve toxicity at > 8 Gy doses) are considered for SRS. Lastly, small residual tumors may be monitored and not treated unless significant growth occurs.

19. What endocrine complications occur in the perioperative period?

Abnormalities of fluid and sodium balance are common after TSS because of antidiuretic hormone (ADH) dysregulation from pituitary stalk and/or posterior pituitary gland manipulation. Transient diabetes insipidus (DI), caused by impaired ADH secretion, may occur in the first 1 to 2 postoperative days in ~ 20% to 30% of TSS patients; DI presents as high-volume, and dilute, urine output (> 250 cc/hr for > 2 to 3 consecutive hours, or > 3 L/day in adults). A second phase, which typically occurs during postoperative days 5 to 10, is characterized by the syndrome of inappropriate ADH release (SIADH), during which time patients are at risk for developing hyponatremia. Very rarely, permanent DI develops (< 2%) after ADH stores are exhausted, and only if there is significant destruction (> 85%) of the hypothalamic ADH neurons. The classic triphasic, DI–SIADH–DI, response is relatively rare. More commonly, isolated SIADH occurs without antecedent DI (20%–25%) and necessitates close follow-up during the first 2 weeks after TSS. Additional new-onset pituitary hormone deficiencies are also uncommon after TSS, particularly at experienced neurosurgery centers (5% to 7%), although adrenal insufficiency should be considered in patients with early and persistent hyponatremia.

20. What is the differential diagnosis and management of postoperative polyuria?

The differential diagnosis for postoperative polyuria includes (1) fluid mobilization from perioperative fluid administration; (2) central DI; (3) osmotic diuresis (i.e., glycosuria); or (4) GH salt and water mobilization after resection of a GH-secreting tumor. The hallmark of central DI is high-volume output (> 250 cc/hr for > 2 to 3 consecutive hours, or > 3 L/day in adults) of dilute urine (< 300 mOsm/kg of water, urine specific gravity < 1.005). Mild postoperative DI can be managed with free water replacement or hypotonic fluids. More severe or persistent DI cases, particularly if associated with hypernatremia, can be treated with desmopressin (trade name DDAVP). Desmopressin, a synthetic analogue of ADH, has advantages over ADH of a longer half-life and an absence of vasopressor effects. In the post-operative setting, low-dose DDAVP can be administered as a single 0.5-1.0 mcg dose, intravenously or subcutaneously, as needed to normalize polyuria and possible hypernatremia. Patients with persistent DI symptoms at the time of hospital discharge can be treated judiciously with PRN (as needed) night-time DDAVP (starting with either a 10-mcg intranasal spray or 0.1-mg oral tablets). In anticipation of spontaneous recovery, patients should be counseled to hold the nighttime DDAVP dose periodically to assess for continued need.

21. What is the management of post-operative SIADH?

Hyponatremia resulting from isolated SIADH is the most common cause for 30-day rehospitalization after TSS. It occurs in upward of 25% of TSS cases, with severe, symptomatic hyponatremia (i.e., sodium [Na] < 125 mEq/L) occurring in ≈ 7% of cases. Nadir sodium levels occur most commonly between postoperative days 5 to 9 when patients are unmonitored at home. Fluid restriction has been the mainstay of treatment for mild SIADH for many years and recent studies now support this approach in post-operative TSS patients. Specifically, in TSS patients without evidence of DI at the time of hospital discharge, recent studies support the implementation of a 1-week 1 to 1.5 L/day fluid restriction, and a routine 1-week postoperative serum sodium level check (as has been recommended by other pituitary experts/guidelines). On the basis of the serum sodium levels at the 1 week postoperative blood test and the patient's symptoms, additional fluid adjustments can be made, using various published protocols.

The diagnosis of SIADH is based on the following criteria: serum sodium < 135 mEq/L, low serum osmolality (< 275 mOsm/kg of water), inappropriately high urine osmolality (> 100 mOsm/kg of water), high urinary sodium (> 40 mEq with normal salt intake), euvolemic status, and normal renal function. In addition, other endocrinopathies associated with hyponatremia, specifically hypothyroidism and adrenal insufficiency, should be excluded. Once in the hospital, patients are routinely placed on fluid restriction and monitored closely neurologically and with serial sodium levels (every 4 hours). A spot urine sodium, urine potassium and urine osmolality tests are recommended at the time of admission to assess for possible superimposed hypovolemia (as best indicated by a spot urine sodium <40 mEq/L) and/or refractoriness to fluid restriction. Specifically, a high urinary osmolality (> 500 mOsm/Kg of water) and a low renal electrolyte-free water clearance (i.e., Urine sodium + Urine potassium/ Serum sodium > 1) predict failure to fluid restriction. An important caveat, however, is that diuretic use, adrenal insufficiency, and renal insufficiency may also present with high urine sodium and osmolality levels.

For patients with hyponatremia with significant neurologic symptoms (from cerebral edema), such as seizures, altered mental status, or coma, hypertonic saline (3%) should be given for a targeted serum sodium correction of 4-6 mEq/L over the first few hours, or until life-threatening symptoms improve. This usually correlates with a serum sodium level in a 'safe' range, generally defined as > 120 to 125 mEq/L. In general, in cases of chronic hyponatremia (> 48 hours' duration), the correction of hyponatremia should be limited to < 10 to 12 mEq/L in the first 24 hours, and even slower correction rates (< 8 mEq/L/first 24 hr) when other risk factors are present for osmotic demyelination syndrome (i.e., hypokalemia, liver disease, alcoholism, or poor nutritional status). Lastly, although generally not prescribed by endocrinologists, vasopressin receptor antagonists (tolvaptan or conivaptan) can be considered in cases of refractory euvolemic hyponatremia.

22. What endocrine problems may occur during long-term follow-up?
Long-term pituitary hormone deficiencies, after the 3 month perioperative period, are generally only associated with recurrent tumors or radiation therapy. The risk of hypopituitarism after conventional radiation therapy is estimated to be ≈ 30% to 60% at 10 years and may be lower for SRS. The development of hypopituitarism generally follows a predictable pattern of hormone loss (GH ≈ LH/FSH > TSH ≈ ACTH > PRL). Posterior pituitary gland deficiencies (i.e., ADH and oxytocin) do not generally occur after radiation therapy. Expectant management for patients after radiation should consist of biannual clinical assessment and biochemical testing for pituitary hormones, and initiation of hormone therapy for any identified deficiencies.

In general, physiologic hormone replacement for any resulting gonadotroph, thyrotroph, growth hormone and corticotroph deficiencies and appropriate monitoring are important to avoid iatrogenic endocrine complications. For example, with central hypothyroidism, the adequacy of thyroid hormone replacement is best assessed with a free T_4 level (not TSH) and should be adjusted to the mid-normative range. For complete corticotroph deficiency, typical glucocorticoid replacement doses include prednisone (≈ 5 mg/day) or hydrocortisone (≈ 15–20 mg/day in 2–3 divided doses). Chronically higher glucocorticoid doses may result in Cushing's syndrome–related complications (e.g., diabetes, hypertension, osteoporosis, and metabolic syndrome). Sex steroid replacement should also be given in a physiologic- and age-appropriate manner. Lastly, GH replacement is sometimes considered in adults with persistent symptoms of hypopituitarism/GH deficiency (e.g., central weight gain, fatigue, hypertension, etc.) after optimal replacements of the other pituitary hormones.

23. Summarize the long-term management of pituitary insufficiency.
See Table 23.1.

24. Describe the presentation, diagnosis, and treatment of pituitary carcinomas.
Pituitary carcinomas are extremely rare (< 0.2% of pituitary tumors) and most commonly arise from longstanding, recurrent, and invasive prolactinomas and ACTH-secreting macroadenomas. Pituitary carcinoma is defined by the presence of a pituitary tumor that either (1) is noncontiguous with the primary sellar tumor, or 2) has spread to distant sites, such as spinal lesions, lymph nodes, bones, or liver. Multimodal therapy with surgery, radiation, and systemic therapy is often required. For patients with symptomatic mass effects, palliative surgical debulking

Table 23.1. Long-Term Management of Pituitary Insufficiency.

HORMONE DISORDER	MANAGEMENT
Adrenal insufficiency	Physiologic glucocorticoid replacement
Hypothyroidism	Levothyroxine replacement
Hypogonadism (men)	Androgen gels, patches, or injections
Hypogonadism (women)	Oral or transdermal contraceptives, or postmenopausal hormone replacement
Growth hormone	Growth hormone replacement
Diabetes insipidus	Desmopressin nasal spray or oral tablets

followed by radiation therapy is usually recommended. In addition, TMZ, an orally-active alkylating agent, has proven efficacy as monotherapy in pituitary carcinomas. A positive response to TMZ has been associated with a downregulation of the DNA-repair enzyme O_6-methylguanine-DNA methyltransferase (MGMT), although variable methods of MGMT quantitation limit its current utility. Lastly, the diagnosis of pituitary carcinoma carries a poor prognosis, with a mean survival of < 4 years.

25. **Which cancers metastasize to the pituitary gland?**
Metastatic disease to the pituitary gland occurs in approximately 3% to 5% of patients with systemic carcinoma of many different types. In a systemic review of 425 published cases of pituitary metastases, the most common primary tumors metastatic to the pituitary gland were (in relative order): breast (37%), lung (24%), prostate (5%), renal (5%), melanoma (3%), thyroid (3%), colon (3%), and unknown primary (3%) cancers. DI is the most common manifestation of metastatic disease ($\approx 45\%$), presumably because of the direct systemic blood supply from the inferior hypophyseal artery to the posterior pituitary gland. Additional clinical features included: CN deficits/palsies (26%), anterior pituitary deficiencies (partial or total, 27%), and headaches (20%). The prognosis usually depends on the course of underlying primary tumors, but is generally poor.

KEY POINTS: NONFUNCTIONING PITUITARY TUMORS AND INCIDENTALOMAS

- Nonfunctioning pituitary tumors can cause symptoms primarily from mass effects, including pituitary hormone deficiencies, hyperprolactinemia, vision defects, ophthalmoplegia, and headaches.
- Nonfunctioning pituitary macroadenomas may elevate serum prolactin levels modestly because of pituitary stalk compression and interrupted dopamine delivery.
- Myriad sellar lesions can resemble a pituitary adenoma and most commonly include Rathke's cleft cysts, craniopharyngiomas, meningiomas, and pituitary hyperplasia (pseudotumors).
- Transsphenoidal surgery (TSS) is first-line treatment for nonfunctioning adenomas complicated by mass effects and functional adenomas (except prolactinomas). Radiation therapy is considered as adjuvant therapy for incompletely resected tumors.
- Nonfunctional pituitary adenomas and incidentalomas that do not meet criteria for surgical resection should be routinely monitored with imaging and possible repeat hormone testing, depending on the clinical assessment and any interval tumor growth.
- Silent and plurihormonal pituitary adenomas are characteristically aggressive, invasive, and frequently recurrent tumors that may later transform to functionally active tumors.
- Abnormalities of fluid and sodium balance from antidiuretic hormone dysregulation are common after TSS and require close monitoring in the 2-week perioperative period.

BIBLIOGRAPHY

Arafah, B. M., Kailani, S. H., Nekl, K. E., Gold, R. S., & Selman W. R. (1994). Immediate recovery of pituitary function after transsphenoidal resection of pituitary macroadenomas. *Journal of Clinical Endocrinology and Metabolism, 79,* 348–354.

Arafah, B. M., Prunty, D., Ybarra, J., Hlavin, M. L., & Selman, W. R. (2000). The dominant role of increased intrasellar pressure in the pathogenesis of hypopituitarism, hyperprolactinemia, and headaches in patients with pituitary adenomas. *Journal of Clinical Endocrinology and Metabolism, 85,* 1789–1793.

Barker, F. G. 2nd., Klibanski, A., Swearingen, B. (2003). Transsphenoidal surgery for pituitary tumors in the United States 1996–2000: mortality, morbidity, and effects of hospital and surgeon volume. *Journal of Clinical Endocrinology and Metabolism, 88,* 4709–4719.

Cortet-Rudelli, C., Bonneville, J. F., Borson-Chazot, F., Clavier, L., Coche Dequéant, B., Desailloud, R., . . . Chanson, P. (2015). Post-surgical management of non-functioning pituitary adenomas. *Annealues d'Endocrinologie, 76,* 228–238.

Deaver, K. E., Catel, C. P., Lillehei, K. O., Wierman, M. E., & Kerr, J. M. (2018). Strategies to reduce readmissions for hyponatremia after transsphenoidal surgery for pituitary adenomas. *Endocrine, 62*(2), 333–339.

Dekkers, O. M., Pereira, A. M., & Romijn, J. A. (2008). Treatment and follow-up of clinically non-functioning pituitary macroadenomas. *Journal of Clinical Endocrinology and Metabolism, 93,* 3717–3726.

Ellison, D. H., & Berl, T. (2007). Clinical practice. The syndrome of inappropriate antidiuresis. *New England Journal of Medicine, 356,* 2064–2072.

Fernandez-Balsells, M. M., Murad, M. H., Barwise, A., Gallegos-Orozco, J. F., Paul, A., Lane, M. A., . . . Montori, V. M. (2011). Natural history of nonfunctioning pituitary adenomas and incidentalomas: a systematic review and metaanalysis. *Journal of Clinical Endocrinology and Metabolism, 96,* 905–912.

Freda, P. U., Beckers, A. M., Katznelson, L., Molitch, M. E., Montori, V. M., Post, K. D., . . . Endocrine Society. (2011). Pituitary incidentalomas: an endocrine society clinical practice guideline. *Journal of Clinical Endocrinology and Metabolism, 96,* 894–904.

Galland, F., Vantyghem, M. C., Cazabat, L., Boulin, A., Cotton, F., Bonneville, J. F., . . . Chanson, P. (2015). Management of nonfunctioning pituitary incidentaloma. *Annals of Endocrinology* (Annales D'Endocrinologie, English Edition), *76,* 191–200

Gnanalingham, K. K., Bhattacharjee, S., Pennington, R., Ng, J., & Mendoza, N. (2005). The time course of visual field recovery following transphenoidal surgery for pituitary adenomas: predictive factors for a good outcome. *Journal of Neurology, Neurosurgery, and Psychiatry, 76,* 415–419.

Hannon, J. M., Finucane, F. M., Sherlock, M., Agha, A., & Thompson, C. J. (2012). Clinical review: disorders of water homeostasis in neurosurgical patients. *Journal of Clinical Endocrinology and Metabolism, 97,* 1423–1433.

He, W., Chen, F., Dalm, B., Kirby, P. A., & Greenlee, J. D. (2014). Metastatic involvement of the pituitary gland: a systemic review with pooled individual patient data analysis. *Pituitary, 18,* 159–168.

Loeffler, J. S., & Shih, H. A. (2011). Radiation therapy in the management of pituitary adenomas. *Journal of Clinical Endocrinology and Metabolism, 96,* 1992–2003.

Lopes, M. B. (2017). The 2017 World Health Organization classification of tumors of the pituitary gland: a summary. *Acta Neuropathologica, 134,* 521–535.

Lucas, J. W., Bodach, M. E., Tumialan, L. M., Oyesiku, N. M., Patil, C. G., Litvack, Z., . . . Zada, G. (2016). Congress of neurological surgeons. Systematic review and evidence-based guideline on primary management of patients with nonfunctioning pituitary adenomas. *Neurosurgery, 79,* E533–E535.

Molitch, M. E. (2012). Management of incidentally found nonfunctional pituitary tumors. *Neurosurgery Clinics of North America, 23,* 543–553.

Ntali, G., & Wass, J. A. (2018). Epidemiology, clinical presentation and diagnosis of non-functioning pituitary adenomas. *Pituitary, 21,* 111–118.

Ramirez, C., Cheng, S., Vargas, G., Asa, S. L., Ezzat, S., Gonzalez, B., . . . Mercado, M. (2012). Expression of Ki-67, PTTG1, FGFR4, and SSTR 2, 3, and 5 in nonfunctioning pituitary adenomas: a high throughput TMA, immunohistochemical study. *Journal of Clinical Endocrinology and Metabolism, 97,* 1745–1751.

Raverot, G., Burman, P., McCormack, A., Heany, A., Petersenn, S., Popovic, V., . . . Dekkers, O. M. (2018). European Society of Endocrinology Clinical Practice Guidelines for the management of aggressive pituitary tumours and carcinoma. *European Journal of Endocrinology, 178,* G1–G24.

Scangas, G. A., & Laws, E. R. Jr. (2014). Pituitary Incidentalomas. *Pituitary, 17,* 486–491.

Tampourlou, M., Ntali, G., Ahmed, S., Arlt, W., Ayuk, J., Byrne, J. V., . . . Karavitaki, N. (2017). Outcome of nonfunctioning pituitary adenomas that regrow after primary treatment: a study from two large UK centers. *Journal of Clinical Endocrinology and Metabolism, 102,* 1889–1897.

Wilson, C. B. (1997). Extensive personal experience: surgical management of pituitary tumors. *Journal of Clinical Endocrinology and Metabolism, 82,* 2381–2385.

Woodmansee, W. W., Carmichael, J., Kelly, D., Katznelson, L. (2015). American Association of Clinical Endocrinologists and American College of Endocrinology Disease State clinical review: postoperative management following pituitary surgery. *Endocrine Practice, 21,* 832–838.

Zatelli, M. C. (2018). Pathogenesis of non-functioning pituitary adenomas. *Pituitary, 21,* 130–137.

CHAPTER 24

PITUITARY STALK LESIONS

Janice M. Kerr

1. **What is the size of a normal pituitary stalk?**
   In adults, the normal pituitary stalk anteroposterior diameter is 3.35 $\pm$ 0.44 mm at the level of the optic chiasm, and tapers to 2.16 mm $\pm$ 0.39 mm at the level of the pituitary gland. In general, a stalk thickness $\geq$ 4 mm is considered abnormal. The pituitary stalk, or infundibulum, lacks a blood–brain barrier and thus enhances intensely with gadolinium. Slight deviation of the pituitary stalk is common and does not necessarily imply an underlying disease.

2. **How common are pituitary stalk abnormalities?**
   The incidence of pituitary stalk lesions is not well characterized but generally accounts for < 2% of all sellar lesions.

3. **What are the main causes of pituitary stalk thickening?**
   The spectrum of pituitary diseases is diverse and includes lesions that arise from the pituitary stalk or from pituitary/hypothalamic–associated tumors. The four main causes of pituitary stalk abnormalities include: congenital, inflammatory, infectious, and neoplastic etiologies.

   The spectrum of pituitary stalk lesions differs between children and adults, and between those with and those without diabetes insipidus. Congenital stalk abnormalities, germ cell tumors, and Langerhans cell histiocytosis are most likely to manifest during childhood and adolescence. Conversely, hypophysitis and many neoplasms typically present in young to middle-aged adults (age 21–65 years). Lastly, metastases to the pituitary gland from a wide variety of solid organ malignancies (e.g., breast, lung, prostate, colon, renal, etc.) and central nervous system (CNS) lymphoma are more likely in older patients (age > 65 years).

4. **What is pituitary stalk interruption syndrome?**
   Pituitary stalk interruption syndrome (PSIS) is characterized by the association of an absent or thin pituitary stalk, an absent or hypoplastic anterior pituitary lobe, and/or an ectopic posterior pituitary lobe. PSIS is a frequent cause of congenital hypopituitarism (50% of cases). Patients with PSIS are usually diagnosed with hypoglycemia during the neonatal period and growth hormone (GH) deficiency during childhood. Much less commonly, it is detected in adulthood as a sequela of traumatic brain/sheering injury. PSIS is either isolated (non-syndromic) or associated with extrapituitary malformations (syndromic), such as midline defects (i.e., craniofacial abnormalities) or optic nerve hypoplasia.

5. **What is hypophysitis?**
   Hypophysitis is an inflammatory condition resulting from infiltration of the pituitary gland and/or stalk. It can involve the anterior pituitary gland only (lymphocytic adenohypophysitis), the posterior pituitary gland and stalk (lymphocytic infundibuloneurohypophysitis), or both the anterior and posterior lobes (lymphocytic panhypophysitis). Hypophysitis can also be divided into primary and secondary etiologies.

6. **What are the main types of primary hypophysitis and their characteristics?**
   Primary hypophysitis affects an estimated 1.9 million people in the United States and is considered an autoimmune disorder. It is subclassified by the primary inflammatory cell sub-type and includes the following main causes and characteristics:
   1. *Lymphocytic hypophysitis:* The most common form of hypophysitis and is characterized by lymphocytic infiltrates of the pituitary gland and/or stalk. It was initially thought to occur almost exclusively in young females during the peripartum period, but additional studies showed that this entity also affects males and comprises $\approx$ 30% of all hypophysitis cases. Preferential deficiencies of adrenocorticotropic hormone (ACTH)– and thyroid-stimulating hormone (TSH)–secreting cells have been described in many, but not all, reports.
   2. *Plasma cell (immunoglobulin G4-related disease [IgG4-RD]) hypophysitis:* A newly-described entity since 2011, and a common cause of primary hypophysitis ($\approx$ 30%). Histologically, it is characterized by infiltration with plasma cells, which produce IgG4, although IgG4 antibodies are not considered pathogenic by themselves. Infiltration of the pituitary is often associated with infiltration of other organs, such as the pancreas (autoimmune pancreatitis), thyroid (Hashimoto's and Riedel's thyroiditis), lungs (interstitial pneumonia). It can also cause retroperitoneal fibrosis, sclerosing cholangitis, and retroorbital pseudotumor, among other disorders.
   3. *Granulomatous hypophysitis:* The third most common type of primary hypophysitis. This condition is characterized histologically by infiltration with histiocytes and giant cells.
   4. *Xanthomatous hypophysitis:* Generally considered the rarest type of primary hypophysitis. It is characterized by the presence of xanthomatous cells (macrophages) and may be associated with progression to xanthogranulomas.

Table 24.1. Secondary Hypophysitis.

	SARCOIDOSIS	GRANULOMA-TOSIS WITH POLYANGIITIS	LANGERHANS CELL HISTIO-CYTOSIS (LCH)	ERDHEIM-CHESTER DISEASE
Age, gender, incidence	Young adults, African American females, 1:100,000	40–60 years of age; M > F = 2:1	Children (< 1:200,0000) > Adults	Middle age (> 50s) M = F
Clinical presentation	Multivisceral (lungs, heart, eyes, skin, sinuses), neuro-sarcoidosis: 5%, hypopituitarism/ DI: 30%	Systemic vasculitis (kidneys, lungs, sinuses, otitis media), DI	Children – DI/GHD Adults – DI (25%) and diffuse dis-ease (bone, skin, lungs)	Multivisceral (osteosclerosis: knees + ankles, heart, kidneys, liver, lungs, spleen, thyroid)
Evaluation (in addition to pituitary hormones)	Serum/CSF ACE, CXR, +/− Chest CT	c-ANCA, PR3-ANCA, CXR, Chest and abdomen CT	CXR, Chest CT, bone scan, FDG-PET, bone mar-row aspiration	Bone scan, Chest and Abdomen CT
Tissue biopsy results	Noncaseating epithelioid cell granulomas	Necrotizing granulomas	Langerhans/ dendritic cells	Non–Langerhans cell histiocytosis
Treatment	Supraphysiologic prednisone: start 1 mg/kg/day × 2 weeks, then taper	Steroids, rituximab, methotrexate	Focal versus systemic chemotherapy and steroids, XRT	Steroids, chemotherapy, surgery, XRT, vemurafenib

ACE, Angiotensin-converting enzyme; *c-ANCA,* cytoplasmic anti-neutrophil cytoplasmic antibody; *CSF,* cerebrospinal fluid; *CT,* computed tomography; *CXR,* chest x-ray; *DI,* diabetes insipidus; *FDG-PET,* fluorodeoxyglucose positron emission tomography; *GHD,* growth hormone deficiency; *PR3-ANCA,* proteinase 3-ANCA; *XRT,* radiation therapy.

5. *Mixed forms of hypophysitis:* Lymphogranulomatous hypophysitis and xanthogranulomatous hypophysitis are mixed forms of hypophysitis.

7. What are the main inflammatory and infectious causes of secondary hypophysitis?
Secondary hypophysitis may be caused by an underlying systemic inflammatory disease, usually multivisceral, or an infectious disease that also involves the pituitary gland and/or stalk. The most common etiologies, and their characteristics, are shown in Table 24.1.
   In addition, some sellar lesions (e.g., Rathke's cleft cyst, meningioma, and germinomas) can be associated with secondary inflammatory cellular reactions consistent with hypophysitis.
Potential infectious etiologies (very rare): Bacterial (most commonly gram-positive bacteria), granulomatous diseases (e.g., tuberculosis [TB], syphilis, brucellosis), fungal infections (aspergillosis, coccidioidomycosis), and Whipple's disease.
Risk factors for pituitary infections: Immunocompromised patients, hematologic/parasellar infections, cavernous sinus thrombosis, and previous pituitary surgery.
Clinical presentation: Most commonly presents with mass effects (e.g., headaches, hypopituitarism, vision defects, and diabetes insipidus [DI]), and less commonly (< 30%) with classic features of infection (e.g., fever, leukocytosis, meningismus).
Radiographic features: Pituitary abscess and TB may present as cystic lesions with gadolinium ring enhancement, although often are radiographically nondiagnostic.
Diagnosis: Usually made during drainage in transsphenoidal surgery (TSS) and follow-up evaluations for infectious etiologies.
Treatment: Parental antibiotics are generally recommended for infectious causes, depending on etiology and drug sensitivities.

8. What types of autoimmune disorders are associated with primary hypophysitis?
Autoimmune diseases are associated with primary hypophysitis in approximately 20% to 25% of cases. Based on a large series of patients with primary hypophysitis (n = 376), the most commonly associated autoimmune diseases included: Hashimoto's thyroiditis (7.4%), autoimmune polyglandular syndrome type 2 (1.8%), Graves' disease (1.6%), systemic lupus erythematosus (1.3%), Sjogren's syndrome (0.8%), type 1 diabetes mellitus (0.8%), sarcoidosis (0.5%), pernicious anemia (0.5%), and Addison's disease (0.5%). As such, upon diagnosis of hypophysitis, patients with signs and symptoms of these autoimmune diseases should be screened and treated accordingly.

9. What is a common clinical presentation of hypophysitis?
   Hypophysitis often presents as a mass lesion of the pituitary gland/stalk that simulates a pituitary adenoma, clinically and radiographically. Clinically, most patients present with headaches (> 70%), vision defects (> 40%), and variable degrees of anterior pituitary hormone deficiencies (50%–70%; most commonly gonadotroph (hypogonadism) > Corticotroph (adrenal insufficiency) > Thyrotroph (hypothyroidism). In addition, and unlike pituitary adenomas, primary and secondary hypophysitis commonly present with central DI (> 50%).

10. What imaging is helpful in evaluating pituitary stalk lesions?
    Ideally, high-resolution, thin-cut, gadolinium-enhanced, pituitary-dedicated magnetic resonance imaging (MRI) should be performed to best characterize the pituitary/stalk lesions and their proximity to adjacent structures. On MRI, the normal posterior pituitary gland is hyperintense/'bright spot' on T1-weighted, non–contrast-enhanced images, because of the neurosecretory granules. The presence of a posterior pituitary hyperintense signal makes central DI unlikely (< 5%), although ≈ 10% to 15% of normal subjects will not demonstrate a posterior gland 'bright spot', so a negative finding does not exclude the diagnosis.
    With regard to potential extrapituitary/stalk MRI image findings, neurosarcoidosis may also demonstrate periventricular lesions and leptomeningeal enhancement. Similarly, TB infection may demonstrate meningeal enhancement, intracranial abscesses, and paranasal sinus involvement. Germinomas may uniquely present with a concomitant pituitary stalk/gland lesion and a pineal gland tumor (Table 24.2).

11. How should patients with pituitary stalk lesions be evaluated?
    A comprehensive history and physical examination should be performed, including medication review, travel history, evaluation for constitutional symptoms, and examination for possible extrapituitary manifestations of systemic disease. The following biochemical evaluation, as guided by clinical context, are also recommended:
    1. Measurement of anterior pituitary hormones and the hormones they regulate, including: ACTH, cortisol, GH, insulin-like growth factor-1, TSH, free thyroxine, follicle-stimulating hormone, luteinizing hormone, testosterone (in men), estradiol (in women), and prolactin
    2. Complete blood count, comprehensive metabolic panel, erythrocyte sedimentation rate, and C-reactive protein

Table 24.2. MRI Characteristics of Hypophysitis versus Pituitary Macroadenomas.

MRI RADIOGRAPHIC FEATURES	HYPOPHYSITIS	MACROADENOMA
Asymmetric mass	−	+
Stalk thickening	+	−
Homogenous enhancement with contrast	+	−
Suprasellar extension	+	+
Stalk displacement	−	+
Loss of posterior pituitary gland hyperintensity	+ (except medication-related hypophysitis)	−

+, More common; −, less common; *MRI,* magnetic resonance imaging.

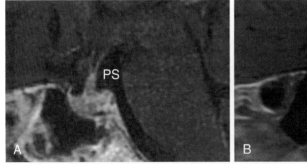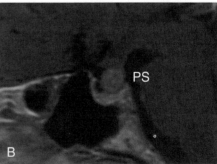

Fig. 24.1. Pituitary stalk thickening. **(A)** Magnetic resonance imaging (MRI) contrast-enhanced, sagittal view of an early pituitary stalk (PS) thickening (4 mm). **(B)** A follow-up MRI, 2 years later, showed diffuse pituitary stalk thickening (8 mm).

3. Suspected sarcoidosis—serum calcium, angiotensin-converting enzyme (ACE), 1,25-dihydroxy vitamin D, $+/-$ 24-hour urinary calcium excretion
4. Suspected germinoma—serum alpha fetoprotein and beta-human chorionic gonadotropin levels
5. Suspected granulomatosis with polyangiitis (formerly Wegener's granulomatosis)—cytoplasmic antineutrophil cytoplasmic antibody (c-ANCA) and proteinase 3 ANCA.
6. Suspected TB—Quantiferon Gold in the presence of risk factors for TB (e.g., immunocompromised or infection with human immunodeficiency virus [HIV], travel to endemic areas)
7. Suspected IgG4-related disease—serum or CSF IgG4 levels.
8. Suspected Langerhans cell histiocytosis (LCH) disease (children)—radiographic skeletal survey, chest radiography, and positron emission tomography/computed tomography (PET/CT) scans to assess for extracranial granulomas which may be amenable to biopsy
9. Suspected CNS lymphoma (systemic or primary)—serum lactate dehydrogenase and HIV serology, CSF analysis (with flow cytometry)
10. Suspected infectious etiologies—lumbar puncture for CSF analyses, culture and sensitivity, $+/-$ polymerase chain reaction (PCR)

   Depending on the clinical context, initial biochemical evaluation, and MRI findings, additional imaging may include contrast-enhanced CT imaging of the neck, chest ($+/-$ chest radiography), abdomen and pelvis are *generally* recommended to evaluate for possible systemic disease and to potentially identify sites for tissue biopsy. In addition, whole-body fluorodeoxyglucose positron emission tomography (FDG-PET) scans are recommended for presumed CNS lymphoma and LCH for staging and to monitor disease activity.

12. How useful are serum ACE, IgG4, and antipituitary antibody (APA) levels for diagnosing hypophysitis?
Sarcoidosis and IgG4-related diseases generally require a tissue sample for diagnosis. A serum or CSF ACE level is a highly specific (95%), but insensitive (25%–76%) marker for neurosarcoidosis. Similarly, for IgG4 hypophysitis, elevated serum/CSF concentrations of IgG4 are found in only $\approx$ 70% of patients. Lastly, investigations of APAs and antihypothalamus antibodies have been studied, but these tests currently have insufficient sensitivities and specificities for diagnostic utility.

   In general, the diagnosis of hypophysitis is difficult as no preoperative laboratory test currently exists. In most cases, the diagnosis is suspected/presumed, and definitive diagnosis of hypophysitis, particularly if indicated by progressive disease, is determined through histologic examination of biopsied tissue.

13. What are the natural history and treatment options for primary hypophysitis?
The natural history of hypophysitis typically involves progressive pituitary inflammation, followed by atrophy, fibrosis, and hypopituitarism. Partial spontaneous recovery of both anterior and posterior pituitary function can occur, but persistent hypopituitarism is more common.

   In cases of suspected, noninfectious hypophysitis (primary/secondary) and neurosarcoidosis, particularly with symptomatic and progressive disease, an empiric trial of high-dose glucocorticoids (prednisone $\approx$ 1 mg/kg/day for $\sim$ 2 to 4 weeks) can be considered, followed by a gradual taper to a physiologic replacement dose. Infectious etiologies should be excluded before committing to a prolonged course of steroids. Glucocorticoids can be effective in reducing mass effects, pituitary/pituitary stalk thickening, and restoring hormone deficiencies, particularly for disease of short duration (< 3–6 months), although randomized, controlled studies that demonstrate clear benefit are lacking. Subsequent steroid dosages and duration are dependent on the disease severity and treatment response. In addition, various other adjuvant immunomodulatory agents, such as rituximab, azathioprine, and methotrexate, have been tried with variable degrees of success.

14. What immunotherapeutic agents may cause hypophysitis/pituitary stalk inflammation?
Hypophysitis is the most common immune-related adverse reaction (IRAE) associated with the immunotherapeutic agents/immune checkpoint inhibitors used to treat melanoma and lung cancer. See Chapter 64 for the pathogenesis of immune therapy-induced hypophysitis. The agents most commonly implicated are ipilimumab, an IgG1 antibody directed against cytotoxic T-lymphocyte antigen 4; pembrolizumab and nivolumab, IgG4 antibodies directed against programmed cell death receptor protein (PD-1) and atezolizumab, durvalumab, and avelumab; programmed cell death receptor ligand (PD-L1) inhibitors. The incidence of hypophysitis is highest for ipilimumab ($\sim$ 3.2% versus 12%–15% at high doses) compared with the PD-1 agents ($< 0.5\%$), and PD-L1 inhibitors ($< 0.1\%$). Higher rates are associated with combination (CTLA-4 and PD-1) therapy (6.4%).

15. What is the clinical presentation for ipilimumab-induced hypophysitis (IH)?
The diagnosis of IH is presumptive and based on the presence of new-onset hypopituitarism in medically-treated patients, and without an alternative etiology. It is most commonly observed in older males (mean age 55 years) and after $\approx$ 3 months (or 3–4 cycles) of treatment. Clinically, patients typically present with headaches (84%), fatigue (66%), and hyponatremia (56%). Biochemically, central hormone deficiencies are commonly observed for the thyroid (93%), gonadal (85%), and adrenal (75%) axes, and less commonly for GH (28%), and prolactin (25%).

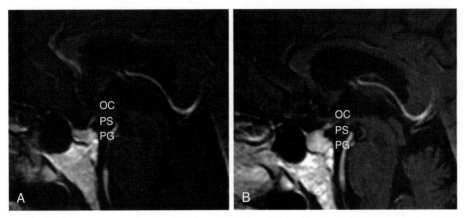

Fig. 24.2. Pituitary magnetic resonance imaging (MRI) changes with ipilimumab-induced hypophysitis (IH). **(A)** Postcontrast, sagittal view of a normal pituitary gland, including: optic chiasm (OC), pituitary stalk (PS), and pituitary gland (PG). **(B)** Postcontrast, sagittal view of a pituitary gland with hypophysitis, demonstrating a hyper-enhancing and enlarged pituitary gland and stalk.

Conversely, ADH deficiency is very rarely observed (< 1%). The absence of DI is a distinct clinical feature of IH, in contrast to other forms of hypophysitis and metastatic disease of the posterior pituitary gland/stalk. Radiographically, heterogeneous mild pituitary gland enhancement, or stalk thickening are common (see Fig. 24.2), although the MRI may also be normal.

On a positive note, the development of IH generally predicts a more effective anticancer response and survival is improved in patients with melanoma treated with ipilimumab who develop IH.

16. Is a biopsy necessary to distinguish IH from progressive metastatic cancer?
No, a biopsy is not recommended for immunotherapy-associated hypophysitis if the condition is temporally associated with the recent initiation of therapy (i.e., after 3–4 cycles). In addition, unlike IH, metastatic cancer in the pituitary gland/stalk would more likely present with DI.

17. What is the treatment options for and natural history of IH?
Physiologic or supraphysiologic glucocorticoid therapy has been frequently used to treat IH, although evidence is lacking that this changes the natural history of the inflammatory process, or improves long-term pituitary function. In general, a brief course of higher dose steroids is recommended for hypophysitis associated with severe headaches, significant hyponatremia, adrenal crisis or pituitary enlargement associated with optic nerve compression (or for other IRAEs which may require high-dose steroids, such as colitis, hepatitis, pneumonitis, etc.). Otherwise, physiologic glucocorticoid therapy (e.g., prednisone 5 mg/day or hydrocortisone 15–20 mg/day) is recommended for central adrenal insufficiency, which is commonly associated with ipilimumab-induced hypophysitis. Importantly the use of high-dose glucocorticoids, but not physiologic glucocorticoids, adversely affects the anticancer response to therapy. Lastly, in addition to possible glucocorticoid replacement, other pituitary deficiencies should be replaced as appropriate.

Resolution of radiographic pituitary/stalk enlargement occurs in the vast majority of cases and usually within several weeks to months of onset. In addition, a reduced pituitary volume or empty sella are commonly observed. With regard to hypopituitarism, a portion of patients with IH may recover some anterior pituitary function, although persistent central adrenal insufficiency, central hypothyroidism, and central hypogonadism are common in an estimated 85%, 40%, and 40% of cases, respectively.

18. What neoplasms can cause pituitary stalk thickening?
Possible neoplastic etiologies of abnormal pituitary stalk thickening are multiple and include:
1. Craniopharyngiomas
2. Posterior pituitary tumors—pituicytomas, spindle cell oncocytomas, ependymomas
3. Neuronal/paraneuronal tumors—gangliocytomas, neurocytomas, paragangliomas, neuroblastomas
4. Germ cell tumors—germinomas, mixed germ-cell tumors, nongerminomatous tumors
5. Metastatic cancers—most commonly lung or breast primary cancers

In conjunction with clinical context (e.g., age, clinical presentation) and biochemical evaluation, the tumor characteristics on MRI (size, sellar/suprasellar extension; cystic components; contrast enhancement; intraparenchymal, leptomeningeal, and/or pineal gland involvement) may help narrow the diagnosis. Diagnostic uncertainly

Table 24.3. Indications for Biopsy of Pituitary Stalk Lesions.

1. Pituitary stalk lesions (> 6.5 mm)
2. Central diabetes insipidus and/or hypopituitarism, or progressive clinical or radiographic disease
3. Diagnosis unclear from extensive investigations
4. Lack of alternative tissue sites for biopsy

is less likely with metastatic tumors to the pituitary gland, as patients usually have widespread cancer at the time of diagnosis.

19. What is a pituicytoma?

Pituicytoma is a rare tumor of the sellar and suprasellar regions (< 0.5% of sellar tumors) originating from specialized glial cells in the neurohypophysis and the infundibulum. These slow growing, benign stalk tumors generally occur in females > males and in the fourth to sixth decades of life. Patients typically present with mass effects (e.g., headaches, vision loss, and hypopituitarism). Surgical resection is usually the first-line therapy for pituicytomas.

20. How should patients with pituitary stalk lesions be monitored?

For relatively smaller pituitary stalk lesions not associated with immunomodulatory drugs or significant mass effects, clinical review and repeat pituitary hormone testing within 3 to 6 months are recommended. Pituitary MRI re-imaging is also recommended every ≈ 6 to 12 months during the first 2 to 3 years. In general, spontaneous resolution of pituitary stalk abnormalities on MRI is most often seen with inflammatory/autoimmune conditions, whereas tumor progression is more likely related to a neoplasm (Fig. 24.1) or LCH (in children).

21. When is biopsy/resection of a pituitary stalk lesion indicated?

In general, biopsy of the pituitary stalk is recommended for the indications listed in Table 24.3.

22. How should biopsy/resection of a pituitary stalk lesion be performed?

The TSS approach to resection/biopsy of a pituitary stalk lesion should only be performed by an experienced neurosurgeon. Depending on the suspected pathology, the neurosurgical approach might include a planned gross total resection, a subtotal/decompressive surgery, or biopsy alone. Complete resection of a presumed inflammatory lesion/hypophysitis should be avoided because surgery is unlikely to be curative and may be associated with increased endocrine and neurosurgical risks. Specifically, with pituitary stalk lesion resection, there is an increased risk of central DI, CSF leak, and hypopituitarism. Lastly, there is ≈ 10% risk of a negative/nondiagnostic biopsy result.

In cases of suspected pituitary stalk neoplasms in adults (e.g., pituicytoma, spindle cell oncocytoma, craniopharyngioma, etc.), the risks and benefits of a gross total resection versus a subtotal resection followed by radiation therapy must be individually assessed. The goal is to control tumor growth and minimize mass effects while also preserving pituitary/hypothalamic function, whenever possible.

23. Summarize the treatment options for pituitary stalk lesions.

Because of the rarity of hypophysitis and pituitary stalk lesions, much of the treatment recommendations are based on nonrandomized, retrospective series and are as follows (Table 24.4):

Table 24.4. Treatment Recommendations for Pituitary Stalk Lesions.

PITUITARY STALK LESIONS	TREATMENT RECOMMENDATIONS
Congenital lesions	• No treatment indicated • Replete deficient pituitary hormones, as indicated
Pituitary stalk neoplasms (e.g., pituicytoma, germinoma, craniopharyngioma, etc.)	• Subtotal or gross total resection, as indicated • Radiation for residual tumors • Replete deficient pituitary hormones
Hypophysitis (primary and secondary)	• Glucocorticoids, alternative immunosuppressive agents, or treatment of systemic diseases • Biopsy/Decompression as indicated (see Table 24.3)
Immunotherapeutic drugs (e.g., ipilimumab > pembrolizumab, nivolumab > atezolizumab, avelumab and durvalumab)	• Glucocorticoids • Replete additional deficient pituitary hormones, as needed • *Biopsy rarely needed*

KEY POINTS: PITUITARY STALK LESIONS

- In adults, a pituitary stalk thickness $\geq$ 4 mm is considered abnormal.
- The four main causes of pituitary stalk abnormalities vary by age and include: congenital, inflammatory, infectious, and neoplastic etiologies.
- Hypophysitis can be divided into primary (autoimmune-mediated) and secondary (systemic- inflammatory-, and infectious-mediated) etiologies.
- Autoimmune disease is associated with primary hypophysitis in upward of 20% to 25% of cases, most commonly Hashimoto's disease, autoimmune polyglandular syndrome type 2, and Graves' disease.
- For progressive and clinically-significant hypophysitis (primary or secondary) and neurosarcoidosis, an empiric trial of glucocorticoids, or directed therapies, are recommended.
- Ipilimumab-induced hypophysitis (IH) is the most common immune-related adverse reaction caused by immunomodulatory cancer drugs, occurring in upwards of 15% of ipilimumab-treated patients.
- IH, unlike most other etiologies of pituitary stalk lesions and metastatic diseases to the pituitary gland, almost never causes diabetes insipidus, but often causes persistent central adrenal insufficiency.
- Biopsy is recommended for pituitary stalk lesions > 6.5 mm, progressive tumor growth, hypopituitarism, an unclear diagnosis, and/or lack of alternative tissue sites for biopsy. Transsphenoidal surgery can also be considered for a presumed pituitary stalk neoplasm or tumor decompression.

BIBLIOGRAPHY

Bar, C., Zadro, C., Diene, G., Oliver, I., Pienkowski, C., Jouret, B., ... Edouard, T. (2015). Pituitary stalk interruption syndrome from infancy to adulthood: clinical, hormonal, and radiological assessment according to the initial presentation. *PLoS One, 10*, e0142354.

Barroso-Sousa, R., Barry, W. T., Garrido-Castro, A. C., Hodi, F. S., Min, I., Krop, I. E., & Tolaney, S. M. (2018). Incidence of endocrine dysfunction following the use different immune checkpoint inhibitor regimens: a systemic review and meta-analysis. *JAMA Oncol, 4*, 173–182.

Carmichael, J. D. (2012). Update on the diagnosis and management of hypophysitis. *Current Opinions in Endocrinology, Diabetes, and Obesity, 19*, 314–321.

Catford, S., Wang, Y. Y, & Wong, R. (2016). Pituitary stalk lesions: systematic review and clinical guidance. *Clinical Endocrinology, 85*, 507–521.

Caturegli, P., Newschaffer, C., Olivi, A., Pomper, M. G., Burger, P. C., & Rose, N. R. (2005). Autoimmune hypophysitis. *Endocrine Reviews, 26*, 599–614.

De Parisot, A., Puéchal, X., Langrand, C., Raverot, G., Gil, H., Perard, L., ... Sève, P.; French Vasculitis Study Group (2015). Pituitary involvement in granulomatosis with polyangiitis. *Medicine, 94*, 1–13.

Di logro, N., Morana, G., & Maghnie, M. (2015). Pituitary stalk thickening on MRI: when is the best time to re-scan and how long should we continue re-scanning for? *Clinical Endocrinology (Oxford), 83*, 449–455.

Faje, A. T. (2016). Immunotherapy and hypophysitis: clinical presentation, treatment and biological insight. *Pituitary, 19*, 82–92.

Faje, A. T., Sullivan, R., Lawrence, D., Tritos, N. A., Fadden, R., Klibanski, A., & Nachtigall, L. (2014). Ipilimumab-induced hypophysitis: a detailed longitudinal analysis in a large cohort of patients with metastatic melanoma. *Journal of Clinical Endocrinology and Metabolism, 99*, 4078–4085.

Falorni, A., Minarelli, V., Bartoloni, E., Alunno, A., & Gerli, R. (2014). Diagnosis and classification of autoimmune hypophysitis. *Autoimmune Reviews, 13*, 412–416.

Hamilton, B. E., Salzman, K. L., & Osborn, A. G. (2007). Anatomic and pathologic spectrum of pituitary infundibulum lesions. *American Journal of Roentgenology, 188*, 223–232.

Howlett, T. A., Levy, M. J., & Robertson, I. J. (2010). How reliably can autoimmune hypophysitis be diagnosed without pituitary biopsy. *Clinical Endocrinology, 73*, 18–21.

Lopes, M. B. (2017). The 2017 World Health Organization classification of tumors of the pituitary gland: a summary. *Acta Neuropathology, 134*, 521–535.

Rupp, D., & Molitch, M. (2008). Pituitary stalk lesions. *Current Opinions in Endocrinology, Diabetes, and Obesity, 15*, 339–345.

Satogami, N., Miki, Y., Koyama, T., Kataoka, M., & Togashi, K. (2010). Normal pituitary stalk: high-resolution MR imaging at 3T. *American Journal of Neuroradiology, 31*, 355–359.

Tritos, N. A., Byrne, T. N., Wu, C. L., & Klibanski, A. (2011). A patient with diabetes insipidus, anterior hypopituitarism and pituitary stalk thickening. *Nature Reviews in Endocrinology, 7*, 54–59.

Turcu, A. F., Erickson, B. J., Lin, E., Guadalix, S., Schwartz, K., Scheithauer, B. W., Atkinson, J. L., & Young, W. F., Jr. (2013). Pituitary stalk lesions: the Mayo Clinic experience. *Journal of Clinical Endocrinology and Metabolism, 98*, 1812–1818.

Umehara, H., Okazaki, K., Masaki, Y., Kawano, M., Yamamoto, M., Saeki, T., ... Inoue, D. (2012). A novel clinical entity, IgG4-related disease (IgG4RD): general concept and details. *Modern Rheumatology, 22*, 1–14.

Zygourakis, C. C., Rolston, J. D., Lee, H. S., Partow, C., Kunwar, S., & Aghi, M. K. (2015). Pituicytomas and spindle cell oncocytomas: modern case series from the University of California, San Francisco. *Pituitary, 18*, 150–158.

CHAPTER 25

PROLACTIN-SECRETING PITUITARY TUMORS

Virginia Sarapura

1. Describe the normal control of prolactin secretion and how it is altered in prolactin-secreting tumors?

   Multiple factors affect prolactin secretion (Fig. 25.1). However, the principal influence on prolactin secretion is tonic inhibition by dopamine input from the hypothalamus. Dopamine interaction with receptors of the D2 subtype on pituitary lactotroph membranes activates the inhibitory G-protein, leading to decreased adenylate cyclase activity and decreased levels of cyclic adenosine monophosphate (cAMP). In prolactin-secreting pituitary adenomas, a monoclonal population of prolactin-producing cells escapes the normal physiologic input of dopamine from the hypothalamus, apparently by acquiring a peripheral blood supply. In almost all cases, responsiveness to a pharmacologic dose of dopamine is maintained.

2. What are the normal levels of serum prolactin? Are they different in men and women? What levels are seen in patients with prolactin-secreting tumors?

   The normal serum prolactin level is < 15 or 30 ng/mL, depending on the laboratory. Women tend to have slightly higher levels than men, probably because of estrogen stimulation of prolactin secretion. In patients with prolactin-secreting tumors, the levels are usually > 100 ng/mL but may be as low as 30 to 50 ng/mL if the tumor is small. A level > 200 ng/mL is almost always indicative of a prolactin-secreting tumor. Very high prolactin levels may be found to be falsely normal because of the high-dose hook effect of the assay; if clinically indicated, the sample should be assayed again after dilution.

3. What are the physiologic causes of an elevated prolactin level that must be considered in the differential diagnosis of prolactin-secreting tumors? What levels can be reached under these circumstances?

   The most important physiologic states in which prolactin is found to be elevated are pregnancy and lactation. During the third trimester of pregnancy, the prolactin level may reach 200 to 300 ng/mL. It then gradually decreases during postpartum week 1 despite continued lactation but may continue to rise acutely at the time of breastfeeding. Prolactin values are also elevated during sleep, strenuous exercise, stress, and nipple stimulation. In these cases, the elevation is mild, < 50 ng/mL.

4. List the abnormal causes of an elevated serum prolactin value other than a prolactin-secreting tumor, and state the mechanisms underlying the abnormal prolactin production.

   See Table 25.1.

5. What are the typical levels of serum prolactin associated with these causes?

   The prolactin level is usually mildly elevated, 30 to 50 ng/mL, and rarely above 100 ng/mL, when the cause of the elevated prolactin is not a prolactin-secreting tumor.

6. How does prolactin elevation result in gonadal dysfunction? What are the symptoms associated with gonadal dysfunction?

   Elevated prolactin levels suppress the hypothalamic–pituitary–gonadal axis primarily by interfering with the secretion of gonadotropin-releasing hormone in the hypothalamus, resulting in decreased circulating levels of gonadotropins and estrogen or testosterone. Symptoms include infertility, loss of libido, menstrual irregularity and amenorrhea in women, and loss of libido and impotence in men.

7. What is galactorrhea? Do most patients with prolactin-secreting tumors present with this symptom?

   Galactorrhea is the discharge of milk from the breast not associated with pregnancy or lactation. Although a typical symptom of prolactin-secreting tumors, it may be absent in up to 50% of women, particularly when estrogen levels are very low. Galactorrhea is uncommon in men but may be seen in conjunction with gynecomastia when decreased gonadal function results in a low ratio of testosterone to estrogen.

8. Why do men with prolactin-secreting tumors often present with more advanced disease compared with women?

   The major symptoms of elevated prolactin values in men are decreased libido and impotence. These symptoms may be ignored or attributed to psychological causes. Many years may go by before an evaluation is sought, often

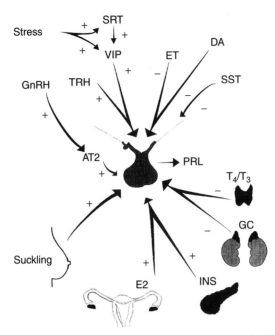

Fig. 25.1. The multiple pathways controlling prolactin secretion. Plus (+), stimulatory effect; minus (−), inhibitory effect. Input from above the pituitary gland *(depicted)* arises in the hypothalamus; input from below arises in the breast nipple, ovary, pancreas, adrenal gland, and thyroid gland, as depicted. *AT2,* Angiotensin 2; *DA,* dopamine; *E2,* estradiol; *ET,* endothelin; *GC,* glucocorticoids; *GnRH,* gonadotropin-releasing hormone; *INS,* insulin; *PRL,* prolactin; *SRT,* serotonin; *SST,* somatostatin; T_4/T_3, thyroxine/triiodothyronine; *TRH,* thyrotropin-releasing hormone; *VIP,* vasoactive intestinal peptide.

Table 25.1. Abnormal Causes of Elevated Serum Prolactin Level Other than Prolactin-Secreting Tumors and Underlying Mechanism of Abnormal Prolactin Production.

CAUSES	MECHANISM
Pituitary stalk interruption Trauma Surgery Pituitary, hypothalamic, or parasellar tumor Infiltrative disorders of the hypothalamus	Interference with the hypothalamic–pituitary pathways: Prolactin production increases because the tonic inhibition of prolactin secretion is interrupted; often accompanied by hypopituitarism
Pharmacologic agents: Phenothiazines Tricyclic antidepressants Alpha-methyldopa Metoclopramide Cimetidine Estrogens	Specific interference with dopaminergic input to the pituitary gland
Hypothyroidism	Increased thyrotropin-releasing hormone that stimulates prolactin release
Renal failure and liver cirrhosis	Decreased metabolic clearance of prolactin; also, increased production in chronic renal failure
Intercostal nerve stimulation Chest wall lesions Herpes zoster	Mimicking of the stimulation caused by suckling

when the patient experiences headaches and visual field defects related to the mass effect of the enlarging tumor. Women are more likely to seek evaluation early in the disease process, when infertility or menstrual irregularities prompt an evaluation of their hormonal status. Interestingly, studies have suggested that large ($\geq$10 mm) and small ($<$ 10 mm) tumors may be biologically different at their onset. There appears to be no difference in the prevalence of large tumors between men and women; however, there is a much higher prevalence of small tumors in women. This difference suggests that factors in women, possibly estrogen, may promote the appearance of prolactin-secreting tumors, but when these appear, they may be smaller and less aggressive.

9. What is the imaging technique of choice when a prolactin-secreting tumor is suspected? Why?
Magnetic resonance imaging (MRI) of the pituitary with a contrast agent, such as gadolinium, is the imaging technique of choice for the evaluation of pituitary tumors. In particular, discrimination of small tumors is improved. Computed tomography allows better visualization of bone structures, such as the floor of the sella, in cases of large tumors. However, the relationship of the tumor to other soft tissue structures, such as the cavernous sinuses and carotid arteries, is best visualized with MRI. Skull radiography and tomography are not helpful.

10. Bone metabolism is altered when prolactin values are elevated. What is the mechanism for this effect? Is it reversible?
The resulting decrease in circulating estrogen or testosterone levels causes a corresponding decrease in osteoblastic bone formation and an increase in osteoclastic bone resorption. Consequently, there is a decrease in bone mineral density and progression to osteoporosis. Studies have suggested that normalization of prolactin levels restores bone density in most but not all patients, particularly those affected at an early age, before reaching peak bone mass in the third decade of life.

KEY POINTS: PROLACTIN-SECRETING PITUITARY TUMORS

- When a mild prolactin elevation is found (30–50 ng/mL), physiologic, pathologic, and iatrogenic causes must be excluded before the diagnosis of a small prolactin-secreting tumor can be made.
- A prolactin level > 200 ng/mL is almost always indicative of a prolactin-secreting tumor, except during pregnancy.
- Elevated prolactin values cause galactorrhea and suppress the hypothalamic–pituitary–gonadal axis, resulting in hypogonadism and a progressive decrease in bone mineral density.
- Untreated prolactin-secreting tumors grow very slowly; < 5% of small tumors are noticeably larger after 2 to 5 years.
- Treatment with dopamine agonists is well tolerated and quickly effective in normalizing the prolactin level and shrinking the tumor mass of even very large prolactin-secreting tumors.

11. If a prolactinoma is left untreated, what is the risk of tumor enlargement?
Many longitudinal studies agree that progression of the disease is rare and occurs at a slow pace. This is particularly true of small prolactin-secreting tumors ($<$ 10 mm), $<$ 5% of which enlarge significantly over 25 years of observation. There is no reliable way to predict which tumors will show progression. Spontaneous resolution, attributed to necrosis, has also been described in some patients, particularly after pregnancy.

12. Is medical treatment available for prolactin-secreting tumors? What is the mode of action?
Medical treatment with dopamine agonists has been available since the early 1980s. The most commonly used drugs are bromocriptine and cabergoline; pergolide and hydergine are also commercially available dopamine agonists, but they are not approved by the U.S. Food and Drug Administration specifically for treatment of prolactin-secreting tumors. Both bromocriptine and cabergoline are highly effective in reducing both prolactin levels and tumor size.

13. Describe the mode of action of dopamine agonists.
Dopamine agonists bind to the pituitary-specific D2 dopamine receptors on the cell membrane of prolactin-secreting cells, decreasing intracellular levels of cAMP and calcium. This process inhibits the synthesis and release of prolactin. An increase in cellular lysosomal activity causes involution of the rough endoplasmic reticulum and Golgi apparatus. The action of dopamine agonists on D1 dopamine receptors in the brain is the reason for the side effects of nausea and dizziness; dopamine agonists with more D2 specificity, such as cabergoline, are less likely to cause these side effects.

14. If a woman with a prolactin-secreting tumor becomes pregnant while undergoing medical treatment, should the treatment be interrupted? Should she breastfeed her infant?
Even though many studies have found that maternal treatment with dopamine agonists is safe for the fetus, it is recommended that the drug be stopped as soon as pregnancy is diagnosed. The risk of tumor reexpansion is low, $<$ 5% for small prolactin-secreting tumors and 15% to 35% for large tumors. Assessment of symptoms,

particularly headaches, and visual field tests should be performed every 1 to 3 months; any evidence of tumor reexpansion should prompt the reinstitution of treatment. Breastfeeding does not appear to add any significant risk for these patients, but close follow-up should be continued. Once breastfeeding ends, the prolactin level should be measured 2 to 3 months later and treatment with a dopamine agonist should be restarted if the prolactin level is high.

15. How long does it take for medical treatment to reduce the serum prolactin level? To reduce the size of the tumor?
    The onset of action of dopamine agonists is rapid; because prolactin has a serum half-life of 50 minutes, a decrease in the prolactin level may be noted within 2 hours. However, normalization of prolactin levels may take weeks or months, with the maximal decrease usually seen by 3 months. Tumor size reduction can occur within 48 hours and may be demonstrated by improvement in visual fields when these are affected by the tumor. Tumor shrinkage is usually evident by 3 months; for larger tumors, it is recommended that MRI be performed again at this time, to ensure that there is an adequate response to the treatment. Maximal tumor shrinkage, however, is not usually observed until after at least 12 months of treatment. Repeat MRI after 1 year of treatment is, therefore, recommended.

16. How long is medical treatment of prolactin-secreting tumors required? Why?
    Lifelong treatment is usually required because prolactin levels rise, and tumors reexpand when treatment is interrupted, suggesting that the effect is mostly cytostatic. More recent reports, however, suggest that $\approx$ 20% of cases may be cured after 2 to 5 years of treatment (longer time may be required for larger tumors), and some evidence suggests that dopamine agonists may have a cytolytic effect in these cases.

17. When is surgical removal of a prolactin-secreting tumor indicated?
    With the availability of dopamine agonists, surgery has become a secondary choice in the treatment of prolactin-secreting tumors, particularly because the long-term surgical cure rate for large tumors is only 25% to 50%. The principal indications for surgical treatment of a prolactin-secreting tumor are intolerance or resistance to dopamine agonists and acute hemorrhage into the tumor. A cerebrospinal fluid leak resulting from erosion of the floor of the sella turcica is another indication for surgical debulking and repair.

18. When is radiotherapy indicated to treat a prolactin-secreting tumor?
    Radiotherapy has rarely been used because hypopituitarism is a common side effect, generally occurring within a few years. This complication is of critical concern, particularly in patients undergoing treatment for infertility. However, radiotherapy may be a useful adjunct in patients who require additional treatment after surgery and who do not tolerate dopamine agonists. Some experts advocate the use of radiotherapy 3 months before attempting pregnancy in women with large tumors to avoid tumor reexpansion during pregnancy. Stereotactic radiosurgical techniques, such as the gamma knife, may improve outcomes and minimize radiation side effects.

19. What is a giant prolactinoma?
    Giant prolactinomas are defined as prolactinomas > 4 cm in size. Cabergoline is usually the initial treatment of choice, although high doses may be required; surgery is indicated for cabergoline-resistant cases, and radiation therapy can be added if the tumor progresses. If progression continues despite these measures, temozolomide, an alkylating agent that depletes a DNA repair enzyme, can be considered.

20. Are prolactinomas ever malignant?
    Malignant prolactinomas account for about 1 to 2 per 1000 pituitary adenomas. Features that may suggest malignancy are loss of responsivity to dopamine agonists in a previously responsive tumor, rapid regrowth after surgery, repeated operations for tumor growth and rising prolactin levels, the development of metastases, and high Ki-67 labeling. Aside from surgery, other treatment measures that may be effective are radiation therapy and/or temozolomide, an alkylating agent that depletes a DNA repair enzyme.

⊕ WEBSITES

1. National Institute for Diabetes, Digestive and Kidney Disorders: http://www.endocrine.niddk.nih.gov/pubs/prolact/prolact.htm.
2. UpToDate: Patient information: https://www.uptodate.com/contents/high-prolactin-levels-and-prolactinomas-beyond-the-basics.
3. Pituitary Society: Information for patients: Prolactinoma: http://www.pituitarysociety.org/patient-education/pituitary-disorders/prolactinoma/what-is-prolactinoma.

BIBLIOGRAPHY

Glezer, A., Bronstein, M. D. (2015). Prolactinomas. *Endocrinology and Metabolism Clinics of North America, 44,* 71–78.

Kaltsas, G. A., Nomikos, P., Kontogeorgos, G., Buchfelder, M., & Grossman, A. B. (2005). Clinical review: diagnosis and management of pituitary carcinomas. *Journal of Clinical Endocrinology and Metabolism, 90,* 3089–3099.

Kars, M., Roelfsema, F., Romijn, J. A., & Pereira, A. M. (2006). Malignant prolactinoma: case report and review of the literature. *European Journal of Endocrinology, 155,* 523–534.

Lim, S., Shahinian, H., Maya, M. M., Yong, W., & Heaney, A. P. (2006). Temozolomide: a novel treatment for pituitary carcinoma. *Lancet Oncology, 7*(6), 518–520.

Melmed, S., Casanueva, F. F., Hoffman, A. R., Kleinberg, D. L., Montori, V. M., Schlechte, J. A., & Wass, J. A. (2011). Diagnosis and treatment of hyperprolactinemia: an Endocrine Society clinical practice guideline. *Journal of Clinical Endocrinology and Metabolism, 96,* 273–288.

Molitch, M. E. (2015). Endocrinology in pregnancy: management of the pregnant patient with a prolactinoma. *European Journal of Endocrinology, 172,* R205–R213.

Molitch, M. E. (2014). Management of medically refractory prolactinoma. *Journal of Neurooncology, 117,* 421–428.

Neff, L. M., Weil, M., Cole, A., Hedges, T. R., Shucart, W., Lawrence, D., . . . Lechan, R. M. (2007). Temozolomide in the treatment of an invasive prolactinoma resistant to dopamine agonists. *Pituitary, 10*(1), 81–86.

CHAPTER 26

GROWTH HORMONE–SECRETING PITUITARY TUMORS

Mary H. Samuels

1. **What is the normal function of growth hormone (GH) in children and adults?**
   In children, GH is responsible for linear growth. In children and adults, GH has many effects on intermediary metabolism, including protein synthesis and nitrogen balance, carbohydrate metabolism, lipolysis, and calcium homeostasis.

2. **How are levels of GH normally regulated?**
   Pituitary secretion of GH is primarily regulated by two hypothalamic hormones: stimulatory GH-releasing hormone (GHRH) and inhibitory somatostatin. Secretion of GH is also affected by adrenergic and dopaminergic hormones, as well as by other central nervous system and peripheral factors. GH is secreted from the pituitary gland in pulses and has a short plasma half-life, so GH levels can vary markedly with repeated measurements in healthy as well as disease states.

3. **Does GH directly affect peripheral tissues?**
   No. Most (although not all) effects of GH are mediated by another hormone called insulin-like growth factor-1 (IGF-1). IGF-1 is made by the liver and other organs in response to stimulation by GH. IGF-1 feeds back to the pituitary gland and suppresses GH secretion. Unlike GH, IGF-1 has a long half-life in plasma; thus, plasma IGF-1 levels are generally more helpful than GH levels in the diagnosis of GH abnormalities.

4. **What are the clinical features of excessive production of GH in children?**
   In children who have not yet undergone puberty and whose long bones still respond to GH, excessive GH causes accelerated linear growth. The result is gigantism.

5. **Describe the clinical features of excessive production of GH in adults.**
   In adults, excessive GH causes acromegaly. Acromegaly is rare, with an incidence of approximately five cases per million people per year, and often progresses gradually and insidiously. The pathologic and metabolic effects of acromegaly are summarized in Table 26.1.

6. **What is the single best clue in examining a patient suspected of having acromegaly?**
   An old driver's license picture or other old photographs provide the best clues. Patients with acromegaly are often unaware of the gradual disfigurement caused by the disease or attribute it to aging. Comparing serial photographs can help establish the diagnosis and date its onset.

7. **What is the cause of death in patients with acromegaly?**
   Acromegaly increases cardiovascular and metabolic risk factors, including hypertension, glucose intolerance, cardiomyopathy, and sleep apnea. The mortality from inadequately treated acromegaly is about double the expected rate in healthy age-matched subjects. Major causes of death include hypertension, cardiovascular disease, heart failure, and diabetes. Improved treatment has decreased this risk, but there is still a 30% increased risk of mortality in patients with acromegaly.

8. **The husband of a patient with acromegaly complains that he cannot sleep because his wife snores. Is this relevant?**
   Sleep apnea occurs in 50% to 70% of patients with acromegaly. It can result from soft tissue overgrowth of the upper airway or to altered central respiratory control. Sleep apnea may contribute to morbidity and mortality in acromegaly by producing hypoxia and pulmonary hypertension.

9. **If you suspect that a patient may have acromegaly, what test should you order?**
   The single best screening test for acromegaly is the plasma level of IGF-1. Unlike GH levels, which are pulsatile and higher at night, samples can be drawn any time of day. In adults, acromegaly is essentially the only condition that causes elevated IGF-1 levels. In children, IGF-1 levels are more difficult to interpret because growing children normally have high levels. IGF-1 levels may be less accurate in mild acromegaly, malnutrition, or hepatic or renal disease.

Table 26.1. Clinical Effects of Acromegaly.

CLINICAL EFFECT	CAUSE
Coarse features	Periosteal formation of new bone
Enlarged hands and feet	Soft tissue hypertrophy
Excess sweating	Hypertrophy of sweat glands
Deepened voice	Hypertrophy of larynx
Skin tags	Hypertrophy of skin
Upper airway obstruction and sleep apnea	Hypertrophy of tongue and upper airway
Osteoarthritis	Hypertrophy of joint cartilage and osseous overgrowth
Carpal tunnel syndrome	Hypertrophy of joint cartilage and osseous overgrowth
Hypertension, congestive heart failure	Cardiac hypertrophy
Hypogonadism	Multifactorial
Diabetes mellitus, glucose intolerance	Insulin antagonism, other factors
Colonic polyps	Colonic hypertrophy

10. The patient's IGF-1 level is not elevated, but you still think that she may have acromegaly. What other test should you order?
    The gold standard test to rule out acromegaly is the measurement of serum GH levels in the fasting state and after glucose suppression. Healthy subjects suppress GH levels to < 1 mcg/L 2 hours after an oral glucose load (75 g), whereas patients with acromegaly show insufficient suppression in GH levels. This test may be unreliable in patients with diabetes mellitus, hepatic or renal disease, obesity, pregnancy, or in patients receiving estrogen therapy.

11. After the biochemical diagnosis of acromegaly or gigantism is made, what is the next step?
    Excessive secretion of GH is almost always caused by a benign pituitary tumor. Therefore, the next step is to obtain a radiologic study of the pituitary gland. The optimal study is magnetic resonance imaging (MRI) with special cuts through the pituitary gland. MRI can help assess tumor size, location, and invasiveness, which are all important for the pituitary surgeon.

12. What causes GH-secreting pituitary tumors?
    GH-secreting pituitary tumors are monoclonal, indicating that a spontaneous somatic mutation is a key event in neoplastic transformation of somatotrophs. Further studies have clarified the nature of the mutation in some GH tumors that appear to have an altered stimulatory subunit (G_S) of the G-proteins that regulate adenylate cyclase activity. In a mutated cell, alterations in the G_S subunit cause autonomous adenylate cyclase activity and elevated secretion of GH. However, the mutant G_S is found only in about 40% of patients with acromegaly. The mechanism of GH regulation and tumor growth differs in other patients with acromegaly.

13. Are some GH-producing tumors more aggressive than others, and is there a way to tell?
    GH-producing tumors causing acromegaly are often characterized histologically as being densely granulated or sparsely granulated. Sparsely granulated GH-producing tumors are less well-differentiated tumors, are generally more locally aggressive, respond less well to somatostatin analogues, and have a worse prognosis.

14. Are other endocrine syndromes possible in patients with acromegaly or gigantism?
    Yes. Otherwise acromegaly and gigantism would not be endocrine disorders. Three endocrine syndromes include acromegaly (Table 26.2).

15. Do other tumors besides pituitary tumors make GH and cause acromegaly or gigantism?
    Yes. Rare tumors of the pancreas, lung, ovary, and breast may produce GH.

16. Do tumors ever cause acromegaly or gigantism by making excessive GH-RH?
    Yes. Rare cases of GHRH production by various tumors have been described in the lung, gastrointestinal tract, or adrenal glands. They cause acromegaly by stimulating pituitary secretion of GH. The clinical and biochemical features of acromegaly are indistinguishable from those of acromegaly caused by a pituitary adenoma. Pituitary enlargement also occurs as a result of hyperplasia of somatotrophs. Some patients have had inadvertent trans-sphenoidal surgery (TSS) before the correct diagnosis was made. Therefore the plasma level of GHRH should be

Table 26.2. Endocrine Syndromes Associated with Acromegaly.

SYNDROME	MAJOR INVOLVED ORGANS	CLINICAL FINDINGS	OTHER CLUES
Multiple endocrine neoplasia type 1 (MEN 1)	Pituitary tumors Parathyroid hyperplasia Islet cell tumors	Hypercalcemia (most) Peptic ulcer disease (if gastrinoma) Hypoglycemia (if insulinoma)	Autosomal dominant Check calcium levels in patients with acromegaly
McCune-Albright syndrome	Bones Skin Gonads Others	Polyostotic fibrous dysplasia Café-au-lait spots Sexual precocity	Mostly in girls
Carney's complex	Heart Skin Adrenals Others	Cardiac myomas Pigmented skin lesions	
Pigmented nodular adrenal hyperplasia	Many other tumors		Autosomal dominant

measured in any patient with acromegaly as well as an extrapituitary abnormality or hyperplasia on pituitary pathology.

17. If MRI of the pituitary confirms a tumor in the patient with acromegaly, what issues other than the metabolic effects of excessive GH should be considered?
    1. *Is the tumor making any other pituitary hormones besides GH?* For example, many GH-secreting tumors also produce prolactin; rare tumors also make thyroid-stimulating hormone or other pituitary hormones. In patients with acromegaly, prolactin levels should be measured, as well as other hormones when clinically indicated.
    2. *Is the tumor interfering with the normal function of the pituitary gland?* Specifically, does the patient have impaired thyroid, adrenal, and gonadal function? Does the patient have diabetes insipidus? It is important to diagnose and treat pituitary insufficiency before therapy for the excessive secretion of GH, especially if the patient is scheduled for surgery.
    3. *Is the tumor causing effects owing to its size and location?* Possible effects include headache, visual field disturbances, and extraocular movement abnormalities. Formal visual fields examination should be carried out in patients with large pituitary tumors.

18. How big are GH-secreting pituitary tumors?
    GH-secreting tumors vary considerably in size, but most are > 1 cm in diameter when diagnosed (i.e., macroadenomas), and some can be very large. Tumor size is an important issue because it determines success rates of treatment.

19. How should acromegaly or gigantism be treated?
    Goals of therapy for GH-secreting tumors include reduction of mortality risk, tumor shrinkage, and control of GH hypersecretion. The treatment of choice for GH-secreting tumors is TSS performed by an experienced pituitary surgeon. Most patients with microadenomas are cured, and larger tumors are debulked. In experienced hands, surgical complications are unusual. Significant reduction in GH levels and improvement in symptoms typically follow surgery, even when further treatment is required. Certain patients may benefit from medical therapy before surgery to reduce surgical risks, including patients with congestive heart failure, severe sleep apnea, intubation problems, or other comorbidities of acromegaly. There are no conclusive data that preoperative treatment improves cure rates, however.

20. What are the options for medical therapy of acromegaly?
    Approximately 40% to 60% of GH macroadenomas are not controlled by surgery alone, and adjuvant therapy is indicated. There are three drug classes available for the treatment of acromegaly: somatostatin analogues (octreotide, lanreotide, pasireotide); the GH receptor antagonist pegvisomant; and dopamine agonists (cabergoline, bromocriptine). In patients with significant residual disease after surgery, either a somatostatin analogue or pegvisomant is recommended as the first-line medical therapy. In patients with modest residual disease, an initial trial of a dopamine agonist is appropriate, although the response to cabergoline appears to decrease with time. When patients do not respond adequately to single agents, combination therapy with two or all three of these agents may improve efficacy and reduce side effects.

21. Discuss the mechanism of action of somatostatin analogues.
    Most GH-secreting tumors have somatostatin receptors and respond to exogenous somatostatin with decreases in GH levels. The development of long-acting somatostatin analogues (octreotide long-acting release, lanreotide autogel/depot, and pasireotide) was a major advance in the treatment of acromegaly.

22. How effective are somatostatin analogues?
    Somatostatin analogues markedly decrease GH levels in most patients with acromegaly, with alleviation of many of the symptoms and side effects of acromegaly. Approximately 20% to 35% of patients receiving somatostatin analogues achieve biochemical remission, although additional patients experience symptomatic improvement with partial biochemical responses. Significant tumor shrinkage occurs in approximately 60% of patients. However, these agents do not cure acromegaly; stopping the drug usually leads to increases in GH levels and tumor re-growth. Somatostatin analogues are commonly used indefinitely after surgery has failed to achieve biochemical control of GH hypersecretion. They can also be used before surgery to improve comorbidities, temporarily after surgery while waiting for radiation therapy to take effect (see below), or instead of surgery in carefully selected patients. Common side effects include gastrointestinal symptoms and gallstone formation.

23. Describe the mechanism of action of pegvisomant.
    Pegvisomant is a human GH receptor antagonist that competes with endogenous GH for binding to its receptor and blocks production of IGF-1. This improves the clinical effects and metabolic defects in acromegaly. Pegviso-mant controls IGF-1 levels in about two thirds of patients. It does not appear to affect tumor size in the great majority of patients, but tumor size should be monitored, given the drug's mechanism of action. It is usually used in patients who are resistant to or do not tolerate somatostatin analogues, or in combination with somatostatin analogues to improve biochemical control. The main side effect of pegvisomant is liver function abnormalities, which are usually transient. Note that IGF-1 remains an accurate biomarker for acromegaly control in pegviso-mant-treated patients, but GH levels cannot be monitored because of the persistence of GH hypersecretion.

24. What about radiation therapy for acromegaly?
    Conventional radiation therapy of GH-secreting tumors causes a gradual decline in GH levels over many years, with maximal effect occurring at 10 to 15 years. Therefore, it is generally reserved as a third-line therapy for acromegaly. It may also increase the long-term risk of mortality. Stereotactic radiotherapy consists of applying a highly concentrated high-energy radiation therapy beam to the tumor and may be more effective and work more quickly than conventional radiation therapy for pituitary tumors. However, stereotactic radiotherapy still takes months to years to work. If radiation therapy is deemed necessary in acromegaly, stereotactic radiotherapy is generally preferred unless there is significant residual tumor, or the tumor is too close to the optic chiasm. Many patients eventually develop hypopituitarism from radiation therapy, and there may also be small risks of vision deficits, secondary tumors, cerebrovascular events, or cognitive effects.

25. How can one tell whether a patient has been cured of acromegaly?
    Older studies defined cure as a random GH level < 5 mcg/L. More recent studies have shown that this criterion is inadequate, and more rigorous criteria have been developed as GH assays have become more sensitive. For complete control of GH secretion, patients should have normal age-adjusted IGF-1 levels and random GH levels < 1.0 mcg/L.

26. The patient has undergone TSS for acromegaly and now has normal IGF-1 and GH levels, as well as suppressed levels of GH after oral glucose administration. How should the patient be monitored?
    It appears that the patient is cured, but GH tumors can slowly regrow over years. At the least, measurements of GH and IGF-1 should be repeated every 6 to 12 months. Some physicians measure GH levels after glucose admin-istration as well. Tumor mass should be monitored at intervals with pituitary MRI. The patient also requires an evaluation for colonic neoplasia, as some studies suggest the incidence of premalignant colonic lesions may be increased in acromegaly. In addition, it is important to assess whether the surgery damaged normal pituitary function by evaluating the patient's thyroid, adrenal, gonadal, and posterior pituitary function. The effects of surgery on visual fields should be assessed, especially if the patient had preoperative defects.

27. The patient asks which symptoms and physical abnormalities will improve after cure is confirmed. What is the appropriate answer?
    Most soft tissue changes improve, including coarsening of facial features, increased size of hands and feet, upper airway hypertrophy, carpal tunnel syndrome, osteoarthritis, and excessive sweating. Unfortunately, bony overgrowth of the facial bones does not regress after treatment. Hypertension, cardiovascular disease, and diabetes also improve. However, not all comorbidities resolve with successful treatment of GH hypersecretion; hypertension, cardiac dysfunction, diabetes, hyperlipidemia, osteoarthritis, and sleep apnea may require additional management.

28. For bonus points, name an actor with acromegaly and the movie in which he starred.

André René Roussimoff, popularly known as Andre the Giant, starred as Fezzik in *The Princess Bride*.

KEY POINTS: ACROMEGALY

- Acromegaly leads to gradual soft tissue enlargement and disfigurement over many years, and the patient may be unaware of the changes.
- Acromegaly causes damage to bones, joints, the heart, and other organs, and is associated with considerable morbidity and excess mortality.
- The best screening test for acromegaly is measurement of insulin-like growth factor type 1 level.
- The best initial treatment for acromegaly is usually surgery, performed by an experienced pituitary surgeon.
- There are new medical treatments for acromegaly that are effective in controlling the metabolic effects of excess growth hormone secretion.

BIBLIOGRAPHY

Cuevas-Ramos, D., Carmichael, J. D., Cooper, O., Bonert, V. S., Gertych, A., Mamelak, A. N., & Melmed, S. (2015). A structural and functional acromegaly classification. *Journal of Clinical Endocrinology and Metabolism, 100,* 122–131.

Lim, D. S., & Fleseriu, M. (2017). The role of combination medical therapy in the treatment of acromegaly. *Pituitary, 20,* 136–148.

Katznelson, L., Laws, E. R., Jr., Melmed, S., Molitch, M. E., Murad, M. H., Utz, A., & Wass, J. A. (2014). Acromegaly: an endocrine society clinical practice guideline. *Journal of Clinical Endocrinology and Metabolism, 99,* 3933–3951.

Maffexxoni, F., Formenti, A. M., Mazziotti, G., Frara, S., & Giustina, A. (2016). Current and future medical treatments for patients with acromegaly. *Expert Opinion on Pharmacotherapy, 17,* 1631–1642.

CHAPTER 27

CUSHING'S SYNDROME

Mary H. Samuels

1. Describe the normal function of cortisol in healthy people.
   Cortisol and other glucocorticoids have many effects as physiologic regulators. They increase glucose production, inhibit protein synthesis and increase protein breakdown, stimulate lipolysis, and affect immunologic and inflammatory responses. Glucocorticoids are important for maintenance of blood pressure and form an essential part of the body's response to stress.

2. How are cortisol levels normally regulated?
   Adrenal production of cortisol is stimulated by the pituitary hormone adrenocorticotropin (ACTH). ACTH production is stimulated by the hypothalamic hormones corticotropin-releasing hormone (CRH) and vasopressin (ADH). Cortisol feeds back to the pituitary and hypothalamus to suppress levels of ACTH and CRH. Under nonstress conditions, cortisol is secreted with a pronounced circadian rhythm, with higher levels early in the morning and lower levels late in the evening. Under stressful conditions, secretion of CRH, ACTH, and cortisol increases, and the circadian variation is blunted. Because of the wide variation in cortisol levels over 24 hours and appropriate elevations during stressful conditions, it may be difficult to distinguish normal secretion from abnormal secretion. For this reason, the evaluation of a patient with suspected Cushing's disease is often complex and confusing.

3. What are the clinical symptoms of excessive levels of cortisol?
   Prolonged and inappropriately high levels of cortisol lead to Cushing's syndrome, characterized by:
   - Obesity, especially central (truncal) obesity, with wasting of the extremities, moon facies, supraclavicular fat pads, and "buffalo hump"
   - Thinning of the skin, with facial plethora, easy bruising, and violaceous striae
   - Muscular weakness, especially proximal muscle weakness, and atrophy
   - Hypertension, atherosclerosis, congestive heart failure, and edema
   - Gonadal dysfunction and menstrual irregularities
   - Psychological disturbances (e.g., depression, emotional lability, irritability, sleep disturbances)
   - Osteoporosis and fractures
   - Increased rate of infections and poor wound healing

4. All of my clinic patients look like they have Cushing's syndrome. Are some clinical findings more specific for Cushing's syndrome than others?
   Some manifestations of Cushing's syndrome are common but nonspecific, whereas others are less common but quite specific. The clinical findings are listed in Table 27.1, with the more specific findings listed first, followed by the more common but less specific findings.

5. A patient presents with a history of obesity, hypertension, irregular menses, and depression. Does she have excessive production of cortisol?
   Excessive cortisol is highly unlikely. Although the listed findings are consistent with glucocorticoid excess, they are nonspecific; most patients with such findings do not have Cushing's syndrome (see Table 27.1). True Cushing's syndrome is uncommon, with an incidence of two to three cases per million people per year, although it may be higher in patients with hypertension, diabetes, osteoporosis, or incidental adrenal masses.

6. The patient also complains of excessive hair growth and has increased terminal hair on the chin, along the upper lip, and on the upper back. Is this finding relevant?
   Hirsutism is a common, nonspecific finding in many female patients. However, it is also consistent with Cushing's syndrome. If it is caused by Cushing's syndrome, hirsutism results from excessive production of adrenal androgens under ACTH stimulation. Thus, hirsutism in a patient with Cushing's syndrome is a clue that the disorder is caused by excessive production of ACTH. (The only other condition associated with excessive production of glucocorticoids and androgens is adrenal cancer, which is usually obvious on presentation.)

7. The patient also has increased pigmentation of the areolae, palmar creases, and an old surgical scar. Are these findings relevant?
   Hyperpigmentation is a sign of elevated production of ACTH and related peptides by the pituitary gland. It is uncommon (but possible) in Cushing's syndrome caused by benign pituitary tumors because levels of ACTH do not usually rise high enough to cause hyperpigmentation. It is more common in the ectopic ACTH syndrome because

Table 27.1. Symptoms and Signs of Cushing's Syndrome.

MORE SPECIFIC, LESS COMMON	MORE COMMON, LESS SPECIFIC
Easy bruising, thin skin (in young patient)	Hypertension
Facial plethora	Obesity/Weight gain
Violaceous striae	Abnormal glucose tolerance or diabetes mellitus
Proximal muscle weakness	Depression, irritability
Hypokalemia	Peripheral edema
Osteoporosis (in young patient)	Acne, hirsutism
	Decreased libido, menstrual irregularities

ectopic tumors produce more ACTH and other peptides. The combination of Cushing's syndrome and hyperpigmentation may be an indication of a serious condition.

8. **What is the cause of death in patients with Cushing's syndrome?**
Patients with inadequately treated Cushing's syndrome have a markedly increased mortality rate (two- to fivefold above normal), usually from cardiovascular disease or infections. Hypertension, impaired glucose tolerance, dyslipidemia, and visceral obesity all contribute to the excess risk for cardiovascular mortality. This excess mortality improves with adequate therapy.

9. **What causes Cushing's syndrome?**
Cushing's syndrome is a nonspecific name for any source of excessive glucocorticoids. There are four main causes, which are further detailed in Table 27.2:
1. Exogenous glucocorticoids (ACTH independent)
2. Pituitary Cushing's syndrome (ACTH dependent)
3. Ectopic production of ACTH (ACTH dependent)
4. Adrenal tumors (ACTH independent)

10. **Of the various types of Cushing's syndrome, which is the most common?**
Overall, exogenous Cushing's syndrome is most common. It rarely presents a diagnostic dilemma because the physician usually knows that the patient is receiving glucocorticoids. Of the endogenous causes of Cushing's syndrome, pituitary Cushing's disease accounts for about 70% of cases. Ectopic secretion of ACTH and adrenal tumors causes approximately 15% of cases each (see Table 27.2 for frequencies).

Table 27.2. Causes of Cushing's Syndrome and their Relative Frequency.

ACTH DEPENDENT (80%)	ACTH INDEPENDENT (20%)
Pituitary (85%)	Adrenal tumors
Corticotroph adenoma	Adrenal adenoma
Corticotroph hyperplasia (rare)	Adrenal carcinoma (rare)
Ectopic ACTH syndrome (15%)	Micronodular hyperplasia (rare)
Oat-cell carcinoma (50%)	Macronodular hyperplasia (rare)
Foregut tumors (35%)	Exogenous glucocorticoids (common)
Bronchial carcinoid	Therapeutic (common)
Thymic carcinoid	Factitious (rare)
Medullary thyroid carcinoma	
Other tumors (10%)	
Islet-cell tumors	
Pheochromocytoma	
Ectopic CRH ($<$ 1%)	

ACTH, Adrenocorticotropin; *CRH,* corticotropin-releasing hormone.

11. Do age and gender matter in the differential diagnosis of Cushing's syndrome?

Of patients with Cushing's disease (pituitary tumors), 80% are women, whereas the ectopic ACTH syndrome is more common in men. Therefore, in a male patient with Cushing's syndrome, the risk of an extrapituitary tumor is increased. The age range in Cushing's disease is most frequently 20 to 40 years, whereas ectopic ACTH syndrome has a peak incidence at 40 to 60 years. Therefore, the risk of an extrapituitary tumor is increased in an older patient with Cushing's syndrome. Children with Cushing's syndrome have a higher risk of malignant adrenal tumors.

12. The patient with obesity, hypertension, irregular menses, depression, and hirsutism looks like she may have Cushing's syndrome. What should I do?

There are three widely used screening tests for Cushing's syndrome that have comparable sensitivity and specificity, and each can be used in the initial evaluation of a patient with suspected Cushing's syndrome (Fig. 27.1):

1. *The overnight low-dose dexamethasone suppression test:* The patient takes 1 mg of dexamethasone at 11 PM and her serum cortisol level is measured at 8 AM the next morning. In healthy subjects who are not stressed, dexamethasone (a potent glucocorticoid that does not cross-react with the cortisol assay) suppresses production of CRH, ACTH, and cortisol. In contrast, patients with endogenous Cushing's syndrome should not suppress cortisol production (serum cortisol remains > 1.8 mcg/dL) when given 1 mg of dexamethasone.
2. *Measurement of cortisol in saliva samples collected on two separate evenings between 11 pm and midnight:* Salivary cortisol levels are low in subjects without stress late at night but are high in those with Cushing's syndrome because of loss of the normal diurnal rhythm in cortisol production.
3. *Urine free cortisol (UFC) levels, measured in a 24-hour collection of urine:* UFC is elevated in most patients with Cushing's syndrome, but only a value fourfold above the normal range is diagnostic of Cushing's syndrome because milder elevations can be seen in stress or illness.

13. The patient had a cortisol level drawn after a 1-mg dose of dexamethasone. The level is 7 mcg/dL. Does she have Cushing's syndrome?

Probably not. Acute or chronic illnesses, depression, and alcohol abuse activate the hypothalamic–pituitary–adrenal (HPA) axis because of stress and make the patient resistant to dexamethasone suppression. In fact, because Cushing's syndrome is so rare, a nonsuppressed cortisol level after dexamethasone is more likely to be a false-positive result, rather than truly indicating the presence of Cushing's syndrome. Similar limitations exist for the other two screening tests. Further evaluation is best performed by an endocrinologist and may include performing the alternate screening tests to see if they are concordant, as well as additional biochemical tests (see Fig. 27.1). In some mild or cyclic cases, repeated testing over time is required to definitively diagnose Cushing's syndrome.

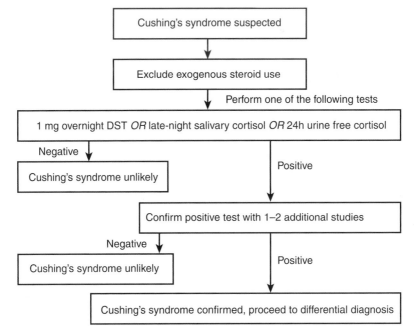

Fig. 27.1 Diagnosis of Cushing's syndrome.

14. Further biochemical testing confirms that the patient has Cushing's syndrome. What should I do next?

After you have made the biochemical diagnosis of Cushing's syndrome, the next step is to determine whether she has ACTH-dependent disease or ACTH-independent disease. This distinction is made by measuring plasma levels of ACTH. Measurements should be repeated a number of times because secretion of ACTH is variable. Dehydroepiandrosterone sulfate (DHEAS) is an adrenal hormone that is secreted from the adrenal cortex solely in response to stimulation by ACTH; it has a much longer half-life than ACTH and, therefore, is a useful surrogate marker of ACTH secretion. Recent studies have indicated that serum DHEAS measurement can provide supportive evidence for ACTH dependence or ACTH independence in patients being evaluated for Cushing's syndrome.

15. The patient's ACTH level is "normal." Was the original suspicion of Cushing's syndrome incorrect?

No. A normal or slightly elevated ACTH level is the usual finding in ACTH-secreting pituitary adenomas. More marked elevations of ACTH levels suggest ectopic secretion of ACTH, although small carcinoid tumors also have normal or mildly elevated levels of ACTH. Suppressed ACTH levels (< 10 pg/mL), in contrast, suggest a cortisol-producing adrenal tumor. If ACTH levels are indeterminate, measurements of ACTH during stimulation with CRH can be helpful. As discussed above, serum DHEAS levels may also be informative in this situation.

16. After the diagnosis of ACTH-dependent Cushing's syndrome, what is the next step?

Because the most common site of excessive secretion of ACTH is a pituitary tumor, radiologic imaging of the pituitary gland is the next step. The best study is high-resolution magnetic resonance imaging (MRI) of the pituitary gland.

17. The pituitary MRI in the patient with ACTH-dependent Cushing's syndrome is normal. Is the next step a search for a carcinoid tumor, under the assumption that the pituitary is not the source of excessive ACTH?

No. At least half of pituitary MRI scans are negative in proven pituitary-dependent Cushing's syndrome because most corticotroph adenomas are tiny and may not be visible on MRI.

18. The pituitary MRI shows a 3-mm hypodense area in the lateral aspect of the pituitary gland. Is it time to call the neurosurgeon?

Again, no. This finding is nonspecific; 10% of healthy adults have pituitary lesions of ≤ 6 mm that are visible on MRI. It is highly likely that the patient has an ACTH-secreting pituitary tumor, but the MRI does not prove this. The MRI is diagnostic only if it shows a larger tumor (> 6 mm).

19. So, what is the next step?

One option is to proceed directly to pituitary surgery because a patient with an abnormal MRI has a 90% chance of having an ACTH-secreting pituitary tumor. To achieve more diagnostic certainty, one has to perform bilateral simultaneous inferior petrosal sinus sampling (IPSS) for ACTH levels. Catheters are advanced through the femoral veins into the inferior petrosal sinuses, which drain the pituitary gland, and blood samples are obtained for ACTH levels. If ACTH levels in the petrosal sinuses are significantly higher than those in peripheral samples, the pituitary gland is the source of excessive ACTH. If there is no gradient between petrosal sinus and peripheral levels of ACTH, the patient probably has a carcinoid tumor somewhere. The accuracy of the test is further increased if ACTH responses to injection of exogenous CRH are measured. Bilateral IPSS should be performed by experienced radiologists at referral centers.

20. IPSS shows no gradient in ACTH levels. What is the next step?

Start the search for a carcinoid tumor. Because the most likely location is the lung, computed tomography (CT) of the lungs should be ordered. If the results are negative, CT of the abdomen should be ordered because carcinoids also occur in the pancreas, intestinal tract, and adrenal glands.

21. IPSS shows a marked central-to-peripheral gradient in ACTH levels. What should be done next?

Transsphenoidal surgery (TSS) should be scheduled with an experienced neurosurgeon who is well versed in examining the pituitary for small adenomas. ACTH levels from the right and left petrosal sinuses obtained during the sampling study may tell the neurosurgeon in which side of the pituitary gland the tumor is likely to be found, but this information is not 100% accurate.

22. What if surgery is unsuccessful?

Approximately 75% of adults with small pituitary tumors causing Cushing's syndrome (termed *Cushing's disease*) achieve remission with TSS. However, initial remission rates are lower for macroadenomas (> 1 cm) and recurrence rates are significant for all tumor sizes (15%–65%). If TSS does not cure a patient with Cushing's disease or if it recurs, repeat TSS may be considered. Additional therapies may also be required because patients with inadequately treated hypercortisolism have increased morbidity and mortality rates. Of the various options after failed surgery, none is ideal. Patients may require repeat pituitary surgery, radiation therapy, medical therapy to block cortisol secretion or action, bilateral adrenalectomy, or a combination of these.

23. What medical treatment options are available for Cushing's syndrome?

There are three main classes of drugs for the medical treatment of Cushing's syndrome: (1) steroidogenesis inhibitors that block cortisol production from the adrenal gland (ketoconazole, metyrapone, mitotane, etomidate), (2) pituitary-directed therapies to lower ACTH secretion (cabergoline, pasireotide), and (3) glucocorticoid receptor–directed therapy to block cortisol effects on other organs (mifepristone). There are pros and cons for each drug, including efficacy, adverse effects, costs, availability, induction of adrenal insufficiency, drug-to-drug interactions, teratogenicity, and difficulties with monitoring and dose titration. These decisions should be made by an experienced endocrinologist.

24. Why not just take out the patient's adrenal glands?

Bilateral adrenalectomy can be safely performed via a laparoscopic approach, with low morbidity in experienced hands. However, this leads to lifelong adrenal insufficiency and dependence on exogenous glucocorticoids and mineralocorticoids. The other main drawback is the development of Nelson's syndrome in approximately 20% of patients after adrenalectomy. Nelson's syndrome is the appearance, sometimes years after adrenalectomy, of an aggressive corticotroph pituitary tumor. Despite these risks, bilateral adrenalectomy is a viable option for patients who have failed initial surgery, with continued monitoring for the emergence of Nelson's syndrome.

25. What are the correct diagnostic and treatment options for patients with ACTH-independent (adrenal) Cushing's syndrome?

Such patients usually have either an adrenal adenoma or carcinoma, so adrenal CT should be ordered. A mass is usually present, and surgery should be planned. Most cases of adrenal Cushing's syndrome are caused by benign unilateral adrenal adenomas, which should be excised by an experienced adrenal surgeon. If the mass is obviously cancer, surgery may still help in debulking the tumor and improving the metabolic consequences of hypercortisolemia. If there are multiple adrenal nodules, the patient may have a rare form of Cushing's syndrome (bilateral macronodular adrenal hyperplasia, primary pigmented nodular adrenal disease, Carney's complex) and should be evaluated by an endocrinologist. As a caveat, there is also a high prevalence of incidental, nonfunctioning adrenal adenomas in the general population (up to 5%) and, therefore, CT findings may not be conclusive.

26. What happens to the HPA axis after a patient undergoes successful removal of an ACTH-secreting pituitary adenoma or a cortisol-secreting adrenal adenoma?

The HPA axis is suppressed, and the patient develops clinical adrenal insufficiency, unless he or she is given gradually decreasing doses of exogenous glucocorticoids until the HPA axis recovers. This usually requires 6 to 12 months postoperatively. Despite the use of glucocorticoids, many patients suffer from glucocorticoid withdrawal symptoms during this period and must be warned that this is common and expected.

27. What would be the most likely diagnosis if the original patient had all the signs of Cushing's syndrome but *low* urinary and serum levels of cortisol?

The most likely scenario is that the patient is surreptitiously or accidentally ingesting a glucocorticoid that gives all the findings of glucocorticoid excess but is not measured in the cortisol assay. The patient and family members should be questioned about possible access to medications, and special assays can measure the various synthetic glucocorticoids.

28. Besides treatment of Cushing's syndrome itself, what common comorbidities should be addressed in these patients?

Diabetes associated with Cushing's syndrome should be treated with the usual lifestyle interventions and diabetes medications; in addition, mifepristone, a glucocorticoid receptor blocker, has been shown to reduce insulin resistance, blood glucose levels, and hemoglobin A_{1c} (HbA_{1c}) values in patients with Cushing's syndrome and is approved by the U.S. Food and Drug Administration for treatment of diabetes in patients with Cushing's syndrome. Bone densitometry testing is advisable to detect osteopenia or osteoporosis; all patients with Cushing's syndrome should be advised on lifestyle measures for osteoporosis prevention (adequate intake of calcium and vitamin D and regular exercise, as tolerated) and strong consideration should be given to the addition of osteoporosis medications if their fracture risk is sufficiently high. Hypertension, hyperlipidemia, and glaucoma should also be addressed as needed.

29. Should prevention of venous thromboembolic events and infectious complications also be a part of the management plan?

Cushing's syndrome is associated with a significantly increased risk of developing venous thromboembolism (VTE) events. The cause appears to be an increase in plasma levels of clotting factors, especially factor VIII and Von Willebrand factor complex and a reduction in plasma fibrinolytic activity. Patients with Cushing's syndrome should be evaluated for their overall VTE risk. Perioperative VTE prophylaxis is recommended in all patients and, if the VTE risk is sufficiently high, chronic prophylaxis may be warranted until the disorder is cured or controlled.

Because of the increased risk of infections resulting from hypercortisolism, it is recommended that clinicians discuss and offer age-appropriate vaccinations, especially those for influenza, pneumococcal pneumonia, and herpes zoster, to these patients. Prophylaxis against *Pneumocystis jiroveci* pneumonia (PJP) has been recommended for patients receiving glucocorticoid therapy at a dose equivalent to 20 mg prednisone for 1 month or more. Although it has not reached the level of a clinical practice recommendation, it is, nonetheless, reasonable to consider PJP prophylaxis in patients with chronic poorly controlled Cushing's syndrome; the antibiotics of choice for this are sulfamethoxazole-trimethoprim, atovaquone, and dapsone.

30. Do tumors ever cause Cushing's syndrome by making excessive CRH?
   Yes. Occasionally patients who undergo TSS for a presumed corticotroph adenoma have corticotroph hyperplasia instead. At least some of these cases are secondary to ectopic production of CRH from a carcinoid tumor in the lung, abdomen, or other location. Therefore, levels of serum CRH should be measured in patients with Cushing's syndrome and corticotroph hyperplasia. If the levels are elevated, a careful search should be performed for possible ectopic sources of CRH.

KEY POINTS: CUSHING'S SYNDROME

- The clinical manifestations of Cushing's syndrome can be subtle or nonspecific.
- Most patients who look like they might have Cushing's syndrome do not.
- Screening biochemical tests for Cushing's syndrome can be misleading, and repeated testing or more extensive confirmatory testing is often necessary.
- Most patients with Cushing's syndrome have a small pituitary tumor producing adrenocorticotropin.
- Patients with pituitary tumors causing Cushing's syndrome should undergo pituitary surgery by an experienced neurosurgeon because none of the other treatment options are ideal.

BIBLIOGRAPHY

Carroll, T. B., & Findling, J. W. (2010). The diagnosis of Cushing's syndrome. *Reviews in Endocrine & Metabolic Disorders, 11,* 147–153.
Creemers, S. G., Hofland, L. J., Lamberts, S. W., & Feelders, R. A. (2015). Cushing's syndrome: an update on current pharmacotherapy and future directions. *Expert Opinion on Pharmacotherapy, 16,* 1829–1844.
Dennedy, M. C., Annamalai, A. K., Prankerd-Smith, O., Freeman, N., Vengopal, K., Graggaber, J., Koulouri O, ... Gurnell, M. (2017). Low DHEAS: a sensitive and specific test for the detection of subclinical hypercortisolism in adrenal incidentalomas. *Journal of Clinical Endocrinology and Metabolism, 102,* 786–792.
Fleseriu, M. (2012). Medical management of persistent and recurrent cushing disease. *Neurosurgery Clinics of North America, 23*(4), 653–668.
Fleseriu, M., Biller, B. M., Findling, J. W., Molitch, M. E., Schteingart, D. E., & Gross, C. (2012). Mifepristone, a glucocorticoid receptor antagonist, produces clinical and metabolic benefits in patients with Cushing's syndrome. *Journal of Clinical Endocrinology and Metabolism, 97,* 2039–2049.
Nieman, L. K., Biller, B. M. K., Findling, J. W., Newell-Price, J., Savage, M. O., Stewart, P. M., & Montori, V. M. (2008). The diagnosis of Cushing's syndrome: an Endocrine Society clinical practice guideline. *Journal of Clinical Endocrinology and Metabolism, 93,* 1526–1540.
Nieman, L. K., Biller, B. M. K., Findling, J. W. Murad, M. H., Newell-Price, J., Savage, M. O., & Tabarin, A. (2015). Treatment of Cushing's Syndrome: an Endocrine Society clinical practice guideline. *Journal of Clinical Endocrinology and Metabolism, 100,* 2807–2831.

CHAPTER 28

GLYCOPROTEIN-SECRETING PITUITARY TUMORS

Majlinda Xhikola, Shon Meek, and Robert C. Smallridge

1. **What are glycoprotein hormones?**
   The glycoprotein hormones include thyroid-stimulating hormone (TSH), luteinizing hormone (LH), follicle-stimulating hormone (FSH), and chorionic gonadotropin (CG), which are composed of two noncovalently bound subunits. The alpha subunit (alpha-SU) is similar among all four hormones. In contrast, the beta subunit (beta-SU) is unique both immunologically and biologically for each hormone.

2. **Name two types of glycoprotein-secreting pituitary tumors and secretory products.**
   1. Gonadotropinomas: LH, FSH, LH-beta, FSH-beta, alpha-SU
   2. Thyrotropinomas (TSH-omas): TSH, alpha-SU

3. **Do pituitary tumors secrete only a single hormone?**
   No. Many tumors make two or more hormones or subunits. At times, sufficient quantities of multiple hormones are secreted to produce clinical symptoms characteristic of several syndromes within the same patient.

4. **Under what circumstances should a TSH-secreting tumor be considered?**
   - Suspected hyperthyroidism
   - Increased serum free thyroxine (T_4) or free triiodothyronine (T_3) with detectable TSH
   - Pituitary tumors

5. **Describe the differential diagnosis for patients with a transient increase in serum T_4 and detectable or elevated TSH.**

EXOGENOUS

- L-Thyroxine (L-T_4) therapy (noncompliant patient who took L-T_4 just before blood was drawn)
- Other drugs (amiodarone, amphetamines, heparin, nonsteroidal antiinflammatory drugs [NSAIDs])

ENDOGENOUS (SUBGROUP OF NONTHYROIDAL ILLNESS)

- Acute psychiatric illness
- Acute liver disease

6. **Describe the differential diagnosis for patients with a permanent increase in serum total T_4 and detectable or elevated level of serum TSH.**

BINDING PROTEIN DISORDERS

- Excessive thyroxine-binding globulin (TBG)
- Abnormal thyroxine-binding prealbumin (TBPA) (transthyretin)
- Familial dysalbuminemic hyperthyroxinemia (FDH)
- T_4 or T_3 antibodies (leading to artefactual high thyroid hormone levels in analogue assays)
- TSH heterophile antibodies to mouse immunoglobulins (requires separate cause for T_4 elevation)

INAPPROPRIATE TSH SECRETION

- Resistance to thyroid hormone (generalized, central)
- TSH-secreting pituitary adenoma

7. **What tests aid in the differential diagnosis in a patient with elevated serum total T_4 and detectable or elevated TSH?**
   The history and physical examination usually rule out medications and nonthyroidal illnesses. The most important laboratory test is the free T_4. A normal free T_4 with an elevated total T_4 strongly suggests one of the binding

protein disorders. An elevated free T_4, in contrast, generally narrows the differential to two disorders: a thyroid hormone resistance syndrome or a TSH-secreting pituitary tumor. Clinical thyrotoxicosis is commonly present in patients with either condition but can also be absent in patients with thyroid hormone resistance syndromes. Abnormal test results should be confirmed in a second laboratory before initiating a workup for these uncommon disorders.

8. How can one distinguish between a patient with hyperthyroidism who has thyroid hormone resistance and one with a pituitary tumor?

Patients with a TSH-secreting pituitary adenoma will usually show biochemical evidence of hyperthyroidism, including an elevated sex hormone–binding globulin (SHBG) level, and will have a high serum alpha-SU level, abnormally high alpha-SU/TSH molar ratio, and lack of TSH response to stimulation by thyrotropin-releasing hormone (TRH) or suppression by T_3. Patients with thyroid hormone resistance have normal SHBG levels, alpha-SU levels, and alpha-SU/TSH molar ratios; their TSH levels respond significantly to stimulation by TRH and suppression by T_3. Dynamic testing for the diagnosis of TSH-secreting pituitary adenomas is limited because of lack of commercial availability of TRH preparations in the United States and the possible cardiovascular risks of T_3 suppression testing (which is contraindicated in the elderly or patients with known cardiovascular disease). Genetic testing for mutations of the thyroid hormone receptor beta-SU is available and is positive in approximately 85% of patients with thyroid hormone resistance syndromes. Genetic testing may be particularly advisable in patients with either a microadenoma or no obvious sellar lesion on magnetic resonance imaging (MRI) (to rule out thyroid hormone resistance). Dynamic MRI, sampling of inferior petrosal sinus blood, or somatostatin receptor scintigraphy (OctreoScan) are also helpful in diagnosing TSH-secreting tumors.

9. Describe how to calculate an alpha-SU/TSH molar ratio.

See Table 28.1.

10. Name the treatment of choice for TSH-secreting tumors.

Transsphenoidal pituitary surgery is the treatment of choice and produces remission in up to 50% of patients. Results are somewhat better if surgery is followed by radiation therapy. Because more microadenomas are being identified, results are improving.

11. How effective is radiation as the sole therapy?

Surgery remains the first-choice treatment for TSH-secreting tumors. When surgery is unsuccessful or contraindicated, somatostatin analogues and radiotherapy are effective in controlling hyperthyroidism and tumor growth in the majority of patients. The effects of radiotherapy on TSH secretion and tumor mass are greater within the first years after treatment, whereas pituitary deficiencies may occur several years later.

12. List the medical therapies used for TSH-secreting tumors.

Somatostatin analogues (octreotide or lanreotide) decrease serum TSH levels in > 90% of cases and normalize free T_4 in 75% of cases; tumor size decreases and vision improves. Dopamine agonists (bromocriptine or cabergoline) have shown limited success in this condition. Dexamethasone reduces TSH secretion, but its side effects exclude long-term use. Antithyroid medications (methimazole or propylthiouracil) and beta-adrenergic receptor antagonists may be used to control hyperthyroidism preoperatively.

13. Summarize the role of thyroid gland ablation in the treatment of TSH-secreting tumors.

Thyroidectomy and iodine-131 (^{131}I) therapy should be avoided. They do not control TSH secretion and may enhance pituitary activity and growth; however, two patients who have been followed up for 8 and 12 years have been reported to have had no tumor growth.

Table 28.1. Alpha-SU/TSH Molar Ratios	
Molar ratio = [alpha-SU (ng/mL)/TSH (mU/)] $\times$ 10	
The following are normal alpha-subunit/TSH molar ratios:	
If TSH is normal:	Molar ratio < 5.7 in normogonadotropic individuals
	Molar ratio < 29.1 in hypergonadotropic individuals
If TSH is elevated:	Molar ratio < 0.7 in normogonadotropic individuals
	Molar ratio < 1.0 in hypergonadotropic individuals
TSH and alpha-SU values are expressed as milliunits per liter (mU/L) and nanograms per milliliter (ng/mL), respectively.	

SU, Subunit; *TSH,* thyroid-stimulating hormone.

14. Do all patients with an enlarged pituitary gland and an elevated level of serum TSH have TSH-secreting tumors?

No. Patients with longstanding hypothyroidism may develop pituitary hyperplasia and a pseudotumor (Fig. 28.1). The mass can extend into the suprasellar region, causing visual field defects. In contrast to TSH-secreting tumors, serum T_4 is always low in this situation. The reported incidence of pituitary hyperplasia in patients with hypothyroidism varies from 25% to 81%; a high incidence (70%) is reported in patients with TSH levels $\geq$ 50 mU/L. Shrinkage of the enlarged gland usually occurs with levothyroxine therapy. Hyperplasia of lactotrophs may also occur, causing elevated prolactin levels. No patient should undergo pituitary gland surgery without preoperative measurement of both serum T_4 and TSH.

15. What clinical features raise suspicion of a TSH-secreting pseudotumor?

Almost all patients have symptoms of hypothyroidism, and the serum T_4 level is always low. The underlying abnormality is usually autoimmune thyroiditis. About 80% of cases of pituitary enlargement with hypothyroidism have occurred in women, whereas only 55% of true TSH tumors occurred in women. Thyroid antibodies are present in > 75% of cases with pseudotumor, compared with $\approx$ 10% of patients with TSH-secreting pituitary tumors that produce hyperthyroidism.

16. Does the presence of abnormal visual fields help distinguish between patients with pituitary hyperplasia caused by primary hypothyroidism and those with TSH-secreting tumors?

No. Abnormal visual fields have been reported in 28% of patients with hypothyroidism-induced pituitary hyperplasia versus 42% with TSH-secreting pituitary tumors. In contrast, patients with thyroid hormone resistance syndromes have normal vision.

17. Does family history provide any clues in distinguishing among these disorders?

In pseudotumor from thyrotroph hyperplasia, the family history may be positive for autoimmune diseases (e.g., Hashimoto's thyroiditis, Graves' disease, type 1 diabetes mellitus, rheumatoid arthritis, lupus erythematosus, Sjögren's syndrome, vitiligo, Addison's disease, pernicious anemia). In TSH-secreting tumors, a family history of these is usually absent. Most cases of generalized thyroid hormone resistance are familial with autosomal dominant inheritance (e.g., 50% of the family have the abnormality).

18. Which hormones are elevated in the serum of patients with gonadotroph adenomas?

Serum FSH is increased much more often than LH. An increase in alpha-SU is not specific for gonadotrophs because it may also derive from thyrotrophs. Furthermore, an alpha-SU/LH (or FSH) molar ratio has not been clinically useful.

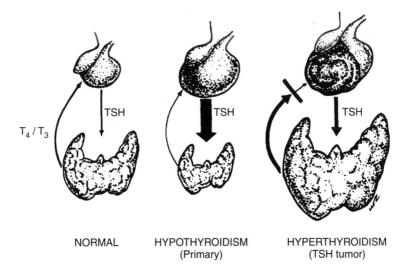

TSH	TSH	TSH
T_4 / T_3		
NORMAL	HYPOTHYROIDISM (Primary)	HYPERTHYROIDISM (TSH tumor)

Fig. 28.1 Pituitary–thyroid axis in normal persons and patients with thyroid-stimulating hormone (TSH)–secreting pituitary tumors. On the left is the appropriate feedback loop in euthyroid persons, with the width of the arrows representing the normal serum concentration of TSH and thyroxine (T_4). The middle figure depicts a small thyroid gland caused by primary hypothyroidism. The low T_4 levels result in markedly increased secretion of TSH and, in some patients, a generalized hyperplasia of the anterior pituitary gland. On the right is an autonomous pituitary tumor secreting TSH. Serum TSH levels may vary greatly but in all cases are sufficiently biologically active to increase levels of T_4 above normal. The elevated T_4 level has little, if any, ability to suppress tumor function.

KEY POINTS: GLYCOPROTEIN-SECRETING PITUITARY TUMORS

- Glycoprotein-secreting pituitary tumors include thyroid-stimulating hormone (TSH)–secreting adenomas and gonadotropinomas (luteinizing hormone– or follicle-stimulating hormone–secreting tumors).
- Hyperthyroid patients with detectable serum TSH levels should always be evaluated for inappropriate TSH secretion (either a TSH-secreting tumor or thyroid hormone resistance).
- TSH tumors are managed by transsphenoidal surgery and possibly a somatostatin analogue.
- Hypothyroidism can produce thyrotroph hyperplasia and pituitary pseudotumors.
- Gonadotropinomas may present with neurologic symptoms as a result of mass effect and require pituitary surgery.

19. List the presenting symptoms of patients with gonadotropinomas.
    See Table 28.2.

20. When gonadotropin levels are elevated, how can one distinguish a gonadotroph adenoma from primary hypogonadism?
    Pituitary gonadotroph adenomas must be considered in the differential diagnosis of women in the reproductive age group presenting with the clinical symptom triad of new-onset oligomenorrhea, bilateral cystic adnexal masses (ovarian hyperstimulation), and elevated estradiol and FSH levels with normal or suppressed levels of LH. This distinction can be challenging in postmenopausal women because they usually have increased levels of LH and FSH. Historically, men with such tumors would have experienced normal puberty and may have fathered children. On examination, testicular size may be normal or increased because of FSH hypersecretion, and testosterone levels may be elevated because of hypersecretion of intact LH. In contrast, men with hypogonadism may have had abnormal pubertal development or a history of testicular injury, and the testes are small.

21. What laboratory tests are helpful?
    In primary hypogonadism, both FSH and LH are increased, whereas in patients with gonadotropinomas FSH is elevated but LH is usually normal. When LH is high in men with gonadotropinomas, testosterone is also high, rather than low, as in hypogonadism. For unclear reasons, about one third of patients with a tumor have an anomalous rise in serum FSH or LH-beta when given a TRH injection. MRI of the pituitary reveals a large tumor. Occasionally, a patient with longstanding hypogonadism may have some degree of pituitary enlargement as a result of gonadotroph hyperplasia.

22. How are gonadotropinomas treated?
    Pituitary surgery is the treatment of choice. Although cure is often impossible, substantial reduction in tumor size and hormone secretion are common. Reduced hormone secretion provides a convenient marker for monitoring tumor recurrence; an abrupt increase in FSH or alpha-SU should prompt repeat imaging. Radiation therapy is often given after surgery to prevent tumor recurrence.

23. Is medical therapy effective?
    Medical therapies have been used in a few cases, but they have not been associated with tumor shrinkage, and their use as a primary therapeutic approach is generally not recommended. Dopamine agonists have reduced FSH levels and improved ovarian hyperstimulation syndrome in a limited number of cases, and it is generally accepted that they are not beneficial in controlling the tumor itself or the clinical syndrome. Somatostatin analogues were used with success in one case of a female patient, and it led to normalization of estradiol and ovarian volumes but not tumor shrinkage. Gonadotropin-releasing hormone (GnRH) agonists have shown limited benefit and also increase the risk of further stimulation of gonadotropin secretion and increase in tumor size. GnRH antagonists (Nal-Glu-GnRH) are used in some cases with inconsistent results.

Table 28.2. Presenting Symptoms of Patients with Gonadotropinomas.

MASS EFFECT (COMMON)	ENDOCRINE EXCESSES (UNCOMMON)
Large tumors with extrasellar growth	Ovarian hyperstimulation
Visual impairment/diplopia	Testicular enlargement
Headaches	Precocious puberty
Apoplexy	
Hypopituitarism	

24. Are pituitary tumors malignant?

Pituitary carcinomas are extremely rare. It is currently unclear whether they develop as de novo carcinomas or pituitary adenomas that gradually gain malignant features. The majority of the cases arise from prolactin and adrenocorticotropic hormone (ACTH)–secreting cells, and, more rarely, growth hormone–, TSH-, or LH/FSH-secreting cells.

25. What causes pituitary tumors?

The key mechanisms involved in the pituitary tumorigenic process are oncogene activation and tumor suppressor gene inactivation. These can occur either independently or in combination. Selected genes that may be involved in the molecular pathogenesis of pituitary adenomas are included in Table 28.3.

Table 28.3. Selected Genes that may be Involved in the Molecular Pathogenesis of Pituitary Adenomas.

	ONCOGENES	TUMOR SUPPRESSOR GENES
Somatotroph adenoma	*CCND1* (Cyclin D1), *CREB*	
Lactotroph adenoma	*FGF4*, *TGFα*	BMP4
Corticotroph adenoma	*CCNE1 (Cyclin E), HDAC2*	*SmarcA4*
Thyrotroph adenoma	Pit-1 factor	(TR)-beta gene
Gonadotroph adenoma	STF1, GATA2	RASSF1A
Nonfunctioning adenoma	*PRKCA, AKT1, AKT2,*	*DKC1, MEG3*, PLAGL1 (ZAC1)

WEBSITE

Thyroid disease manager: http://www.thyroidmanager.org.

BIBLIOGRAPHY

Al-Gahtany, M., Horvath, E., & Kovacs, K. (2003). Pituitary hyperplasia. *Hormones, 2,* 149–158.

Amlashi, F. G., Tritos, N. A. (2016). Thyrotropin-secreting pituitary adenomas: epidemiology, diagnosis and management. *Endocrine, 52*(3), 427–440.

Azzalin, A., Appin, C. L., Schniederjan, M. J., Constantin, T., Ritchie, J. C., Veledar, E., ... Ioachimescu, A. G. (2016). Comprehensive evaluation of thyrotropinomas: single-center 20-year experience. *Pituitary, 19*(2), 183–193.

Beck-Peccoz, P., Lania, A., Beckers, A., Chatterjee, K., & Wemeau, J. L. (2013). European thyroid association guidelines for the diagnosis and treatment of thyrotropin-secreting pituitary tumors. *European Thyroid Journal, 2*(2), 76–82.

Beck-Peccoz, P., Persani, L., & Lania, A. (2019). Thyrotropin-secreting pituitary adenomas. In K. R. Feingold, B. Anawalt, A. Boyce, et al. (Eds.), *Endotext* [Internet]. PMID: 25905212.

Beck-Peccoz, P., Persani, L., Mannavola, D., & Campi, I. (2009). TSH-secreting adenomas. *Best Practice & Research. Clinical Endocrinology & Metabolism, 23,* 597–606.

Brown, R. L., Muzzafar, T., Wollman, R., & Weiss, R. E. (2006). A pituitary carcinoma secreting TSH and prolactin: a non-secreting adenoma gone awry. *European Journal of Endocrinology, 154,* 639–643.

Chaidarun, S. S., & Klibanski, A. (2002). Gonadotropinomas. *Seminars in Reproductive Medicine, 20,* 339–348.

Clarke, M. J., Erickson, D., Castro, M. R., & Atkinson, J. L. (2008). Thyroid-stimulating hormone pituitary adenomas. *Journal of Neurosurgery, 109,* 17–22.

Cooper, O., Geller, J. L., & Melmed, S. (2008). Ovarian hyperstimulation syndrome caused by an FSH-secreting pituitary adenoma. *Nature Clinical Practice Endocrinology & Metabolism, 4*(4), 234–238.

Cote, D. J., Smith, T. R., Sandler, C. N., Gupta, T., Bale, T. A., Bi, W. L., ... Laws, E. R. Jr. (2016). Functional gonadotroph adenomas: case series and report of literature. *Neurosurgery, 79*(6), 823–831.

Dahlqvist, P., Koskinen, L. O., Brännström, T., & Hägg, E. (2010). Testicular enlargement in a patient with a FSH-secreting pituitary adenoma. *Endocrine, 37*(2), 289–293.

Daousi, C., Foy, P. M., & MacFarlane, I. A. (2007). Ablative thyroid treatment for thyrotoxicosis due to thyrotropin-producing pituitary tumours. *Journal of Neurology, Neurosurgery, and Psychiatry, 78,* 93–95.

Davis, J. R., McNeilly, J. R., Norris, A. J., Pope, C., Wilding, M., McDowell, G., ... McNeilly, A. S. (2006). Fetal gonadotroph cell origin of FSH-secreting pituitary adenoma – insight into human pituitary tumour pathogenesis. *Clin Endocrinol (Oxf), 65,* 648–654.

Dong, B. J. (2000). How medications affect thyroid function. *Western Journal of Medicine, 172*(2), 102–106.

Elhadd, T. A., Ghosh, S., Teoh, W. L., Trevethick, K. A., Hanzely, Z., Dunn, L. T, ... Collier, A. (2009). A patient with thyrotropinoma cosecreting growth hormone and follicle-stimulating hormone with low alpha-glycoprotein: a new subentity. *Thyroid, 19*(8), 899–903.

Garmes, H. M., Grassiotto, O. R., Fernandes, Y. B., Queiroz Lde, S., Vassalo, J., de Oliveira, D. M., & Benetti-Pinto, C. L. (2012). A pituitary adenoma secreting follicle-stimulating hormone with ovarian hyperstimulation: treatment using a gonadotropin-releasing hormone antagonist. *Fertility and Sterility, 97,* 231–234.

Karapanou, O., Tzanela, M., Tamouridis, N., & Tsagarakis, S. (2012). Gonadotroph pituitary macroadenoma inducing ovarian hyperstimulation syndrome: successful response to octreotide therapy. *Hormones, 11*, 199–202.

Khawaja, N. M., Taher, B. M., Barham, M. E., Naser, A. A., Hadidy, A. M., Ahmad, A. T., … Ajlouni, K. M. (2006). Pituitary enlargement in patients with primary hypothyroidism. *Endocrine Practice, 12*, 29–34.

Knoepfelmacher, M., Danilovic, D. L., Rosa Nasser, R. H., & Mendonca, B. B. (2006). Effectiveness of treating ovarian hyperstimulation syndrome with cabergoline in two patients with gonadotropin-producing pituitary adenomas. *Fertility and Sterility, 86*(3), 719.e15–18.

Malchiodi, E., Profka, E., Ferrante, E., Sala, E., Verrua, E., Campi, I., … Mantovani, G. (2014). Thyrotropin-secreting pituitary adenomas: outcome of pituitary surgery and irradiation. *Journal of Clinical Endocrinology and Metabolism, 99*(6), 2069–2076.

Mannavola, D., Persani, L., Vannucchi, G., Zanardelli, M., Fugazzola, L., Verga, U., … Beck-Peccoz, P. (2005). Different responses to chronic somatostatin analogues in patients with central hyperthyroidism. *Clinical Endocrinology, 62*, 176–181.

Narumi, S., & Hasegawa, T. (2015). TSH resistance revised. *Endocrine Journal, 62*(5), 393–398.

Nicholas, A., & Tritos, M. D. (2011). Thyrotropin-secreting pituitary adenomas: pitfalls in diagnosis and management. *Neuroendocrine Clinical Center Bulletin, 18*(1), 1–3.

Ntali, G., Capatina, C., Grossman, A., & Karavitaki, N. (2014). Functioning gonadotropin adenomas. *Journal of Clinical Endocrinology and Metabolism, 99*(12), 4423–4433.

Ónnestam, L., Berinder, K., Burman, P., Dahlqvist, P., Engström, B. E., Wahlberg, J., & Nyström, H. F. (2013). National incidence and prevalence of TSH-secreting pituitary adenomas in Sweden. *Journal of Clinical Endocrinology and Metabolism, 98*(2), 626–635.

Refetoff, S., Weiss, R. E., & Usala, S. J. (1993). The syndromes of resistance to thyroid hormone. *Endocrine Reviews, 14*, 348–399.

Rotermund, R., Riedel, N., Burkhardt, T., Matschke, J., Schmidt, N. O., Aberle, J., & Flitsch, J. (2017). Surgical treatment and outcome of TSH-producing pituitary adenomas. *Acta Neurochirurgica, 159*(7), 1219–1226.

Simard, M. F. (2003). Pituitary tumor endocrinopathies and their endocrine evaluation. *Neurosurgery Clinics of North America, 14*, 41–54.

Smallridge, R. C. (2000). Thyrotropin and gonadotropin producing tumors. In S. G. Korenman, & M. E. Molitch, (Ed.), *Atlas of clinical endocrinology: neuroendocrinology and pituitary disease* (pp. 95–113). Philadelphia: Blackwell Science.

Smallridge, R. C. (2001). Thyrotropin-secreting pituitary tumors: clinical presentation, investigation, and management. *Current Opinion in Endocrinology & Diabetes, 8*, 253–258.

Smallridge, R. C., Czervionke, L. F., Fellows, D. W., & Bernet, V. J. (2000). Corticotropin and thyrotropin secreting pituitary microadenomas: detection by dynamic magnetic resonance imaging. *Mayo Clinic Proceedings, 75*, 521–528.

Socin, H. V., Chanson, P., Delemer, B., Tabarin, A., Rohmer, V., Mockel, J., … Beckers, A. (2003). The changing spectrum of TSH-secreting pituitary adenomas: diagnosis and management in 43 patients. *European Journal of Endocrinology, 148*, 433–442.

van Varsseveld, N. C., Bisschop, P. H., Biermasz, N. R., Pereira, A. M., Fliers, E., & Drent, M. L. (2013). A long-term follow-up study of eighteen patients with thyrotrophin-secreting pituitary adenomas. *Clinical Endocrinology, 80*(3), 395–402.

Young, W. F. Jr., Scheithauer, B. W., Kovacs, K. T., Horvath, E., Davis, D. H., & Randall, R. V. (1996). Gonadotroph adenoma of the pituitary gland: a clinicopathologic analysis of 100 cases. *Mayo Clinic Proceedings, 71*, 649–656.

CHAPTER 29

WATER METABOLISM

Leonard R. Sanders

1. **What is the water composition of the human body?**

   Water composition of the body depends on age, sex, muscle mass, body habitus, and fat content. Various body tissues have the following water percentages: lungs, heart, and kidneys (80%); skeletal muscle and brain (75%); skin and liver (70%); bone (20%); and adipose tissue (10%). Clearly, people with more muscle than fat have more water. Generally, thin people have less fat and more water. By weight, men's bodies are 60% water, and women's bodies are 50% water. Older people have more fat and less muscle. The average man and woman age > 60 years are made up of 50% and 45% water, respectively (Table 29.1). Most discussions of total body water (TBW) consider a man with 60% body water, weight 70 kg, and height 69 inches (175 cm).

2. **Where is water located within the body?**

   TBW comprises water located inside the cells (intracellular fluid [ICF]) and outside the cells (extracellular fluid [ECF]). TBW is 60% of body weight—40% ICF (two thirds) and 20% ECF (one third). Of the ECF, interstitial fluid (ISF) makes up approximately three fourths, and intravascular fluid (IVF) makes up one fourth. IVF is a major component of the total blood volume necessary to maintain effective vascular pressure. ISF makes up 15% of body weight and IVF 5% of body weight. In a 70-kg man, TBW = 42 L; ICF water = 28 L; and ECF water = 14 L. ISF is 10.5 L, and IVF (plasma) is 3.5 L. Tight regulation of the relatively small volume of IVF maintains blood pressure and avoids symptomatic hypovolemia and congestive heart failure. Normal plasma is 93% water and 7% proteins and lipids. The arterial volume is only 15% of IVF. Although arterial volume is small, its integrity is most important for maintaining the effective circulation and preventing abnormalities of water balance (Fig. 29.1).

3. **What is transcellular water (TCW)?**

   TCW is water formed by cellular transport activities and is located in various ducts and spaces throughout the body. This water includes cerebrospinal fluid (CSF) and aqueous humor; secretions in the sweat, salivary, and lacrimal glands; secretions in the pancreas, liver, biliary, gastrointestinal, and respiratory tracts; and peritoneal, pleural, and synovial fluids.

4. **What is the significance of TCW?**

   TCW carries secretions to specific sites for enzymatic and lubricant activity and usually is quite small—1.5% of body weight. In disease states, excess or deficiency of TCW can cause dysfunction. Marked excess of TCW formation—called *third spacing*—may decrease effective circulating volume (ECV), stimulate antidiuretic hormone (ADH) and aldosterone release, increase retention of salt and water, and cause edema and hyponatremia.

5. **What controls the distribution of body water?**

   With few exceptions (e.g., ascending loop of Henle [LOH] and distal nephron), water moves freely across cell membranes, depending on tonicity. Because tonicity depends on impermeable solutes, such as sodium (Na), disorders of water metabolism are reflected by changes in solute concentrations. In addition to changes in water distribution, changes in TBW, blood volume, and ECV affect overall water balance. A thorough understanding of disorders of water metabolism requires a clear understanding of changes in plasma Na (P_{Na}) concentration, plasma osmolality (P_{osm}), and ECV.

KEY POINTS: WATER METABOLISM

- Changes in body water or distribution are usually reflected by changes in plasma sodium concentration (P_{Na}) and may occur in states of low, normal, or high total body sodium. Low P_{Na} reflects high total body water (TBW), and high P_{Na} reflects low TBW.
- Water always moves across cell membranes from lower to higher osmolality. This movement is determined by the concentration of effective osmotic solute in the intracellular or extracellular fluid and is responsible for the neurologic symptoms and signs associated with changes in P_{Na}.
- Hyponatremia may occur with low, normal, or high osmolality, whereas hypernatremia is always associated with hyperosmolality.
- The water content of the body is a balance of input and output.
- Water balance is controlled by thirst, access to water, solute intake, antidiuretic hormone (ADH), cortisol, aldosterone, natriuretic peptides, baroreceptor sensors, ADH receptors, renal water channels (called *aquaporins*), level of kidney function, and drugs.

Table 29.1. Water as a Percent of Body Weight.			
Body Habitus	**Percentage Body Weight**		
	INFANT	**MAN**	**WOMAN**
Thin	80	65	55
Medium	70	60	50
Obese	65	55	45

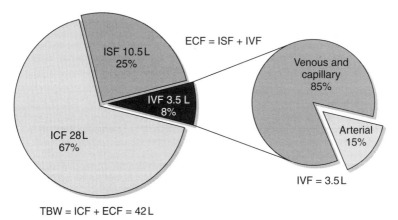

TBW = ICF + ECF = 42 L

Fig. 29.1 *Left,* Distribution of body water; *right,* total blood volume. *ECF,* Extracellular fluid; *ICF,* intracellular fluid; *ISF,* interstitial fluid; *IVF,* intravascular fluid; *TBW,* total body water.

6. What is ECV?
ECV is the arterial volume required to maintain normal baroreceptor pressure that is appropriate for a given level of vascular resistance. ECV is also called *effective arterial blood volume* (EABV). By inducing changes in baroreceptor tone, alterations in ECV have a significant impact on water balance. Low ECV causes renal salt and water retention, whereas high ECV causes renal salt and water loss. Depending on the patient's water intake, these changes may produce significant hyponatremia. Maintaining normal ECV preserves circulatory homeostasis.

7. How do baroreceptors affect ECV?
Baroreceptors are the major sensors of changes in ECV (Fig. 29.2). However, their main role is to maintain normal pressure (not volume) at the level of the baroreceptor sensors located primarily in the carotid sinus, aortic arch, atria, pulmonary veins, and afferent renal arterioles. These anatomic locations are important because perfusion to these areas affects the three main effectors of circulatory homeostasis and ECV—brain, heart, and kidneys.

8. How does vascular pressure, as sensed by the baroreceptors, relate to ECV and hyponatremia?
Baroreceptors maintain tonic inhibition of vasoconstrictor nerves and natriuretic hormone release but tonic stimulation of cardiac vagal nerves. A drop in ECV decreases effective vascular pressure (EVP), baroreceptor tone, tonic inhibition, and tonic stimulation, resulting in vasoconstriction; increased heart rate; increased secretion of renin, aldosterone, angiotensin II, and ADH; and decreased secretion of atrial natriuretic peptide (ANP), brain natriuretic peptide (BNP), and urodilatin. These changes enhance renal Na and water retention. Therefore, decreased ECV/EVP predisposes to water retention and hyponatremia. The venous system, through atrial stretch receptors, has similar effects and responds to changes in ECV earlier compared with the arterial system.

9. How does osmolality differ from tonicity, and what are their effects on water movement?
Osmolality is the concentration of osmotically active particles of a substance in solution. Tonicity is effective osmolality—the concentration of osmotically active particles restricted to one side of the cell membrane that generates the osmotic pressure responsible for water movement between the ECF and ICF compartments. Effective osmoles are at least partially restricted to one side of the cell membrane, contribute to both osmolality and tonicity, may cause a difference in osmolality between the ECF and ICF (tonicity), and promote water flow. Effective osmoles include Na, glucose, mannitol, sorbitol, glycerol, and glycine. Ineffective osmoles freely cross cell membranes, distribute evenly in TBW, contribute equally to osmolality between the ECF and ICF, and do not change tonicity or water flow. Ineffective osmoles include urea, ethanol, and methanol. Water always moves across cell membranes

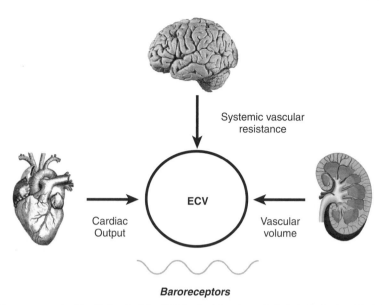

Fig. 29.2 Primary components of the effective circulation (ECV). By stimulating changes in the brain, the heart, and the kidney, baroreceptors have a major impact on vascular pressure and volume and overall water balance. *ECV,* Effective circulating volume.

from lower osmolality to higher osmolality until osmolality on the two sides is equal. At equilibrium, the following is always true:

$$ICF\ osmolality = ECF\ osmolality = P_{osm}$$

10. What formulas are useful in evaluating osmolality and tonicity?

$$ECF\ osmolality = 2P_{Na} + \frac{glucose}{18} + \frac{blood\ urea\ nitrogen\ (BUN)}{2.8}$$

$$Normal\ osmolality = 2(140) + \frac{90}{18} + \frac{14}{2.8} = 280 + 5 + 5 = 290\ mOsm/kg$$

$$ECF\ tonicity\ (effective\ osmolality) = 2P_{Na} + \frac{glucose}{18}$$

$$Normal\ tonicity = 2(140) + \frac{90}{18} = 280 + 5 = 285\ mOsm/kg$$

The normal range for P_{osm} (275–295 mOsm/kg) varies with the normal ranges for P_{Na}, glucose, and urea. The difference between measured osmolality (Osm_m) and calculated osmolality (Osm_c) = the osmolar gap. The normal osmolar gap ($Osm_m - Osm_c$) is < 10 mOsm/Kg. An increased osmolar gap (> 10) indicates that unmeasured osmoles are contributing to osmolarity and, if they are effective osmoles, contributing to tonicity. Correction factors for some effective solutes (osmoles) are mannitol/18, sorbitol/18, and glycerol/9. Correction factors for some ineffective solutes (osmoles) are ethanol/4.6 and methanol/3.2.

11. How does P_{Na} relate to TBW, osmolality, and tonicity?
The following formulas are useful for understanding the relationship of P_{Na}, plasma potassium (P_K), total body sodium and potassium [$Na^+ + K^+$], and TBW. [$Na^+ + K^+$] estimates total body solute:

$$P_{Na} \cong \frac{total\ body\ [Na^+ + K^+]}{TBW}$$

$$TBW \cong \frac{[Na^+ + K^+]}{P_{Na}}$$

$$P_{Na} \cong P_{osm} \cong [total\ body\ osmolality] \cong [total\ body\ solutes] \cong \frac{1}{TBW}$$

Thus, P_{Na} is proportional to $[Na^+ + K^+]$ and inversely proportional to TBW. An increase or decrease in total plasma Na particles can proportionately change the P_{Na}. However, in clinical medicine, changes in P_{Na} usually reflect changes in plasma water. When P_{Na} is high, plasma water is low. When P_{Na} is low, plasma water is high. Low P_{Na} may occur with low, normal, or high osmolality, whereas high P_{Na} is always associated with hyperosmolality.

12. **How does P_K relate to P_{Na} and TBW?**
    Although 98% of K^+ is intracellular, a K^+ infusion increases P_{Na} by the following mechanisms: In hypokalemia, infused K^+ enters cells. To preserve electroneutrality, Na^+ leaves or chloride (Cl^-) enters cells. ECF water follows K^+ and Cl^- into cells because of increased ICF osmolality. Both mechanisms (Na efflux from cells and water movement into cells) increase the P_{Na}. Patients with hypokalemia infused with equal amounts of potassium chloride (KCl) or sodium chloride (NaCl) have equal increases in P_{Na}. Thus, the addition of KCl to isotonic saline makes hypertonic saline, and infusion of saline with KCl may correct hyponatremia too rapidly (see questions 36 and 44).

13. **Describe the input and output of water in an average adult.**
    TBW is a balance of input (including endogenous production) and output. In an average adult, input approximates 1600 mL (liquids), 700 mL (foods), and 200 mL (metabolic oxidation of carbohydrate and fat) for a total of 2500 mL/day. Average water losses are 1500 mL (kidneys), 500 mL (skin [400 mL evaporation and 100 mL perspiration]), 300 mL (lung—respiration), and 200 mL from the gastrointestinal tract (stool) for a total of 2500 mL/day. Large losses of water (increased output) occur with excessive sweating, respiration (exercise), burns, diarrhea, vomiting, and diuresis. Decreased water input occurs when defects in thirst and altered mental or physical function (especially in the elderly) prevent access to water.

14. **What are the normal limits of urine output?**
    Water intake and osmotic products of metabolism determine the usual daily output of urine. When on an average diet, an adult must excrete 800 to 1000 mOsm of solute per day. The normal range of renal concentrating function is 50 to 1200 mOsm/kg. On this basis, the obligate water excretion varies from 0.8 to 20 L/day. The calculations are as follows:

$$1000 \text{ mOsm/day} \div 1200 \text{ mOsm/L} = 0.8 \text{ L/day at maximal concentration}$$

$$1000 \text{ mOsm/day} \div 50 \text{ mOsm/L} = 20 \text{ L/day at maximal dilution}$$

Note that higher solute loads (e.g., dietary) require more water excretion. For example, bodybuilders consuming high-protein and high-carbohydrate diets with 1400 mOsm solute/day require a urine output of (1400/1200) to (1400/50) or 1.2 to 28 L/day. Alternatively, a low solute intake (starvation) with high water intake predisposes to water retention and water intoxication. This combination exists in binge beer drinkers, in whom the solute load may be only 300 mOsm/day. Low solute intake may also occur in starvation and elderly people on a "tea and toast diet." The range of urine output would drop to (300/1200) − (300/50) or 0.25 to 6 L/day in such patients.

15. **What are the main factors controlling water metabolism?**
    The nervous system, baroreceptors, thirst, and hormonal and renal mechanisms are tightly integrated for control of water metabolism (see Fig. 29.2).

16. **What are the stimuli of thirst?**
    Osmoreceptors in the organum vasculosum of the anterior hypothalamus respond to increasing plasma tonicity and stimulate thirst at an osmotic threshold 5 mOsm/kg higher than that needed to stimulate ADH release. Oropharyngeal receptors are also important in thirst regulation. A dry mouth increases thirst, whereas drinking and swallowing water decrease thirst without changing P_{osm}. Volume depletion changes afferent baroreceptor input and increases angiotensin II—both changes increase thirst. An unusual, idiosyncratic effect of angiotensin-converting enzyme (ACE) inhibitors may cause central polydipsia, increase ADH release, and promote hyponatremia.

17. **What hormonal mechanisms are involved in the control of body water?**
    Although natriuretic peptides, aldosterone, angiotensin II, prostaglandins, and neurohumoral changes affect renal water retention and excretion, ADH is most important hormonal influence. ADH is also called *arginine vasopressin* (AVP). Supraoptic and paraventricular nuclei in the hypothalamus secrete ADH in response to increased osmolality and decreased volume. ADH attaches to vasopressin 2 receptors (V2-Rs) on the basolateral membrane of renal collecting tubular cells. This activates cyclic adenosine monophosphate (cAMP) and protein kinase A, causing intracellular water channels called *aquaporins* (AQPs) to insert into the luminal membrane. Water moves down osmotic gradients from the tubular lumen through AQP channels into the cell and the interstitium. At least seven AQP isoforms (AQP1–4,

AQP6–8) are present in the kidney. AQP1 is constitutively expressed in the proximal tubule and descending LOH and is essential for isotonic fluid reabsorption and water conservation. The collecting duct has high concentrations of AQP2 that serve as the primary target for ADH-mediated water reabsorption. Abnormalities of the V2-R cause most cases of nephrogenic diabetes insipidus (DI), but some are caused by abnormalities of AQP2. Increased AQP2 may cause water retention in conditions such as pregnancy and congestive heart failure. Twenty percent of ADH receptors in the collecting tubular cells are vasopressin 1 receptors (V1-Rs). At very high levels only, ADH activates V1-Rs that increase prostaglandin E2 and prostacyclin and oppose the antidiuretic effects of excessive ADH.

18. What physiologic changes affect ADH secretion?

ADH functions to maintain both osmotic and volume homeostasis. ADH secretion starts at an osmotic threshold of 280 mOsm/kg and increases proportionately with further rises in tonicity. Maximum diuresis (urine dilution) occurs at ADH levels of < 0.5 pmol/L, and maximum reabsorption (urine concentration) occurs at ADH levels of 3 to 4 pmol/L. A 1% to 2% increase in plasma osmolality stimulates ADH secretion, whereas an 8% to 10% drop in intravascular volume is required for the same effect. Through action on baroreceptors, increased ECV raises the osmotic threshold for ADH secretion, whereas decreased ECV lowers this threshold. Severe volume depletion and hypotension may completely override the hypoosmotic inhibition of ADH secretion. This finding has been called the "law of circulating volume." In severe volume depletion and hypotension, ADH secretion continues despite low osmolality, thereby worsening the hyponatremia.

19. What clinical conditions cause excess ADH secretion?

Clinical conditions that increase ADH secretion include hyperosmolality, hypovolemia, nausea, pain, stress, human chorionic gonadotropin as in pregnancy (reset osmostat), hypoglycemia, corticotropin-releasing hormone (CRH), central nervous system (CNS) infections, CNS tumors, CNS vascular catastrophes (thrombosis, hemorrhage), and ectopic ADH secretion of malignancy (carcinomas of the lung [primarily small cell], duodenum, pancreas, ureter, bladder, and prostate, and lymphoma). ADH secretion may also be increased by any major pulmonary disorder, including pneumonia, tuberculosis, asthma, atelectasis, cystic fibrosis, positive pressure ventilation, and adult respiratory distress syndrome. Human immunodeficiency virus (HIV) infection may have a multifactorial role by causing CNS dysfunction, pulmonary disease, and malignancy. Nausea, pain, and stress (as seen postoperatively) are potent stimuli of ADH release and may cause life-threatening hyponatremia if hypotonic fluid is given. This is particularly true if patients with these symptoms receive hypotonic fluid with drugs, such as pain relievers that potentiate the release or action of ADH. Excessive exogenous ADH or desmopressin acetate (DDAVP) in patients with DI directly increases ADH effect. Oxytocin also has significant ADH activity in the large dosages used to induce labor. Other drugs that affect ADH secretion and action are listed in Table 29.2.

KEY POINTS: SYNDROMES AND TREATMENT OF WATER DYSFUNCTION

- Clinical syndromes of water dysfunction include syndrome of inappropriate secretion of antidiuretic hormone, diabetes insipidus, and changes in effective circulating volume (ECV) that can cause marked retention of salt and water, pulmonary and peripheral edema, and severe neurologic dysfunction.
- Effective correction of water problems requires correcting abnormalities of plasma sodium (P_{Na}) and a clear understanding of changes in plasma and urine osmolality (U_{osm}), urine sodium (U_{Na}), urine potassium (U_K), and ECV. Additionally, a thorough assessment of patient volume and neurologic symptoms is essential.
- If neurologic symptoms occur rapidly or are severe, correction of P_{Na} toward normal should be rapid; if symptoms are absent, there is no urgency, and P_{Na} correction should occur more slowly.
- Depending on the water disturbance, treatment includes water restriction or administration; hypertonic, isotonic, or hypotonic saline; sodium; diuretics; antidiuretic hormone; and aquaretics or other medications.

20. How does the kidney handle salt and water?

For the kidney to correct for excess or deficient water intake, there must be an adequate glomerular filtration rate (GFR) and delivery of filtrate to the LOH and distal nephron. Solute is separated from water in the ascending limb of the LOH, distal convoluted tubule (DCT), and cortical connecting segment; normal action of ADH then allows controlled reabsorption of water in the cortical and medullary collecting ducts. The proximal convoluted tubule reabsorbs 65%, and the descending limb of the LOH absorbs 25% of filtered solute and water isotonically. The ascending limb is impermeable to water but removes solute, resulting in dilution of the luminal filtrate, concentration of the interstitium (important for ADH action), and delivery of 10% of the filtrate to the cortical collecting ducts with an osmolality of 100 mOsm/kg. In the absence of ADH, this fluid ($\approx$ 18 L/day) would be lost in the urine and cause marked dehydration. In the presence of ADH, the collecting duct becomes permeable to water and reabsorbs all but 1% of the filtrate. Thus, the final urine volume is only 1.5 to 2.0 L/day. Because the normal GFR is 125 mL/min, normal kidneys filter 180 L of plasma each day and reabsorb 99%. In normal adults, 99% of all Na and water filtered is reabsorbed.

Table 29.2. Drugs that Affect Antidiuretic Hormone (ADH) Secretion and Action.[a]

Increase ADH Secretion	**Antidepressants**
	Amitriptyline
	Protriptyline
	Desipramine
	Selective serotonin reuptake inhibitors
	Duloxetine
	Antipsychotics[a]
	Fluphenazine
	Haloperidol
	Thioridazine
	Phenothiazines
	Butyrophenones
	Monoamine oxidase inhibitors
	Other
	Ecstasy
	Nicotine
	Bromocriptine
	Carbamazepine
	Chlorpropamide
	Clofibrate
	Cyclophosphamide
	Ifosfamide
	Morphine
	Nicotine
	Vincristine
	Angiotensin-converting enzyme inhibitors
	Amiodarone
	Methyldopa
Increase ADH Effect	Acetaminophen
	Carbamazepine
	Chlorpropamide
	Cyclophosphamide
	Nonsteroidal antiinflammatory drugs
	Tolbutamide
Decrease ADH Secretion	Ethanol
	Phenytoin
Decrease ADH Effect	Demeclocycline
	Lithium
	Acetohexamide
	Tolazamide
	Glyburide
	Methoxyflurane
	Propoxyphene
	Colchicine
	Amphotericin
	Vinblastine
	Prostaglandin E2
	Prostacyclin

[a]Because psychosis itself may cause the syndrome of inappropriate secretion of ADH (SIADH), one must question the true ADH-stimulatory effect of the antipsychotic drugs. Changes in ADH secretion may be direct or indirect.

21. What are the causes and consequences of decreased renal water excretion?
   Any reduction in water excretion predisposes to hyponatremia and hypoosmolality. Conditions that impair GFR, the delivery of tubular fluid to the distal nephron, or the ability of the distal nephron to separate solute from water, or that increase the permeability of the collecting tubule to water, impair water excretion include renal failure, decreased ECV, diuretics (thiazides and loop), and excessive ADH or ADH action.

22. How do hypothyroidism and adrenal insufficiency cause hyponatremia?

Hypothyroidism and adrenal insufficiency reduce cardiac output and thereby decrease ECV and increase ADH secretion. The hypothyroidism-associated decrease in ECV reduces renal blood flow, glomerular filtration, and maximal solute-free water excretion. Failure to dilute urine maximally results from nonosmotic ADH release and increased ADH-mediated AQP2 receptors and action. The main effect of glucocorticoid deficiency is altered systemic hemodynamics, and not salt and water loss. Low cortisol impairs cardiac output and the systemic vascular responses to catecholamines, reducing both blood pressure and ECV. The resulting drop in absolute and effective vascular filling pressure reduces stretch on the arterial baroreceptors and thereby decreases tonic vagal and glossopharyngeal inhibition of ADH release. These baroreceptor changes override the hypoosmotic inhibition of ADH release, and consequently, ADH secretion increases. The decreased ECV also lowers GFR, thereby reducing delivery of filtrate to the distal nephron and enhancing proximal tubular water reabsorption. Normally, CRH and ADH are cosecreted from the same neurons in the paraventricular nuclei of the hypothalamus, and both hormones work synergistically to release adrenocorticotropic hormone (ACTH) from the anterior pituitary—ADH via the vasopressin V1b receptor. Cortisol feeds back negatively at the hypothalamus and pituitary to inhibit the release of both CRH and ADH. Cortisol deficiency decreases this negative feedback and increases ADH release to enhance water reabsorption. Unlike secondary adrenal insufficiency, mineralocorticoid deficiency associated with primary adrenal insufficiency causes a hyperkalemic nonanion gap metabolic acidosis. This is caused by retention of K^+ and hydrogen (H^+) normally excreted under aldosterone influence. The aldosterone deficiency also causes renal NaCl loss and associated volume (ECF) depletion. The resulting low ECV stimulates ADH release. There is also upregulation of collecting duct AQP2 and AQP3, which enhances ADH action. The combination of increased ADH secretion and augmented ADH responsiveness promotes the development of hyponatremia. A high-sodium diet can compensate for the mineralocorticoid deficiency and improve the hyponatremia. Although hyponatremia may occur with both primary and secondary adrenal insufficiency, it occurs more commonly and is more severe in primary adrenal insufficiency. This fact emphasizes the importance of aldosterone deficiency in renal salt wasting, volume depletion, and ADH secretion. All of these events combined with continued water intake synergistically contribute to hyponatremia.

23. What P_{Na} concentrations are causes for concern?

The seriousness of hyponatremia or hypernatremia depends on the rapidity of development. Acute changes in P_{Na} (within 48 hours) are always of more concern. Normal P_{Na} ranges from 135 to 145 mEq/L. Patients with a P_{Na} value of 115 or 165 mEq/L may not show any clinical features if the problem develops over several days to weeks. However, both conditions may produce major neurologic dysfunction if they develop over hours to days. As a rule, however, Na concentrations of 125 to 155 mEq/L are not usually associated with symptoms. P_{Na} values outside these limits and occasionally rapidly developing disturbances within these limits may be of major concern. With appropriate care, patients have been reported to survive with PNa as low as 85 mEq/L and as high as 274 mEq/L without permanent sequelae. Although elderly individuals with chronic P_{Na} levels of 120 to 125 mEq/L may appear asymptomatic, they may have associated gait disturbances and may be at increased risk for falls and fractures. These complications have also been reported with milder hyponatremia ($P_{Na} < 135$ mEq/L). Thus, treatment of this mild hyponatremia may benefit this group.

24. What causes the symptoms and signs of increased or decreased TBW?

The main symptoms and signs of TBW excess (decreased P_{Na}) or TBW deficiency (increased P_{Na}) result from brain swelling and contraction, respectively. If TBW changes occur more rapidly than the brain can adapt, symptoms and signs occur. The severity of the symptoms and signs depends on the degree and rapidity of the TBW change. After adaptation occurs, correcting the disturbance in body water too rapidly may be more deleterious than the initial disturbance.

25. What are the symptoms and signs of hyponatremia and hypernatremia?

The severity of symptoms and signs of hyponatremia or hypernatremia are proportional to the degree and rapidity of changes in P_{Na}.
- *Hyponatremia:* Headache, confusion, muscle cramps, weakness, lethargy, apathy, agitation, nausea, vomiting, anorexia, altered levels of consciousness, seizures, depressed deep tendon reflexes, hypothermia, Cheyne-Stokes respiration, respiratory depression, coma, and death.
- *Hypernatremia:* Weakness, irritability, lethargy, confusion, somnolence, muscle twitching, seizures, respiratory depression, paralysis, and death.

26. How does the brain adapt to hyponatremia?

Because ICF and ECF osmolalities must always be equal, developing hyponatremia and decreased P_{osm} immediately shift water into the brain, raising intracranial pressure (ICP). Increased ICP causes loss of ICF NaCl into CSF. Over the next several hours, there is also loss of intracellular K^+ and, over the next few days, loss of organic solute. These changes lower ICF osmolality and return the brain volume toward normal. However, if severe hyponatremia occurs too rapidly, there is not enough time for cerebral adaptation. Brain edema occurs, further increasing ICP; the brain may herniate, and the patient may die.

27. How does the brain adapt to hypernatremia?

With acute hypernatremia and increased P_{osm}, water immediately shifts out of the brain and decreases ICP. Decreased ICP promotes movement of CSF with NaCl into the brain ICF, partially correcting the volume loss. Within hours, further brain adaptation occurs, increasing brain ICF K^+, Na^+, and Cl^-. The resulting increase in osmolality pulls water from the ECF and restores about 60% of the brain volume. Over the next several days, the brain accumulates organic solutes (osmolytes), previously called *idiogenic osmoles*, which return the brain volume to a near-normal level. These solutes include glutamine, taurine, glutamate, myoinositol, and phosphocreatine. If the brain has no time to adapt to rapidly developing hypernatremia, it shrinks, retracts from the dura, and tears vessels, causing intracranial hemorrhage, increased ICP, compressive injury, herniation, and death.

28. How should you approach the patient with hyponatremia?

Hyponatremia occurs in 1% of outpatients, > 4% to 15% of hospitalized patients, 18% of elderly nursing home residents, and nearly 30% of intensive care unit (ICU) patients. For hyponatremia evaluation, first clinically assess the patient's volume status—whether hypovolemic, euvolemic, or hypervolemic. Begin with a history and physical examination. Inquire about diuretics, other medications (see Table 29.2), cathartics, diarrhea, excessive urination, nausea, vomiting, diabetes, kidney disease, and liver disease. Ask about dizziness or loss of balance. Because total body volume is proportional to total body Na, a thorough assessment of the patient's volume status helps determine ECV and therapy. Patients whose neck veins are flat while they are supine and who have postural changes in blood pressure (BP) and pulse (standing BP decreases by > 20/10 mm Hg and pulse increases by > 20 beats/min) are hypovolemic, and invariably saline (NaCl and water) depleted. Patients with distended neck veins and edema are hypervolemic and have salt and water (saline) excess. Patients with hyponatremia with no postural changes and no edema are clinically euvolemic, but volume may be subclinically increased or decreased. After the history and physical, assess the acuity and severity of symptoms. Hyponatremia ($P_{Na} < 135$ mEq/L) may be classified as mild (> 129 mEq/L), moderate (125–129 mEq/L), and severe (< 125 mEq/L). The treatment depends on symptoms, and if symptoms are severe, the hyponatremia requires immediate treatment before extensive assessment (see question 25). To evaluate the patient further, consider if the hyponatremia is hypertonic, isotonic, or hypotonic by measuring the P_{osm}. Also, measure the U_{osm} and the osmolar gap. If P_{osm} is elevated (hypertonic hyponatremia with $P_{osm} > 295$ mOsm/kg) with a high osmolar gap (> 10 mOsm/kg), ECF is high in osmotically active substances other than sodium, glucose, and urea, such as maltose, glycine, and mannitol. The patient may have a recent history of treatment for increased ICP, recent prostate or uterine surgery, or intravenous immunoglobulin (IVIG) administration. When P_{osm} is normal (isotonic hyponatremia with P_{osm} 280–295 mOsm/kg) with a high osmolar gap, there may be displacement of water in the assay volume by excess lipid (hypertriglyceridemia) or protein (multiple myeloma), causing pseudohyponatremia. With pseudohyponatremia, the measured P_{osm} is normal, and the osmolar gap is increased to > 10 mOsm/kg. Measurement of P_{Na} without dilution with a direct Na-selective electrode gives a true P_{Na} concentration that is normal. Last, when P_{osm} is low (hypotonic hyponatremia with $P_{osm} < 280$ mOsm/kg), the P_{osm} is considered appropriate for the P_{Na}, and the osmolar gap is usually normal. Measuring U_{osm} is helpful in the differential diagnosis. If $U_{osm} < 100$ mOsm/kg consider primary polydipsia, beer potomania, a tea-and-toast diet, or malnutrition (see questions 45 and 48). However, most patients with hypotonic hyponatremia have a $U_{osm} > 100$ mOsm/kg (> 200 mOsm/Kg in advanced chronic kidney disease [CKD]). This is compatible with a diluting defect and an ADH effect (appropriate or not). Here, the initial assessment of volume status is important to correct the underlying disorder, as outlined in Tables 29.3 and 29.4. Measurement of urine sodium is critical to diagnosis and treatment as well. $U_{Na} < 30$ mEq/L suggests decreased ECV and $U_{Na} \geq 30$ mEq/L suggests normal or increased ECV. If patients have lost saline, give them saline. If they have retained too much water, restrict their water. If they have retained too much salt and water but more water than salt, restrict their salt and water, with water restricted more than salt. It sounds simple. However, sometimes it is difficult to determine the subtle changes in volume status that are key to this assessment (see question 29). Carefully use loop diuretics in patients with hypervolemia and 3% saline in acutely symptomatic patients (see question 47).

29. What is the importance of an initial thorough volume assessment in patients with hyponatremia?

A thorough volume assessment is essential to help determine the underlying cause of hyponatremia (see Table 29.3) and to guide treatment (see Table 29.4). The volume status is best assessed by looking at neck veins, orthostatic vital signs, and edema. At times, even the best clinician cannot make a good evaluation of ECV, but central venous catheterization is rarely necessary. U_{Na} and edema are other valuable ECV clues. Body weight should be measured daily, and orthostatic vital signs should be assessed serially as necessary. Initial laboratory tests should include P_{osm}, general blood chemistry panel (Na, K, Cl, carbon dioxide [CO_2], creatinine [Cr], blood urea nitrogen [BUN], glucose, albumin, calcium [Ca], Mg); U_{Na}, U_{Cl}, U_{Cr}, U_{osm}; and fractional excretion of Na. The presence or absence of edema and the U_{Na} value are most helpful.

30. How should you characterize and diagnose the patient with SIADH?

SIADH, which has also been called *SIAD* or *syndrome of inappropriate antidiuresis*, occurs when there is evidence of continued secretion of ADH in the absence of an appropriate osmotic or volume stimulus. Clinical euvolemia, hypotonic plasma, and less than maximally dilute urine are the clues to SIADH. The patient should be approached

Table 29.3. Causes of Hyponatremia.[a]

PATHOPHYSIOLOGY	ASSOCIATED CONDITIONS
Renal saline loss and decreased ECV urine sodium (U_{Na}) > 30 mEq/L	Diuretics Osmotic diuresis (glucose, urea, mannitol) Primary adrenal insufficiency Renal tubular acidosis ($NaHCO_3$ loss) Salt-losing nephritis Ketonuria Cerebral salt wasting
Nonrenal saline loss and decreased ECV U_{Na} < 30 mEq/L	Vomiting Diarrhea Pancreatitis, rhabdomyolysis, burns Peritonitis, bowel obstruction
Water excess U_{Na} > 30 mEq/L	SIADH Drugs (see Table 24.2) Secondary adrenal insufficiency Hypothyroidism
Sodium (Na) and water excess with decreased ECV U_{Na} < 30 mEq/L	Congestive heart failure Cirrhosis Nephrotic syndrome
Na and water excess with increased ECV U_{Na} > 30 mEq/L	Acute renal failure Chronic renal failure Pregnancy

[a]Hyponatremia always means too much plasma water relative to Na. Thorough volume assessment is crucial. Volume loss (renal or nonrenal) usually means saline (salt > water) loss and is associated with decreased ECV. Volume excess (hypervolemic) usually means saline (water > salt) excess with associated edema and may be associated with decreased or increased ECV. Water excess usually causes mild excess of volume that affects baroreceptor activity. U_{Na} reflects renal perfusion, tubular integrity, and hormonal status. When U_{Na} > 20–30 mEq/L, the kidney contributes to Na loss; and when U_{Na} < 20–30 mEq/L, the kidney is conserving Na. *ECV,* Effective circulating volume; *SIADH,* syndrome of inappropriate antidiuretic hormone.

Table 29.4. Approach to Hyponatremia.[a]

CONDITION	POSTURAL SIGNS	EDEMA	U_{Na} (mEq/L)	TREATMENT
Renal saline loss	Yes	No	> 30	Give isotonic saline
Nonrenal saline loss	Yes	No	< 30	Give isotonic saline
Water excess	No	No	> 30	Restrict water
Sodium (Na) and water excess	No	Yes	< 30	Restrict water > salt
Na and water excess	No	Yes	> 30	Restrict water > salt

[a]Marked hyperlipidemia or hyperproteinemia causes pseudohyponatremia and artifactually lowers the standard measurement for plasma sodium (P_{Na}). Measuring P_{Na} undiluted with direct Na-selective electrodes corrects for the excess lipid and protein, and provides a true P_{Na} reading. However, routine measurement or prior dilution give falsely low results for the P_{Na}. Measuring Posm helps differentiate pseudohyponatremia. Osmometer-measured plasma osmolality (P_{osm}) measures only the osmotic activity of plasma water that excludes lipids and proteins. Measured P_{osm} is normal in pseudohyponatremia, and the osmolar gap is increased to >10 mOsm/kg as a result of artifactually low measured P_{Na}. Use loop diuretics carefully to treat edema and 3% saline for symptomatic acute hyponatremia.

as discussed in question 28. It is important to establish normovolemia by physical examination. Then, P_{osm}, U_{osm}, P_{Na}, U_{Na}, and U_K should be ordered. Finally, pituitary, adrenal, and thyroid dysfunction must be excluded before a diagnosis of SIADH can be made. Confirmatory criteria of SIADH include low P_{Na} (< 135 mEq/L), low P_{osm} (< 280 mOsm/kg), U_{osm} > 100 mOsm/kg, U_{Na} > 40 mEq/L, and $[U_{Na} + U_K] > P_{Na}$. Patients with SIADH are usually said to have normal volume status. However, they, in fact, have excess TBW. Unlike excess saline, which is limited to ECF, excess water distributes two thirds to the ICF and one third to the ECF (see Fig. 29.1). Thus, ECF excess is minor and not usually perceptible by clinical examination. Nonetheless, patients with SIADH have mildly increased ECV, which is sensed by the kidneys. The GFR is increased, causing low serum levels of uric acid (< 4 mg/dL), BUN, and creatinine. The increased ECV also increases secretion of ANP, which, along with the increased GFR, promotes natriuresis. These are the classic findings in SIADH. SIADH does not protect against dehydration and other conditions that can obscure the classic presentation. For example, a patient with ectopic

ADH from lung cancer may present with dehydration from diarrhea, lack of food intake (solute), and lack of water intake from debilitation. In this instance, the U_{Na} and U_{Cl} may be < 20 mEq/L; directly measuring ADH may be helpful in this situation.

31. How do you treat the patient with SIADH?

SIADH should be treated initially with water restriction (500–1000 mL/day). However, the fluid restriction needed to correct the hyponatremia is often not tolerated, especially when $[U_{Na} + U_K]$ is significantly $> P_{Na}$. The combination of a high-sodium (4–8 g/day) diet, high-protein (≥ 2 g/kg/day) diet, a loop diuretic (e.g., furosemide 20 mg twice daily), and water restriction may be more practical. If dietary modification and water restriction are not tolerated or insufficient, oral urea 15 to 60 g/day may help correct the hyponatremia by increasing osmotic excretion of free water and decreasing natriuresis. Demeclocycline and lithium carbonate both act on the collecting tubule to diminish the response to ADH and improve hyponatremia. Demeclocycline and lithium carbonate are both dosed orally at 600 to 1200 mg/day in two to four divided doses. Because lithium carbonate can cause neurologic, cardiovascular, and other toxicities, it should be avoided, unless there are no other therapeutic options. Both drugs may cause nephrotoxicity and demeclocycline may cause severe renal failure in patients with cirrhosis. Thus demeclocycline is contraindicated in patients with cirrhosis and severe liver disease, and lithium should be avoided if the GFR is < 30 mL/min per 1.73 m^2. V2-R antagonists (vaptans) given orally (tolvaptan) or intravenously (conivaptan) have also proven useful for SIADH treatment (see question 42). Although careful monitoring of P_{Na} is important and the expense of these aquaretics may be prohibitive, vaptans may be needed to treat hyponatremia when other interventions fail. Because of the slow response time for change in P_{Na} (days), vaptans are not indicated for the treatment of neurologic symptoms related to acute hyponatremia. They are also contraindicated in severe liver disease and are not indicated for chronic therapy (> 30 days). When possible, it is important to correct the underlying abnormality or contributory causes of the SIADH (see questions 18 and 19). The treatment of markedly symptomatic hyponatremia is discussed in question 40.

32. What are the four patterns of SIADH?

The four patterns of SIADH are distinguished according to responses of ADH to P_{osm}.
- *Type A:* Unregulated and erratic ADH secretion with no predictable response to P_{osm}
- *Type B:* ADH leak with selective loss of ADH suppression and continued secretion when Posm is low but normal suppression and secretion when P_{osm} is normal to high
- *Type C:* Reset osmostat with normal relationship of ADH to Posm but with a lower threshold for ADH release (e.g., 260–275 mOsm/kg or P_{Na} 125–135 mEq/L)
- *Type D:* ADH-dissociated antidiuresis at low P_{osm} with appropriately low or undetectable ADH (possibly from increased renal sensitivity to ADH or unknown ADH-like substance)

33. What are the main causes of polyuria?

Polyuria is a urine output > 3.0 L/day. Four main disorders cause polyuria: (1) central neurogenic DI (defect in ADH secretion), (2) nephrogenic DI (defect in ADH action on the kidney), (3) psychogenic polydipsia (psychosis), and (4) dipsogenic DI (defect in thirst center). All forms of DI may be partial or complete. In general, patients with DI have $U_{osm} < P_{osm}$, and often the U_{osm} is < 100 mOsm/kg. Polyuria also may occur from osmotic diuresis in such conditions as diabetes mellitus (glucose), recovery from renal failure (urea), and intravenous (IV) infusions (saline, mannitol). In the latter cases, the diagnosis is usually clear from the history and U_{osm} is $> P_{osm}$. See Table 29.2 for drugs and conditions that decrease ADH secretion and action. Causes of acquired nephrogenic DI include chronic renal disease, electrolyte abnormalities (hypokalemia, hypomagnesemia, hypercalcemia), drugs (lithium, demeclocycline, cisplatinum), sickle cell disease (damaged medullary interstitium), diet (increased water and decreased solute—beer, starvation), and inflammatory or infiltrative renal diseases (multiple myeloma, amyloidosis, sarcoidosis). DI may also be associated with specific genetic abnormalities. Hereditary central DI is usually autosomal dominant and manifests in childhood rather than at birth. Wolfram's syndrome results from a familial defect on the short arm of chromosome 4 and has associated central DI, and diabetes mellitus, optic atrophy, and deafness (DIDMOAD). Congenital nephrogenic DI results from abnormalities of the V2-R or AQP2 channels; in these conditions, symptoms of polyuria and dehydration appear in the first week of life. Most cases of congenital nephrogenic DI (90%) are related to abnormalities of the V2-R and are X-linked; therefore, they are almost always limited to expression in males. Greater than 150 mutations have been noted to cause DI related to V2-R abnormalities. Nephrogenic DI related to abnormalities of AQP2 (10%) may be autosomal dominant or recessive. When recessive and in a female, the DI is likely caused by a mutation on chromosome 12.

34. How do you distinguish patients with polyuria and the various forms of DI from patients with excessive water drinking?

In excessive water drinking, P_{Na}, BUN, and uric acid are all relatively low. In DI, P_{Na} and uric acid are relatively high, and BUN is relatively low. Central DI often has an abrupt onset resulting from loss of a critical amount of ADH caused by the destruction of $> 80\%$ to 90% of the ADH-secreting hypothalamic neurons at a critical point in time. Patients with central DI also prefer ice-cold water. Often, the cause of polyuria is clear from the history and basic laboratory values. If the diagnosis is in doubt, a water restriction test (WRT) can be performed. Other names for the WRT are *dehydration test* and *water deprivation test*. The test may take 6 to 18 hours, depending on the initial state of hydration. The WRT should not be performed in patients with hypovolemia, hypothyroidism, adrenal insufficiency, uncontrolled diabetes mellitus, or renal insufficiency.

35. How is the WRT performed?
- Office testing is acceptable unless the patient cannot be watched closely, in which case hospitalization may be required.
- Measure baseline weight, P_{osm}, P_{Na}, PBUN, plasma glucose, urine volume, U_{osm}, U_{Na}, and U_K. During the test, measure hourly weight, urine volume, and U_{osm}.
- Allow no food or water.
- Watch the patient closely for signs of dehydration (hypotension, tachycardia) and surreptitious water drinking.
- End the WRT when U_{osm} has not increased by > 30 mOsm/kg for 3 consecutive hours, P_{osm} has reached 295 to 300 mOsm/kg, the patient has lost 3% to 5% of body weight, or hypotension has developed. If weight loss exceeds 3% to 5% of body weight, further dehydration is unsafe.
- At P_{osm} of 295 to 300 mOsm/kg, endogenous ADH levels should be $\geq$ 5 pg/mL, and the kidneys should respond with maximal urinary concentration.
- Repeat all baseline measurements toward and at the end of the WRT.
- Give 5 units of aqueous AVP or 2 mcg of desmopressin (DDAVP) subcutaneously.
- Repeat the baseline tests at 30, 60, and 120 minutes.
- Calculate the U_{osm}/P_{osm} and $[U_{Na} + U_K]/P_{Na}$ ratios as a check on measured U_{osm}/P_{osm}.

36. How do you interpret the results of the WRT?
Table 29.5 summarizes the expected results of the WRT. The WRT stimulates maximal endogenous ADH release by increasing P_{osm} and evaluates the kidneys' concentrating ability by measuring U_{osm}. Giving exogenous ADH allows for evaluation of the renal concentrating response to ADH if dehydration-induced ADH production is impaired. Baseline and end-test plasma samples should be saved and frozen for later ADH measurement if the WRT results are equivocal. Expected normal values for P_{ADH} are < 0.5 pg/mL for P_{osm} < 280 mOsm/kg, and > 5 pg/mL for P_{osm} > 295 mOsm/kg.

37. What are the expected plasma ADH concentrations and urinary osmolality in patients with polyuria after water restriction?
See Table 29.6.

38. How should you evaluate the patient with hypernatremia?
Hypernatremia is uncommon in comparison with hyponatremia, occurring in < 1% of hospitalized patients. Indeed, unless patients have an abnormality of thirst or do not have access to water, they usually maintain near-normal P_{Na} by drinking water in proportion to water loss. However, as many as 5% to 10% of ICU patients may have some degree of hypernatremia. Loss of water is the usual cause of hypernatremia, and almost all patients require water for treatment (Table 29.7). As discussed in questions 28 and 29, the patient's volume status must be assessed carefully. After laboratory results are obtained, the patient should be approached as outlined in Table 29.8. If the patient has polyuria, the approach described in questions 33 and 34 should be included.

Table 29.5. Values Before and After Water Restriction.[a]

	Before Restriction			After Restriction		
	P_{osm}	P_{Na}	U_{osm}/P_{osm}	U_{osm}/P_{osm} + ADH[b]	PADH
Normals	Normal	Normal	> 1	> 1 (< 10%)	↑
Psychogenic polydipsia/ Dipsogenic DI	↓	↓	> 1	> 1 (< 10%)	↑ or NL
Complete central DI	↑	↑↑	< 1	> 1 (> 50%)	—
Partial central DI	↑	↑	> 1	> 1 (10%–50%)	↓
Complete nephrogenic DI	↑	↑	< 1	< 1 (< 10%)	↑↑
Partial nephrogenic DI	↑	↑	> 1	> 1 (< 10%)	↑↑

[a]Recall that when U_{osm} > P_{osm}, there is antidiuresis, and the kidney is retaining free water. The same is true when $[U_{Na} + U_K]$ > P_{Na}, and these measurements are more easily obtainable. When U_{osm} < P_{osm} or $[U_{Na} + U_K]$ < P_{Na}, there is a net loss of free water with little net clinical ADH effect.

[b]The values in parentheses indicate the percentage changes in U_{osm} (not the U_{osm}/P_{osm} ratios) after 5 units of subcutaneous aqueous vasopressin or 2 μg of desmopressin acetate.

↓, Low-to-normal; ↑↑, high; ↑, high-to-normal; —, undetectable; *ADH*, antidiuretic hormone; *DI*, diabetes insipidus; *NL*, normal.

Table 29.6. Expected Values for ADH and U_{osm} after Water Restriction.

CAUSE OF POLYURIA	ADH (pg/mL)	U_{OSM} (mOsm/kg)
Normal	> 2	> 800
Primary polydipsia	< 5	> 500
Complete central DI	Undetectable	< 300
Partial central DI	< 1.5	300–800
Nephrogenic DI	> 5	300–500

ADH, Antidiuretic hormone; *DI,* diabetes insipidus; U_{osm}, urine osmolality.

Table 29.7. Causes of Hypernatremia.[a]

PATHOPHYSIOLOGY	ASSOCIATED CONDITION
Renal water loss > Na loss, U_{Na} > 20 mEq/L	Osmotic diuretics Loop diuretics Renal disease Postobstructive diuresis
Nonrenal water loss > Na loss, U_{Na} < 20 mEq/L	Osmotic diarrhea Vomiting Sweating Diarrhea Burns
Excess Na > water, U_{Na} > 20 mEq/L	Cushing's syndrome Primary hyperaldosteronism Excessive intake of sodium chloride (NaCl) or sodium bicarbonate ($NaHCO_3$) Hypertonic saline and bicarbonate Hypertonic dialysis
Renal water loss, U_{Na} > 20 mEq/L	Central diabetes insipidus Nephrogenic diabetes insipidus
Nonrenal water loss U_{Na} < 20 mEq/L	Increased sensible loss No access to water

[a]Hypernatremia always means too little plasma water relative to sodium (Na). With access to water, hypernatremia usually does not occur or is mild. However, unattended patients who are too old, too young, or too sick may not have adequate access to water, and hypernatremia may be severe. Thorough volume assessment is crucial. Volume loss (hypovolemic) usually means renal or nonrenal saline (water > salt) loss and is usually treated with 0.9% to 0.45% saline to correct the volume deficit, followed by water. Volume excess (hypervolemic) usually means saline (salt > water) excess with high total body Na and is treated with water and restriction of salt. A loop diuretic may also be necessary to treat volume overload. Euvolemic hypernatremia results from water loss and is treated with free water replacement, and vasopressin is used if water loss is caused by diabetes insipidus.

Table 29.8. Approach to Hypernatremia.

CONDITION	POSTURAL SIGNS	EDEMA	U_{Na} (mEq/L)	U_{osm}	TREATMENT
Renal water > Na loss	Yes	No	> 20	↓–	0.9%–0.45% saline
Nonrenal water > Na loss	Yes	No	< 20	↑	0.9%–0.45% saline
Na excess	No	Yes/No	> 20	↑–	Free water/diuretics
Renal water loss	No	No	> 20	↓↑–	Free water
Nonrenal water loss	No	No	< 20	↑	Free water

Free water = 5% dextrose in water infusion or water orally. Infuse saline to restore the volume deficit when patients show signs of severe volume depletion, such as hypotension or postural changes in blood pressure and pulse. This is appropriate when isotonic (0.9%) saline with an osmolality of 308 mOsm/kg is lower than plasma osmolality. This corrects both the volume deficit and the hypernatremia. After the volume deficit has improved, switch to 0.45% saline and eventually 5% dextrose in water. Loop diuretics are used to treat Na excess.
↑, Hypertonic; ↓, hypotonic; –, isosmotic.

39. **How should you diagnose and manage the patient with DI?**

Patients with DI have excessive renal water loss resulting from decreased ADH secretion (central DI) or renal unresponsiveness to ADH (nephrogenic DI). The hallmark of DI is polyuria with hypotonic urine. Mild hypernatremia, low BUN, and relatively high uric acid are suggestive of DI. ADH and oxytocin neurosecretory vesicles are responsible for the normal finding of a high-signal-intensity posterior pituitary lobe that appears as a bright spot on T1-weighted magnetic resonance imaging (MRI). In patients with idiopathic central DI, this normal posterior pituitary bright spot is absent. However, the posterior pituitary bright spot also decreases with age and may be absent in a majority of elderly patients without DI. Abrupt onset of polyuria is also suggestive of central DI. Little ADH is necessary for urinary concentration, and therefore, 80% to 90% of the ADH-secreting neurons would have to be lost before polyuria develops. As described in questions 33 and 34, DI must first be distinguished from primary polydipsia and identified as being central or nephrogenic. Water should then be given to prevent dehydration until further evaluation suggests definitive therapy. Mild cases of DI require no treatment other than adequate fluid intake. A patient with DI will probably self-treat with water unless there is a thirst deficit or there is no access to water. Central DI is treated with DDAVP as a nasal spray or oral tablet. DDAVP is available for oral use (0.1 mg or 0.2 mg tablets) with a starting dose of 0.05 mg once or twice daily and increasing to a maximum of 0.4 mg every 8 hours as necessary. The tablet is 5% absorbed, and absorption is further decreased by as much as 50% with meals. At least one dose should be given at bedtime. Oral DDAVP is preferred if sinusitis develops from use of the nasal preparation. DDAVP nasal spray (100 mcg/mL solution) is given every 12 to 24 hours, as needed, for thirst and polyuria. It may be administered nasally through a metered-dose inhaler (0.1 mL/spray) or through a plastic calibrated tube. The starting dosage is 0.05 to 0.1 mL once or twice daily, and the dosage is titrated up to acceptable urine output. Parenteral DDAVP (4 mcg/mL) may be given intravenously, intramuscularly, or subcutaneously at 1 to 2 mcg every 12 to 24 hours to hospitalized patients. Nephrogenic DI may be partial or incomplete and, therefore, may respond to DDAVP. If possible, the underlying cause should be corrected or ameliorated (see question 33).

A low-sodium and low-protein diet that does not compromise nutritional needs should be recommended. Regular voiding to avoid overdistending the bladder and to prevent bladder dysfunction should be emphasized. Both central DI and nephrogenic DI respond partially to hydrochlorothiazide (25 mg once or twice daily). Amiloride 5 to 10 mg once or twice daily may be used as an adjunct to thiazides and is especially useful for lithium nephrotoxicity. Nephrogenic DI may respond to combination therapy if one agent is ineffective. Combinations may include indomethacin with hydrochlorothiazide, indomethacin with DDAVP, or indomethacin with amiloride. Although oral indomethacin 25 to 50 mg every 8 hours has been effective, other nonsteroidal antiinflammatory drugs (NSAIDs; tolmetin and ibuprofen) may be less effective.

40. **How quickly should you correct states of water excess or deficiency?**

The main concern in therapy for abnormal TBW is prevention of devastating neurologic complications. An understanding of cerebral adaptation to changes in TBW, as outlined in questions 25 and 26, emphasizes the need for urgent therapy only in the symptomatic patient. The three useful rules in treating disturbances of water (measured by changes in P_{Na}) are as follows:

1. Return P_{Na} to normal at a speed relative to that by which it became abnormal. If the change in P_{Na} was slow (days), correct it slowly (days). If the change was rapid (minutes to hours), correct it rapidly (minutes to hours).
2. If there are no symptoms of water or Na imbalance (see question 24), there is no immediate urgency. If there are symptoms, there is urgency. Questions 25 and 26 outline the cerebral adaptations to altered tonicity that may cause devastating changes in brain volume. These adaptations also cause the patient's symptoms. Thus symptoms should drive the clinician to correct the altered tonicity rapidly.
3. The degree of rapid P_{Na} correction should be toward normal (until symptoms abate), not to normal.

These concepts—speed, symptoms, and degree of P_{Na} correction—apply to both hyponatremia and hypernatremia (see question 47).

41. **What is the significance of the $[U_{Na} + U_K]/P_{Na}$ ratio?**

The $[U_{Na} + U_K]/P_{Na}$ ratio allows for calculation of electrolyte-free water excreted per day and is useful in deciding how much water can be consumed without lowering P_{Na}. If the $[U_{Na} + U_K]/P_{Na}$ ratio is > 1, the patient is excreting no free water. Thus, all water given to the patient is being retained, and free water clearance is negative. Any water consumed would lower P_{Na}. If the ratio is < 1, the patient is excreting free water and may consume some free water without decreasing P_{Na}.

For example, if patient A makes 2 L of urine daily and has a U_{Na} value of 20 mEq/L, a UK value of 20 mEq/L, and a P_{Na} value of 135 mEq/L, the patient excretes 1.4 L of electrolyte-free urine. If insensible loss is 800 mL, then patient A could consume 1.4 L + 0.8 L = 2.2 L without a change in the P_{Na}. If patient A had a 1000-mL fluid restriction, the net fluid balance would be 1000 mL − 2200 mL = 1200 mL lost.

However, if patient B makes 2 L of urine and has a U_{Na} value of 130 mEq/L, a U_K value of 60 mEq/L, and a P_{Na} value of 125 mEq/L, patient B makes −1.04 L or retains free water; therefore, there is no free water loss. If patient B has the same insensible loss of 800 mL, patient B will retain 204 mL if no additional fluid were allowed. Given the same 1000-mL fluid restriction, patient B would have 1000 mL + 204 mL = 1204 mL net gain in fluid.

This net free water retention would make the hyponatremia worse. The calculations for free water clearance in patient A and B are as follows:

The formula for free water clearance is:

$$CH_2O = V\left(1 - \frac{[U_{Na} + U_K]}{P_{Na}}\right)$$

Patient A:

$$CH_2O = 2L\left(1 - \frac{[20 + 20]}{135}\right) = 2\,L(1 - 0.30) = 2\,L \times 0.70 = 1.4\,L$$

Patient B:

$$CH_2O = 2L\left(1 - \frac{[130 + 60]}{125}\right) = 2\,L(1 - 1.52) = 2\,L \times (-0.52) = -1.04\,L$$

42. What are vasopressin receptor antagonists, and when would you use them for hyponatremia therapy?
The conventional treatment of hyponatremia—water restriction or saline administration—is still appropriate therapy for most patients with hyponatremia. Conivaptan is a first-in-class vasopressin receptor antagonist (VRA) available for treatment of hospitalized patients with hyponatremia and normal extracellular fluid volume (SIADH). Conivaptan prevents AVP binding to V1a and V2 receptors located within the vasculature and renal tubules, respectively. Blocking the V2-R decreases free water reabsorption and increases excretion. Blocking the V1a receptor not only may cause vasodilatation, reducing afterload in congestive heart failure (CHF), but also may cause negative hemodynamics in cirrhosis. Conivaptan is available in 20-mg/5-mL glass ampules. The recommended dosage is a 20-mg loading dose administered intravenously over 30 minutes followed by 20 mg infused continuously over 24 hours for an additional 2 to 4 days. If the serum sodium fails to rise at the desired rate, the dosage is increased to 40 mg/day by continuous infusion. The infusion should not exceed 4 days in duration. Tolvaptan is a pure V2-R antagonist available in 15-mg and 30-mg tablets for once-daily oral dosing. The dose can be increased by 15 to 30 mg daily to a maximum dose of 60 mg daily. Like conivaptan, tolvaptan produces selective water diuresis, with no effect on Na and K excretion. The term *aquaretic drugs* (or *aquaretics*) has been coined for these medications to highlight the fact that they have different mechanisms of action from those of the saluretic diuretic furosemide. Blocking the ADH effect on the V2-R may allow rapid correction of hyponatremia to occur; therefore, judicious monitoring of P_{Na} changes is important to prevent excessively rapid correction of P_{Na}. Vaptans are proven to be beneficial in short- and long-term studies in hyponatremic patients with SIADH, cirrhosis, and CHF. However, these drugs are contraindicated for use in chronic liver disease, and the U.S. Food and Drug Administration (FDA) has issued a general warning against the use of tolvaptan for longer than 30 days. Additionally, the 30-day cost of tolvaptan is about $13,000.

43. What is the appropriate P_{Na} correction factor for hyperglycemia?
The standard correction factor is a 1.6-mEq/L decrease in P_{Na} for each 100-mg/dL increase in plasma glucose concentration above 100 mg/dL up to 400 mg/dL. If patients have glucose values > 400 mg/dL, the correction factor is 2.4 mEq/L.

CLINICAL PROBLEMS IN WATER METABOLISM

44. A 75-year-old woman presents with confusion but no focal neurologic signs. She has type 2 diabetes mellitus. Blood pressure is 110/54 mm Hg. Pulse is 96 beats/min. Neck veins are not visualized in the supine position. Plasma glucose = 900 mg/dL, P_{Na} = 135 mEq/L, CO_2 = 20 mEq/L, P_{Cr} = 3.0 mg/dL, BUN = 50 mg/dL, U_{Na} = 40 mEq/L; urine glucose is 4+ and urine ketones 3+. What is her fluid and volume status and treatment?
Glucose remains in the ECF because of insulin deficiency and increases ECF tonicity. Greater tonicity pulls water from ICF to ECF, concentrating ICF and diluting ECF until ICF and ECF osmolalities are equal. The osmotic pressure of 900 mg/dL glucose (900 ÷ 18 = 50 mOsm/kg) is the driving force for water movement from ICF to ECF. Water movement from ICF to ECF dilutes the ECF and decreases P_{Na} (translocation hyponatremia). Each 100-mg/dL rise in plasma glucose above 100 mg/dL decreases P_{Na} by 1.6 mEq/L. In this patient, the predicted decrease in P_{Na} = (900 − 100) ÷ 100 × 1.6 = 13 mEq/L. The predicted P_{Na} would be 140 − 13 = 127 mEq/L. However, a more accurate correction factor for elevated glucose values over 400 mg/dL would be 2.4 mEq/L (see question 43). Thus, the predicted decrease in P_{Na} would be (900 − 100) ÷ 100 × 2.4 = 19 mEq/L. The predicted P_{Na} would be 140 − 19 = 121 mEq/L. But this patient's P_{Na} is 135 mEq/L, suggesting that there has been further water loss from osmotic diuresis and significant dehydration. The effective osmolality is 2(135) + 900 ÷ 18 = 320 mOsm/kg and is compatible with hyperosmolar coma. Because this woman has decreased TBW, decreased blood pressure, and a BUN/Cr ratio that suggests prerenal azotemia, you might expect her to have low U_{Na} and high U_{osm}. However, osmotic diuresis caused by urine glucose, ketones, and urea increases U_{Na} and water, making U_{Na} and U_{osm} less useful markers of dehydration. The flatness of neck veins in the supine position usually results from intravascular

volume depletion. Rapid lowering of her glucose to 100 mg/dL will quickly decrease P_{osm}, shift water to ICF, increase P_{Na} by 13 to 19 mEq/L, and potentially cause cerebral edema and cardiovascular collapse. This patient has the hyperglycemic hyperosmolar state (HHS) with mild ketosis, confusion, volume depletion, and an effective osmolarity of 320 mOsm/Kg. Recommendations include ICU admission and administration of 0.9% saline at 500 to 1000 mL/hr for 2 to 4 hours to replace volume with careful monitoring to avoid volume overload. Then, if glucose does not decrease by 50 to 70 mg/dL per hour with fluid management, an IV bolus (0.1 units/kg body weight) of regular insulin should be added, followed by a continuous infusion of regular insulin at 0.1 units/kg per hour, and adjust IV fluids (usually a switch to 0.45% saline) and insulin to avoid changes in $P_{osm} > 3$ mOsm/kg/hr. Follow the protocol for the treatment of HHS.

45. You admit a 35-year-old patient with schizophrenia because of a change in mental function and excessive urine output. $U_{osm} = 70$ mOsm/kg. $P_{osm} = 280$ mOsm/kg. 24-hour urine output $= 12$ L/day. How much free water is the patient excreting each day?
CH_2O is the amount of solute-free water excreted per day. Osmolar clearance (C_{osm}) is the amount of urine excreted per day that contains all the solute that is isosmotic to plasma. When urine is hypotonic to plasma, the total urine volume consists of two components: one part that is free of solute (CH_2O) and the other that is isosmotic to plasma (C_{osm}). To measure how much of the urine is pure (free) water, calculate the CH_2O. To do so, you need to know the C_{osm} and the urine volume (V). The formula for clearance of any substance (including osmoles) is always the same:

$$C = \frac{UV}{P}$$

where C is the volume of plasma cleared of the substance per unit time, U is the urinary concentration of the substance, P is plasma concentration of the substance, and V is total urinary volume per unit time. The calculations for this patient follow:

$$V = C_{osm} + CH_2O$$

$$CH_2O = V - C_{osm}$$

$$C_{osm} = \frac{U_{osm} V}{P_{osm}}$$

$$C_{osm} = \frac{(70 \text{ mOsm/kg} \times 12 \text{ L/day})}{280 \text{ mOsm/kg}} = 3.0 \text{ L/day}$$

$$CH_2O = V - C_{osm} = 12 \text{ L/day} - 3 \text{ L/day} = 9 \text{L/day}$$

Manipulation of formula (2) offers another means of calculating free water clearance, as follows:

$$CH_2O = V\left(1 - \frac{U_{osm}}{P_{osm}}\right)$$

$$CH_2O = 12 \text{ L/day}\left(1 - \frac{70}{280}\right) = 9 \text{ L/day}$$

Thus, the patient's daily urine output contains 9 L/day of pure (free) water and 3 L/day that is isotonic to plasma. This information does not distinguish primary polydipsia from DI. However, the low P_{osm} (280 mOsm/kg) suggests primary polydipsia.

46. A 45-year-old-man with a 30-pack-year history of smoking presents with cough, dyspnea, fatigue, and a 15-lb weight loss. Chest radiography shows mediastinal adenopathy and right atelectasis with pleural effusion. $P_{osm} = 270$ mOsm/kg. $P_{Na} = 125$ mEq/L. $U_{osm} = 470$ mOsm/kg. $U_{Na} = 130$ mEq/L. $U_K = 60$ mEq/L. Urine volume $= 1$ L/day. How much free water is the patient excreting each day? What is the likely pulmonary lesion?
Urine is hypertonic to plasma if the U_{osm} exceeds P_{osm} or the $U_{[Na + K]}$ exceeds P_{Na}. Urine hypertonic to plasma contains two parts: (1) the volume that would be required to contain all solute and remain isosmotic to plasma is the osmolar clearance (C_{osm}); and (2) the volume of free water that was removed from the isotonic glomerular filtrate to make U_{osm} higher than P_{osm} or $U_{[Na + K]}$ higher than P_{Na} is the negative free water clearance (T^{CH_2O}; see next paragraph). There are two ways to calculate free water clearance: one method uses osmolality, as in question 45; the other uses electrolytes (Na and K). Electrolyte-free water clearance more accurately estimates free water clearance and negative free water clearance, especially when urine contains large numbers of nonelectrolyte osmolytes, such as urea, that increase osmolality unrelated to free water clearance. To calculate electrolyte

free-water clearance, the U_{Na} and U_K concentrations and the P_{Na} are used. Because $U_{[Na + K]}$ is $> P_{Na}$—$(130 + 60)$ > 130—the net urinary excretion of free water is negative, and therefore, free water clearance is negative. Calculations for osmolar and electrolyte-free water clearances in this patient follow:

Calculations for classic osmolar (negative) free water clearance:

$$V = C_{osm} - T^{CH_2O}$$

$$T^{CH_2O} = C_{osm} - V$$

$$C_{osm} = 1 \, L/day \left[\frac{470}{270} \right] = 1.74 \, L/day$$

$$T^{CH_2O} = 1.74 \, L/day - 1 \, L/day = 0.74 \, L/day$$

Manipulation of formula 2 offers another means of calculating negative free water clearance, as follows:

$$T^{CH_2O} = V \left[\frac{U_{osm}}{P_{osm}} - 1 \right]$$

$$T^{CH_2O} = 1 \, L/day \left[\frac{470}{270} - 1 \right] = 0.74 \, L/day$$

Calculations for electrolyte-free water clearance (negative free water clearance) are as follows:

$$T^{CH_2O} = C_{[Na+K]} - V$$

$$C_{[Na+K]} = \left[\frac{U_{[Na+K]}}{P_{Na}} \times V \right]$$

$$C_{[Na+K]} = \left[\frac{190 \, mEq/L}{125 \, mEq/L} \times 1 \, L/day \right] = 1.52 \, L/day$$

$$T^{CH_2O} = 1.52 \, L/day - 1 \, L/day = 0.52 \, L/day$$

Thus, the patient's kidneys add (by water reabsorption) 520 to 740 mL of free water to plasma each day. With a low P_{osm}, it is inappropriate to retain water. This finding suggests SIADH. Volume depletion, adrenal insufficiency, and hypothyroidism must be excluded before making the diagnosis of SIADH. This patient had small cell carcinoma of the lung with ectopic ADH secretion. SIADH develops in 15% of patients with small cell carcinoma of the lung. This tumor is highly associated with smoking and accounts for 15% to 25% of lung cancer. Other lung cancers rarely secrete ADH.

47. A 34-year-old, 60-kg woman presents 12 hours after discharge following cholecystectomy. She has a head-ache, confusion, muscle cramps, weakness, lethargy, agitation, nausea, and vomiting. She had no symptoms at discharge. P_{Na} is 110 mEq/L. What has caused the hyponatremia, and how quickly should you treat it? The patient's hyponatremia was likely caused by drinking too much free water after her surgery, along with ADH release induced by pain and postoperative medications. According to this history, hyponatremia developed acutely (< 48 hours), and the patient presents with severe symptoms of hyponatremia. Risk of cerebral edema is high, and risk of osmotic demyelination syndrome from treatment is low. Therefore, treatment should begin immediately in the emergency department, and then the patient should be transferred to the ICU. In this setting of acute symptomatic hyponatremia, the goal of therapy is to increase P_{Na} rapidly by 4 to 6 mEq/L and then more gradually, once the symptoms have improved, to a P_{Na} of about 130 mEq/L. This is best done by administering 2 to 3 boluses (100 cc each) of 3% saline intravenously over 10 minutes, each bolus followed by 3% saline at 1 to 2 mL/kg/hr until P_{Na} increases to the expected goal. A 1- to 2-mL/kg/hr infusion of 3% saline will usually increase P_{Na} by about 1 to 2 mEq/hr. P_{Na} should be measured every 2 to 4 hours to monitor progress and to guide therapy. To guide replacement of water and electrolyte losses in urine, U_{Na} and U_K measurements should be ordered, as needed, especially if P_{Na} is not changing at the expected rate. In acute hyponatremia, if the patient's symptoms are mild to moderate, a slower rate of correction with fluid restriction and/or 3% saline at 1 to 2 mL/kg/hr until P_{Na} is 130 mEq/L would be reasonable,

followed by fluid restriction with increased oral sodium intake until P_{Na} returns to normal. The calculations for water excess and the amount of 3% saline necessary to correct the P_{Na} to 120 mEq/L in this patient are as follows:

$$\text{Water excess} = \left(\frac{\text{normal } P_{Na} - \text{observed } P_{Na}}{\text{normal } P_{Na}} \right) \times TBW$$

$$= \left(\frac{140-110}{140} \right) \times 0.5 \times 60 \text{ kg}$$

$$= 0.21 \times 30 \text{ L}$$

$$= 6.3 \text{ L excess in TBW}$$

$$\text{Na deficit} = (\text{desired } P_{Na} - \text{observed } P_{Na})$$

$$= (120-110) \times 0.5 \times 60 \text{ kg}$$

$$= 10 \text{ mEq/L} \times 30 \text{ L}$$

$$= 300 \text{ mEq Na}$$

Knowing the Na deficit is useful clinically because Na can be replaced at a controlled rate to improve the hyponatremia. The Na in 3% saline is 513 mEq/L:

$$\frac{300 \text{ mEq Na}}{513 \text{ mEq/L}} = 0.585 \text{ L}$$

Assuming no Na or water would be lost in urine, giving 585 mL of 3% saline will correct this patient's P_{Na} to 120 mEq/L. A similar calculation for 3% saline to infuse to increase P_{Na} by 6 mEq/L is as follows: A 6 mEq/L increase in P_{Na} in a woman with a weight of 60 kg, which is 50% water, would require: 6 mEq/L $\times$ 0.5 $\times$ 60 kg = 180 mEq Na. Because 3% saline has 513 mEq/L sodium, 0.351L (180 mEq Na ÷ 513 mEq/L) or 351 mL of 3% saline would be required to increase the P_{Na} by 6 mEq/L. Thus, three boluses of 100 cc of 3% saline empirically given over 10 minutes each would correct P_{Na} by about 6 mEq/L over the 30 to 40 minutes needed to give the three boluses.

48. An 80-year-old woman who rarely leaves her home is brought to the hospital after being found in a confused state. Three weeks ago, she had seen her physician, who started her on a diuretic for systolic hypertension. On arrival, her P_{Na} is 110 mEq/L. What is the cause of her hyponatremia?
As a consequence of aging, elderly patients lose GFR, concentrating ability, and diluting ability. Thus, an 80-year-old woman may have a normal (for age) renal-concentrating range of 100 to 700 mOsm/kg. However, maximal U_{osm} in the elderly may be as low as 350 mOsm/kg. This woman's average diet may generate only 600 mOsm/day. Her normal range of urine output would then be 0.9 to 6.0 L/day. If her dietary intake fell to 300 mOsm/day, her maximal urine output would fall to 3 L/day, calculated as follows:

$$300 \text{ mOsm/day} \div 100 \text{ mOsm/kg} = 3 \text{ L/day}$$

Given free access to water and a thiazide diuretic, which impairs urinary dilution, she could easily become water intoxicated and hyponatremic. The mechanism of hyponatremia in beer potomania and the "tea-and-toast diet" is low total osmolar intake and relatively increased water intake. The decreased osmotic load for excretion limits the amount of water excreted. This patient's hyponatremia is probably chronic; however, her only symptom is confusion—so she is considered mild to moderately symptomatic. The mild symptoms with severe hyponatremia also suggest chronicity. If the duration is known to be > 48 hours or if the duration of the hyponatremia is not clear in an outpatient setting, it is likely that the symptoms are chronic, and it would be safest to treat for chronic hyponatremia, given the high risk for osmotic demyelination syndrome (ODS). Computed tomography (CT) or MRI would be appropriate modalities to use in this patient in a confused state, and might change therapy if the presence of cerebral edema is revealed. To avoid ODS in this patient and in high-risk individuals, the rate of P_{Na} correction to a goal of 130 mEq/L should be slow and average no more than 4 to 6 mEq/L during the first 24 hours and 8 mEq/L per each additional 24-hour period. For normal-risk individuals, correction rates can be 4 to 8 mEq/L in the first 24 hours and 9 mEq/L in any subsequent 24-hour period. Treatment of this patient should consist of discontinuation of the thiazide diuretic and fluid restriction until symptoms further improve or the P_{Na} is 130 mEq/L. Symptoms, signs, and P_{Na} should be assessed frequently. Remember: elderly women taking thiazide diuretics, those who have alcoholism, malnourished patients, those with hypokalemia, and burn victims are at particular risk for ODS.

⊕ WEBSITES

American Academy of Family Physicians: Diagnosis and management of sodium disorders: hyponatremia and hypernatremia: https://www.aafp.org/afp/2015/0301/p299.html
EMedicine: SIADH review: http://www.emedicine.com/ped/topic2190.htm.
EMedicine: Hyponatremia review: http://www.emedicine.com/med/topic1130.htm.
EMedicine: Lithium nephropathy review: http://www.emedicine.com/med/topic1313.htm.
EMedicine: Diabetes insipidus review: http://www.emedicine.com/med/topic543.htm.

BIBLIOGRAPHY

Adrogue, H. J., & Madias, N. E. (2000). Hypernatremia. *New England Journal of Medicine, 342*, 1493–1499.
Adrogue, H. J., & Madias, N. E. (2000). Hyponatremia. *New England Journal of Medicine, 342*, 1581–1589.
Berl, T. (2015). Vasopressin antagonists. *New England Journal of Medicine, 372*, 2207-2216.
Berl, T., & Schrier, R. W. (2018). Disorders of water metabolism. In R. W. Schrier, (Ed.), *Renal and electrolyte disorders* (8th ed., p. 1). Philadelphia: Wolters Kluwer; 2018.
Braun, M. M., Barstow, C. H., & Pyzocha, N. J. (2015). Diagnosis and management of sodium disorders: hyponatremia and hypernatremia. *American Family Physician, 91*(5), 299–307.
Chawla, A., Sterns, R. H., Nigwekar, S. U., & Cappuccio J. D. (2011). Mortality and serum sodium: do patients die from or with hyponatremia? *Clinical Journal of the American Society of Nephrology, 6*, 960–965.
Ellison, D. H., & Berl, T. (2007). The syndrome of inappropriate antidiuresis. *New England Journal of Medicine, 356*, 2064–2072.
Filippatos, T. D., Makri, A., Elisaf, M. S., & Liamis, G. (2017). Hyponatremia in the elderly: challenges and solutions. *Clinical Interventions in Aging, 12*, 1957–1965.
Hannon, M. J., Finucane, F. M., Sherlock, M., Agha, A., & Thompson, C. J. (2012). Disorders of water homeostasis in neurosurgical patients. *Journal of Clinical Endocrinology and Metabolism, 97*, 1423–1433.
Hoorn, E. J., & Zietse, R. (2017). Diagnosis and treatment of hyponatremia: compilation of the guidelines. *Journal of the American Society of Nephrology, 28*(5), 1340–1349.
Knepper, M. A., Kwon, T. H., & Nielsen, S. (2015). Molecular physiology of water balance. *New England Journal of Medicine, 372*, 1349–1358.
Maesaka, J. K., Imbriano, L. J., & Miyawaki, N. (2017). Application of established pathophysiologic processes brings greater clarity to diagnosis and treatment of hyponatremia. *World Journal of Nephrology, 6*(2), 59–71.
Pasquel, F. J., & Umpierrez, G. E. (2014). Hyperosmolar hyperglycemic state: a historic review of the clinical presentation, diagnosis, and treatment. *Diabetes Care, 37*, 3124–3131.
Piper, G. L., & Lewis, J. K. (2012). Fluid and electrolyte management for the surgical patient. *Surgery Clinics of North America, 92*, 189–205.
Robinson, A. G., & Verbalis, J. G. (2016). Posterior pituitary. In S. Melmed, K. S. Polonsky, P. R. Larsen, & H. M. Kronenberg, (Eds.), *Williams textbook of endocrinology* (13th ed., p. 300). Philadelphia: Elsevier; 2016.
Robinson, A. G. (2018). The posterior pituitary (neurohypophysis). In D. G. Gardner, & D. Shoback (Eds.), *Greenspan's Basic & Clinical Endocrinology* (10th ed., p. 121). New York: McGraw-Hill Education.
Sterns, R. H. (2018). Treatment of severe hyponatremia. *Clinical Journal of the American Society of Nephrology, 13*(4), 641–649.
Verbalis, J. G., Goldsmith, S. R., Greenberg, A., Korzelius, C., Schrier, R. W., Sterns, R. H., . . . Thompson, C. J. (2013). Diagnosis, evaluation, and treatment of hyponatremia: expert panel recommendations. *American Journal of Medicine, 126*, S1–S42.
Verbalis, J. G. (2018). Hyponatremia and hypoosmolar disorders. In S. J. Gilbert, D. E. Weiner, A. S. Bomback, M. A. Perazella, M. & Tonelli, (Eds.), *Primer on Kidney Diseases* (7th ed. p. 68). Philadelphia: Elsevier.
Yee, A. H., Burns, J. D., & Wijdicks, E. F. (2010). Cerebral salt wasting: pathophysiology, diagnosis, and treatment. *Neurosurgery Clinics of North America, 21*, 339–352.
Zeidel, M. L. (2010). Hyponatremia: mechanisms and newer treatments. *Endocrine Practice, 16*, 882–887.

CHAPTER 30

DISORDERS OF GROWTH

Philip Zeitler

1. Summarize normal growth velocity in children until the pubertal growth spurt.
   - First 6 months—16 to 17 cm
   - Second 6 months—approximately 8 cm
   - Second year—just over 10 cm
   - Third year—approximately 8 cm
   - Fourth year—7 cm
   - Later childhood until puberty (5–10 years)—growth averages 5 to 6 cm/year

2. Summarize growth velocity during the pubertal growth spurt.
   Maximum growth rate is 11 to 13 cm/year. In girls, growth spurt occurs early in puberty (breast Tanner stage II). Growth spurt is later in boys (pubic hair Tanner stage III-IV, testicular volume 12–15 mL). Some children may experience a transient period of slow growth just before the onset of puberty (prepubertal slowing).

3. How is height measured accurately?
   - The most essential tool for the detection of growth abnormalities is the ability to obtain accurate and reproducible measurements. This requires the availability of appropriate equipment as well as proper positioning of the patient.
   - At all ages, children should be measured at full stretch with a straight spine because this is the only position that will be reproducible.
   - Children should be shoeless, and hair decorations or braids need to be removed if they interfere with positioning of the stadiometer.
   - Scales with floppy arms are unreliable.

4. What technique is used in infants up to age 2 years?
   Supine length should be measured in infants and children up to age 2 years. Accurate measurement requires a supine stadiometer, a box-like structure with a headboard and movable footplate. Two people are needed, with one holding the infant's head against the headboard, while the other straightens the legs and places the ankles at 90 degrees against the movable footplate. The length is read from the attached measuring device, or marks are made for measurement by tape measure.

5. Describe the technique for children age ≥ 2 years.
   1. Standing height is measured. Accurate measurement requires a stadiometer with a rigid headboard, footplate, and backboard.
   2. The child stands against the backboard, with heels, buttocks, thoracic spine, and head touching.
   3. The measurer exerts upward pressure on the patient at the angle of the jaw to bring the spine into full stretch, and the headboard is lowered until it touches the top of the head. A counter reads the measurement.
   4. If a stadiometer is not available, the child should stand against a wall in the same position as used for a stadiometer. A rigid right angle is moved downward to touch the top of the head, and a mark is made and measured.
   5. Weight and head circumference (when appropriate) should be recorded.

6. How is height recorded?
   The second critical tool for evaluation of growth is the standardized growth curve, and all measurements should be plotted rather than just recorded in the chart. A carefully constructed and up-to-date growth curve is critical to the recognition of growth abnormalities. Furthermore, the more the points that are plotted on the curve, the greater is the understanding of the child's growth. Thus, efforts should be made to obtain growth measurements at all patient contacts, including illness visits, because well-child visits are infrequent during the middle childhood years when growth abnormalities are most common.

7. List the common errors in plotting growth charts.
   Errors in plotting of growth points are a frequent cause of apparent growth abnormalities. Common errors include:
   - Plotting the wrong height (e.g., plotting inches instead of centimeters)
   - Not plotting the patient's height at the exact chronologic age (height should be plotted to the nearest month or decimal age)
   - Use of an inappropriate growth chart

8. What is meant by "appropriate growth chart"?

A number of growth charts are available, and careful consideration should be given to the appropriate chart for a particular patient at a particular time. Commonly available growth charts include:
- Charts for plotting supine length (the 0–36-month charts in common use)
- Charts for plotting stature (i.e., standing height; 2–18-year charts)

Other specific growth charts are available and should be used, when appropriate. These include:
- Ethnicity-specific charts
- Growth charts specific for common syndromes (e.g., Turner's syndrome, Down's syndrome, achondroplasia) should be used, when appropriate

9. How do age and position affect growth measurements?
- A patient measured in the supine position is slightly longer than the same patient measured in the standing position.
- Charting of a standing patient on a supine chart gives the erroneous impression of decreased growth velocity. This is a common cause of apparent growth abnormality in children ages 2 to 3 years when measured standing up for the first time but whose measurements continue to be plotted on the supine chart.

10. What historic information is necessary for interpreting a growth chart?
- Birth history and birth weight
- Attainment of developmental milestones
- History of chronic illnesses
- Medication exposure
- History of surgery or trauma
- Current symptoms, if any
- Height of biologic parents and family history of significant short stature
- Timing of parental puberty and family history of significant pubertal delay

11. What physical examination findings help interpret a growth chart?
- Signs of chronic illness
- Stigmata of a syndrome
- Specific signs of hormonal abnormality (thyroid deficiency, growth hormone [GH] deficiency, glucocorticoid excess)

12. How does radiologic imaging help interpret growth chart measurements?

A bone-age film can provide important information about skeletal maturity. The degree of skeletal maturity is an important determinant of remaining growth potential and can help estimate expected height in children developing more slowly or more rapidly than their peers.

KEY POINTS: GENERAL GROWTH

- Proper evaluation of growth depends on accurate measurement of height and correct plotting of measurements on the appropriate growth curve.
- Common errors in plotting include plotting the wrong height, not plotting the patient's height at the exact chronologic age, and use of an inappropriate growth chart.
- An abnormal growth velocity for age generally distinguishes growth abnormalities from normal growth variants.
- Apparent abnormalities in growth are most frequently because of normal growth variants. Poor growth secondary to chronic medical illness is the next most frequent cause. Hormonal causes are less frequent.
- A radiograph of the left hand and wrist is obtained in children ages > 2 years and maturation of epiphyseal centers is compared with available standards.

13. Explain the significance of parental target height or "midparental height."

Parental height helps determine expected adult height on the basis of genetic potential. Add both parents' heights in centimeters; add 13 cm if the child is male, and subtract 13 cm if the child is female; then, divide by two. The resulting midparental height ±5 cm gives the expected 10th to 90th percentile for the offspring of those parents.

14. What is the most important factor in identifying an abnormal growth curve?

An abnormal growth velocity for age generally distinguishes growth abnormalities from normal growth variants. Although there are many causes of short stature, including genetic factors, normal children who are short grow normally, whereas children with a problem almost always have an abnormal growth velocity. For example, a child with stature in the fifth percentile who is growing with a normal growth velocity is less worrisome than the child whose stature has fallen from the 90th to the 75th percentile, even though the latter is taller than the former. Growth velocity abnormalities may, however, be subtle.

15. What causes abnormal growth in children?

Abnormalities in growth most frequently result from either normal growth variants (familial short stature or constitutional delay of growth and puberty) or underlying chronic medical illness, either recognized or unrecognized. Hormonal causes are less frequent.

16. Which syndromes are associated with abnormal growth?
   - Down's syndrome
   - Prader-Willi syndrome
   - Turner's syndrome
   - Noonan's syndrome
   - Other chromosomal abnormalities

17. List nonendocrine diseases and treatments that may be associated with poor growth.
   - Malnutrition
   - Pulmonary disease (cystic fibrosis, asthma)
   - Cardiac disease
   - Rheumatologic disease
   - Gastrointestinal disease (Crohn's disease, inflammatory bowel disease)
   - Neurologic disease (ketogenic diet, stimulant medications)
   - Renal disease
   - Anemia
   - Neoplasia
   - Long-term glucocorticoid use

18. Using the tools of growth curve, bone age, and height, how does one distinguish between familial (genetic) short stature and other causes?

Children with familial short stature grow at a normal velocity for age but with stature below the normal curve. They also grow within the expected target height percentile (i.e., they are as tall as expected for their genetic potential). If a child's projected height (by extrapolation of the growth curve along the current percentile) falls within the target range, the likelihood is high that current height is explained by genetic factors. Children with familial short stature also have a bone age approximately equal to chronologic age.

19. Give an example of distinguishing familial short stature from other causes of short stature.

A 5-year-old whose height is below the third percentile, whose growth has traced a line parallel to the third percentile, whose height projects within the parental target range, and whose bone age is also 5 years is likely to have familial short stature. However, if the growth velocity is abnormal or projected height falls below the predicted range, other factors may be involved in the short stature (Figs. 30.1 and 30.2).

20. Other than familial short stature, what is the most common cause of short stature?

Constitutional delay of growth (constitutional short stature or "late bloomer"), which affects up to 2% of children, is characterized by short stature and delayed bone age, and represents a normal growth pattern simply shifted to a later age. Affected children typically have a period of subnormal growth between 9 and 30 months of age, followed by normal growth velocity throughout the remainder of childhood. In accord with the delayed developmental pattern, bone age is delayed. The continuing growth delay also results in a delay in pubertal development and physical maturity. Such children (more often boys) generally have a family history of a similar growth pattern and may have a more dramatic deceleration of growth velocity before they enter puberty than normal children. They complete their growth at a later age, reaching an adult height within the expected genetic potential (Fig. 30.3).

21. How is the diagnosis of constitutional delay of growth made?

The diagnosis of constitutional delay of growth based on the following criteria does not require further laboratory support:
   - Period of slowed growth in the second year of life with downward crossing of percentile.
   - Normal growth velocity during childhood but with stature below the expected percentile for family
   - Delayed bone age
   - Height prediction appropriate for family (Plot the current height at the patient's bone age, and follow the resulting percentile to adult height. In constitutional delay, this generally leads to a projected height within the parental target range.)
   - Positive family history, delayed dentition, and delayed puberty in adolescence

22. What is the effect of testosterone therapy on boys with constitutional delay of growth?

Short-term testosterone therapy for boys with constitutional delay (75–100 mg of long-acting testosterone esters given once a month for 6 months) accelerates growth and stimulates pubertal development without compromising

Girls: 2–18 years
Physical growth

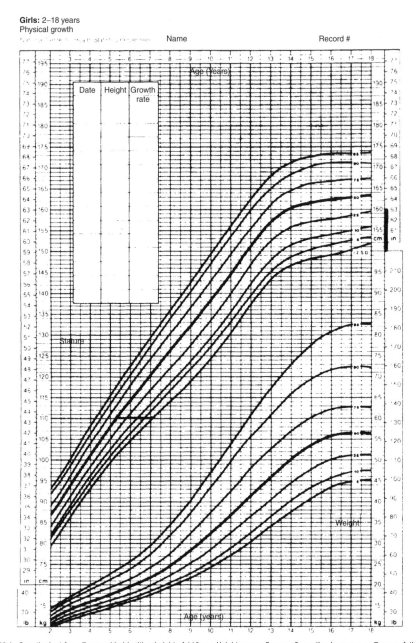

Fig. 30.1. Growth chart for a 7-year-old girl with a height of 110 cm. Height age ≈ 5 years, 3 months; bone age ≈ 7 years; father's height ≈ 65 inches (165 cm); mother's height ≈ 62 inches (157 cm); corrected midparental height (± 1 standard deviation [SD]) ≈ 155 ± 5 cm; predicted adult height ≈ 60 inches. The child has a predicted adult height within genetic potential and a bone age equal to chronologic age. She has genetic or familial short stature.

Girls: 2–18 years
Physical growth

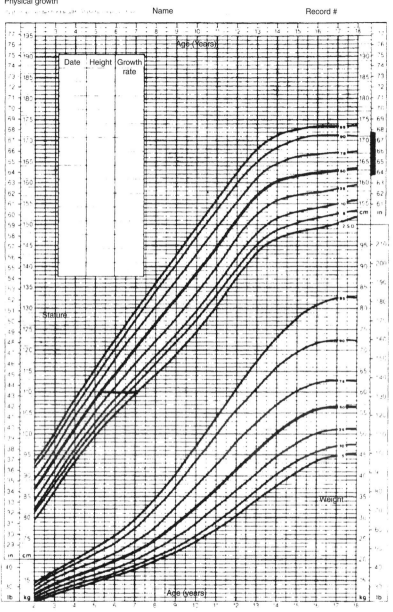

Fig. 30.2. Growth chart for a 7-year-old girl with a height of 110 cm. Height age ≈ 5 years, 3 months; bone age ≈ 5 years; father's height ≈ 70 inches (178 cm); mother's height ≈ 66 inches (168 cm); corrected midparental height (± 1 SD) ≈ 167.5 ± 5 cm. The child is growing below the fifth percentile, but extrapolation of her growth curve to adult height gives a final height below genetic potential. Clearly, her height cannot be attributed to genetic short stature alone.

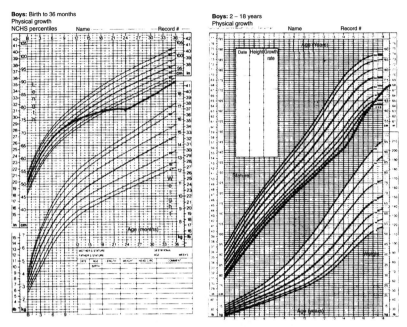

Fig. 30.3. Growth charts for a patient with constitutional delay of growth. Subnormal velocity during the second year of life *(left chart)* followed by normal velocity through childhood and a prolonged growth period with eventual achievement of normal adult height *(right chart)*.

final adult height or advancing bone age. Clinically, these boys experience pubertal changes, including genital enlargement (but not testicular growth), growth of pubic and axillary hair, deepening of voice, body odor, and acne. There may be personality changes characteristic of early puberty as well.

23. List the endocrine causes for short stature in children, in order of prevalence.
    - Hypothyroidism: congenital or acquired
    - GH deficiency
    - Glucocorticoid excess: iatrogenic or endogenous (less common)
    - Pseudohypoparathyroidism

24. What laboratory measurements should be considered in evaluating a patient for short stature?
    Laboratory tests should be designed to achieve two goals: (1) exclusion of undiagnosed chronic illness; and (2) exclusion of specific disorders associated with poor growth.

25. Which laboratory tests help exclude undiagnosed chronic illness?
    - Electrolyte measurements
    - Blood urea nitrogen/creatinine measurement
    - Liver transaminase measurements
    - Complete blood count
    - Erythrocyte sedimentation rate (ESR) measurement

26. Which laboratory tests help exclude gastrointestinal disorders associated with poor growth?
    Because symptoms may be limited, the following tests are recommended:
    - Celiac antibody (antitissue transglutaminase) test
    - Inflammatory bowel disease screen if child has an elevated ESR or anemia

27. List the laboratory tests for genetic disorders associated with poor growth.
    - Karyotype—for Turner's syndrome; consider in all short girls
    - Fluorescence in situ hybridization—for Prader-Willi syndrome
    - Genetic test for *PTPN11* mutation—for Noonan's syndrome

28. Which hormonal disorders should be excluded by laboratory results?
    - Thyroid deficiency (thyroid-stimulating hormone and total or free thyroxine)
    - GH deficiency (see question 30)

29. Describe the causes of GH deficiency.
    Most cases of GH deficiency are isolated and idiopathic. Idiopathic GH deficiency affects as many as 1:10,000 to 1:15,000 children. It is sporadic in the great majority of cases, but a rising number of specific gene mutations involved in the synthesis of GH or the regulation of its secretion is being reported. The other important underlying causes are listed in the answers for the following questions.

30. How is GH deficiency diagnosed?
    The diagnosis of GH deficiency is primarily a clinical one, aided by laboratory support, rather than a diagnosis based on definitive testing. Most important is identifying the patient in whom such a diagnosis would be appropriate. Children with subnormal growth should be evaluated for GH deficiency only after a thorough search fails to reveal any other cause for growth delay.

31. List the components of the laboratory evaluation for GH deficiency.
    - Measurement of the serum level of insulin-like growth factor 1 (IGF-1)
    - Measurement of IGF-binding protein 3 (IGFBP3). (May be useful in limited specific clinical situations [infancy, poor nutritional state] because IGF-1 may be low for reasons other than GH deficiency in these circumstances.)
    - GH stimulation testing

32. Why is the serum level of IGF-1 important?
    IGF-1 is a GH-dependent protein that is produced in target tissues in response to GH. The serum level of IGF-1 reflects production of the protein by the liver and gives an indirect indication of GH secretion. The following characteristics of IGF-1 should be kept in mind when its serum level is assessed:
    - The concentration of IGF-1 remains constant during the day, unlike the GH level.
    - The concentration of IGF-1 varies with age, and the reported value must be compared with appropriate age-specific and pubertal stage-specific norms available from performing laboratories.
    - A low serum level of IGF-1 ($>$ 2 standard deviations below the mean for age) is 70% to 80% predictive of low values on more rigorous tests of GH secretion, as long as other causes of low IGF-1 (e.g., poor nutrition, hypo-thyroidism, liver disease) have been excluded.

33. Does a normal level of IGF-1 exclude GH deficiency?
    No. A normal IGF-1 level is reassuring but does not rule out GH deficiency in a suggestive clinical context.

34. Does a low serum level of IGF-1 confirm the diagnosis of GH deficiency?
    No. Poor nutrition, chronic disease, and hypothyroidism suppress IGF-1 concentrations. In addition, before age 6 years, the IGF level is low, and the overlap between normal and GH-deficient levels renders its measurement highly insensitive. Measurement of IGFBP3 may be useful in this situation, although this test is less sensitive than IGF-1 in identifying likely GH deficiency.

35. How is GH testing done?
    Because secretion of GH is episodic, random measurements are not helpful for the diagnosis of GH deficiency. GH must be formally measured in response to a series of stimuli. Various pharmacologic agents are used, but there is no consensus about which one is optimal. The child must have fasted overnight, must be euthyroid, and must have no underlying chronic disease. In addition, at least two tests using different stimulating agents are generally performed.

36. How are the results of GH testing interpreted?
    The normal GH response to stimulation testing depends on the stimulation test and the type of GH assay used. Failure of response to all tests with values equal to or greater than those expected for normal children is consistent with the diagnosis of classic GH deficiency.
    Criteria for the diagnosis of partial GH deficiency and of neurosecretory dysfunction (normal pituitary response to stimuli, but low IGF-1, suggesting that endogenous GH secretion is impaired) are less well established.

37. How is idiopathic GH deficiency diagnosed?
    GH deficiency can be isolated or associated with other pituitary hormone deficiencies. It can be congenital or can result from trauma or an intracranial neoplasm. All patients diagnosed with GH deficiency should undergo cranial imaging unless the cause of the deficiency is previously known. Isolated GH deficiency without identifiable anatomic or physiologic etiology is considered idiopathic.

38. How is GH deficiency treated?

GH for administration is available through recombinant DNA technology; the majority of children are treated with six or seven daily shots per week at a total weekly dose of 0.18 to 0.30 mg/kg administered subcutaneously. Because the effect of GH wanes after several years of therapy, it is common to see dramatic catch-up growth ($\approx$ 10–12 cm/yr) in the first or second year of therapy, followed by velocities ranging from normal to 1.5 times normal in subsequent years.

39. What is the prognosis for adult height in treated children with GH deficiency?

Although nearly all treated children reach an adult height significantly better than predicted before therapy is initiated, many do not reach their predicted genetic potential. Children diagnosed and treated at earlier ages have better height prognoses than those whose therapy is initiated later. Similarly, the more mature the skeleton at diagnosis, the poorer is the final outcome.

40. When is GH therapy discontinued?

In children with GH deficiency, the point of diminishing benefit of therapy correlates with skeletal maturity, rather than chronologic age or duration of therapy. Therapy often is discontinued at a bone age of 15 years (96% of growth) to 16 years (98% of growth) in boys and 14 years (98% of growth) in girls. However, given what is known about the effects of GH deficiency in adulthood, some patients with severe deficiency may require lifelong hormonal replacement.

41. What other syndromes are considered indications for GH therapy?

GH is now approved by the U.S. Food and Drug Administration (FDA) for the treatment of short stature in the following conditions:

1. Chronic renal insufficiency before transplantation
2. Turner's syndrome (45,XO or mosaic variants)
3. Acquired immunodeficiency syndrome–related wasting syndrome
4. Prader-Willi syndrome
5. Noonan's syndrome
6. Short stature caused by intrauterine growth retardation in the absence of catch-up growth
7. Idiopathic short stature in boys with predicted adult height < 63 inches and girls with predicted height < 59 inches (normal GH secretion)

   Indications 2 through 6 do not require demonstration of GH deficiency. The use of GH for treatment of idiopathic short stature remains controversial among pediatric endocrinologists.

42. What is the prognosis for girls with Turner's syndrome treated with GH?

Girls with Turner's syndrome generally demonstrate a significant increase in predicted adult height, with an average increase of 8.8 cm. The overall effectiveness of GH therapy, like that in GH deficiency, depends on chronologic age and bone age at initiation of treatment and on duration of treatment. Because GH therapy in Turner's syndrome normalizes height in younger girls, estrogen replacement therapy can be initiated at an age similar to the age of puberty of the patient's peers.

43. What are the potential risks of GH therapy?

The side effects of GH therapy can be divided into three categories: (1) common but clinically unimportant, (2) uncommon with potential clinical importance, and (3) rare or theoretical.

44. List the common but clinically unimportant side effects of GH therapy.

- Acute correction of body water deficit after initiation of GH in deficient patients may lead to transient peripheral edema, headache, and joint aches and stiffness
- Increased average glucose concentration
- Increased systolic blood pressure

45. List the uncommon side effects with potential clinical importance.

- Pseudotumor cerebri
- Slipped capital femoral epiphysis
- Overt glucose intolerance
- Worsening of underlying scoliosis

46. What rare or theoretical side effects may be associated with GH therapy?

- *Risk for tumor recurrence or development of a secondary neoplasm*—the most recent analyses indicate no increase in the risk of tumor recurrence or development of secondary neoplasms in childhood cancer survivors treated with GH.
- A possible increase in cancer-related mortality in adults treated with GH as children—as suggested by analysis of a large French database. This report is not yet confirmed, and the regulatory agencies have not changed labeling in response to this report.

47. Should children with idiopathic short stature (without GH deficiency) be treated with GH?

    The FDA has approved the use of GH in children with idiopathic short stature with a predicted adult height < 63 inches (160 cm) for boys and < 59 inches (150 cm) for girls. However, the use of GH in children in whom no hormonal abnormality can be demonstrated continues to be controversial among pediatric endocrinologists. Short-term studies involving small cohorts have demonstrated a consistent increase in growth velocity with GH therapy in such children. Several studies that monitored children to final height disagreed about the overall effectiveness of therapy. However, most studies agree that the increase in final adult height is limited and can be obtained only at significant financial cost. The decision to use GH in such children should be carefully considered and requires a thoughtful discussion among the child, his or her family, and an experienced pediatric endocrinologist who knows the child well.

48. How does the pattern of growth in children with excessive glucocorticoids differ from the pattern in children with exogenous obesity?

    Glucocorticoid excess, whether iatrogenic (common) or intrinsic (rare), results in impairment of linear growth. The mechanism reflects increased protein catabolism, increased lipolysis, and a decline in collagen synthesis. Glucocorticoids also suppress the pulsatile release of GH from the pituitary gland and the production of IGF-1 at the target organ. The net result is that children with steroid excess are frequently short. They also have an increased weight-to-height ratio and appear obese. Children with exogenous obesity, on the other hand, generally show accelerated linear growth; thus, they are not only obese but also tall for their age.

49. What conditions are associated with excessive growth in childhood?

    Relatively few conditions result in overgrowth during childhood. These include familial tall stature (stature appropriate for parental target), constitutional advanced growth, hormonal causes, and genetic syndromes.

50. Explain constitutional advanced growth.

    Constitutional advanced growth is associated with advanced bone age, accelerated growth, and early puberty, with predicted adult height appropriate for parental target (see question 21). Obesity and familial factors may be involved.

51. List the hormonal causes of excessive growth.
    - Hyperthyroidism
    - Androgen excess
    - GH excess (pituitary gigantism)
    - Estrogen excess

52. Summarize the characteristics of GH excess in childhood.

    GH excess is rare in children, in whom it causes tall stature (gigantism), rather than the bony overgrowth seen in adults (acromegaly). Diagnosis is based on the following laboratory results:
    - Elevated values on random measurements of GH
    - Extremely high levels of IGF-1
    - Lack of suppression of GH during a standard glucose tolerance test

53. With what findings is androgen excess associated?
    - Precocious puberty in boys
    - Congenital adrenal hyperplasia
    - Androgen-producing tumors

54. With what findings is estrogen excess associated?
    - Precocious puberty in girls
    - Estrogen-producing tumors

55. List the genetic syndromes associated with excessive growth.
    - Klinefelter's syndrome (47,XXY)—tall stature, small testes, delay of puberty
    - Connective tissue disorders
    - Marfan's syndrome—tall stature, arachnodactyly, joint laxity, lens displacement
    - Stickler's syndrome
    - Soto's syndrome (cerebral gigantism)—macrocephaly, progressive macrosomia, dilated ventricles, retardation, advanced bone age
    - Beckwith-Wiedemann syndrome—macroglossia, umbilical hernia, hypoglycemia, macrosomia in infancy
    - Homocystinuria—arachnodactyly, retardation, homocysteine in urine

KEY POINTS: GROWTH VARIANTS

- Children with familial short stature grow at a normal velocity for age and within their expected target height percentile and have a bone age approximately equal to chronologic age.
- Children with constitutional delay of growth have a period of slow growth in the second year of life but then grow with a normal growth velocity.
- Children with constitutional delay of growth also have delayed bone age, height prediction appropriate for family, and delayed entry into puberty.
- The diagnosis of a growth variant does not require laboratory confirmation, but growth should be monitored over time to confirm the initial impression.

KEY POINTS: GROWTH HORMONE DEFICIENCY

- Growth hormone (GH) deficiency is a clinical diagnosis.
- Other causes of poor growth should be excluded.
- Laboratory testing is supportive and confirmatory.
- Laboratory measures include measurement of serum insulin-like growth factor-1 and GH stimulation testing.

BIBLIOGRAPHY

Carel, J. C. (2006). Management of short stature with GnRH agonist and co-treatment with growth hormone: a controversial issue. *Molecular and Cellular Endocrinology, 254*, 226–233.

Clayton, P. E., Cianfarani, S., Czernichow, P., Johannsson, G., Rapaport, R., & Rogol, A. (2007). Management of the child born small for gestational age through to adulthood: a consensus statement of the International Societies of Pediatric Endocrinology and the Growth Hormone Research Society. *Journal of Clinical Endocrinology and Metabolism, 92*, 804–810.

Cytrynbaum, C. S., Smith, A. C., Rubin, T., Weksberg, R. (2005). Advances in overgrowth syndromes: clinical classification to molecular delineation in Soto's syndrome and Beckwith-Wiedemann syndrome. *Current Opinion in Pediatrics, 17*, 740–746.

Davenport, M. L. (2006). Evidence for early initiation of growth hormone and transdermal estradiol therapies in girls with Turner syndrome. *Growth Hormone and IGF Research, 16*, 591–597.

Lee, M. M. (2006). Clinical practice. Idiopathic short stature. *New England Journal of Medicine, 354*, 2576–2582.

Myers, S. E., Carrel, A. L., Whitman, B. Y., & Allen, D. B. (2000). Sustained benefit after 2 years of growth hormone on body composition, fat utilization, physical strength and agility, and growth in Prader-Willi syndrome. *Journal of Pediatrics, 137*, 42–49.

Quigley, C. A. (2007). Growth hormone treatment of non-growth hormone-deficient growth disorders. *Endocrinology Metabolism Clinics of North America, 36*, 131–186.

Rosenbloom, A. L., & Connor, E. L. (2007). Hypopituitarism and other disorders of the growth hormone-insulin like growth factor-1 axis. In F. Lifshitz (Ed.), *Pediatric endocrinology* (Vol. 2., pp. 65–100). New York, NY: Informa Healthcare.

Zeitler, P. S., Meacham, L. R., & Allen, D. B. (2005). *Principles and practice of pediatric endocrinology* (pp. 857–910). Springfield, IL: Charles C. Thomas.

CHAPTER 31

GROWTH HORMONE USE AND ABUSE

Carlos A. Torres and Homer J. LeMar, Jr.

Growth hormone (GH) plays an essential role in human growth and development; deficiency results in short stature and other defects, whereas high levels can cause excessive growth and acromegaly. In addition to recognized medical indications for replacement, GH has come to public attention because of its use by athletes to enhance performance. This chapter will cover the most recent evidence about GH physiology, therapeutic use, abuse, and detection.

1. What is GH?

   GH is the most abundant hormone produced by the anterior pituitary gland; it is a single-chain peptide hormone produced and secreted by somatotroph cells in the anterior pituitary gland in two molecular forms: the 22-kDa GH is more abundant than the 20-kDa form, but both have similar biologic activity. Measurement of individual GH isoforms plays a key role in the detection of doping in athletes. Endogenous GH production is highest during puberty and by middle age decreases to only about 15% of peak levels.

2. How does GH secretion occur?

   GH is secreted in a pulsatile fashion, mostly at night. Factors that increase secretion include sleep, exercise, trauma, and sepsis. Obesity and increasing age decrease GH secretion.

3. How is the release of GH regulated?

   GH secretion is stimulated by GH-releasing hormone (GH-RH) and inhibited by somatostatin, both from the hypothalamus. Ghrelin, a gastric-derived peptide, also stimulates GH release. Another major regulator of GH production is insulin-like growth factor-1 (IGF-1), which acts at the pituitary to directly inhibit GH production, and at the hypothalamus to inhibit the production of GH-RH and to stimulate somatostatin.

4. List the actions of GH.

   As the name implies, GH stimulates both linear growth and growth of internal organs (Table 31.1).

5. Does GH exert all of its effects directly?

   No. Many of the effects are mediated by IGF-1, which is also called *somatomedin C*. GH stimulates the production of IGF-1 in peripheral tissues, particularly the liver. In patients with GH resistance, often caused by GH receptor mutations, some effects of GH can be achieved by IGF-1 administration; IGF-1 has been approved for treatment of GH-resistant patients.

6. What causes excessive GH secretion, and what are the consequences?

   The major cause of excessive GH secretion is a GH-producing pituitary tumor. GH excess during childhood results in gigantism. Numerous historical examples have been noted, including Robert Wadlow, the "Alton giant," who reached a height of just over 8 feet 11 inches and wore size 37AA shoes. GH excess after epiphyseal closure results in acromegaly.

7. What conditions are associated with GH deficiency?

   GH deficiency can be congenital (genetic mutations) or may result from damage to the pituitary gland from intracranial tumors, surgery, radiation therapy, trauma, and a variety of infiltrative and infectious diseases. Adult-onset GH deficiency is much less common than that occurring during infancy and childhood and is often related to a preceding event, such as radiation exposure or trauma.

8. What are some common signs and symptoms of GH deficiency?

   GH deficiency in childhood results in short stature; similar effects are seen in GH resistance. GH deficiency in adults causes increased adiposity, decreased lean body mass, decreased bone density, decreased extracellular water, reduced cardiac function, decreased muscle force and strength, and diminished exercise performance. Patients have reduced exercise capacity and strength levels, and often complain of lethargy and fatigue. Quality of life may be diminished, with manifestations of depression, anxiety, mental fatigue, and decreased self-esteem. Excessive intraabdominal fat is associated with an increased risk of cardiovascular disease, which is the predominant cause of mortality in patients with GH deficiency.

Table 31.1. Actions of Growth Hormone at Specific Sites.

TARGET SYSTEM	ACTIONS
Liver and muscle	Increases nitrogen retention, amino acid uptake, and protein synthesis
Cardiovascular	Increases cardiac muscle mass and increases cardiac output at rest and during maximal exercise
Hematologic	Increases plasma volume and red blood cell mass
Skeletal tissue	Increases bone mineral density and bone turnover
Connective tissue	Increases collagen turnover at nonskeletal sites, including tendons
Metabolism	Increases rates of sweating and thermal dispersion during exercise
Endocrine—acute	Increases the uptake and utilization of glucose by muscle; antagonizes the lipolytic effect of catecholamines on adipose tissue
Endocrine—chronic	Reduces glucose utilization, enhances lipolysis, and increases lean body mass

9. Where do we get the GH used therapeutically?
   Historically, GH was derived from human cadavers; however, modern techniques have allowed for abundant production of biosynthetic GH, which is identical to the endogenous form.

10. Besides availability, what problem was associated with GH derived from human cadavers?
    Creutzfeldt-Jakob disease, an uncommon, rapidly progressive, and fatal spongiform encephalopathy, has been reported to result from iatrogenic transmission through human cadaver pituitary tissue. More than 30 young adults who had received human cadaver pituitary products have died of this disease, and at least 60 to 70 cases of Creutzfeldt-Jakob disease have been identified in recipients.

11. What are some uses of GH approved by the U.S. Food and Drug Administration?
    Historically, the only approved indication for GH therapy was treatment of short stature in children with GH deficiency. Currently, GH is also approved for treatment of short stature that is idiopathic, or associated with Turner's syndrome, Prader-Willi syndrome, Noonan's syndrome, and progressive chronic renal insufficiency in children. GH is also approved for treating wasting in patients with acquired immunodeficiency syndrome and for replacement in adults with GH deficiency.

12. What are some other potential uses of GH?
    GH use has other potential indications: (1) Russell-Silver syndrome, (2) chondrodysplasia in children, (3) steroid-induced growth suppression, (4) short stature associated with myelomeningocele, (5) any severe wasting state (e.g., wounds, burns, cancer), (6) normal aging, (7) non–islet cell tumor hypoglycemia, (8) gonadal dysgenesis, (9) Down's syndrome, (10) short stature associated with neurofibromatosis, (11) human immunodeficiency virus–associated adipose redistribution syndrome, and (12) osteoporosis.

13. How does GH help adults with GH deficiency?
    The reported beneficial effects in adults with GH deficiency are an increase in muscle mass and function, reduction of total body fat mass, and increased plasma volume, and improved peripheral blood flow. Reductions in serum total and low-density lipoprotein cholesterol, reduction in diastolic blood pressure, a trend toward reduction in systolic blood pressure, and beneficial effects on bone metabolism and skeletal mass have also been documented. In addition, an improvement in psychological well-being and quality of life can occur with GH replacement.

14. How is GH administered?
    GH is administered through subcutaneous injection. In children, the dose can be divided into regimens of two or three times weekly, or daily. Daily injections appear to result in greater growth velocity compared with less frequent administration. In adults with GH deficiency, replacement is usually given daily.

15. Why is GH used as an ergogenic aid by athletes?
    Some athletes have used GH in an effort to improve performance. Supraphysiologic doses of GH have been reported to increase lean body mass and reduce body fat in trained athletes. In 2010, a clinical research facility in Sydney, Australia, performed the largest randomized control trial to date to determine the effect of GH on body composition and measures of performance. The study showed that GH in both men and women significantly reduced body fat mass, increased lean body mass, and improved sprint capacity, but not strength, power, or endurance. The effects were even greater when GH was coadministered with testosterone.

16. **What recent developments have been made in testing for GH abuse?**
    Before 2004, there was no reliable method to detect exogenous GH administration because of difficulties in distinguishing it from endogenous hormone. After years of study and international collaboration, scientists developed a test that has been endorsed by the World Anti-Doping Association. In February 2010, the test caught its first doper, a British rugby player, who was banned from competition for 2 years for the infraction. The test was used experimentally in 2004 and became widely available by 2010, with expanded testing starting during the 2012 Olympic Games. The test's limitations include the need for a blood sample and its inability to detect use > 1 to 2 days before testing.

17. **Why was GH abuse so difficult to detect in the past?**
    GH was difficult to detect in the past because exogenously administered GH is identical in structure to endogenous hormone, so simply detecting GH on a blood sample was not evidence of doping. Additionally, endogenous GH is secreted in a pulsatile manner; therefore, an increased level detected on random testing could simply reflect a natural peak because GH secretion is stimulated by acute exercise. Cadaveric GH has also been used for doping purposes and is difficult to detect because of the normal ratios of GH isomers.

18. **How can GH abuse in athletes be detected?**
    GH doping can be detected by two distinct methods. The first method measures the ratio of the two isoforms of GH, and the second method measures the markers of GH action, such as IGF-1 and propeptide of type III procollagen.

19. **How prevalent is GH use among athletes?**
    The prevalence is not known, but it is thought to be widespread. Its use is probably not as extensive as that of anabolic–androgenic steroids. One limiting factor is the expense. Even a 1-month supply may cost several thousand dollars, depending on dosages.

20. **What are the adverse effects of the therapeutic use of GH in adults?**
    Fluid retention causing edema and carpal tunnel syndrome are common in adults, but not in children. Arthralgias, myalgias, paresthesias, and worsening glucose tolerance are also common and may be present in up to one third of patients taking GH. Other potential side effects include gynecomastia, pancreatitis, behavioral changes, worsening of neurofibromatosis, scoliosis and kyphosis, and hypertrophy of tonsils and adenoids.

21. **What are the adverse effects of GH in children?**
    Intracranial hypertension has been reported in children; this is most common in children with renal disease, although it has also been observed in children with GH deficiency and in girls with Turner's syndrome. GH therapy is associated with an increased risk of slipped capital femoral epiphysis in the same three groups of children. Children with GH deficiency caused by deletion of the *GH* gene may develop antibodies to GH with secondary growth deceleration. This phenomenon is rare in other children.

22. **What adverse effects occur in athletes using GH?**
    Little is known about side effects of GH use in athletes. Chronic abuse of supraphysiologic GH doses may lead to features of acromegaly; osteoarthritis; irreversible bone and joint deformities; increased vascular, respiratory, and cardiac abnormalities; hypertrophy of other organs; hypogonadism; diabetes mellitus; abnormal lipid metabolism; increased risk of breast and colon cancers; and muscle weakness caused by myopathy. Use of GH in combination with anabolic–androgenic steroids may increase left ventricular mass and cause cardiac remodeling.

23. **Can GH reverse the natural aging process?**
    No. However, alternative medicine companies promote products alleged to stimulate increased production of GH in hopes of reversing normal aging. This theory has been sustained partly by a study that suggested that diminished secretion of GH is responsible for the effects of aging, including increased adipose tissue, decreased lean body mass, and thinning of the skin. Although GH replacement has a role in individuals with GH deficiency, no studies have shown that supplemental GH can reverse physiologic aging.

KEY POINTS: GROWTH HORMONE USE AND ABUSE

- Growth hormone (GH) secretion is stimulated by exercise, sleep, stress, trauma, and signaling by growth hormone-releasing hormone and grehlin. Inhibition occurs by feedback from somatostatin and insulin-like growth factor-1.
- GH abuse is thought to be prevalent in athletes to enhance performance, but little evidence supports meaningful performance enhancement, except for some increase in anaerobic exercise capacity.
- Large-scale detection of GH doping has recently become possible, including at the Olympic Games. Current testing relies on either altered GH isoform ratios or altered markers of GH action.
- Long-term effects of supratherapeutic doses of GH in athletes are not known, but there is concern about multiple possible negative effects.

⊕ WEBSITES

Human Growth Foundation: http://www.hgfound.org
Mayo Clinic Article about performance-enhancing medications: http://www.mayoclinic.com/health/performance-enhancing-drugs/HQ01105
World Anti-Doping Agency: http://www.wada-ama.org/

BIBLIOGRAPHY

Althobiti, S. D., Alqurashi, N. M., Alotaibi, A. S., Alharthi, T. F., & Alswat, K. A. (2018). Prevalence, attitude, knowledge, and practice of anabolic androgenic steroid (AAS) use among gym participants. *Materia Socio-Medica, 30*(1), 49–52.

Anderson, L. J., Tamayose, J. M., & Garcia, J. M. (2018). Use of growth hormone, IGF-I, and insulin for anabolic purpose: pharmacological basis, methods of detection, and adverse effects. *Molecular and Cellular Endocrinology, 464*, 65–74.

Berrgren, A., Ehrnborg, C., Rosén, T., Ellegård, L., Bengtsson, B. A., & Caidahl, K. (2005). Short-term administration of supraphysiological growth hormone does not increase maximum endurance exercise capacity in healthy, active young men and women with normal GH-insulin-like growth factor I axes. *Journal of Clinical Endocrinology and Metabolism, 90*, 3268–3273.

Bidlingmaier, M., & Strasburger, C. J. (2007). Technology insight: detecting growth hormone abuse in athletes. *Nature Clinical Practice. Endocrinology & Metabolism, 3*(11), 769–777.

Bildlingmaier, M., & Manolopoulou, J. (2010). Detecting growth hormone abuse in athletes. *Endocrinology and Metabolism Clinics of North America, 39*, 25–32.

Blackman, M. R., Sorkin, J. D., Münzer, T., Bellantoni, M. F., Busby-Whitehead, J., Stevens, T. E., ... Harman, S. M. (2002). Growth hormone and sex steroid administration in healthy aged women and men: a randomized controlled trial. *JAMA, 288*, 2282–2292.

Bouillanne, O., Raenfray, M., Tissandier, O., Nasr, A., Lahlou, A., Cnockaert, X., & Piette, F. (1996). Growth hormone therapy in elderly people: an age delaying drug? *Fundamental & Clinical Pharmacology, 10*, 416–430.

Cooke, D. W., Divall, S. A., & Radovick, S. (2011). Normal and aberrant growth. In S. Melmed, K. S. Polonsky, P. R. Larsen, & H. M. Kronenberg, (Ed.), *Williams Textbook of Endocrinology* (12th ed., pp. 935–1053). W.B. Saunders: Philadelphia.

Cummings, D. E., & Merriam, G. R. (2003). Growth hormone therapy in adults. *Annual Review of Medicine, 54*, 513–533.

Dean, H. (2002). Does exogenous growth hormone improve athletic performance? *Clinical Journal of Sport Medicine, 12*, 250–253.

Hermansen, K., Bengtsen, M., Kjær, M., Vestergaard, P., & Jørgensen, J. O. L. (2017). Impact of GH administration on athletic performance in healthy young adults: a systematic review and meta-analysis of placebo-controlled trials. *Growth Hormone & IGF Research, 34*, 38–44.

Holt, R. I. (2011). Detecting growth hormone abuse in athletes. *Analytical and Bioanalytical Chemistry, 401*, 449–462.

Hurel, S. J., Koppiker, N., Newkirk, J., Close, P. R., Miller, M., Mardell, R., ... Kendall-Taylor, P. (1999). Relationship of physical exercise and ageing to growth hormone production. *Clinical Endocrinology, 51*, 687–691.

Jenkins, P. J. (1999). Growth hormone and exercise. *Clinical Endocrinology, 50*, 683–689.

Karila, T. A., Karjalainen, J. E., Mäntysarri, M. J. Viitasalo, M. T., & Seppälä, T. A. (2003). Anabolic androgenic steroids produce dose-dependent increase in left ventricular mass in power athletes, and this effect is potentiated by concomitant use of growth hormone. *International Journal of Sports Medicine, 24*, 337–343.

Laron, Z. (2004). Laron syndrome (primary growth hormone resistance or insensitivity): the personal experience 1958–2003. *Journal of Clinical Endocrinology and Metabolism, 89*, 1031–1044.

Meinhardt, A. U., Nelson, A. E., Hansen, J. L. Birzniece, V., Clifford, D., Leung, K. C., ... Ho, K. K. (2010). The effects of growth hormone on body composition and physical performance in recreational athletes. *Annals of Internal Medicine, 152*, 568–577.

Melmed, S., Jameson, J. L. (2011). Disorders of the anterior pituitary and hypothalamus. In D. L. Longo, D. L. Kasper, J. L. Jameson, A. S. Fauci, S. L. Hauser, J. Loscalzo. *Harrison's Principles of Internal Medicine* (18th ed., pp. 339, 2876–2902). McGraw Hill.

Melmed, S., Kleinberg, D., Ho, K. (2011). Pituitary physiology and diagnostic evaluation. In S. Melmed, K. S. Polonsky, P. R. Larsen, H. M. Kronenberg, (Ed.), *Williams Textbook of Endocrinology* (12th ed., pp. 175–228). Philadelphia: W.B. Saunders.

Molitch, M. E., Clemmons, D. R., Malozowski, S., Merriam, G. R., Vance, M. L. (2006). Evaluation and treatment of adult growth hormone deficiency: an Endocrine Society clinical practice guideline. *Journal of Clinical Endocrinology and Metabolism, 91*, 1621–1634.

Murray, R. D., Skillicorn, C. J., Howell, S. J., Lissett, C. A., Rahim, A., Smethurst, L. E., & Shalet, S. M. (1999). Influences on quality of life in growth hormone-deficient adults and their effect on response to treatment. *Clinical Endocrinology, 51*, 565–573.

Nelson, A. E., Meinhardt, U., Hansen, J. L., Walker, I. H., Stone, G., Howe, C. J., ... Ho, K. K. (2008). Pharmacodynamics of growth hormone abuse biomarkers and the influence of gender and testosterone: a randomized double-blind placebo-controlled study in young recreational athletes. *Journal of Clinical Endocrinology and Metabolism, 93*(6), 2213–2222.

Robinson, N., Sottas, P. E., & Schumacher, Y. O. (2017). The athlete biological passport: how to personalize anti-doping testing across an athlete's career? *Medicine and Sport Science, 62*, 107–118.

Rodrigues–Arnao, J., Jabbar, J., Fulcher, K., Besser, G. M. & Ross, R. J. (1999). Effects of growth hormone replacement on physical performance and body composition in growth hormone-deficient adults. *Clinical Endocrinology, 51*, 53–60.

Rudman, D., Feller, A., Nagraj, H., Gergans, G. A., Lalitha, P. Y., Goldberg, A. F., ... Mattson, D. E. (1990). Effects of growth hormone in men 60 years old. *New England Journal of Medicine, 323*, 1–6.

Travis, J. (2010). Pharmacology, Growth hormone test finally nabs first doper. *Science, 327*, 1185.

Wallace, J. D., & Cuneo, R. C. (2000). Growth hormone abuse in athletes: a review. *Endocrinologist, 10*, 175–184.

Weber, M. M. (2002). Effects of growth hormone on skeletal muscle. *Hormone Research, 58*(Suppl. 3), 43–48.

IV

ADRENAL DISORDERS

CHAPTER 32

PRIMARY ALDOSTERONISM

John J. Orrego

1. Define primary aldosteronism (PA).

PA, first recognized by Jerome Conn in 1954, refers to a group of disorders characterized by excessive and autonomous aldosterone secretion by one or both adrenal glands; the aldosterone secretion is independent of the renin–angiotensin system, plasma adrenocorticotropic hormone (ACTH) levels, and serum potassium concentrations (the major physiologic regulators of aldosterone production), and is nonsuppressible by sodium loading. There are five clinical entities that are included under PA:
- Idiopathic hyperaldosteronism (IHA)—bilateral hyperplasia of the zona glomerulosa
- Aldosterone-producing adenoma (APA) or Conn's syndrome
- Primary adrenal hyperplasia (PAH)—unilateral hyperplasia of the zona glomerulosa
- Adrenocortical carcinoma (ACC)
- Glucocorticoid-remediable aldosteronism (GRA)

2. How common is PA?

The most common manifestation of excess aldosterone secretion is hypertension. Cross-sectional and prospective studies around the world have substantiated that 5% to 13% of patients with hypertension, both in general and in specialty clinics, have PA.

3. What are the clinical manifestations of PA?

Aldosterone normally acts at the renal distal convoluted tubule to stimulate reabsorption of sodium ions (Na^+), as well as secretion of potassium (K^+) and hydrogen ions (H^+), and at the cortical and medullary collecting ducts to cause direct secretion of H^+. Excessive secretion of aldosterone in PA results in hypertension, hypokalemia, and metabolic alkalosis; hypomagnesemia may also occur. In general, patients with APA have more severe hypertension and hypokalemia compared with their IHA counterparts. In one series, the mean blood pressure was 184/112 mm Hg in the former group and 161/105 mm Hg in the latter group. Although resistant hypertension is common in patients with PA, malignant hypertension is rare. Spontaneous hypokalemia is actually an uncommon presenting manifestation of PA. Symptoms are usually those associated with hypertension (headaches and dizziness) or with hypokalemia (muscle weakness and cramping, paresthesias, palpitations, polyuria, and polydipsia). Patients with PA have a higher prevalence of cardiovascular morbidity and mortality compared with age- and gender-matched patients with primary hypertension and the same degree of blood pressure elevation. They are also more likely to have type 2 diabetes mellitus and metabolic syndrome.

4. Is hypokalemia a *sine qua non* for PA?

No. Different series have documented hypokalemia in only 9% to 37% of patients with PA. In a large single study published in 2006, almost 50% of patients with APA had hypokalemia, whereas only 17% of those with IHA did. Therefore, normokalemic severe hypertension is the most common presentation of PA.

5. What is the differential diagnosis of mineralocorticoid hypertension?

Hypertension with hypokalemia and suppression of plasma renin activity (PRA) is known as *mineralocorticoid hypertension*. The most common cause of mineralocorticoid hypertension is PA. The plasma aldosterone concentration (PAC) is always elevated in PA, whereas all the other types of mineralocorticoid hypertension are characterized by suppressed PAC because of activation of the mineralocorticoid receptor by other compounds or from constitutive activation of collecting tubule sodium channels:
1. Deoxycorticosterone (a precursor of aldosterone with mineralocorticoid activity):
   - Congenital adrenal hyperplasia, caused by 11beta-hydroxylase deficiency and 17alpha-hydroxylase deficiency
   - Deoxycorticosterone-secreting adrenocortical tumors
   - Glucocorticoid-receptor resistance (glucocorticoid receptor mutations, mifepristone)
2. Cortisol (severe hypercortisolemia overwhelms renal 11beta-hydroxysteroid dehydrogenase type 2 and results in spillover to the mineralocorticoid receptor):
   - Apparent mineralocorticoid excess
   - Licorice and carbenoxolone ingestion
   - Ectopic ACTH syndrome
3. Mutations in genes that encode the beta and delta subunits of the collecting tubule sodium channels preventing their removal from the cell surface:
   - Liddle's syndrome

6. Why is it important to detect PA?

The primary reason is that hypertension accompanying PA is potentially curable. The most important reason, however, is that patients with PA have a higher prevalence of cardiovascular morbidity and mortality compared with age- and gender-matched patients with primary hypertension and the same degree of blood pressure elevation. Specifically, patients with PA, compared with those with primary hypertension, have increased left ventricular mass and decreased left ventricular function, and a higher risk of atrial fibrillation, stroke, and myocardial infarction. These effects seem to be mediated through activation of mineralocorticoid receptors in the heart and blood vessels, with subsequent impairment of endothelial function. Therefore, timely detection and treatment (surgery or mineralocorticoid receptor antagonists) can reduce the impact of aldosterone on these tissues.

7. Which patients with hypertension should be investigated for PA?

Case detection should be targeted to the following groups of patients:

1. Sustained blood pressure > 150/100 mm Hg[a]
2. Sustained blood pressure > 140/90 mm Hg despite the use of three antihypertensive medications, including a thiazide diuretic (resistant hypertension)[a]
3. Controlled blood pressure < 140/90 mm Hg on ≥ four antihypertensive medications[a]
4. Hypertension and spontaneous or diuretic-induced hypokalemia
5. Hypertension and an adrenal incidentaloma
6. Hypertension and sleep apnea
7. Hypertension and family history of hypertension or cerebrovascular disease at age < 40 years old
8. All hypertensive first-degree relatives of patients with PA

8. What tests are recommended to detect possible cases of PA (case detection)?

The diagnosis of PA is based on the demonstration of inappropriately high PAC with concomitantly suppressed PRA. The most reliable screening test is the aldosterone/renin ratio (ARR). This test is more sensitive when concomitant PAC (in ng/dL) and PRA (in ng/mL/hr) samples are collected in the morning, with the patient out of bed for at least 2 hours and seated for 5 to 15 minutes. Preparation before ARR testing includes correction of hypokalemia (as hypokalemia reduces aldosterone secretion), sodium-unrestricted diet, and withdrawal of mineralocorticoid receptor antagonists (spironolactone and eplerenone), renin inhibitors, and amiloride (if > 5 mg per day) 4 to 6 weeks before testing, if clinically feasible. ARR > 20 with PAC > 15 ng/dL strongly suggests PA. However, because 10% to 40% of patients with confirmed PA have PAC in the 10- to 15-ng/dL range, ARR > 30 is suggestive of PA in these patients.

9. What medications affect the ARR?

Medications do not cause false-positive results for PA; this is the only condition that can cause a frankly elevated PAC and suppressed PRA. Therefore, when suspicion is high that a patient has PA, screening can be done no matter what medications the patient is taking; if the diagnostic criteria are met, screening does not need to be repeated off medications. However, medications can cause false-negative results, either by raising the PRA (most often) or suppressing the PAC. Thus, if testing is borderline or negative and PA is still suspected, medications may need to be discontinued and the tests repeated. Or the medications can be stopped proactively before initial testing. These are the most common medications that cause false-negative test results:

- Mineralocorticoid receptor antagonists, renin inhibitors, and high-dose amiloride can all elevate the PRA, causing a falsely negative ARR. If discontinuation of these is indicated, they should be stopped 4 to 6 weeks before ARR testing. When this is not safe, PA-related testing can still be pursued; if the PRA level is suppressed on these medications, they will not affect the test.
- Angiotensin-converting enzyme (ACE) inhibitors, angiotensin receptor blockers (ARBs), and diuretics can also sometimes elevate the PRA and cause a false-negative ARR. Thus, in cases where the ARR is borderline or negative but PA is still suspected, these medications should be discontinued briefly (1–2 weeks) and testing repeated. However, if the PRA is suppressed, these medications will not produce false results.
- Beta-adrenergic receptor blockers and central alpha-2 agonists (clonidine, alpha-methyldopa) suppress PRA and, to a lesser degree, PAC in individuals with normal levels; therefore, although ARR may increase modestly in hypertensive patients without PA treated with these medications, PAC remains < 15 ng/dL and test interpretation is not usually affected.
- Calcium-channel blockers belonging to the dihydropyridine family can elevate the PRA and slightly decrease PAC, also causing a false-negative ARR.
- Verapamil slow-release, hydralazine, prazosin, doxazosin, and terazosin have little effect on the ARR and may be substituted for temporary control during case finding and confirmatory testing.

---

[a]These blood pressure cut-offs were recommended before the 2017 American College of Cardiology/American Heart Association High Blood Pressure Guidelines were released

10. What tests are recommended to confirm PA (case confirmation)?

Most, but not all, patients with a positive ARR should undergo one or more confirmatory tests to definitively confirm or exclude the diagnosis. There are several tests which confirm PA:

- *Oral sodium loading test:* Intravascular volume expansion should normally suppress aldosterone secretion. In the oral sodium loading test, the patient consumes > 200 mmol (6 g) of dietary sodium for 3 days and from day 3 through day 4, 24-hour urine samples for aldosterone, sodium, and creatinine are collected. Urinary excretion of aldosterone (high-performance liquid chromatography [HPLC]–tandem mass spectrometry) > 12 mcg/day confirms a diagnosis of PA. Urinary sodium of at least 200 mmol/day ensures adequacy of the test. Hypertension and hypokalemia should be controlled before this test is performed.
- *Saline infusion test:* An alternative test is acute volume expansion by administering 2 liters of normal saline intravenously over 4 hours, while the patient stays in the recumbent position, with measurement of PAC at baseline and at the end of the saline infusion. Postinfusion PAC > 10 ng/dL confirms the diagnosis. PAC < 5 ng/dL rules out PA, and levels between 5 and 10 ng/dL are indeterminate; another confirmatory test may be considered.

11. When is confirmatory testing not needed?

Confirmatory testing (oral sodium loading or intravenous saline infusion) is not considered necessary when all three of the following criteria are met:

- Spontaneous hypokalemia
- PRA suppressed
- PAC > 20 ng/dL

 Confirmatory testing is not needed in this situation because nothing else besides PA can cause this picture. Adrenal imaging can now be pursued.

12. Are any other tests used for case confirmation?

Additional testing to confirm the diagnosis is seldom necessary. Less commonly used confirmatory tests include the fludrocortisone suppression test and the captopril challenge test. In the former, the patient takes 0.1 mg of fludrocortisone and slow-release potassium chloride (KCl) supplements orally every 6 hours and a high-sodium diet for 4 days. Upright PAC > 6 ng/dL on day 4 at 10 am confirms PA, provided PRA is < 1 ng/mL/h and cortisol is lower than the value obtained at 7 AM. In the latter, the patient receives 25 to 50 mg of captopril orally after sitting or standing for at least 1 hour. Blood is drawn 2 hours later while the patient is seated. PAC is normally suppressed > 30% by captopril. In patients with PA, PAC remains elevated, and PRA remains suppressed.

13. What is the most common form of PA?

IHA is the most common form of PA, accounting for 60% to 70% of cases in most series. IHA is characterized by bilateral hyperplasia (diffuse and focal) of the zona glomerulosa layer of both adrenal glands. Although the cause has not yet been determined, it has been hypothesized that there is supranormal sensitivity of the zona glomerulosa to physiologic concentrations of angiotensin II in affected adrenal glands. However, the hyperaldosteronism in these patients is not reversed with angiotensin II inhibitors. IHA is generally a milder disease with less aldosterone hypersecretion and, therefore, milder hypertension and mild or no hypokalemia.

14. What is the second most common cause of PA?

APAs comprise 30% to 40% of PA cases. Patients with APA are usually younger (< 50 years) and have higher PAC, resulting in more severe hypertension and hypokalemia. APAs are small (< 2 cm), occur more commonly in the left adrenal gland, and are composed of zona glomerulosa cells, zona reticularis cells, and hybrid cells with characteristics of both layers. APAs are also known as Conn's syndrome.

15. What other features differ between APAs and IHA?

APAs produce greater amounts of aldosterone compared with IHA and other forms of PA; consequently, the degree of hypertension and biochemical abnormalities (hypokalemia and PAC levels) tend to be more severe in patients with an APA. APAs also demonstrate partial responses to ACTH stimulation, whereas the adrenal glands in IHA remain primarily under the control of angiotensin II. PAC in patients with APAs, therefore, parallels the normal circadian rhythm of ACTH secretion (highest in the AM and lowest in the PM), whereas PAC in patients with IHA does not show diurnal variation but increases with upright posture. This is the basis for the (seldom used) posture test in which PAC levels are drawn at baseline in the AM and after 4 hours of upright posture; during this test PAC decreases in patients with an APA and increases in patients with IHA.

16. Why is it important to differentiate between these two conditions?

APAs are a surgically curable form of PA. IHA, in contrast, cannot be cured with surgery and requires chronic medical management.

17. What should be the initial imaging study once PA is confirmed (subtype classification)?

High-resolution adrenal computed tomography (CT) is the recommended initial study to determine the subtype once a diagnosis of PA is confirmed. Magnetic resonance imaging (MRI) has no advantage over CT in subtype evaluation of PA because MRI is more expensive, scan time is longer, and it has less spatial resolution than CT. If the patient is interested in surgery (if an APA is found) and the results of cross-sectional imaging are not clear-cut (normal-appearing glands, unilateral or bilateral adrenal limb thickening, or micro- or macroadenomas), the next step should be bilateral adrenal vein sampling (AVS) by an experienced interventional radiologist.

18. Why is AVS the "gold-standard" test for subtype classification?

Nonfunctional adrenal incidentalomas are common, true APAs may be very small, and the adrenal enlargement seen in IHA can be asymmetric. For these reasons, adrenal imaging alone can lead to significant diagnostic errors and unnecessary surgery. In most cases, therefore, when surgical cure is being considered, AVS is a fundamental diagnostic step to accurately differentiate between unilateral and bilateral adrenal hyperaldosteronism. In a large series of patients with PA who underwent AVS at the Mayo Clinic, CT scan, was accurate in only 53% of patients. On the basis of CT findings, 22% of patients would have been incorrectly excluded as candidates for adrenalectomy and 25% might have had unnecessary or inappropriate surgery.

19. How is AVS performed?

Catheters are introduced into the left and right adrenal veins and the inferior vena cava (IVC). Plasma aldosterone and serum cortisol levels are obtained from these sites at baseline and following a continuous cosyntropin (synthetic ACTH) infusion. Cortisol levels are obtained to ensure that the adrenal veins are properly catheterized; the adrenal vein to IVC cortisol ratio is typically > 10:1. Dividing the right and left adrenal vein aldosterone levels by their respective cortisol level corrects for the dilutional effect of the inferior phrenic vein flow into the left adrenal vein ("cortisol-corrected" ratios). APAs produce large amounts of aldosterone; the normal adrenal vein aldosterone level is 100 to 400 ng/dL, whereas APAs may generate concentrations of 1000 to 10,000 ng/dL. A cortisol-corrected aldosterone ratio from the high side to the low side > 4:1 is indicative of unilateral aldosterone hypersecretion. Uncommon complications of this procedure include adrenal hemorrhage and adrenal vein dissection.

20. Why should adrenal venous sampling be performed by an experienced interventional radiologist?

Collection of blood for measurement of aldosterone and cortisol from the left adrenal gland is relatively simple because the venous effluent drains directly into the left renal vein. The venous flow from the right adrenal, however, flows directly into the IVC. Catheterization of the right adrenal vein is more difficult because of its smaller size and greater angulation compared with the contralateral vein. The success rate for right adrenal vein catheterization increases from 74% to 96% in experienced hands.

21. When is AVS not needed in patients with documented PA?

AVS is not considered necessary when all three of the following criteria are all met:
- Age < 35 years
- PAC markedly elevated
- Unilateral cortical adenoma on CT

When these three criteria are met, and the patient is interested in surgery, AVS is not necessary before proceeding to surgery for PA. AVS is also not necessary when the evaluation strongly supports a diagnosis of IHA or if the patient is not otherwise interested in or unable to undergo surgery.

22. Are there any other diagnostic tests?

These are mainly of historical interest. If both adrenal veins are not successfully catheterized, a posture stimulation test or iodocholesterol scintigraphy (NP-59 scan), if available, may be informative in patients with a unilateral adrenal mass. In most patients with APA, the PAC is relatively unaffected by increasing angiotensin II levels upon standing, whereas in most patients with IHA, the hyperplastic zona glomerulosa of both adrenal glands has enhanced sensitivity to angiotensin II. Therefore, PAC levels increase with upright posture in patients with IHA and decrease or remain unchanged in patients with APAs. The NP-59 scan, which is no longer used in the United States, demonstrates tracer uptake in APAs > 1.5 cm.

23. What is PAH?

This is an uncommon cause of PA characterized by unilateral micronodular or macronodular hyperplasia of the zona glomerulosa layer. The clinical presentation and outcome of these patients is similar to those with APAs. The treatment is laparoscopic adrenalectomy of the affected gland.

24. How is aldosterone synthesis regulated in the zona glomerulosa?

Humans possess two mitochondrial 11 beta-hydroxylase isoenzymes that are responsible for cortisol and aldosterone synthesis (designated CYP11B1 and CYP11B2, respectively). Both are encoded on chromosome 8. CYP11B1, which is responsible for conversion of 11-deoxycortisol to cortisol, is expressed only in the zona fasciculata. CYP11B2, which is responsible for the conversion of corticosterone to aldosterone, is expressed only in the zona glomerulosa. CYP11B2 activity is stimulated by ACTH, whereas CYP11B2 is stimulated by angiotensin II or hypokalemia.

25. What is GRA?

GRA, also known as *familial hyperaldosteronism type I* (FH-I), is responsible for 1% of PA cases. The disorder is inherited in an autosomal-dominant fashion. The presentation of GRA is variable, with some patients having normal blood pressure and others manifesting severe and refractory hypertension at a young age. Less than 50% of patients with GRA have spontaneous hypokalemia. Strokes, mainly hemorrhagic, resulting from a ruptured intracranial aneurysm, occur in almost 20% of affected individuals. The genetic abnormality in these patients is a fusion of two genes, *CYP11B1/CYP11B2*, forming a chimeric gene product, which results in ACTH-sensitive aldosterone synthesis in the zona fasciculata. Genetic testing is now preferred over dexamethasone suppression testing for making the diagnosis of GRA. The treatment for this condition is physiologic doses of glucocorticoids.

26. Explain the genetic basis of GRA.

GRA results from a heritable mutation that causes the fusion of the promoter (regulatory) region of the *CYP11B1* gene with the structural (coding) region of the *CYP11B2* gene. The resulting chimeric gene product synthesizes aldosterone and its precursors in the zona fasciculata in response to ACTH (instead of angiotensin II). The metabolites (18-hydroxycortisol and 18-oxocortisol) can serve as biochemical markers that facilitate identification of affected family members. The excessive aldosterone secretion can usually be inhibited by administration of glucocorticoids that suppress ACTH secretion by the pituitary.

27. Can adrenal carcinoma cause PA?

ACC as a cause of PA is rare. The tumors are very large (> 6 cm) and commonly metastatic at the time of diagnosis. All cases of PA should be imaged with CT to exclude this rare cause of PA.

28. What patients with PA should be treated medically?

Patients with IHA, GRA, and those with an APA unwilling or unfit to undergo surgery should be treated with chronic medical therapy. Patients with an APA who are planning surgery should also be treated medically before their surgery. Treatment goals are normalization of blood pressure and serum potassium without the need for potassium supplementation and maintenance of the PRA within the normal range.

29. What medications are used to treat PA?

The medications of choice are mineralocorticoid receptor antagonists (MRAs; spironolactone and eplerenone). Spironolactone doses are usually 25 to 200 mg per day; eplerenone doses are usually 25 to 50 mg twice daily. However, higher doses are often required. MRA doses should be titrated up until blood pressure is controlled, PRA is in the normal range and serum potassium levels are normal without the need for potassium supplements. Hypokalemia is corrected immediately, whereas hypertension responds after 4 to 8 weeks.

Because spironolactone interferes with the action of androgens, side effects can include decreased libido, impotence, and gynecomastia in men and menstrual irregularities in women. Eplerenone has 50% of the potency of spironolactone and is more expensive but does not have many of the side effects seen with spironolactone. To avoid the dose-related side effects of spironolactone and reduce the cost of using eplerenone, some providers use a combination of lower doses of the two medications. If blood pressure is not controlled with adequate doses of an MRA, additional blood pressure medications should be added.

30. What other pharmacologic options are available?

In patients intolerant to MRAs, amiloride (5–15 mg twice daily), an epithelial sodium channel antagonist, corrects hypokalemia within several days. A concomitant antihypertensive agent is usually necessary to reduce blood pressure. Success also has been reported in IHA treated with calcium channel blockers (calcium is involved in the final common pathway for aldosterone production) and ACE inhibitors (IHA appears to be sensitive to low concentrations of angiotensin II).

31. What patients with PA should be referred to surgery?

Unilateral laparoscopic adrenalectomy is the procedure of choice for patients with benign unilateral hyperaldosteronism. Fifty percent of patients with APA are able to stop their blood pressure medications postoperatively, and the other half achieves better blood pressure control with a reduced number of blood pressure medications. Nearly all patients remain normokalemic after MRAs are discontinued following successful adrenalectomy. The following three groups of patients should be referred to surgery:

- Patients with unequivocal lateralization of aldosterone hypersecretion on AVS
- Patients with hypertension age < 35 years with spontaneous hypokalemia, PAC > 30 ng/dL, and a unilateral adrenal macroadenoma (1–2 cm) with normal contralateral adrenal morphology (AVS is not needed in this subgroup)
- Patients with aldosterone-producing adrenocortical carcinoma (open adrenalectomy)

32. How should medications for PA be managed in the postoperative period?

The following are general guidelines for postoperative management after successful surgical removal of an APA:
- Reduce all blood pressure medications by 50%.
- Stop all medications that can cause hyperkalemia: spironolactone, eplerenone, ACE inhibitors, ARBs, potassium supplements.

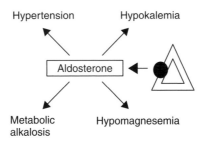

Fig. 32.1 Proposed algorithm for the evaluation and management of primary aldosteronism. (Adapted from Funder, J. W., Carey, R. M., Mantero, F., Murad, M. H., Reincke, M., Shibata, H., ... & Young, W. F., Jr. (2016). The management of primary aldosteronism: case detection, diagnosis, and treatment: an Endocrine Society clinical practice guideline. *Journal of Clinical Endocrinology and Metabolism, 101,* 1889–1916.).

- Monitor blood pressure daily.
- Check serum potassium weekly for 4 weeks.
- Start fludrocortisone if serum K > 5.2 mEq/L.

33. What are other familial forms of PA?
    - Familial hyperaldosteronism type II (FH-II) is an autosomal dominant disorder characterized by unilateral (APA) or bilateral (IHA) excessive aldosterone secretion, which does not suppress with dexamethasone. Patients with this condition are clinically indistinguishable from those with sporadic PA. FH-II is more common than FH-I (GRA). Although the molecular basis for FH-II has not been elucidated, GRA mutation testing is negative in these patients.
    - Familial hyperaldosteronism type III (FH-III) is caused by a mutation in the *KCNJ5* gene coding for the potassium channel Kir3.4, which affects the ion selectivity of the channel, which, in turn, results in increased sodium conductance and chronic cell depolarization. These changes lead to opening of voltage-dependent calcium channels and enhanced calcium signaling, resulting in constitutive aldosterone production and possibly proliferation of glomerulosa cells. Patients with this condition have severe and refractory hypertension requiring bilateral adrenalectomy at a young age for uncontrolled hypertension.

34. Are there any somatic mutations associated with adrenal-producing adenomas?
    In the last few years, somatic mutations in some key proteins in zona glomerulosa cells have been identified in APAs; these mutations constitutively alter the function of potassium and calcium channels and ion pumps. Somatic heterozygous gain-of-function mutations in the *KCNJ5* gene have been shown to cause severe hypertension and hypokalemia. These mutations are more common in women. Likewise, somatic mutations in *ATP1A1*, encoding the alpha-subunit of the Na/K–adenosine triphosphatase (ATPase), and *ATP2B3*, encoding the plasma membrane calcium-transporting ATPase 3 (PMCA3), have also been recently described. These mutations are more common in men. Finally, somatic mutations in the gene *CACNA1D* coding for a voltage-gated calcium channel have been described. These mutation lead to intracellular calcium influx, enhanced calcium signaling, and unilateral hyperaldosteronism (APA).

35. Develop an algorithm for the evaluation and management of patients with PA.
    See Fig. 32.1.

KEY POINTS: PRIMARY ALDOSTERONISM

- Spontaneous hypokalemia in a hypertensive patient should suggest the possibility of primary aldosteronism (PA)—but normokalemic hypertension is the most common presentation.
- PA is usually caused by bilateral adrenal hyperplasia or a small adrenal adenoma.
- The best test for PA case detection is an aldosterone/renin ratio > 20, with a plasma aldosterone concentration > 15 ng/dL.
- PA is confirmed with a 24-hour urine aldosterone > 12 mcg/day after salt loading.
- Because computed tomography and magnetic resonance imaging are often unable to distinguish adenomas from hyperplasia, adrenal venous sampling is often necessary to determine whether the excessive aldosterone secretion is unilateral or bilateral.
- Adenomas are treated surgically; bilateral hyperplasia is treated pharmacologically with aldosterone receptor antagonists (spironolactone and/or eplerenone).
- Glucocorticoid-remediable aldosteronism is treated with physiologic doses of glucocorticoids.

BIBLIOGRAPHY

Choi, M., Scholl, U. I., Yue, P., Björklund, P., Zhao, B., Nelson-Williams, C., , , ... & Lifton, R. P. (2011). K^+ channel mutations in adrenal aldosterone-producing adenomas and secondary hypertension. *Science, 331,* 768–772.

Dluhy, R. G., & Lifton, R. P. (1999). Glucocorticoid-remediable aldosteronism. *Journal of Clinical Endocrinology and Metabolism, 84,* 4341–4344.

Fardella, C. E., Mosso, L., Gomez-Sanchez, C., Cortés, P., Soto, J., Gómez, L., . . . Montero, J. (2000). Primary hyperaldosteronism in essential hypertensives: prevalence, biochemical profile, and molecular biology. *Journal of Clinical Endocrinology and Metabolism, 85,* 1863–1867.

Funder, J. W., Carey, R. M., Mantero, F., Murad, M. H., Reincke, M., Shibata, H., , . . . Young, W. F., Jr. (2016). The management of primary aldosteronism: case detection, diagnosis, and treatment: an Endocrine Society clinical practice guideline. *Journal of Clinical Endocrinology and Metabolism, 101,* 1889–1916.

Jossart, G. H., Burpee, S. E., & Gagner, M. (2000). Surgery of the adrenal glands. *Endocrinology and Metabolism Clinics of North America, 29,* 57–68.

Magill, S. B., Raff, H., Shaker, J. L., Brickner, R. C., Knechtges, T. E., Kehoe, M. E., & Findling, J. W. (2001). Comparison of adrenal vein sampling and computed tomography in the differentiation of primary aldosteronism. *Journal of Clinical Endocrinology and Metabolism, 86,* 1066–1071.

Milliez, P., Girerd, X., Plouin, P. F., Blacher, J., Safar, M. E., & Mourad, J. J. (2005). Evidence for an increased rate of cardiovascular events in patients with primary aldosteronism. *Journal of the American College of Cardiology, 45,* 1243–1248.

Monticone, S., D'Ascenzo, F., Moretti, C., Williams, T. A., Veglio, F., Gaita, F., & Mulatero, P. (2018). Cardiovascular events and target organ damage in primary aldosteronism compared with essential hypertension: a systematic review and meta-analysis. *Lancet Diabetes and Endocrinology, 6,* 41–50.

Mulatero, P., Rabbia, F., Milan, A., Paglieri, C., Morello, F., Chiandussi, L., & Veglio, F. (2002). Drug effects on aldosterone/plasma renin activity ratio in primary aldosteronism. *Hypertension, 40,* 897–902.

Mulatero, P., Stowasser, M., Loh, K., Fardella, C. E., Gordon, R. D., Mosso, L., . . . Young, W. F., Jr. (2004). Increased diagnoses of primary aldosteronism, including surgically correctable forms, in centers from five continents. *Journal of Clinical Endocrinology and Metabolism, 89,* 1045–1050.

Rossi, G. P., Auchus, R. J., Brown, M., Lenders, J. W., Naruse, M., Plouin, P. F., , . . . Young, W. F., Jr. (2014). An expert consensus statement on use of adrenal vein sampling in primary aldosteronism. *Hypertension, 63,* 151–160.

Rossi, G. P., Bernini, G., Caliumi, C., Desideri, G., Fabris, B., Ferri, C., ,... Mantero, F. (2006). A prospective study of the prevalence of primary aldosteronism in 1,125 hypertensive patients. *Journal of the American College of Cardiology, 48,* 2293–2300.

Rossi, G., Bernini, G., Desideri, G., Fabris, B., Ferri, C., Giacchetti, G., Letizia C... Mantero, F. (2006). Renal damage in primary aldosteronism: Results of the PAPY study. *Hypertension, 48,* 232–238.

Rossi, P. (2011). Diagnosis and treatment of primary aldosteronism. *Endocrinology and Metabolism Clinics of North America, 40,* 313–332.

Scholl, U. I., Goh, G., Stölting, G., de Oliveira, R. C., Choi, M., Overton, J. D., , . . . Lifton, R. P. (2013). Somatic and germline CADNA1D calcium-channel mutations in aldosterone-producing adenomas and primary aldosteronism. *Nature Genetics, 45,* 1050–1054.

Schwartz, G. L. (2011). Screening for adrenal-endocrine hypertension: overview of accuracy and cost-effectiveness. *Endocrinology and Metabolism Clinics of North America, 40,* 279–294.

Schwartz, G. L., & Turner, S. T. (2005). Screening for primary aldosteronism in essential hypertension: diagnostic accuracy of the ratio of plasma aldosterone concentration to plasma renin activity. *Clinical Chemistry, 51,* 386–394.

Tanabe, A., Naruse, M., Takagi, S., Tsuchiya, K., Imaki, T., & Takano, K. (2003). Variability in the renin/aldosterone profile under random and standardized sampling conditions in primary aldosteronism. *Journal of Clinical Endocrinology and Metabolism, 88,* 2489–2492.

Tiu, S. C, Choi, C. H., Shek, C. C., Ng, Y. W., Chan, F. K., Ng, C. M., & Kong, A. P. (2005). The use of aldosterone-renin ratio as a diagnostic test for primary hyperaldosteronism and its test characteristics under different conditions of blood sampling. *Journal of Clinical Endocrinology and Metabolism, 90,* 72–78.

Whelton, P. K., Carey, R. M., Aronow, W. S., Casey, D. E., Jr., Collins, K. J., Dennison Himmelfarb, C., . . . Wright, J. T., Jr. (2018). 2017 ACC/AHA/AAPA/ABC/ACPM/AGS/APhA/ASH/ASPC/NMA/PCNA Guideline for the prevention, detection, evaluation, and management of high blood pressure in adults: a report of the American College of Cardiology/American Heart Association Task Force on Clinical Practice Guidelines. *Journal of the American College of Cardiology, 71,* 127–248.

CHAPTER 33

PHEOCHROMOCYTOMAS AND PARAGANGLIOMAS

John J. Orrego

1. What are catecholamine-secreting tumors?

   A pheochromocytoma (PHEO) is an adrenal medullary tumor that arises from chromaffin cells and secretes one or more catecholamines, including epinephrine (EPI), norepinephrine (NE), and dopamine. Approximately 80% to 85% of catecholamine-secreting tumors are PHEOs.

   A paraganglioma (PGL) is an extraadrenal tumor derived from chromaffin cells of the sympathetic paravertebral ganglia of the chest, abdomen, and pelvis, capable of secreting catecholamines. Between 15% and 20% of catecholamine-secreting tumors are PGLs. Nonfunctioning PGLs arising from parasympathetic ganglia located along the vagal and glossopharyngeal nerves in the neck and skull base are termed *head and neck (HN) PGLs*.

   Other neoplasms of the sympathetic ganglia that also arise from neural crest–derived cells, such as neuro-blastomas and ganglioneuromas, may produce similar amines and peptides, but these will not be covered here.

2. How common are catecholamine-secreting tumors?

   PHEOs and functioning PGLs are rare, affecting 0.2% to 0.6% of patients with hypertension in general outpatient clinics. The annual incidence of PHEO is 0.8 per 100,000 person-years. Autopsy studies reveal undiagnosed tumors in 0.05% to 0.1% of people, indicating that many catecholamine-secreting neoplasms go unnoticed during life. About 5% to 10% of patients with adrenal incidentalomas prove to have a PHEO.

3. What are common clinical manifestations of catecholamine-secreting tumors?

   PHEOs and sympathetic PGLs occur with equal frequency in men and women, mainly in the third to fifth decades. About 50% of patients with PHEO/PGL are actually asymptomatic. Symptomatic patients usually have episodic and paroxysmal symptoms including anxiety, diaphoresis, headaches, palpitations, dyspnea, epigastric and chest pain, nausea, and tachycardia. These spells may be either spontaneous or precipitated by postural change, exercise, medications, or maneuvers that increase intraabdominal pressure, and tend to be stereotypical for each patient. The classic triad of sudden severe headaches, diaphoresis, and palpitations is present in a minority of patients and is not pathognomonic of these tumors. Although the most common sign of PHEO is sustained or paroxysmal hypertension, 5% to 15% of patients are normotensive.

   Additional clinical and biochemical manifestations of PHEO/PGLs include orthostatic hypotension (caused by hypovolemia and impaired arterial and venous constriction responses), papilledema, blurred vision, weight loss, constipation (megacolon may be the presenting symptom), livedo reticularis, Raynaud's phenomenon, hyperglyce-mia, leukocytosis, polycythemia, and stress-induced cardiomyopathy. Given the broad variety of clinical manifesta-tions affecting such a variety of organ systems, PHEO/PLGs are known as the "great mimickers."

4. What is the "rule of 10" for PHEOs?

   This rule has been quoted for describing the characteristics of PHEOs: 10% are extraadrenal (PGLs), 10% are multiple or bilateral, 10% are malignant, 10% occur in children, and 10% are familial. Because current estimates indicate that 15% to 20% of PHEOs are extraadrenal, 10% to 20% are malignant, 10% to 20% occur in pediatric patients, and up to 40% are hereditary, the "rule of 10" for PHEOs has become obsolete.

5. Discuss the cardiovascular manifestations of PHEOs and PGLs.

   Cardiovascular manifestations of PHEO/PGLs include arrhythmias and catecholamine-induced cardiomyopathy (Takotsubo cardiomyopathy). Atrial and ventricular fibrillation commonly result from precipitous release of cate-cholamines during surgery or from therapy with tricyclic antidepressants, phenothiazines, metoclopramide, opioid analgesics, and neuromuscular blocking agents. Although pulmonary edema may result from cardiomyopathy, noncardiogenic pulmonary edema may also occur as a result of transient pulmonary vasoconstriction and increased capillary permeability. Blood pressure lability, a common manifestation of these tumors, is caused by episodic catecholamine secretion, chronic hypovolemia, and impaired sympathetic reflexes.

6. Describe the intracerebral symptoms related to PHEOs and PGLs.

   Seizures, altered mental status, and cerebral infarctions may occur as a result of intracerebral hemorrhage or embolization. Malignant hypertension with papilledema, decreased mentation, and cerebral edema has also been described. Rarely, patients have presented with reversible cerebral vasoconstriction or vasculitis.

7. What are some of the nonclassic manifestations of catecholamine-secreting tumors?

Signs and symptoms of other endocrine disorders may dominate the presentation of a PHEO/PGL. Tumors may elaborate corticotropin (adrenocorticotropic hormone) with resultant manifestations of Cushing's syndrome and hypokalemic alkalosis. Vasoactive intestinal peptide may be produced, causing severe diarrhea and hypokalemia. Hyperglycemia, resulting from catecholamine-induced antagonism of insulin release, and hypercalcemia, caused by adrenergic stimulation of the parathyroid glands or elaboration of parathyroid hormone-related peptide, have also been described. Lactic acidosis may occur as a result of catecholamine-associated disturbance in tissue oxygen delivery.

8. Can PHEOs and PGLs metastasize?

Yes. Demonstration of a metastatic focus in tissue normally devoid of chromaffin cells is the only accepted indication that a PHEO/PGL is malignant. Local invasion into surrounding tissues or organs or distant metastases occur in 10% to 20% of PHEOs and 15% to 35% of sympathetic PGLs. The most common sites of distant metastases are regional lymph nodes, liver, bone, lung, and muscle. Mutations of succinate dehydrogenase subunit B (SDHB) lead to metastatic disease in 40% of affected individuals.

9. Where are PHEOs located?

Approximately 80% to 85% of catecholamine-secreting tumors arise within the adrenal glands, whereas 15% to 20% are extraadrenal (sympathetic PGLs). Nearly 95% of PHEO/PGLs are found in the abdomen. Sporadic, solitary PHEOs are located more commonly in the right adrenal gland, whereas familial forms tend to be bilateral and multicentric. Bilateral adrenal tumors raise the possibility of multiple endocrine neoplasia 2A or 2B (MEN 2A or MEN 2B) syndromes.

10. Where are PGLs located?

Sympathetic PGLs have ubiquitous distribution and can originate along the entire sympathetic paraganglia chain, from the skull base to the pelvic floor. Most PGLs arise in the abdomen, most often at the junction of the vena cava and the left renal vein, or at the organ of Zuckerkandl, which resides at the aortic bifurcation near the take-off of the inferior mesenteric artery. Other locations are the thorax, including the pericardium, the bladder, and the prostate gland.

11. What do PHEOs and PGLs elaborate?

Catecholamine-secreting tumors synthetize NE, EPI, and dopamine. Most PHEOs and PGLs secrete NE. Tumors that produce EPI are more commonly intraadrenal because the extraadrenal sympathetic ganglia do not contain the enzyme phenylethanolamine N-methyltransferase (PNMT), which converts NE to EPI. Dopamine is most commonly associated with PGLs and malignant tumors.

PHEO/PGLs can be classified in noradrenergic, adrenergic, and dopaminergic phenotypes, based on predominant production of respective normetanephrine, metanephrine, and 3-methoxytyramine relative to combined production of all three metabolites. The location, the presence or absence of metastases, and the specific phenotype of the PHEO/PGL can be used to generate a decisional algorithm for genetic testing.

12. How are catecholamines synthetized?

Catecholamines are synthetized from tyrosine, which enters chromaffin cells by active transport. Tyrosine is converted to dopa by tyrosine hydroxylase, the rate-limiting step in catecholamine synthesis. Dopa is decarboxylated to dopamine by aromatic L-amino acid decarboxylase. Dopamine is actively transported into granulated vesicles where it is hydroxylated to NE by dopamine beta-hydroxylase. In the adrenal medulla, NE is released into the cytoplasm where it is converted to EPI by PNMT. EPI is then transported back into storage vesicles. In the extraadrenal sympathetic ganglia, which do not contain PNMT, NE cannot be converted to EPI.

13. How are catecholamines metabolized?

Catecholamines are cleared from the circulation either by reuptake in sympathetic nerve terminals or by metabolism through two enzymatic pathways, followed by sulfate conjugation and renal excretion. Catechol-O-methyltransferase (COMT) converts EPI to metanephrine and NE to normetanephrine. Metanephrine and normetanephrine are oxidized to vanillylmandelic acid (VMA) by monoamine oxidase (MAO). EPI and NE are also oxidized by MAO to dihydroxymandelic acid, which is then converted to VMA by COMT. Dopamine is metabolized by COMT to 3-methoxytyramine, which is subsequently converted to homovanillic acid (HVA) by MAO.

14. Describe the adrenergic receptors that bind circulating catecholamines.

There are two types and five subtypes of adrenergic receptors that mediate the biologic actions of catecholamines:
- Alpha-1 is a postsynaptic receptor that, when stimulated, causes vasoconstriction and increases blood pressure. Alpha-2 is a presynaptic receptor that, when activated, decreases blood pressure by inhibiting NE secretion and reducing central sympathetic outflow.
- Beta-1 mediates cardiac effects; stimulation causes positive inotropic and chronotropic effects on the heart, increased renin secretion in the kidney, and lipolysis in adipocytes. Beta-2 mediates bronchial and vascular

effects; stimulation causes bronchodilation, vasodilation in skeletal muscle, glycogenolysis, and increased NE release from sympathetic nerve endings. Beta-3 regulates energy expenditure and lipolysis.

15. Why is the blood pressure response among patients with PHEOs so variable?
    1. PHEOs elaborate different biogenic amines. NE is a direct-acting adrenergic agonist with activity at both alpha-1 and beta-1 receptors. It is similar to EPI except that NE lacks the beta-2-effect of EPI and has much stronger alpha-1 activity. EPI, however, has more affinity for the alpha-2 receptor compared with NE. Most PHEOs/PGLs produce NE, thus causing chronic or episodic hypertension in many of them. Less than 10% of PHEOs secrete predominantly EPI, which may cause postural hypotension or episodic bouts of hypertension alternating with hypotension.
    2. Tumor size indirectly correlates with plasma catecholamine concentrations. Large tumors ($>$ 50 g) manifest slow turnover rates and release catecholamine degradation products, whereas small tumors ($<$ 50 g) with rapid turnover rates elaborate more active catecholamines.
    3. Tissue responsiveness to ambient catecholamine concentrations does not remain constant. Prolonged exposure of tissue to increased plasma catecholamines causes downregulation of alpha-1 receptors and tachyphylaxis. Plasma catecholamine levels, therefore, do not correlate with mean arterial pressure.

16. How are catecholamine-secreting tumors diagnosed?
    The diagnosis of PHEOs/PGLs depends on the demonstration of excessive plasma or urine catecholamine levels or urine degradation products. Despite consistently high plasma concentrations of normetanephrine or metanephrine, some patients with PHEO/PGL have normal plasma concentrations of catecholamines or only have high concentrations during paroxysmal attacks. The silent or intermittently secreting tumors in these patients are, therefore, continuously metabolizing catecholamines to metanephrines, without consistently secreting the parent amines into the circulation. This is why it is recommended to measure plasma free metanephrines or urinary fractionated metanephrines for initial biochemical testing. Normal plasma or urinary metanephrines reliably exclude PHEO/PGL. Three- to fourfold elevations of plasma free metanephrines are associated with nearly 100% probability of a catecholamine-secreting tumor. Plasma free metanephrines should be drawn from an indwelling catheter with the patient supine for 30 minutes after an overnight fast. When plasma or urine fractionated metanephrine levels are equivocal, further testing is warranted. In the rare cases of PGLs that produce predominantly or exclusively dopamine, because these tumors are often deficient in dopamine beta-hydroxylase, the enzyme that converts dopamine to NE, fasting plasma free methoxytyramine, should be obtained.

17. What is the differential diagnosis of hyperadrenergic spells?
    Other psychological, neurologic, pharmacologic, endocrine, and cardiovascular etiologies of hyperadrenergic spells include panic disorder, hyperventilation, postural orthostatic tachycardia syndrome, diencephalic epilepsy, migraine headaches, cocaine ingestion, withdrawal of adrenergic inhibitor, sympathomimetic drug ingestion, hypoglycemia, thyrotoxicosis, labile primary hypertension, orthostatic hypotension, paroxysmal cardiac arrhythmia, idiopathic flushing, and diaphoretic spells.

18. What medications may cause falsely elevated plasma or urinary metanephrines?
    False-positive results for plasma or urinary metanephrines may result from taking medications that directly interfere with measurement methods (acetaminophen, mesalamine, and sulfasalazine in liquid chromatography electrochemical detection methods) or that interfere with the disposition of catecholamines (tricyclic antidepressants, cocaine, sympathomimetics, and MAO inhibitors).

19. What medications may cause interference with measurements of catecholamines?
    - Tricyclic antidepressants block NE reuptake, raising urinary NE, normetanephrine, and VMA.
    - Levodopa is metabolized by enzymes that also metabolize catecholamines.
    - Caffeine, nicotine, and sympathomimetics increase plasma and urinary catecholamines.
    - Calcium-channel blockers increase plasma catecholamines as a result of sympathetic activation.
    - Phenoxybenzamine blocks presynaptic alpha-2 adrenoreceptors, causing increases in plasma and urinary NE, normetanephrine, and VMA.

20. What is the clonidine suppression test?
    In cases in which plasma normetanephrine levels are only mildly elevated because of increased sympathetic activity rather than secondary to a catecholamine-secreting tumor, a clonidine suppression test may be indicated. This test employs a centrally acting alpha-2 adrenoreceptor agonist that inhibits neuronal NE release in patients without PHEO/PGL but not in patients with autonomous tumoral catecholamine secretion. Sympatholytic drugs (i.e., beta-blockers) must be discontinued at least 48 hours before testing. After 20 minutes of supine rest, baseline plasma free fractionated metanephrines are obtained from an indwelling venous catheter. Clonidine 0.3 mg is administered and blood pressure and pulse are measured every 30 minutes. A second blood sample is drawn 3 hours into the test. A positive test is obtained when the plasma normetanephrine level at 3 hours does not drop by $>$ 40% compared with the initial value.

21. What is the best diagnostic method to localize a PHEO or PGL?

It is important to emphasize that imaging studies should only be ordered when the diagnosis of PHEO/PGL has been clearly established. The majority of tumors are > 3 cm, rendering them detectable by computed tomography (CT) or magnetic resonance imaging (MRI). CT of the abdomen and pelvis is advocated as the initial localizing procedure (95% are intraabdominal). The use of nonionic contrast is safe and, therefore, can be used in these patients without adrenergic receptor blockade. CT is the most cost-effective means of localization. MRI is recommended in patients with metastatic PHEO/PGL, in patients with an allergy to CT contrast, in children and pregnant women, and for detection of skull base and neck PGLs. Advantages of MRI include the lack of radiation exposure and a characteristic hyperintense image on T2-weighted scans.

22. What other modalities are useful for localization of PHEOs?

Scintigraphic localization with ^{123}I-metaiodobenzylguanidine (MIBG) may also reveal unsuspected metastases. MIBG is actively concentrated by sympathomedullary tissue and is subject to interference by drugs that block reuptake of catecholamines (tricyclic antidepressants, calcium-channel blockers, labetalol).

Fluorodeoxyglucose positron emission tomography/CT (^{18}F-FDG PET/CT) is the preferred imaging study over ^{123}I-MIBG scintigraphy in patients with known metastatic PHEO/PGL.

PHEO/PGL express somatostatin receptors, enabling imaging with ^{68}Ga-DOTA-coupled peptides such as DOTATATE. ^{68}Ga-DOTATATE PET/CT has significantly greater lesion-to-background contrast compared with ^{18}F-FDG PET/CT.

23. What patients with PHEO or PGL should undergo genetic testing?

Many experts in the field recommend genetic testing in all patients presenting with PHEOs/PGLs. The rationale for this is that 30% to 40% of patients with these tumors have disease-causing germ-line mutations; therefore, confirming a hereditary syndrome in the proband may result in early detection in relatives. In view of the financial costs, however, genetic counseling and genetic testing could also be limited to patients with bilateral PHEOs, multiple PGLs, positive family history, and young age at presentation.

PHEO/PGL susceptibility genes include *NF1*, *RET*, *VHL*, *SDHA*, *SDHB*, *SDHC*, *SDHD*, *SDHAF2*, *EPAS1*, *TMEM127*, and *MAX*.

24. How are PHEOs and PGLs treated?

Surgical resection is the only definitive therapy. Laparoscopic adrenalectomy is recommended for most PHEOs. Open resection is recommended for large or invasive PHEOs to ensure complete tumor resection and prevent tumor rupture.

For PGLs, although open resection is suggested, laparoscopic resection can be an option in patients with small and noninvasive PGLs in surgically favorable locations.

25. Why is preoperative preparation with alpha blockade recommended?

Alpha blockade, started 10 to 14 days before surgery, reduces the incidence of serious and potentially life-threatening catecholamine-induced perioperative complications, including hypertensive crises, cardiac arrhythmias, cardiac ischemia, and pulmonary edema. With adequate pretreatment, perioperative mortality has fallen to less than 3%. Retrospective studies support the use of alpha-blockers as the first-choice drug class. Either phenoxybenzamine (longer acting, noncompetitive alpha-blocker) or doxazosin (shorter acting, competitive alpha-blocker) are the first-line therapy. Phenoxybenzamine is started at 10 mg twice daily and advanced up to 80 to 100 mg/day as needed and tolerated. Doxazosin is started at 2 to 4 mg per day, and advanced up to 32 mg daily.

26. Discuss the role of beta-blockers and other agents in the preoperative period.

The use of beta-blockers is indicated to control tachycardia only after administration of alpha-blockers. The initiation of the former in the absence of the latter may precipitate a hypertensive crisis resulting from unopposed stimulation of alpha-adrenergic receptors. Both beta-1-selective and nonselective beta-adrenergic receptor blockers can be used. Atenolol 25 to 50 mg per day or propranolol 20 to 40 mg three times per day should be started at least 3 days after alpha-blockers have been initiated.

Calcium channel blockers are the most often used add-on drug class to further improve blood pressure control in patients already taking alpha-blockers. Labetalol, which has more potent beta than alpha antagonistic activity, should be avoided as initial therapy. Intraoperative hypertension associated with tumor manipulation may be controlled with either phentolamine or nitroprusside.

Postoperative hypotension may be minimized by high fluid intake and a diet rich in sodium, started 3 to 4 days before surgery.

27. What are the goals of preoperative therapy?

The goals of preoperative therapy include blood pressure reduction to $< 130/80$ mm Hg while seated and systolic blood pressure > 90 mm Hg while standing, with a heart rate of 60 to 70 beats per minute seated and 70 to 80 beats per minute standing.

28. **How are malignant PHEOs treated?**
There are no curative treatments for metastatic PHEO/PGLs. Alpha- and beta-blockade are used to control symptoms of catecholamine excess. Surgical resection or debulking is the therapy of choice. For patients with unresectable disease, other treatment modalities are available, including external beam radiation therapy for painful bone metastases, percutaneous radiofrequency ablation or transarterial chemoembolization for liver metastases, and cryoablation or percutaneous ethanol injection for metastatic lesions at a variety of sites.

29. **Discuss the role of ^{131}I-MIBG ablation and chemotherapy.**
Treatment with ^{131}I-MIBG should be considered in patients with a positive ^{123}I-MIBG scan by dosimetry when there are unresectable progressive tumors not amenable to locoregional methods of control. Other therapies for which partial tumor responses have been reported in patients with progressive disease include chemotherapy with cyclophosphamide and vincristine, and peptide receptor radionuclide therapy using ^{177}Lu-Dotatate. Encouraging partial responses have also been recently reported with the tyrosine kinase inhibitors, sunitnib, and cabozantinib.

30. **What is the prognosis for malignant PHEOs and PGLs?**
The clinical course of patients with malignant PHEOs/PGLs is extremely variable, with some patients living > 50 years after diagnosis. Recent data suggest that overall 5- and 10-year survival rates are 85% and 72.5%, respectively. Rapid disease progression is associated with male gender, older age, larger tumor size, synchronous metastases, elevated dopamine, and not resecting the primary tumor.

31. **What is the molecular taxonomy of catecholamine-secreting tumors?**
    1. *Pseudohypoxic PHEO/PGL:* Under pseudohypoxia (a situation where oxygen is present but cannot be processed because of an alteration in oxygen-sensing pathways), hypoxia-inducible factors are produced in large amounts leading to transcription of hypoxia-responsive genes, which are involved in tumorigenesis.
        * *TCA cycle related:* A majority of patients have familial PGLs associated with mutations in SDHx (x = A, B, C, D, or AF2). Mutations of these genes prevent the oxidation of succinate to fumarate, affecting the respiratory electron transfer chain. A minority of patients have pathogenic mutations in fumarate hydratase, which prevent the conversion from fumarate to malonate.
        * *VHL/EPAS1 related:* Patients with germline mutations in VHL and germline or mosaic gain-of-function mutations in *EPAS1* have von Hippel-Lindau syndrome and Pacak-Zhuang syndrome, respectively.
    2. *Wnt signaling PHEO/PGL:* These patients have sporadic disease associated with mutually exclusive somatic mutations in CSDE1 or somatic gene fusions of *UBTF-MAML3* in chromaffin cells that activate the Wnt and Hedgehog signaling pathways, leading to tumorigenesis.
    3. *Kinase signaling PHEO/PGL:*
        * *Germline mutations:* The most common syndrome in this subgroup is MEN 2, which is caused by gain-of-function mutations in *RET*. A minority of patients have pathogenic mutations in *NF1* (neurofibromatosis type 1) and *TMEM127* and *MAX* (familial paraganglioma syndromes). These cases result from activation of kinase signaling pathways that induce tumorigenesis: RAS-RAF-MEK and PI3K-AKT-mTOR (RET), NF1, TMEM127, and MYC-MAX (MAX)
        * *Somatic mutations:* Some sporadic cases have been found to have gain-of-function mutations in the *HRAS* protooncogene.

32. **What syndromes are associated with PHEOs and PGLs?**
    * *MEN 2A:* Medullary thyroid carcinoma (MTC), primary hyperparathyroidism, and PHEO
    * *MEN 2B:* MTC, PHEO, marfanoid habitus, mucosal neuromas, and intestinal ganglioneuromatosis
    * *von Hippel-Lindau (VHL) syndrome type 2:* cerebellar, spinal, and retinal hemangioblastoma, clear-cell renal cell carcinoma, pancreatic neuroendocrine tumor, endolymphatic sac tumor of the middle ear, serous cystadenoma of the pancreas, and PHEO/PGL
    * *NF1:* Peripheral neurofibromas, café-au-lait spots, axillary freckling, optic glioma, Lisch's nodules, and PHEO. One percent of patients with NF1 have PHEOs
    * *Familial PGL syndromes type 1 to 5:* different combinations of multiple thoracic and abdominal PGLs, head and neck PGLs, and PHEOs.
    * *Carney triad:* PGL, gastrointestinal stromal tumor (GIST), and pulmonary chondroma
    * *Carney-Stratakis syndrome:* PGL and GIST
    * *Pacak-Zhuang syndrome:* PGL, somatostatinoma, and polycythemia
    * *Hereditary leiomyomatosis and renal cell cancer:* some patients also have PGLs

KEY POINTS: PHEOCHROMOCYTOMA

* Paroxysmal hyperadrenergic spells (headache, diaphoresis, palpitations, pallor, and anxiety) in a hypertensive patient suggest pheochromocytoma/paraganglioma (PHEO/PGL).
* About 80% to 85% of catecholamine-secreting tumors are PHEOs, and 15% to 20% are PGLs.

KEY POINTS: PHEOCHROMOCYTOMA—cont'd

- The best screening tests for PHEO/PGLs are fractionated urinary or plasma free metanephrines.
- Tumor localization is accomplished with computed tomography (most cost effective) or magnetic resonance imaging.
- Therapy is surgical resection after administration of alpha blockade followed by beta blockade.
- About 30% to 40% of patients with PHEO/PGL have a disease-causing germline mutation.

BIBLIOGRAPHY

Crona, J., Taieb, D., & Pacak, K. (2017). New perspectives on pheochromocytoma and paraganglioma: toward a molecular classification. *Endocrinology Review, 38*, 489–515.

Eisenhofer, G., Goldstein, D. S., Sullivan, P., Csako, G., Brouwers, F. M., Lai, E. W., . . . Pacak, K. (2005). Biochemical and clinical manifestations of dopamine-producing paragangliomas: utility of plasma methoxytyramine. *Journal of Clinical Endocrinology and Metabolism, 90*, 2068–2075.

Fishbein, L., Leshchiner, I., Walter, V., Danilova, L., Robertson, A. G., Johnson, A. R., . . . Wilkerson, M. D. (2017). Comprehensive molecular characterization of pheochromocytoma and paraganglioma. *Cancer Cell, 31*, 181–193.

Hamidi, O., Young, W. F., Jr., Iniguez-Ariza, N. M., Kittah, N. E., Gruber, L., Bancos, C., . . . Bancos, I. (2017). Malignant pheochromocytoma and paraganglioma: 272 patients over 55 years. *Journal of Clinical Endocrinology and Metabolism, 102*, 3296–3305.

Jossart, G. H., Burpee, S. E., & Gagner, M. (2000). Surgery of the adrenal glands. *Endocrinology and Metabolism Clinics of North America, 29*, 57–68.

Krane, N. K. (1986). Clinically unsuspected pheochromocytomas: experience at Henry Ford Hospital and a review of the literature. *Archives of Internal Medicine, 146*, 54–57.

Kudva, Y. C., Sawka, A. M., & Young, W. F. (2003). The laboratory diagnosis of adrenal pheochromocytoma: the Mayo Clinic experience. *Journal of Clinical Endocrinology and Metabolism, 88*, 4533–4539.

Lenders, J. W., Pacak, K., Walther, M. M., Linehan, W. M., Mannelli, M., Friberg, P., . . . Eisenhofer, G. (2002). Biochemical diagnosis of pheochromocytoma: which test is best? *Journal of the American Medical Association, 287*, 1427–1434.

Lenders, J. W. M., Duh, Q. Y., Eisenhofer, G., Gimenez-Roqueplo, A. P., Grebe, S. K., Murad, M. H., . . . Young, W. F., Jr.; (2014). Pheochromocytoma and paraganglioma: an Endocrine Society clinical practice guideline. *Journal of Clinical Endocrinology and Metabolism, 99*, 1915–1942.

Neumann, H. P., & Eng, C. (2009). The approach to the patient with paraganglioma. *Journal of Clinical Endocrinology and Metabolism, 94*, 2677–2683.

Pacak, K. (2007). Preoperative management of the pheochromocytoma patient. *Journal of Clinical Endocrinology and Metabolism, 92*, 4069–4079.

Prys-Roberts, C. (2000). Phaeochromocytoma—recent progress in its management. *British Journal of Anaesthesiology, 85*, 44–57.

Schwartz, G. L. (2011). Screening for adrenal-endocrine hypertension: overview of accuracy and cost-effectiveness. *Endocrinology and Metabolism Clinics of North America, 40*, 279–294.

Wittles, R. M., Kaplan, E. L., & Roizen, M. F. (2000). Sensitivity of diagnostic and localization tests for pheochromocytoma in clinical practice. *Archives of Internal Medicine, 160*, 2521–2524.

Xekouki, P., & Stratakis, C. A. (2011). Pheochromocytoma. *Translational Endocrinology Metabolism, 2*, 77–127.

Zuber, S. M., Kantorovich, V., & Pacak, K. (2011). Hypertension in pheochromocytoma: characteristics and treatment. *Endocrinology and Metabolism Clinics of North America, 40*, 295–311.

CHAPTER 34

ADRENAL INCIDENTALOMAS

Michael T. McDermott

1. What is the definition of adrenal incidentaloma?

   Adrenal incidentalomas are adrenal masses > 1 cm in largest dimension that are discovered incidentally during abdominal imaging procedures that are ordered for unrelated reasons. Adrenal incidentalomas may be unilateral or bilateral.

2. How common are incidentally discovered adrenal masses?

   Adrenal incidentalomas have been estimated, on the basis of findings from large studies, to be present in approximately 4% of all people undergoing abdominal computed tomography (CT). They are more common in older individuals, with an estimated prevalence of 10%. Unilateral adrenal masses account for 85% to 90% of incidentalomas, whereas 10% to 15% are bilateral.

3. What are the most common etiologies of a unilateral adrenal incidentaloma?

   Unilateral adrenal incidentalomas most often are caused by benign adrenal cortical adenomas, pheochromocytomas, adrenocortical carcinomas, metastatic cancer, and myelolipomas.

4. What are the most common causes of bilateral adrenal incidentalomas?

   Bilateral adrenal incidentalomas are most often a result of metastatic cancer, congenital adrenal hyperplasia, nonfunctioning adrenal adenomas, primary aldosteronism (PA; bilateral adrenal hyperplasia and other bilateral conditions), pheochromocytoma (especially familial), adrenocorticotropic hormone (ACTH)–dependent Cushing's syndrome (ACTH-secreting pituitary adenomas, ectopic ACTH-secreting tumors), bilateral macronodular adrenal hyperplasia, adrenal hemorrhage (most often in the setting of systemic anticoagulation), tuberculosis, deep fungal infections, lymphomas, and infiltrative diseases (amyloidosis, hemochromatosis).

5. What are the goals of the diagnostic evaluation of adrenal incidentalomas?

   The goal for evaluating unilateral adrenal incidentalomas is to determine whether the adrenal mass is malignant or if the mass is secreting adrenal cortical or medullary hormones. Approximately 2% of adrenal incidentalomas are malignant, and about 10% secrete excess hormones. For bilateral adrenal masses, the goal is to rule in or out these same conditions in addition to the disorders, listed above, that cause enlargement or masses in both adrenal glands.

6. What imaging studies are most useful in the evaluaton of adrenal incidentalomas?

   A non–contrast-enhanced CT (NCCT) of the abdomen is the best overall imaging test to assess incidentally discovered adrenal masses. Features on CT that suggest a benign adenoma are size < 4 cm, homogeneity, smooth borders, and high lipid content. Lipid content is assessed by signal attenuation, expressed in Hounsfield units (HUs); low HUs (< 10) are indicative of high lipid content (benign adenoma). In contrast, adrenocortical cancers, pheochromocytomas, and metastatic cancers are characterized by low lipid content and high HUs (> 20). Other features that suggest adrenocortical cancer are size > 4 cm, heterogeneity, calcifications, irregular borders, local invasion, and lymphadenopathy. Alternatively, magnetic resonance imaging (MRI) may be used for this evaluation.

   Table 34.1 shows a more extensive adrenal mass. A CT protocol is employed in many institutions utilizing NCCT, followed by contrast-enhanced CT, delayed contrast-enhanced CT (10–15 minutes postcontrast injection), and calculation of relative washout percentage (RWP).

   Table 34.2 shows features of various adrenal masses found on MRI. Adrenal adenomas are bright on in-phase imaging but lose the signal on out-of-phase images. Adenomas show mild enhancement and rapid washout with gadolinium diethylene pentaacetic acid administration, whereas malignant tumors show rapid, robust enhancement, and slower washout.

7. What are the most common hormone syndromes caused by functioning adrenal incidentalomas?

   Approximately 10% of adrenal incidentalomas secrete adrenal cortical or medullary hormones. The most common hormone syndromes among these are Cushing's syndrome ($\approx$ 6%), pheochromocytoma ($\approx$ 3%), and PA ($\approx$ 0.6%).

8. What are the best tests to evaluate for excess cortisol secretion by an adrenal incidentaloma?

   An overnight 1-mg dexamethasone suppression test is considered the best overall test to assess for autonomous cortisol secretion. Dexamethasone 1 mg is given at bedtime, and serum cortisol is drawn at 8 AM the next morning. A normal serum cortisol value the morning after taking dexamethasone is < 1.8 mcg/dL. Serum cortisol

Table 34.1. CT Adrenal Mass Protocol.

	NCCT	CECT	DCECT	RWP
Adenoma	< 10 HU	Enhances	< 30 HU	> 50%
Carcinoma	> 20 HU		> 30 HU	< 50%
Pheochromocytoma	> 20 HU		> 30 HU	< 50%
Metastatic cancer	> 20 HU		> 30 HU	< 50%

CT, Computed tomography; *CECT,* contrast-enhanced CT; *DCECT,* delayed contrast-enhanced CT; *HU,* Hounsfield unit; *NCCT,* non–contrast-enhanced CT; *RWP,* relative washout percentage.

Table 34.2. Magnetic Resonance Imaging of Adrenal Mass (Compared with Liver: T1 / T2 Weighted Images).

Adenoma	Intensity versus liver: isodense (T1 and T2); chemical shift, indicative of high lipid content
Carcinoma	Intensity versus liver: lower (T1); high/intermediate (T2)
Pheochromocytoma	Intensity versus liver: high (T2)
Metastatic cancer	Intensity versus liver: isodense or low (T1); high/intermediate (T2)

values > 5 mcg/dL indicate autonomous cortisol secretion. Borderline serum cortisol values of 1.8 to 5.0 mcg/dL merit repeat testing later.

Dehydroepiandrosterone sulfate (DHEAS) is secreted by the adrenal glands under the regulation of ACTH; the half-life of DHEAS is 10 to 16 hours. DHEAS, therefore, represents a durable indicator of endogenous ACTH secretion. Excess cortisol production from an adrenal adenoma suppresses ACTH secretion, resulting in a low serum DHEAS level. A 2017 study demonstrated that a DHEAS ratio ≤ 1.12 (DHEAS ratio—divide DHEAS level by the lower limit of the DHEAS reference range) has 99% sensitivity and 92% specificity for autonomous cortisol secretion. This test, therefore, appears to be useful and complementary to the dexamethasone suppression test.

9. What tests are recommended to determine whether an adrenal incidentaloma is a pheochromocytoma?
   Pheochromocytomas often have a characteristic imaging phenotype on CT and MRI (see above). If imaging features are suggestive of a pheochromocytoma (high pretest probability), a test with high sensitivity is preferred; plasma metanephrines (sensitivity 95%–98%; specificity 89%–95%) is the preferred test in this situation. If imaging is not strongly suggestive of a pheochromocytoma (low-to-moderate pretest probability), a test with higher specificity is best. Measurement of 24-hour urinary metanephrines and catecholamines are recommended in this situation.

10. When and how should a patient with an adrenal incidentaloma be assessed for PA?
    Testing for PA in the setting of an adrenal incidentaloma is recommended only in patients who also have hypertension. In this situation, plasma aldosterone and plasma renin activity should be measured.

11. Summarize the overall hormone evaluation for an adrenal incidentaloma.
    An outline of the recommended evaluation is shown in Table 34.3.

Table 34.3. Recommended Hormone Evaluation for Adrenal Incidentalomas.

All Patients
Overnight dexamethasone suppression test (1 mg)
Dehydroepiandrosterone sulfate (DHEAS)

Hypertension Present
Plasma aldosterone and plasma renin activity

Imaging Suggestive of Pheochromocytoma (Pretest Probability High)
Plasma metanephrines

Imaging Not Strongly Suggestive of Pheochromocytoma
24-hour urine metanephrines and catecholamines

Table 34.4. Recommended Management of Adrenal Incidentalomas.

Surgery Recommended or Should be Strongly Considered
Adrenocortical carcinoma diagnosed or suspected
Cushing's syndrome with clinical features (diabetes, hypertension, osteoporosis)
Pheochromocytoma diagnosed or suspected
Primary aldosteronism diagnosed
Mass > 4 cm
Mass increases by > 1 cm during serial monitoring

Surgery or Monitoring May be Considered
Subclinical Cushing's syndrome without clinical features (diabetes, hypertension, osteoporosis)

12. When should biopsy of an adrenal mass be performed?
A biopsy should be considered when an adrenal mass is discovered in a patient who has another primary malignancy with known metastases to determine whether the adrenal mass is metastatic cancer. Biopsy of an adrenal mass should be strictly avoided if suspicion for adrenocortical carcinoma or pheochromocytoma is moderate to high. Biopsy of an adrenocortical carcinoma poses a significant risk of malignant cell spillage from the tumor. Biopsy of a pheochromocytoma can precipitate a hypertensive crisis because of sudden release of large amounts of catecholamines from the tumor.

13. How should the incidentally discovered adrenal mass be managed?
An outline of the recommended management is shown in Table 34.4.

14. When surgery is not performed, how should an adrenal incidentaloma be monitored?
Surgery is not recommended if an adrenal incidentaloma appears to be a benign adenoma that does not exhibit hormone secretion. In these cases, repeat cross-sectional imaging (CT, MRI) is recommended 6 to 12 months after the initial evaluation. If there is no growth, further imaging may not be necessary, but clinical judgment must be used. If the mass enlarges by > 1 cm surgery is recommended because it may be an adrenocortical carcinoma diagnosed at an early stage. It is now recommended that the overnight 1-mg dexamethasone suppression test be repeated yearly for 4 years because autonomous cortisol secretion can be subtle and often increases over time. If other hormone testing was normal on the initial evaluation, repeat testing for hormone excess, other than cortisol, is not necessary.

KEY POINTS

- Incidentally discovered adrenal masses are most often benign nonfunctioning adrenal cortical adenomas.
- The goal of evaluation of adrenal incidentaloma is to determine whether the mass is malignant or is secreting excess adrenal hormones.
- The different types of adrenal masses often have characteristic phenotypes on cross-sectional imaging that make or strongly suggest a specific diagnosis.
- The most common hormonal abnormality seen with adrenal incidentalomas is autonomous cortisol secretion.
- Adrenal biopsies should not be done if there is any suspicion that the adrenal mass is an adrenocortical carcinoma or pheochromocytoma.
- Surgery is indicated for adrenal incidentalomas when they are diagnostic of or suspicious for adrenocortical carcinoma or pheochromocytoma, if they secrete excess adrenal hormones, if they are > 4 cm in size, or if they grow by > 1 cm on follow-up imaging studies.

BIBLIOGRAPHY

Dennedy, M. C., Annamalai, A. K., Prankerd-Smith, O., Freeman, N., Vengopal, K., Graggaber, J., . . . & Gurnell, M. (2017). Low DHEAS: a sensitive and specific test for the detection of subclinical hypercortisolism in adrenal incidentalomas. *Journal of Clinical Endocrinology and Metabolism, 102*, 786–792.

Dinnes, J., Bancos, I., Ferrante di Ruffano, L., Chortis, V., Davenport, C., Bayliss, S., . . . Arlt, W. (2016). Management of endocrine disease: Imaging for the diagnosis of malignancy in incidentally discovered adrenal masses: a systematic review and meta-analysis. *European Journal of Endocrinology, 175*, R51–R64.

Fassnacht, M., Arlt, W., Bancos, I., Dralle, H., Newell-Price, J., Sahdev, A., . . . Dekkers, O. M. (2016). Management of adrenal incidentalomas: European Society of Endocrinology clinical practice guideline in collaboration with the European Network for the Study of Adrenal Tumors. *European Journal of Endocrinology, 175*, G1–G34.

Morelli, V., Reimondo, G., Giordano, R., Della Casa, S., Policola, C., Palmieri, S., . . . Chiodoni, I. (2014). Long-term follow-up in adrenal incidentalomas: an Italian multicenter study. *Journal of Clinical Endocrinology and Metabolism, 99*, 827–834.

Nieman, L. K., Biller, B. M., Findling, J. W., Newell-Price, J., Savage, M. O., Stewart, P. M., & Montori, V. M. (2008). The diagnosis of Cushing's syndrome: an Endocrine Society Clinical Practice Guideline. *Journal of Clinical Endocrinology and Metabolism, 93*, 1526–1540.

Nieman, L. K. (2010). Approach to the patient with an adrenal incidentaloma. *Journal of Clinical Endocrinology and Metabolism, 95*, 4106–4113.

Terzolo, M., Stigliano, A., Chiodini, I., Loli, P., Furlani, L., Arnaldi, G., . . . & Tabarin, A.; Italian Association of Clinical Endocrinologists. (2011). AME position statement on adrenal incidentaloma. *European Journal of Endocrinology, 164*, 851–870.

Vanderveen, K. A., Thompson, S. M., Callstrom, M. R., Young, W. F. Jr., Grant, C. S., Farley, D. R., . . . Thompson, G. B. (2009). Biopsy of pheochromocytomas and paragangliomas: potential for disaster. *Surgery, 146*, 1158–1166.

Young, W. F. Jr. (2007). Clinical practice. The incidentally discovered adrenal mass. *New England Journal of Medicine, 356*, 601–610.

CHAPTER 35

ADRENAL MALIGNANCIES

Michael T. McDermott

1. What types of cancer occur in the adrenal glands?

   Adrenocortical carcinomas arise in the adrenal cortex, and malignant pheochromocytomas develop in the adrenal medulla. Metastatic cancer from primary malignancies in other organs may also be seen in the vascular adrenal glands. Adrenocortical carcinoma is a rare cancer, affecting approximately 1 to 2 adults per million population per year. Malignant pheochromocytomas are similarly rare and difficult to diagnose.

2. How do adrenocortical carcinomas present clinically?

   Adrenocortical carcinomas may present with symptoms and signs of excess steroid hormone secretion ($\approx$ 40%–60%), with tumor mass effects of abdominal or flank pain ($\approx$ 33%), or as an incidentally discovered adrenal mass found during abdominal imaging procedures ordered for unrelated reasons ($\approx$ 20%–30%).

3. What clinical features are seen with steroid hormone-secreting adrenocortical carcinomas?

   Functioning adrenocortical carcinomas secrete cortisol, androgens, aldosterone, or estrogens—alone or sometimes in combination. Cortisol overproduction is most common ($\approx$ 45%) and results in Cushing's syndrome. Androgen secretion ($\approx$ 25%), most commonly dehydroepiandrosterone sulfate (DHEAS), causes hirsutism and virilization in women and precocious puberty in children. Aldosterone secretion causes hypertension and hypokalemia (Conn's syndrome). Estrogen production (rare) causes menstrual disturbances in women and gynecomastia and hypogonadism in men (Fig. 35.1). Combined hormone secretion is particularly suggestive of an adrenocortical carcinoma rather than a benign adrenal adenoma.

4. What imaging features are most suggestive of an adrenocortical carcinoma?

   A non–contrast-enhanced abdominal computed tomography (NCCT) is the best overall imaging test to assess an adrenal mass. Features that most strongly suggest adrenocortical carcinoma are size > 4 cm, heterogeneity, calcifications, irregular borders, local invasion, lymphadenopathy, and decreased lipid content. Lipid content is assessed by signal attenuation, expressed in Hounsfield units (HU); low HU are indicative of high lipid content and high HU are indicative of low lipid content. Adrenocortical carcinomas typically have very low lipid content, yielding a HU score > 20 on NCCT.

   An adrenal mass CT protocol is employed in many institutions utilizing NCCT, followed by contrast-enhanced CT (CECT), delayed contrast-enhanced CT (DCECT; 10–15 minutes postcontrast injection), and calculation of relative washout percentage (RWP). Adrenocortical carcinomas typically show HU > 20 on NCCT, HU > 30 on DCECT, and < 50% RWP. Magnetic resonance imaging (MRI) can also be used to assess the size, features, and lipid content of adrenal masses. Fluorodeoxyglucose positron emission tomography (FDG-PET) or positron emission tomography (PET)/CT fusion scanning may also be useful, especially to distinguish adrenocortical carcinoma from other masses with high HU or low RWP on CT (pheochromocytomas, metastatic cancers).

5. Should a biopsy of adrenal masses suspicious for adrenocortical carcinoma be performed?

   Biopsy of potentially resectable masses for which there is moderate-to-high suspicion for adrenocortical carcinoma should not be performed because of the risk of spillage of malignant cells from the tumor. A biopsy should be considered when an adrenal mass is present in a patient who has another primary malignancy with known metastases to determine whether the adrenal mass is metastatic cancer from the other tumor.

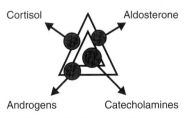

Fig. 35.1. Functioning adrenal tumors.

6. What histologic features are characteristic of an adrenocortical carcinoma?

The Weiss Scoring System is most commonly used. This system evaluates nine characteristics: nuclear grade, mitotic rate, atypical mitosis, clear cell component, diffuse architecture, tumor necrosis, venous invasion, sinus structure invasion, and capsule invasion. Adrenocortical carcinoma is diagnosed when ≥ three of these features are present. Adrenocortical carcinomas are further classified as low grade (< 20 mitoses per 50 high-power fields or Ki67 expression < 10%) and high grade (> 20 mitoses per 50 high-power fields or Ki67 expression > 10%).

7. What inherited or acquired genetic abnormalities might cause adrenocortical carcinoma?

In adults, approximately 10% of adrenocortical carcinomas are associated with germline P53 mutations, and 3% are associated with mutations in mismatch repair genes (Lynch's syndrome). Somatic mutations that have been identified include P53, B-catenin, insulin-like growth factor-2 (IFG-2), glucose transporter 1 (GLUT1), steroidogenic factor 1 (SF1), excision repair cross-complement 1 (ERCC1), and serum/glucocorticoid regulated kinase 1 (SGK1). Adrenocortical carcinoma in children often occurs in the setting of germline P53 mutations (Li Fraumeni's syndrome) or IGF-2 locus imprinting defects (Beckwith-Weidemann syndrome).

8. Describe the most commonly used staging systems for adrenocortical carcinoma.

Adrenocortical carcinomas are first classified by their Tumor Node Metastasis (TNM) status. T refers to the primary tumor: TX – cannot be assessed; T0 – no evidence of primary tumor; T1 – tumor < 5 cm, no extra-adrenal disease; T2 – tumor > 5 cm, no extra-adrenal disease; T3 – tumor any size, local invasion but not into local organs; T4 – tumor any size, invades local organs or large vessels. N refers to regional lymph nodes: NX – cannot be assessed; N0 – nodes absent; N1 – nodes present. M refers to distant metastases: M0 – metastases absent; M1 – metastases present.

Tumors are then staged by their TNM status. The American Joint Committee on Cancer (AJCC) stages tumors as follows: Stage 1: T1N0M0; Stage 2: T2N0M0; Stage 3: T1N1M0, T2N1M0, T3AnyNM0, T4AnyNM0; Stage 4: M1. The European Network for the Study of Adrenal Tumors (ENSAT) uses a slightly different staging system: Stage 1: T1N0M0; Stage 2: T2N0M0; Stage 3: T3/T4N0M0, T1/T2/T3/T4N1M0; Stage 4: M1.

9. What is the distribution of adrenocortical carcinoma stages at diagnosis?

Stage 1: 14%
Stage 2: 45%
Stage 3: 27%
Stage 4: 24%

10. Describe the preferred initial treatment for adrenocortical carcinoma.

Surgical resection is the only option that is potentially curative and is, therefore, the initial treatment of choice for all resectable stage I–III disease. Surgery is best done by surgical oncology teams at centers where there is significant experience with this condition. Open adrenalectomy is recommended over laparoscopic adrenalectomy by most authorities. Removal of suspicious lymph nodes encountered during surgery is recommended, but there is insufficient evidence at present to recommend prophylactic lymph node exploration. Even in patients with stage I–III disease, recurrence is common, probably because of the presence of undetected micrometastases.

11. When and what type of adjuvant therapy is recommended after resection of an adrenocortical carcinoma?

Because of the high recurrence rate (60%–80%), adjuvant therapy with mitotane is recommended for all patients who have adrenocortical carcinoma with incomplete resections, tumor fracture or spillage during the resection, low-grade large tumors with capsular invasion, or high-grade pathology (> 20 mitoses per 50 high-power fields or Ki67 expression > 10%). Combination adjuvant therapy using mitotane plus cisplatin-based chemotherapy, such as etoposide, doxorubicin, and cisplatin (EDC), has been suggested for those at high risk for early recurrence based on extensive vascular invasion or high-grade pathology. Adjuvant tumor bed radiation therapy is also advised for patients who have incompletely resected tumors, tumor fracture or spillage during surgery, or high-grade pathology.

12. What is mitotane, and how is it used?

Mitotane is an adrenocorticolytic agent with significant antitumor efficacy against adrenocortical carcinoma. The starting dose is 500 mg twice daily with dose escalation to 6 g daily over the ensuing 4 to 12 weeks. Mitotane metabolism shows significant interindividual variability, and therefore, serum mitotane level monitoring every 2 to 3 weeks is strongly recommended with a goal of maintaining serum mitotane in the 14 to 20 mcg/mL range. Nausea, which can be a limiting factor in achieving a therapeutic dose, can usually be managed with metoclopramide or ondansetron.

13. What effect does mitotane have on adrenal function, and how is this managed?

Mitotane causes atrophy and destruction of the adrenal cortex. As a result, it causes adrenocortical insufficiency in virtually all adrenocortical carcinoma patients except those with cortisol-producing tumors. Therefore, glucocorticoid replacement therapy should be started at the same time mitotane therapy is initiated. Mitotane potently induces cytochrome P450 enzymes that metabolize cortisol, hydrocortisone, dexamethasone, and fludrocortisone. Therefore, higher glucocorticoid replacement doses are needed in mitotane-treated patients than in those with adrenal insufficiency of other causes. Typically, hydrocortisone 30 to 40 mg divided into two times daily or three times daily dosing schedules (or equivalent doses of other glucocorticoids) should be started right away; even higher doses ($\geq$ three fold above usual glucocorticoid replacement doses) may be required later as mitotane dosing is escalated. Mitotane also raises cortisol-binding globulin levels, rendering serum cortisol values inaccurate. Monitoring the adequacy of hydrocortisone dosing is best done by regular measurements of 24-hour urine cortisol excretion. Mineralocorticoid replacement is often not needed initially but regular monitoring of blood pressure, serum potassium and sodium, and plasma renin levels is recommended with the addition of fludrocortisone therapy if the patient develops hypotension, hyperkalemia, hyponatremia, or elevated plasma renin.

14. What other endocrine effects does mitotane have?
Mitotane suppresses pituitary thyroid-stimulating hormone (TSH) secretion, resulting in central hypothyroidism (low TSH and low free thyroxine [T_4]); it also increases serum T_4-binding globulin levels, which can further lower serum free T_4 levels. Levothyroxine replacement should be given to patients who develop central hypothyroidism. Mitotane also causes hypogonadism in men, often severe enough to require testosterone replacement; because it also increases sex hormone–binding globulin levels, measurement of total testosterone may underestimate the severity of the testosterone deficiency. In women taking mitotane, elevations of both luteinizing hormone and follicle stimulating hormone and the development of large ovarian cysts have been reported.

15. How does the management of cortisol-producing adrenal cancers differ from other adrenocortical carcinomas?
Cortisol excess predisposes patients to infections, sepsis, thromboembolic events, poor wound healing, hypergly-cemia, and other glucocorticoid effects. Mitotane alone is not usually sufficient to control the hypercortisolism. Metyrapone, a steroidogenic enzyme inhibitor, is the most effective agent for reducing cortisol production; the starting dose is 250 mg every 6 hours, with subsequent dose escalation up to a total daily dose of 6 g in divided doses. When metyrapone does not lower cortisol levels sufficiently, ketoconazole, also an enzyme inhibitor, can be added with a starting dose of 200 mg three times daily with titration up to a target dose of 400 mg three times daily. If hypercortisolism persists on these two agents, the glucocorticoid receptor antagonist mifepristone can also be added; this medication will not serum lower cortisol levels but will block glucocorticoid action at the tissue receptor level. Etomidate, an 11-hydroxylase inhibitor that is administered intravenously, can be given, starting with a dose of 0.3 mg/kg/hr in patients who cannot take oral medications or when serum cortisol levels must be lowered acutely. If primary and adjuvant therapy are effective in reducing the tumor burden, adrenal insufficiency may eventually develop, resulting in a requirement for glucocorticoid and mineralocorticoid replacement therapy, as discussed above.

16. What type and frequency of monitoring is recommended after treatment for adrenocortical carcinomas?
Follow-up imaging with CECT or MRI of the chest, abdomen, and pelvis is recommended every 3 months for 2 to 3 years and then every 4 to 6 months for 5 years. FDG-PET/CT imaging at 6-month intervals is recommended by some, but high-quality evidence supporting its routine use is lacking. Regular monitoring of specific steroid hormone production for the hormone-secreting tumors is advocated by some, but others suggest testing these only if clinical signs of hormone excess recur. Patients on mitotane should also have regular assessments of serum mitotane levels (target: 14–20 mcg/mL) and 24-hour urine cortisol excretion to guide mitotane and hydrocortisone dose adjustments.

17. How should unresectable, recurrent, and metastatic adrenal cortical carcinomas be managed?
Primary therapy with mitotane, usually in combination with EDC chemotherapy, is recommended for patients with unresectable adrenocortical carcinomas. Radiofrequency ablative therapy may offer additional benefit in select cases. Targeted therapies utilizing tyrosine or multikinase inhibitors and growth factor receptor (IGF-1R, epidermal growth factor receptor) inhibitors have also shown some promise. Referral to centers doing clinical trials of investigative agents should, therefore, also be considered. For locally recurrent disease, surgical resection followed by mitotane $+/-$ EDC chemotherapy and/or radiation therapy are the best options. For distant metastatic disease, radiation therapy to specific lesions may also be beneficial.

18. What is the prognosis for patients with adrenocortical carcinoma?
The mean survival is 15 months. The 5-year survival rate is $<$ 30%. Prognosis is improved with young age, small tumor size, localized disease, complete tumor resection, and nonfunctioning tumors. The two most significant prognostic factors are disease stage and completeness of the initial surgical resection. Grading (low versus high grade) based on the Weiss Scoring System adds additional prognostic information. Oncogene and tumor marker assessment are currently being evaluated, but as yet, sufficient data to ascribe specific prognostic predictability to these molecular markers are not available. The 5-year disease-free survival rates by disease stage are shown in Table 35.1.

19. How often are pheochromocytomas malignant?
Approximately 15% to 25% of pheochromocytomas and paragangliomas are malignant.

Table 35.1. Five-Year Disease-Free Survival for Adrenocortical Carcinoma According to European Network for the Study of Adrenal Tumors (ENSAT) 2008 Staging System.

STAGE	5-YEAR DISEASE-FREE SURVIVAL
I	82%
II	61%
III	50%
IV	13%

20. What are the clinical features of malignant pheochromocytomas?

Pheochromocytomas, benign and malignant, usually cause hypertension, headaches, sweating, and palpitations, but some are asymptomatic. They are diagnosed by finding increased plasma or urinary levels of metanephrine or catecholamines; plasma and urinary metanephrines have the highest sensitivities and specificities of all available tests. Pheochromocytomas also have a characteristic phenotype on cross-sectional imaging. Malignant pheochromocytomas usually do not differ clinically or histologically at presentation from those that are benign.

21. What clues suggest that a pheochromocytoma is malignant?

Malignancy is most strongly suggested by tumor size > 6 cm, evidence of extraadrenal spread (usually to the lymph nodes, liver, lungs, or bones), and elevated plasma or urinary dopamine levels. Because malignant pheochromocytomas cannot be distinguished from benign ones histologically, the malignant character of some tumors may not become apparent until metastatic disease appears.

KEY POINTS: ADRENAL MALIGNANCIES

- Adrenocortical carcinomas present with features of excess cortisol, androgens, aldosterone, or estrogens; with abdominal or flank pain; or as an incidentally discovered adrenal mass.
- Malignant pheochromocytomas often present with features similar to those of benign pheochromocytomas (hypertension, headaches, palpitations, sweating).
- Features suggesting that an adrenal tumor is malignant are size > 4 cm, heterogeneity, calcifications, irregular borders, local invasion, lymphadenopathy, decreased lipid content (Hounsfield units [HU] > 20), or elevated levels of serum androgens or urinary or plasma dopamine.
- Surgery is the treatment of choice for all malignant adrenal tumors; mitotane +/− chemotherapy and tumor bed radiation therapy are recommended adjuvant therapies for adrenocortical carcinomas.

22. Which of the familial pheochromocytoma/paraganglioma syndromes is most commonly associated with malignancy?

Table 35.2 lists the four well-recognized familial pheochromocytoma and paraganglioma syndromes. Of the succinate dehydrogenase (SDH) mutations, SDHB is most often associated with malignant paragangliomas.

23. What are the best tests to localize metastatic pheochromocytomas and paragangliomas?

Cross-sectional imaging with CT or MRI will localize most metastatic pheochromocytomas and paragangliomas, and are the initial imaging procedure of choice in most circumstances. When cross-sectional imaging is negative, when there is an adrenal pheochromocytoma ≥ 10 cm in size, or when dealing with paragangliomas, functional imaging should be performed next. Somatostatin receptor-based imaging [68-Ga DOTATATE, In-111 Pentetreotide (OctreoScan)] and PET/CT scanning have been shown to be superior to and have largely replaced ^{123}I-metaiodobenzylguanidine (MIBG) scans. A 2016 study reported a better metastatic lesion detection rate with 68-Ga Dotatate PET/CT (97.6%), compared with CT/MRI (81.6%), ^{18}F-FDG PET/CT (77.7%), ^{18}F-FDOPA PET/CT (74.8%), and ^{18}F-FDG PET/CT (49.2%). Therefore, 68-Ga Dotatate PET/CT is currently the most accurate imaging technique available for the detection of metastatic pheochromocytomas and paragangliomas.

Table 35.2. Genetic Syndromes Associated with Pheochromocytomas and/or Paragangliomas.

Syndrome (Gene Mutation)
  Multiple endocrine neoplasia 2 (Ret)
  Von Hippel-Lindau syndrome (VHL)
  Neurofibromatosis 1 (NF-1)
  Succinate dehydrogenase (SDH)

24. What is the treatment for malignant pheochromocytomas and paragangliomas?

Surgery is the treatment of choice, when possible. Preoperatively, alpha-adrenergic blocking agents (phenoxybenzamine, prazosin, terazosin, doxazosin) or calcium channel blockers are given to control blood pressure and to replete intravascular volume. Beta-blockers may then be added for reflex tachycardia or persistent hypertension. Therapies for which partial tumor responses have been reported include chemotherapy with cyclophosphamide, vincristine, and dacarbazine, and radionuclide therapy with ^{131}I-MIBG. Peptide receptor radionuclide therapy using ^{177}Lu-DOTATATE has also shown promising results. Similarly, encouraging responses have also been recently reported with the tyrosine kinase inhibitor cabozantinib.

     If curative therapy is not possible or successful, the therapeutic goals are blood pressure and symptom control. Alpha-blockers, calcium channel blockers, and the catecholamine synthesis inhibitor alpha-methyltyrosine are the best agents for long-term management.

25. What is the prognosis for malignant pheochromocytomas and paragangliomas?

A 2017 study at the Mayo Clinic reported a mean overall survival of 24.6 years and mean disease-specific survival of 33.7 years. Shorter survival was predicted with male gender, older age, large primary tumor size, synchronous metastases at diagnosis, elevated dopamine levels, and not undergoing primary tumor resection. They reported patients having metastases that were stable for over 40 years and metastases being discovered > 50 years after the primary diagnosis was made. Therefore, pheochromocytomas and paragangliomas require lifelong surveillance, and malignant pheochromocytomas and paragangliomas are managed much like any other chronic illness, with attention focused on controlling blood pressure and symptoms of catecholamine excess.

26. What tumors metastasize to the adrenal glands?

The vascular adrenal glands are a frequent site of bilateral metastatic spread from cancers of the lung, breast, stomach, pancreas, colon, and kidney, and from melanomas and lymphomas.

27. What is the clinical significance of metastatic disease to the adrenal glands?

Acute adrenal crises are rare. However, up to 33% of patients may have subtle adrenal insufficiency manifested by nonspecific symptoms and an inadequate response (peak cortisol level < 18 mcg/dL) to a 250-mcg cosyntropin stimulation test. These patients may experience improvement in well-being when given physiologic glucocorticoid replacement.

BIBLIOGRAPHY

Assié, G., Letouze, E., Fassnacht, M., Jouinot, A., Luscap, W., Barreau, O., . . . Bertherat, J. (2014). Integrated genomic characterization of adrenocortical carcinoma. *Nature Genetics, 46*, 607–612.

Berruti, A., Grisanti, S., Pulzer, A., Claps, M., Daffara, F., Loli, P., . . . Terzolo, M. (2017). Long-term outcomes of adjuvant mitotane therapy in patients with radically resected adrenocortical carcinoma. *Journal of Clinical Endocrinology and Metabolism, 102*, 1358–1365.

Beuschlein, F., Weigel, J., Saeger, W., Kroiss, M., Wild, V., Daffara, F., . . . Fassnacht, M. (2015). Major prognostic role of Ki67 in localized adrenocortical carcinoma after complete resection. *Journal of Clinical Endocrinology and Metabolism, 100*, 841–849.

Dinnes, J., Bancos, I., Ferrante di Ruffano, L., Chortis, V., Davenport, C., Bayliss, S., . . . Arlt, W. (2016). Management of endocrine disease: imaging for the diagnosis of malignancy in incidentally discovered adrenal masses: a systematic review and meta-analysis. *European Journal of Endocrinology, 175*, R51–R64.

Else, T., Kim, A. C., Sabolch, A., Raymond, V. M., Kandathil, A., Caolili, E. M., . . . Hammer, G. D. (2014). Adrenocortical carcinoma. *Endocrine Reviews, 35*, 282–326.

Else, T., Williams, A. R., Sabolch, A., Jolly, S., Miller, B. S., & Hammer, G. D. (2014). Adjuvant therapies and patient and tumor characteristics associated with survival of adult patients with adrenocortical carcinoma. *Journal of Clinical Endocrinology and Metabolism, 99*, 455–461.

Fassnacht, M., Kroiss, M., & Allolio, B. (2013). Update in adrenocortical carcinoma. *Journal of Clinical Endocrinology and Metabolism, 98*, 4551–4564.

Fassnacht, M., Berruti, A., Baudin, A., Demeure, M. J., Gilbert, J., Haak, H., . . . Hammer, G. D. (2015). Linsitinib (OSI-906) versus placebo for patients with locally advanced or metastatic adrenocortical carcinoma: a double-blind, randomized, phase 3 study. *Lancet Oncology, 16*, 426–435.

Habra, M. A., Ejaz, S., Feng, L., Das, P., Deniz, F., Grubbs, E. G., . . . Vassilopoulou-Sellin, R. (2013). A retrospective cohort analysis of the efficacy of adjuvant radiotherapy after primary surgical resection in patients with adrenocortical carcinoma. *Journal of Clinical Endocrinology and Metabolism, 98*, 192–197.

Hamidi, O., Young, W. H., Iniquez-Ariza, N., Kittah, N. E., Gruber, L., Bancos, C., . . . Bancos, I. (2017). Malignant pheochromocytomas and paragangliomas: 272 patients over 55 years. *Journal of Clinical Endocrinology and Metabolism, 102*, 3296–3305.

Janssen, I., Chen, C. C., Millo, C. M., Ling, A., Taieb, D., Lin, F. I., . . . Pacak, K. (2016). PET/CT comparing 68Ga-Dotatate and other radiopharmaceuticals and in comparison with CT/MRI for the localization of sporadic metastatic pheochromocytoma and paraganglioma. *European Journal of Nuclear Medicine and Molecular Imaging, 43*, 1784–1791.

Kerkhofs, T. M., Derijks, L. J., Ettaieb, M. H., Eekhoff, E. M., Neef, C., Gelderblom, H., . . . Haak, H. R. (2014). Short-term variation in plasma mitotane levels confirms the importance of trough level monitoring. *European Journal of Endocrinology, 171*, 677–683.

Kong, G., Grozinsky-Glasberg, S., Hofman, M. S., Callahan, J., Meirovitz, A., Maimon, O., . . . Hicks, R. J. (2017). Efficacy of peptide receptor radionuclide therapy for functional metastatic paraganglioma and pheochromocytoma. *Journal of Clinical Endocrinology and Metabolism, 102*, 3278–3287.

Lenders, J. W., Duh, Q. Y., Eisenhofer, G., Gimenez-Roqueplo, A. P., Grebe, S. K., Murad, M. H., . . . Young, W. F. Jr. (2014). Pheochromocytoma and paraganglioma: an Endocrine Society clinical practice guideline. *Journal of Clinical Endocrinology and Metabolism, 99*, 1915–1942.

Miller, B. S., Gauger, P. G., Hammer, G. D., & Doherty, G. M. (2012). Resection of adrenocortical carcinoma is less complete and local recurrence occurs sooner and more often after laparoscopic adrenalectomy than after open adrenalectomy. *Surgery, 152*, 1150–1157.

Miller, B. S., & Else, T. (2017). Personalized care of patients with adrenocortical carcinoma: a comprehensive approach. *Endocrine Practice, 23*, 705–715.

Naing, A., Lorusso, P., Fu, S., Hong, D., Chen, H. X., Doyle, L. A., . . . Kurzrock, R. (2013). Insulin growth factor receptor (IGF-1R) antibody cixutumumab combined with mTOR inhibitor temsirolimus in patients with metastatic adrenocortical carcinoma. *British Journal of Cancer, 108*, 826–830.

Phan, A. T., Grogan, R. H., Rohren, E., & Perrier, N. D. (2017). Adrenal cortical carcinoma. In M. B. Amin (Ed.), *AJCC Cancer Staging Manual* (8th ed., p. 911). New York: Springer.

Russo, M., Scollo, C., Pellegriti, G., Cotta, O. R., Squatrito, S., Frasca, F., . . . Gullo, D. (2016). Mitotane treatment in patients with adrenocortical carcinoma causes central hypothyroidism. *Clinical Endocrinology, 84*, 614–619.

Sabolch, A., Else, T., Griffith, K. A., Ben-Josef, E., Williams, A., Miller, B. S., . . . Jolly, S. (2015). Adjuvant radiation therapy improves local control after surgical resection in patients with localized adrenocortical carcinoma. *International Journal of Radiation Oncology, Biology, Physics, 92*, 252–259.

Salenave, S., Bernard, V., Do Cao, C., Guignat, L., Bachelot, A., Leboulleux, S., . . . Young, J. (2015). Ovarian macrocysts and gonadotrope-ovarian axis disruption in premenopausal women receiving mitotane for adrenocortical carcinoma or Cushing's disease. *European Journal of Endocrinology, 172*, 141–149.

Sgourakis, G., Lanitis, S., Kouloura, A., Zaphiriadou, P., Karkoulias, K., Raptis, D., . . . Caraliotas, C. (2015). Laparoscopic versus open adrenalectomy for stage I/II adrenocortical carcinoma: meta-analysis of outcomes. *Journal of Investigation Surgery, 28*, 145–152.

Taieb, D., Jha, A., Guerin, C., Pang, Y., Adams, K. T., Chen, C. C., . . . Pacak, K. (2018). 18F-DOPA PET/CT imaging of MAX related pheochromocytoma. *Journal of Clinical Endocrinology and Metabolism, 103*, 1574–1582.

Terzolo, M., Angeli, A., Fassnacht, M., Daffara, F., Tauchmanova, L., Conton, P. A., . . . Berruti, A. (2007). Adjuvant mitotane treatment for adrenocortical carcinoma. *New England Journal of Medicine, 356*, 2372–2380.

Terzolo, M., Baudin, A. E., Ardito, A., Kroiss, M., Leboulleux, S., Daffara, F., . . . Berruti, A. (2013). Mitotane levels predict the outcome of patients with adrenocortical carcinoma treated adjuvantly following radical resection. *European Journal of Endocrinology, 169*, 263–270.

Yan, Q., Bancos, I., Gruber, L. M., Bancos, C., McKenzie, T. J., Babovic-Vuksanovic, D., & Young, W. F. Jr. (2018). When biochemical phenotype predicts genotype: pheochromocytoma and paraganglioma. *American Journal of Medicine, 131*, 506–509.

Zhang, J., Walsh, M. F., Wu, G., Edmonson, M. N., Gruber, T. A., Easton, J., . . . Downing. J. R. (2015). Germline mutations in predisposition genes in pediatric cancer. *New England Journal of Medicine, 373*, 2336–2346.

Zheng, S., Cherniack, A. D., Dewal, N., Moffitt, R. A., Danilova, L., Murray, B. A., . . . Verhaak, R. G. W. (2016). Comprehensive pan-genomic characterization of adrenocortical carcinoma. *Cancer Cell, 29*, 1–14.

CHAPTER 36

ADRENAL INSUFFICIENCY

Emily B. Schroeder and Cecilia C. Low Wang

1. **What is adrenal insufficiency, and how is it categorized?**
   Adrenal insufficiency is the term used to describe inadequate production of glucocorticoids, mineralocorticoids, or both by the adrenal glands. This can occur because of dysfunction or complete destruction of the adrenal cortex (primary adrenal insufficiency), inadequate adrenocorticotropic hormone (ACTH) production by the pituitary (secondary adrenal insufficiency), or inadequate corticotropin-releasing hormone (CRH) production by the hypothalamus (tertiary adrenal insufficiency).

2. **What are common causes of adrenal insufficiency?**
   Autoimmune adrenalitis (Addison's disease) is the most common cause of primary adrenal insufficiency and is associated with increased levels of 21-hydroxylase antibodies. Addison's disease can occur in isolation or in combination with other endocrine deficiencies as part of an autoimmune polyglandular syndrome. The most common cause of central (secondary/tertiary) adrenal insufficiency is withdrawal of glucocorticoids after long-term use. Central adrenal insufficiency can also occur as part of panhypopituitarism from large pituitary tumors or their treatment with surgery and/or radiation therapy. See Table 36.1 for other causes of adrenal insufficiency.

3. **What are common symptoms of adrenal insufficiency?**
   Most patients report nonspecific symptoms, such as weakness, fatigue, and anorexia. Many also complain of gastrointestinal symptoms, such as nausea, vomiting, vague abdominal pain, or constipation. Psychiatric symptoms and symptoms of orthostatic hypotension, arthralgias, myalgias, and salt craving are also reported.

4. **How does adrenal insufficiency usually present?**
   Weight loss is a common presenting sign. Hyperpigmentation, particularly of the buccal mucosa and gums, is noted in most patients with primary adrenal insufficiency. Patients should be examined for darkening of the palmar creases, nail beds, and scars forming after onset of ACTH excess. Hyperpigmentation occurs because production of proopiomelanocortin (POMC), a prohormone that is cleaved into ACTH, melanocyte-stimulating hormone, and other hormones, is increased and leads to increased melanin production. Orthostasis is common in both primary insufficiency and central adrenal insufficiency.

5. **What laboratory abnormalities can be found in adrenal insufficiency?**
   The classic laboratory abnormalities are hyponatremia and hyperkalemia. The hyperkalemia is caused by mineralocorticoid deficiency, whereas the hyponatremia occurs mainly because of glucocorticoid deficiency. Hyponatremia is the result of elevated vasopressin levels with free water retention, shift of extracellular sodium

Table 36.1. Causes of Adrenal Insufficiency.

PRIMARY	SECONDARY	TERTIARY
• Autoimmune	• Pituitary tumors including craniopharyngioma	• Withdrawal of long-term suppressive glucocorticoid therapy
• Bilateral adrenal hemorrhage or thrombosis: coagulopathy, meningococcal sepsis	• Metastases to the pituitary	• Hypothalamic tumors
• Metastases: lung, breast, renal, gastrointestinal, lymphoma	• Pituitary surgery or irradiation	• Metastases to the hypothalamus
• Infectious: tuberculosis, HIV, CMV, fungal	• Lymphocytic hypophysitis: idiopathic, drug induced	• Infiltrative diseases affecting the hypothalamus
• Adrenoleukodystrophy and other congenital disorders	• Infiltrative diseases: hemochromatosis, sarcoidosis, histiocytosis X	• Cranial irradiation
• Adrenalectomy	• Infection (e.g., tuberculosis, histoplasmosis, syphilis)	• Traumatic brain injury
• Infiltrative: amyloidosis, hemochromatosis	• Sheehan's syndrome (massive peripartum blood loss leading to shock)	• Infections (e.g., tuberculosis)
• Congenital adrenal hyperplasia	• Traumatic brain injury disrupting the pituitary stalk or pituitary gland	
• Drugs (see text)		

CMV, Cytomegalovirus; *HIV,* human immunodeficiency virus.

into cells, and decreased delivery of filtrate to the diluting segments of the nephron resulting from decreased glomerular filtration rate. Azotemia can be seen because of hypovolemia. Patients often develop a normocytic normochromic anemia and may have eosinophilia and lymphocytosis. Mild-to-moderate hypercalcemia may occur. Fasting blood glucose is usually low-normal, but occasionally patients can develop fasting or postprandial hypoglycemia. Patients with coexisting type 1 diabetes mellitus and adrenal insufficiency may develop increased frequency and severity of hypoglycemic episodes.

6. How do the clinical presentations of primary insufficiency and central adrenal insufficiency differ?
Hyperpigmentation and hyperkalemia are not observed in secondary/tertiary adrenal insufficiency. Otherwise, the clinical presentations are similar.

7. How is adrenal insufficiency usually diagnosed biochemically?
In the outpatient setting, a low morning cortisol ($<$ 3 mcg/dL) is sufficient to diagnose adrenal insufficiency, and a high morning cortisol ($>$ 18 mcg/dL) excludes the diagnosis. Levels between 3 and 18 mcg/dL are equivocal; this usually requires that a dynamic test, the cosyntropin stimulation test, is also performed. This test determines whether the adrenals are able to respond to maximal stimulation by synthetic ACTH. The test can also be used in the diagnosis of central adrenal insufficiency, as long as sufficient time has elapsed for the adrenal cortex to atrophy in response to lack of ACTH stimulation.

The standard cosyntropin test is performed by drawing a baseline serum cortisol level, administering 250 mcg of cosyntropin (brand names Cortrosyn or Synthacten) intravenously or intramuscularly, then drawing a serum cortisol level 30 and 60 minutes later. An abnormal result is defined as a stimulated cortisol at either 30 or 60 minutes of $<$ 18 to 20 mcg/dL ($<$ 450–500 nmol/L). This test can be performed at any time during the day. If an individual is receiving glucocorticoid therapy, the dose should be held (12 hours for hydrocortisone, 24 hours for prednisone) before the test is performed to avoid detecting synthetic glucocorticoids in the cortisol assay (Fig. 36.1).

Other dynamic testing includes the insulin tolerance test, metyrapone test, glucagon stimulation test, and CRH stimulation test. The insulin tolerance test evaluates the hypothalamic–pituitary–adrenal (HPA) axis in response to insulin-induced hypoglycemia (blood glucose $<$ 40 mg/dL). This test should only be performed in experienced centers with trained staff and should not be performed if the individual has significant coronary artery disease or an uncontrolled seizure disorder. Metyrapone blocks the final step in cortisol biosynthesis, which decreases cortisol levels and increases ACTH secretion.

8. What about the low-dose cosyntropin stimulation test?
It has been argued that mild cases of primary adrenal insufficiency may be missed with the standard-dose cosyntropin stimulation test because the dose of ACTH administered in this test is quite supraphysiologic. Data from studies examining the potential role of low-dose cosyntropin stimulation testing, in which 1 mcg cosyntropin is administered, do not clearly establish that the low-dose test is better than the standard test. There are several potential problems with performing the test, including false-positive results caused by inaccurate or irreproducible dilution of cosyntropin, the need for intravenous (IV) administration, and the need for carefully timed sampling for serum cortisol levels. It is unclear whether abnormal results from this test are clinically relevant. Therefore, the standard dose test should be used in most instances.

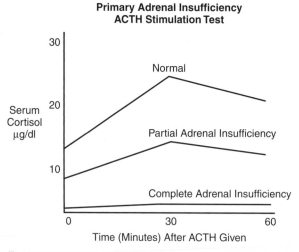

**Primary Adrenal Insufficiency
ACTH Stimulation Test**

Fig. 36.1. Interpretation of the adrenocorticotropic hormone (ACTH) stimulation test.

9. **What testing can be used to distinguish primary from central adrenal insufficiency?**
   In primary adrenal insufficiency, the plasma ACTH level is elevated, whereas ACTH is "abnormally normal" (i.e., not elevated in response to low cortisol) or frankly low in central adrenal insufficiency.

10. **When can the results of the ACTH stimulation test be misleading?**
    Partial ACTH deficiency and recent ACTH deficiency are situations that may lead to false-negative results of the cosyntropin stimulation test. Insulin-induced hypoglycemia (insulin tolerance testing) or metyrapone testing may be used in these situations.

11. **When are imaging tests appropriate?**
    After the biochemical diagnosis of adrenal insufficiency, imaging may be performed in certain instances to help determine the cause. In cases of central adrenal insufficiency, magnetic resonance imaging of the pituitary and hypothalamus is indicated if exogenous glucocorticoids have not been implicated. If a primary adrenal process is suspected, abdominal computed tomography can be performed with thin cuts through the adrenals. Imaging should not be performed before a biochemical diagnosis is made because of the high incidence of incidental findings without clinical significance. As a general rule, bilateral small glands are usually seen in patients who have autoimmune adrenalitis (Addison's disease), and adrenoleukodystrophy and large adrenal glands are found in most other causes of adrenal insufficiency.

12. **Develop an algorithm for the evaluation of adrenal insufficiency.**
    See Fig. 36.2.

13. **When should the diagnosis of adrenal crisis be considered?**
    Adrenal crisis should be suspected in patients with unexplained catecholamine-resistant hypotension or other severe signs or symptoms consistent with adrenal insufficiency. Symptoms of adrenal crisis are often nonspecific, such as weakness, fatigue, nausea, vomiting, abdominal pain, fever, and altered mental status. Acute adrenal hemorrhage should be suspected if there is a constellation of abdominal/flank pain, hypotension/shock, fever, and hypoglycemia in a deteriorating patient. Adrenal crisis is more common in primary adrenal insufficiency than central adrenal insufficiency.

14. **How is adrenal crisis managed?**
    If adrenal crisis is suspected, it should be treated aggressively because, if left untreated, it can be fatal. A formal diagnosis of adrenal insufficiency can be performed later. The patient can receive a dose of IV dexamethasone initially (4 mg) while the basal cortisol and the cosyntropin stimulation test are performed; empiric treatment with IV hydrocortisone can then be initiated (Table 36.2). Dexamethasone is not detected in standard serum cortisol assays. In addition, treatment should include IV saline and glucose to correct volume depletion, dehydration, and hypoglycemia. Patients often need intensive care unit-level supportive care. A search for precipitating factors and the underlying cause needs to be performed.

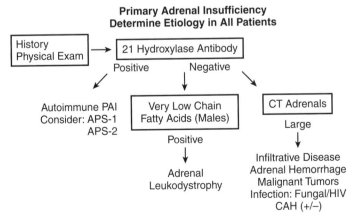

Fig. 36.2. Evaluation to determine the cause of adrenal insufficiency. *APS,* Autoimmune polyendocrine syndrome; *CAH,* congenital adrenal hyperplasia; *HIV,* human immunodeficiency virus; *PAI,* primary adrenal insufficiency. (Modified from Bornstein, S. R. (2016). *Journal of Clinical Endocrinology and Metabolism, 101,* 364–389, Fig. 1; Husebye, E. S., et al. (2014). Consensus statement on the diagnosis, treatment and follow-up of patients with primary adrenal insufficiency. *Journal of Internal Medicine, 275,* 104–115 (181), Fig. 1, John Wiley & Sons, Inc.)

Table 36.2. Treatment of an Adrenal Crisis.

Primary Adrenal Insufficiency
Treatment of Adrenal Crisis

AGENT	DOSE
Hydrocortisone (Solu-Cortef)	100 mg IV, then 200 mg/24 hr infusion $\times$ 24 hr, then 100 mg/24 hr infusion $\times$ 24 hr
Normal Saline ($+/-$D5)	1 L over 1 hour, then guided by individual needs

D5, 5% Dextrose solution; *IV,* intravenous.
Data from Bornstein, S. R. (2016). Clinical practice guidelines—Endocrine Society. *Journal of Clinical Endocrinology and Metabolism,*
101, 364–389.

15. How is adrenal insufficiency diagnosed in the critical care setting?

Because the diurnal rhythm of ACTH and cortisol secretion is disrupted in acute illness and because severe stress should stimulate cortisol production, a random cortisol can be drawn to diagnose complete or relative adrenal insufficiency in the critical care setting. Patients who are hemodynamically unstable and unresponsive to vasopressors despite adequate fluid resuscitation and patients with signs or symptoms suggestive of adrenal insufficiency should have a random cortisol level determined and a cosyntropin stimulation test performed immediately afterward. However, the benefits of formal testing for adrenal insufficiency in critically ill patients continue to be debated.

The cortisol level at which adrenal insufficiency should be diagnosed in this setting (a random level of < 20 mcg/dL, some other value, such as < 25 mcg/dL, and/or an increment of 9 mcg/dL after cosyntropin administration) is controversial. This is because of concerns about the existence of a cortisol-resistant state in critically ill patients caused by inflammatory cytokines, a reduction in binding affinity to cortisol binding globulin, and proinflammatory transcription factors. Some in this field believe that a cortisol level that is adequate in an ambulatory setting may not be adequate in the setting of severe stress or prolonged or complicated surgical procedures; this is referred to as "relative" adrenal insufficiency, "functional" adrenal insufficiency, or "critical illness-related corticosteroid insufficiency."

16. When and how should glucocorticoids be used in the critical care setting?

There is considerable debate about the most appropriate use of glucocorticoids in the critical care setting. Although clinical trials of glucocorticoid treatment for sepsis without proven adrenal insufficiency have shown mixed results, a systematic review of 33 trials showed that treatment with corticosteroids in sepsis reduced 28-day mortality and increased the resolution of shock. However, there is marked heterogeneity among trial results. The ADRENAL (Adjunctive Corticosteroid Treatment in Critically Ill Patients with Septic Shock) trial empirically treated individuals with severe septic with hydrocortisone and found faster resolution of shock, but no change in overall mortality. In contrast, the APROCCHSS (Activated Protein C and Corticosteroids for Human Septic Shock) trial did find a mortality benefit from the use of hydrocortisone and fludrocortisone.

Most groups currently advocate for treating individuals with severe septic shock that does not respond to adequate fluid resuscitation and vasopressor therapy with IV hydrocortisone at doses of 200 to 400 mg a day (50 mg every 6 hours or 100 mg IV every 8 hours). These dosages should be tapered quickly as the patient's clinical status improves and the underlying illness resolves.

17. How do you manage chronic adrenal insufficiency, and when should you consider prescribing fludrocortisone?

All patients with chronic adrenal insufficiency require replacement with glucocorticoids, and occasionally with a mineralocorticoid. Hydrocortisone is frequently used in primary adrenal insufficiency because it has some mineralocorticoid activity and can be dosed in a way that mimics, although not perfectly, the normal diurnal variation of serum cortisol levels. The usual dosage of hydrocortisone is 10 to 15 mg every morning and 5 to 10 mg in the afternoon. When prednisone is used, typical doses are 2.5 to 5 mg daily. If additional mineralocorticoid effect is necessary for persistent hyperkalemia and/or orthostatic hypotension, fludrocortisone 0.05 to 0.2 mg once a day may be added.

18. What are some deficiencies in the current approach to treating adrenal insufficiency?

Many individuals with adrenal insufficiency experience significantly reduced subjective health status and quality of life, increased fatigue, and depression. Some of this may be because current treatment regimens do not replicate the physiologic diurnal cortisol profile or because most female patients do not receive replacement of adrenal androgens. Work is being done to develop sustained-release glucocorticoid formulations that better approximate the natural diurnal cortisol pattern; one of these preparations is already available in Europe, marketed under the trade name Plenadren.

19. Should you recommend dehydroepiandrosterone (DHEA) replacement to patients with adrenal insufficiency?

DHEA and dehydroepiandrosterone sulfate are the main androgens produced by the adrenals. Both are weak androgens, but they are converted to the more potent androgens, testosterone and 5α-dihydrotestosterone, peripherally. This peripheral conversion is a significant source of androgens in women. Oral DHEA supplementation

Table 36.3. Relative Potencies of Selected Steroid Formulations.

COMPOUND	PHYSIOLOGIC REPLACEMENT DOSE, MG	GLUCOCORTICOID ACTIVITY[a] RELATIVE TO HYDROCORTISONE	MINERALOCORTICOID ACTIVITY RELATIVE TO HYDROCORTISONE	DURATION OF ACTION
Hydrocortisone[b]	15–25	1	1.0	Short
Methylprednisolone	4	4	0.5	Short
Prednisone	5	4	0.75	Longer
Prednisolone	5	4	0.75	Longer
Dexamethasone	0.25–0.50	17	0.0	Long

[a]Suppression of hypothalamic–pituitary–adrenal axis
[b]Hydrocortisone is the synthetic form of cortisol

at a dose of 25 to 50 mg/day normalizes circulating levels of androgens in women with adrenal insufficiency. A meta-analysis of 10 randomized, placebo-controlled trials showed a small improvement in health-related quality of life and depression after treatment with DHEA, with no significant improvement in anxiety or sexual well-being. The data are insufficient to recommend DHEA therapy for all women with adrenal insufficiency, but it may be tried in women who continue to have significantly impaired well-being despite optimal glucocorticoid and mineralocorticoid treatment. In the United States, DHEA is classified as a dietary supplement and, therefore, is not subject to the same quality control as medications.

20. What are the relative potencies of available glucocorticoids?
    See Table 36.3.

21. How is treatment for chronic adrenal insufficiency monitored?
    Adequate treatment for chronic adrenal insufficiency is monitored by taking a focused history regarding overall well-being and symptoms suggestive of orthostasis, and obtaining blood pressure, weight, and electrolytes. It is important to avoid having patients on excessive dosages of replacement glucocorticoids, which can lead to iatrogenic Cushing's syndrome and could result in needless weight gain, osteoporosis, hypertension, hyperglycemia, glaucoma, or avascular necrosis. The goal should be to use the smallest replacement dosage of glucocorticoids possible while maintaining normal electrolytes and good quality of life. Serum cortisol and plasma ACTH levels are not useful for monitoring treatment of adrenal insufficiency.

22. When do individuals with chronic adrenal insufficiency require "stress dose" glucocorticoids and what doses should be used?
    Any medical stress, including febrile illnesses, trauma, labor and delivery, and diagnostic or surgical procedures, can precipitate an acute adrenal crisis in patients with chronic adrenal insufficiency. Supplemental steroids should be used to prevent an adrenal crisis, but care should be taken to avoid unnecessary supplemental doses of glucocorticoids. Typically, the usual replacement dose is doubled or tripled for mild-to-moderate infections and during labor and delivery. Doses should also be doubled or tripled for approximately 24 hours for dental surgeries, minor surgeries (cataract, laparoscopic), and invasive diagnostic procedures. See Table 36.4.

Table 36.4. Stress Dosing of Glucocorticoids to Avoid an Adrenal Crisis.

Primary Adrenal Insufficiency
Prevention of Adrenal Crisis

CONDITION	SUGGESTED ACTION
Home illness with fever	T > 38°C (100.4°F) 2 × dose for 2–3 days T > 39°C (102.2°F) 3 × dose for 2–3 days
Same but no oral intake	Hydrocortisone 100 mg SQ or IM
Surgery: Minor/Moderate	Hydrocortisone 25–75 mg/24hr
Surgery: Major, trauma, medical intensive care	Hydrocortisone 100 mg IV, then 50 mg every 6 hours IV or IM

IM, Intramuscular; *IV*, intravenous; *SQ*, subcutaneous.
Modified from Bornstein, S. R. (2016). *Journal of Clinical Endocrinology and Metabolism 11*, 354–389, T4; Bancos, I, et al. (2015). Diagnosis and management of adrenal insufficiency. *Lancet Diabetes Endocrinology 3*, 216–226 (122), Elsevier Limited.

Patients with adrenal insufficiency should wear a medical alert bracelet or necklace identifying them as individuals with adrenal insufficiency in case they are incapable of providing an adequate history. An alternative form of hydrocortisone or dexamethasone can be provided so that patients will still be able to receive glucocorticoids intramuscularly (hydrocortisone, methylprednisolone, or dexamethasone) or per rectum (hydrocortisone) in an emergency situation.

23. **What drugs can cause adrenal insufficiency?**
The most common cause of central adrenal insufficiency is glucocorticoid therapy. Glucocorticoids can cause exogenous Cushing's syndrome, leading to suppression of the HPA axis. Patients may then be unable to mount an adequate cortisol response to stress or may develop adrenal insufficiency or an adrenal crisis if the steroid dose is abruptly stopped or tapered. Exogenous Cushing's syndrome can result from oral, ocular, inhaled, transdermal, rectal, or parenteral glucocorticoids. Some injected glucocorticoids for musculoskeletal disorders can last for weeks to months. Glucocorticoids are also found in some herbal or complementary/alternative therapies. Protease inhibitors and other drugs slow metabolism of glucocorticoids via interactions with the CYP3A4 enzyme. Thus, when protease inhibitors and glucocorticoids are used to together, exogenous Cushing's disease with HPA suppression can result even at low glucocorticoid doses.

High-dose progestins, such as megestrol acetate and medroxyprogesterone acetate, have enough glucocorticoid activity to cause exogenous Cushing's syndrome and HPA axis suppression. Opioids can also significantly suppress the HPA axis and can sometimes result in very low levels of serum cortisol and plasma ACTH. Drugs that can cause primary adrenal sufficiency include the azole antifungal agents, the anesthetic etomidate, the antiparasitic suramin, and steroid synthesis inhibitors, such as aminoglutethimide, metyrapone, and mitotane. Mifepristone, a progesterone antagonist, antagonizes the glucocorticoid receptor; it can, therefore, cause symptoms of adrenal insufficiency without concomitant low serum cortisol levels.

24. **How should steroids be tapered in patients on pharmacologic doses of steroids to treat nonadrenal diseases?**
Patients may be placed on glucocorticoids to treat a variety of autoimmune, neoplastic, or inflammatory disorders. Discontinuing glucocorticoid therapy can be challenging because of (1) worsening of the disorder for which the glucocorticoid is being used; (2) suppression of the HPA axis with resulting secondary adrenal insufficiency upon discontinuation of the glucocorticoid; and (3) steroid withdrawal syndrome.

The initial tapering of glucocorticoids from pharmacologic to physiologic doses depends on the underlying illness for which the steroids are being used. If the illness worsens during this period of tapering, the dosage needs to be increased and continued until the symptoms stabilize before another attempt at more gradual tapering. When the patient is on a near-physiologic dosage, she or he can be switched to a shorter acting glucocorticoid, such as hydrocortisone, and tapering continued to below physiologic dosages; alternate-day therapy may be helpful in certain instances.

Testing should be performed when patients have been at physiologic doses or below for at least 1 month, to ensure that adrenal suppression has resolved and that normal responsiveness of the HPA axis has returned. A morning cortisol measurement should be drawn 12 to 24 hours after the last dose of glucocorticoid (12 hours for short-acting synthetic glucocorticoids, such as hydrocortisone, and 24 hours for longer acting ones, such as prednisone). A plasma cortisol level < 3 mcg/dL is consistent with adrenal insufficiency, so the glucocorticoid should be continued for 4 to 6 weeks before retesting. A level > 18 mcg/dL is consistent with return of adrenal function, and glucocorticoids can be discontinued. A level between 3 and 18 mcg/dL is equivocal, and further testing is needed, usually with a cosyntropin stimulation test. It may take months for the HPA axis to respond normally to ACTH.

Central adrenal insufficiency should be suspected in individuals with a clinical presentation suggestive of adrenal insufficiency and who have received the equivalent of 20 mg prednisone for 5 days or physiologic dosages of glucocorticoid for at least 30 days in the past 12 months. These patients should receive stress doses of glucocorticoids during moderate-to-severe illness or surgeries.

KEY POINTS: CLASSIFICATION AND DIAGNOSIS OF ADRENAL INSUFFICIENCY

- Adrenal insufficiency is classified as primary (failure of adrenals to produce cortisol), secondary (failure of pituitary to produce adrenocorticotropic hormone [ACTH]), or tertiary (failure of hypothalamus to produce corticotropin-releasing hormone).
- Adrenal insufficiency should be suspected in outpatients who have received supraphysiologic doses of glucocorticoids for >1 month, intensive care unit patients who are hemodynamically unstable despite aggressive fluid resuscitation or have septic shock, and any patient with signs or symptoms suggesting adrenal insufficiency.
- Adrenal insufficiency is diagnosed by using a 30- or 60-minute cortisol level < 18 mcg/dL in a standard-dose cosyntropin stimulation test.

KEY POINTS: TREATMENT OF ADRENAL INSUFFICIENCY

- Treatment of adrenal insufficiency depends on the condition of the patient.
- Nonstressed outpatients should be treated with replacement doses of hydrocortisone or prednisone with or without fludrocortisone, depending on the type of adrenal insufficiency.
- Stressed patients should receive supplemental glucocorticoids tailored to the degree of stress.
- Adrenal crisis should be treated aggressively using intravenous (IV) saline and dextrose, IV glucocorticoids (dexamethasone if treating before drawing random cortisol and ACTH, hydrocortisone afterward), other supportive care, and a search for the precipitating illness.

BIBLIOGRAPHY

Alkatib, A. A., Cosma, M., Elamin, M. B., Erickson, D., Swiglo, B. A., Erwin, P. J., & Montori, V. M. (2009). A systemic review and meta-analysis of randomized placebo-controlled trials of DHEA treatment effects on quality of life in women with adrenal insufficiency. *Journal of Clinical Endocrinology and Metabolism, 94,* 3676–3681.

Annane, D., Bellissant, E., Bollaert, P. E., Briegel, J., Keh, D., & Kupfer, Y. (2015). Corticosteroids for treating sepsis. *Cochrane Database of Systematic Reviews, 12,* CD002243.

Annane, D., Pastores, S. M., Rochwerg, B., Arlt, W., Balk, R. A., Beishuizen, A., Briegel J, ... Van den Berghe, G. (2017). Guidelines for the diagnosis and management of critical illness-related corticosteroid insufficiency (CIRCI) in critically ill patients (Part 1): Society of Critical Care Medicine (SCCM) and European Society of Intensive Care Medicine (ESICM) 2017. *Intensive Care Medicine, 43,* 1751–1763.

Annane, D., Renault, A., Brun-Buisson, C., Megarbane, B., Quenot, J. P., Siami, S., ... Bellissant, E. (2018). Hydrocortisone plus fludrocortisone for adults with septic shock. *New England Journal of Medicine, 378,* 809–818.

Axelrod, L. (2003). Perioperative management of patients treated with glucocorticoids. *Endocrinology and Metabolism Clinics of North America, 32,* 367–383.

Bornstein, S. R. (2009). Predisposing factors for adrenal insufficiency. *New England Journal of Medicine, 360,* 2328–2339.

Bornstein, S. R., Allolio, B., Arlt, W., Barthel, A., Don-Wauchope, A., Hammer, G. D., ... Torpy, D. J. (2016). Diagnosis and treatment of primary adrenal insufficiency: an Endocrine Society clinical practice guideline. *Journal of Clinical Endocrinology and Metabolism, 101,* 364–389.

Bouillon, R. (2006). Acute adrenal insufficiency. *Endocrinology and Metabolism Clinics of North America, 35,* 767–775.

Carroll, T. B., Aron, D. C., Findling, J. W., Tyrrell, J. B. (2018). Chapter 9: Glucocorticoids and adrenal androgens. In D. G. Gardner & D. Shoback. (Eds.), *Greenspan's basic and clinical endocrinology* (10th ed.). Chicago, Il: McGraw-Hill.

Fleseriu, M., Hashim, I. A., Karavitaki, N., Melmed, S., Murad, M. H., Salvatori, R., & Samuels, M. H. (2016). Hormonal replacement in hypopituitarism in adults: an Endocrine Society clinical practice guideline. *Journal of Clinical Endocrinology and Metabolism, 101,* 3888–3921.

Grossman, A. B. (2010). The diagnosis and management of central hypoadrenalism. *Journal of Clinical Endocrinology and Metabolism, 95,* 4855–4863.

Hopkins, R. L., & Leinung, M. C. (2005). Exogenous Cushing's syndrome and glucocorticoid withdrawal. *Endocrinology and Metabolism Clinics of North America, 34,* 371–384.

Meikle, A. W., & Tyler, F. H. (1977). Potency and duration of action of glucocorticoids: effects of hydrocortisone, prednisone and dexamethasone on human pituitary-adrenal function. *American Journal of Medicine, 63,* 200–207.

Neary, N., & Nieman, L. (2010). Adrenal insufficiency: etiology, diagnosis and treatment. *Current Opinion in Endocrinology, Diabetes & Obesity, 17,* 217–223.

Rhodes, A., Evans, L. E., Alhazzani, W., Levy, M. M., Antonelli, M., Ferrer, R., ... Dellinger, R. P. (2017). Surviving Sepsis Campaign: international guidelines for management of sepsis and septic shock: 2016. *Critical Care Medicine, 45,* 486–552.

Stewart, P. M., & Newell-Price, J. D. C. (2016). Chapter 15: The adrenal cortex. In S. Melmed, K. S. Polonsky, P. R. Larsen & H. M. Kronenberg (Eds.), *Williams Textbook of Endocrinology* (13th ed., pp. 489–555). Philadelphia, PA: Elsevier.

Venkatesh, B., Finfer, S., Cohen, J., Rajbhandari, D., Arabi, Y., Bellomo, R. ... Myburgh, J. (2018). Adjunctive glucocorticoid therapy in patients with septic shock. *New England Journal of Medicine, 378,* 797–808.

CHAPTER 37

CONGENITAL ADRENAL HYPERPLASIA

Harris M. Baloch, Nicole Vietor, and Robert A. Vigersky

1. Define congenital adrenal hyperplasia (CAH).

   CAH is a group of autosomal recessive disorders involving a partial or complete defect in cortisol synthesis, aldosterone synthesis, or both, resulting in varying degrees of deficiency in one or both hormones.

2. How common is CAH?

   CAH is one of the most common inherited diseases. The most common form of CAH, 21-hydroxylase deficiency, has an incidence of 1:14,000 to 1:18,000 births. The prevalence of this disorder varies greatly among different ethnic groups and is highest among the Ashkenazi Jewish population of Eastern Europe. The nonclassic 21-hydroxylase deficiency occurs in approximately 0.2% of the general Caucasian population but more frequently (1%–2%) in certain populations, such as Ashkenazi Jews. Because of its high prevalence, newborn screening for CAH is performed in most countries.

3. What is the normal steroidogenesis pathway in the adrenal cortex?

   There are six enzymes required for the synthesis of cortisol from cholesterol in the adrenal cortex (Fig. 37.1). The first is the protein steroidogenic acute regulator (StAR), which is essential in transporting cholesterol to the mitochondria. The p450 side-chain cleavage (CYP11A1) is responsible for cholesterol side-chain cleavage, forming pregnenolone. 3beta-hydroxysteroid dehydrogenase converts the delta5-steroids (pregnenolone, 17-hydroxypregnenolone, dehydroepiandrosterone [DHEA]) to the delta4-steroids (progesterone, 17-hydroxyprogesterone, androstenedione). And, finally, the three hydroxylases CYP17A1 (17alpha-hydroxylase), CYP21A1 (21-hydroxylase), and CYP11B1 (11-hydroxylase) convert specific precursors to steroids in the cortisol pathway. These pathways are stimulated by

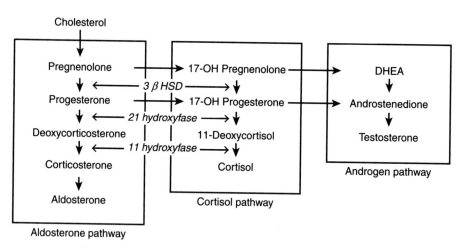

Fig. 37.1. Steroidogenic pathway in the adrenal cortex. *DHEA,* Dehydroepiandrosterone.

The views expressed in this manuscript are those of the authors and do not reflect the official policy of the Department of the Army, Navy, the Department of Defense, the National Institutes of Health, or the United States Government. Dr. Baloch and Dr. Vietor are military service members. This work was prepared as part of our official duties. Title 17 U.S.C. 105 provides the "Copyright protection under this title is not available for any work of the United States Government." Title 17 U.S.C. 101 defines a U.S. Government work as a work prepared by a military service member or employee of the U.S. Government as part of that person's official duties. We certify that all individuals who qualify as authors have been listed; each has participated in the conception and design of this work, the analysis of data (when applicable), the writing of the document, and/or the approval of the submission of this version; that the document represents valid work; that if we used information derived from another source, we obtained all necessary approvals to use it and made appropriate acknowledgements in the document; and that each takes public responsibility for it.

adrenocorticotropic hormone (ACTH) from the anterior pituitary gland. Knowledge of this pathway is critical to recognizing and predicting the effects of each enzyme deficiency.

4. Explain why adrenal hyperplasia develops.
   The process of adrenal hyperplasia begins in utero. Reduced production of cortisol in the fetus caused by decreased activity of one of the enzymes needed for cortisol synthesis results in lowered levels of serum cortisol. Cortisol normally acts through a negative feedback loop to inhibit the secretion of ACTH by the pituitary gland and corticotropin-releasing hormone (CRH) by the hypothalamus. Thus, the low serum cortisol levels that occur in a person with CAH increase the secretion of CRH and ACTH in an attempt to stimulate the adrenal glands to overcome the enzyme block and to return the serum cortisol level to normal. As this process continues over time, the elevated levels of serum ACTH stimulate growth of the adrenal glands, leading to hyperplasia. It has been shown that the adrenal volume correlates positively with 17-hydroxyprogesterone (17-OHP) levels in patients with 21-hydroxylase deficiency (Fig. 37.2).

5. Describe the functions of the three hydroxylases.
   - CYP17A1 (17alpha-hydroxylase) is essential in converting progesterone to 17-OHP and pregnenolone to 17-hydroxypregnenolone. This enzyme also includes a 17,20-lyase activity, which converts 17-hydroxypregnenolone to dehydroepiandrosterone.
   - CYP21A2 (21-hydroxylase) converts progesterone to deoxycorticosterone (DOC) and 17-OHP to 11-deoxycortisol.
   - CYP11B1 (11beta-hydroxylase) converts DOC to corticosterone (which then goes on to aldosterone) and 11-deoxycortisol to cortisol.

6. How is CAH inherited?
   All of the enzyme defects leading to CAH are autosomal recessive disorders; hence, both copies of the involved gene must be abnormal for the condition to occur.

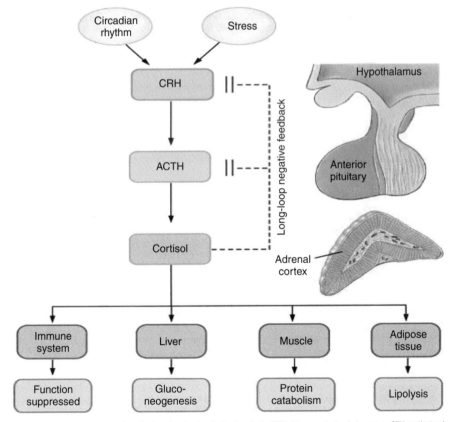

Fig. 37.2. Hypothalamic–pituitary–adrenal axis and systemic effects of cortisol. *ACTH,* Adrenocorticotropic hormone; *CRH,* corticotropin-releasing hormone.

7. What is the most common form of CAH?

By far, the most common form is 21-hydroxylase (CYP21A2) deficiency, which accounts for 90% of cases and leads to deficiencies of the salt-retaining hormones DOC and aldosterone in both genders, and/or virilization of genetic females. Both of these are considered "classic" CAH.

8. What percentage of the population at large are heterozygote carriers of the 21-hydroxylase defect?

Less than 2% of Americans are heterozygote carriers of the 21-hydroxylase defect. However, higher carrier rates are observed in persons of Eastern European descent (approximately 10%); these carriers have an abnormality in one of the two copies of the 21-hydroxylase gene. They appear normal in all respects but may have elevated serum 17-OHP levels with ACTH stimulation testing.

9. Which genes encode for 21-hydroxylase?

Two genes encode for 21-hydroxylase: *CYP21A1* (pseudogene) and *CYP21A2* (true gene), both of which are located in a 35-kb region on the short arm of chromosome 6 (6p21.3). Both genes are located downstream of the gene coding for complement factor 4 (C4A and C4B). *CYP21A1* and *CYP21A2* have 98% nucleotide sequence identity, but the former has accumulated several mutations that totally inactivate its gene product. *CYP21A1* is thus an inactive pseudogene, whereas the *CYP21A2* gene codes for the active 21-hydroxylase enzyme.

10. What causes most of the genetic events responsible for *CYP21A2* deficiencies?

Most of the genetic events responsible for *CYP21A2* deficiencies result from the similarity between *CYP21A1* and *CYP21A2*. This similarity leads to two types of recombination events between *CYP21A2* and the pseudogene. Seventy-five percent of these events represent deleterious mutations found in the pseudogene that are transferred to *CYP21A2* during mitosis. This process is termed *gene conversion*. Twenty percent are meiotic recombinations producing a nonfunctional chimeric pseudogene. Greater than 100 additional mutations account for the remaining 5%.

11. What determines the patient's phenotype for 21-hydroxylase deficiency?

Clinical manifestations of the disease are related to the degree of cortisol deficiency, aldosterone deficiency, or both, and the accumulation of precursor hormones. Greater than 100 *CYP21A2* mutations are known. The patient's phenotype is generally based on the specific genetic alteration of the *CYP21A2* gene and can be grouped into three categories:

- Patients with no enzyme activity typically have large deletions or splicing mutations and predominantly have the salt-wasting form of the disorder.
- Patients with a nonconservative amino substitution in exon 4 usually have 1% to 2% of enzyme activity and typically have the simple virilizing form of the disease.
- Patients with a point mutation in exon 7 have 20% to 50% of normal enzyme activity and most often have the nonclassic form of the disease.
- Patients who are heterozygotes have mild abnormalities but no clinically important endocrine disorder.

12. What is the second most common cause of CAH?

The second most common cause of CAH (7% of all cases) is deficiency of the 11beta-hydroxylase enzyme (CYP11B1), which is also an autosomal recessive defect caused by a mutation on the short arm of chromosome 8 (8q24.3). The result of this deficiency is an increased level of DOC, which may cause hypertension through activation of the mineralocorticoid receptor, leading to sodium retention and hypokalemic alkalosis. The enzyme deficiency also results in increased production of androgens and their precursors, which causes ambiguous genitalia in genetic females.

13. How common is 11beta-hydroxylase deficiency?

11beta-hydroxylase deficiency, the second most frequent form of CAH, occurs in 1:100,000 births in the general population but in 1:5,000 births in Jews of Moroccan decent. CAH caused by defects of the other enzymes listed here is extremely rare.

14. Summarize the rarer forms of CAH.

The rarer forms of CAH are 17alpha-hydroxylase and 3beta-hydroxysteroid dehydrogenase deficiency. There have been fewer than 200 reported cases of 17alpha-hydroxylase deficiency with 40 described mutations of *CYP17A1* that span an 8.7-kb region on the short arm of chromosome 10 (10q24.3). The consequences of this deficiency are hypertension caused by sodium retention and hypokalemia resulting from DOC excess (associated with suppressed renin and aldosterone), along with deficiency of androgens and androgen precursors, which causes pseudohermaphroditism in genetic males and delayed puberty in both genders.

15. What is the most serious clinical consequence of CAH?

Adrenal crisis in newborns is the most serious consequence of CAH caused by 21-hydroxylase deficiency. This occurs with those genetic defects that cause severely reduced or absent 21-hydroxylase activity, resulting in absolute or near-absolute aldosterone, DOC, and cortisol deficiencies. This is especially insidious in genetic males, who do not have ambiguous genitalia as an earlier and critical clue to this diagnosis. Overall, about two thirds of people with 21-hydroxylase deficiency have the salt-wasting form. These newborns produce very low or no levels of aldosterone and DOC, resulting in severe renal salt wasting, hypotension, and hypovolemic shock; in addition, their increased levels of progesterone and 17-OHP exacerbate the effects of aldosterone deficiency because progesterone and 17-OHP are mineralocorticoid antagonists. This situation leads to volume depletion, hypotension, hyponatremia, hyperkalemia, and increased renin activity. Cortisol deficiency contributes to poor cardiac function, poor vascular response to catecholamines, decreased glomerular filtration rate, and increased secretion of antidiuretic hormone.

16. What are other clinical consequences of CAH in females?
Many of the precursors and metabolites that build up behind the blocked enzymes 21-hydroxylase, 11beta-hydroxylase, or 3beta-hydroxysteroid dehydrogenase are androgen precursors. They may cause the following:
- Masculinization of the external genitalia of a genetic female fetus, leading to ambiguous genitalia at birth (female pseudohermaphroditism)
- Behaviors more typical of boys during childhood in terms of toy preference, rough play, and aggressiveness (however, most females are heterosexual and their sexual identity is invariably female.)
- Rapid growth during early childhood, with ultimate short stature as an adult because of early closure of epiphyses
- Infertility in 20% of females with simple virilizing disease and approximately 40% of females with salt-wasting disease
- Osteopenia as young adults in 45% of women with salt wasting
- Obesity
- Lower quality of life scores compared with age- and gender-matched controls
- Variable and subtle hyperpigmentation

17. What are other clinical consequences of CAH in males?
Newborn males with CAH caused by deficiency of 21-hydroxylase or 11beta-hydroxylase do not have ambiguous genitalia. Because of the typical normal physical appearance, it is often difficult to detect an affected male, especially when symptoms of salt wasting occur after the first week of life.
    Later in childhood or in early adulthood, males may present with the following:
- No overt signs
- Premature puberty
- Variable and subtle hyperpigmentation
- Advanced height in early childhood with ultimate short stature
- Acne
- Testicular enlargement caused by adrenal rests, which may produce adrenal-specific hormones
- Oligospermia and/or infertility
- Lower quality-of-life scores compared with age- and gender-matched controls

18. Are patients with CAH at increased risk for cardiovascular disease?
Cardiovascular risk factors that have been identified in patients with CAH include increased body mass index, higher blood pressure, and more insulin resistance compared with age-matched controls. They also have endothelial dysfunction similar to other patients who are obese. These effects are especially prominent in males > 30 years of age.

19. How do patients with 11beta-hydroxylase deficiency present?
In 11beta-hydroxylase deficiency, the enzyme defect blocks synthesis of both aldosterone and cortisol. As such, these patients are at risk of adrenal insufficiency. However, they do not have mineralocorticoid deficiency because they oversecrete the aldosterone precursor 11-DOC, which is itself a powerful mineralocorticoid. Excess precursors also drive production of androgens and patients present with:
- Cortisol deficiency
  - Adrenal insufficiency
- Mineralocorticoid excess
  - Hypertension
  - Hypokalemia
- Androgen excess
  - Increased penile size in males
  - Ambiguous genitalia, including clitoral enlargement and labioscrotal fusion in females (female pseudohermaphroditism)

20. How do patients with 17alpha-hydroxylase deficiency present?
In 17alpha-hydroxylase deficiency, the enzyme defect blocks the synthesis of cortisol and androgens but leads to excess mineralocorticoids. Thus, patients present with:
- Cortisol deficiency
  - Adrenal insufficiency
- Mineralocorticoid excess
  - Hypertension
  - Hypokalemia

- Androgen deficiency
  - Undervirilization in males
  - Absence of secondary characteristics and primary amenorrhea in females

21. How do patients with 3beta–hydroxysteroid dehydrogenase type 2 deficiency present?
    In 3beta–hydroxysteroid dehydrogenase type 2 deficiency, the enzyme defect blocks synthesis of aldosterone, cortisol, and androgens. As such, these patients are at risk of deficiency in all three pathways. However, in peripheral tissue (liver and skin) 3beta–hydroxysteroid dehydrogenase type 1 converts DHEA to androstenedione, providing mild levels of androgens. These levels are enough to cause clitoral enlargement, acne, and hirsutism in females but not enough to lead to proper male development. Hence, these patients present with:
    - Cortisol deficiency
      - Adrenal insufficiency
    - Mineralocorticoid deficiency
      - Hypotension
      - Hyperkalemia
    - Androgen excess
      - Ambiguous genitalia in males
      - Mild-to-moderate clitoral enlargement, hirsutism, and acne in females
      Generally, these patients present as neonates or early infants with feeding difficulties, vomiting, volume depletion, and the problems listed above.

22. How do patients with nonclassic CAH present?
    Patients with nonclassic CAH (also called *late-onset CAH*) produce normal amounts of cortisol and aldosterone at the expense of mild-to-moderate overproduction of sex hormone precursors. The prevalence of nonclassic CAH in women presenting with hyperandrogenic signs and symptoms has been shown to be 2.2%. Thus, follicular-phase 17-OHP should be included in the evaluation of any female patient with hyperandrogenic symptoms. Usually, these patients are asymptomatic and have normal external genitalia but may present with the following:
    - Premature puberty
    - Severe cystic acne—occurring in 33% of patients
    - Hirsutism—most common symptom, occurring in 60% of symptomatic females
    - Oligomenorrhea and polycystic ovaries—second most common, occurring in 54% of patients
    - Infertility—occurring in 13% of patients

23. Summarize the relationship between adrenal "incidentalomas" and CAH.
    Adrenal incidentalomas are more common in patients with CAH and in heterozygotes. Conversely, 60% of patients with incidentalomas have exaggerated 17-OHP responses to ACTH stimulation testing.

24. Describe the clinical features that suggest the possibility of CAH.
    Adrenal crisis or severe salt wasting in the newborn period suggests the possibility of CAH. CAH also must be considered prominently in the differential diagnosis of any newborn with ambiguous genitalia. Because adrenal crisis and salt wasting in CAH may be fatal if not treated, the finding of ambiguous genitalia in a newborn should trigger a rapid attempt to confirm or exclude CAH. Most males with CAH do not have ambiguous genitalia; consequently, many cases go unrecognized at birth unless there is a documented family history of the disorder.

25. What clinical clues help to support or refute the diagnosis of CAH in a newborn with ambiguous genitalia?
    The overwhelming majority of genetic males with CAH have unambiguous external genitalia at birth; conversely, CAH is an uncommon cause of ambiguous genitalia in a genetic male. Thus, determination that the infant with ambiguous genitalia is a genetic male makes CAH unlikely and decreases the diagnostic urgency because the disorders giving rise to ambiguous genitalia in genetic males are rarely associated with a fatal outcome. For example, the finding of palpable gonads in the scrotal or inguinal area suggests that the infant is a genetic male because such palpable gonads are almost always testes. Conversely, the detection of a uterus in an infant with ambiguous genitalia, through either physical examination or ultrasonography, strongly suggests that the infant is a genetic female, thus heightening the possibility of CAH.

26. Discuss the role of molecular biology techniques in the diagnosis of CAH.
    Molecular biology techniques can rapidly confirm the genetic sex of a newborn without the prolonged wait for a traditional chromosome analysis. Because of the potentially severe consequences of CAH, it is probably prudent to assume that any genetic female with ambiguous genitalia has CAH, until proven otherwise. Furthermore, it is probably best to wait to assign gender until molecular testing is done because gender misassignment may cause long-term psychological problems in such children and their families. Early diagnosis and appropriate therapy also help avoid the progressive effects of excess adrenal androgens, which will cause short stature, gender confusion in girls, and psychosexual disturbances in both boys and girls.

27. How is the diagnosis of CAH confirmed?

Because one does not know which enzyme is deficient in a newborn with suspected CAH (unless the family has a documented history of a particular enzyme defect), serum levels of all steroids that may be in the affected biosynthetic pathway can be measured before and after the administration of 250 mcg of synthetic ACTH. Urinary measurement of these steroids with the use of gas chromatography/mass spectroscopy has recently become economically feasible. Plasma renin activity and aldosterone levels should also be measured to assess the adequacy of aldosterone synthesis. Determination of which steroid levels are supranormal and which are low facilitates localization of the exact enzyme block.

28. How are specific genetic defects confirmed?

Specific genetic defects may be confirmed with molecular genetic testing. Polymerase chain reaction amplification for the rapid simultaneous detection of the 10 mutations that are found in approximately 95% of 21-hydroxylase deficiency alleles is used for rapid results. Molecular genetic analysis of CYP21 is not essential for diagnosis but may be helpful to:

- Confirm the basis of the defect
- Aid in genetic counseling
- Establish the disease in certain cases

29. What should be done when nonclassic CAH is suspected at a later age?

When nonclassic CAH is suspected in the preteen, teenage, or adult patient, an early-morning 17-OHP level should be obtained; if 17-OHP levels are < 200 ng/dL, then CAH is excluded, and levels > 1000 ng/dL confirm CAH. If 17-OHP levels are 200 to 1000 ng/dL, ACTH stimulation testing is the next step. ACTH stimulation testing should be done with 250 mcg (not 1 mcg) of synthetic ACTH; measurement of 17-OHP, 17-OH pregnenolone, and cortisol should be done before and 60 minutes after the ACTH injection. Stimulated levels of 17-OHP with classic CAH are typically > 10,000 ng/dL, whereas patients with nonclassic CAH will usually have 17-OHP levels in the range of 1000 to 10,000 ng/dL. Hyperandrogenism can be assessed in women by measuring serum levels of testosterone, androstenedione, and 3alpha-androstanediol glucuronide (Fig. 37.3).

30. Describe the tests used for newborn screening.

The screening process for newborns is divided into first-tier screening and second-tier screening tests. First-tier screening for CAH focuses on the rapid detection of classic 21-hydroxylase deficiency on Guthrie cards (filter paper on which blood samples are collected, dried, and transported) and measured by automated time-resolved dissociation-enhanced lanthanide fluoroimmunoassay. This screening method measures 17-OHP. Basal 17-OHP usually exceeds 10,000 ng/dL in affected infants, whereas the levels in normal infants are below 100 ng/dL. To have a high level of sensitivity, cut-off values are set low in order to have 1% of all tests reported as positive, thus leading to several false-positive results. Infants that are premature, sick, or stressed will have higher levels of 17-OHP. Second-tier testing includes molecular genetic testing or biochemical testing that measures steroid ratios through liquid chromatography followed by mass spectrometry. As of 2009, all 50 states in the United States and at least 12 other countries screen for CAH at birth. Fig. 37.4 outlines the algorithm normally used.

31. What other tests may be used?

If CAH is suspected in the newborn and filter paper screening is not available, ACTH stimulation with steroid precursor measurements should be done after the first 24 hours of life. Adrenal ultrasonography can also be

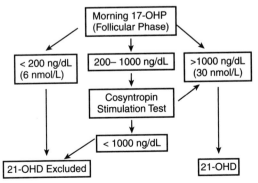

Fig. 37.3. Algorithm for diagnosing nonclassic congenital adrenal hyperplasia (CAH). *21-OHD,* 21-Hydroxylase; *17-OHP,* 17-hydroxyprogesterone. (From Speiser, P., Arlt, W., Auchus, R., Baskin, L. S., Conway, G. S., Merke, D. P., Meyer-Bahlburg, H. F. L., ... White, P. C. (2018). Congenital adrenal hyperplasia due to steroid 21-hydroxylase deficiency: an Endocrine Society clinical practice guideline. *Journal of Clinical Endocrinology and Metabolism, 103*(11), 4043–4088.)

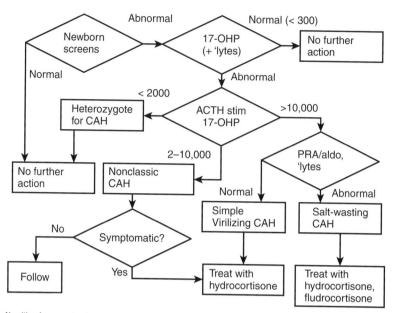

Fig. 37.4. Algorithm for screening for congenital adrenal hyperplasia (CAH) in neonates. *ACTH,* Adrenocorticotropic hormone; *17-OHP,* 17-hydroxyprogesterone; *PRA,* . (From White, P., Spieser, P. (2000). Congenital adrenal hyperplasia due to 21-hydroxylase deficiency. *Endocrine Reviews, 21*(3), 245–291.)

used as a potential screening test for neonates with CAH and ambiguous genitalia and/or salt-wasting crisis by detecting > 4 mm adrenal limb width.

32. How is CAH treated in neonates?

The most important goal of treatment is to prevent salt-wasting and adrenal crisis in the newborn period. This goal requires the prompt administration of glucocorticoids and, in many cases, mineralocorticoids, as well as careful monitoring of salt intake. This treatment not only replaces the deficient hormones but also suppresses elevated serum ACTH levels, thereby reducing adrenal production of androgenic precursors and metabolites. Such treatment may be given presumptively while awaiting the results of definitive laboratory tests and then discontinued if the tests rule out CAH.

33. What is the appropriate hydrocortisone formulation in infants and children unable to take a tablet?

The hydrocortisone tablet and suspension are not bioequivalent and the suspension may have uneven distribution. Infants and children unable to take a tablet should be given crushed hydrocortisone tablets in liquid.

34. When is surgical correction of ambiguous genitalia carried out?

Surgical correction of ambiguous genitalia in girls consists of genitoplasty of the clitoris and labia and vaginoplasty. Single-stage surgery is now implemented between 2 and 6 months of life.

35. Describe the treatment for CAH in children.

The preferred glucocorticoid for chronic replacement is hydrocortisone at doses of 10 to 15 mg/m^2/day in three divided doses. Hydrocortisone is preferred because of its short half-life, which minimizes growth suppression and other Cushing-like side effects. It is sometimes extremely difficult or impossible to find a dosage of glucocorticoid that normalizes production of androgen and maintains normal growth and weight gain. In such situations, mineralocorticoids (fludrocortisone) and/or spironolactone/flutamide (androgen receptor blockers that prevent virilization) in combination with the aromatase inhibitor testolactone (which prevents estrogen-induced epiphyseal fusion) may be useful adjunctive therapy in combination with nonsuppressive replacement doses of glucocorticoids. Rarely, adrenalectomy has been used for difficult-to-control CAH because treatment of adrenal insufficiency is relatively much simpler. All patients with salt-wasting CAH should be treated with fludrocortisone, with recommended dosing of 0.05 to 0.2 mg/day given once or twice a day.

36. How is CAH treated in adolescents and adults?

The use of growth hormone, gonadotropin-releasing hormone analogues, antiandrogens, and aromatase inhibitors, alone or in various combinations, may improve the final predicted height, particularly in those whose predicted height is ≤ 2.25 Standard Deviations (SD). However, such treatment should be done under the auspices of an institutional review board (IRB)–approved protocol, because both the necessity and the long-term consequences of such an approach have yet to be determined. Prednisone (5–7.5 mg daily in two divided doses) or dexamethasone (0.25–0.5 mg daily) may be used once growth is complete. Because of the potency of dexamethasone, intermediate doses can be achieved by using liquid dexamethasone (1 mg/mL) which is generally used for other conditions in infants and children. Patients should be monitored carefully for signs of iatrogenic Cushing's syndrome and ultrasonography should be used in males to detect testicular adrenal rests.

37. **What is the role of glucocorticoid treatment in nonclassic CAH?**
    Glucocorticoid therapy is not recommended in asymptomatic patients because they are unlikely to suffer from adrenal insufficiency. Considerations for initiation of glucocorticoid therapy in patients with nonclassic CAH include:
    - Evidence has shown that women with nonclassic CAH on glucocorticoid therapy have lower miscarriage rates compared with women not on glucocorticoids.
    - If a patient has an inappropriately early onset and rapid progression of pubarche/bone age *or* excess virilization, glucocorticoids can be initiated and then discontinued after adult height is attained.
    - If a patient has significant hyperandrogenism, therapy can be considered.
    - Glucocorticoid therapy may benefit women with infertility or those with a history of miscarriage.
    - Testicular adrenal rest tumors are rare in male patients with nonclassic CAH; thus, glucocorticoid therapy is not indicated for prevention.

38. **What factors favor the achievement of predicted adult height?**
    - Early diagnosis
    - Lower doses of hydrocortisone in the first year of life
    - Use of hydrocortisone rather than prednisone or dexamethasone during the pubertal growth spurt
    - Mineralocorticoid treatment in all patients who are genetically determined to be "salt-wasters," even if they are not so clinically.

39. **What changes in therapy are necessary as a result of medically significant stress?**
    Patients with CAH who have been on steroid therapy should wear a medical alert bracelet or necklace, and should be provided with an emergency kit of hydrocortisone or dexamethasone for intramuscular use. For medically significant stress, the following measures are recommended (Table 37.1):
    - Triple the oral dose of glucocorticoids
    - Intramuscular (or intravenous) steroids if the patient is unable to consume oral medications. (Hydrocortisone is the preferred glucocorticoid because of its mineralocorticoid properties.)
    - Sodium chloride 1 to 2 g/day may be necessary in infants
    - Higher doses of fludrocortisone acetate (Florinef) are not recommended during severe stress. (The mineralocorticoid effects of hydrocortisone are sufficient.)
    - Successive intravenous hydrocortisone doses should be given as maintenance doses three to four times per day, every 6 hours.

40. **What changes in therapy are necessary during pregnancy for patients with classic CAH?**
    - Previous dosage of glucocorticoids can be continued but the dose may be adjusted if symptoms of glucocorticoid insufficiency occur.
    - Glucocorticoids that do not traverse the placenta, such as hydrocortisone or prednisone (placental 11B-HSD2 degrades these glucocorticoids), should be used rather than dexamethasone, which passes through the placenta unmetabolized.
    - Dose should be increased during the third trimester by 20% to 40%.
    - Stress doses of steroids should be used during labor and delivery.

Table 37.1. Recommended Initial Treatment for Patients with Congenital Adrenal Hyperplasia (CAH) Exposed to Clinically Significant Medical Stress.

PATIENT'S AGE	INITIAL PARENTERAL HYDROCORTISONE DOSE
Infants and preschool children	25 mg
School-age children	50 mg
Adults	100 mg

From Speiser, P., Arlt, W., Auchus, R., Baskin, L. S., Conway, G. S., Merke, D. P., Meyer-Bahlburg, H. F. L., ... White, P. C. (2018). Congenital adrenal hyperplasia due to steroid 21-hydroxylase deficiency: an Endocrine Society clinical practice guideline. *Journal of Clinical Endocrinology and Metabolism, 103*(11), 4043–4088.

41. **What changes in therapy are necessary during pregnancy for patients with nonclassic CAH?**
Current recommendations are to consider treatment with glucocorticoids if patients have had a previous miscarriage. Use of dexamethasone is *not* recommended for the reasons stated above. Stress dosing is usually not necessary unless patients have had a documented suboptimal response to ACTH stimulation testing previously (peak cortisol < 14–18 mcg/dL).

42. **How is treatment monitored?**
The goals of treatment are to prevent symptoms of adrenal insufficiency and to suppress ACTH and adrenal androgen production. For the latter, it is most appropriate to monitor the levels of the key precursors immediately behind the blocked enzyme (e.g., 17-OHP and androstenedione in the case of 21-hydroxylase deficiency). The goal is not to normalize the 17-OHP level because this will lead to iatrogenic Cushing's syndrome. Monitoring should be done every 3 months initially and then every 4 to 12 months. The goal is to maintain normal serum sodium, potassium, testosterone, and androstenedione levels. In women attempting to get pregnant, follicular-phase progesterone levels should be < 0.6 ng/mL.

43. **What other monitoring tools may be beneficial?**
Androgen levels should be monitored during treatment. These include testosterone, androstenedione, and 3alpha-androstanediol glucuronide. In addition, plasma renin activity should be monitored in patients with salt-wasting CAH. Children must have annual bone age determinations, and their height should be carefully monitored. Because patients with CAH have an increased number of cardiovascular risk factors, they should be routinely monitored and treated, if needed, for cardiovascular disease, which may begin earlier than expected. Adult men with CAH are prone to developing testicular adrenal rests and may have reduced fertility. This can be monitored by using serial ultrasonography and semen analysis, if appropriate.

44. **What genetic counseling is appropriate for a couple who have had a child with CAH?**
Because all forms of CAH are autosomal recessive disorders, both parents of a child with CAH are obligate hetero-zygote carriers of the gene defect. Consequently, the chance that another child of the same couple will have CAH is one in four; 50% of the children will be heterozygote carriers. Genetic counseling should be given to all parents who have a child with CAH. Modern genetic techniques and chorionic villus sampling of fetal DNA at 9 weeks' gestation allow for the diagnosis of CAH during the first trimester of pregnancy. The other use for genotypic identification includes the prediction of the phenotype (i.e., severity of the disease). There appears to be a good relationship between genotype and phenotype in classic CAH but not in nonclassic CAH.

45. **Are any prenatal treatments available for the fetus with CAH?**
Glucocorticoid treatment of the fetus with 21-hydroxylase deficiency should be regarded as experimental at this time and only provided in the context of an IRB-approved protocol. Earlier recommendations for such treatment were based on small, uncontrolled studies. The potential adverse effects of glucocorticoid therapy in this setting may outweigh any benefits.

KEY POINTS: CAH

- Congenital adrenal hyperplasia (CAH), the most common inherited disease, is a group of autosomal recessive disorders, the most frequent of which is 21-hydroxylase deficiency.
- The most serious consequences of CAH are neonatal salt wasting, ambiguous genitalia in females at birth, short stature, and premature puberty.
- CAH is diagnosed through measurement of cortisol precursors before and 1 hour after the intravenous adminis-tration of 250 mcg of synthetic ACTH.
- Predicted adult height can be achieved through early diagnosis, lower doses of corticosteroids in the first year of life and during puberty, and the use of fludrocortisone, even in those who are "salt wasters" genetically but not clinically.
- CAH is a rare cause of ambiguous genitalia in a genetic male.
- The most common symptom in nonclassic CAH in females is hirsutism.
- Prenatal treatment with dexamethasone and height-enhancing treatment with growth hormone and/or gonadotropin-releasing hormone analogues (GNRHa) should be done only under institutional review board-approved protocols in centers of excellence.

⊕ WEBSITES

http://www.endocrine.org

BIBLIOGRAPHY

Arlt, W., Willis, D., Wild, S., Krone, N., Doherty, E. J., Hahner, S., … Ross, R. J. (2010). Health status of adults with congenital adrenal hyperplasia: a cohort study of 203 patients. *Journal of Clinical Endocrinology and Metabolism, 95*, 5110–5121.

Balsamo, A., Cicognani, A., Baldazzi, L., Barbaro, M., Baronio, F., Gennari, M., … Cacciari, E. (2003). CYP21 genotype, adult height, and pubertal development in 55 patients treated for 21-hydroxylase deficiency. *Journal of Clinical Endocrinology and Metabolism, 88*, 5680–5688.

Bidet, M., Bellanne-Chantelot, C., Galand-Portier, M., Golmard, J. L., Tardy, V., Morel, Y., … Kuttenn, F. (2010). Fertility in women with nonclassical congenital adrenal hyperplasia due to 21-hydroxylase deficiency. *Journal of Clinical Endocrinology and Metabolism, 95*,1182–1190.

Cabrera, M. S., Vogiatzi, M. G., & New, M. I. (2001). Long term outcome in adult males with classic congenital adrenal hyperplasia. *Journal of Clinical Endocrinology and Metabolism, 86*, 3070–3078.

Chrousos, G. P., Loriaux, D. L., Mann, D. L., Cutler, G. B. Jr. (1982). Late-onset 21-hydroxylase deficiency mimicking idiopathic hirsutism or polycystic ovarian disease: an allelic variant of congenital virilizing adrenal hyperplasia with a milder enzymatic defect. *Annals of Internal Medicine, 96*, 143–148.

Claahsen-van der Grinten, H., Otten, B. J., Sweep, F., Span, P. N., Ross, H. A., Meuleman, E., Hermus, R. (2007). Testicular tumors in patients with congenital adrenal hyperplasia due to 21-hydroxylase deficiency show functional features of adrenocortical tissue. *Journal of Clinical Endocrinology and Metabolism, 92*, 2674–3680.

Deneux, C., Veronique, T., Dib, A., Mornet, E., Billaud, L., Charron, D., … Kuttenn, F. (2001). Phenotype–genotype correlation in 56 women with nonclassical congenital adrenal hyperplasia due to 21-hydroxylase deficiency. *Journal of Clinical Endocrinology and Metabolism, 86*, 207–213.

Escobar-Morreale, H., Sanchón, R., & Millán, Jose. (2008). A prospective study of the prevalence of nonclassical congenital adrenal hyperplasia among women presenting with hyperandrogenic symptoms and signs. *Journal of Clinical Endocrinology and Metabolism, 93*, 527–533.

Falhammar, H., Nyström, H. F., Ekström, U., Granberg, S., Wedell, A., & Thorén, M. (2012). Fertility, sexuality and testicular adrenal rest tumors in adult males with congenital adrenal hyperplasia. *European Journal of Endocrinology, 166*, 441–449.

Falhammar, H., Nyström, H. F., Wedell, A., & Thorén, M. (2010). Cardiovascular risk, metabolic profile, and body composition in adult males with congenital adrenal hyperplasia due to 21-hydroxylase deficiency. *European Journal of Endocrinology, 164*(2), 285–293. doi:10.1530/eje-10-0877.

Forest, M. G., Bétuel, H., & David, M. (1989). Prenatal treatment in congenital adrenal hyperplasia due to 21-hydroxylase deficiency: Update 88 of the French multicenter study. *Endocrine Research, 15*, 277–301.

Harrington, J., Peña, A. S., Gent, R., Hirte, C., & Couper, J. (2012). Adolescents with congenital adrenal hyperplasia due to 21-hydroxylase deficiency have vascular dysfunction. *Clinical Endocrinology, 76*, 837–842.

Hirvikoski, T., Lindholm, T., Lindblad, F., Ritzén, M., Wedell, A., & Lajic, S. (2007). Cognitive functions in children ar risk for congenital adrenal hyperplasia treated prenatally with dexamethasone. *Journal of Clinical Endocrinology and Metabolism, 92*, 542–548.

Hirvikoski, T., Nördenstrom, A., Ritzén, M., Wedell, A., & Lajic, S. (2012). Prenatal dexamethasone treatment of children at risk for congenital adrenal hyperplasia: the Swedish experience and standpoint. *Journal of Clinical Endocrinology and Metabolism, 97*, 1881–1883.

King, J., Wisniewski, A., Bankowski, B., Carson, K. A., Zacur, H. A., & Migeon, C. J. (2006). Long-term corticosteroid replacement and bone mineral density in adult women with classical congenital adrenal hyperplasia. *Journal of Clinical Endocrinology and Metabolism, 91*, 865–869.

Levine, L. (2000). Congenital adrenal hyperplasia. *Pediatric Rev, 21*, 159–171.

Lin-Su, K., Vogiatzi, M., Marshall, I., Harbison, M. D., Macapagal, M. C., Betensky, B., … New, M. I. (2005). Treatment with growth hormone and luteinizing hormone releasing hormone analog improves final adult height in children with congenital adrenal hyperplasia. *Journal of Clinical Endocrinology and Metabolism, 90*, 3318–3325.

Lin-Su, K., Harbison, M., Lekarev, O., Vogiatzi, M. G., & New, M. I. (2011). Final adult height in children with congenital adrenal hyperplasia treated with growth hormone. *Journal of Clinical Endocrinology and Metabolism, 96*, 1710–1717.

Linder, B., Esteban, N., Yergey, A., Winterer, J. C., Loriaux, D. L., & Cassorla, F. (1991). Cortisol production rate in childhood and adolescence. *Journal of Pediatrics, 117*, 892–896.

Lo, J., Schwitzgebel, V., Tyrrell, J., Fitzgerald, P. A., Kaplan, S. L., Conte, F. A., & Grumbach, M. M. (1999). Normal female infants born of mothers with classic congenital adrenal hyperplasia due to 21-hydroxylase deficiency. *Journal of Clinical Endocrinology and Metabolism, 84*, 930–936.

Merke, D., Keil, M., Jones, J., Fields, J., Hill, S., & Cutler, G. Jr. (2000). Flutamide, testolactone, and reduced hydrocortisone dose maintain normal growth velocity and bone maturation despite elevated androgen levels in children with congenital adrenal hyperplasia. *Journal of Clinical Endocrinology and Metabolism, 85*, 1114–1120.

Merke, D. P., & Bornstein, S. R. (2005). Congenital adrenal hyperplasia. *Lancet, 365*, 2125–2136.

Miller, W. (2012). The syndrome of 17,20 lyase deficiency. *Journal of Clinical Endocrinology and Metabolism, 97*, 59–67.

Mnif, M. F., Kamoun, M., Mnif, F., Charfi, N., Kallel, N., Ben Naceur, B., … Abid, M. (2012). Long-term outcome of patients with congenital adrenal hyperplasia due to 21-hydroxyase deficiency. *American Journal of Medical Sciences, 344*, 363–373.

Mulaikal, R. M., Migeon, C. J., & Rock, J. A. (1987). Fertility rates in female patients with congenital adrenal hyperplasia due to 21-hydroxylase deficiency. *New England Journal of Medicine, 316*, 178–182.

Muthusamy, K., Elamin, M., Smushkin, G., Murad, M. H., Lampropulos, J. F., Elamin, K. B., … Montori, V. M. (2010). Adult height in patients with congenital adrenal hyperplasia: a systematic review and metaanalysis. *Journal of Clinical Endocrinology and Metabolism, 95*, 4161–4172.

New, M. I., Carlson, A., Obeid, J., Marshall, I., Cabrera, M. S., Goseco, A., … Wilson, R. C. (2001). Prenatal diagnosis for congenital adrenal hyperplasia in 532 pregnancies. *Journal of Clinical Endocrinology and Metabolism, 86*, 5651–5657.

Nordenström, A., Frisén, L., Falhammar, H., Filipsson, H., Holmdahl, G., Janson, P. O., … Nordenskjöld, A. (2010). Sexual function and surgical outcome in women with congenital adrenal hyperplasia due to CYP21A2 deficiency: clinical persepctive and the patients' perception. *Journal of Clinical Endocrinology and Metabolism, 95*, 3633–3640.

Nordenström, A., Servin, A., Bohlin, G,. Larsson, A., & Wedell, A. (2002). Sex-typed toy play behavior correlates with the degree of prenatal androgen exposure assessed by CYP21 genotype in girls with congenital adrenal hyperplasia. *Journal of Clinical Endocrinology and Metabolism, 87*, 5119–5124.

Nordenskjöld, A., Holmdahl, G., Frisén, L., Falhammar, H., Filipsson, H., Thorén, M., ... Hagenfeldt, K. (2008). Type of metation and surgical procedure affect long-term quality of life for women with congenital adrenal hyperplasia. *Journal of Clinical Endocrinology and Metabolism, 93*, 380–386.

Pang, S. (1997). Congenital adrenal hyperplasia. *Endocrinology and Metabolism Clinics of North America, 26*, 853–891.

Reisch, N., Scherr, M., Flade, L., Bidlingmaier, M., Schwarz, H. P., Muller-Lisse, U., ... Beuschlein, F. (2010). Total adrenal volume but not testicular adrenal rest tumor volume is associated with hormonal control in patients with 21-hydroxylase deficiency. *Journal of Clinical Endocrinology and Metabolism, 95*, 2065–2072.

Sherman, S. L., Aston, C. E., Morton, N. E., Speiser, P. W., & New, M. I. (1988). A segregation and linkage study of classical and nonclassical 21-hydroxylase deficiency. *American Journal of Human Genetics, 42*, 830–838.

Speiser, P. W., Arlt, W., Auchus, R. J., Baskin, L. S., Conway, G. S., Merke, D. P., ... Oberfield, S. E. (2018). Congenital adrenal hyperplasia due to steroid 21-hydroxylase deficiency: an Endocrine Society clinical practice guideline. *Journal of Clinical Endocrinology and Metabolism, 103* (11), 4043–4088.

Speiser, P. W., Azziz, R., Baskin, L. S., Ghizzoni, L., Hensle, T. W., Merke, D. P., ... White, P. C. (2010). Congenital adrenal hyperplasia due to steroid 21-hydroxylase deficiency: an endocrine soceity clinical practice guidelines. *Journal of Clinical Endocrinology and Metabolism, 95*, 4133–4160.

Speiser, P., & White, P. (2003). Congenital adrenal hyperplasia. *New England Journal of Medicine, 349*, 776–788.

Therrell, B. Jr., Berenbaum, S. A., Manter-Kapanke, V., Simmank, J., Korman, K., Prentice, L., ... Gunn, S. (1998). Results of screening 1.9 million Texas newborns for 21-hydroxylase-deficient congenital adrenal hyperplasia. *Pediatrics, 101*, 583–590.

Trapp, C. M., & Oberfield, S. E. (2012). Recommendations for treatment of nonclassic congenital adrenal hyperplasia (NCCAH): an update. *Steroids, 77*, 342–346.

Urban, M. D., Lee, P. A., & Migeon, C. J. (1978). Adult height and fertility in men with congenital virilizing adrenal hyperplasia. *New England Journal of Medicine, 299*, 1392–1396.

Van Wyk, J. J., & Ritzen, E. M. (2003). The role of bilateral adrenalectomy in the treatment of congenital adrenal hyperplasia. *Journal of Clinical Endocrinology and Metabolism, 88*, 2993–2998.

Wedell, A. (1998). Molecular genetics of congenital adrenal hyperplasia (21-h/ydroxylase deficiency): implications for diagnosis, prognosis and treatment. *Acta Paediatrica, 87*, 159–164.

White, P., New, M., & Dupont, B. (1986). Structure of the human 21-hydroxylase gene. *Proceedings of the National Academy of Sciences of the United States of America, 83*, 5111.

White, P. C., & Spieser, P. W. (2000). Congenital adrenal hyperplasia due to 21-hydroxylase deficiency. *Endocrine Reviews, 21*(3), 245–291.

V

THYROID DISORDERS

CHAPTER 38

THYROID TESTING

Michael T. McDermott

1. What is the single best test to screen for abnormal thyroid gland function?

   Serum thyroid-stimulating hormone (TSH) measurement is the best initial test for assessing thyroid function because the vast majority of thyroid dysfunction is caused by primary thyroid disease, to which the pituitary gland responds with predictable changes in TSH secretion. Situations in which serum TSH levels do not accurately reflect thyroid function include pituitary–hypothalamic disorders, nonthyroidal illnesses, and the use of certain medications, such as glucocorticoids, dopamine, mitotane, and somatostatin analogues. Measurement of serum thyroxine (T_4) and triiodothyronine (T_3) are useful when TSH levels are outside the reference range (Fig. 38.1).

2. How do you interpret the serum TSH level?

   TSH is the primary regulator of thyroid hormone synthesis and secretion. The hypothalamic–pituitary unit exerts exquisite control over the thyroid system, resulting in a log-linear relationship between serum TSH levels and serum free T_4 levels. Accordingly, small changes in T_4 production result in large changes in serum TSH levels. Abnormal serum TSH values appear long before serum T_4 and T_3 levels are outside their reference ranges. If the TSH is elevated, the patient almost always has primary hypothyroidism; this should prompt ordering of a serum free T_4 level. When TSH is low, primary hyperthyroidism is the usual cause; this finding should be followed by measurement of serum free T_4 and total T_3. When interpreting serum TSH values, it should be kept in mind that TSH secretion has a diurnal pattern, with the highest serum TSH levels occurring in the late afternoon and evening.

3. Explain how serum TSH is used to manage patients on thyroid hormone therapy.

   Thyroid hormone therapy is usually given to patients for one of two purposes: (1) replacement therapy for hypothyroidism or (2) suppression therapy for thyroid cancer. When replacement is the goal, the dosage should be adjusted to maintain the serum TSH level within the reference range. When suppression is the goal, the dosage should be adjusted to maintain the serum TSH level in the low-normal or slightly low range for most patients and in the undetectable range for those with aggressive or metastatic thyroid cancer.

4. What do total T_4 and T_3 assays measure?

   Approximately 99.98% of circulating T_4 and 99.70% of T_3 are bound to proteins, such as thyroxine-binding globulin (TBG), thyroxine-binding prealbumin (or transthyretin), and albumin (Fig. 38.2). Total T_4 and T_3 assays measure the total amounts of T_4 and T_3 (protein bound and free) in the circulation. Serum total T_4 and T_3 levels can be altered significantly by protein-binding disorders.

5. Discuss the advantages of free thyroid hormone assays.

   Free T_4 and T_3 assays determine the amounts of unbound, bioactive thyroid hormones in the circulation. Free thyroid hormone tests fall into two main categories: (1) equilibrium dialysis and (2) analogue assays. Equilibrium

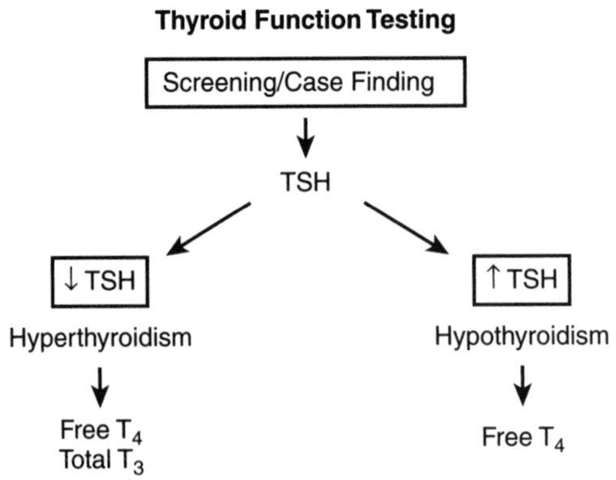

Thyroid Function Testing

Screening/Case Finding

↓

TSH

↙   ↘

↓ TSH   ↑ TSH

Hyperthyroidism   Hypothyroidism

↓   ↓

Free T_4 Free T_4
Total T_3

Fig. 38.1. Thyroid hormone testing strategy. *T_3*, Thyroxine; *T_4*, triiodothyronine; *TSH*, thyroid-stimulating hormone.

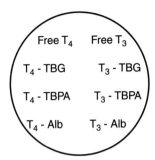

	Bound	Free
T_4	99.98%	0.02%
T_3	99.70%	0.30%

Assay Accuracy 2018	
Adequate	Not Accurate
Free T_4	Free T_3
Total T_4	
Total T_3	

Fig. 38.2. Protein-bound and free thyroid hormones in the circulation. *Alb*, Albumin; T_3, Thyroxine; T_4, triiodothyronine; *TBG*, thyroxine-binding globulin; *TBPA*, thyroxine-binding prealbumin (transthyretin).

dialysis methods are more accurate because they are not affected by serum thyroid hormone-binding protein abnormalities, but they are expensive. Analogue methods, which are used by most commercial laboratories, are variably affected by protein binding. Currently, free T_4 assays are considered reasonably good, but the accuracy of commercially available free T_3 assays remains problematic. This is why total T_3 assays are preferred over free T_3 assays by most experts in the field.

6. What is reverse T_3, and when should it be measured?

T_4 is the primary hormone secreted by the thyroid gland. Circulating T_4 is converted into T_3 in the liver and kidneys by an enzyme deiodinase 1 (D1), generating the majority of circulating T_3, and in the brain by deiodinase 2 (D2) to provide most of the T_3 required by the brain. T_4 can also be converted into Reverse T3 (RT3) by deiodinase 3 (D3) (see Chapter 45, Fig. 45.1, and Table 45.1).

RT3 is considered an inactive thyroid metabolite; compared with T_3, RT3 has a 100-fold lower affinity for the T_3 receptor. During nonthyroidal illnesses, serum T_3 decreases significantly and RT3 rises because of decreased activity of D1. Conversely, in hypothyroidism of any type, D1 activity is enhanced, promoting more conversion of T_4 to T_3 and less conversion to RT3. As a result, RT3 is usually low in hypothyroidism. RT3 measurement, although not indicated for evaluation of other thyroid conditions, can sometimes be helpful in distinguishing thyroid hormone changes associated with nonthyroidal illnesses (euthyroid sick syndrome) from central hypothyroidism. Serum TSH, free T_4, and total T_3 can be low in both conditions but RT3 is usually high in euthyroid sick syndrome and low in central hypothyroidism.

7. Name the major disorders of thyroid hormone-binding proteins.

Pregnancy, estrogen use, congenital TBG excess, and familial dysalbuminemic hyperthyroxinemia (FDH) are the most common. FDH is an inherited disorder in which albumin has enhanced affinity for T_4, resulting in increased levels of total T_4 but not T_3. Protein binding of T_4 and T_3 is reduced by androgens and congenital TBG deficiency.

A T_3 resin uptake (T_3RU) measurement helps distinguish protein-binding disorders from true thyroid diseases. The T_3RU is inversely proportional to the protein-binding capacity; accordingly, T_3RU is low when T_4 protein binding is increased and high when protein binding is reduced. Table 38.1 shows how these tests are used to make the correct diagnosis.

8. What antithyroid antibody tests are clinically useful?

Antithyroid peroxidase (TPO) and antithyroglobulin antibodies are present in the sera of most patients with Hashimoto's thyroiditis. Either test can establish a diagnosis of Hashimoto's disease, but the TPO antibodies are

Table 38.1. Diagnosing Disorders of Thyroid Hormone-Binding Proteins.

	TOTAL T_4	TOTAL T_3	T_3RU
Hyperthyroidism	↑	↑	↑
Increased protein-binding state	↑	↑	↓
Hypothyroidism	↓	↓	↓
Decreased protein-binding state	↓	↓	↑

T_3, Triiodothyronine; T_3RU, triiodothyronine resin uptake; T_4, thyroxine.

more sensitive. TSH receptor antibodies (TRAb) and thyroid-stimulating immunoglobulins are detectable in the sera of most patients with Graves' disease; their measurement is not necessary when the diagnosis of Graves' disease is obvious, but they may be helpful when the diagnosis is in question.

9. How useful are thyroglobulin (TG) measurements?

TG is the major iodoprotein constituent of thyroid follicles. Serum TG levels are mildly increased in many thyroid diseases, but marked elevations are seen mainly with active thyroid cancer and in destructive thyroiditis (subacute, postpartum, or silent thyroiditis). TG measurements are useful for monitoring patients with thyroid cancer. When a patient has been treated and is cancer free, the serum TG should be undetectable. Normal or rising serum TG levels in such patients suggest the presence of residual or metastatic thyroid cancer. Most TG assays are not reliable in patients who have positive anti-TG antibodies because these antibodies interfere with the method of TG measurement.

10. When should a serum calcitonin level be measured?

Calcitonin is made by thyroid parafollicular C cells rather than by follicular cells. Serum calcitonin is elevated in medullary carcinoma of the thyroid (MCT) and in its familial precursor lesion, C-cell hyperplasia. Because MCT is an uncommon thyroid neoplasm, serum calcitonin measurements should not be used in the routine evaluation of most thyroid nodules. They are indicated, however, if a patient exhibits a feature that is characteristic of MCT, such as familial occurrence or associated diarrhea.

11. Discuss the utility and interpretation of the radioactive iodine uptake (RAIU) test.

Thyroid follicular cells have sodium iodine symporters that bring iodine into the cells for thyroid hormone synthesis. The activity of these symporters can be assessed by measuring the RAIU. The normal 24-hour RAIU is approximately 10% to 25% in the United States, but this value varies according to location because of geographic differences in dietary iodine intake. The RAIU test is most useful in the differential diagnosis of thyrotoxicosis by separating cases into two distinct categories: high-RAIU thyrotoxicosis and low-RAIU thyrotoxicosis. See Table 38.2.

12. When and why should a thyroid scan be ordered?

A thyroid scan helps distinguish among the three most common types of high-RAIU thyrotoxicosis: (1) Graves' disease, which is characterized by diffuse tracer uptake; (2) toxic multinodular goiter, which is characterized by multiple discrete areas of increased uptake; and (3) the solitary toxic adenoma, which is characterized by a single area of intense uptake. The scan is not helpful in low-RAIU thyrotoxicosis. A thyroid scan is no longer recommended in the evaluation of thyroid nodules unless the serum TSH level is low, in which case the scan can detect the presence of functioning (hot) nodules.

13. How does biotin interfere with assessment of thyroid function?

Biotin is a reagent used in many hormone assays, including those for TSH, free T_4, and TRAb. It must be present in these assays in precise amounts to provide an accurate measurement of the analyte. High-dose biotin supplements, as commonly used for cosmetic skin, nail, and hair conditions, result in significant circulating biotin levels. Thyroid disorders, such as Graves' disease, can be erroneously diagnosed in patients taking biotin supplements, depending on the assay techniques used. This situation can be resolved by asking patients to repeat their thyroid testing after at least 2 days of abstinence from the biotin supplements.

14. How can heterophile antimouse antibodies (HAMAs) interfere with assessment of thyroid function?

HAMAs sometimes develop in people who are regularly exposed to rodents, such as laboratory workers, farm workers, and other people who spend a lot of time outdoors, including homeless people. HAMAs can interfere with the measurement of several hormones, including TSH and TG. When TSH or TG values are not consistent with the clinical picture, interference by HAMA should be suspected and the patient questioned about possible sources of rodent exposure. When a laboratory is alerted to the possibility of HAMA interference, assay conditions can be altered to minimize or eliminate the misleading results.

Table 38.2. High-RAIU Thyrotoxicosis and Low-RAIU Thyrotoxicosis Categories.

HIGH-RAIU THYROTOXICOSIS	LOW-RAIU THYROTOXICOSIS
Graves' disease	Factitious thyrotoxicosis
Toxic multinodular goiter	Iodine-induced thyrotoxicosis
Solitary toxic adenoma	Subacute thyroiditis
TSH-secreting tumor	Postpartum thyroiditis
HCG-induced thyrotoxicosis	Silent thyroiditis

HCG, Human chorionic gonadotropin; RAIU, radioactive iodine uptake; TSH, thyroid-stimulating hormone.

KEY POINTS: THYROID TESTING

- Serum thyroid-stimulating hormone (TSH) measurement is the best overall test to screen and evaluate patients for thyroid disease and to monitor thyroid hormone replacement therapy.
- Serum free thyroxine (T_4) should be measured in all patients whose TSH is elevated, and serum free T_4 and total triiodothyronine should be measured in patients whose TSH is suppressed.
- Antithyroid peroxidase antibodies are the most accurate test to establish a diagnosis of chronic lymphocytic thyroiditis (Hashimoto's disease).
- Serum thyroglobulin is useful for monitoring for recurrence of differentiated thyroid cancer and for assisting in the diagnosis of destructive thyroiditis.
- The radioactive iodine uptake (RAIU) test is used primarily to determine whether patients with thyrotoxicosis have a high RAIU or a low RAIU disorder.
- A thyroid scan is used mainly to distinguish among the three most common types of high-RAIU thyrotoxicosis: Graves' disease, toxic multinodular goiter, and a solitary toxic adenoma.
- Biotin supplements and human antimouse antibodies can cause significant interference with assays used to evaluate the thyroid system.

BIBLIOGRAPHY

Andersen, S., Pedersen, K. M., Bruun, N. H., & Laurberg, P. (2002). Narrow individual variations in serum T_4 and T_3 in normal subjects: a clue to the understanding of subclinical thyroid disease. *Journal of Clinical Endocrinology and Metabolism, 87,* 1068–1072.

Baloch, Z., Carayon, P., Conte-Devolx, B., Demers, L. M., Feldt-Rasmussen, U., Henry, J. F., ... Stockigt, J. R. (2003). Laboratory medicine practice guidelines: laboratory support for the diagnosis and monitoring of thyroid disease. *Thyroid, 13,* 3–126.

Elston, M., Shegal, S., Du Toit, S., Yarndley, T., & Conaglen, J. V. (2016). Factitious Graves' disease due to biotin immunoassay interference—a case and review of the literature. *Journal of Clinical Endocrinology and Metabolism, 101,* 3251–3255.

Li, D., Radulescu, A., Shrestha, R. T., Root, M., Karger, A. B., Killeen, A. A., ... Burmeister, L. A. (2017). Association of biotin ingestion with performance of hormone and non-hormone assays in healthy adults. *Journal of the American Medical Association, 318,* 1150–1160.

Nelson, J. C., Wang, R., Asher, D. T., & Wilcox, R. B. (2004). The nature of analogue-based free thyroxine estimates. *Thyroid, 14,* 1030–1036.

Nicoloff, J. T., & Spencer, C. A. (1990). The use and misuse of the sensitive thyrotropin assays. *Journal of Clinical Endocrinology and Metabolism, 71,* 553–558.

Preissner, C. M., Dodge, L. A., O'Kane, D. J., Singh, R. J., & Grebe, S. K. (2005). Prevalence of heterophilic antibody interference in eight automated tumor marker immunoassays. *Clinical Chemistry, 51,* 208–210.

Preissner, C. M., O'Kane, D. J., Singh, R. J., Morris, J. C., & Grebe, S. K. (2003). Phantoms in the assay tube: heterophile antibody interferences in serum thyroglobulin assays. *Journal of Clinical Endocrinology and Metabolism, 88,* 3069–3074.

Schmidt R. L., LoPresti J. S., McDermott M. T., Zick S. M., Straseski J. A. (2018). Is reverse triiodothyronine ordered appropriately? Data from reference lab shows wide practice variation in orders for reverse triiodothyronine. *Thyroid, 28,* 842–848.

Wang, R., Nelson, J. C., Weiss, R. M., & Wilcox, R. B. (2000). Accuracy of free thyroxine measurements across natural ranges of thyroxine binding to serum proteins. *Thyroid, 10,* 31–39.

CHAPTER 39

HYPERTHYROIDISM

Thanh D. Hoang and Henry B. Burch

1. What is the difference between thyrotoxicosis and hyperthyroidism?

   Thyrotoxicosis is the general term for the presence of increased levels of thyroxine (T_4), triiodothyronine (T_3), or both, from any cause. It does not imply that a patient is markedly symptomatic or "toxic." *Hyperthyroidism* refers to causes of thyrotoxicosis in which the thyroid is actively overproducing thyroid hormone.

2. Define the term "autonomy" as it applies to thyroid hyperfunction.

   Thyroid autonomy refers to the spontaneous production and secretion of thyroid hormone, independent of thyroid-stimulating hormone (TSH).

3. What is subclinical thyrotoxicosis?

   Subclinical thyrotoxicosis is defined as a low serum TSH level with free T_4 and T_3 levels that are still within the reference range. The low TSH concentration can result from either excessive ingestion of thyroid hormone or excessive release of endogenous thyroid hormone. Free T_4 or T_3 levels are frequently in the high-normal range in affected individuals. Clinical symptoms and signs are generally absent or nonspecific.

4. What are the long-term consequences of subclinical thyrotoxicosis?

   Some studies have linked subclinical thyrotoxicosis to (1) progression to clinical thyrotoxicosis; (2) skeletal effects, including decreased bone mineral density, accelerated bone loss, and increased fracture risk, particularly in post-menopausal women; and (3) cardiac effects, such as a two- to threefold higher risk of atrial fibrillation, impaired left ventricular diastolic filling, and impaired ventricular ejection fraction response to exercise. A recent extensive meta-analysis by Collet et al. found an increased rate of both cardiovascular and all-cause mortality in patients with subclinical hyperthyroidism. A TSH value < 0.1 mU/L is more likely to be associated with adverse consequences than a TSH value in the 0.1 to 0.5 mU/L range.

5. Does subclinical hyperthyroidism require treatment?

   The 2016 American Thyroid Association (ATA) Guidelines for Diagnosis and Management of Hyperthyroidism and Other Causes of Thyrotoxicosis suggest that patients with TSH < 0.1 mU/L who are older than age 65 years or who are younger but with symptomatic disease or comorbidities that may be aggravated by mild hyperthyroidism (i.e., coronary heart disease, osteoporosis, menopausal symptoms) should be actively treated. Patients with TSH values between 0.1 and 0.4 mU/L should at least be *considered* for therapy if greater than age 65 years or younger but with comorbidities as above.

6. List the three most common causes of hyperthyroidism.

   - Graves' disease
   - Toxic multinodular goiter (TMNG)
   - Toxic adenomas or autonomously functioning thyroid nodules (AFTNs)

7. Define Graves' disease.

   Graves' disease is an autoimmune disease in which autoantibodies directed against the TSH receptor result in continuous stimulation of thyroid hormone production and secretion as well as thyroid growth (goiter). Extrathyroidal manifestations of Graves' disease include orbitopathy (manifest as proptosis, periorbital edema, extraocular muscle dysfunction, and optic neuropathy), dermopathy (pretibial myxedema), and thyroid acropachy (digital clubbing and edema).

The views expressed in this manuscript are those of the authors and do not reflect the official policy of the Department of the Army, Navy, the Department of Defense, the National Institutes of Health, or the United States Government. We are military service members or employees of the U.S. Government. This work was prepared as part of our official duties. Title 17 U.S.C. 105 provides the "Copyright protection under this title is not available for any work of the United States Government." Title 17 U.S.C. 101 defines a U.S. Government work as a work prepared by a military service member or employee of the U.S. Government as part of that person's official duties. We certify that all individuals who qualify as authors have been listed; each has participated in the conception and design of this work, the analysis of data (when applicable), the writing of the document, and/or the approval of the submission of this version; that the document represents valid work; that if we used information derived from another source, we obtained all necessary approvals to use it and made appropriate acknowledgments in the document; and that each takes public responsibility for it.

8. Explain TMNG.

TMNG generally arises in the setting of a longstanding multinodular goiter, in which certain individual nodules have developed autonomous function and secrete thyroid hormone independent of stimulation by TSH.

9. What are AFTNs?

AFTNs, or toxic adenomas, are benign tumors that have constitutive activation of the TSH receptor or its signal-transduction apparatus. These tumors frequently produce subclinical thyrotoxicosis and may have a predilection for spontaneous intranodular hemorrhage or degeneration. AFTNs generally must be > 3 cm in diameter before attaining sufficient secretory capacity to produce overt thyrotoxicosis. Often, inefficient iodine processing leads to an excess of T_3 relative to T_4 in AFTNs.

10. What is the Jod-Basedow phenomenon?

The Jod-Basedow phenomenon is named after the German physician Dr. Karl Adolph Von Basedow, who first described the phenomenon, and the German word for iodine, "Jod." The term refers to thyrotoxicosis that can occur after exposure to large quantities of iodine (typically in iodinated radiographic contrast agents for computed tomography or angiography, but also with the antiarrhythmic drug amiodarone). Historically, it was first described following iodine supplementation in people living in regions of endemic iodine deficiency, which is associated with the development of autonomous thyroid nodules.

11. What are some rare causes of hyperthyroidism?

Rare causes of hyperthyroidism include TSH-secreting pituitary adenomas; stimulation of TSH receptors by high levels of human chorionic gonadotropin, most often in choriocarcinomas in women or germ cell tumors in men; struma ovarii (ectopic thyroid hormone production in thyroid tissue–containing ovarian teratomas); and functional metastatic follicular or papillary thyroid carcinoma. Thyroiditis (postpartum, subacute, painless, radiation, or palpation) and ingestion of excessive exogenous thyroid hormone (iatrogenic, inadvertent, or surreptitious) are causes of thyrotoxicosis but not hyperthyroidism (see question 1).

12. How do patients with thyrotoxicosis present clinically?

Common symptoms include palpitations, anxiety, agitation, restlessness, insomnia, impaired concentration/memory, irritability or emotional lability, weight loss, heat intolerance, sweating, exertional dyspnea, fatigue, hyperdefecation, amenorrhea, oligomenorrhea, hypomenorrhea, anovulation, and hair thinning. Occasionally, patients may experience weight gain rather than loss during thyrotoxicosis, presumably owing to polyphagia.

13. What is apathetic hyperthyroidism?

Older patients with hyperthyroidism may lack typical symptoms and signs of sympathetic activation and present instead with apathy or depression, weight loss, atrial fibrillation, shortness of breath, worsening angina pectoris, or congestive heart failure.

14. Describe the physical signs of thyrotoxicosis.

Tremors, tachycardia, flow murmurs, systolic hypertension, warm and moist skin, thin and fine hair, hyperreflexia with rapid relaxation phases, lid lag/lid retraction (stare), and goiter may be found in patients with thyrotoxicosis. Some patients with Graves' disease also present with orbitopathy, pretibial myxedema, acropachy, and a thyroid bruit. Eye findings in thyrotoxicosis are discussed in question 15.

15. How does hyperthyroidism cause eye disease?

Lid retraction and stare can be seen with any cause of thyrotoxicosis and are caused by sympathetic/adrenergic overactivity. True orbitopathy is unique to Graves' disease and is thought to be caused by thyroid autoantibodies that cross-react with antigens in fibroblasts, preadipocytes, and adipocytes of the retroorbital tissues. Insulin-like growth factor-1 receptor signal transduction may also contribute to orbitopathy. Common manifestations of orbitopathy include proptosis, diplopia, eye irritation, excessive tearing, eye or retroorbital discomfort, blurred vision, and inflammatory changes, such as conjunctival injection and periorbital edema.

16. What laboratory testing should be performed to confirm thyrotoxicosis?

Measurement of serum TSH with a third-generation assay (with detection limits of 0.01 mU/L) is the most sensitive means for detecting thyrotoxicosis. Serum free T_4 and T_3 levels should be measured to determine the degree of biochemical thyrotoxicosis. Other associated laboratory findings may include mild leukopenia, normochromic normocytic anemia, hepatic transaminitis, elevated serum alkaline phosphatase and osteocalcin (increased bone turnover), mild hypercalcemia, hyperphosphatemia, and low serum levels of albumin and total cholesterol.

17. When is thyroid antibody testing needed in patients with thyrotoxicosis?

The cause of thyrotoxicosis usually can be determined with history, physical examination, and radionuclide studies. Testing for TSH receptor antibodies can be used to diagnose Graves' disease during pregnancy, when radionuclide imaging is contraindicated. It is also useful in (1) pregnant women with current or previously treated Graves' disease to determine the risk of fetal and neonatal thyroid dysfunction resulting from transplacental passage of stimulating or blocking antibodies; (2) biochemically euthyroid patients with orbitopathy; (3) patients with alternating periods of hyper- and hypothyroidism as a result of fluctuations in blocking and stimulating TSH receptor antibodies; and (4) atypical cases when differentiation of Graves' disease from toxic multinodular goiter is challenging and therapeutically essential. The 2016 American Thyroid Association Guidelines for Diagnosis and Management of Hyperthyroidism and Other Causes of Thyrotoxicosis suggest that TSH-receptor antibody testing may be used as a diagnostic alternative to radioiodine uptake measurement to make the diagnosis of Graves' disease in a patient with thyrotoxicosis.

18. What is the difference between a thyroid scan and an uptake test?
    A radioactive iodine uptake (RAIU) test uses radioiodine (^{131}I) or iodine-123 (^{123}I) to assess quantitatively the functional status of the thyroid gland. A small dose of radioisotope is given orally followed by measurement of radioactivity over the thyroid in 4 to 24 hours. Often, two measurements are taken, at 4 to 6 hours and at 24 hours. A high uptake confirms hyperthyroidism, whereas a low (nearly absent) radioiodine uptake indicates either destruction of thyroid tissue with release of preformed hormone into the circulation or an extrathyroidal source of iodine or thyroid hormone (Table 39.1). A thyroid scan provides a two-dimensional image showing the distribution of isotope trapping within the thyroid gland. Uniform distribution in a hyperthyroid patient suggests Graves' disease, patchy distribution suggests TMNG, and unifocal activity corresponding to a nodule, with suppression of the rest of the thyroid, suggests a toxic adenoma.

19. Can thyroid ultrasonography be used to determine the etiology of thyrotoxicosis?
    Assessment of thyroid blood flow by Doppler ultrasonography can distinguish between the increased flow seen with active Graves' disease, sometimes referred to as "thyroid inferno," and the normal vascular flow pattern seen in patients with thyrotoxicosis caused by destructive thyroiditis.

20. How should hyperthyroidism be treated?
    The three main treatment options are antithyroid drugs (ATDs), radioiodine (^{131}I) ablation, and surgery. ATDs available in the United States include methimazole (MMI) and propylthiouracil (PTU). MMI is almost always the preferred agent. Because of concerns about severe hepatotoxicity, PTU is recommended only in (1) the first trimester of pregnancy (MMI has been linked to embryopathy when used during the first trimester); (2) thyroid storm therapy, because of the ability of PTU to block T_4-to-T_3 conversion; and (3) patients with minor reactions to MMI who refuse ^{131}I therapy or surgery. Unless contraindicated, most patients should receive beta-blockers for heart rate control and symptomatic relief. Although most patients in the United States have historically been treated with radioactive iodine rather than long-term ATDs or surgery, a growing percentage of patients and providers are choosing long-term ATD therapy. Patients scheduled to receive ^{131}I should be advised to avoid pregnancy for 4 to 6 months and should be cautioned that oral contraceptives may not be fully effective in the hyperthyroid state because of increased levels of sex hormone–binding globulin and increased clearance of the contraceptive.

21. When is surgery indicated for hyperthyroidism?
    Surgery is generally not the treatment of choice for hyperthyroidism. It is most often used (1) in patients with symptomatic compression or large goiters ($\geq$ 80 g) who are less likely to respond to ATDs or ^{131}I; (2) in patients with relatively low RAIU; (3) when thyroid cancer is documented or suspected; (4) in patients with large nonfunctioning, photopenic, or hypofunctioning nodules (> 4 cm); (5) in pregnant patients allergic to or intolerant of ATDs

Table 39.1. Radioactive Iodine Uptake (RAIU) Differentiation of Hyperthyroidism.

HIGH RAIU	LOW RAIU
Common	Common
Graves' disease	Postpartum thyroiditis
Toxic multinodular goiter	Subacute thyroiditis
Toxic solitary adenoma	
Rare	Rare
Thyroid-stimulating hormone (TSH)–producing pituitary adenoma	Painless thyroiditis
Human chorionic gonadotropin (hCG)–producing choriocarcinoma	Surreptitious (intravenous radiographic contrast, amiodarone) or accidental levothyroxine (LT_4) or liothyronine (LT_3)
	Struma ovarii

(^{131}I is contraindicated in pregnancy); (6) in patients with coexisting hyperparathyroidism requiring surgery; (7) in female patients who plan a pregnancy in < 6 months provided normal thyroid hormone levels, especially if TSI antibody levels are high; and (8) in patients who wish to avoid ^{131}I exposure and potential side effects of long-term ATDs. Surgery may also be preferred when there is moderate-to-severe active Graves' orbitopathy because ^{131}I has been linked to worsening eye disease in these patients. Patients should be euthyroid before surgery (with ATD pretreatment, with or without beta-adrenergic blockade) to decrease the risk of arrhythmias and the risk of postoperative thyroid storm. Preoperative potassium iodide (KI), saturated solution of potassium iodide (SSKI), or Lugol's solution is often given before surgery to decrease thyroid blood flow, vascularity, and intraoperative blood loss during thyroidectomy (see question 22).

22. **What is the role of iodine in the treatment of hyperthyroidism? What is the Wolff-Chaikoff effect?**
    Inorganic iodine rapidly decreases the synthesis and release of T_4 and T_3. The transient inhibition of thyroid hormone synthesis by excess iodine is known as the *Wolff-Chaikoff effect*. However, because escape from this effect often occurs after 10 to 14 days, iodine is generally used only after ATDs have been started to prepare a patient rapidly for surgery or as an adjunctive measure in patients with "thyroid storm." Iodine is also used in some centers to decrease the vascularity of the thyroid before thyroidectomy for Graves' disease. Typical doses are Lugol's solution (8 mg iodide/drop) 5 to 7 drops (0.25–0.35 mL) or SSKI (50 mg iodide/drop) 1 to 2 drops (0.05–0.1 mL) three times daily mixed in water or juice for 10 days before surgery.

23. **Are other treatments available to lower thyroid hormone levels?**
    Yes. Two iodine-containing oral cholecystographic agents, ipodate and iopanoic acid, cause dramatic reductions in serum T_3 and T_4 through inhibition of T_4 5'-monodeiodinase. Neither of these agents is currently available in the United States. Other agents occasionally used to treat hyperthyroidism include lithium, which decreases thyroid hormone release, and potassium perchlorate, which inhibits thyroid uptake of iodine. Cholestyramine interferes with enterohepatic recycling of thyroid hormone and, when given with MMI, lowers serum T_4 and T_3 more rapidly than MMI alone.

24. **Which medications block peripheral conversion of T_4 to T_3?**
    PTU, propranolol, glucocorticoids, iopanoic acid, ipodate, tyropanoate, and amiodarone inhibit the peripheral conversion of T_4 to T_3.

25. **How effective are ATDs?**
    Ninety percent of patients taking ATDs become euthyroid without significant side effects. Approximately half of patients attain a remission from Graves' disease after a treatment course of 12 to 18 months. However, only 30% maintain a long-term remission; the remainder experience recurrence of Graves' disease within 1 to 2 years after the drugs are withdrawn. TMNG and AFTNs are not autoimmune diseases; therefore, patients with these diseases do not go into remission. The role of ATDs in these two disorders is only to render a patient euthyroid before surgery or when pretreatment is necessary before ^{131}I therapy (see question 27). The usual starting doses for moderate thyrotoxicosis are MMI, 10 to 20 mg/day, or PTU, 50 to 150 mg three times/day. MMI is recommended for all patients who select ATD therapy for Graves' disease, except in the clinical circumstances listed in question 20.

26. **What side effects are associated with ATDs?**
    - Agranulocytosis is a rare but life-threatening complication of ATD therapy (incidence 0.11%–0.27%), occurring in approximately 1 in every 500 to 900 patients treated with ATDs, usually within 1 to 3 months of starting ATD. Patients should be instructed to promptly report fever, sore throat, or minor infections that do not resolve quickly. Agranulocytosis appears to be dose related with MMI but not with PTU. Patients developing agranulocytosis on one ATD should not be exposed to another.
    - Hepatotoxicity with occasional progression to fulminant hepatic necrosis can occur with PTU; cholestatic jaundice has been reported with MMI. Recent findings suggested similar low frequency of cholestatic or hepatocellular hepatotoxicity for both MMI and PTU (0.03%). Patients should be instructed to report right upper quadrant pain, anorexia, nausea, jaundice, light-colored stool or dark urine, and new-onset pruritus, while taking ATDs.
    - Rashes occur in approximately 2% of patients (more common with PTU or higher dose MMI > 30 mg/day) and can range from limited erythema to an exfoliative dermatitis. Dermatologic reactions to one ATD do not preclude the use of another, although cross-sensitivity occurs in approximately 50% of cases.
    - Arthropathy or a lupus-like syndrome can rarely be seen with either PTU or MMI.
    - Antineutrophil cytoplasmic antibody–positive vasculitis has been associated with PTU use (rarely MMI).
    - Potential teratogenicity (so-called *MMI embryopathy*) can be associated with MMI; this includes rare fetal scalp defects (aplasia cutis), choanal atresia, omphalocele, omphalomesenteric duct anomaly, patent vitellointestinal duct, and tracheoesophageal fistulas. Mild birth defects, such as preauricular sinuses/cysts and urinary tract abnormalities, can be observed with use of PTU.
    - Insulin autoimmune syndrome with symptomatic hypoglycemia has rarely been reported with use of MMI.
    - Baseline blood tests (complete blood count and liver function test) should be obtained before starting ATD therapy. One should reconsider ATD therapy if the baseline absolute neutrophil count is $< 1000/mm^3$ or liver transaminase enzyme levels $>$ three fold above the upper limit of normal.

27. **What laboratory tests should be monitored in patients taking ATDs?**

Serum free T_4 and total T_3 should be retested about 2 weeks after initiation of an ATD and the dose adjusted accordingly. TSH may remain suppressed for several months and, therefore, free T_4 and T_3 levels are more reliable for assessing thyroid hormone status during this time. Thyroid tests should thereafter be monitored every 4 to 8 weeks until euthyroidism is achieved with a goal of using the lowest effective ATD dose. Routine monitoring of the white blood cell (WBC) count and liver function, though commonly done in clinical practice, has not been shown to prevent agranulocytosis or hepatotoxicity. A WBC count and differential should be assessed during any febrile illness and at the onset of sore throat/pharyngitis in all patients taking ATDs. Liver function tests should be ordered in patients who experience a pruritic rash, jaundice, light-colored stools or dark urine, arthralgias, abdominal pain or bloating, anorexia, nausea, or fatigue. The ATD therapy should be discontinued if transaminase levels are > three times the upper limit of normal or progressively increasing from an elevated baseline level. Liver function tests should be monitored every week until resolution of transaminitis after discontinuing the ATD.

28. **How does radioactive iodine work?**

Thyroid cells trap and concentrate iodine and use it to make thyroid hormone. [131]I is utilized in the same manner as inorganic iodine. Because ^{131}I emits locally destructive beta particles, extensive local thyrocyte damage and ablation of thyroid function occurs over a period of approximately 6 to 18 weeks after treatment. Dosages of ^{131}I should be high enough to cause permanent hypothyroidism and are usually based on the size of the thyroid gland and the pretreatment RAIU. A typical dose for Graves' disease is 10 to 15 millicuries (mCi); for TMNG, higher doses of 25 to 30 mCi are often given. These doses are effective in 90% to 95% of patients.

29. **When is pretreatment with ATDs indicated before ^{131}I ablation?**

The use of ATDs before and after ^{131}I therapy may be considered in (1) patients who are extremely symptomatic or have free T_4 levels that are three to four times the upper normal limit; (2) the elderly; and (3) those with substantial comorbidities, such as atrial fibrillation, heart failure, pulmonary hypertension, renal failure, infection, trauma, poorly controlled diabetes mellitus, and cerebrovascular or pulmonary disease. These patients should also be medically stable and treated with beta-adrenergic blocking drugs before ^{131}I therapy.

Pretreatment with ATDs helps deplete the thyroid of preformed hormones and thereby to theoretically reduce the risk of ^{131}I-induced thyroid storm. When pretreatment with ATDs is used, the drugs are generally continued until the patient is euthyroid and then discontinued before ^{131}I is given. Abrupt discontinuation of ATDs is associated with a rapid increase in thyroid hormone levels, and therefore, current recommendations favor a brief discontinuation of only 2 to 3 days before ablation therapy is given. Nonpretreated patients usually experience a rapid decrease in thyroid hormone levels after ^{131}I therapy, therefore most otherwise healthy patients do not require or benefit from ATD pretreatment.

30. **How long after ^{131}I treatment should women wait before becoming pregnant or resuming breastfeeding?**

Pregnancy should be deferred for at least 4 to 6 months after ^{131}I ablation to ensure successfully cured hyperthyroidism and corrected hypothyroidism before conception. In addition, patients should be on a stable dose of thyroid hormone replacement and free of active orbitopathy. Breast milk radioactivity, measured in one study after an 8.3-mCi therapeutic dose of ^{131}I, remained unacceptably high for 45 days, prohibiting resumption of breastfeeding after ^{131}I therapy. If [99m]Technetium or ^{123}I is used for diagnostic studies, breastfeeding may be resumed in 2 to 3 days, with pumping and disposal of breast milk in the interim.

31. **Does ^{131}I cause or worsen orbitopathy in Graves' disease?**

The natural history of Graves' disease is such that up to 25% of patients develop clinically apparent orbitopathy, but < 5% develop severe eye involvement. The majority of orbitopathy cases arise in the period from 18 months before to 18 months after the onset of thyrotoxicosis. Thus, a fair number of new cases can be expected to coincide with the timing of ^{131}I ablation. However, three randomized clinical trials have shown that ^{131}I therapy is more likely to be associated with new or worsened orbitopathy compared with either ATDs or thyroidectomy. [131]I therapy results in a sustained increase in TSH receptor antibodies that may be important in exacerbating orbitopathy. Patients with preexisting eye disease, those who smoke cigarettes, and those with higher levels of thyroid hormone and high titers of TSH-receptor antibodies are more likely to experience worsening. It is, therefore, prudent to avoid ^{131}I in patients with active moderate-to-severe Graves' orbitopathy. In patients with initially mild eye involvement, concurrent use of oral glucocorticoids can be used to prevent an exacerbation during ^{131}I therapy, particularly in the presence of other risk factors for worsening orbitopathy.

32. **How is thyrotoxicosis managed in pregnancy?**

Caution must be exercised in interpreting thyroid laboratory results during pregnancy, because low TSH values are not uncommon in the first trimester, and total T_4 and total T_3 levels are elevated by increased thyroxine-binding globulin levels. Free T_4 levels, using equilibrium dialysis or an assay with trimester-specific reference ranges, are the best indicators of thyroid function during pregnancy. Symptomatic women with marked elevation in trimester-specific free T_4 levels or those with total T_4 and/or total T_3 above 1.5 times the upper normal limit should be considered for treatment. Pregnant women with subclinical hyperthyroidism (low TSH, normal free T_4)

and asymptomatic or mild hyperthyroidism may be monitored without treatment by measuring TSH and free T_4 every 4 to 6 weeks. Beta-adrenergic blockers (propranolol or metoprolol, but not atenolol) can be used cautiously and should be weaned once hyperthyroidism is controlled by ATDs because of the risks of fetal growth restriction, hypoglycemia, respiratory depression, and bradycardia. Nuclear medicine testing with RAIU or thyroid scanning is contraindicated in pregnancy because of the risk of fetal exposure to isotopes. Because ^{131}I therapy is also contra-indicated during pregnancy, treatment options are limited to ATDs or surgery. The ATA and the U.S. Food and Drug Administration (FDA) recommend that PTU be used in the first trimester because of the potentially serious terato-genic effects of MMI during organogenesis of the first trimester (aplasia cutis, choanal atresia, and tracheoesoph-ageal fistulas). Upon reaching the second trimester, patients are frequently switched to MMI, but alternatively, PTU may be continued if concerns about loss of control are deemed to outweigh the risk of hepatic dysfunction. A 100-mg dose of PTU is roughly equivalent to 5 to 10 mg of MMI. Thyroid function tests should be obtained 2 to 4 weeks after switching ATDs to ensure maintenance of euthyroidism. The lowest possible dose of ATD should be used to keep the mother's thyroid hormone levels at or slightly above the reference range and TSH slightly suppressed. Pregnant patients with Graves' disease require close follow-up to ensure adequate control and to prevent hypothyroidism caused by overtreatment with ATDs because Graves' disease frequently remits during the course of pregnancy. TSH receptor antibodies, which cross the placenta after 26 weeks, should be measured at the time of diagnosis of pregnancy, and if elevated, the assessment should be repeated at 18 to 22 weeks, and again at 30 to 34 weeks of gestation to assess the risk of neonatal thyroid dysfunction. Fetal assessment should include monitoring for tachycardia in mothers with persistent elevations in TSH receptor antibodies, and fetal ultrasonography to assess for evidence of fetal goiter or growth restriction.

Surgery (thyroidectomy) should only be performed when medical management has been unsuccessful or ATDs cannot be used, if possible during the second trimester because of teratogenic effects associated with anesthetic agents and increased risk of fetal loss in the first trimester and high risk of preterm labor in the third trimester.

33. What are the treatments for Graves' orbitopathy?

Patients with Graves' orbitopathy should be treated according to the severity of their eye disease. The general approach to treatment includes reversal of hyperthyroidism, smoking cessation, and reduction of ocular surface irritation and periorbital inflammation. Those with only mild eye involvement may generally be treated with local measures alone, such as tinted lenses for photosensitivity, artificial tears (methylcellulose eye drops), raising the head of the bed to prevent worsening retroocular edema in the recumbent position overnight, and eye patching or prisms for diplopia. Active, moderate eye involvement with lid erythema and edema, conjunctival erythema, and edema (chemosis) generally requires glucocorticoid therapy. Additional medications being investigated in patients with Graves' orbitopathy include rituximab and teprotumumab, but neither are approved by the FDA for this indi-cation. Severe orbitopathy including advanced proptosis or extraocular muscle dysfunction often requires initial immunomodulatory medication followed by surgical rehabilitation. Sight-threatening orbitopathy is a medical emergency, occurring as a result of optic nerve compression by enlarged extraocular muscles at the apex of the orbit, or because of corneal ulceration. In the former case, pulse intravenous glucocorticoids should be given immediately, and patients should be admitted to the hospital for possible urgent orbital decompression surgery.

KEY POINTS: HYPERTHYROIDISM

- The three most common causes of hyperthyroidism are Graves' disease, toxic multinodular goiter, and toxic adenoma.
- Thyroiditis can cause severe thyrotoxicosis but generally resolves without intervention and may be followed by a hypothyroid phase.
- Routine diagnostic testing for hyperthyroidism includes thyroid-stimulating hormone (TSH), free thyroxine, and triiodothyronine. The diagnosis may be confirmed with the radioactive iodine uptake test, thyroid radionuclide scanning, and measurement of TSH-receptor antibodies, or with the use of color-flow Doppler ultrasonography by experienced technicians.
- The major treatment choices for hyperthyroidism are radioiodine, antithyroid drugs (usually methimazole), and thyroidectomy. Beta-blockers can significantly improve adrenergic symptoms of thyrotoxicosis and do not inter-fere with testing or later treatment.
- Treatment is generally indicated in all patients when TSH is < 0.1 mU/L.

BIBLIOGRAPHY

Andersen, S. L., Olsen, J., & Laurberg, P. (2016). Antithyroid drug side effects in the population and in pregnancy. *Journal of Clinical Endocrinology and Metabolism, 101,* 1606–1614.

Bahn, R. S., Burch, H. B., Cooper, D. S., Garber, J. R., Greenlee, C. M., Klein, I. L., ... Stan, M. N. (2009). The role of propylthiouracil in the management of Graves' disease in adults: report of a meeting jointly sponsored by the American Thyroid Association and the Food and Drug Administration. *Thyroid, 19,* 673–674.

Bahn, R. S. (2010). Graves' ophthalmopathy. *New England Journal of Medicine, 362,* 726–738.

Biondi, B., & Cooper, D. S. (2008). The clinical significance of subclinical thyroid dysfunction *Endocrinolgy Review, 29,* 76–131.

Boelaert, K., Torlinska, B., Holder, R. L., & Franklyn, J. A. (2010). Older subjects with hyperthyroidism present with a paucity of symptoms and signs: a large cross-sectional study. *Journal of Clinical Endocrinology and Metabolism, 95,* 2715–2726.

Burch, H. B., & Cooper, D. S. (2015). Management of Graves' disease: a review. *Journal of the American Medical Association, 314*(23), 2544–2554.

Burch, H. B., Solomon, B. L., Cooper, D. S., Ferguson, P., Walpert, N., & Howard, R. (2001). The effect of antithyroid drug pretreatment on acute changes in thyroid hormone levels after ^{131}I ablation for Graves' disease. *Journal of Clinical Endocrinology and Metabolism, 86,* 3016–3021.

Collet, T. H., Gussekloo, J., & Bauer, D. C. (2012). Subclinical hyperthyroidism and the risk of coronary heart disease and mortality. *Archives of Internal Medicine, 172,* 799–809.

Cooper, D. S. (2005). Antithyroid drugs. *New England Journal of Medicine, 352,* 905–917.

Luton, D., Le Gac, I., Vuillard, E., Castanet, M., Guibourdenche, J., Noel, M., ... Polak, M. (2005). Management of Graves' disease during pregnancy: the key role of fetal thyroid gland monitoring. *Journal of Clinical Endocrinology and Metabolism, 90,* 6093–6098.

Mai, V. Q., & Burch, H. B. (2012). A stepwise approach to the evaluation and management of subclinical hyperthyroidism. *Endocrine Practice, 18,* 772–780.

McDermott, M. T., & Ridgway, E. C. (1998). Central hyperthyroidism. *Endocrinology and Metabolism Clinics of North America, 27,* 187–203.

Ross, D. S., Burch, H. B., Cooper, D. S., Greenlee, M. C., Laurberg, P., Maia, A. L., ... Walter, M. A. (2016). American Thyroid Association guidelines for diagnosis and management of hyperthyroidism and other causes of thyrotoxicosis. *Thyroid, 26,* 1343–1421.

Stagnaro-Green, A., Abalovich, M., Alexander, E., Azizi, F., Mestman, J., Negro, R., ... Wiersinga, W. (2011). Guidelines of the American Thyroid Association for the diagnosis and management of thyroid disease during pregnancy and postpartum. *Thyroid, 21,* 1081–1125.

Surks, M. I., Ortiz, E., Daniels, G. H., Sawin, C. T., Col, N. F., Cobin, R. H., ... Weissman, N. J. (2004). Subclinical thyroid disease: scientific review and guidelines for diagnosis and management. *Journal of the American Medical Association, 291,* 228–239.

Wang, M. T., Lee, W. J., Huang, T. Y., Chu, C. L., & Hsieh, C. H. (2014). Antithyroid drug-related hepatotoxicity in hyperthyroidism patients: a population-based cohort study. *British Journal of Clinical Pharmacology, 78,* 619–629.

Yang, J., Li, L. F., Xu, Q., Zhang, J., Weng, W. W., Zhu, Y. J., & Dong, M. J. (2015). Analysis of 90 cases of antithyroid drug-induced severe hepatotoxicity over 13 years in China. *Thyroid, 25,* 278–283.

CHAPTER 40

HYPOTHYROIDISM

Katherine Weber and Bryan R. Haugen

1. **What is hypothyroidism?**
   Hypothyroidism is a condition that results from inadequate production or action of thyroid hormone, most commonly as a result of primary hypothyroidism or the failure of the thyroid gland itself. Hypothyroidism can be overt, with a frank decrease in serum thyroxine (T_4) levels and a compensatory increase in thyroid-stimulating hormone (TSH) levels. It is more commonly seen in subclinical hypothyroidism (also called *mild thyroid failure*), in which the TSH is mildly elevated, but T_4 levels are normal. Subclinical hypothyroidism often presents with few or no symptoms, but hypercholesterolemia and subtle cardiac abnormalities can be seen.

2. **How common is hypothyroidism?**
   Hypothyroidism is a common condition. The prevalence of overt hypothyroidism in the United States is estimated at 0.3% to 0.4%, whereas the prevalence of subclinical hypothyroidism is much higher (4%–8%). The mean age at diagnosis is the mid-50s. Hypothyroidism is much more common in women, with a female-to-male ratio of 3:1. Postpartum hypothyroidism, a transient hypothyroid phase after pregnancy, occurs in 5% to 10% of women.

3. **What are the two most common causes of hypothyroidism?**
   Although many disorders can cause hypothyroidism, the two most common causes are chronic lymphocytic thyroiditis (Hashimoto's disease), an autoimmune form of thyroid destruction, and radioiodine-induced hypothyroidism after treatment of Graves' disease (autoimmune hyperthyroidism).

4. **List the less common causes of hypothyroidism.**
   - Thyroidectomy
   - Thyroiditis (viral, postpartum, silent)
   - External irradiation to the neck
   - Medications (antithyroid drugs, amiodarone, lithium, bexarotene, tyrosine kinase inhibitors, immune checkpoint inhibitors, and interferon)
   - Infiltrative diseases
   - Central (pituitary/hypothalamic) hypothyroidism (Fig. 40.1)
   - Congenital defects
   - Endemic (iodine-deficient) goiter, which is fairly common outside the United States

5. **List the symptoms commonly experienced in hypothyroidism.**
   Hypothyroidism commonly presents with nonspecific symptoms, such as fatigue, cold intolerance, depression, weight gain, weakness, joint aches, constipation, dry skin, hair loss, and menstrual irregularities.

6. **What findings on physical examination are consistent with hypothyroidism?**
   Physical examination may be normal with mild thyroid failure and should not deter further workup if clinical suspicions are high. Common signs of moderate-to-severe hypothyroidism include:
   - Hypertension (diastolic hypertension is a clue)
   - Bradycardia
   - Coarse hair
   - Periorbital swelling
   - Yellow skin (caused by elevated levels of beta-carotene)
   - Carpal tunnel syndrome
   - Delayed relaxation of the deep tendon reflexes

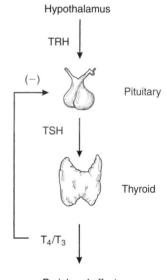

Hypothalamus

TRH

$(-)$

Pituitary

TSH

Thyroid

T_4/T_3

Peripheral effects

Fig. 40.1. Hypothalamic–pituitary–thyroid axis. T_3, Triiodothyronine; T_4, thyroxine; *TRH*, thyrotropin-releasing hormone; *TSH*, thyroid-stimulating hormone.

7. **What does palpation of the thyroid reveal?**
   The thyroid may be enlarged, normal, or small in hypothyroidism, but thyroid consistency is usually firm.

8. Summarize the unusual presentations of hypothyroidism.

   The unusual presentations of hypothyroidism include megacolon, cardiomegaly, pericardial effusion, and congestive heart failure (CHF). In one reported case, the patient was scheduled for cardiac transplantation for severe CHF, but before transplantation could be undertaken, the CHF resolved with thyroid hormone replacement alone.

9. Describe the laboratory tests that may be abnormal during hypothyroidism.

   Laboratory clues to hypothyroidism include normochromic, normocytic anemia (menstruating women may also have iron-deficiency anemia caused by excessive bleeding resulting from irregular menses), hyponatremia, hypercholesterolemia, and elevated levels of creatine phosphokinase.

10. What tests best confirm the diagnosis of hypothyroidism in the outpatient setting?

    Many thyroid function tests are available to the clinician, including assessments of TSH, T_4, triiodothyronine (T_3), T_3 resin uptake (T_3RU), free T_4, free T_3, and reverse T_3 (RT_3). In the outpatient setting, only one test is usually necessary—that is, the TSH test. TSH, which is synthesized and secreted from the anterior pituitary gland, is the most sensitive indicator of thyroid function in the nonstressed state. Basically, if the TSH is normal (range: 0.45–4.5 mU/L), the patient is euthyroid; if the TSH is elevated (> 4.5 mU/L), the patient has primary gland failure. In the unusual case where central hypothyroidism is suspected, a free T_4 test is the best screening test.

11. How should total T_4 levels be interpreted?

    Care must be taken in interpreting total T_4 levels (occasionally performed on health screening panels). Many conditions unrelated to thyroid disease cause low or elevated levels of total T_4 because $> 99\%$ of T_4 is protein bound, and total T_4 levels depend on the amount of thyroid-binding proteins, which may vary greatly. Total T_4 levels must always be interpreted with the T_3RU, which reflects the amount of thyroid hormone–binding protein.

KEY POINTS: HYPOTHYROIDISM

- Thyroid-stimulating hormone (TSH) test is the best screening test for primary hypothyroidism in the outpatient setting.
- Levothyroxine administration is the preferred initial treatment for hypothyroidism and in healthy young patients can be started at a dose of 1.6 mcg/kg/day.
- The goal TSH for treatment of primary hypothyroidism is 0.5 to 2.0 mU/L.
- Subclinical hypothyroidism (elevated TSH but normal thyroxine/triiodothyronine) is common, and treatment can alleviate symptoms, as well as cardiac and lipid abnormalities.

12. Explain why thyroid function tests are more difficult to interpret in acutely ill inpatients.

    Interpretation of thyroid function tests in acutely ill inpatients is more difficult when hypothyroidism is suspected. Acute nonthyroidal illness may cause reversible suppression of the total T_4, free T_4, total T_3, free T_3, and TSH levels; TSH may then be elevated in the recovery phase (see Chapter 45). Medications, such as dopamine and glucocorticoids, may also suppress the TSH.

13. How do you diagnose hypothyroidism in acutely ill inpatients?

    When hypothyroidism is suspected in the stressed, hospitalized patient, a combination of clinical signs (inappropriate bradycardia, puffy facies, dry skin, and delayed relaxation of deep tendon reflexes) and laboratory tests (TSH and free T_4 levels) is necessary to exclude or confirm the diagnosis of hypothyroidism. If these tests are equivocal, the RT_3 level, which is normal or elevated in nonthyroidal illness and low in hypothyroidism, may prove helpful. Inpatient TSH testing also may be confounded by normal diurnal variations in TSH. TSH levels in euthyroid individuals may exceed the reference range at night, when patients are frequently admitted. A morning test may help to clarify the significance of a mildly elevated TSH.

14. Who should be treated for hypothyroidism?

    All patients with overt hypothyroidism should be treated. Treatment is also generally recommended for subclinical hypothyroidism, especially for patients with persistent TSH levels > 10 mU/L because with treatment, patients often experience improvement in their sense of well-being and alleviation of their cardiac and lipid abnormalities. Thyroid antibodies, an indicator of autoimmune thyroid disease, may help predict which patients with subclinical hypothyroidism will progress to overt hypothyroidism; testing is recommended for patients with minimally elevated TSH levels.

15. Which thyroid hormone preparation should you use?

    Since 1891, when sheep thyroid extract was first used to treat myxedema, many preparations have been developed and are still available. Currently, the best replacement regimen is levothyroxine (LT_4).

16. What other thyroid hormone preparations are available?

Other thyroid hormone preparations include liothyronine (LT_3), which is reserved for special cases because of its potency and short half-life, and desiccated thyroid hormone preparations, which give unpredictable serum thyroid hormone concentrations because of variable content and bioavailability.

17. What is the recommended dose of LT_4 for replacement therapy in a patient with hypothyroidism?

Otherwise healthy, young patients may be started on full replacement doses of LT_4 (1.6 mcg/kg/day). Elderly patients and those with known or suspected cardiac disease should be started on low LT_4 doses (25–50 mcg/day), which are increased by 25 mcg/day every 4 to 6 weeks until the TSH reaches normal levels. In patients with subclinical hypothyroidism, consider starting the patient on 50% to 75% of the predicted full replacement dose.

18. What is the appropriate goal for TSH in the treatment of primary hypothyroidism?

Traditionally, the target TSH level in treated hypothyroid patients has been 0.5 to 2.0 mU/L, representing the lower end of the normal range reported by most laboratories. This was based on the fact that when the usual reference ranges for TSH were developed, they included subjects with antithyroid antibodies suggestive of occult autoimmune thyroid disease. The "normal" ranges are, therefore, thought to be skewed toward higher TSH values. When normal subjects with no antithyroid antibodies are evaluated, most have TSH values < 2.5 mU/L. However, there are little data to support the idea that a low-normal TSH is clinically superior to a TSH in the high-to-normal reference range.

19. Discuss the evidence supporting combination T_4/T_3 therapy.

The medical and lay literature has taken a renewed interest in combination therapy. Animal studies have shown that T_4 therapy alone does not restore tissue levels of T_4 and T_3 to euthyroid levels, even when the TSH level is normalized. Some hypothyroid patients continue to report symptoms despite normal TSH values on LT_4 alone. Although these observations are provocative, most studies evaluating combination therapy, including a large meta-analysis, have shown no demonstrable difference in symptoms or weight with LT_4 monotherapy versus combination therapy. (Some patients in the studies did report their preference for combination therapy despite lack of objective measurable benefit.) Most experts agree that more information is needed before combination T_4/T_3 therapy can be recommended for most patients. Our current approach is to discuss this information openly with inquiring patients.

20. When should you consider combination T_4/T_3 therapy?

We suggest a trial of LT_4 alone to normalize TSH within the low-normal range (0.5–2.0 mU/L) for a period of 2 to 4 months. Many patients do extremely well with this approach. Patients who have low-normal TSH while taking LT_4 and still feel "hypothyroid" require further evaluation before LT_3 therapy is considered. We generally exclude anemia and vitamin B_{12} deficiency (associated with Hashimoto's thyroiditis) and inquire about sleep apnea. If this assessment is negative, we decrease the LT_4 by 12 to 25 mcg and add 5 mcg of liothyronine (LT_3) in the morning. The goal is to see whether the patient's symptoms improve without persistent suppression of the serum TSH (measured in the morning before taking medication). There are no data to clearly support or refute this position; we believe that it is a position of "good" medical practice.

21. What are the consequences of treating patients with hypothyroidism with excess doses of thyroid hormone?

The consequences of overtreatment of hypothyroidism can be both acute and chronic. Acute complications include symptoms of thyrotoxicosis: anxiety, tremors, palpitations, insomnia, and so on. Chronic complications of thyroid hormone excess that are well documented include a significantly increased risk of atrial fibrillation, osteoporosis with skeletal fractures, and premature mortality. These risks are especially high in patients age > 60 years.

22. How should the clinician approach surgery in the patient with hypothyroidism?

There are two broad categories to consider: emergent/cardiac surgery and elective surgery. Hypothyroidism is associated with minor postoperative complications—gastrointestinal (prolonged constipation, ileus), as well as neuropsychiatric (confusion, psychosis); in addition, the incidence of fever in response to infections is lower. Patients scheduled for elective surgery should wait until the TSH level is normalized because of the potential postoperative complications associated with hypothyroidism. However, rates of mortality and major complications (blood loss, arrhythmias, and impaired wound healing) are similar to the rates in euthyroid patients.

23. Summarize the current recommendations for emergent surgery.

Current recommendations are to proceed with emergent surgery in the hypothyroid patient and to monitor for potential postoperative complications while giving replacement therapy with LT_4. Patients with ischemic coronary artery disease requiring surgery should proceed without LT_4 replacement because T_4, if given before surgery, increases myocardial oxygen demands and may precipitate worsening cardiac symptoms. Postoperatively, the patient should receive replacement therapy with LT_4 at a slow rate and be monitored for CHF (the risk for which is increased in patients with hypothyroidism undergoing cardiac surgery).

24. How does myxedema differ from hypothyroidism?

Myxedema is a severe, uncompensated form of prolonged hypothyroidism. Complications include hypoventilation, cardiac failure, fluid and electrolyte abnormalities, and coma (see Chapter 44). Myxedema coma is frequently precipitated by an intercurrent systemic illness, surgery, or narcotic/hypnotic drugs. Patients with myxedema coma should receive replacement therapy with 300 to 500 mcg of intravenous LT_4, followed by 50 to 100 mcg each day. Because conversion of T_4 to T_3 (active hormone) is decreased with severe illness, patients with profound cardiac failure that requires pressors or patients unresponsive to 1 to 2 days of LT_4 therapy should be given LT_3 at 12.5 mcg intravenously every 6 hours.

 WEBSITE

http://www.nacb.org

BIBLIOGRAPHY

Almandoz, J. P., & Gharib, H. (2012). Hypothyroidism: etiology, diagnosis, and management. *Medical Clinics of North America, 96*, 203–221.

Arem, R., & Patsch, W. (1990). Lipoprotein and apolipoprotein levels in subclinical hypothyroidism. Effect of levothyroxine therapy. *Archives of Internal Medicine, 150*, 2097–2100.

Boeving, A., Paz-Filho, G., Radominski, R. B., Graf, H., & Amaral de Carvalho G. (2011). Low-normal or high-normal thyrotropin target levels during treatment of hypothyroidism: a prospective, comparative study. *Thyroid, 21*, 355–360.

Bunevicius, R., Kazanavicius, G., Zalinkevicius, R., & Prange, A. J. (1998). Effects of thyroxine as compared with thyroxine plus triiodothyronine in patients with hypothyroidism. *New England Journal of Medicine, 340*, 424–429.

Canaris, G. J., Manowitz, N. R., Mayor, G., & Ridgway, E. C. (2000). The Colorado thyroid disease prevalence study. *Archives of Internal Medicine, 104*, 526–534.

Celi, F., Zemskova, M., Linderman, J., Smith, S., Drinkard, B., Sachdev, V., … Pucino, F. (2011). Metabolic effects of liothyronine therapy in hypothyroidism: a randomized, double-blind, crossover trial of liothyronine versus levothyroxine. *Journal of Clinical Endocrinology and Metabolism, 96*, 3466–3474.

Chaker, L., Bianco, A. C., Jonklass, J., Peeters, R. P. (2017). Hypothyroidism. *Lancet, 390*, 1550–1562.

Cooper, D. S. Halpern, R., Wood, L. C., Levin, A. A., & Ridgway, E. C. (1984). L-thyroxine therapy in subclinical hypothyroidism. A double-blind, placebo-controlled trial. *Annals of Internal Medicine, 101*, 18–24.

Demers, L. M. & Spencer, C. A. (2003). Laboratory medicine practice guidelines: laboratory support for the diagnosis and monitoring of thyroid disease. *Thyroid, 13*, 45–56.

Elder, J., McLelland, A., O'Reilly, S. J., Packard, C. J., Series, J. J., & Shepherd, J. (1990). The relationship between serum cholesterol and serum thyrotropin, thyroxine, and tri-iodothyronine concentrations in suspected hypothyroidism. *Annals of Clinical Biochemistry, 27*, 110–113.

Grozinsky-Glasberg, S., Fraser, A., Nahshoni, E., Weizman, A., & Leibovici, L. (2006). Thyroxine-triiodothyronine combination therapy versus thyroxine monotherapy for clinical hypothyroidism: meta-analysis of randomized controlled trials. *Journal of Clinical Endocrinology and Metabolism, 91*, 2592–2599.

Hay, I. D., Duick, D. S. Vliestra, R. E., Maloney, J. D., & Pluth, J. R. (1981). Thyroxine therapy in hypothyroid patients undergoing coronary revascularization: a retrospective analysis. *Annals of Internal Medicine, 95*, 456–457.

Hollowell, J. G., Staehling, N. W., Flanders, W. D., Hannon, W. H., Gunter, E. W., Spencer, C. A., & Braverman, L. E. (2002). Serum TSH, T_4, and thyroid antibodies in the United States population (1988 to 1994): National Health and Nutrition Examination Survey (NHANES III). *Journal of Clinical Endocrinology and Metabolism, 87*, 489–499.

Ladenson, P. W. (1990). Recognition and management of cardiovascular disease related to thyroid dysfunction. *American Journal of Medicine, 88*, 638–641.

Ladenson, P. W., Levin, A. A., Ridgway, E. C., & Daniels, G. H. (1984). Complications of surgery in hypothyroid patients. *American Journal of Medicine, 77*, 262–266.

Mandel, S. J., Brent, G. A., & Larsen, P. R. (1993). Levothyroxine therapy in patients with thyroid disease. *Annals of Internal Medicine, 119*, 492–502.

Panicker, V., Saravanan, P., Vaidya, B., Evans, J., Hattersley, A. T., Frayling, T. M., & Dayan, C. M. (2009). Common variation in the *DIO2* gene predicts baseline psychological well-being and response to combination thyroxine plus triiodothyronine therapy in hypothyroid patients. *Journal of Clinical Endocrinology and Metabolism, 94*, 1623–1629.

Patel, R., & Hughes, R. W. (1992). An unusual case of myxedema megacolon with features of ischemic and pseudomembranous colitis. *Mayo Clinic Proceedings, 67*, 369–372.

Rosenthal, M. J., Hunt, W. C., Garry, P. J., & Goodwin, J. S. (1987). Thyroid failure in the elderly: microsomal antibodies as discriminant for therapy. *Journal of the American Medical Association, 258*, 209–213.

Roti, E., Minelli, R., Gardini, E., Braverman, L. E. (1993). The use and misuse of thyroid hormone. *Endocrine Reviews, 14*, 401–423.

Walsh, J., Ward, L., Burke, V., Bhagat, C. I., Shiels, L., Henley, D., … Stuckey, B. G. (2006) Small changes in thyroxine dosage do not produce measurable changes in hypothyroid symptoms, well-being, or quality of life: results of a double-blind, randomized clinical trial. *Journal of Clinical Endocrinology and Metabolism, 91*, 2624–2630.

CHAPTER 41

THYROIDITIS

Ayesha F. Malik, Robert C. Smallridge, and Ana Chindris

1. What is thyroiditis?

   Thyroiditis is inflammation of the thyroid and can be caused by various conditions. Destructive thyroiditis, which includes acute, subacute, postpartum, and painless thyroiditis, involves a transient destruction of thyroid follicles, leading to release of excessive amounts of thyroxine (T_4) and triiodothyronine (T_3) into the circulation. Thyroid hormone abnormalities may or may not resolve with time. Hashimoto's thyroiditis, an autoimmune disorder, is characterized by lymphocytic infiltration and a progressive course toward hypothyroidism. Other causes include certain drugs, Riedel's struma, radiation, and trauma.

2. Give the differential diagnosis for thyroiditis.
   1. Infectious
      a. Acute (suppurative)
      b. Subacute (also known as *granulomatous*, *non-suppurative*, or *de Quervain's*)
   2. Autoimmune
      a. Chronic lymphocytic (Hashimoto's)
      b. Atrophic
      c. Immunoglobulin G_4 (IgG_4)
      c. Juvenile (goitrous or atrophic)
      d. Postpartum
   3. Painless (non-postpartum)
   4. Drug induced (lithium, amiodarone, tyrosine kinase inhibitors, checkpoint inhibitor immunotherapy, iodinated contrast material)
   5. Riedel's struma (fibrous)
   6. Radiation induced (radioiodine and external radiation)
   7. Trauma or palpation induced
   8. Tumor embolization

3. How does acute thyroiditis present, and what causes it?

   Patients may present with anterior neck pain after a respiratory infection. It sometimes presents with symptoms of thyrotoxicosis or abnormal thyroid hormone levels.

   This rare disease has an infectious etiology, with the most commonly reported pathogens being *Staphylococcus*, *Streptococcus*, and *Mycobacterium* species. Fungal, parasitic, or syphilitic infections have been reported, and immunocompromised patients may be at increased risk. Rarely, metastatic disease to the thyroid gland can present as acute thyroiditis.

4. How is acute thyroiditis managed?

   Treatment involves incision and drainage of the abscess or surgical excision and antimicrobials. Children often have a pyriform sinus fistula, which should be surgically repaired.

5. Describe the four stages of subacute thyroiditis.
   - *Stage I:* Patients have pain and unilateral or bilateral tenderness of the thyroid that may radiate to the ears or jaw. Systemic symptoms (fatigue, malaise, fever) may be present. Inflammatory destruction of thyroid follicles permits release of T_4 and T_3 into blood, and thyrotoxicosis may ensue.
   - *Stage II:* A transitory period (several weeks) of euthyroidism occurs after the T_4 is cleared from the body.
   - *Stage III:* With severe disease, patients may become hypothyroid until the thyroid gland repairs itself.
   - *Stage IV:* Euthyroid state usually returns, but 5% to 15% of patients remain hypothyroid.

6. What causes subacute thyroiditis?

   Subacute thyroiditis is a granulomatous inflammation, probably viral in origin. Agents implicated include the mumps virus, Coxsackie virus, influenza, or adenoviruses. Although patients almost always recover clinically, serum thyroglobulin (Tgb) levels remain elevated, and intrathyroidal iodine content is low for many months (Fig. 41.1). Such findings suggest persistent subclinical abnormalities after an episode of subacute thyroiditis. Up to 4% of patients have a second episode many years later.

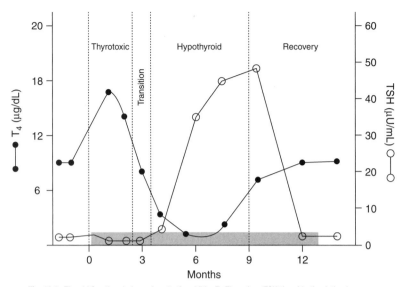

Fig. 41.1. Thyroid function during subacute thyroiditis. T_4, Thyroxine; *TSH*, thyroid-stimulating hormone.

7. **How is subacute thyroiditis managed?**
   Nonsteroidal antiinflammatory drugs (NSAIDs) are the first-line treatment in mild-to-moderate cases, whereas
   steroids may be needed when the condition is more severe. Patients requiring steroids are more likely to become
   hypothyroid at a later time.

8. **What is the most common cause of thyroiditis?**
   Autoimmune thyroid disease is recognized by the presence of thyroid peroxidase (TPO) antibody and, less frequently,
   Tgb antibody in serum. The prevalence of these antibodies is about 10% in women of reproductive age, about
   19% in older women, and 5% in men.

9. **Describe the clinical characteristics of autoimmune thyroid disease.**
   Chronic lymphocytic thyroiditis (Hashimoto's disease) usually presents as a euthyroid goiter in a female. It progresses
   to hypothyroidism at a rate of 5% per year. Progressive disease may lead to a small thyroid gland causing atrophic
   thyroiditis. Some evidence suggests that thyroid growth–inhibitory antibodies may account for the lack of a goiter
   in atrophic thyroiditis. Those with juvenile thyroiditis usually present with a goiter. IgG_4 thyroiditis is thought to be
   on the spectrum of Hashimoto's thyroiditis and is characterized by a greater degree of stromal fibrosis, lympho-
   plasmacytic infiltration, and hypothyroidism.

10. **Does postpartum thyroiditis follow a clinical course different from those of other types of autoimmune
    thyroiditis?**
    Yes. Postpartum disease develops in women between the third and ninth months after delivery, sometimes even
    1 year later. It typically follows the stages seen in patients with subacute thyroiditis, although histologically
    patients have lymphocytic infiltration.

11. **How common is postpartum thyroiditis?**
    After delivery, 5% to 10% of women develop biochemical evidence of thyroid dysfunction. Approximately one third
    of affected women develop symptoms (hyperthyroidism, hypothyroidism, or both) and benefit from 6 to 12 months
    of therapy with levothyroxine (LT_4) if it is hypothyroidism. Up to 70% of patients will develop recurrence with
    subsequent pregnancies. The frequency of each clinical presentation is depicted in Fig. 41.2.

12. **Which patients with postpartum thyroiditis should be treated?**
    Postpartum thyroiditis is a destructive process; therefore, antithyroid drugs (methimazole or propylthiouracil) are
    not effective. If hyperthyroid symptoms are present, beta-blockers can be used. Patients with hypothyroidism
    who have severe symptoms and those who desire conception should receive treatment with LT_4. In these cases,
    however, tapering off the medication should be tried 6 to 12 months after initiation, in the attempt to eventually
    discontinue therapy.

Types of postpartum thyroid dysfunction

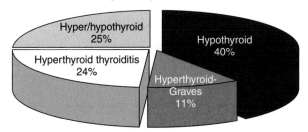

Fig. 41.2. Frequency of clinical presentations of postpartum thyroiditis.

Table 41.1. Subacute Versus Postpartum Thyroiditis.

	SUBACUTE THYROIDITIS	POSTPARTUM THYROIDITIS
Thyroid pain	Yes	No
Sedimentation rate	Increased (> 50 mm/hr)	Normal
TPO antibody	Transient increase only	Positive
HLA status	B-35	DR3, DR5
Histology	Giant cells, granulomas	Lymphocytes

HLA, Human leucocyte antigen; *TPO,* thyroid peroxidase.

13. Summarize the differences between subacute and postpartum thyroiditis.
    See Table 41.1.

14. Why does thyroiditis develop after delivery?
    Women with postpartum thyroiditis have underlying, usually asymptomatic, autoimmune thyroiditis. During pregnancy, the maternal immune system is partially suppressed, with a dramatic rebound rise in thyroid antibodies after delivery. Although TPO or Tgb antibodies are not believed to be cytotoxic, they are currently the most reliable marker of susceptibility to postpartum disease.

15. Does thyroid function in patients with postpartum thyroiditis return to normal as it does in subacute thyroiditis?
    Not always. Approximately 20% of women become permanently hypothyroid, and a similar number of them have persistent mild abnormalities. An annual TSH test is, therefore, recommended.

16. What factors identify women at increased risk for postpartum thyroiditis?
    Women with a higher TPO antibody titer have a higher risk for postpartum thyroiditis. In approximately 25% of women with type 1 diabetes mellitus, thyroiditis develops after delivery. For high-risk patients, screening for thyroid antibodies and careful monitoring of thyroid function at 3 to 6 months after delivery are indicated.

17. What is painless thyroiditis?
    Both men and non-postpartum women may present with transient thyrotoxic symptoms. As with subacute thyroiditis, these patients often experience subsequent hypothyroidism. Unlike subacute disease, this disorder is painless. It has been given a variety of names, including *hyperthyroiditis, silent thyroiditis, transient painless thyroiditis with hyperthyroidism,* and *lymphocytic thyroiditis with spontaneously resolving hyperthyroidism.* This disease was first described in the 1970s and reached its peak incidence in the early 1980s. It seems to occur less often now.

18. What causes painless thyroiditis?
    Some investigators believe that it is a variant of subacute thyroiditis because a small percentage of patients with biopsy-proven subacute (granulomatous) disease have had no pain (they may have fever and weight loss, and may be misdiagnosed as having systemic disease or malignancy). Others believe that it is a variant of Hashimoto's disease because of similar histology. Hashimoto's thyroiditis can occasionally present with thyroid pain; rarely, surgery is necessary to relieve symptoms.

19. What is the natural history of destructive thyroiditis?

    It is similar to the stages of subacute thyroiditis. It may present with hyperthyroidism in the first 6 weeks, followed by 4 weeks of euthyroid state and another 4 to 6 weeks of hypothyroidism, and ultimately the euthyroid state returns.

20. When a patient presents with hyperthyroid symptoms, an elevated free T_4 level, and suppressed TSH, what test should be ordered next?

    A 24-hour RAIU should be performed. When the thyroid is overactive (as in Graves' disease or toxic nodular disease), the RAIU level is elevated. In destructive thyroiditis, the RAIU level is low, as a result of both suppression of TSH by the acutely increased level of serum T_4 and the diminished ability of damaged thyroid follicles to trap and organify iodine.

21. What is the appropriate therapy for patients with any type of destructive thyroiditis?

    In the thyrotoxic stage, beta-blockers relieve adrenergic symptoms. All forms of antithyroid therapy (drugs, radioactive iodine ablation, and surgery) are absolutely contraindicated. NSAIDs or aspirin may provide prompt relief of thyroid pain. If there is no improvement in 2 to 3 days, then the NSAID treatment should be discontinued and prednisone 40 mg daily should be started. Some studies have also shown improvement with prednisolone 15 mg daily. For the hypothyroid phase, thyroid hormone may be used to relieve symptoms of hypothyroidism and should be continued for 6 to 12 months, depending on severity of disease. Some patients require no therapy.

22. Which drugs can induce thyroiditis?

    Amiodarone, an iodine-containing antiarrhythmic drug, may cause thyroid damage and thyrotoxicosis in about 5% to 20% of cases by inhibitory or cytotoxic mechanisms, or precipitation of underlying autoimmune disease.

    Lithium therapy used for bipolar disease has been associated with granulomatous thyroiditis, as well as with destructive thyroiditis without lymphocytic infiltration, causing hypothyroidism more commonly than hyperthyroidism.

    Interferon-alpha, used commonly for treatment of hepatitis C (less commonly, interferon-beta), and interleukin-2, used for metastatic cancer and leukemia (e.g., denileukin diftitox), can cause both hyperthyroidism and hypothyroidism.

    Tyrosine kinase inhibitors (e.g., sunitinib, sorafenib, cabozantinib) have been noted to cause hypothyroidism in 50% to 70% of patients, potentially by causing destructive thyroiditis. Hyperthyroidism has also been reported.

    Checkpoint inhibitor immunotherapies (ipilimumab, nivolumab, pembrolizumab, atezolizumab) are used commonly for metastatic melanoma and multiple other malignancies. They have been found to cause many endocrinopathies, including hypophysitis and destructive thyroiditis, which causes hypothyroidism.

    Nonionic contrast materials (e.g., ioxaglate [Hexabrix]) were reported to cause destructive thyroiditis.

23. How does amiodarone-induced thyroiditis present?

    Amiodarone contains 37% iodine by weight, and about 3000 mcg of iodine is released into the systemic circulation per 100 mg of amiodarone. The daily recommended allowance of iodine is 150 mcg for men and nonpregnant women and 220 mcg for pregnant women. Because of the large amount of iodine in this drug, it can cause either hypothyroidism or hyperthyroidism. Distinguishing hyperthyroidism caused by iodine excess (type 1 disease) from amiodarone-induced destructive thyroiditis (type 2 disease) can be difficult. Some differentiating features are listed in Table 41.2. Absence of blood flow on Doppler ultrasonography is particularly helpful in confirming type 2 disease.

24. What is Riedel's struma?

    Riedel's struma is a rare disorder in which the thyroid becomes densely fibrotic and hard. Local fibrosis of adjacent tissues may produce obstructive symptoms that require surgery. In some cases, fibrosis of other tissues (fibrosing retroperitonitis, orbital fibrosis, or sclerosing cholangitis) may occur.

Table 41.2. Type 1 Versus Type 2 Amiodarone-Induced Thyroiditis.

	TYPE 1	TYPE 2
Thyroid size	Goiter; nodules	Normal
RAIU	↓, normal, ↑	↓↓
Thyroid antibodies	↑ negative	Negative
Interleukin-6	Normal, ↑	↑↑
Ultrasound Doppler flow	↑	↓
Therapy	Antithyroid drugs, potassium perchlorate; thyroidectomy	Antithyroid drugs (?), steroids

RAIU, Radioactive iodine uptake; ↓, low; ↑, high; ↓↓, very low; ↑↑, very high.

25. How is Riedel's thyroiditis treated?

Surgical removal of the thyroid isthmus may relieve constrictive symptoms. Glucocorticoids have been helpful, as has tamoxifen, which inhibits fibroblast growth by stimulating transforming growth factor-beta. Treatment with a combination of mycophenolate mofetil and prednisone has been reported.

26. Are there any other causes of thyroiditis?

Yes. High-dose external radiation can cause painless thyrotoxic thyroiditis. Various forms of neck trauma (neck surgery, cyst aspiration, seat-belt injury) and tumor emboli have also been reported. Infiltration by sarcoidosis or amyloid may also cause thyroiditis.

⊕ WEBSITE

http://www.thyroidmanager.org

BIBLIOGRAPHY

Alexander, E. K., Pearce, E. N., Brent, G. A., Brown, R. S., Chen, H., Dosiou, C., . . . Sullivan, S. (2017). 2017 Guidelines of the American Thyroid Association for the diagnosis and management of thyroid disease during pregnancy and the postpartum. *Thyroid, 27*(3), 315–389.

Bogazzi, F., Bartalena, L., & Martino E. (2010). Approach to the patient with amiodarone-induced thyrotoxicosis. *Journal of Clinical Endocrinology and Metabolism, 95,* 2529–2535.

Calvi, L., & Daniels, G. H. (2011). Acute thyrotoxicosis secondary to destructive thyroiditis associated with cardiac catheterization contrast dye. *Thyroid, 21*(4), 443–449.

Hennessey, J. V. (2011). Riedel's thyroiditis: a clinical review. *Journal of Clinical Endocrinology and Metabolism, 96,* 3031–3041.

Jimenez-Heffernan, J., Perez, F., Hornedo, J., Perna, C., & Lapuente, F. (2004). Massive thyroid tumoral embolism from a breast carcinoma presenting as acute thyroiditis. *Archives of Pathology & Laboratory Medicine, 128,* 804–806.

Kottahachchi, D., & Topliss, D. J. (2016). Immunoglobulin G4-related thyroid diseases. *European Thyroid Journal, 5*(4), 231–239.

Kubota, S., Nishihara, E., Kudo, T., Ito, M., Amino, N., & Miyauchi. A. (2013). Initial treatment with 15 mg of prednisolone daily is sufficient for most patients with subacute thyroiditis in Japan. *Thyroid, 23*(3), 269–272.

Lazarus, J. H. (2009). Lithium and thyroid. *Best Practice & Research. Clinical Endocrinology & Metabolism, 23,* 723–733.

Mammen, J. S., Ghazarian, S. R., Pulkstenis, E., Subramanian, G. M., Rosen, A., & Ladenson, P. W. (2012). Phenotypes of interferon-α-induced thyroid dysfunction among patients treated for hepatitis C are associated with pretreatment serum TSH and female sex. *Journal of Clinical Endocrinology and Metabolism, 97*(9), 3270–3276.

Meek, S. E., & Smallridge, R. C. (2008). Thyroiditis and other more unusual forms of hyperthyroidism. In D. S. Cooper (Ed.), *Medical management of thyroid disease* (pp. 101–144). New York: Informa Healthcare.

Melme, S., Polonsky, K. S., Larsen, P. R., & Kronenberg, H. M. (2016). *Williams textbook of endocrinology* (13th ed.). Philadelphia, PA. Elsevier.

Nagayama, T. (2017). Radiation-related thyroid autoimmunity and dysfunction. *Journal of Radiation Research, 59* (Suppl. 2), ii98–ii107.

Nicholson, W. K., Robinson, K. A., Smallridge, R. C., Ladenson, P. W., & Powe, N. R. (2006). Prevalence of postpartum thyroid dysfunction: a quantitative review. *Thyroid, 16,* 573–582.

Paes, J. E., Burman, K. D., Cohen, J., Franklyn, J., McHenry, C. R., Shoham, S., & Kloos, R. T. (2010). Acute bacterial suppurative thyroiditis: a clinical review and expert opinion. *Thyroid, 20*(3), 247–255.

Ross, D. S., Burch, H. B., Cooper, D. S., Greenlee, M. C., Laurberg, P., Maia, A. L., . . . Walter, M. A. (2016). American Thyroid Association guidelines for diagnosis and management of hyperthyroidism and other causes of thyrotoxicosis. *Thyroid, 26*(10), 1343–1421.

Rotondi, M., Capelli, V., Locantore, P., Pontecorvi, A., & Chivovato, L. (2017). Painful Hashimoto's thyroiditis: myth or reality? *Journal of Endocrinological Investigation, 40*(8), 815–818.

Samuels, M. H. (2012). Subacute, silent and postpartum thyroiditis. *Medical Clinics of North America, 96,* 223–233.

Smallridge, R. C. (2002). Hypothyroidism and pregnancy. *Endocrinologist, 12,* 454–464.

Smallridge, R. C. (2000). Postpartum thyroid disease: a model of immunologic dysfunction. *Clinical and Applied Immunology Reviews*, *1*, 89–103.

Vanderpump, M. P. J. (2005). The epidemiology of thyroid disease. In L. E. Braverman, & R. D. Utiger (Eds.), *Werner and Ingbar's the thyroid: a fundamental and clinical text* (9th ed., pp. 398–406). Philadelphia, PA: Lippincott Williams and Wilkins.

Yavuz, S., Apolo, A. B., Kummar, S., del Rivero, J., Madan, R. A., Shawker, T., . . . Celi, F. S. (2014). Cabozantinib-induced thyroid dysfunction: a review of two ongoing trials for metastatic bladder cancer and sarcoma. *Thyroid, 24*(8), 1223–1231.

THYROID NODULES AND GOITER

Michele B. Glodowski and Sarah E. Mayson

CHAPTER 42

1. **What is thyroid nodule?**

   Thyroid nodule, a lesion or growth in the thyroid gland, is radiographically distinct from the surrounding thyroid parenchyma. It may or may not be palpable on clinical examination. The differential diagnosis of thyroid nodule includes both benign and malignant etiologies. Benign lesions include cysts, inflammatory nodules, colloid nodules, and follicular and Hürthle's cell adenomas. Thyroid nodules can also represent nonthyroidal lesions (e.g., parathyroid adenoma). Malignant lesions constitute only a small percentage of all thyroid nodules. The most common malignant lesions, representing > 90% of all thyroid carcinomas, are papillary and follicular carcinomas (together referred to as *differentiated thyroid carcinomas*), but medullary, anaplastic, and metastatic nonthyroidal carcinomas and thyroid lymphomas are also seen.

2. **How common are thyroid nodules?**

   Thyroid nodules are fairly common, but the prevalence depends on the population studied and the methods used to detect them. For nodules discovered on palpation, the prevalence is 1% to 6%. With the use of thyroid ultrasonography, the prevalence increases to 19% to 68%, and on autopsy the prevalence is 8% to 65%. Nodules are more common with increasing age, in women, in those living in geographic areas with iodine deficiency, and in individuals exposed to ionizing radiation.

3. **What is a goiter?**

   Goiter refers to a clinically or radiographically enlarged thyroid gland. It can be diffusely enlarged or nodular (either with a single nodule or multiple nodules, termed *multinodular goiter*). It can be toxic (with autonomous thyroid hyperfunction) or nontoxic (normal thyroid function). The most common cause of goiter worldwide is iodine deficiency. In the United States, more common etiologies of goiter include autoimmune thyroid disease (Hashimoto's thyroiditis or Graves' disease), simple nodular goiter, and thyroid carcinoma.

4. **What are the clinical manifestations of a simple nodular goiter?**

   The clinical relevance of a simple (nonfunctioning) nodular goiter is mainly related to its size and association with compressive symptoms. Both cervical and substernal (those that extend through the thoracic outlet) goiters can cause compression of surrounding structures, such as the trachea, esophagus, and recurrent laryngeal nerves, leading to dyspnea, cough, dysphagia, globus sensation, and voice changes. In addition, nodular goiters carry the same risk of cancer as does a single nonfunctioning nodule. Therefore, malignancy needs to be ruled out in multinodular goiters by using the same approach as that for a single nodule.

5. **What is the role of iodine in the formation of goiters?**

   Iodine is an essential dietary micronutrient and a key structural component of thyroxine (T_4) and triiodothyronine (T_3). Iodine deficiency leads to decreased production of these thyroid hormones. This, in turn, leads to increased production of thyroid-stimulating hormone (TSH), which binds to TSH receptors on thyroid follicular cells and causes an increase in the size of the thyroid gland, resulting in both diffuse growth and nodular growth.

6. **What is the evaluation of a patient with compressive symptoms related to a goiter?**

   When a patient complains of symptoms suggestive of compression related to a goiter, further diagnostic studies may be warranted. Spirometry is noninvasive and provides an assessment of airflow during both inspiration and expiration, creating a flow volume loop curve. The shape of the flow volume loop curve allows for identification of respiratory tract obstruction. Barium swallow with esophagography can be used to evaluate thyroid mass effects on the esophagus. Computed tomography (CT) or chest radiography can be useful to evaluate the extent of a large goiter and assess for deviation or narrowing of the trachea or esophagus. However, radioiodinated contrast materials should usually be avoided because of the risk of iodine-induced thyrotoxicosis.

7. **What is Pemberton's sign?**

   Pemberton's sign, first described by Dr. Hugh Pemberton in 1946, is useful for evaluating possible thoracic outlet obstruction by a substernal goiter. The patient is asked to elevate both arms overhead until they touch the sides of the face. Diffuse neck and facial congestion occur if the goiter obstructs the thoracic inlet by a "cork effect." Imaging is important to delineate the goiter; however, as mentioned above, contrast-enhanced studies should be avoided because of the risk of iodine-induced thyrotoxicosis (Jod-Basedow disease).

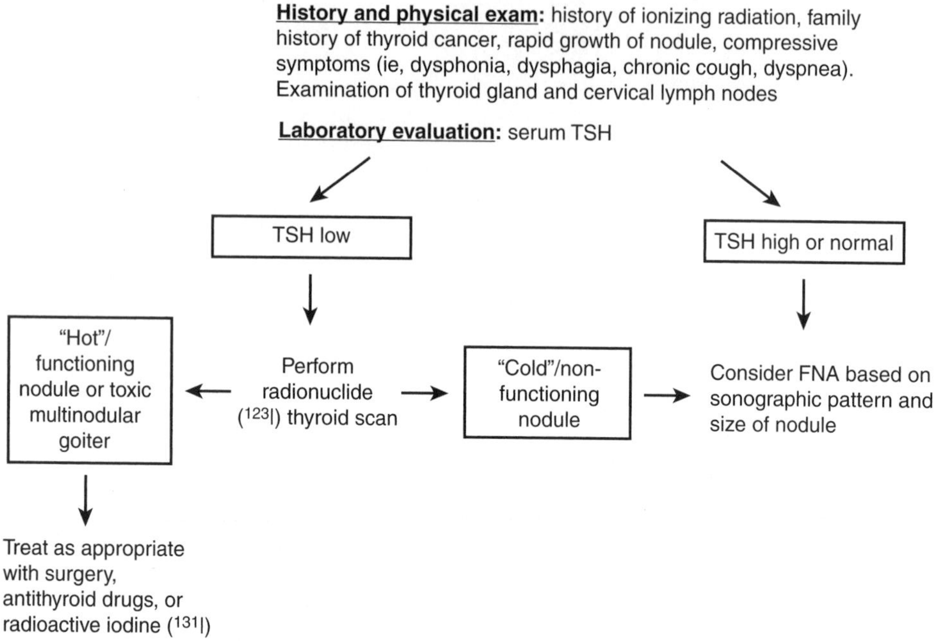

History and physical exam: history of ionizing radiation, family history of thyroid cancer, rapid growth of nodule, compressive symptoms (ie, dysphonia, dysphagia, chronic cough, dyspnea). Examination of thyroid gland and cervical lymph nodes

Laboratory evaluation: serum TSH

TSH low

TSH high or normal

"Hot"/ functioning nodule or toxic multinodular goiter

Perform radionuclide (^{123}I) thyroid scan

"Cold"/non-functioning nodule

Consider FNA based on sonographic pattern and size of nodule

Treat as appropriate with surgery, antithyroid drugs, or radioactive iodine (^{131}I)

Fig. 42.1. Algorithm for the evaluation of thyroid nodules. *FNA*, Fine-needle aspiration; *TSH*, thyroid-stimulating hormone.

8. What is the initial approach to a patient with a newly discovered thyroid nodule?

   The initial approach to a patient with a newly discovered thyroid nodule is also outlined in Fig. 42.1. The first step in the evaluation of a thyroid nodule or nodules is to perform a complete history and physical examination. The history should note any factors that may increase the risk of or be indicative of thyroid cancer, including a history of ionizing radiation exposure (especially in childhood), family history of thyroid cancer, rapid growth of the nodule, or presence of compressive symptoms (dyspnea, cough, dysphagia, globus sensation, and voice hoarseness). Examination should include a thorough neck assessment, including palpation of the thyroid gland and cervical lymph nodes. Serum TSH level should then be checked. If the TSH level is normal or elevated, ultrasonography of the thyroid gland and cervical lymph nodes should be performed to determine if fine-needle aspiration (FNA) biopsy should be done. If the TSH level is low, serum free T$_4$ should be measured and radionuclide thyroid imaging should be ordered.

9. What is the difference between a hot nodule and a cold nodule?

   One of the first steps in the initial evaluation of a thyroid nodule is to determine thyroid function by measuring serum TSH. If the TSH level is low, indicating overt or subclinical hyperthyroidism, the next step is to measure serum free T$_4$ and to perform a thyroid uptake and scan using radioiodine (typically ^{123}I). A hot nodule is identified as a focal area of increased radiotracer uptake in association with decreased uptake in the remainder of the gland, indicating autonomous nodular function. A cold nodule is one with decreased radiotracer uptake. A toxic (autonomous) multinodular goiter will have mildly increased, heterogeneous uptake. Biopsy of hot nodules is not recommended because of the very low likelihood ($< 1\%$) of malignancy.

10. Why is FNA performed under ultrasound guidance?

    The main purpose of FNA is to identify malignant thyroid nodules and thereby select patients who require surgery. Several studies have shown that ultrasound-guided FNA, as opposed to conventional FNA guided by palpation, results in more precise and adequate sampling, with lower rates of nondiagnostic findings and lower rates of false-negative cytology. It, therefore, improves surgical selectivity and cost of care.

11. What is the approach to selecting thyroid nodules for FNA when multiple nodules are detected in a single gland?

    When there are multiple nodules in a single gland, each nodule should be considered for FNA independently in terms of its size and ultrasonographic pattern.

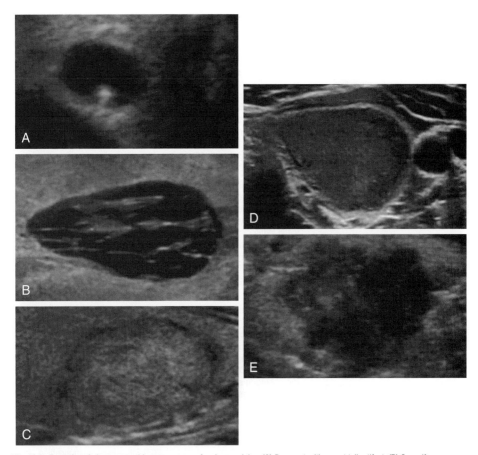

Fig. 42.2. Examples of ultrasonographic appearances of various nodules. **(A)** Pure cyst with comet tail artifact. **(B)** Spongiform. **(C)** Isoechoic solid. **(D)** Hypoechoic solid. **(E)** Hypoechoic solid with irregular/infiltrative margins.

12. How are the characteristics of a thyroid nodule demonstrated on ultrasonography?

When evaluating a thyroid nodule, we consider its composition (solid, cystic, mixed solid and cystic, or spongiform [comprising > 50% microcystic components]); echogenicity (relative to the surrounding thyroid tissue); shape (taller than wide or wider than tall on transverse view); margins (regular, irregular, infiltrative, or spiculated); and the presence or absence of echogenic foci (macro- and microcalcifications). The nodule's size in three dimensions and location in the thyroid gland should also be noted. Other characteristics that are considered include the presence of a sonolucent halo and its appearance (thin and regular versus thick and irregular), nodule vascularity, rim calcification, and presence of extrathyroidal extension. The cervical lymph nodes should also be evaluated. Examples of thyroid nodule ultrasonographic images are shown in Fig. 42.2.

13. Does every thyroid nodule have the same risk of cancer?

Several studies have shown that certain ultrasonographic patterns correlate with thyroid carcinoma, specifically with papillary thyroid carcinoma (PTC). We therefore use thyroid ultrasonography to determine a nodule's risk of malignancy. Features associated with PTC include microcalcifications, hypoechogenicity, shape taller than wide, irregular margins, extrathyroidal extension, interrupted rim calcification with soft tissue extrusion, and presence of any abnormal-appearing lymph nodes.

14. Which thyroid nodules need to be biopsied?

The decision to biopsy a thyroid nodule is based on the size and sonographic appearance of the nodule, which correspond to its risk of malignancy. The American Thyroid Association, the American Association of Clinical Endocrinologists, and the American College of Radiology all have published recommendations describing when to consider FNA of a thyroid nodule. These criteria are summarized in Table 42.1.

Table 42.1. Comparison of Guidelines for Thyroid FNA.

ATA	AACE/ACE-AME	ACR
High Suspicion Hypoechoic + one of the following: Taller than wide, microcalcifications, irregular margins, extrathyroidal extension, interrupted rim calcification with soft tissue extrusion, suspicious lymph nodes **Biopsy when ≥ 1 cm**	High Risk At least one of the following: Marked hypoechogenicity, spiculated or microlobulated margins, microcalcifications, taller than wide, extrathyroidal growth, pathologic adenopathy **Biopsy when ≥ 1 cm** **Consider biopsy when 5–10 mm**	Highly Suspicious ≥ 7 points based on composition, echogenicity, shape, margins, and echogenic foci **Biopsy when ≥ 1 cm**
Intermediate Suspicion Hypoechoic (without features described above) **Biopsy when ≥ 1.5 cm**	Intermediate Risk Slightly hypoechoic or isoechoic with ovoid-to-round shape and smooth or ill-defined margins, intranodular vascularization, elevated stiffness at elastography, macro- or continuous rim calcifications, hyperechoic spots of uncertain significance **Biopsy when ≥ 2 cm**	Moderately Suspicious 4–6 points based on composition, echogenicity, shape, margins, and echogenic foci **Biopsy when ≥ 1.5 cm**
Low Suspicion Hyperechoic, isoechoic, partially cystic with eccentric solid area (without features described above) **Biopsy when ≥ 1.5 cm** Very Low Suspicion Spongiform, partially cystic (without features described above) **Biopsy when ≥ 2.0 cm[a]**	Low Risk Cysts (> 80%), mostly cystic (> 50%) with reverberating artifacts (without suspicious ultrasonographic signs), isoechoic spongiform **Biopsy when ≥ 2 cm only when increasing in size or in special circumstances**	Mildly Suspicious 3 points based on composition, echogenicity, shape, margins, and echogenic foci **Biopsy when ≥ 2.5 cm** Not Suspicious 2 points based on composition, echogenicity, shape, margins, and echogenic foci **Biopsy not recommended**
Benign Pure cyst **Biopsy not recommended**		Benign 0 points based on composition, echogenicity, shape, margins, and echogenic foci **Biopsy not recommended**

[a]Can consider clinical and ultrasonographic follow-up in lieu of FNA biopsy.
AACE/ACE/AME, American Association of Clinical Endocrinologists/American College of Endocrinology/Associazione Medici Endocrinologi; *ACR,* American College of Radiology; *ATA,* American Thyroid Association; *FNA,* fine-needle aspiration.

15. How is thyroid cytology interpreted?

When an FNA is performed, the cytology is generally reported by using the Bethesda System for Reporting Thyroid Cytopathology, which was initially proposed in 2007 and updated in 2017. An FNA sample of a thyroid nodule is considered adequate when it comprises at least six groups of 10 to 15 follicular cells each. Based on certain features, an FNA sample is classified into one of six categories, each of which has a corresponding risk of malignancy. These categories are: I = nondiagnostic or unsatisfactory; II = benign; III = atypia of undetermined significance or follicular lesion of undetermined significance (AUS/FLUS); IV = follicular neoplasm or suspicious for follicular neoplasm (FN/SFN); V = suspicious for malignancy; and VI = malignant.

16. What is the management of a thyroid nodule that is found to have benign cytology on FNA?

Benign thyroid cytology carries a 0% to 3% risk of malignancy, and thus, no immediate follow-up testing is warranted. It is recommended that clinical follow-up be scheduled and repeat neck ultrasonography performed in 12 to 24 months, depending on the ultrasonographic appearance of the nodule on the initial examination. If the nodule is unchanged on the repeat ultrasonography, another examination can be considered after a longer interval. If, on repeat ultrasonography, there is evidence of growth (≥ 50% change in volume or ≥ 20% increase in at least two dimensions with a minimal increase of 2 mm), then repeat FNA can be considered. If a nodule has had two benign FNA results, no additional FNA sampling is warranted.

17. What is the management of an indeterminate thyroid nodule?
Indeterminate thyroid nodules are nodules with Bethesda categories III (AUS/FLUS), IV (FN/SFN), or V (suspicious for malignancy) cytology results. With Bethesda III cytology, the ultrasonographic pattern and patient risk factors and preferences are taken into consideration to determine the need for surgery versus repeat FNA or clinical and ultrasonographic surveillance. Molecular diagnostic testing may be used adjunctively to help inform clinical decision making. With Bethesda IV cytology, either diagnostic surgery (lobectomy) or molecular testing is appropriate. The management of Bethesda V nodules is the same as for nodules with malignant cytology (Bethesda VI).

18. What is the role of molecular testing in thyroid nodule management?
Molecular diagnostic testing can be useful in the evaluation of thyroid nodules with indeterminate cytology (Bethesda III, IV, or V). Molecular diagnostic tests include messenger ribonucleic acid (mRNA) or micro-RNA gene expression classifiers and gene panels that evaluate for the presence of genetic alterations (mutations, insertions/deletions, gene fusions, copy number alterations, or gene expression alterations). Tests with high sensitivity and negative predicative value are used to rule out thyroid cancer, and those with high specificity and positive predictive value are used to rule in thyroid cancer. Both positive predictive value and negative predictive value are dependent on the prevalence of malignancy in the population and must be calculated by each institution/region.

19. What is the management of a thyroid nodule that is found to be suspicious for malignancy or is malignant after FNA?
Classification of malignant (Bethesda VI) on cytology carries a 94% to 96% risk of malignancy, and classification of suspicious for malignancy (Bethesda V) carries a 45% to 60% risk of malignancy. Surgical resection (near total thyroidectomy or lobectomy) is recommended for both.

20. What is the management of a thyroid nodule that does not meet the criteria for FNA?
The follow-up of a nodule that does not meet the criteria for FNA depends on its initial ultrasonographic appearance. For nodules that raise high suspicion on ultrasonography but do not meet biopsy criteria because of the small size, a repeat ultrasonographic examination should be performed in 6 to 12 months. Nodules that did not have suspicious features and did not meet the criteria for biopsy can be reimaged in 12 to 24 months. Cysts and small spongiform nodules do not require routine imaging follow-up.

KEY POINTS

- Thyroid nodules are common, and only a small percentage of nodules are malignant.
- The initial evaluation of a thyroid nodule involves measurement of serum thyroid-stimulating hormone (TSH) and ultrasonography of the thyroid gland and cervical nodes. A subnormal TSH should prompt diagnostic radionucleotide scanning.
- The decision to biopsy a thyroid nodule depends on its size and ultrasonographic features.
- Molecular testing can be useful in the management of thyroid nodules with indeterminate cytology, specifically those with Bethesda III and IV cytology.

BIBLIOGRAPHY

Abu-Shamra, Y., & Cuny, T. (2018). Pemberton's sign in a patient with a goiter. *New England Journal of Medicine, 378*, (22):e31.
Ali, S. Z., & Cibas, E. S. (2010). *The Bethesda system for reporting thyroid cytopathology: definitions, criteria, and explanatory notes.* New York: Springer.
Allen, B. C., Baker, M. E., & Falk, G. W. (2009). Role of barium esophagography in evaluating dysphagia. *Cleveland Clinic Journal of Medicine, 76*, 105–111.
Basaria, S., & Salvatori, R. (2004). Pemberton's sign. *New England Journal of Medicine, 350*, 1338.
Brito, J. P., Gionfriddo, M. R., Al Nofal, A., Boehmer, K. R., Leppin, A. L., Reading, C., . . . Montori, V. M. (2014). The accuracy of thyroid nodule ultrasound to predict thyroid cancer: systematic review and meta-analysis. *Journal of Clinical Endocrinology and Metabolism, 99*, 1253–1263.
Cibas, E. S., & Ali, S. Z. (2017). The 2017 Bethesda system for reporting thyroid cytopathology. *Thyroid, 27*, 1341–1346.
Cramer, H. (2000). Fine-needle aspiration cytology of the thyroid: an appraisal. *Cancer, 90*, 325–329.
Dean, D. S., & Gharib, H. (2008). Epidemiology of thyroid nodules. *Best Practice & Research. Clinical Endocrinology & Metabolism, 22*, 901–911.
Geraghty, J. G., Coveney, E. C., Kiernan, M., & O'Higgins, N. J. (1992). Flow volume loops in patients with goiters. *Annals of Surgery, 215*, 83–86.
Gharib, H., Papini, E., Garber, J. R., Duick, D. S., Harrell, R. M., Hegedüs, L., . . . Vitti, P. (2016). American Association of Clinical Endocrinologists, American College of Endocrinology, and Associazione Medici Endocrinologi medical guidelines for clinical practice for the diagnosis and management of thyroid nodules – 2016 Update. *Endocrine Practice, 22*, 622–639.
Hanson, G. A., Komorowski, R. A., Cerletty, J. M., & Wilson, S. D. (1983). Thyroid gland morphology in young adults: normal subjects versus those with prior low-dose neck irradiation in childhood. *Surgery, 94*, 984–988.

Haugen, B. R., Alexander, E. K., Bible, K. C., Doherty, G. M., Mandel, S. J., Nikiforov, Y. E., . . . Wartofsky, L. (2016). 2015 American Thyroid Association Management Guidelines for Adult Patients with Thyroid Nodules and Differentiated Thyroid Cancer: The American Thyroid Association Guidelines Task Force on Thyroid Nodules and Differentiated Thyroid Cancer. *Thyroid, 26*, 1–133.

Hegedus, L., Bonnema, S. J., & Bennedbaek, F. N. (2003). Management of simple nodular goiter: current status and future perspectives. *Endocrine Reviews, 24*, 102–132.

Hegedüs, L. (2004). Clinical practice. The thyroid nodule. *New England Journal of Medicine, 351*, 1764–1771.

Jeh, S. K., Jung, S. L., Kim, B. S., & Lee, Y. S. (2007). Evaluating the degree of conformity of papillary carcinoma and follicular carcinoma to the reported ultrasonographic findings of malignant thyroid tumor. *Korean Journal of Radiology, 8*, 192–197.

Katlic, M. R., Wang, C. A., & Grillo, H. C. (1985). Substernal goiter. *Annals of Thoracic Surgery, 39*, 391–399.

Mandel, S. J. (2004). A 64-year-old woman with a thyroid nodule. *Journal of the American Medical Association, 292*, 2632–2642.

Pearce, E. N., & Braverman, L. E. (2004). Pemberton's sign. *New England Journal of Medicine, 351*, 196.

Sarkar, S. D. (2006). Benign thyroid disease: what is the role of nuclear medicine? *Seminars in Nuclear Medicine, 36*, 185–193.

Sorensen, J. R., Hegedüs, L., Kruse-Andersen, S., Godballe, C., & Bonnema, S. J. (2014). The impact of goitre and its treatment on the trachea, airflow, oesophagus and swallowing function. A systematic review. *Best Practice & Research. Clinical Endocrinology & Metabolism, 28*, 481–494.

Steward, D. L., Carty, S. E., Sippel, R. S., Yang, S. P., Sosa, J. A., Sipos, J. A., . . . Nikiforov, Y. E. (2018). Performance of a multigene genomic classifier in thyroid nodules with indeterminate cytology: a prospective blinded multicenter study. *JAMA Oncology*, doi:10.1001/jamaoncol.2018.4616. [Epub ahead of print].

Vanderpump, M. P. (2011). The epidemiology of thyroid disease. *British Medical Bulletin, 99*, 39–51.

CHAPTER 43

THYROID CANCER

Veena R. Agrawal and Sarah E. Mayson

INTRODUCTION

1. **How common is thyroid cancer?**

   In the United States, thyroid cancer is the 12th most common cancer, with an estimated lifetime prevalence of 1.2%. It is the fifth most common cancer in women, and the most common cancer among women age 20 to 34 years. The incidence of thyroid cancer has been rising by about 3% per year, largely because of identification of incidental thyroid nodules on screening or on imaging performed for other reasons. This steady increase in diagnosis has also been seen worldwide. Overall mortality rates from thyroid cancer have been decreasing, although there has been an increase in the incidence-based mortality rate (2.9% per year) of advanced-stage papillary thyroid carcinoma. The median age at diagnosis is 51 years.

2. **What are the types of thyroid cancer?**

   The most common type of thyroid cancer is differentiated thyroid cancer (DTC), which comprises > 90% of all thyroid cancers and includes papillary thyroid carcinoma (PTC), follicular thyroid carcinoma (FTC), Hurthle cell carcinoma (HCC), and poorly differentiated thyroid cancer (PDTC). Other types of thyroid cancer include medullary and anaplastic thyroid cancers. Rarely, other tumor types including lymphoma, salivary gland tumors, and metastases from nonthyroid malignancies (e.g., breast, renal cell cancers) can be seen in the thyroid gland.

3. **How does thyroid cancer present?**

   Thyroid cancer is often identified when patients present with a palpable thyroid nodule. Thyroid nodules may also be identified on imaging performed for evaluation of other thyroid disorders or incidentally on imaging performed for unrelated reasons. Diagnostic workup typically includes measurement of serum thyroid-stimulating hormone (TSH), neck ultrasonography, and, if indicated, fine-needle aspiration biopsy (see Chapter 42).

DIFFERENTIATED THYROID CANCER

4. **What is DTC?**

   DTC arises from thyroid follicular epithelial cells. PTC is the most common type of DTC and is associated with nuclear changes (e.g., pseudoinclusions, grooves) on pathology. Several PTC subtypes can be seen, the most common of which are the classic and follicular variants. Some PTC subtypes demonstrate more aggressive clinical behavior (e.g., tall cell and hobnail variants). The encapsulated follicular variant of PTC, when lacking invasion, necrosis, or high mitotic activity, has been renamed noninvasive follicular thyroid neoplasm with papillary-like nuclear features and is no longer considered a malignancy. FTC, the second-most common DTC, is distinguished from a benign follicular adenoma by the presence of capsular and/or vascular invasion. HCC comprises predominantly Hurthle cells and also features capsular and/or vascular invasion. PDTC is thought to devolve from well-differentiated thyroid cancer; it is associated with more aggressive behavior and a poorer prognosis.

5. **What are risk factors for DTC?**

   Thyroid cancer is more common in women than in men. Most DTC arises sporadically; however, approximately 5% to 10% may have a familial association, although the genetic drivers of this association are not well understood. Several genetic syndromes are also associated with DTC, including phosphatase and tensin homolog (PTEN) hamartoma tumor syndrome (also known as Cowden's disease), familial adenomatous polyposis, Carney's complex, and Werner's syndrome or progeria. A history of ionizing radiation exposure (> 10 rads), including childhood head and neck irradiation or environmental radiation exposure, increases the risk of thyroid cancer.

6. **What staging is used for DTC?**

   Ten-year disease-specific survival (DSS) is based on stage at diagnosis according to the *American Joint Committee on Cancer (AJCC) Staging,* 8th edition, system (Table 43.1). Of note, age is one of the factors used to determine stage in DTC. For patients < 55 years of age, the highest stage is II, which indicates the presence of distant metastases. For patients ≥ 55 years of age, the stages are I through IV. Estimated 10-year DSS is ≥ 98% for stage I; 85% to 95% for stage II; 60% to 70% for stage III; and < 50% for stage IV.

Table 43.1. Differentiated Thyroid Cancer Staging System.

Primary Tumor (T)	
TUMOR (T) CATEGORY	**DEFINITION**
TX	Cannot be assessed
T0	No evidence of primary tumor
T1a	Tumor $\leq$ 1 cm, limited to thyroid
T1b	Tumor > 1 cm but $\leq$ 2 cm, limited to thyroid
T2	Tumor > 2 cm but $\leq$ 4 cm, limited to thyroid
T3a	Tumor > 4 cm, limited to thyroid
T3b	Gross extrathyroidal extension to strap muscles
T4a	Gross extrathyroidal extension to subcutaneous soft tissue, larynx, trachea, esophagus, or recurrent laryngeal nerve
T4b	Gross extrathyroidal extension to prevertebral fascia, carotid artery, or mediastinal vessels
Regional Lymph Node (N)	
NODE (N) CATEGORY	**DEFINITION**
NX	Cannot be assessed
N0a	Cytology- or histology-confirmed benign lymph nodes
N0b	No clinical or radiologic evidence of lymph node metastasis
N1a	Central (level VI or VII) lymph node metastases
N1b	Lateral (level I–V) or retropharyngeal lymph node metastases
Distant Metastasis (M)	
METASTASIS (M) CATEGORY	**DEFINITION**
M0	No distant metastasis
M1	Distant metastasis present
Staging	
STAGE	**CRITERIA**
I	Age < 55: Any T, Any N, M0 Age $\geq$ 55: T1–2, N0, M0
II	Age < 55: Any T, Any N, M1 Age $\geq$ 55: T1–2, N1, M0 T3, Any N, M0
III	Age $\geq$ 55: T4a, Any N, M0
IVA	Age $\geq$ 55: T4b, Any N, M0
IVB	Age $\geq$ 55: Any T, Any N, M1

7. What is the preoperative evaluation of patients with DTC?

All patients should undergo preoperative neck ultrasonography to carefully evaluate cervical lymph nodes. The anatomic levels of the neck are shown in Fig. 43.1. The central neck includes levels VI and VII, and the lateral neck the remaining neck zones. Ultrasonographically suspicious lymph nodes should be subjected to biopsy prior to surgery to guide surgical planning. Computed tomography (CT) or magnetic resonance imaging (MRI) of the neck can be considered if invasive disease is suspected. It is also recommended that serum calcium be measured prior to thyroid surgery to rule out concomitant primary hyperparathyroidism, another common endocrine disorder

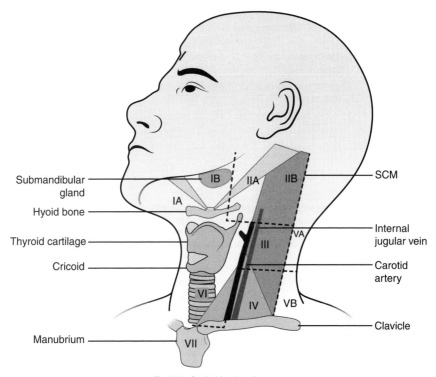

Fig. 43.1. Cervical lymph node zones.

that can be addressed at the time of thyroid surgery (see Chapter 18). Laboratory assessment of serum thyroglobulin (Tg) and antithyroglobulin antibodies (TgAbs) prior to surgery may allow identification of TgAb positivity, which causes negative interference with serum Tg measurement in immunometric assays. Although Tg is a sensitive tumor marker after thyroidectomy, absolute serum Tg levels prior to surgery do not correlate with prognosis because normal thyroid tissue also produces Tg (see question 13, below).

8. What type of surgery should patients with DTC undergo?

Surgery is the mainstay of DTC treatment. The exception is papillary thyroid microcarcinoma (tumors ≦ 1 cm) without evidence of extrathyroidal extension, lymph node involvement, or distant metastases, for which active surveillance may be an appropriate option. Most evidence supports that either hemithyroidectomy (lobectomy) or total thyroidectomy yield equivalent outcomes for tumors ≦ 4 cm without evidence of extrathyroidal extension, nodal involvement, or distant metastases. Thyroidectomy is preferred for tumors not meeting these criteria. Therapeutic central and/or lateral neck dissections should be performed for clinically or histologically confirmed lymph node involvement in the relevant compartment. Prophylactic central neck dissections are also performed when there is lateral nodal involvement or suspected extrathyroidal extension. See also the chapter on thyroid surgery (chapter 66).

9. What is the role of levothyroxine administration in the treatment of DTC?

Following thyroidectomy, thyroid hormone administration (oral levothyroxine) is required because of loss of endogenous thyroid hormone production. Under normal physiologic conditions, binding of TSH to TSH receptors on thyroid follicular cells mediates growth. Because DTC cells usually express the TSH receptor, supraphysiologic levothyroxine doses may be administered to suppress serum TSH, thereby preventing TSH-mediated stimulation of thyroid cancer cell growth and potentially reducing the risk of thyroid cancer recurrence. In general, low-risk patients with an excellent response to therapy have a goal TSH of 0.5 to 2.0 mU/L; high-risk patients or those with structural incomplete responses have a goal TSH of < 0.1 mU/L; and the remainder have a goal TSH of 0.1 to 0.5 mU/L. Less strict TSH goals may later be set for patients with a sustained excellent response to therapy. In all patients, the potential cancer benefit must be weighed against the risks of subclinical hyperthyroidism, especially bone loss and risk of arrhythmia in older patients.

Table 43.2. Radioactive Iodine (RAI) Approaches.

RAI STRATEGY	TARGET	PURPOSE	DOSE
Remnant ablation	Remaining normal thyroid tissue	Facilitate posttreatment follow-up	30 mCi
Adjuvant therapy	Suspected but undocumented residual disease	Reduce risk of recurrence	Up to 150 mCi
Therapy	Persistent/metastatic disease	Improve survival	100–200 mCi (consider reduced dose in elderly or dosimetry)

10. When should radioactive iodine be offered to patients with DTC?

As DTC usually expresses the sodium–iodide symporter, radioactive iodine (RAI; ^{131}I) administered postoperatively may be taken up by and destroy thyroid cancer cells as well as any residual normal thyroid tissue. General RAI treatment approaches are outlined in Table 43.2. However, these indications must be balanced against the potential risks of RAI, including sialadenitis, dental caries, nasolacrimal duct obstruction, and increased relative risk of secondary malignancies (e.g., leukemia). In general, RAI is not indicated for low-risk thyroid cancer, can be considered in intermediate-risk patients, and should be given to high-risk patients. When RAI is administered, a posttherapy whole-body scan should be completed to document sites of RAI-avid disease.

11. How is RAI given?

To increase the uptake of RAI into cells, patients are placed on a low-iodine diet for 1 to 2 weeks prior to treatment, and the TSH level is deliberately elevated. The latter has traditionally been accomplished by stopping thyroid hormone therapy 3 to 4 weeks before RAI administration. In patients without distant metastases, recombinant human thyrotropin (rhTSH) can be administered instead of withdrawing thyroid hormone. The use of rhTSH in preparation for RAI therapy has not been rigorously evaluated in the setting of distant metastases. Patients should be counseled about isolation precautions after RAI administration to minimize potential radiation exposure to other people and animals. Women of reproductive age should have a serum pregnancy test prior to RAI administration and be advised to avoid pregnancy for 6 to 12 months after RAI treatment because of the associated risk of ablation of the fetal thyroid and the recommendation to have stable thyroid function prior to pregnancy.

12. In addition to clinical staging, how is prognosis assessed in patients with DTC?

The American Thyroid Association (ATA) guidelines for the management of DTC recommend classifying patients as having low, intermediate, or high risk of thyroid cancer recurrence based on the clinical, pathologic, and radiologic findings at the time of initial diagnosis and treatment. High-risk features include distant metastases, gross extrathyroidal extension or residual tumor, FTC with extensive vascular invasion ($>$ four foci), extranodal extension, or lymph node metastases $>$ 3 cm in size. Risk of recurrence is intermediate in the setting of aggressive PTC subtypes, PTC with vascular invasion, clinically apparent adenopathy, $>$ five involved lymph nodes, or persistent RAI-avid metastatic foci in the neck after initial RAI administration. Risk of recurrence is low for patients lacking these features. Prognosis is reevaluated at every visit by designating a patient's response to therapy as excellent, biochemically incomplete, structurally incomplete, or indeterminate based on the results of serum Tg testing and imaging (Table 43.3).

Table 43.3. Response to Therapy.

CATEGORY	FEATURES
Excellent	Negative imaging, and Suppressed Tg $<$ 0.2 ng/mL or stimulated Tg $\leqq$ 1 ng/mL
Indeterminate	Suppressed or stimulated Tg not meeting definition for another category, or Stable or declining TgAb levels, or Nonspecific findings on imaging
Biochemical incomplete	Negative imaging, and Suppressed Tg $\geqq$ 0.2 ng/mL, stimulated Tg $>$ 1 ng/mL, or rising TgAb
Structural incomplete	Imaging suggestive of or biopsy-proven residual or recurrent disease

Tg, Thyroglobulin; *TgAb*, antithyroglobulin antibody.

13. How should patients with DTC be followed up to detect recurrence?

Patients with DTC should be followed up with physical examination, Tg and TgAb measurements, and neck ultra-sonography. The frequency of follow-up is dictated by the patient's risk of recurrence and response to therapy. Tg is a protein precursor to thyroid hormone made by intact thyroid tissue but is also made by most DTCs. Serum Tg can be used as a DTC tumor marker in patients who have undergone thyroidectomy. TgAbs are present in up to 30% of patients with DTC, however, and interfere with standard immunometric Tg measurements, causing falsely low serum Tg levels. In patients with any level of detectable TgAb, nonimmunometric methods of Tg measure-ment, such as radioimmunoassay or liquid chromatography-tandem mass spectrometry, should be considered. As the most common site of PTC recurrence is in the cervical lymph nodes, combining Tg/TgAb measurement with neck ultrasonography detects recurrences in most patients. In patients with rising Tg but no evidence of disease on neck ultrasonography, additional imaging (of the chest, abdomen, bone, and brain) may be required to identify sites of disease.

14. Define radioiodine-refractory thyroid cancer.

RAI-refractory thyroid cancer is considered to be present if it meets any of the following conditions: malignant tis-sue that never concentrates RAI, malignant tissue that loses the ability to concentrate RAI, only some of the tissue concentrates RAI, and malignant tissue grows despite concentrating RAI.

15. What treatment modalities are used for recurrent and/or metastatic DTC?

In general, treatment modalities for recurrent and/or metastatic DTC fall into four categories: close observation, directed therapies, systemic therapies, and, where applicable, clinical trials. In a patient with low-volume, slowly progressive disease, close observation with TSH suppression and regular clinical, laboratory, and radiologic sur-veillance may be reasonable. Directed therapies, such as surgery, external beam radiotherapy (EBRT), and ethanol, radiofrequency, or laser ablation of lymph node metastases, may be considered for localized disease. RAI can be used even in the metastatic setting for disease that retains the ability to concentrate and respond to iodine, but not in patients with RAI-refractory disease. Patients with high-volume, progressive, RAI-refractory disease may be treated with multikinase inhibitors such as lenvatinib and sorafenib, which have response rates of up to 65%. However, adverse events are common with these agents, so the risks of untreated progressive disease must be weighed against the risks of therapy. Denosumab or bisphosphonates should be added in patients with bone metastases to reduce the frequency of adverse skeletal events.

KEY POINTS: DIFFERENTIATED THYROID CANCER

- Differentiated thyroid cancer (DTC) is the most common type of thyroid cancer and includes papillary, follicular, Hurthle cell, and poorly differentiated thyroid cancers.
- Prognosis of DTC is determined by initial staging, risk stratification, and ongoing assessment of response to therapy.
- The main modalities of treatment of DTC are surgery and thyroid-stimulating hormone suppression, with or without radioactive iodine therapy.

ANAPLASTIC THYROID CANCER

16. What is anaplastic thyroid cancer?

Anaplastic thyroid cancer (ATC) comprises approximately 1% to 2% of all thyroid cancers but carries the worst prognosis, with a median survival of 3 to 6 months. In contrast to DTC, patients are usually older at diagnosis and frequently present with a rapidly enlarging neck mass and compressive symptoms. Although derived from thyroid follicular cells, ATC cells are dedifferentiated and no longer express the TSH receptor or sodium–iodide symporter; TSH suppression and RAI therapy are, therefore, not components of ATC management. On pathology, high degrees of necrosis and mitotic activity are frequently seen, and traditional markers of thyroid tissue are typically absent on immunostaining. ATC is frequently found in conjunction with or in patients with a history of DTC and is gener-ally thought to devolve from DTC as more mutations, such as p53, are acquired.

17. How is ATC staged?

Definitions of primary tumor, regional lymph node involvement, and distant metastases are the same as in DTC (see Table 43.1). However, all ATC is considered stage IV disease, as depicted in Table 43.4. Unlike DTC, age is not a component of the staging system. Expedited imaging with neck ultrasonography, cross-sectional imaging of the neck and chest, and possibly [18]fluorodeoxyglucose–positron emission tomography should be performed as part of the initial staging workup.

18. How is ATC treated?

ATC should be managed under the care of a multidisciplinary team. If disease is considered resectable (e.g., stage IVA and some IVB), surgery (total thyroidectomy with therapeutic central and lateral neck dissection) should be

Table 43.4. Anaplastic Thyroid Cancer Staging System.

STAGE	CRITERIA
IVA	T1–T3a, N0, M0
IVB	T1–T3a, N1, M0
	T3b–T4, any N, M0
IVC	Any T, any N, M1

M, Metastasis; *N*, node; *T*, tumor.

undertaken on an urgent basis. In general, surgery is followed by adjuvant EBRT, with or without systemic chemotherapy. Patients with unresectable locoregional disease (unresectable stage IVB) may receive neoadjuvant EBRT and cytotoxic chemotherapy. If the disease becomes resectable after neoadjuvant therapy, surgery may be reconsidered. Treatment of metastatic ATC (stage IVC) is generally palliative but may include EBRT (especially for symptomatic lesions) and/or chemotherapy. Several different cytotoxic chemotherapy regimens have been described, usually involving doxorubicin, platinum-based agents, and/or taxanes, but all have limited efficacy. However, the combination of dabrafenib and trametinib had an unprecedented 69% response rate in an open-label phase 2 trial in *BRAF*^{V600E}-mutated ATC, leading to the recent approval by the U.S. Food and Drug Administration (FDA) for this indication.

KEY POINTS: ANAPLASTIC THYROID CANCER

- Anaplastic thyroid cancer is a rare, aggressive, undifferentiated form of thyroid cancer, with an extremely poor prognosis.
- Treatment includes surgery in those with resectable disease, palliative or curative-intent external beam radiotherapy, and cytotoxic chemotherapy or targeted therapies, depending on mutational status.

MEDULLARY THYROID CANCER

19. What is medullary thyroid cancer (MTC)?
    Unlike DTC and ATC, MTC arises from parafollicular C-cells within the thyroid gland. As these C-cells develop embryologically from neural crest cells, MTC is considered a neuroendocrine tumor. C-cells produce calcitonin, which can thus be used to identify MTC histologically with immunostains and biochemically as a serum tumor marker to follow disease. Because MTC is not derived from thyroid follicular cells, it does not respond to TSH suppression or RAI therapy. MTC, especially when there is a high tumor burden, can sometimes be associated with watery diarrhea.

20. What genetic syndromes are associated with MTC?
    Although the majority of MTCs are sporadic, about 25% of cases are hereditary. MTC can occur as a component of multiple endocrine neoplasia type 2A (MEN 2A) or type 2B (MEN 2B) (see Chapter 60). MEN 2A, by far more common, comprises several clinical subtypes and may be associated with pheochromocytoma and/or primary hyperparathyroidism. MEN 2B is frequently associated with pheochromocytoma (but not hyperparathyroidism) and a characteristic physical appearance (marfanoid habitus and mucosal neuromas). Both MEN 2A and MEN 2B, as well as about 50% of sporadic MTC, are associated with mutations in the *RET* oncogene and different mutations are associated with specific phenotypes. The *RET* codon M918T mutation is the most common mutation in MEN 2B; the aggressive disease in patients with this mutation tends to present in infancy. Genetic screening of first-degree relatives is recommended for all patients with MCT. Children known to carry high-risk *RET* mutations should undergo prophylactic thyroidectomy.

21. How is MTC staging determined?
    The AJCC staging system for MTC uses the same definitions for primary tumor, regional lymph nodes, and distant metastases as for DTC (see Table 43.1). MTC staging is outlined in Table 43.5. Regional lymph node and distant metastases are common in MTC, present in up to 80% and 10% of patients, respectively.

22. What preoperative evaluation is indicated?
    After confirmation of the diagnosis of MTC (usually based on fine-needle aspiration biopsy of a thyroid nodule), patients should undergo neck ultrasonography for evaluation of suspicious lymph nodes. Preoperative serum calcitonin and carcinoembryonic antigen (CEA) levels should also be measured. If serum calcitonin is > 500 pg/mL or if there is suspicion for invasive local disease, cross-sectional imaging of the neck and chest, dedicated three-phase CT or MRI of the liver, and/or skeletal imaging can be performed. Additionally, patients with suspected hereditary MTC should be evaluated for pheochromocytoma and hyperparathyroidism prior to surgery. Rarely, MTC

Table 43.5. Medullary Thyroid Cancer Staging System.

STAGE	CRITERIA
I	T1, N0, M0
II	T2-3, N0, M0
III	T1-3, N1a, M0
IVA	T1-3, N1b, M0 T4a, any N, M0
IVB	T4b, any N, M0
IVC	Any T, any N, M1

M, Metastasis; *N,* node; *T,* tumor.

can secrete adrenocorticotropic hormone (ACTH) or corticotropin-releasing hormone, causing ectopic Cushing's syndrome (see Chapter 27).

23. What is the recommended extent of surgery for MTC?

Total thyroidectomy with central neck dissection is the primary treatment for MTC. Lateral neck dissection should be performed if there is ultrasonographic evidence of lymph node metastases. As preoperative serum calcitonin and CEA levels are associated with disease extent, some advocate for ipsilateral lateral neck dissection when calcitonin is > 20 pg/mL and contralateral lateral neck dissection when calcitonin is > 200 pg/mL. If distant metastases are present, the initial surgery should be less aggressive (e.g., total thyroidectomy alone) to minimize morbidity. Adjuvant EBRT may be considered in patients at high risk of locoregional recurrence. Postoperatively, patients should be started on replacement doses (~1.6 mcg/kg) of levothyroxine. Also, see the chapter on thyroid surgery (chapter 66).

24. How should patients with MTC be followed up after surgery?

All patients should undergo a physical examination, neck ultrasonography, and serum calcitonin and CEA measurements 6 months after surgery. Low or undetectable calcitonin levels are associated with an excellent prognosis. Postoperative calcitonin levels up to 150 pg/mL are associated with cervical lymph node metastases; levels > 150 pg/mL may be associated with distant metastases and should prompt further imaging to identify sites of metastasis. Calcitonin and CEA doubling times should be calculated during follow-up. Doubling times of < 6 months are associated with a poor prognosis, whereas doubling times of > 2 years are associated with a good prognosis. Tools for calculating the calcitonin and CEA doubling times can be accessed on the ATA website (www.thyroid.org).

25. How is metastatic MTC treated?

Therapy for metastatic MTC may be directed or systemic. Examples of directed therapy include EBRT for bone or brain metastases, and surgery or chemoembolization for limited liver metastases. Bisphosphonates or denosumab should be added for treating bone metastases. As in DTC, systemic treatment of MTC involves multikinase inhibitors. There are two FDA-approved drugs in this setting: vandetanib and cabozantinib. Adverse events are common, however. Additionally, metastatic MTC is frequently associated with diarrhea, which is usually managed with antimotility drugs, such as loperamide.

KEY POINTS: MEDULLARY THYROID CANCER

- Medullary thyroid cancer (MTC) is a neuroendocrine tumor arising from parafollicular C-cells within the thyroid gland.
- MTC may be associated with multiple endocrine neoplasia types 2A and 2B.
- Surgery is the mainstay of treatment; systemic therapies for those with metastatic disease include the multikinase inhibitors vandetanib and cabozantinib.

 WEBSITES

American Thyroid Association: www.thyroid.org

BIBLIOGRAPHY

Brito, J. P., Ito, Y., Miyauchi, A., & Tuttle, R. M. (2016). A clinical framework to facilitate risk stratification when considering an active surveillance alternative to immediate biopsy and surgery in papillary microcarcinoma. *Thyroid, 26*(1),144–149.

Brose, M. S., Nutting, C. M., Jarzab, B., Elisei, R., Siena, S., Bastholt, L., . . . Schlumberger, M. J.; (2014). Sorafenib in radioactive iodine-refractory, locally advanced or metastatic differentiated thyroid cancer: a randomised, double-blind, phase 3 trial. *Lancet, 384*(9940), 319–328.

Cibas, E. S., & Ali, S. Z. (2017). The 2017 Bethesda System for Reporting Thyroid Cytopathology. *Thyroid, 27*(11), 1341–1346.

Elisei, R., Schlumberger, M. J., Muller, S. P., Schöffski, P., Brose, M. S., Shah, M. H., . . . Sherman, S. I. (2013). Cabozantinib in progressive medullary thyroid cancer. *Journal of Clinical Oncology, 31*(29), 3639–3646.

Gartland, R. M., & Lubitz, C. C. (2018). Impact of extent of surgery on tumor recurrence and survival for papillary thyroid cancer patients. *Annals of Surgical Oncology, 25*(9), 2520–2525.

Haugen, B. R., Alexander, E. K., Bible, K. C., Doherty, G. M., Mandel, S. J., Nikiforov, Y. E., . . . Wartofsky, L. (2016). 2015 American Thyroid Association Management Guidelines for Adult Patients with Thyroid Nodules and Differentiated Thyroid Cancer: The American Thyroid Association Guidelines Task Force on Thyroid Nodules and Differentiated Thyroid Cancer. *Thyroid, 26*(1), 1–133.

La Vecchia, C., Malvezzi, M., Bosetti, C., Garavello, W., Bertuccio, P., Levi, F., & Negri. E. (2015). Thyroid cancer mortality and incidence: a global overview. *International Journal of Cancer, 136*(9), 2187–2195.

Lamartina, L., Durante, C., Filetti, S., & Cooper, D. S. (2015). Low-risk differentiated thyroid cancer and radioiodine remnant ablation: a systematic review of the literature. *Journal of Clinical Endocrinology and Metabolism, 100*(5), 1748–1761.

Lim, H., Devesa, S. S., Sosa, J. A., Check, D., & Kitahara, C. M. (2017). Trends in thyroid cancer incidence and mortality in the United States, 1974–2013. *Journal of the American Medical Association, 317*(13), 1338–1348.

National Cancer Institute. (2015). SEER Cancer stat facts: thyroid cancer. Retrieved from https://seer.cancer.gov/statfacts/html/thyro. html.

Nikiforov, Y. E., Seethala, R. R., Tallini, G., Baloch, Z. W., Basolo, F., Thompson, L. D., . . . Gossein, R. A. (2016). Nomenclature revision for encapsulated follicular variant of papillary thyroid carcinoma: a paradigm shift to reduce overtreatment of indolent tumors. *Journal of the American Medical Association Oncology, 2*(8), 1023–1029.

Pozdeyev, N., Gay, L. M., Sokol, E. S., Hartmaier, R., Deaver, K. E., Davis, S., . . . Bowles, D. W. (2018). Genetic analysis of 779 advanced differentiated and anaplastic thyroid cancers. *Clinics in Cancer Research, 24*(13), 3059–3068.

Rosen, J. E., Lloyd, R. V., Brierley, J. D., Grogan, R. H., Haddad, R., Hunt, J. L., . . . Perrier, N. D. (2017). Thyroid—medullary. In American Joint Committee on Cancer (Ed.), *AJCC Cancer Staging Manual* (8th ed., pp. 891–901). Chicago, IL: Springer.

Schlumberger, M., Tahara, M., Wirth, L. J., Robinson, B., Brose, M. S., Elisei, R., . . . Sherman, S. I. (2015). Lenvatinib versus placebo in radioiodine-refractory thyroid cancer. *New England Journal of Medicine, 372*(7), 621–630.

Smallridge, R. C., Ain, K. B., Asa, S. L., Bible, K. C., Brierley, J. D., Burman, K. D., ,. . . Tuttle, R. M.; (2012). American Thyroid Association guidelines for management of patients with anaplastic thyroid cancer. *Thyroid, 22*(11), 1104–1139.

Subbiah, V., Kreitman, R. J., Wainberg, Z. A., Cho, J. Y., Schellens, J. H. M., Soria, J.C., . . . Keam, B. (2018). Dabrafenib and trametinib treatment in patients with locally advanced or metastatic BRAF V600-mutant anaplastic thyroid cancer. *Journal of Clinical Oncology, 36*(1), 7–13.

Tuttle, R. M., Haugen, B. R., & Perrier, N. D. (2017). Updated American Joint Committee on cancer/tumor-node-metastasis staging system for differentiated and anaplastic thyroid cancer (eighth edition): what changed and why? *Thyroid, 27*(6), 751–756.

Tuttle, M. R., Morris, L. F., Haugen, B. R., Shah, J. P., Sosa, J. A., Rohren, E., . . . Perrier, N. D. (2017). Thyroid—differentiated and anaplastic carcinoma. In American Joint Committee on Cancer (Ed.), *AJCC Cancer Staging Manual* (8th ed., pp. 873–890). Chicago, IL: Springer.

Wells, S. A., Jr., Asa, S. L., Dralle, H., Elisei, R., Evans, D. B., Gagel, R. F., . . . Waguespack, S. G. (2015). Revised American Thyroid Association guidelines for the management of medullary thyroid carcinoma. *Thyroid, 25*(6), 567–610.

Wells, S. A., Jr., Robinson, B. G., Gagel, R. F. (2012). Vandetanib in patients with locally advanced or metastatic medullary thyroid cancer: a randomized, double-blind phase III trial. *Journal of Clinical Oncology, 30*(2), 134–141.

CHAPTER 44

THYROID EMERGENCIES

Michael T. McDermott

1. **What is thyroid storm, or thyroid crisis?**
   Thyroid storm, or thyroid crisis, is a life-threatening condition characterized by an exaggeration of the manifestations of thyrotoxicosis. Some prefer the term *decompensated thyrotoxicosis* instead of *thyroid storm*. At the time thyroid storm was first described, the acute mortality rate was nearly 100%. Today, the prognosis is significantly improved if appropriate therapy is initiated early, with recent mortality rates of < 10% being reported.

2. **How does thyroid storm develop?**
   Thyroid storm usually occurs in patients who have unrecognized or inadequately treated thyrotoxicosis and a superimposed precipitating event, such as thyroid surgery, nonthyroidal surgery, infection, or trauma.

3. **What are the clinical manifestations of thyroid storm?**
   Fever (> 102°F [38.9°C]) is the cardinal manifestation. Tachycardia is usually present, and tachypnea is common, but blood pressure is variable. Cardiac arrhythmias, congestive heart failure, and ischemic heart symptoms may develop. Nausea, vomiting, diarrhea, and abdominal pain are frequent features (Fig. 44.1). Central nervous system manifestations include hyperkinesis, psychosis, and coma. A goiter is a helpful finding but is not always present.

4. **What laboratory abnormalities are seen in thyroid storm?**
   Serum thyroxine (total T_4 and free T_4) and triiodothyronine (total T_3 and free T_3) are usually significantly elevated, and serum thyroid-stimulating hormone (TSH) is undetectable. These hormone levels, however, cannot reliably distinguish patients with thyroid storm from those who have uncomplicated thyrotoxicosis. Other common findings include anemia, leukocytosis, hyperglycemia, azotemia, hypercalcemia, and elevated liver enzymes.

5. **How is the diagnosis of thyroid storm made?**
   The diagnosis of thyroid storm must be made on the basis of suspicious but nonspecific clinical findings, supported by laboratory testing if done expeditiously. Table 44.1 provides a useful published and validated scoring system to aid in diagnosis (see article by Burch & Wartofsky et al., 1993). A different scoring system has been proposed by a separate group (see article by Akamizu et al., 2012). Although scoring systems are often helpful, they are no substitute for a careful evaluation and the use of sound clinical judgement by an experienced clinician.

6. **What other conditions may mimic thyroid storm?**
   Similar presentations may be seen with sepsis, pheochromocytoma, and malignant hyperthermia.

7. **What is the treatment for thyroid storm?**
   The immediate goals are to decrease thyroid hormone synthesis, to inhibit thyroid hormone release, to reduce the heart rate, to support the circulation, and to treat the precipitating condition. Because beta$_1$-adrenergic receptors are significantly increased in patients with this condition, beta$_1$-selective blockers are the preferred agents for heart rate control. Table 44.2 lists the medications and doses commonly used to treat thyroid storm.

8. **When traditional therapy fails, what additional options should be considered?**
   Plasma exchange or plasmapheresis can be lifesaving measures in thyroid storm patients who have not adequately responded to the above standard measures.

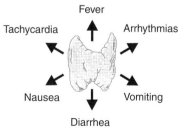

Fig. 44.1. Features of thyroid storm.

Table 44.1. Thyroid Storm Scoring System.

Temperature	
FEVER (°F)	**SCORE**
99–99.9°	5
100–100.9°	10
101–101.9°	15
102–102.9°	20
103–103.9°	25
≧ 104°	30
Central Nervous System	
AGITATION	**SCORE**
Absent	0
Mild	10
Moderate	20
Severe	30
Cardiovascular System	
HEART RATE	**SCORE**
99–109	5
110–119	10
120–129	15
130–139	20
> 140	25
Atrial fibrillation	10
CONGESTIVE HEART FAILURE	**SCORE**
Absent	0
Mild (edema)	5
Moderate (rales)	10
Severe (pulmonary edema)	15
GASTROINTESTINAL	
SYMPTOMS	**SCORE**
Absent	0
Nausea/Vomiting/Diarrhea/Pain	10
Jaundice	20
PRECIPITANT HISTORY	**SCORE**
Present	10
Thyroid Storm Score Interpretation	
TOTAL SCORE	**THYROID STORM**
< 25	Unlikely
25–44	Suggestive
> 45	Likely

Burch, H. B., & Wartofsky, L. (1993). Life-threatening thyrotoxicosis: Thyroid storm. *Endocrinology and Metabolism Clinics of North America, 22,* 263–278.

Table 44.2. Treatment of Thyroid Storm.

Reduce Thyroid Hormone Synthesis
Propylthiouracil (PO, NG, rectal): 600–1200 mg daily, or
Methimazole (PO, NG, rectal, IV): 60–120 mg daily

Reduce Thyroid Hormone Release
Sodium iodide (IV): 1 g over 24 hours, or
Potassium iodide (SSKI, Lugol's – PO): 5 drops qid

Reduce Heart Rate
Esmolol (IV): 500 mcg over 1 minute, then 50–300 mcg/kg/min, or
Metoprolol (IV): 5–10 mg q2–4 hr, or
Propranolol (PO): 60–80 mg q4 hr, or
Diltiazem (IV): 0.25 mg/kg over 2 minutes, then 10 mg/min, or
(PO): 60–90 mg q6–8 hr

Glucocorticoid Therapy (Stress Doses for 2–3 Days)
Hydrocortisone 200 mg daily, or
Methylprednisolone 40 mg daily, or
Prednisone 50 mg daily, or
Dexamethasone 7.5 mg daily

Support Circulation, Oxygenation and Ventilation
IV fluids
Oxygen

Treat Precipitating Cause (critically important)

IV, Intravenous; *NG,* nasogastric; *PO,* oral; *qid,* four times daily; *SSKI,* potassium iodide oral solution, USP.

9. Define myxedema coma.

Myxedema coma is a life-threatening condition characterized by an exaggeration of the manifestations of hypo-thyroidism. Some prefer the term *decompensated hypothyroidism.* Myxedema coma originally had a mortality rate of 100%. Today, the outlook is much improved for appropriately treated patients; mortality rates in recent studies have ranged from 0% to 45%.

10. How does myxedema coma develop?

Myxedema coma usually occurs in elderly patients who have inadequately treated or untreated hypothyroidism and a superimposed precipitating event. Important events include prolonged cold exposure, infection, trauma, surgery, myocardial infarction, congestive heart failure, pulmonary embolism, stroke, respiratory failure, gastrointestinal bleeding, and administration of various drugs, particularly those that have a depressive effect on the central nervous system.

11. What are the clinical manifestations of myxedema coma?

Hypothermia, bradycardia, and hypoventilation are common. Blood pressure, although generally low, is more variable. Pericardial, pleural, and peritoneal effusions are often found. An ileus is frequently present, and acute uri-nary retention may be seen. Central nervous system manifestations include seizures, stupor, and coma (Fig. 44.2).

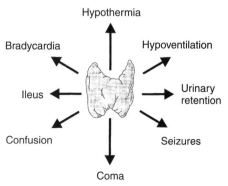

Fig. 44.2. Features of myxedema coma.

Deep tendon reflexes are absent or exhibit a delayed relaxation phase. Typical hypothyroid skin and hair changes are often apparent. A goiter, although frequently absent, is a helpful finding. A thyroidectomy scar may also be an important clue.

12. What laboratory abnormalities are seen in myxedema coma?

Serum T_4 (total and free T_4) and T_3 (total and free T_3) are usually low, and the TSH is significantly elevated. Other frequent abnormalities include anemia, hyponatremia, hypoglycemia, and elevated serum levels of cholesterol and creatine kinase (CK). Arterial blood gases often reveal carbon dioxide retention and hypoxemia. Electrocardiography often shows sinus bradycardia, various types and degrees of heart block, low voltage, and T-wave flattening.

13. How is the diagnosis of myxedema coma made?

The diagnosis of myxedema coma, like thyroid storm, must be made on the basis of suspicious but nonspecific clinical findings, supported by laboratory testing if done expeditiously. Table 44.3 provides a useful published and validated scoring system to aid in diagnosis (see article by Popoveniuc et al., 2014). A different scoring system has been proposed by a separate group (see article by Chiong et al., 2015). Although scoring systems can be useful, a careful evaluation and the use of sound clinical judgement by an experienced clinician are of paramount importance.

Table 44.3. Myxedema Coma Scoring System.

Temperature	
HYPOTHERMIA (°C)	**SCORE**
> 35°	0
32–35°	10
< 32°	20
Cardiovascular–Pulmonary Effects	
FEATURE	**SCORE**
Heart rate > 60	0
Heart rate 50–59	10
Heart rate 40–49	20
Heart rate < 40	30
Hypotension	20
Cardiomegaly	15
Pulmonary edema	15
Pericardial/Pleural effusion	10
Hypoxemia	10
Hypercarbia	10
Other ECG changes[a]	10
Central Nervous System Effects	
FEATURE	**SCORE**
Absent	0
Somnolent/Lethargic	10
Obtunded	15
Stupor	20
Coma/Seizures	30
Gastrointestinal Effects	
FEATURE	**SCORE**
Anorexia/Pain/Constipation	5
Decreased motility	15
Paralytic ileus	20

Table 44.3. Myxedema Coma Scoring System. *(Continued)*

Metabolic/Renal Disorders

FEATURE	SCORE
Hypoglycemia	10
Hyponatremia	10
Decreased GFR	10

Precipitating Event

FEATURE	SCORE
Present	10

Myxedema Coma Score Interpretation

TOTAL SCORE	MYXEDEMA COMA
< 24	Unlikely
25–59	Suggestive
> 60	Likely

[a]Other electrocardiography (ECG) changes: QT prolongation, low voltage, BBB, non-specific ST-T wave changes.

GFR, Glomerular filtration rate.

Adapted from Popoveniuc, G., Chandra, T., Sud, A., Sharma, M., Blackman, M. R, Burman, K. D., Mete, M., ... & Wartofsky, L. (2014). A diagnostic scoring system for myxedema coma. *Endocrine Practice, 20,* 808–817.

Table 44.4. Treatment of Myxedema Coma.

Thyroid Hormone Replacement (Rapid)
Levothyroxine 200–300 mcg IV over 5 minutes, or
Triiodothyronine 5–10 mcg IV every 6–12 hours, then
Levothyroxine 50–100 mcg daily PO or IV
Glucocorticoid Therapy (Stress Doses for 2–3 Days)
Hydrocortisone 200 mg daily, or
Methylprednisolone 40 mg daily, or
Prednisone 50 mg daily, or
Dexamethasone 7.5 mg daily
Support Circulation, Oxygenation and Ventilation
IV fluids
Oxygen
Mechanical ventilation (if needed)
Passive rewarming (if severely hypothermic)
Treat Precipitating Cause (critically important)

IV, Intravenous; *PO,* oral.

14. What is the treatment for myxedema coma?
   The goals are to rapidly replace the depleted thyroid hormone pool, to replace glucocorticoids, to support vital functions, and to treat any precipitating conditions. The normal total body pool of T_4 is about 1000 mcg (500 mcg in the thyroid, 500 mcg in the rest of the body). Table 44.4 lists the medications and doses commonly used to treat myxedema coma.

KEY POINTS: THYROID EMERGENCIES

- Thyroid storm is a life-threatening form of severe thyrotoxicosis that usually has a precipitating factor and a high mortality rate if not treated promptly and appropriately.
- When thyroid storm is diagnosed or suspected, treatment with antithyroid drugs, cold iodine, beta-blockers, and stress doses of glucocorticoids, along with management of any precipitating factors, should be promptly initiated.

KEY POINTS: THYROID EMERGENCIES—cont'd

- Myxedema coma is a life-threatening form of severe hypothyroidism that often has a precipitating cause and a high mortality rate if not promptly and adequately treated.
- When myxedema coma is diagnosed or suspected, management should include rapid repletion of thyroid hormones, stress glucocorticoid doses, and treatment of any precipitating causes.

BIBLIOGRAPHY

Angell, T. E., Lechner, M. G., Nguyen, C. T., Salvato, V. L., Nicoloff, J. T., & LoPresti, J. S. (2015). Clinical features and hospital outcomes in thyroid storm: a retrospective cohort study. *Journal of Clinical Endocrinology and Metabolism, 100,* 451–459.

Akamizu, T., Satoh, T., Isozaki, O., Suzuki, A., Wakino, S., Iburi, T., Tsuboi K,... Mori, M. (2012). Diagnostic criteria, clinical features, and incidence of thyroid storm based on nationwide surveys. *Thyroid, 22,* 661–679.

Beynon, J., Akhtar, S., & Kearney, T. (2008). Predictors of outcome in myxedema coma. *Critical Care, 12,* 111.

Burch, H. B., & Wartofsky, L. (1993). Life-threatening thyrotoxicosis: thyroid storm. *Endocrinology and Metabolism Clinics of North America, 22,* 263–278.

Chaker, L., Bianco, A. C., Jonklass, J., & Peeters, R. P. (2017). Hypothyroidism. *Lancet, 390,* 1550–1562.

Chiong, Y. V., Brammerlin, E., & Mariash, C. N. (2015). Development of an objective tool for the diagnosis of myxedema coma. *Translational Research, 166,* 233–243.

Cooper, D. S. (2005). Antithyroid drugs. *New England Journal of Medicine, 352,* 905–917.

Fliers, E., & Wiersinga, W. M. (2003). Myxedema coma. *Reviews in Endocrine and Metabolic Disorders, 4,* 137–141.

Hodak, S. P., Huang, C., Clarke, D., Burman, K. D., Jonklaas, J., & Janicic-Kharic, N. (2006). Intravenous methimazole in the treatment of refractory hyperthyroidism. *Thyroid, 16,* 691–695.

Klubo-Gwiezdzinska, J., & Wartofsky, L. (2012). Thyroid emergencies. *Medical Clinics of North America, 96,* 385–403.

Koball, S., Hickstein, H., Gloger, M., Hinz, M., Henschel, J., Stange, J., & Mitzner, S. (2010). Treatment of thyrotoxic crisis with plasmapheresis and single pass albumin dialysis: a case report. *Artificial Organs, 34,* E55–E58.

Kokuho, T., Kuji, T., Yasuda, G., & Umemura, S. (2004). Thyroid storm-induced multiple organ failure relieved quickly by plasma exchange therapy. *Therapeutic Apheresis and Dialysis, 8,* 347–349.

Martin, G. (Ed.). (2018). *Endocrine and metabolic medical emergencies. A clinician's guide* (2nd ed.). New York: Wiley Blackwell.

Nguyen, C., Angell, T., Wu, K., & LoPresti, J. An evaluation of the clinical and laboratory changes after treatment with 500 mcg IV L-thyroxine in 45 patients with myxedema coma. Presented: 84th Annual Meeting of The American Thyroid Association, Coronado, CA, Oct 29–Nov 4, 2014 (Poster 134).

Popoveniuc, G., Chandra, T., Sud, A., Sharma, M., Blackman, M. R, Burman, K. D., Mete M... Wartofsky, L. (2014). A diagnostic scoring system for myxedema coma. *Endocrine Practice, 20,* 808–817.

Sarlis, N. J., & Gourgiotis, L. (2003). Thyroid emergencies. *Reviews in Endocrine and Metabolic Disorders, 4,* 129–136.

CHAPTER 45

EUTHYROID SICK SYNDROME

Michael T. McDermott

1. What are euthyroid sick syndrome and nonthyroidal illness syndrome?

   Euthyroid sick syndrome (ESS), also commonly called *nonthyroidal illness syndrome (NTIS)*, refers to changes in serum thyroid-stimulating hormone (TSH), serum thyroid hormone, and tissue thyroid hormone levels that occur in patients with various nonthyroidal illnesses and starvation. It is not a primary thyroid disorder; instead, it results from changes in thyroid hormone secretion, transport, and metabolism induced by nonthyroidal illness.

2. When should thyroid tests be ordered in seriously ill patients?

   Thyroid tests should be ordered in patients with serious illnesses only when the presence of hyperthyroidism or hypothyroidism is considered likely. Serious nonthyroidal illnesses cause changes in thyroid hormone levels that can easily be confused with thyroid disorders, especially central hypothyroidism. Furthermore, during recovery from serious illnesses, thyroid hormone changes can be mistaken for primary hypothyroidism. Therefore, it is generally best to avoid thyroid testing during or in the first few weeks after recovery from a significant nonthyroidal illness. Considerable experience is often necessary to interpret thyroid tests in these settings.

3. When thyroid testing is necessary in seriously ill patients, which tests are recommended?

   When thyroid testing is deemed necessary, a serum TSH level alone is not adequate to distinguish euthyroid sick syndrome from true thyroid disorders. Serum TSH, total triiodothyronine (T_3) and free thyroxine (T_4) or total T_4 with T_3 resin uptake (T_3RU) should be ordered in this situation. Reverse T_3 (RT_3) measurement, although not indicated for evaluation of other thyroid conditions, can sometimes be helpful in distinguishing euthyroid sick syndrome from central hypothyroidism.

4. What thyroid hormone changes occur in patients with mild-to-moderate nonthyroidal illnesses?

   Even in mild-to-moderate nonthyroidal illnesses in the ambulatory setting, serum total T_3 can decrease to low-normal or frankly low levels because of reduced T_4 to T_3 conversion as a result of reduced hepatic deiodinase type 1 activity. The magnitude of the serum T_3 reduction correlates well with the severity of the nonthyroidal illness. Serum free T_4, total T_4, and TSH levels usually remain within the reference range in the mildest form of this condition (Fig. 45.1).

5. Describe the thyroid hormone changes that are seen in patients with moderate-to-severe nonthyroidal illnesses.

   In more severe nonthyroidal illnesses, serum total T_3 drops to very low levels, generally in proportion to the underlying illness severity. Serum total T_4 levels also become low and T_3RU rises, both as a result of reduced binding of thyroid hormones to their transport proteins because of impaired hepatic protein synthesis and the presence of circulating inhibitors of protein binding. Serum TSH levels also decrease below the reference range at this stage because of cytokine-mediated suppression of thyrotropin-releasing hormone (TRH) and TSH secretion. TSH secretion can also be inhibited by numerous medications, most notably glucocorticoids and dopamine. Reduced TSH secretion further decreases T_3 and T_4 levels. Free T_4 values are highly variable (normal, decreased, or increased), depending on the underlying illness, concomitant medications, and the assay technique. The most common pattern, therefore, is low TSH, low total T_4 or free T_4, and very low total T_3 (Fig. 45.1).

6. Describe the thyroid hormone changes associated with recovery from severe nonthyroidal illnesses.

   When patients begin to recover from severe nonthyroidal illnesses, serum TSH levels increase and may become transiently elevated above the reference range. Serum total T_3 and total T_4 levels begin to increase but may remain low for a while, and free T_4 often decreases because of recovery of hepatic production of thyroid hormone–binding proteins. A relatively common pattern during this transition is mildly elevated serum TSH, low total T_4 or free T_4, and low total T_3 (Fig. 45.1).

7. How can euthyroid sick syndrome be distinguished from central hypothyroidism?

   In severe nonthyroidal illnesses, total T_3 is reduced proportionately far more compared with total T_4 and free T_4 levels; in contrast, total T_4 and free T_4 levels are reduced more compared with total T_3, relative to their respective reference ranges, in any type of hypothyroidism. Furthermore, in euthyroid sick syndrome, T_3RU and RT_3 are usually increased, whereas both T_3RU and RT_3 tend to be low in hypothyroidism. Therefore, a diagnosis of euthyroid sick syndrome is supported by low TSH, very low total T_3, and elevated T_3RU and RT_3 levels, whereas central hypothyroidism is indicated by low TSH, low-normal or mildly low T_3, proportionately lower total T_4 and free T_4,

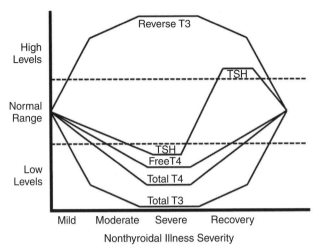

Fig. 45.1. Changes in thyroid hormone levels in patients with nonthyroidal illnesses of varying severity and during recovery. *TSH*, Thyroid-stimulating hormone.

and decreased T_3RU and RT_3 levels. Suspicion of central hypothyroidism should lead to computed tomography (CT) or magnetic resonance imaging (MRI) of the hypothalamic–pituitary region and further investigations to determine if central adrenal insufficiency may also be present.

8. How can recovery from euthyroid sick syndrome be distinguished from primary hypothyroidism?
   Thyroid hormone tests during recovery from nonthyroidal illnesses can show an elevated serum TSH level (transiently), along with low levels of free T_4, total T_4, and total T_3, making this condition difficult to distinguish from mild primary hypothyroidism. Serum T_3RU and RT_3 levels are not likely to be helpful in the differentiation at this point. Considering the transient nature of thyroid hormone changes during recovery from euthyroid sick syndrome and the lack of urgency for immediate treatment of mild primary hypothyroidism, it is best to simply repeat the thyroid testing 2 to 3 months after full recovery from the nonthyroidal illness.

9. What is the pathophysiology of euthyroid sick syndrome?
   Euthyroid sick syndrome is believed to be caused by increased circulating cytokines and other inflammation mediators resulting from the underlying nonthyroidal illness. These mediators inhibit the thyroid axis at multiple levels, including the hypothalamus (decreased TRH secretion), pituitary gland (decreased TSH secretion), thyroid gland (decreased T_4 and T_3 responses to TSH), transport proteins (decreased thyroid hormone binding), and peripheral tissues (decreased T_4 to T_3 conversion by tissue deiodinases).

10. What is the function of deiodinase enzymes?
    Deiodinases are selenocysteine enzymes that activate and deactivate thyroid hormones by removing iodine molecules. Deiodinase enzymes have three major subtypes: deiodinase 1 (D1), deiodinase 2 (D2), and deiodinase 3 (D3) (Table 45.1 and Fig. 45.2). D1 converts T_4 to T_3 in the liver and kidneys, producing the majority of circulating T_3, and converts RT_3 to diiodothyronine (T_2); D1 has a higher affinity for RT_3 than for T_4. D2 converts T_4 to T_3

Table 45.1. Deiodinase Enzymes: Selenocysteine Enzymes that Deiodinate Thyroid Hormones.

	DEIODINASE 1 (D1)	DEIODINASE 2 (D2)	DEIODINASE 3 (D3)
Substrate	$RT_3 \gg T_4$	$T_4 \gg RT_3$	$T_4 + T_3$
Tissue	Liver	Brain	Placenta
	Kidney	Pituitary	Brain
		Fat	
Function	Clear RT_3	↑ Cellular T_3	Protect fetus
	↑ Serum T_3	↑ Serum T_3	↓ Cellular T_3
			Clear $T_4 + T_3$

DEIODINASES

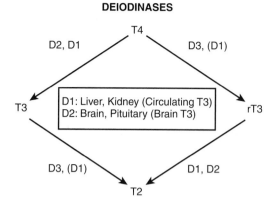

Fig. 45.2. Deiodinase function. *D1*, Deiodinase 1; *D2*, deiodinase 2; *D3*, deiodinase 3; *RT₃*, reverse triiodothyronine; *T₂*, diiodothyronine; *T₃*, triiodothyronine; *T₄*, thyroxine.

in the brain and pituitary gland, producing the majority of intracellular T_3 in these tissues; D2 has a higher affinity for T_4 than for RT_3. D3 converts T_4 to RT_3 and T_3 to T_2 (Fig. 45.2).

11. What changes in deiodinase function are seen in euthyroid sick syndrome?
    D1 activity is significantly reduced, and D3 activity is enhanced in euthyroid sick syndrome. These changes are responsible for the low serum T_3 and high serum RT_3 levels that are characteristic of this condition.

KEY POINTS: EUTHYROID SICK SYNDROME

- Euthyroid sick syndrome is not a thyroid disorder but is instead a group of changes in serum thyroid-stimulating hormone (TSH) and thyroid hormones that result from cytokines and inflammatory mediators produced during nonthyroidal illnesses.
- Mild euthyroid sick syndrome is characterized by low serum triiodothyronine (T_3) levels as a result of reduced conversion of thyroxine (T_4) to T_3 by deiodinase enzymes in the liver and other tissues.
- More severe nonthyroidal illnesses cause decreased serum TSH, very low T_3, low total T_4, variable changes in free T_4, increased T_3 resin uptake (T_3RU) and increased reverse T_3 (RT_3) as a result of suppressed pituitary TSH secretion, reduced thyroid hormone binding to transport proteins, and changes in tissue deiodinase activity.
- Transient elevation of serum TSH is often seen as patients recover from a nonthyroidal illness.
- Euthyroid sick syndrome appears to be an adaptive response to reduce tissue metabolism and preserve energy during systemic illnesses; therefore, treatment with thyroid hormone is not generally recommended but may be beneficial in patients with chronic heart failure.

12. Is euthyroid sick syndrome an adaptive mechanism, or is it a harmful condition?
    Most experts consider euthyroid sick syndrome to be an adaptive mechanism developed to reduce peripheral tissue energy expenditure during nonthyroidal illness. Conversely, some argue that the alterations in circulating thyroid hormone levels may be harmful and may accentuate the effects of nonthyroidal illness. The majority favors the former view, but the issue is likely to remain controversial for years to come.

13. Should patients with euthyroid sick syndrome be treated with thyroid hormones?
    Management of euthyroid sick syndrome is also controversial. Interventional studies have not reported consistent or convincing evidence of benefit from treating euthyroid sick syndrome patients with either liothyronine (LT_3) or levothyroxine (LT_4), and there is some evidence that thyroid hormone treatment may be harmful. LT_3 therapy was shown to improve ventricular performance and neuroendocrine profiles in patients with chronic heart failure in a randomized controlled trial. Experts agree that large, prospective studies in a variety of settings are needed. Therefore, thyroid hormone therapy cannot, at present, be recommended for patients with euthyroid sick syndrome, except possibly those with chronic heart failure.

14. Does euthyroid sick syndrome have any prognostic significance?
    Low serum T_3 and T_4 levels have been shown to have significant prognostic value in a variety of serious nonthyroidal illnesses. The degree of serum T_3 reduction predicts a poor prognosis in patients with ischemic heart disease,

heart valve disease, congestive heart failure, meningococcal sepsis, and numerous illnesses in the intensive care setting. Patients with extremely low serum T_3 levels have a high mortality rate.

15. Are levels of thyroid hormone ever elevated in patients with nonthyroid diseases?

The serum T_4 may be transiently elevated in patients with acute psychiatric illnesses and various acute medical illnesses. The mechanisms underlying such elevations of T_4 are not well understood but may be mediated by alterations in neurotransmitters or cytokines. This condition must be distinguished from true thyrotoxicosis.

BIBLIOGRAPHY

Adler, S. M., & Wartofsky, L. (2007). The nonthyroidal illness syndrome. *Endocrinology and Metabolism Clinics of North America, 36,* 657–672.

Boonen, E., & Van den Berghe, G. (2014). Endocrine responses to critical illness: novel insights and therapeutic implications. *Journal of Clinical Endocrinology and Metabolism, 99,* 1569–1582.

Debaveye, Y., Ellger, B., Mebis, L., Darras, V. M., & Van den Berghe, G. (2008). Regulation of tissue iodothyronine deiodinase activity in a model of prolonged critical illness. *Thyroid, 18,* 551–560.

den Brinker, M. , Joosten, K. F., Visser, T. J., Hop, W. C., de Rijke, Y. B., Hazelzet, J. A., ... Koelega, A. C. (2005). Euthyroid sick syndrome in meningococcal sepsis: the impact of peripheral thyroid hormone metabolism and binding proteins. *Journal of Clinical Endocrinology and Metabolism, 90,* 5613–5620.

Fliers, E., Bianco, A. C., Langouche, L., & Boelen, A. (2015). Thyroid function in critically ill patients. *Lancet Diabetes & Endocrinology, 3,* 816–825.

Huang, S. A., & Bianco, A. C. (2008). Reawakened interest in type III iodothyronine deiodinase in critical illness and injury. *Nature Clinical Practice. Endocrinology & Metabolism, 4,* 148–154.

Iervasi, G., Pingitore, A., Landi, P., Raciti M., Ripola A., Scarlattini M., L'Abbate A., Donato L. (2003). Low serum free triiodothyronine values predict mortality in patients with cardiac disease. *Circulation, 107,* 708–711.

Kaptein, E. M., Sanchez, A., Beale, E., & Chan, L. S. (2010). Clinical review: thyroid hormone therapy for postoperative nonthyroidal illnesses: a systematic review and synthesis. *Journal of Clinical Endocrinology and Metabolism, 95,* 4526–4534.

Kimura, T., Kanda, T., Kotajima, N., Kuwabara, A., Fukumura, Y., & Kobayashi, I. (2000). Involvement of circulating interleukin-6 and its receptor in the development of euthyroid sick syndrome in patients with acute myocardial infarction. *European Journal of Endocrinology, 143,* 179–184.

Langouche, L., Vander Perre, S., Marques, M., Boelen, A., Wouters, P. J., Casaer, M. P., & Van den Berghe, G. (2013). Impact of early nutrition restriction during critical illness on the nonthyroidal illness syndrome and its relation with outcome: a randomized, controlled clinical study. *Journal of Clinical Endocrinology and Metabolism, 98,* 1006–1013.

Liu, J., Wu, X., Lu, F., Zhao, L., Shi, L., & Xu, F. (2016). Low T3 syndrome is a strong predictor of poor outcomes in patients with community-acquired pneumonia. *Scientific Reports, 6,* 22271.

Nagaya, T., Fujieda, M., Otsuka, G., Yang, J. P., Okamoto, T., & Seo, H. (2000). A potential role of activated NF-kappa B in the pathogenesis of euthyroid sick syndrome. *Journal of Clinical Investigation, 106,* 393–402.

Pasqualetti, G., Calsolaro, V., Bernardini, S., Linsalata, G., Bigazzi, R., Caraccio, N., & Monzani, F. (2018). Degree of peripheral thyroxin deiodination, frailty, and long-term survival in hospitalized older patients. *Journal of Clinical Endocrinology and Metabolism, 103,* 1867–1876.

Peeters, R. P., Wouters, P. J., Kaptein, E., van Toor, H., Visser, T. J., & Van den Berghe, G. (2003). Reduced activation and increased inactivation of thyroid hormone in tissues of critically ill patients. *Journal of Clinical Endocrinology and Metabolism, 88,* 3202–3211.

Peeters, R. P., Wouters, P. J., van Toor, H., Kaptein, E., Visser, T. J., & Van den Berghe, G. (2005). Serum 3, 3′, 5′-triiodothyronine and 3, 5, 3′-triiodothyronine/rT3 are prognostic markers in critically ill patients and are associated with tissue deiodinase activities. *Journal of Clinical Endocrinology and Metabolism, 90,* 4559–4565.

Peeters, R. P., Kester, M. H. A., Wouters, P. J., Kaptein. E., van Toor, H., Visser, T. J., & Van den Berghe, G. (2005). Increased thyroxine sulfate levels in critically ill patients as a result of a decreased hepatic type I deiodinase activity. *Journal of Clinical Endocrinology and Metabolism, 90,* 6460–6465.

Peeters, R. P., van der Geyten, S., Wouters, P. J., Darras, V. M., van Toor, H., Kaptein, E.,... Van den Berghe, G. (2005). Tissue thyroid hormone levels in critical illness. *Journal of Clinical Endocrinology and Metabolism, 90,* 6498–6507.

Pingitore, A., Landi, P., Taddei, M. C., Ripoli, A., L'Abbate, A., & Iervasi, G. (2005). Triiodothyronine levels for risk stratification of patients with chronic heart failure. *American Journal of Medicine, 118,* 132–136.

Pingitore, A., Galli, E., Barison, A., Iervasi, A., Scarlattini, M., Nucci, D., ... Iervasi, G. (2008). Acute effects of triiodothyronine (T3) replacement therapy in patients with chronic heart failure and Low-T3 syndrome: a randomized, placebo-controlled study. *Journal of Clinical Endocrinology and Metabolism, 93,* 1351–1358.

Plikat, K., Langgartner, J., Buettner, R., Bollheimer L. C., Woenckhaus U., Scholmerich J., Wrede C. E. (2007). Increasing thyroid dysfunction is correlated with degree of illness and mortality in intensive care unit patients. *Metabolism, 56,* 239–244.

Rothberger, G. D., Gadhvi, S., Michelakis, N., Kumar, A., Calixte, R., & Shapiro, L. E. (2017). Usefulness of serum triiodothyronine (T3) to predict outcomes in patients hospitalized with acute heart failure. *American Journal of Cardiology, 119,* 599–603.

Schmidt R. L., LoPresti J. S., McDermott M. T., Zick S. M., Straseski J. A. (2018). Is reverse triiodothyronine ordered appropriately? Data from reference lab shows wide practice variation in orders for reverse triiodothyronine. *Thyroid* 28:842-848.

Spratt, D. I., Frohnauer, M., Cyr-Alves, H., Kramer, R. S., Lucas, F. L., Morton, J. R., ... Devlin, J. T. (2007). Triiodothyronine replacement does not alter the hemodynamic, metabolic, and hormonal responses to coronary artery surgery. *American Journal of Physiology. Endocrinol and Metabolism, 293,* E310–E315.

Van den Berghe, G. (2014). Non-thyroidal illnesses in the ICU: a syndrome with different faces. *Thyroid, 24,* 1456–1465.

Vanhorebeek, I., Langouche, L., & Van den Berghe, G. (2006). Endocrine aspects of acute and prolonged critical illness. *Nature Clinical Practice. Endocrinology & Metabolism, 2,* 20–31.

Zhang, K., Meng, X., Wang, W., Zheng, J., An, S., Wang, S., ... Tang, Y. D. (2018). Prognostic value of free triiodothyronine level in patients with hypertrophic obstructive cardiomyopathy. *Journal of Clinical Endocrinology and Metabolism, 103,* 1198–1205.

CHAPTER 46

THYROID DISEASE IN PREGNANCY

Meghan Donnelly and Linda A. Barbour

1. **How does normal pregnancy affect maternal thyroid function?**

   The profound hormonal influences that alter maternal physiology and the increased metabolic demands of the fetus cause significant changes in thyroid hormone synthesis, secretion, and transport (Table 46.1). In women, thyroid hormone (TH) production increases significantly during pregnancy because of the following factors:
   - Plasma volume expands by 30% to 40%, requiring expansion of the TH pool.
   - Placental type 3 deiodinase (D3) activity results in increased thyroxine (T_4) metabolism to reverse triiodothyronine (RT_3).
   - Transfer of T_4 across the placenta to the fetus occurs.
   - High thyroxine-binding globulin (TBG) levels decrease the levels of free TH.
   - Renal clearance of TH increases.
   - Absorption of exogenous TH may be impaired by iron in prenatal vitamins.

2. **Why must thyroid function tests be interpreted cautiously, and what are the pregnancy norms?**

   The influence of estrogen and human chorionic gonadotropin (hCG) on circulating TH levels lead to normal alterations in thyroid function tests compared with the nonpregnant norms. Estrogen increases TBG by two- to threefold beginning a few weeks after conception. The result is an approximately 50% increase in total thyroxine (TT_4) and total triiodothyronine (TT_3) levels because circulating T_4 and T_3 are highly protein bound to TBG. Throughout pregnancy, the range for both total hormone levels should be approximately 1.5 times the nonpregnant range. Measurement of the T_3 resin uptake (T_3RU), which is inversely related to serum thyroid-binding capacity, is correspondingly low, so that the calculated free T_4 index (FT_4 index; product of multiplying TT_4 by T_3RU) is usually normal. Although the normal ranges for free T_4 (FT_4) and free T3 (FT_3) levels are usually unchanged in pregnancy, they must be interpreted with caution because the reference ranges provided by manufacturers have been established using pools of sera from the nonpregnant population. Only 0.03% of serum TT_4 is unbound to serum proteins, and this is the FT_4 available for tissue uptake; the case is similar for TT_3 and FT_3. Furthermore, the very high TBG levels, the low albumin levels, and the high nonesterified fatty acids in pregnancy may all affect the FT_4 and FT_3 immunoassays. The FT_3 assay is especially unreliable in pregnancy, so TT_3 levels are often used (adding 50% to the normal nonpregnancy range). These effects can be mitigated by the use of an equilibrium dialysis assay or online solid-phase extraction–liquid chromatography/tandem mass spectrometry (LC/MS/MS), but these methods are expensive and often not readily available. A slightly low FT_4 in the late second or third trimester may be normal or may represent true hypothyroidism and should be interpreted in the context of the serum thyroid-stimulating hormone (TSH) and TT_4 levels. If TSH is < 4 mU/L and TT_4 is 1.5-fold elevated, it is unlikely that the patient has true hypothyroidism (in an iodine-sufficient region). If possible, pregnancy and trimester-specific norms for TSH, FT_4, and FT_3 should be established by the laboratory, but these are not typically provided (see Table 46.1).

3. **How do TSH levels change throughout the course of pregnancy?**

   The beta-subunit of hCG has 85% sequence homology in the first 114 amino acids with TSH and can, thus, bind to and stimulate the TSH receptor. Levels of hCG $> 50,000$ IU/L, which may be seen when hCG peaks at the end of the first trimester, can, therefore, increase the FT_4 level enough (but typically still within the reference range) to suppress the serum TSH level. This is especially commonly seen with multifetal pregnancies. The upper and lower TSH normative limits are, therefore, shifted lower because of the thyrotropic effect of hCG. In one large series, the 95% confidence limits were as low as 0.03 mU/L in the first and second trimesters and 0.13 mU/L in the third trimester. Although previous recommendations by the Endocrine Society and American Thyroid Association (ATA) suggested TSH upper norms of 2.5 mU/L in the first trimester and 3 mU/L in the second and third trimesters, the 2017 ATA guidelines have reestablished the upper limit of normal for TSH in all trimesters to be 4 mU/L (or, for most assays, a reduction of the upper limit of normal TSH level by about 0.5 mU/L). The lower limit is suggested as 0.4 mU/L less than the nonpregnant range (≈ 0.1 mU/L). This change was based on the Treatment of Subclinical Hypothyroidism or Hypothyroxinemia Study performed by the Maternal-Fetal Medicine Units Network, which screened the thyroid function of $> 97,000$ pregnant women before 20 weeks' gestation. This study established that the 97.5th percentile TSH level in the first 15,000 women to be screened was 4 mU/L, prompting the new recommended definition for an upper limit of normal TSH level in pregnancy. Although the serum TSH is likely to be lower in the first trimester or early second trimester when hCG peaks, trimester-specific ranges were not established and there are insufficient data that treatment of a TSH value < 4 mU/L improves pregnancy outcomes. Ethnicity-related differences are also significant; Black and Asian women have TSH values

Table 46.1. Thyroid Function Tests During Normal Pregnancy.

	FIRST TRIMESTER	SECOND TRIMESTER	THIRD TRIMESTER
Total T4	$1.5\times\uparrow$	$1.5\times\uparrow$	$1.5\times\uparrow$
Total T3	$1.5\times\uparrow$	$1.5\times\uparrow$	$1.5\times\uparrow$
T3RU	$\downarrow$	$\downarrow$	$\downarrow$
Free T4 index	Normal	Normal	Normal
TSH	$\downarrow$ or normal	$\downarrow$ or normal	Slight $\downarrow$ or normal
Free T4	Usually normal	Usually normal	Usually normal or slight $\downarrow$

$\uparrow$ Increased; $\downarrow$, decreased; *T3*, triiodothyronine; T_3RU, T_3 resin uptake; T_4, thyroxine; *TSH*, thyroid-stimulating hormone.

that are, on average, 0.4 mU/L lower than in Caucasian women. Given all of these variables, it is important that the TSH also be interpreted in the context of the actual thyroid hormone levels. If TT_4 and TT_3 are < 1.5-fold elevated compared with the nonpregnancy range, and FT_4 and FT_3 are not increased, the suppressed TSH may simply reflect the effect of hCG, but this could also be caused by subclinical hyperthyroidism from Graves' diseases or a hot nodule. However, no matter the etiology, a suppressed TSH alone (subclinical hyperthyroidism) does not warrant treatment in pregnancy. As hCG levels fall with advancing pregnancy, the TSH level may be slightly less suppressed in the second trimester than the first, but by the third trimester, it is usually within the normal range.

4. What factors may compromise maternal ability to increase thyroid hormone production?
Women with limited thyroid reserve because of chronic thyroiditis, partial ablation, or surgical resection may be unable to increase thyroid hormone production during pregnancy and often develop hypothyroidism at this time. Women with inadequate iodine intake may also develop hypothyroidism and a goiter because iodine requirements increase by approximately 40% to 50% in pregnancy.

5. What is the iodine requirement in pregnancy, and what happens if iodine intake is insufficient?
Iodine requirements increase markedly during pregnancy as a result of increased urinary iodine losses secondary to the 50% to 100% increase in the glomerular filtration rate (GFR) during pregnancy, the diversion of iodine to the fetus for TH synthesis and increased maternal TH requirements. If iodine intake is insufficient, TH production drops, resulting in increased secretion of TSH, which then stimulates thyroid gland growth. Thyroid volume commonly increases by $\geq$ 30% during pregnancy in iodine-deficient regions and often does not completely regress after delivery (goiter of pregnancy). In iodine-replete areas, such as the United States, thyroid gland volume may increase by 10% to 15%, primarily as a result of pregnancy-induced vascular swelling of the gland, but this usually cannot be appreciated by palpation. Therefore, any goiter found during pregnancy in an iodine-replete area should be evaluated in the same manner as a goiter occurring outside of pregnancy. Many European countries and developing countries with endemic iodine deficiency do not supplement with iodine; therefore, women are at risk of iodine-deficiency goiters during pregnancy. When iodine intake is severely deficient, overt hypothyroidism results in both the mother and the fetus. Endemic cretinism occurs if severe hypothyroidism secondary to iodine deficiency goes unrecognized and untreated at birth. The World Health Organization (WHO)/ATA recommendations for iodine intake are 250 mcg/day during pregnancy and lactation and 150 mcg/day in the nonpregnant state. Iodine insufficiency is an increasing problem in the United States as a result of the availability of deiodinated salt and is estimated at 5% to 10%. Because most prenatal vitamins do not contain iodine, women of childbearing age should be instructed to use only iodinated salt or to make sure to ingest a prenatal vitamin containing iodine.

6. Do thyroid hormones, TSH, thyrotropin-releasing hormone (TRH), and iodine cross the placenta?
It is known that significant amounts of T_4 cross the placenta because fetuses with complete thyroid agenesis have approximately 30% to 40% of the normal amount of TH at birth. However, transplacental passage of TH is limited partly because of the high placental activity of the type 3 monodeiodinase (D3) that converts T_4 to RT_3 and T_3 to diiodothyronine (T_2). Maternal TH transported across the placenta is critical for development of the fetal brain, especially prior to 16 to 18 weeks when fetal brain maturation is completely dependent on maternal T_4. Evidence suggests that transthyretin, a circulating thyroid hormone–binding protein synthesized and secreted by the placenta, may provide a mechanism for delivery of TH to the fetus. To date, six TH transporters have been identified in placental tissue. However, T_3 crosses the placenta poorly, and therefore, T_3 preparations should not be used to treat hypothyroidism in pregnancy. Furthermore, the fetal brain primarily has T_4 receptors and not T_3 receptors, underscoring the importance of T_4 in pregnancy. Iodine easily crosses the placenta for use by the fetal thyroid,

which, after 12 to 14 weeks of gestation, takes up iodine even more avidly than does the maternal thyroid. TRH, but not TSH, crosses the placenta and has been used in experimental protocols to attempt to accelerate fetal lung maturity.

7. Summarize the ability of thyroid-related antibodies to cross the placenta.

Immunoglobulin G (IgG) TSH receptor–stimulating antibodies (thyroid-stimulating immunoglobulins [TSIs] and TSH receptor antibodies [TRAbs]) cross the placenta as early as 18 to 20 weeks' gestation and can occasionally cause fetal/neonatal hyperthyroidism in women with Graves' disease when maternal levels are at least ≈ 3-fold elevated. It is recommended that both TSIs and TRAbs be measured in these women, because if either antibody is ≈ 3 times the normal, surveillance for fetal Graves' disease is indicated. Although anti–thyroperoxidase (TPO) antibodies and anti–thyroglobulin (TG) antibodies can also cross the placenta, they usually have no clinically significant effect on fetal thyroid function. Rarely, they may be associated with thyrotropin receptor–blocking antibodies that can cause transient neonatal hypothyroidism.

8. List the medications commonly used to treat hyperthyroidism that cross the placenta.

Propylthiouracil (PTU), methimazole (MMI), beta-blockers, and dexamethasone commonly used to treat hyperthyroidism cross the placenta.

9. Describe fetal thyroid function and brain development.

At approximately 12 to 14 weeks' gestation, the fetal thyroid gland develops, and the hypothalamic–pituitary–thyroid axis begins to function. Before 16 weeks, however, the fetus relies solely on transplacental delivery of T_4 from the mother. Significant amounts of T_4 cross the placenta in the first trimester and early second trimester before the fetal thyroid begins functioning; thus, in early pregnancy, when adequate fetal TH is crucial for normal neurologic development, fetal brain T_4 levels reflect maternal levels. TH and type 2 deiodinase (D2) have been observed in the fetal cerebral cortex by 5 to 7 weeks. T_4 binds to T_4 receptors on fetal brain astrocytes and is deiodinated to T_3 by D2. The fetal brain thus depends on an adequate supply of maternal T_4 because of the presence of primarily fetal brain T_4 receptors. Consequently, maternal T_3 supplementation cannot be utilized for an adequate supply of fetal brain T_3. These findings emphasize the importance of maternally derived T_4 conversion to T_3 in the fetal brain in influencing neuronal and astrocyte proliferation and migration early in pregnancy, and the importance of treating maternal hypothyroidism with T_4 because of lack of bioavailability of exogenous T_3 to the developing fetal brain. Babies born with very low T_4 levels as a result of iodine deficiency or complete thyroid agenesis are usually grossly neurologically normal as long as T_4 is immediately given at birth, but subtle cognitive changes may persist.

10. Is fetal thyroid hormone production independent of the mother?

After 16 to 18 weeks, the fetal hypothalamic–pituitary–thyroid axis is fairly independent of the mother, with the exception of its dependence on adequate maternal iodine stores. Antithyroid drugs or high levels of TSIs or TRAbs may, however, affect fetal thyroid function or cause goiter development at this stage. TH and TBG levels increase in the fetus and plateau at about 35 to 37 weeks' gestation. High fetal levels of RT_3 and low T_3 levels are maintained throughout the pregnancy as a result of the high placental D3 activity. The fetal pituitary–thyroid axis is relatively immature, however, considering the increased fetal TSH levels relative to the low level of T_4 production at birth. At the time of labor and in the early neonatal period, there are dramatic increases in TSH and T_4 levels and in the capacity of the liver to convert T_4 to T_3. This TSH surge at birth may not be possible if the fetal pituitary has been exposed to chronic overt maternal hyperthyroidism because the pituitary thyrotropic cells have been suppressed, resulting in neonatal central hypothyroidism.

11. What are the most common causes of overt hyperthyroidism in pregnancy? During what period of gestation is hyperthyroidism most likely to occur?

Overt hyperthyroidism from causes not related to pregnancy complicates pregnancy in 0.3% of women. Graves' disease, the most common cause of hyperthyroidism in pregnancy, accounts for nearly 85% of the cases. Autoimmune thyroid disease is most likely to manifest in the first trimester or the postpartum period because the immune suppression of pregnancy has been shown to decrease thyroid antibody levels significantly during the second and third trimesters. Other causes include toxic multinodular goiters, solitary toxic adenomas, iodine-induced hyperthyroidism, subacute thyroiditis and gestational transient thyrotoxicosis (GTT).

12. What is GTT, or thyrotoxicosis in hyperemesis gravidarum?

GTT, diagnosed in 1% to 3% of pregnancies, refers to maternal hyperthyroidism caused by elevated levels of hCG, which binds to the TSH receptor and stimulates TH release. Posttranslational modification of the sialylation of hCG can change its affinity for the TSH receptor and its half-life in the circulation, thus resulting in elevated TH levels in the first half of pregnancy. hCG levels > 75,000 IU/mL, which may be seen in women with hyperemesis gravidarum, multifetal gestations, and especially molar pregnancies, can often cause hyperthyroidism; however, no cut-off level of hCG can predict or rule out GTT. Women with hyperemesis gravidarum (characterized by persistent nausea and vomiting accompanied by electrolyte derangements and at least a 5% weight loss) commonly have abnormal thyroid function tests and, in one series, half the study patients had elevated FT_4 levels. There is no goiter associated with GTT, unlike with Graves' disease or a toxic multinodular goiter. GTT usually resolves without antithyroid treatment by approximately 18 weeks of pregnancy when hCG levels decline, so it is rarely necessary to treat with beta-blockers or antithyroid drugs (ATDs). Hyperthyroidism is probably not the cause of the nausea; instead the nausea is likely caused by a direct effect of hCG.

13. Summarize the diagnostic approach to the pregnant woman with suspected hyperthyroidism.
    Normal pregnancy can produce clinical features that mimic hyperthyroidism, such as heat intolerance, mild tachycardia, increase in cardiac output, a systolic flow murmur, peripheral vasodilatation, and a widened pulse pressure. Weight loss may be obscured by the weight gain of pregnancy. As in the nonpregnant state, hyper-thyroidism in pregnancy is usually characterized by low serum TSH levels and increased serum FT_4 and/or TT_3 levels; it must be kept in mind that in normal pregnancies TSH levels are often lower and that TT_4 and TT_3 levels are $\approx$ 50% elevated compared with the nonpregnant ranges. Radioisotope scans are contraindicated during pregnancy, and therefore, the differential diagnosis of hyperthyroidism in pregnancy must be based on history, physical examination, and laboratory values. Obstetric ultrasonography may be indicated to exclude a hydatidiform mole or to identify multifetal gestation.

14. What findings help distinguish Graves' disease from GTT, and why is it important to do so?
    If a woman is actively vomiting, the distinction between early Graves' disease and gestational hyperthyroidism accompanied by hyperemesis gravidarum (GTT) may be particularly difficult. A prior history of thyroid dysfunc-tion, symptoms predating pregnancy, and physical examination findings, such as goiter, orbitopathy, or pretibial myxedema, are suggestive of Graves' disease or toxic multinodular goiter, rather than GTT. Elevated levels of TRAbs and TSIs point to Graves' disease and are positive in about 95% of patients with active Graves' hyper-thyroidism. Indications to measure TRAbs or TSIs include (1) hyperthyroidism of uncertain cause, (2) a history of hyperthyroidism previously treated with radioiodine or total thyroidectomy, and (3) a history of delivering an infant with hyperthyroidism. Importantly, TT_3 levels are generally higher in Graves' disease because hyperemesis gravidarum results in a compromised nutritional state and decreased conversion of T_4 to T_3 in peripheral tissues. It is extremely important to differentiate between GTT and Graves' disease because GTT commonly resolves by $\approx$ 18 to 20 weeks with supportive care alone, whereas Graves' disease often requires ATD therapy to prevent maternal and fetal complications of thyrotoxicosis.

15. Why is the woman's original country of residence significant in evaluating hyperthyroidism?
    Women who have goiters from areas of endemic iodine deficiency and who move to the United States may develop iodine-induced hyperthyroidism when they suddenly become iodine replete. Hot nodules are also more common in these women, and, in contrast to Graves' disease, hot nodules do not improve with the immune sup-pression of the later stages of pregnancy. Furthermore, T_3 is synthesized in preference to T_4 in iodine deficiency states; as a result, although rare, a low free T_4 level may occur without elevated TSH because the higher T_3 levels feedback on TSH, potentially causing it to be relatively normal in spite of overt hypothyroxinemia (low FT_4).

16. What are the risks of hyperthyroidism to the pregnant woman?
    - Inadequately treated maternal hyperthyroidism can result in weight loss, tachycardia, proximal muscle weakness, anxiety, and atrial fibrillation, as well as increase the risk for preeclampsia and preterm labor. Left ventricular dysfunction can occur with high output failure. This cardiac condition may place the pregnant woman at risk for congestive heart failure, especially in the presence of superimposed preeclampsia, infection, and anemia or at the time of delivery. Thyroid storm can also occur in these women.

17. What are the risks to the fetus/neonate from maternal hyperthyroidism in pregnancy?
    Pregnancy outcomes are directly related to the control of maternal hyperthyroidism in pregnancy. Inadequately treated maternal hyperthyroidism can result in fetal loss, fetal tachycardia, intrauterine growth restriction, premature delivery, and a ninefold increased incidence of low birth weight in the infants. Congenital malformations are probably not increased in babies born to mothers with either treated or untreated hyperthyroidism. Inadequately treated maternal hyperthyroidism can cause suppression of the fetal hypothalamic–pituitary–thyroid axis, resulting in temporary central hypothyroidism in the neonate and the inability of the neonate to mount an appropriate TSH response at birth. Other data suggest that poorly controlled maternal hyperthyroidism may be associated with a risk of seizure disorders to the fetus/neonate and neurobehavioral disorders later in life.

18. How do Graves' disease antibodies impact the fetus during gestation?
    In $\approx$ 5% of cases of Graves' disease in pregnancy, fetal or neonatal thyroid dysfunction can develop as a result of very high levels of maternal TSH receptor–stimulating antibodies as measured by TSI or TRAb assays. Maternal levels of these antibodies may remain high even after ablation therapy, with greater elevations after radioiodine therapy compared with thyroidectomy. Because transplacental passage of IgG is limited, fetal thyroid dysfunction rarely occurs unless the maternal titers of TSIs (functional assay measuring cyclic adenosine monophosphate [cAMP]) or TRAbs (TSH receptor antibodies by radioimmunoassay) are at least threefold elevated during the

second and third trimesters; maternal levels this high or above may increase the risk for fetal or neonatal thyroid dysfunction by as much as 30%. If TRAb or TSI levels are threefold higher, fetuses should be screened for thyroid dysfunction by evaluating for the presence of a goiter on prenatal ultrasonography starting at 20 to 24 weeks' gestation and every 4 weeks, or as clinically indicated. Fetal hyperthyroidism may also be accompanied by intra-uterine growth restriction, fetal tachycardia, fetal hydrops, craniosynostosis, or advanced bone maturation. All pregnant women with Graves' disease or a history of Graves' disease should be tested for TSIs and TRAbs at 18 to 20 weeks' gestation. Numerous cases of fetal Graves' disease have been reported in mothers previously treated with ablative doses of iodine-131 (^{131}I) and who are taking thyroid replacement. TSI or TRAb are some-times high in the first trimester and then fall to < 3 times the normal by 18 weeks with the increasing immuno-suppression of pregnancy. If these antibodies are < 3-fold elevated by 18 weeks, the risk of fetal or neonatal Graves' disease is negligible.

19. What is the treatment for fetal hyperthyroidism caused by maternal Graves' disease?

    Fetal thyroid dysfunction should be confirmed by percutaneous fetal umbilical blood sampling (PUBS) and direct thyroid assays if the cause of the fetal goiter is in doubt, because TRAbs can be either stimulating (fetal hyperthy-roidism) or, rarely, blocking (fetal hypothyroidism). However, in most cases where the mother is hyperthyroid, the antibodies are stimulating. In addition, ATDs used to treat maternal hyperthyroidism can also cross the placenta and render a fetus hypothyroid, resulting in a goiter; this is especially likely if the minimum amount of the ATD is not being used to keep the mother's FT_4 at the upper limit of the normal range.

    Treatment of fetal hyperthyroidism consists of administering high doses of PTU to the mother so that a sufficient amount of medication is delivered into the fetal circulation. MMI is poorly studied for the treatment of fetal Graves' disease. Mothers who are already hypothyroid as a result of previous ablation or surgery will also require supplementation with T_4, which crosses the placenta less well compared with PTU. Thus, both medications are sometimes required when the fetus has hyperthyroidism and the mother has postablative or postoperative hypothyroidism. Maternal–fetal medicine experts should be consulted in any women with TRAB/TSI levels that are > 3-fold elevated or when there are any concerns about fetal Graves' disease.

20. Why is neonatal hyperthyroidism more common than fetal hyperthyroidism, and how does it manifest?

    Neonatal hyperthyroidism is more common because of the high activity of placental D3, the relatively low serum T_3 levels in utero, and the effects of maternal ATDs on the fetus. TSIs and TRAbs pass transplacentally and remain at high levels after birth; these antibodies stimulate the neonatal thyroid to produce excess thyroid hormone for up to 3 months because they are IgG antibodies with long half-lives. Neonatal hyperthyroidism may manifest as irritability, failure to thrive, hyperkinesis, diarrhea, poor feeding, jaundice, tachycardia, poor weight gain, thrombocytopenia, and goiter. Less commonly, exophthalmos, cardiac failure, hepatosplenomegaly, hyperviscosity syndrome, or craniosynostosis may occur. If the mother had been receiving ATDs during pregnancy, it may take 5 to 10 days for the neonate to manifest symptoms because of the residual effects of the medication.

21. How serious is neonatal hyperthyroidism, and what is the treatment for hyperthyroidism in infants?

    The neonatal mortality rate may be as high as 30% if the condition is unrecognized. Infants may require ATDs until the antibody levels wane, which usually occurs by 12 weeks.

22. How can pregnant women with Graves' disease be treated safely?

    Treatment of overt hyperthyroidism (suppressed serum TSH and elevated FT_4 levels) is indicated to decrease morbidity in both the mother and fetus. ATDs and the judicious use of beta-blockers until TT_4 is at goal (1.5 times the upper limit of the nonpregnant range) or until FT_4 levels are in the high-to-normal range for pregnancy are the preferred treatment. Unless the patient has severe T_3 thyrotoxicosis, the TT_3 is usually not targeted because normalization of TT_3 without maintaining FT_4 in the upper limit of the normal range has been reported to cause hypothyroidism. Cold iodine is not the first-line treatment, and radioactive iodine is absolutely contraindicated because ^{131}I readily crosses the placenta, is concentrated by the fetal thyroid after 10 to 12 weeks' gestation, and is destructive to the fetal thyroid. Pregnant women with thyroid storm can be safely treated with PTU, followed by cold iodine, along with hydrocortisone (crosses the placenta poorly) and judicious use of beta-blockers.

23. Should subclinical hyperthyroidism be treated during pregnancy?

    No. TSH levels remain suppressed normally in some pregnant women. In a series of > 400 women with subclinical hyperthyroidism, pregnancy outcomes in untreated women were no different from those of women without sup-pressed TSH levels. Furthermore, such treatment risks the unnecessary exposure of the fetus to ATDs, which can render the fetus hypothyroid. Therefore, no matter the cause (Graves' disease versus GTT versus warm nodule), a suppressed TSH level alone without elevated thyroid hormone levels should not be treated during pregnancy.

24. Which is preferable for treating hyperthyroidism in pregnant women, PTU or MMI?

    ATDs should be avoided in the first trimester in cases of very mild overt hyperthyroidism because both PTU and MMI are associated, although uncommonly, with birth defects when there is fetal exposure during organogenesis ($\approx$ 5–10 weeks). PTU is preferred over MMI in the first trimester for moderate-to-severe overt hyperthyroidism because MMI has long been associated with a 2% to 4% risk of congenital malformations, such as aplasia cutis, choanal or esophageal atresia, abdominal wall defects, ventricular septal defects, and eye and urinary abnormalities. PTU has traditionally been considered safer, from a teratogenicity standpoint, in the first trimester; however, a more recent study reported that up to 2% of children exposed to PTU in the first trimester suffer congenital malformations, such as facial and neck cysts and urinary tract abnormalities. These defects that occur (uncommonly) with PTU are felt to be less severe than those associated with MMI, leading to PTU being the preferred drug for use in the first trimester. In 2010, the U.S. Food and Drug Administration (FDA) reported PTU as third on the list of drugs leading to liver transplantation in the United States. The investigators estimated the risk of PTU-related liver injury to be 1:1000 and 1:10,000 for acute liver failure requiring transplantation or causing death. There were two reported cases occurring during pregnancy, and both cases also had evidence of fetal liver injury. Because of this concern, switching to MMI in the second trimester is often recommended if it can be done effectively and without compromising the optimal ATD dose titration. This approach balances the risks of MMI embryopathy in the first trimester with the risk of maternal hepatotoxicity from PTU in the second or third trimesters.

25. How are PTU and MMI doses determined and managed during pregnancy?

Because both PTU and MMI cross the placenta and can cause fetal hypothyroidism with overtreatment, the lowest possible doses should be given, with a goal of maintaining the mother's serum FT_4 level in the high-normal range or the TT_4 level approximately 1.5 times the nonpregnancy range. Serum TSH levels often remain persistently suppressed in women with FT_4 and TT_4 levels in these ranges and should never be used to titrate the dose of ATDs during pregnancy. According to the ATA guidelines, in early pregnancy (< 10 weeks) women with Graves' disease only requiring low doses of medication (MMI $< 5–10$ mg/day; PTU $< 100–200$ mg/day) can consider cessation of medication to reduce the small risk for teratogenicity. In women requiring low doses of PTU in the first trimester, doses can be tapered off later in pregnancy because of the immunosuppression of pregnancy; therefore, switching to MMI may not be necessary. The usual conversion ratio of PTU to MMI is about 20:1 (200 mg PTU is ≈10 mg MMI), but maternal FT_4 or TT_4 levels need to be carefully monitored because responses may vary. If T_3 thyrotoxicosis is the predominant manifestation, PTU may be superior to MMI because PTU also decreases the conversion of T_4 to T_3. Cessation or continued treatment with ATDs should be followed by thyroid function testing every ≈ 2 to 4 weeks initially, with testing intervals increased to ≈ 4 weeks in the second and third trimesters if thyroid function appears stable.

Approximately 1% to 3% of newborns exposed to PTU or MMI in utero develop transient neonatal hypothyroidism or a small goiter when PTU or MMI doses are titrated to maintain FT_4 in the upper normal range, but this is much more common if the maternal FT_4 levels fall into the middle or lower-to-normal range, or if attempts are made to normalize the TSH. Although it is unknown whether monitoring liver function tests is beneficial in preventing severe hepatotoxicity, it is reasonable to have women on PTU undergo liver function tests several times and be advised to report any new symptoms immediately. Both thionamides are associated with a 1% or less risk for agranulocytosis; thus, patients should be counseled to report if they develop a fever or sore throat while on these medications and complete blood count should be done at that time. Typically, ATDs can be decreased by the late second and third trimesters, and sometimes even stopped because of decreasing TRAb levels that accompany the natural immunosuppression of pregnancy. However, it is important to ensure that mothers are not hyperthyroid near delivery to reduce the risk of hyperthyroid complications of the cardiovascular system and suppression of fetal pituitary function, which can result in neonatal central hypothyroidism at birth. Most women have a rebound in their Grave's disease after delivery and need to have ATDs increased or restarted.

26. Discuss the role of beta-blockers during pregnancy.

Beta-blockers are indicated to treat symptomatic hyperadrenergic signs and symptoms until ATD therapy has rendered the patient euthyroid. However, beta-blockers should be discontinued when the patient becomes euthyroid because chronic long-term treatment with these drugs has been associated with intrauterine growth restriction. No compelling data indicate that one beta-blocker is safer than another; however, metoprolol and propranolol are usually favored over atenolol.

27. Why is radioactive iodine administration contraindicated during pregnancy?

Radioactive iodine (RAI) is contraindicated during pregnancy because maternally administered RAI readily crosses the placenta and is highly concentrated in the fetal thyroid after 10 weeks gestation. At ≈ 12 to 14 weeks' gestation, the fetal thyroid gland has avidity for iodine that is 20 to 50 times that of the maternal thyroid, and one dose of RAI will easily ablate the fetal thyroid gland.

28. Can cold iodine be given for hyperthyroidism during pregnancy?

Cold iodine (e.g., Lugol's solution or saturated solution of potassium iodide [SSKI]) should be avoided in pregnancy except in women with thyroid storm or hyperthyroidism refractory to other treatments. If it must be given after 10 to 12 weeks, the fetus should be monitored for the development of a goiter, and the duration should be limited, if possible, to 3 days.

29. Does surgery for hyperthyroidism have a role during pregnancy?

Surgery is rarely indicated for hyperthyroidism during pregnancy but may be necessary in women who are unable to take ATDs (i.e., because of agranulocytosis) or who are refractory to high doses of ATDs. If necessary, it is best to perform surgery in the second trimester before fetal viability. The first trimester may pose a risk of miscarriage, and preterm labor risk is increased when surgery is performed after 24 weeks. However, the overall risks to the pregnancy are low and surgery should not be withheld during pregnancy if it is deemed necessary. Plasmapheresis may be useful to lower TH levels with Graves' disease to allow safe surgery if ATDs cannot be given.

30. Should a woman be counseled to terminate a pregnancy if she inadvertently receives a ^{123}I scan or an ablative dose of ^{131}I?

A woman who receives ^{123}I for a thyroid scan early in pregnancy can be reassured, for the most part, because the fetus has not developed the ability to concentrate iodine before 10 weeks and the radiation exposure from this isotope is very low, with a half-life of only approximately 8 hours. An ablative dose of ^{131}I given early in pregnancy, however, is cause for greater concern because the half-life of ^{131}I is 8 days and the radiation is more destructive to the thyroid gland. Generally, if the dose is given very early, when the fetal thyroid gland is not yet trapping iodine, the risk for fetal hypothyroidism is low. Termination of pregnancy is rarely recommended, but the fetus and neonate should be monitored very closely for evidence of development of a goiter or hypothyroidism.

31. How may the risk to the fetus be minimized if a woman inadvertently has radioiodine therapy during pregnancy?

It may be useful in this situation to give PTU or cold iodine to block the recycling of ^{131}I in the fetal thyroid gland, especially if PTU or cold iodine can be given within 1 week of ^{131}I treatment. If the fetus does develop hypothyroidism, it can be diagnosed in utero by percutaneous umbilical sampling, and T_4 treatment may be given through amniotic fluid injections, although such treatment is not well studied, and a maternal–fetal medicine physician should be consulted. Certainly, all women of childbearing age, regardless of contraceptive measures, should have a pregnancy test before receiving any dose of ^{123}I or ^{131}I, and efficacious contraception should be ensured.

32. How should women with Graves' disease be counseled before conception about treatment alternatives?

Many experts recommend definitive treatment with ^{131}I (after a negative pregnancy test) in a woman of childbearing age who wishes to become pregnant. In several series of women given RAI for thyroid cancer therapy, no significant differences in stillbirths, preterm births, low-birth-weight infants, or congenital malformations were reported in subsequent pregnancies. Effective birth control must be established, and then women should optimally wait for at least 6 months after regaining a stable euthyroid status before trying to conceive. Women with Graves' disease who undergo ablation therapy with ^{131}I may continue to have high (> 3 times normal) TSI or TRAb levels for 1 year, increasing the risk of fetal and neonatal Graves' disease. For women who have very high TRAb levels and require high doses of ATDs and who wish to become pregnant within 6 to 12 months, thyroidectomy may be a reasonable option. In women who are stable on low doses of ATDs, these drugs should not be problematic during pregnancy, but it is highly likely that ATD doses will need to be adjusted during pregnancy and the postpartum period. Women requiring high ATD doses or who have large goiters should be counseled about the benefits of definitive therapy before becoming pregnant.

33. Describe the natural history of Graves' disease in the postpartum period.

Approximately 70% of women have a postpartum relapse or exacerbation of Graves' disease, usually within the first 3 months after delivery. ATDs must almost always be restarted or the dose increased during this time.

34. Does maternal thyroid status impact lactation?

Several case series and cohort studies have demonstrated that both hyperthyroidism and hypothyroidism can negatively impact milk production and the ability to successfully breastfeed, and that lactogenesis improves with appropriate therapy. Therefore, it is recommended that lactating women who are experiencing inadequate milk production without other identifiable causes have their TSH assessed for thyroid dysfunction and treatment offered if it is identified.

35. What treatments can be recommended for women with hyperthyroidism who wish to breastfeed?

Because PTU is more highly protein bound and may cross less efficiently into breast milk than MMI, it was previously recommended that nursing mothers be treated with PTU rather than MMI. However, MMI doses up to 20 mg have been safely used in nursing mothers without any evidence of neonatal hypothyroidism. Therefore, because of concerns about PTU-induced hepatotoxicity, women are usually counseled that they can safely nurse, as long as these MMI doses are not exceeded. Nursing women requiring ATDs should tell their pediatrician. Thyroid function tests in the neonates may be indicated if a woman is taking > 450 mg of PTU or > 20 mg of MMI per day.

36. Can a nursing mother undergo a diagnostic ^{123}I scan to assess the cause of hyperthyroidism?

A diagnostic ^{123}I scan can be performed if the woman is willing to interrupt breastfeeding for 2 to 3 days, when the diagnosis is unclear. Both ^{123}I and technetium-99 (^{99}Tc) pertechnetate are excreted into breast milk with effective half-lives of 5 to 8 hours and 2 to 8 hours, respectively.

37. Can ^{131}I ablative therapy be offered to nursing women?

Ablative therapy with ^{131}I cannot be offered unless the woman is willing to give up nursing altogether for this child, because even a 5-mCi dose requires discontinuation of breastfeeding for at least 56 days. Further, it is recommended that ^{131}I not be given to women until at least 4 weeks after breastfeeding has ceased to avoid high radioisotope levels in breast tissue.

38. Can beta-blockers be used in nursing women?

Beta-blockers can be used, if necessary, in breastfeeding mothers. However, atenolol may produce higher breast milk drug concentrations than other beta-blockers, and there are rare reports of neonatal bradycardia. The lowest doses of propranolol or metoprolol are preferred.

39. When should a nursing woman take antithyroid drugs to minimize exposure to her infant?

It is always best if a mother takes ATDs immediately after nursing to avoid exposing the infant to peak concentrations of the drug.

40. Do overt and subclinical hypothyroidism pose a risk to pregnancy?

Hypothyroidism occurs in approximately 2% to 4% of pregnancies; overt hypothyroidism (defined as an elevated TSH > 4 mU/L with a decreased serum FT_4 concentration; also sometimes considered if TSH > 10 mU/L regardless of the FT_4 level) occurs in approximately 0.5%. Untreated overt hypothyroidism can cause maternal anemia, myopathy, bradycardia, neuropsychologic symptoms, carpal tunnel syndrome, and congestive heart failure. It has also been associated with an increased risk of preterm delivery, pregnancy loss, gestational hypertension, placental abruption, low-birth-weight infants, postpartum hemorrhage, and possible neurodevelopmental delay in the infant.

Subclinical hypothyroidism, defined as elevated serum TSH (usually < 10 mU/L) but with FT_4 level within a normal range, is variably associated with adverse pregnancy outcomes. Heterogeneous definitions of an elevated TSH among studies have contributed to the difficulty in determining the true risk this condition poses to pregnancy. The available evidence most strongly supports an association between subclinical hypothyroidism with pregnancy loss and preterm delivery, with possibly an additive risk associated with TPO antibody-positive status. Most series reporting that subclinical hypothyroidism is not associated with adverse fetal or neonatal outcomes have included primarily women with minimally elevated TSH levels (< 6 mU/L); therefore, it is unclear whether subclinical hypothyroidism characterized by higher TSH levels of 7 to 10 mU/L result in similar outcomes.

41. Should treatment be given to pregnant women with overt and subclinical hypothyroidism?

No prospective randomized controlled trials (RCTs) on the treatment of overt hypothyroidism have been performed in pregnancy or in the nonpregnant population because this is felt to be unethical. Because available retrospective data support the benefits of treatment in preventing both maternal and fetal adverse pregnancy outcomes, overt hypothyroidism in pregnancy should be treated with levothyroxine (LT_4) replacement therapy. Many consider a serum TSH ≥ 10 mU/L as being equivalent to "overt" hypothyroidism even when FT_4 levels are normal.

Available data do not definitively support LT_4 treatment for women with very mild subclinical hypothyroidism in pregnancy; two large multicenter RCTs showed no improvement in pregnancy outcomes or cognitive function in childhood after treatment during pregnancy. The Controlled Antenatal Thyroid Screening study (CATS Study) screened nearly 22,000 women for subclinical hypothyroidism and demonstrated no improvement in pregnancy outcomes or neurocognitive outcomes in children at age 3 years with treatment versus no treatment in those identified as having subclinical hypothyroidism. The more recent Treatment of Subclinical Hypothyroidism or Hypothyroxinemia in Pregnancy Study randomized almost 700 women with subclinical hypothyroidism to treatment with LT_4 versus placebo and reported no differences in obstetric outcomes, neonatal outcomes, or cognitive function of the children at age 5 years between treated and untreated pregnancies. However, this study was limited by late gestational age at randomization (mean ≈ 17 weeks) and a relatively low baseline serum TSH level (mean 4.5 mU/L) in the treatment group. The median TSH treated in the CATS study was only 3.8 mU/L. Additionally, TPO antibody status was unknown for both studies. Thus, the question of whether treatment of subclinical hypothyroidism diagnosed earlier in pregnancy, with an elevated TSH between 6 to 10 mU/L or with positive TPO antibody status, improves outcomes remains unsettled.

The ATA recommends treating any patient with subclinical hypothyroidism during pregnancy if the TSH level is > 10 mU/L; treating if the TSH is between 4 and 10 mU/L, especially with positive TPO antibodies; and considering treatment for TSH levels of 2.5 to 4.0 mU/L with positive TPO antibodies. The American College of Obstetricians and Gynecologists (ACOG) has stated that there is no evidence to support screening for and treating subclinical hypothyroidism, but it does not address TPO antibody status or the degree of TSH elevation. Because a

TSH level of $\geq$ 4 mU/L is definitely abnormal for pregnancy, most health care providers treat patients with this TSH level, whether or not they have positive TPO antibodies. Furthermore, obtaining TPO antibody measurements can delay treatment, and there remains controversy as to the level at which TPO antibodies should be considered positive. Because there has been no demonstrated benefit in treating TPO antibody–positive patients with a TSH level of 2.5 to 4 mU/L, treating patients with TSH values < 4 mU/L is not recommended because it may result in overtreatment. Treatment for patients with a TSH between 4 and 10 mU/L should be with low doses of LT_4 (50 mcg daily) and a goal on-treatment TSH level of 0.5 to 2.5 mU/L.

42. What is the risk of abnormal intellectual development in infants born to mothers who are hypothyroid during the first trimester of pregnancy?

All newborns in the United States are screened for hypothyroidism because it is well established that infants who have severe congenital hypothyroidism but who then receive thyroid hormone therapy at birth appear to have fairly normal intellectual growth and development. As previously mentioned, fetal brain maturation is dependent on maternal thyroid hormone prior to 18 weeks and retrospective studies have suggested that infants born to mothers who had untreated overt hypothyroidism during pregnancy have slightly decreased neurodevelopmental testing results. However, whether subclinical hypothyroidism causes any neurodevelopmental concerns remains a matter of debate, as discussed previously.

43. Should all pregnant women be screened for elevated TSH in early pregnancy?

Because of maternal and fetal concerns, some have advocated universal screening of pregnant women in the first trimester for elevated TSH levels. It has been shown that targeted screening of only high-risk women fails to detect approximately 25% to 35% of women with elevated TSH values. However, given the lack of evidence supporting the treatment of mild subclinical hypothyroidism in pregnancy as discussed above, the ACOG does not recommend universal screening for abnormal TSH levels in pregnancy. In its 2017 guidelines, the ATA stated that there is insufficient evidence either for or against universal screening for abnormal TSH levels early in pregnancy. Currently, the ATA recommends that all pregnant women undergo clinical screening for risk factors for hypothyroidism and that TSH levels be measured in women with the following risk factors:

1. History of hypo- or hyperthyroidism or current signs/symptoms of thyroid dysfunction
2. Known thyroid antibody positivity or presence of a goiter
3. History of head or neck radiation or prior thyroid surgery
4. Age > 30 years
5. Type 1 diabetes (T1D) or other autoimmune disorders
6. History of pregnancy loss, preterm delivery, or infertility
7. Multiple prior pregnancies (> 2)
8. Family history of autoimmune thyroid disease or thyroid dysfunction
9. Morbid obesity (body mass index [BMI] > 40 kg/m^2)
10. Use of amiodarone or lithium, or recent administration of iodinated radiologic contrast
11. Residing in an area of moderate-to-severe iodine insufficiency

44. Should pregnant women with recurrent pregnancy loss be screened for TPO antibodies and, if the antibodies are found, should thyroid hormone be offered despite a normal serum TSH?

Several meta-analyses have found an increased rate of nonrecurrent spontaneous pregnancy loss in TPO antibody-positive (TPO+) women, with odds ratios ranging from 2.3 to 3.9. There are also data linking thyroid autoimmunity with recurrent pregnancy loss (two consecutive pregnancy losses or three total losses). However, a causal relationship has not been established. Several mechanisms explaining the link have been proposed, including decreased thyroid reserve/thyroid hypofunction, altered endometrial cytokine levels, altered trophoblast function, and autoimmunity. However, these antibodies may simply be markers of other autoimmune diseases that could be associated with pregnancy loss. A single RCT by Negro et al. (2006) suggested that treating unselected euthyroid women who were TPO+ with low doses of thyroid hormone could decrease first trimester loss but not loss later in pregnancy. However, many of the losses occurred so early that initiating treatment before the loss would not have been possible, and it is difficult to understand on a mechanistic basis how only several days of treatment could prevent pregnancy loss. A subsequent larger trial by Negro et al. (2016) found no benefit in treatment of TPO+ women who had serum TSH levels < 2.5 mU/L. A trial from China randomized 600 euthyroid TPO+ women who were undergoing in vitro fertilization (IVF) and embryo transfer to treatment with 25 to 50 mcg/day of LT_4 versus no therapy and found no reduction of miscarriage rates or improvement in live birth rates. There are two ongoing RCTs assessing the impact of LT_4 treatment versus placebo on live birth rates. The ongoing Thyroid AntiBodies and LEvoThyroxine study (TABLET) in the United Kingdom is randomizing euthyroid TPO+ women with a history of infertility or recurrent losses, and the ongoing T4Lifetrial in the Netherlands is doing the same in women with a history of recurrent loss. Although the ATA considers that treatment of TPO+ women with a history of recurrent pregnancy loss could be an option, the ACOG has stated that women with recurrent pregnancy loss should not be routinely screened for TPO antibodies. Women who are TPO+ clearly have approximately a 15% risk of developing subclinical hypothyroidism later in pregnancy and a 50% chance of postpartum thyroiditis; therefore, they should be monitored closely for these developments.

KEY POINTS: THYROID DISEASE IN PREGNANCY

- All women at increased risk for thyroid disease should be screened in the first trimester.
- The normal ranges of thyroid-stimulating hormone (TSH), total thyroxine (TT_4) and total triiodothyronine (TT_3) change in pregnancy, and free T_4 and free T_3 assays by analogue methods may be inaccurate. TT_4 and TT_3 increase by $\approx$ 50%, and a TSH reference range of 0.1 to 4.0 mU/L has been recently advocated.
- Gestational transient thyrotoxicosis associated with hyperemesis gravidarum can cause overt hyperthyroidism, but this most often is self-limiting and does not require antithyroid drug (ATD) therapy.
- Graves' disease most commonly manifests in the first trimester with improvement in later pregnancy and treatment can often be tapered, but it usually exacerbates after delivery.
- Women with current Graves' disease or a history of Graves' disease (regardless of history of thyroid ablation or thyroidectomy) should be evaluated for TSH receptor antibodies (TRAbs) and thyroid-stimulating immunoglobulins (TSIs). If levels are $\geq$ 3 times elevated at 18 weeks' gestation or beyond, the fetus should be monitored for the development of fetal and neonatal Graves' disease.
- Subclinical hyperthyroidism (only a suppressed TSH) should *not* be treated in pregnancy.
- Treatment of subclinical hypothyroidism should be offered if TSH is > 4 mU/L; treatment is with low doses of levothyroxine (50 mcg daily) and a goal TSH level of 0.5 to 2.5 mU/L.
- Although thyroperoxidase (TPO) antibodies may be associated with a small increased risk of miscarriage, there is currently insufficient evidence to recommend routine screening for TPO antibodies and treatment of TPO antibody–positive women with a history of recurrent pregnancy loss if they are euthyroid.
- Thyroid hormone requirements usually increase in pregnancy, beginning in the first trimester, and it is reasonable to increase thyroid hormone doses by 25% in athyreotic women as soon as pregnancy is confirmed. Only LT_4 (not T_3) should be used for thyroid hormone replacement and a full replacement dose is estimated at $\approx$ 2 mcg/kg in pregnancy.
- Postpartum thyroiditis occurs in approximately 5% of physiologically normal women and approximately 20% to 25% of women with T1D.

45. How do LT_4 therapy requirements change during pregnancy?

LT_4 dose requirements in treated hypothyroid patients often increase during pregnancy, with up to 75% of pregnant women requiring an increase in dosage of 25% to 30%. One study suggested that athyreotic women requiring full replacement doses should receive a 25% dose increase as soon as pregnancy is confirmed despite a normal TSH, and another study confirmed that 85% of athyreotic pregnant women required an increase in LT_4 of 47% by 16 weeks of pregnancy.

46. What causes the rapid increase in thyroid hormone requirements in early pregnancy?

The rapid increase in TH requirements that occurs in the first trimester may result from the sudden increase in the estrogen-stimulated TBG pool associated with pregnancy. This change can be especially striking in women undergoing assisted reproduction with very high estrogen levels.

47. In women with hypothyroidism, when should TSH be checked in pregnancy, what doses of thyroid hormone should be prescribed, and at what level of TSH should therapy be directed?

The TSH level should be checked as soon as pregnancy is confirmed, and an appropriate increase in the LT_4 dose should be made. Athyreotic women, or those requiring full replacement doses of LT_4, should receive a 25% to 30% dose increase as soon as pregnancy is confirmed. One trial demonstrated that this can be done by adding two tablets of the current LT_4 dose per week to the patient's regimen. As discussed earlier, the TSH may be mildly suppressed in normal women during the first trimester because of the thyrotropic influence of hCG. Therefore, unless a woman is symptomatically hyperthyroid or has frankly elevated serum FT_4 levels, the LT_4 dosage should not be reduced in response to the finding of a low first-trimester TSH.

Women with subclinical hypothyroidism (TSH 4–10 mU/L) can usually be adequately treated with 50 mcg/day of LT_4 or 75 mcg/day if they are heavier and TSH levels are in the 7- to 10-mU/L range. Pregnant women with overt hypothyroidism (elevated TSH; FT_4 below the normal range or TSH > 10 mU/L) should be given full LT_4 replacement doses immediately; this can be estimated at 2 mcg/kg/day in pregnancy. Liothyronine (LT_3) should not be used in pregnancy, given the poor placental passage of T_3 and the fetal brain requirements for T_4. The serum TSH level should be checked 4 weeks after a dose change and every 4 weeks until $\approx$ 18 weeks to target TSH levels between 0.5 and 2.5 mU/L (and ensure TSH is maintained at < 4 mU/L) while the fetus is dependent on maternal TH. Once stable, levels can then be monitored every 4 to 8 weeks for the remainder of pregnancy. In women who have had a thyroidectomy for thyroid cancer, the goal of maintaining a suppressed but detectable serum TSH without rendering them thyrotoxic should be adhered to during pregnancy. The LT_4 dose should be reduced almost immediately after delivery to avoid hyperthyroidism; prepregnancy doses may be resumed as soon as the woman has lost the majority of her pregnancy weight gain. A TSH level should be checked 6 weeks after delivery.

48. Can commonly used supplements, such as biotin, affect thyroid function laboratory assays?

    Patients are increasingly using biotin dietary supplements marketed to improve hair, skin, and nail health. However, excess biotin in blood can affect laboratory assays that utilize biotinylated antibodies and thereby lead to interference and erroneous test results, especially if the patient has taken biotin within several hours of having her sample taken. There are case reports of misdiagnoses of hyperthyroidism in patients taking large doses of biotin, resulting in interference with biotin-sensitive immunoassays, including T_4, T_3, TSH, thyroglobulin, and TRAb assays. In one case, the test results were questioned because the patient had no hyperthyroid symptoms, and the results normalized when the test was repeated after several days of cessation of biotin treatment. All patients being evaluated for thyroid disorders should be questioned on their use of dietary supplements, and biotin-sensitive tests should be avoided in those patients ingesting supplementary biotin. The FT_4 equilibrium dialysis assay should not be affected. Alternatively, biotin-sensitive tests can be accurately performed 2 to 3 days after supplements have been held. Finally, results should be interpreted in the overall clinical context and results questioned if they are not consistent with the patient presentation or symptoms.

49. When should a pregnant woman take her thyroid hormone?

    It is extremely important to advise the pregnant woman to take her LT_4 and prenatal vitamins and/or iron supplements at least 4 hours apart because ferrous sulfate can bind to T_4 and decrease its bioavailability. High doses of calcium and soy can also interfere with LT_4 absorption.

50. How should a thyroid nodule be evaluated during pregnancy?

    Both hormonal effects, likely from estrogen, progesterone, and hCG, and from relative iodine deficiency, likely contribute to the development of thyroid nodules during pregnancy. The evaluation of a solitary or dominant thyroid nodule in a pregnant woman is similar to that in nonpregnant women. Ultrasonography is indicated to evaluate for multiple nodules and for ultrasonographic features suggestive of malignancy (microcalcifications, hypoechoic patterns, irregular margins, nodules that are taller than they are wide, intranodular vascularity, and lymphadenopathy). In patients with a normal or elevated serum TSH, nodules are recommended for fine-needle aspiration biopsy (FNAB) based on size and sonographic appearance. The ATA 2015 guidelines recommend FNAB of nodules consistent with high and intermediate suspicion patterns if > 1 cm in size, low suspicion pattern if > 1.5 cm, and very low suspicion pattern if > 2 cm in size or not at all, with clinical observation being an acceptable alternative. FNAB of purely cystic nodules is not indicated for cytology determination. Abnormal-appearing cervical lymph nodes should also be targeted for biopsy. The ATA does not recommend FNAB for nodules < 1 cm unless associated with pathologic lymphadenopathy, extrathyroidal extension, or a high-risk personal history (rapid onset or growth of nodule, history of head and neck irradiation during childhood, hoarseness, persistent cough). Women who have nodules discovered in the last month of pregnancy can have FNAB delayed until after delivery, but it is often helpful to make the diagnosis of thyroid cancer during pregnancy so that appropriate planning of surgical treatment can be made. Women found to have a thyroid nodule and suppressed TSH may have a warm or hot nodule. Warm or hot nodules are rarely malignant but FNAB is often nondiagnostic. Therefore, pregnant women with a suppressed TSH and a nodule should undergo a radioisotope scan after delivery to determine whether it is a warm or a cold nodule before obtaining an FNAB. FNAB specimens should be evaluated with the same criteria as used for non-pregnant patients.

51. What is the likelihood that thyroid nodules discovered during pregnancy are malignant?

    Data suggest that thyroid nodules discovered during pregnancy may have a higher risk of being malignant compared with nodules in nonpregnant women. However, this finding is likely partly the result of selection or sampling bias because many young women do not have systematic health examinations until they become pregnant. Also, these data have come from tertiary referral centers and, thus, are not likely representative of the general pregnant population. Depending on the patient population, the incidence of benign cytology among biopsied nodules has been > 80%, whereas differentiated thyroid cancer has been found in 5% to 40% of biopsies. Most malignant nodules are papillary thyroid carcinoma. FNA cytology is highly accurate in diagnosing papillary carcinoma, whereas cytology showing follicular or Hürthle cell neoplasms predicts only a 5% to 20% likelihood of malignancy. There are no prospective studies evaluating the outcome and prognosis of thyroid nodules with indeterminate cytology in pregnant women. During pregnancy, surgery is usually deferred until after delivery for nodules with indeterminate or suspicious cytology, unless clinical suspicion is high for aggressive behavior. Molecular genetic testing is not validated in pregnancy because of the unknown influence of pregnancy on signaling biomarkers; therefore, this is not recommended in pregnancy but may be useful after delivery to stratify the risk of malignancy in indeterminate nodules.

52. How should a malignant thyroid nodule be managed during pregnancy?

    If FNA cytology suggests or confirms papillary thyroid cancer, the best time to offer a thyroidectomy is in the second trimester to avoid the risk of miscarriage in the first trimester and preterm labor in the third trimester. The risk of preterm labor or adverse fetal outcomes related to surgery performed in the second trimester is exceedingly low. If the nodule is < 2 cm, has not rapidly increased in size, and the patient has no lymphadenopathy, it may be reasonable to postpone thyroidectomy until after delivery and consider administering LT_4 suppression therapy in the meantime, with careful attention to avoiding elevated T_4 levels. It is appropriate to administer LT_4 to achieve a suppressed but detectable serum TSH level in pregnant women with a recent history of thyroid cancer or thyroid cancer diagnosed during pregnancy, or when there is a highly suspicious thyroid nodule, provided the FT_4 or TT_4 levels are not increased above the normal range for pregnancy. Disease-specific survival has not been shown to be affected by whether thyroidectomy for a malignant nodule is performed during pregnancy or immediately after delivery as long as the nodule shows well-differentiated thyroid cancer and treatment occurs within 1 year of diagnosis. However, some evidence suggests that recurrence, based on serum TG levels or rising TG antibody titers, may be slightly higher in women who wait to have surgery after delivery compared with women who elect to have surgery in the second trimester.

53. How common is postpartum thyroiditis? Who is at risk, and what is the pathology?

Postpartum thyroid dysfunction occurs in approximately 5% to 10% of women, with a much higher incidence in certain populations. In one series, 25% of women with T1D developed postpartum thyroid dysfunction; it is, therefore, recommended that women with T1D be routinely screened during the postpartum period. In another series of 152 TPO+ women detected at 16 weeks, postpartum thyroiditis occurred in 50%. Of these, 19% had hyperthyroidism alone, 49% had hypothyroidism alone, and 32% had hyperthyroidism followed by hypothyroidism. Women known to be TPO+ should have a serum TSH level measured at 6 to 12 weeks and 6 months after delivery, or if they develop symptoms.

The disorder is highly associated with TPO antibodies and the histology is identical to Hashimoto's thyroiditis with diffuse mononuclear cell infiltration and destruction of thyroid follicles.

54. What are the phases of postpartum thyroiditis, and how does the first phase typically present?

Classically, the clinical course consists of three phases (hyperthyroidism, then hypothyroidism, followed by resolution), but not all women manifest each phase.

At 1 to 3 months after delivery, affected women develop mild hyperthyroidism secondary to immunologically mediated destruction of thyroid follicles, resulting in the release of stored TH into the circulation. Such women may experience anxiety, irritability, palpitations, fatigue, and insomnia, but commonly, this phase does not come to clinical attention. Symptomatic patients are best treated with low-dose beta-blockers, which must soon be tapered and discontinued as the thyrotoxic phase resolves spontaneously. The use of PTU or MMI is not indicated because the hyperthyroidism in these patients is caused by inflammatory destruction of thyroid follicles and not by increased TH synthesis.

55. How can phase 1 of postpartum thyroiditis be distinguished from Graves' disease?

Occasionally, there is a question about the cause of the postpartum hyperthyroidism because Graves' disease commonly appears or exacerbates in the first several months after delivery. Distinguishing between the two conditions is facilitated by measurement of a serum TG level and TPO antibodies (both are high in postpartum thyroiditis) and TRAbs or TSIs (often elevated with Graves' disease). However, the most definitive test is a ^{123}I uptake test (low in postpartum thyroiditis and high in Graves' disease), if the mother is willing to interrupt nursing for 2 to 3 days. Ultrasonography can sometimes demonstrate Graves' disease versus lymphocytic thyroiditis on the basis of size, vascularity, and heterogeneity of the gland.

56. Describe phase 2 of postpartum thyroiditis, how it is treated, and the usual course.

More commonly, women present with stage 2 of postpartum thyroiditis, which is characterized by hypothyroidism alone or following transient hyperthyroidism (phase 1), at about 4 to 8 months after delivery. Nonspecific symptoms include fatigue, depression, impaired concentration or memory, dry skin, and weight gain, all of which may be overlooked by the clinician. Symptoms may predate the onset of thyroid function abnormalities in TPO+ women and may persist for some time after a euthyroid state is achieved. Women with abnormal thyroid function tests and symptoms consistent with hypothyroidism should be treated with LT_4 replacement for approximately 6 to 12 months or at least until 1 year after delivery. At that time, discontinuation of LT_4 can be attempted to identify the 70% to 80% of women who will return to the euthyroid state by 12 months after delivery.

However, thyroid function tests should then be performed at least annually in women who become euthyroid. In a series of 43 patients with postpartum thyroiditis, 23% of the women were hypothyroid at 2 to 4 years, and, in a longer series, approximately 50% of women were hypothyroid 7 to 9 years later. Women with the highest TPO antibody titers and the most severe hypothyroidism appear to be at the highest risk of developing permanent hypothyroidism. If a woman becomes euthyroid within a year after delivery, she has a high likelihood (70%) of developing postpartum thyroiditis after a subsequent pregnancy.

BIBLIOGRAPHY

Alexander, E. K., Pearce, E. N., Brent, G. A., Brown, R. S., Chen, H., Dosiou, C., ... Sullivan, S. (2017). 2017 Guidelines of the American Thyroid Association for the Diagnosis and Management of Thyroid Disease During Pregnancy and the Postpartum. American Thyroid Association Taskforce on Thyroid Disease During Pregnancy and Postpartum. *Thyroid, 27,* 315–389.

American College of Obstetricians and Gynecologists. (2015). Practice Bulletin No. 148. Thyroid disease in pregnancy. *Obstetrics and Gynecology, 125,* 996–1005.

Andersen, S. L., Olsen, J., Wu, C. S., & Laurberg, P. (2014). Severity of birth defects after propylthiouracil exposure in early pregnancy. *Thyroid*, *24*, 1533–1540.

Andersen, S. L., Olsen, J., & Laurberg, P. (2015). Foetal programming by maternal thyroid disease. *Clinical Endocrinology*, *83*, 751–758.

Azizi, F., Khoshniat, M., Bahrainian, M., & Hedayati, M. (2000). Thyroid function and intellectual development of infants nursed by mothers taking methimazole. *Journal of Clinical Endocrinology and Metabolism*, *85*, 3233–3238.

Barbesino, G. (2016). Misdiagnosis of Graves' disease with apparent severe hyperthyroidism in a patient taking biotin megadoses. *Thyroid*, *26*, 860–863.

Bilir, B. E., Atile, N. S., Kirkizlar, O., Kömürcü, Y., Akpinar, S., Sezer, A., ... Hekimoğlu, S. (2013). Effectiveness of preoperative plasmapheresis in a pregnancy complicated by hyperthyroidism and anti-thyroid associated angioedema. *Gynecological Endocrinology*, *29*(5), 508–510.

Boucek, J., de Haan, J., Halaska, M. J., Plzak, J., Van Calsteren, K., de Groot, C. J. M., ... Amant, F. (2018). Maternal and obstetrical outcome in 35 cases of well-differentiated thyroid carcinoma during pregnancy. *Laryngoscope*, *128*(6), 1493–1500.

Casey, B. M., Dashe, J. S., Wells, C. E., McIntire, D. D., Leveno, K. J., & Cunningham, F. G. (2006). Subclinical hyperthyroidism and pregnancy outcomes. *Obstetrics and Gynecology*, *107*, 337–341.

Casey, B. M., Thom, E. A., Peaceman, A. M., Varner, M. W., Sorokin, Y., Hirtz, D. G., ... VanDorsten, J. P. (2017). Treatment of subclinical hypothyroidism orhypothyroxinemia in pregnancy. *New England Journal of Medicine*, *376*, 815–825.

De Groot, L., Abalovich, M., Alexander, E., Amino, N., Barbour, L., Cobin, R. H., ... Sullivan, S. (2012). Management of thyroid dysfunction during pregnancy and postpartum: an Endocrine Society clinical practice guideline. *Journal of Clinical Endocrinology and Metabolism*, *97*, 2543–2565.

De Leo, S., & Pearce, E. N. (2018). Autoimmune thyroid disease during pregnancy. *Lancet. Diabetes & Endocrinology*, *6*, 575–586.

Donnelly, M. A., Wood, C., Casey, B., Hobbins, J., & Barbour, L. A. (2015). Earliest case report of severe fetal Graves' disease in a mother previously treated with both thyroid ablation and surgical removal. *Obstetrics and Gynecology*, *25*(5), 1059–1062.

Fang, Y., Yao, L., Sun, J., Zhang, J., Li, Y., Yang, R., ... Tian, L. (2018). Appraisal of clinical practice guidelines on the management of hypothyroidism in pregnancy using the Appraisal of Guidelines for Research and Evaluation II instrument. *Endocrine*, *60*, 4–14.

Haddow, J. E., Cleary-Goldman, J., McClain, M. R., Palomaki, G. E., Neveux, L. M., Lambert-Messerlian, G., ... D'Alton, M. E. (2010). Thyroperoxidase and thyroglobulin antibodies in early pregnancy and preterm delivery. *Obstetrics and Gynecology*, *116*, 58–62.

Haugen, B. R., Alexander, E. K., Bible, K. C., Doherty, G. M., Mandel, S. J, Nikiforov, Y. E., ... Wartofsky, L. (2016). 2015 American Thyroid Association Management Guidelines for Adult Patients with Thyroid Nodules and Differentiated Thyroid Cancer. American Thyroid Association Guidelines Task Force on Thyroid Nodules and Differentiated Thyroid Cancer. *Thyroid*, *26*, 1–133.

Haymart, M. R., & Pearce, E. N. (2017). How much should thyroid cancer impact plans for pregnancy? *Thyroid*, *27*(3), 312–314.

King, J. R., Lachica, R., Lee, R. H., Montoro, M., & Mestman, J. (2016). Diagnosis and management of hyperthyroidism in pregnancy. A review. *Obstetrical & Gynecological Survey*, *71*, 675–685.

Korevaar, T., Tiemeier, H., & Peeters, R. P. (2018). Clinical associations of maternal thyroid function with foetal brain development: epidemiological interpretation and overview of available evidence. *Clinical Endocrinology*, *89*, 129–138.

Laurberg, P., Wallin, G., Tallstedt, L., Abraham-Nordling, M., Lundell, G., & Tørring, O. (2008). TSH-receptor autoimmunity in Graves' disease after therapy with antithyroid drugs, surgery or radioiodine: a 5-year prospective randomized study. *European Journal of Endocrinology*, *156*, 69–75.

Lazarus, J. H., Bestwick, J. P., Channon, S., Paradice, R., Maina, A., Rees, R., ... Wald, N. J. (2012). Antenatal thyroid screening and childhood cognitive function. *New England Journal of Medicine*, *366*, 493–501.

Leiva, P., Schwarze, J. E., Vasquez, P., Ortega, C., Villa, S., Crosby, J., ... Pommer, R. (2017). There is no association between the presence of anti-thyroid antibodies and increased reproductive loss in pregnant women after ART: a systematic review and meta-analysis. *JBRA Assisted Reproduction*, *21*(4), 361–365.

Li, D., Radulescu, A., Shrestha, R. T., Root, M., Karger, A. B., Killeen, A. A., ... Burmeister, L. A. (2017). Association of biotin ingestion with performance of hormone and nonhormone assays in healthy adults. *JAMA*, *318*, 1150–1160.

Lockwood, C. M., Grenache, D. G., & Gronowski, A. M. (2009). Serum human chorionic gonadotropin concentrations greater than 400,000 IU/L are invariably associated with suppressed serum thyrotropin concentrations. *Thyroid*, *19*, 863–868.

Luton, D., Le Gac, I., Vuillard, E., Castanet, M., Guibourdenche, J., Noel, M., ... Polak, M. (2005). Management of Grave's disease during pregnancy: the key role of fetal thyroid gland monitoring. *Journal of Clinical Endocrinology and Metabolism*, *90*, 6093–6098.

Maraka, S., Ospina, N. M., O'Keeffe, D. T., Espinosa De Ycaza, A. E., Gionfriddo, M. R., Erwin, P. J., ... Montori, V. M. (2016). Subclinical hypothyroidism in pregnancy: a systematic review and meta-analysis. *Thyroid*, *26*, 580–590.

Maraka, S., Singh Ospina, N. M., Mastorakos, G., & O'Keeffe, D. T. (2018). Subclinical hypothyroidism in women planning conception and during pregnancy: who should be treated and how? *Journal of Endocrine Society*, *2*(6), 533–546.

Mayson, S., & Barbour, L. A. (2019). Thyroid nodules and cancer in pregnancy. In J. Eaton (Ed.), *Thyroid Disease and Reproduction: A Clinical Guide to Diagnosis and Management* (pp. 137–156). Springer Nature Switzerland AG.

Miranda, A., & Sousa, N. (2018). Maternal hormonal milieu influence on fetal brain development. *Brain and Behavior*, *8*:e00920.

Moog, N. K., Entringer, S., Heim, C., Wadhwa, P. D., Kathmann, N., & Buss, C. (2017). Influence of maternal thyroid hormones during gestation on fetal brain development. *Neuroscience*, *342*, 68–100.

Nachum, Z., Rakover, Y., Weiner, E., & Shalev, I. (2003). Grave's disease in pregnancy: prospective evaluation of a selective invasive treatment protocol. *American Journal of Obstetrics and Gynecology*, *189*, 159–165.

Negro, R., Formoso, G., Mangieri, T., Pezzarossa, A., Dazzi, D., & Hassan, H. (2006). Levothyroxine treatment in euthyroid pregnant women with autoimmune thyroid disease: effects on obstetrical complications. *Journal of Clinical Endocrinology and Metabolism*, *91*, 2587–2591.

Negro, R., Schwartz, A., Gismondi, R., Tinelli, A., Mangieri, T., & Stagnaro-Green, A. (2010). Increased pregnancy loss rate in thyroid antibody negative women with TSH levels between 2.5 and 5.0 in the first trimester of pregnancy. *Journal of Clinical Endocrinology and Metabolism*, *95*, E44–E448.

Negro, R., Schwartz, A., Gismondi, R., Tinelli, A., Mangieri, T., & Stagnaro-Green, A. (2010). Universal screening versus case finding for detection and treatment of thyroid hormonal dysfunction during pregnancy. *Journal of Clinical Endocrinology and Metabolism*, *95*, 1699–1707.

Negro, R., Schwartz, A., & Stagnaro-Green, A. (2016). Impact of levothyroxine in miscarriage and preterm delivery rates in first trimester thyroid antibody positive women with TSH < 2.5 mU/L. *Journal of Clinical Endocrinology and Metabolism*, *101*(10), 3685–3690.

Nguyen, C. T., Sasso, E. B., Barton, L., & Mestman, J. H. (2018). Graves' hyperthyroidism in pregnancy: a clinical review. *Clinical Diabetes and Endocrinology*, *4*, 4.

Okosieme, O. E., Khan, I., & Taylor, P. (2018). Preconception management of thyroid dysfunction. *Clinical Endocrinology, 89*(3), 269–279.

Patel, J., Landers, K., Huika, L., & Richard, K. (2011). Delivery of maternal thyroid hormones to the fetus. *Trends in Endocrinology and Metabolism, 22,* 164–170.

Pearce, E. N., Lazarus, J. H., Moreno-Reyes, R., & Zimmermann, M. B. (2016). Consequences of iodine deficiency and excess in pregnant women: an overview of current knowns and unknowns. *American Journal of Clinical Nutrition, 104*(Suppl. 3), S918–S923.

Pelag, D., Cada, S., Peleg, A., & Ben-Ami, M. (2002). The relationship between maternal serum thyroid-stimulating immunoglobulin and fetal and neonatal thyrotoxicosis. *Obstetrics and Gynecology, 99,* 1040–1043.

Sam, S., & Molitch, M. E. (2003). Timing and special concerns regarding endocrine surgery during pregnancy. *Endocrinology and Metabolism Clinics of North America, 32,* 337–354.

Sapin, R., D'Herbomez, M., & Schlienger, J. L. (2004). Free thyroxine measured with equilibrium dialysis and nine immunoassays decreased in late pregnancy. *Clinical Laboratory, 50,* 581–584.

van der Kaay, D. C., Wasserman, J. D., & Palmer, M. R. (2016). Management of neonates born to mothers with Graves' disease. *Pediatrics, 137*(4), e20151878.

Vannucchi, G., Perrino, N., Rossi, S., Colombo, C., Vicentini, L., Dazzi, D., ... Fugazzola, L. (2010). Clinical and molecular features of differentiated thyroid cancer diagnosed during pregnancy. *European Journal of Endocrinology, 162,* 145–151.

Walker, J. A., Illions, E. H., Huddleston, J. F., & Smallridge, R. C. (2005). Racial comparisons of thyroid function and autoimmunity during pregnancy and the postpartum period. *Obstetrics and Gynecology, 106,* 1365–1371.

Want, H., Gao, H., Chi, H., Zeng, L., Xiao, W., Wang, Y., ... Qiao, J. (2017). Effect of levothyroxine on miscarriage among women with normal thyroid function and thyroid autoimmunity undergoing in vitro fertilization and embryo transfer: a randomized clinical trial. *JAMA, 318*(22), 2190–2198.

Wu, J. X., Young, S., Ro, K., Li, N., Leung, A. M., Chiu, H. K., ... Yeh, M. W. (2015). Reproductive outcomes and nononcologic complications after radioactive iodine ablation for well-differentiated thyroid cancer. *Thyroid, 25*(1), 133–138.

Yassa, L., Marqusee, E., Fawcett, R., & Alexander, E. K. (2010). Thyroid hormone early adjustment in pregnancy (the THERAPY) trial. *Journal of Clinical Endocrinology and Metabolism, 95,* 3234–3241.

Zhou, Y. Q., Zhou, Z., Qian, M. F., & Wang, J. D. (2015). Association of thyroid carcinoma with pregnancy: a meta-analysis. *Molecular and Clinical Oncology, 3*(2), 341–346.

CHAPTER 47

PSYCHIATRIC DISORDERS AND THYROID DISEASE

Roselyn I. Mateo and James V. Hennessey

1. How is hypothyroidism diagnosed—then and now?

For over a century, since the publication of the Clinical Society of London's "Report on Myxoedema" in 1888, it has been recognized that overt clinical thyroid disease may give rise to psychiatric disorders that can be corrected by the reestablishment of normal thyroid hormone levels. In those times, hypothyroidism was fatal. Almost all patients were diagnosed late in the course of their disease and were often besieged with intellectual, neurologic, and psychiatric deficiencies.

Just 50 years later, Asher reemphasized the fact that patients with profound hypothyroidism may present with psychosis and thus coined the term "myxedema madness." He reported that although the presentation is inconsistent, general confusion and disorientation with persecutory delusions and hallucinations were common. Diagnosis was based on the myxedematous appearance of the patient and not the specific mental symptoms. In fact, prior to the advent of routine laboratory measurements of TSH and thyroid hormones, thyroid status was assessed by using tools that may have correlated with thyroid dysfunction but were not sufficiently specific to ensure a definitive diagnosis. Asher would use a photograph taken before and after thyroid treatment, with a recognizable change serving as a confirmatory test. Other markers of diagnostic value, such as blood cholesterol, decreased sleeping heart rate, delay in Achilles' tendon reflex time, and basal metabolic rate, were the standard. Extremely high and low values correlated well with marked hyperthyroidism and hypothyroidism, respectively. However, Asher commented that the presence of mental changes or respiratory obstruction and other diverse conditions, such as acute hospitalization, nonthyroidal illness, pregnancy, cancer, acromegaly, hypogonadism, and starvation, compromised the accuracy of diagnosis.

In current practice, the measurement of serum thyroid-stimulating hormone (TSH) and free thyroxine (FT_4) are the primary tests for diagnosing thyroid dysfunction and evaluation of thyroid hormone replacement in patients with primary hypothyroidism.

2. How is hypothyroidism linked to psychiatric disease?

It is well recognized that overt disturbances in thyroid function may significantly affect mental status, emotion, cognition, and mood. Hypothyroid symptoms, as outlined in the Table 47.1, are nonspecific and often mimic those of depression, whereas those of hyperthyroidism, which include anxiety, dysphoria, emotional lability, and intellectual dysfunction, may be seen in both mania and depression, the latter being especially characteristic among the elderly presenting with (the so-called) apathetic thyrotoxicosis.

3. Which patients with symptoms consistent with the presence of thyroid dysfunction are typically evaluated with TSH and circulating thyroid hormone levels?

Those who are referred for thyroid function testing, based on clinical suspicion of thyroid dysfunction, have been shown to have high rates of psychological distress but are no more likely than asymptomatic subjects to have hypothyroidism. Hence, if mild elevations in TSH, consistent with the presence of "subclinical hypothyroidism," are detected in patients with psychological distress, it is more likely to be a coincidental finding rather than an absolute causal finding. Because of this, such patients would not automatically warrant treatment in the absence of significant hypo- or hyperthyroidism because this would be unlikely to result in clinical improvement.

4. What is the association between subclinical hypothyroidism and depression?

Observational studies have reported an increased prevalence of depression in subjects with subclinical hypothyroidism, defined as a TSH greater than "normal," whereas FT_4 was normal; however, larger and more recent studies have found no difference in depressive symptoms between euthyroid and subclinically hypothyroid subjects at baseline and when monitored over time.

Kim et al. (2018) conducted a large prospective study in a cohort of 220,545 subjects, without a diagnosis of depression at baseline, who underwent at least two comprehensive health examinations between January 1, 2011, and December 31, 2014. TSH, free triiodothyronine (FT_3), and FT_4 levels were measured at baseline, and incident depressive symptoms occurred in 7323 (8%) participants over a mean follow-up period of 2 years. After accounting for covariates, the authors found no association between biochemical subclinical hypothyroidism, defined as a FT_4 within the normal range and TSH > 5 mU/L, and incident depressive symptoms. Sensitivity analyses among the participants with subclinical hypothyroidism (n = 4384), further subdivided by TSH levels, showed similar associations with depression for those with TSH ≤ 10 and TSH > 10 mU/L. Similarly, there was no association between

Table 47.1. Clinical Features Common to Both Thyroid Diseases and Mood Disorders.

	HYPOTHYROIDISM	MOOD DISORDERS	HYPERTHYROIDISM
Depression	Yes	Yes	Yes
Diminished interest	Yes	Yes	Yes
Diminished pleasure	Yes	Yes	No
Decreased libido	Yes	Yes	Sometimes
Weight loss	No	Yes	Yes
Weight gain	Yes	Sometimes	Occasionally
Appetite loss	Yes	Yes	Sometimes
Increased appetite	No	Yes	Yes
Insomnia	No	Yes	Yes
Hypersomnia	Yes	Yes	No
Agitation/anxiety	Occasionally	Yes	Yes
Fatigue	Yes	Yes	Yes
Poor memory	Yes	Yes	Occasionally
Cognitive dysfunction	Yes	Yes	Yes
Impaired concentration	Yes	Yes	Yes
Constipation	Yes	Sometimes	No

Adapted from Hennessey, J. V., & Jackson, I. M. D. (1996). The interface between thyroid hormones and psychiatry. *Endocrinologist, 6*, 214–223.

circulating thyroid hormone levels and the risk of incident depressive symptoms among the euthyroid participants (n = 87,822).

In an older population age 70 to 82 years, Blum et al. (2016) conducted a cross-sectional and longitudinal study involving 606 participants without antidepressant medication use. Geriatric Depression Scale 15 (GDS-15) scores at baseline did not differ among participants with subclinical hypothyroidism (defined as TSH levels $\geq$ 4.5 mU/L and FT_4 within the reference range of 12–18 pmol/L), those with baseline subclinical hyperthyroidism (defined as TSH levels < 0.45 mU/L and FT_4 within the reference range of 12–18 pmol/L), and those designated as the euthyroid controls. After 3 years, changes in GDS-15 scores did not differ for participants considered to have subclinical hypothyroidism at baseline, while those considered subclinically hyperthyroid experienced an increase in GDS-15 scores consistent with the development of depression.

5. What is the impact of mild thyroid dysfunction on performance and survival in old age?

Gussekloo et al. (2004) conducted a study evaluating 599 elderly participants (age 85–89 years at enrollment) who were followed up for a mean of 3.7 years. Results showed that baseline serum levels of TSH and FT_4 were not associated with disability in daily life, depressive symptoms, or cognitive impairment at baseline or during follow-up. Mildly elevated TSH levels were paradoxically associated with decreased all-cause mortality in both men and women, after adjusting for baseline disability and health status, whereas increasing FT_4 levels were associated with increased mortality. Therefore, the general population of the "oldest old" with higher levels of TSH does not appear to experience adverse effects and may have a prolonged life span.

6. What is the association between subclinical hyperthyroidism and depression?

Findings derived from the prospective Caerphilly Prospective Study (CaPS), which consisted of 2269 middle-aged men (age 45–59 years) with thyroid dysfunction and a meta-analysis of population-based studies examining thyroid function and mood have shown a positive association (odds ratio [OR] 1.12) between depression and endogenous circulating T_4 levels and an inverse association with TSH. Another prospective cohort study assessed 1503 elderly Dutch men and women (mean age 70.6 years), who were followed up for 8 years. Those in the lowest TSH tertile (0.3–1.0 mU/L) had more concurrent depressive symptoms and were at a substantially higher risk of developing a depressive syndrome in subsequent years when compared with persons in the highest normal range TSH tertile (1.6–4.0 mU/L).

Interestingly, these studies show that depression seems more closely related to the presence of subclinical hyperthyroidism, where empiric treatment with thyroid hormone would be illogical.

7. What should be considered the normal reference range for serum TSH values?

There are differing opinions and contentions as to what should be accepted as a "normal" TSH reference interval and at what value thyroid treatment should commence. This is of paramount importance for every clinician. Over the years, there have been many studies that have examined the predictive value of various ranges of TSH values to identify abnormal thyroid function and predict a positive response to treatment.

A study by Surks and Hollowell (2007) analyzed the age-specific distribution of serum TSH in a thyroid disease–free population without antithyroid antibodies. In this study, serum TSH concentrations were arbitrarily categorized as < 0.4, 0.4 to 2.49, 2.5 to 4.5, and > 4.5 mU/L. Results from the study showed that the TSH distribution among the age deciles progressively shifted toward higher TSH concentrations with aging: 88.8% of those age 20 to 29 years compared with 61.5% of those age $\geq$ 80 years were in the 0.4 to 2.49 mU/L range; 6.5% compared with 23.9%, respectively, were in the 2.5 to 4.49 mU/L range; 2% compared with 12%, respectively, were in the > 4.5 mU/L range. TSH is redistributed toward higher concentrations with aging in $\approx$ 30% of the disease-free population. It then raises the question whether the currently used upper limit of 4.5 mU/L, derived from a composite of all age groups in the population, is appropriate for elderly people.

Fontes et al. (2013) prospectively evaluated 1200 subjects of both genders stratified by age groups and found the association between TSH and age to be highly significant. The median serum TSH level was 1.5 mU/L in people age < 60 years, increasing to 1.7 mU/L in those age 60 to 79 years, and to 2 mU/L for those age > 80 years. The upper TSH limit (97.5%) increases from 4.3 mU/L for those age < 60 years, to 5.8 mU/L in those age 60 to 79 years and to 6.7 mU/L in those age > 80 years. According to the National Health and Nutrition Examination Survey (NHANES) III, in a thyroid disease–free population, which excluded subjects who self-reported thyroid disease or goiter, the upper normal of serum TSH levels was 4.5 mU/L. A reference population taken from the disease-free population, further excluding pregnancy, those on thyroid active medications, and those having detectable anti-thyroglobulin antibodies (anti-TG) or antithyroperoxidase antibodies (anti-TPO), had an upper normal TSH value of 4.12 mU/L. When age was considered, the upper limit of normal TSH values were as low as 3.24 mU/L for disease-free subjects age 30 to 39 years and as high as 7.84 mU/L for subjects age > 80 years. The 97.5th percentile of serum TSH appears to increase by 0.3 mU/L for every 10-year age increase after 30 to 39 years of age. Thus, very mild "elevations" in TSH levels observed in older individuals may reflect a normal physiologic change in TSH with aging, rather than being diagnostic of subclinical thyroid dysfunction and that the "normal" range may need to be adjusted with increasing age.

These studies demonstrate evidence that TSH distribution progressively shifts with age, and an age-specific reference range should be used to avoid overdiagnosis and overtreatment of thyroid dysfunction in older individuals who are not hypothyroid because we would not expect their nonthyroidal symptoms to respond to thyroid hormone replacement.

8. Are there any effects on quality of life with variations in thyroid function within the age-specific range?

A study by Samuels et al. (2016) examined data from the Osteoporotic Fractures in Men (MrOS) Study, a cohort of community-dwelling men age $\geq$ 65 years in the United States. The study included 539 men who were not on thyroid medications and underwent detailed testing of quality of life, mood, and cognitive function at baseline. This study used gender- and age-adjusted upper reference TSH ranges derived from the NHANES III. The upper limit of normal was 7.48, mU/L for those age 60 to 69 years, 9.80, mU/L for those age 70 to 79 years, and 9.36, mU/L for those age $\geq$ 80 years. FT_4 levels were all within the assay-specific reference range.

At baseline, there were no associations between TSH or FT_4 levels and measures of quality of life, mood, or cognition in the 539 euthyroid men. Over the subsequent 5 to 8 years, they were tested again and median quality of life, mood, and cognitive measures were relatively unchanged. Baseline thyroid function did not predict changes in any of these outcomes over a mean of 6 years in the 193 men reassessed in the longitudinal analysis. Variations in thyroid function within the age-adjusted laboratory reference range were not associated with variations in quality of life, mood, or cognitive function.

9. Does treatment of subclinical hypothyroidism specifically among older individuals lead to resolution of symptoms?

Patients with classical symptoms of hypothyroidism and with elevated serum TSH levels combined with low serum FT_4 levels should be treated with levothyroxine (LT_4), but the decision to treat symptoms of subjects with subclinical hypothyroidism, defined as an elevated serum TSH level with serum FT_4 within the reference range, is controversial. Contrary to traditional thinking, subclinical hypothyroidism is not consistently predictive of a diagnosis which, once treated, is likely to result in clinical improvement. Many patients with depression are screened for thyroid dysfunction and classified as having subclinical hypothyroidism when marginal TSH elevations and normal FT_4 levels are present. Among the general population, the estimated prevalence of subclinical hypothyroidism, based on laboratory-suggested TSH cut-offs, is 3% to 8%, and as the average age of the population increases, so does the diagnosis of subclinical hypothyroidism. The consequences of subclinical hypothyroidism are different for the elderly compared with younger individuals. In current practice, many patients diagnosed with neuropsychiatric symptoms and subclinical hypothyroidism are started on LT_4 treatment. They frequently experience no improvement in symptoms with thyroid hormone replacement, and this, in turn, may lead to multiple increases in LT_4 doses, resulting in exogenous thyrotoxicosis, or consideration of combination treatment with LT_4 and liothyronine (LT_3).

Regardless of these interventions, there is still often a failure to reverse symptoms because they are not due to hypothyroidism.

A study by Jorde et al. (2006) evaluated the relationship of neuropsychological function and subclinical hypothyroidism, defined as a serum TSH of 3.5 to 10 mU/L and normal serum FT_4 and FT_3 levels, and the effect of LT_4 supplementation in a prospective, placebo-controlled, double-blind intervention study over 1 year. Various tests of cognitive function, Beck Depression Inventory, General Health Questionnaire, and a questionnaire on hypothyroid symptoms were used to assess the impact of LT_4 intervention. At the end of the study, there were no significant differences in any parameter of cognitive function, emotional function, or hypothyroid symptoms, either at the start of the intervention or at the end of the study, among 69 subclinically hypothyroid participants.

Another double-blind, placebo-controlled, randomized controlled trial by Parle et al. (2010) was conducted in 94 subjects age $\geq$65 years. Subjects underwent extensive baseline mood and neurocognitive testing, and then were randomized to either LT_4 therapy or placebo; thyroid function tests were performed at 8-weekly intervals for dosage adjustments to achieve TSH within the reference range for subjects in the treatment arm. The serum TSH reference range was 0.4 to 5.5 mU/L. Cognitive tests were administered at baseline and after LT_4 intervention. In the LT_4 group, 82% and 84% of the subjects achieved euthyroidism at 6- and 12-month intervals, respectively. Results revealed no significant changes in any of the measures of cognitive function over time and no between-group differences in cognitive scores at 6 and 12 months, thus strengthening the evidence that treating elderly subjects with subclinical hypothyroidism with LT_4 replacement therapy fails to improve cognitive function.

Stott et al. (2017) conducted a double-blind, randomized, placebo-controlled, parallel-group trial involving 737 adults who were at least 65 years of age. Study subjects had serum TSH levels between 4.60 and 19.99 mU/L and FT_4 levels within the reference range, and were designated as being subclinically hypothyroid. The subjects who were treated with LT_4, compared with those given placebo, showed no change in a hypothyroid symptom score or tiredness score on a thyroid-related quality-of-life questionnaire assessed at 1-year follow-up.

Multiple studies have now shown no benefit to LT_4 treatment of subclinical hypothyroidism diagnosed with non–age-adjusted TSH levels. This may support the concept that using the laboratory TSH cut-offs is not sufficiently specific to identify hypothyroidism as the cause of nonspecific complaints found frequently among those offered thyroid function testing.

10. What is the "labeling effect" seen in patients with known thyroid dysfunction?

Many hypothyroid patients treated with LT_4 report persistent neuropsychiatric symptoms, which may result from a "labeling effect" wherein subjects with self-knowledge of a thyroid condition are more likely to report symptoms. In a population-based study of over 25,000 subjects age $\geq$ 40 years, higher TSH levels were associated with normal or lower levels of depression and anxiety among the subjects not on LT_4, whereas in subjects on LT4 therapy, higher TSH levels were associated with higher degrees of depression and anxiety. Additionally, once a person is labeled as hypothyroid in the face of a minimally elevated TSH, the search for alternative explanations for symptoms commonly ceases.

11. Does LT_4 therapy improve symptoms in symptomatic euthyroid subjects?

Pollock et al. (2001), in a randomized, double-blind, placebo-controlled, crossover trial, showed that treatment with LT_4 was no more effective than with placebo in improving cognitive function and psychological well-being in patients who had symptoms suggestive of hypothyroidism but whose thyroid function tests were within the reference range. Serum FT_4 concentrations increased and TSH decreased in those taking LT_4, confirming compliance with treatment, whereas those on placebo remained unchanged. Nonetheless, LT_4 did not improve cognitive function or psychological well-being in these thyroid-healthy participants. Thyroid hormone treatment clearly does not change hypothyroid-like symptoms when given to those without biochemical evidence of hypothyroidism, underscoring the necessity of confirming the presence of hypothyroidism before diagnosing and treating patients with thyroid hormone therapy.

12. Does titration of thyroid hormone therapy to target TSH values to the high-normal range versus the low-normal range have a beneficial effect on symptoms?

Walsh et al. (2006) studied 56 subjects with primary hypothyroidism rendered euthyroid with at least 100 mcg daily of LT_4. Thyroid hormone doses were then adjusted to achieve high-, mid-, and low-normal TSH levels. Well-being was assessed with the General Health Questionnaire (GHQ-28), short form 36 (SF-36), and a thyroid symptom questionnaire at baseline and after 8 weeks at each TSH level. No measurable differences in outcomes were detected across the normal TSH range.

Samuels et al. (2018) analyzed 138 subjects who had LT_4-treated hypothyroidism and normal TSH levels and underwent testing for measures of quality of life (SF-36, ThyDQoL), mood (Profile of Mood States, Affective Lability Scale), and cognition (executive function, memory). They were then randomly assigned to receive an unchanged, higher, or lower LT_4 dose in a double-blind fashion, targeting 1 of 3 TSH ranges (0.34–2.50, 2.51–5.60, or 5.61–12 mU/L). Doses were adjusted every 6 weeks until TSH was stable and in the target range. TSH levels and baseline neurocognitive measures were reassessed at 6 months. At the end of study, by intention to treat, mean LT_4 doses were 1.50 ± 0.07, 1.32 ± 0.07, and 0.78 ± 0.08 mcg/kg ($P < 0.001$) and achieved mean serum TSH levels of 1.85 ± 0.25, 3.93 ± 0.38, and 9.49 ± 0.80 mU/L ($P < 0.001$) in the three arms. Results of this study showed that altering LT_4 doses to target TSH levels to the low-normal, high-normal, or slightly above-normal ranges does not affect quality of life, mood, or cognition. Despite a lack of objective benefit, the subjects preferred what they perceived to be higher doses.

It is important for physicians to be mindful that not all subclinical hypothyroidism, which is more commonly seen in the elderly, represents true thyroid failure, that not all neurocognitive and neuropsychiatric symptoms should be attributed to subclinical hypothyroidism, and that initiation of treatment with thyroid hormone may not lead to significant symptomatic benefits, and may, in fact, even lead to iatrogenic thyrotoxicosis, which has been well documented to significantly increase the risk of developing atrial fibrillation and skeletal fractures. There is a need to reconsider who should receive thyroid hormone and the impact or lack thereof that thyroid hormone replacement will have on expected clinical outcomes.

13. What abnormalities of thyroid function are found in psychiatric disorders?

Because patients with thyroid disease may manifest frank psychiatric disorders that are reversible with thyroid medications, the thyroid axis has been extensively studied in patients presenting with a wide variety of behavioral disturbances. Various abnormalities of thyroid function have been identified, particularly in depression. In most depressed subjects the basal serum TSH, T_4, and T_3 levels are within the normal range, although in one report, a third of such patients were observed to have suppressed TSH values.

A "blunted" TSH response to thyrotropin-releasing hormone (TRH) administration (defined as a TSH rise < 5 mU/L) is seen in approximately 25% of depressed subjects. The blunted TSH response is said to be observed more often in unipolar than bipolar depression, but differentiating these disorders with TRH testing has been disappointing. The blunted TSH response is a "state" marker that normalizes upon recovery from depression.

14. Describe a mechanism for the blunted TSH response to TRH in affective disorders.

The mechanism for the blunted TSH response to TRH administration in affective disorders is not known; however, glucocorticoids, known to inhibit the hypothalamic–pituitary–thyroid axis, are elevated in depression and could be responsible. This suppressed TSH response is not specific to depression and may be observed in alcohol withdrawal, starvation, normal aging in males, renal failure, acromegaly, Cushing's syndrome, and hypopituitarism. The blunting may also be caused by some medications, such as thyroxine, glucocorticoids, growth hormone, somatostatin, dopamine, and phenytoin, all of which have been reported to diminish this response.

15. Can abnormalities in the TSH circadian rhythm be identified in depression?

In normal subjects, serum TSH levels begin to rise in the evening before the onset of sleep, reaching a peak between 11:00 PM and 4:00 AM. In depression, the nocturnal TSH surge is frequently absent, resulting in reduced thyroid hormone secretion, supporting the view that functional central hypothyroidism might occur in some depressed subjects. Sleep deprivation, which has an antidepressant effect, returns the TSH circadian rhythm to normal. The mechanism for the impaired nocturnal TSH rise is unknown.

16. Is autoimmune thyroid disease frequently present in the patient with depression?

Although the blunted TSH response to TRH administration is well recognized in depression, it is less clearly appreciated that an enhanced TSH response may occur in up to 15% of subjects with depression but normal baseline thyroid function test results. The majority of those patients have antithyroid antibodies. When autoimmunity is tested utilizing the anti-TPO, rather than the less specific antimicrosomal antibody, the prevalence of autoimmune thyroid disease is even higher. Independent of thyroid function, anti-TPO positivity has been associated with depression, anxiety, emotional susceptibility, and impaired social life. Another study involving euthyroid women with a high anti-TPO antibody level of > 121 IU/mL showed an association with symptoms of chronic fatigue, chronic irritability, chronic nervousness, and decreased quality of life. Conversely, not all studies of subjects with depression have found an increased prevalence of antithyroid antibodies compared with matched control groups.

17. What is the frequency of elevated thyroxine values in patients with psychiatric disorders?

Approximately 20% of patients admitted to a hospital with acute psychiatric presentations, including schizophrenia and major affective disorders, but rarely dementia or alcoholism, may demonstrate mild elevations in their serum T_4 levels, and less often T_3 levels. The basal TSH is usually normal but may demonstrate blunted TRH responsiveness in up to 90% of such patients. These findings do not appear to represent thyrotoxicosis, and the abnormalities spontaneously resolve within 2 weeks without specific therapy. Such phenomena may result from central activation of the hypothalamic–pituitary–thyroid axis, resulting in enhanced TSH secretion with consequent elevation in circulating T_4 levels.

18. What is the most consistent abnormality of the thyroid axis in hospitalized patients with depression?

In patients with depression, the most consistent abnormality of the thyroid axis may be an increase in serum total T_4 or FT_4 levels, although usually within the conventional reference range. This generally regresses following successful treatment of the depression.

19. **What is the prevalence of thyroid dysfunction seen in psychiatric populations?**

Thyroid function test abnormalities are common in older individuals. In otherwise normal female subjects age > 60 years, the prevalence of elevated TSH values and/or positive antithyroid antibodies is ≥ 10%. Subjecting apparently asymptomatic individuals with slight elevations of serum TSH but normal T_4 and T_3 levels to a battery of psychological tests has revealed significant differences from control subjects on scales measuring memory, anxiety, somatic complaints, and depression in many, but not all, reported studies. It is becoming increasingly recognized that depression is much more common in elderly individuals. Whether borderline hypothyroidism plays a role in these behavioral disturbances requires clinical attention. Further investigation should also be directed at studying the outcomes of LT_4 intervention in depressed patients with serum TSH levels greater than the age-adjusted normal range. Studies evaluating patients with subclinical hyperthyroidism observed over 3 years have also shown its association with increased depressive symptoms by using the Geriatric Depression Scale (GDS). Among the very elderly and chronic alcoholics and those suffering from anorexia nervosa, suppressed serum T_3 levels with elevations in reverse T_3 (RT_3) and normal TSH values are consistent with the "euthyroid sick syndrome." These findings likely result from caloric deprivation, interference from medications, and physiologic aging.

20. **Which medications affect thyroid function and thyroid function tests?**

Medications commonly used to treat psychiatric illness have been shown to affect thyroid function tests (Table 47.2).

21. **How does lithium affect the pituitary–thyroidal axis?**

Lithium carbonate, used to treat bipolar disorders, interferes with both the release and organification of thyroid hormone. Therapeutic lithium levels diminish both T_3 and T_4 release from the thyroid gland, while at higher (probably toxic) levels iodine uptake and organification may also be inhibited. Following a 3-week therapeutic course of lithium carbonate, suppression of serum T_4 and T_3 levels, elevations of basal serum TSH values, and exaggerated TSH responses to TRH administration may be noted; these abnormalities generally return to normal within 3 to 12 months, even if the medication is continued.

Table 47.2. Impact of Psychotropic Medications on Thyroid Function Tests.

MEDICATION	MECHANISM	TEST FINDINGS
Lithium carbonate	↓ Thyroglobulin hydrolysis	TSH ↑ (transiently)
	↓ T_4 and T_3 release	Hypothyroidism, goiter
ANTIPSYCHOTICS Perphenazine	↑ TBG concentration	↑ T_4, nl FT_4
ANTICONVULSANTS Phenytoin	↑ Hepatic clearance of T_4	↓ T_4, ± ↓ FT_4, nl TSH
Carbamazepine	↓ T_4 binding, ↑ hepatic clearance	↓ T_4, ± ↓ FT_4, nl TSH
Phenobarbital	↑ Hepatic clearance	↓ T_4, ± ↓ FT_4, nl TSH
Valproic acid	↓ T_4 binding (?), ↑ hepatic clearance (?)	↓ T_4, ± ↓ FT_4, nl TSH
NARCOTICS Heroin	↑ TBG concentration	↑ T_4, nl FT_4
Methadone	↑ TBG concentration	↑ T_4, nl FT_4
MISCELLANEOUS Amphetamines	↑ TSH secretion (?)	↑ T_4, ↑ FT_4
Biotin	Competes with biotinylated	↑ T_4
	T_4 competitive assay for binding with streptavidin	
	Competes with the biotinylated sandwich complex for binding with streptavidin	↓TSH

FT_4, Free T_4; *Nl* = normal; T_3, triiodothyronine; T_3RU, T_3 resin uptake; T_4, thyroxine; *TBG*, thyroxine-binding globulin; *TSH*, thyroid stimulating hormone.

Adapted from Hennessy, J. V., & Jackson, I. M. D. (1996). The interface between thyroid hormones and psychiatry. *Endocrinologist, 6*, 214–223; Shrestha, R. T., Malabanan, A., Haugen, B. R., Levy, E. G., & Hennessey, J. V. (2017). Adverse event reporting in patients treated with thyroid hormone extract. *Endocrine Practice, 23*, 566–575.

22. What is the most common thyroid disorder in lithium-treated patients?

Goiter is the most common thyroid disorder occurring in lithium-treated patients. Hypothyroidism can also occasionally develop, particularly in patients who have thyroid glands that have been compromised by disorders such as Hashimoto's thyroiditis and Graves' disease previously treated with ^{131}I therapy. However, it is uncommon for hypothyroidism to occur if pretreatment thyroid function is completely normal and patients are thyroid antibody negative. If considered clinically necessary, lithium may be continued and LT_4 added to treat patients who develop goiter or hypothyroidism.

23. How does phenytoin affect laboratory tests and the function of the thyroid?

The effects of phenytoin (Dilantin), occasionally used for bipolar disorder, on thyroid function are quite complex. Suppressed values of total T_4 and, occasionally, FT_4 are observed in a significant minority of patients who are chronically treated with phenytoin alone and in upward of 75% of those in whom the drug is combined with carbamazepine (Tegretol). The lower total T_4 levels are likely caused by displacement of T_4 from thyroxine-binding globulin (TBG), whereas the reduced FT_4 levels result from enhanced clearance of T_4 through phenytoin-induced hepatic microsomal oxidative enzyme activity. Generally, the suppressed T_4 levels are accompanied by normal total T_3 and FT_3 levels and normal TSH concentrations. Normal basal TSH values with diminished TSH responses to TRH have been attributed to potential phenytoin agonism at the T_3 receptor. However, other studies have suggested that this may be an assay artifact because FT_4 values have been found to be normal or mildly elevated in analyses using undiluted serum.

24. Describe the effects of carbamazepine on thyroid function.

Carbamazepine (Tegretol) is used increasingly in bipolar disorder. Chronic use with maintenance of therapeutic serum levels suppresses serum T_4 values in > 50% of patients. This may be caused by the enhanced hepatic metabolism of T_4. TRH stimulation testing before and after initiation of carbamazepine therapy reveals that TSH responsiveness is reduced by the addition of this drug; this has led to speculation that carbamazepine may inhibit thyroid function through effects on the pituitary gland. Displacement of T_4 from TBG, similar to that seen with phenytoin, has additionally been cited as a potential effect.

25. How do phenobarbital, valproic acid, and other psychotropic medications affect thyroid function?

Both phenobarbital and valproic acid are reported to lower serum levels of T_4 in chronically treated patients, the former via enhanced hepatic T_4 clearance and the latter likely as a result of protein binding changes. Heroin, methadone, and perphenazine commonly increase serum TBG levels and, therefore, may elevate serum total T_4 levels, although TSH and FT_4 values remain normal. Amphetamines induce hyperthyroxinemia through enhanced secretion of TSH, an effect that appears to be centrally mediated.

26. How do antidepressant therapies affect thyroid function?

Antidepressants do not generally cause abnormal peripheral thyroid hormone levels but may affect thyroid hormone metabolism in the central nervous system (CNS). Selective serotonin reuptake inhibitors (SSRIs) and tricyclic antidepressants (TCAs) appear to promote activity of D2, which causes increased conversion of T_4 into T_3 in the brain. Circulating total T_4 and FT_4, but not TT_3, levels often show a modest decline, although still within the normal range, after treatment with various pharmacologic classes of antidepressants; this also occurs with electroconvulsive therapy. There are case reports of sertraline, paroxetine- and escitalopram-related asymptomatic hypothyroidism, but more recent studies evaluating fluoxetine and sertraline have shown no clinically significant changes in thyroid function test results.

27. Are there caveats of antidepressant usage in individuals with thyroid disease?

The use of TCAs in patients with thyrotoxicity should be pursued with caution, as cardiac dysrhythmias may be exacerbated or precipitated. Further, the monoamine oxidase inhibitors may cause hypertension in patients with thyrotoxicity, although they generally do not affect thyroid function or serum thyroid hormone levels.

28. Has thyroxine been used as sole treatment for depression?

Asher's report (1949) on "myxoedema madness" demonstrated that thyroid hormone deficiency resulted in depression that reversed with thyroid extract administration. This led to studies of the role of thyroid hormone therapy alone in the treatment of depression and other psychiatric diseases and open studies of high dose LT_4 for refractory bipolar and unipolar depression. Euthyroid individuals with symptoms suggestive of hypothyroidism and considered depressed on psychological testing do not improve when treated with LT_4. In fact, patients presenting with symptoms of hypothyroidism but with normal thyroid function tests respond more positively to placebo. Although initial reports of LT_3 as single therapy were promising, these studies were methodologically flawed; therefore, the role of thyroid hormone by itself in the treatment of depression in the absence of abnormal thyroid function has not been established. Studies assessing improvement of symptoms with combination LT_4/LT_3 treatment have also been inconclusive.

29. How effective is the combination of LT_4 and LT_3 in the treatment of neuropsychiatric symptoms of hypothyroidism?

Murray introduced thyroid hormone therapy to the English-speaking clinical world in 1891. From the beginning, this was a treatment based on a combination of T_4 and T_3 derived from animal thyroid extracts. Variability of the T_4

and T_3 contents and ratios from batch to batch and brand to brand led to the replacement of "natural" combination therapy with pharmaceutically more precise synthetic LT_4 and LT3. Eventually, the simplicity of LT_4 monotherapy was adopted as usual therapy and found to be safe and effective. The LT_4 dosage was historically titrated on the basis of symptoms until TSH assays became available. During the 1980s, sensitive TSH assays allowed for down-titration of LT_4 therapy to "normal," which resulted in significant dose reductions of as much as 100 mcg/day. Once euthyroid, however, some patients were noted to complain of symptoms consistent with some components of textbook lists of symptoms noted in overt hypothyroidism. Since that time, multiple reports have appeared evaluating the effectiveness of combining LT_3 with LT4 to improve neuropsychological outcomes. The 1999 report of Bunevicius et al., for example, indicated that substituting 12.5 mcg of LT_3 for 50 mcg of the individual's usual LT_4 dose resulted in improvement in mood and neuropsychological function. Multiple double-blind randomized controlled trials designed to correct design flaws of previous trials subsequently failed to reproduce the positive effects reported by Bunevicius et al. and did not demonstrate objective improvement in mood, well-being, or depression scales with the addition of LT_3 to LT_4 therapy. In addition, three meta-analyses by Grozinsky-Glasberg et al. (2006), Joffe et al. (2007), and Escobar et al. (2015) failed to demonstrate differences in cognitive function, quality of life, or subjective satisfaction with treatment, but reported that anxiety scores worsened in some subjects who were treated with the LT_4/LT_3 combination. At this point in time, use of combined LT_4/LT_3 treatment does not appear to be justified in hypothyroid patients who complain of nonspecific depressive symptoms after biochemical euthyroidism is restored with LT_4 therapy. In the few studies where patients preferred LT_4/LT_3 combinations over LT_4 alone, this finding could not be explained by changes in the objective psychological and psychometric tests used, or the biological endpoints that were measured.

30. **Can combination antidepressant medication and thyroid hormone enhance the response to depression treatment?**
Adjuvant therapy has been said to be logical when depression fails to resolve after 6 weeks of adequate anti-depressant medication. Such resistance occurs in about 30% to 45% of cases. The role of adjuvant thyroid hormone with TCAs has been investigated in euthyroid patients with depression for > 25 years. LT_3 doses of 25 to 50 mcg daily increase serum T_3 levels and suppress serum TSH and T_4 values. Two separate therapeutic effects of LT_3 therapy have been studied: first, its ability to accelerate the onset of the antidepressant response; second, its ability to augment antidepressant responses among those considered pharmacologically resistant.

31. **How effective is thyroid hormone for the acceleration of the antidepressant response?**
Given that the antidepressant effect of TCAs is known to be delayed, the role of LT_3 in accelerating the therapeutic onset of these drugs has been investigated. Several reports detailing the clinical outcomes of starting LT_3 (5–40 mcg daily) along with varying doses of TCAs as well as SSRIs at the outset of therapy have appeared in the literature. The study populations were inhomogeneous, consisting of patients with various types of depression. Furthermore, there were important methodologic limitations, including small sample sizes, inadequate medication doses, lack of serum medication level monitoring, and variable outcomes measures. As two relatively large, prospective, randomized placebo-controlled studies have come to opposite conclusions, it still has not been clearly established that LT_3 accelerates the antidepressant effect of TCAs.

32. **Can LT_3 therapy augment the clinical antidepressant response?**
An additional hypothesis is that adding small doses of LT_3 to the antidepressant therapy of patients who have little or no initial response will enhance the clinical effectiveness of the antidepressant. Resistance to antidepressants is defined as inadequate remission after 2 successive trials of monotherapy with different antidepressants in adequate doses, each for 4 to 6 weeks before changing to alternative therapies. However, 8 to 12 weeks of ineffective antidepressant therapy is commonly deemed unacceptable, and strategies designed to augment the response are being sought. Early studies assessing LT_3 effectiveness in augmenting the antidepressant response were neither placebo controlled nor focused on patient populations that could be directly compared. The first placebo-controlled, double-blind, randomized study reported results in 16 outpatients with unipolar depression who had experienced no improvement in their clinical outcomes with TCAs alone. The intervention consisted of adding 25 mcg of LT_3 or placebo daily for 2 weeks before the patients were crossed over to the opposite treatment for an additional 2 weeks. No beneficial effect of LT_3 was apparent. The only other placebo-controlled, randomized, double-blind trial investigating this question involved 33 patients with unipolar depression treated with either desipramine or imipramine for 5 weeks prior to random assignment to placebo or 37.5 mcg of LT_3 daily. After 2 weeks of observation on LT_3, during which TCA levels were monitored, significantly more patients treated with LT_3 (10 of 17; 59%) had a positive response compared with placebo-treated patients (3 of 16; 19%). A subsequent open clinical trial of imipramine-resistant depression, using a prolonged TCA treatment period preceding the addition of LT_3, showed no demonstrable effect of T_3.

33. **What evidence is there that the effect of selective SSRIs and electroconvulsive therapy (ECT) may be enhanced by the addition of LT_3?**
The SSRI group of medications (including fluoxetine and sertraline) is the preferred antidepressant treatment in the United States today. A large, double-blind, placebo-controlled trial to evaluate the role of LT_3 as augmentation therapy did not demonstrate an effect of LT_3 in augmenting the response to paroxetine (an SSRI) therapy in patients with major depressive disorder, but a similar study using sertraline and LT_3 reported a positive response.

Responders in the Cooper-Karaz report appeared to have had lower circulating thyroid hormone levels before treatment and to have had greater decreases in TSH levels in response to the intervention. This may indicate that those benefiting from the addition of LT_3 may have been subtly hypothyroid and the addition of LT_3 compensated for this deficiency. A recent meta-analysis of the available data suggests that coadministration of LT_3 and SSRIs has no significant clinical effect in patients with depression compared with SSRIs alone. More research is necessary to determine if patients with functional type 1 deiodinase (D1) gene polymorphisms may be more responsive to LT_3 cotreatment. Of interest, LT_3 has been reported to augment the antidepressant effect of ECT. However, there is little-to-no evidence to guide the duration of treatment with LT_3, and there are few studies regarding side effects of long-term administration.

34. **Are any psychiatric conditions recognized to respond to pharmacologic doses of LT_4?**
For the 10% to 15% of patients with bipolar disorder who have $\geq$ 4 episodes of manic-depressive psychosis yearly (rapid cyclers), the prevalence of autoimmune thyroid disease is as high as 50% or more. Therapeutic interventions with standard therapy, such as lithium, are frequently disappointing. In open-label studies, treatment of such patients with LT_4 in pharmacologic doses, sufficient to suppress serum TSH and elevate T_4 levels to approximately 150% of normal, has decreased the manic and depressive phases in both amplitude and frequency and has led to remission in some patients. Given these encouraging results, controlled studies on the efficacy of LT_4 or LT_3 seem warranted.

35. **Are mechanisms of thyroid hormone action on the brain known?**
Thyroid hormones play a critical role in the development and function of the CNS. T_3 receptors are widely distributed throughout the brain, and there is much evidence that thyroid hormone regulates brain function through interaction with the catecholaminergic system. Thyroid hormone action in brain tissue is accomplished through the binding of T_3 to its nuclear receptors. Brain T_3 is derived from T_4 by the action of D2, which is located throughout the CNS.

36. **Should LT_4 or LT_3 be used in treating the patient with depression?**
Most studies using thyroid hormone as adjuvant therapy for depression have utilized LT_3 rather than LT_4; in those reports where the advantages of one over the other were assessed, LT_3 was considered superior. In a randomized trial combining LT_4 or LT_3 with antidepressants, only 4 of 21 patients (19%) treated with 150 mcg/day of LT_4 for 3 weeks improved, whereas 9 of 17 (53%) responded with 37.5 mcg/day of LT_3. Additional studies of open-label LT_4 treatment in antidepressant-resistant patients have appeared, but the lack of controls makes outcome interpretation difficult. One of these indicated that responders to LT_4 had significantly lower pretreatment serum T_4 and reverse T_3 levels, leading the authors to speculate that the responders might have been subclinically hypothyroid. Adjuvant therapy with LT_4 rather than LT_3 may be indicated when subclinical hypothyroidism or rapid-cycling bipolar disease is present. Because LT_4 equilibrates in tissues more slowly compared with LT_3, treatment with LT_4 for at least 6 to 8 weeks, and preferably longer, would be necessary to determine its efficacy in this situation.
  It has been postulated that there may be a subset of patients that will benefit from LT_3 supplementation. To explore predictive markers for success with combination therapy, various studies evaluating deiodinase gene polymorphisms that encode the enzymes that convert T_4 to T_3 have been conducted. So far, results have been inconclusive.

37. **Are there genes that may be implicated in the response to treatment?**
As personalized medicine evolves, therapies will inevitably become more directed. Initial research investigating D1, which is important for hepatic and renal conversion of T_4 to T_3 to provide T_3 for the circulation, had suggested that certain D1 polymorphisms may be associated with significant LT_3 potentiation of SSRIs. Patients with certain alleles have inherently lower D1 enzyme activity, and, therefore, have naturally lower serum T_3 levels. Compared with those given placebo, these patients had improved depression scores after 8 weeks of LT_3 supplementation in combination with sertraline.
  Nonetheless, reported results, so far, have been inconclusive. An earlier study focusing on the Thr92Ala polymorphism in the deiodinase 2 gene (*D2*) showed an association with worse baseline General Health Questionnaire (GHQ) scores in LT_4-treated patients who had this polymorphism; furthermore, these subjects had significant improvement on LT_4/LT_3 combination therapy compared with LT_4 alone, although there was no effect on serum thyroid hormone levels. More recent studies on both the D2-Thr92Ala and the D2-ORFa-Gly3Asp polymorphisms, however, have shown no association with measures of health-related quality of life, neurocognitive functioning, or preference for combined LT_4/LT_3 therapy.
  There is emerging evidence that specific subsets of patients may not respond to LT_3 potentiation. Molecular biology studies have identified an organic anion transporting polypeptide (OATP), which is considered to be key in delivery of T_4 to the brain. Polymorphisms in the *OATP1C1* gene appear to be linked to increased depressive symptoms among patients with hypothyroidism. These patients do not appear to have any decrease in depressive scores with LT_3 supplementation compared with controls. The clinical significance of these findings has yet to be determined but may have a meaningful impact on the future of depression treatment.

38. **Describe the proposed mechanisms linking thyroid function and depression.**
It has been postulated that D2 activity in the CNS is deficient in depression, giving rise to a state of relative brain hypothyroidism coexisting with systemic euthyroidism. Alternatively, D2 activity could be suppressed by the

elevated serum cortisol levels that occur in depression and stress, promoting preferential conversion of T_4 to RT3 by type 3 deiodinase (D3) activity; this would result in decreased serum and brain T_3 levels and increased RT3 levels. Interestingly, LT_3 treatment could potentially be beneficial because T_3 is not dependent on transport by transthyretin (which is low in depression), and therefore, exogenous LT_3 therapy could ensure adequate T_3 delivery across the blood–brain barrier to the brain.

39. Do antidepressant medications have a mechanistic connection to the action of thyroid hormone in the brain?
It has been shown that desipramine, a TCA, and fluoxetine, an SSRI, both enhance D2 activity in the CNS, and, therefore, may presumably increase the availability of T_3 in the brain. This could conceivably account for the clinical efficacy of these classes of drugs.

40. What recommendations can be made for the thyroid evaluation in patients with psychiatric disorders?
It seems prudent to check thyroid function tests in those patients with psychiatric disorders who are at increased risk for thyroid disease. Women age > 45 years, patients with known autoimmune diseases, individuals with a family history of thyroid disease, and those receiving lithium or suffering from dementia should be screened for underlying thyroid abnormalities. Patients receiving medications known to influence the interpretation of thyroid function tests should have these considered when interpreting the results of testing.

41. Who should receive thyroid hormone for alleviation of psychiatric symptoms?
It is recommended that LT_4 therapy be offered to any depressed patient with significantly elevated serum TSH levels (> 10 mU/L), especially if accompanied by increased anti-TPO titers and/or low serum FT_4 levels (overt hypothyroidism). Thyroid hormone replacement may alleviate the symptoms of depression in these individuals. However, antidepressant therapy, if required, may be ineffective prior to normalization of thyroid axis parameters in subjects without overt hypothyroidism. Patients who have *D2* gene polymorphisms may be predicted to benefit from the addition of LT_3 according to one study, but prospective trials in this situation have not yet been conducted, and genetic testing is not currently recommended for clinical purposes. Adjuvant LT_3 lacks clear evidence of effectiveness in patients with depression refractory to treatment but who have normal systemic thyroid function.

KEY POINTS

- The symptoms of hypothyroidism are very nonspecific and often mimic those of depression, while those of hyperthyroidism may be confused with mania or depression.
- Mild elevations in serum thyroid-stimulating hormone (TSH) levels, consistent with a diagnosis of subclinical hypothyroidism, detected in patients with psychological distress are more likely to be a coincidental finding rather than an absolute causal finding.
- More recent studies have found no difference in depressive symptoms between euthyroid subjects and those with subclinical hypothyroidism when followed over time; some studies have even shown that depression seems more closely related to subclinical hyperthyroidism.
- Not all neurocognitive and neuropsychiatric symptoms should be attributed to subclinical hypothyroidism when present.
- Thyroid hormone treatment may not provide significant symptomatic benefits in those diagnosed with subclinical hypothyroidism and may, in fact, lead to iatrogenic thyrotoxicosis with proven risks.
- The use of age-adjusted TSH ranges will likely prevent overdiagnosis of subclinical hypothyroidism and may pave the way to better patient selection for thyroid hormone replacement.
- Normalization of the serum TSH level with levothyroxine (LT_4) therapy may completely reverse the neuropsychiatric features of overt hypothyroidism but is far less likely to be effective if the symptoms are not caused by the underlying hypothyroidism.
- Approximately 20% of patients admitted to the hospital with acute psychiatric presentations, including schizophrenia and major affective disorders, but rarely dementia or alcoholism, may demonstrate mild elevations in their serum T_4 levels and, less often, in their T_3 levels; these usually resolve within 2 weeks without specific thyroid therapy.
- On the basis of the results of prospective controlled studies, it would not appear justified to utilize combined LT_4 and liothyronine (LT_3) treatment in hypothyroid patients who complain of depressive symptoms after biochemical euthyroidism is restored with LT_4 therapy. Recent guidelines suggest consideration of a wide spectrum of different diagnostic alternative explanations of the symptoms before consideration of additional treatment with LT_3 is contemplated.
- Although a large double-blind, placebo-controlled study to determine the role of LT_3 therapy as augmentation to antidepressant therapy did not demonstrate an effect of LT_3 in enhancing the response to paroxetine therapy in patients with major depressive disorder, a more recent meta-analysis of the available data on LT_3 augmentation demonstrated very mixed results. Therefore, it is difficult to make strong recommendations for or against augmentation therapy.
- It is recommended that LT_4 therapy be offered to any patient with depression who has a reproducibly elevated serum TSH level, especially if accompanied by positive anti-TPO antibody titers and/or low serum FT_4 levels.

BIBLIOGRAPHY

Appelhof, B. C., Peeters, R. P., Wiersinga, W. M., Visser, T. J., Wekking, E. M., Huyser, J., . . . Fliers, E. (2005). Polymorphisms in type 2 deiodinase are not associated with well-being, neurocognitive functioning, and preference for combined thyroxine/3,5,3'-triiodothyronine therapy. *Journal of Clinical Endocrinology and Metabolism, 90*(11), 6296–6299.

Applehof, B. C., Brouwer, J. P., van Dyck, R., Fliers, E., Hoogendijk, W. J., Huyser, J., . . . Wiersinga, W. M. (2004). Triiodothyronine addition to paroxetine in the treatment of major depressive disorder. *Journal of Clinical Endocrinology and Metabolism, 89*(12), 6271–6276.

Asher, R. (1949). Myxoedematous madness. *British Medical Journal, 2*(4627), 555–562.

Bauer, M., & Whybrow, P. C. (1988). Thyroid hormones and the central nervous system in affective illness: interactions that may have clinical significance. *Integrity Psychiatry, 6*, 75–100.

Bauer, M., Baur, H., Berghöfer, A., Ströhle, A., Hellweg, R., Müller-Oerlinghausen, B., & Baumgartner, A. (2002). Effects of supraphysiological thyroxine administration in healthy controls and patients with depressive disorders. *Journal of Affective Disorders, 68*(2–3), 285–294.

Blum, M. R., Wijsman, L. W., Virgini, V. S., Bauer, D. C., den Elzen, W. P., Jukema, J. W., . . . Rodondi, N. (2016). Subclinical thyroid dysfunction and depressive symptoms among the elderly: a prospective cohort study. *Neuroendocrinology, 103*(3–4), 291–299.

Bocchetta, A., & Loviselli, A. (2006). Lithium treatment and thyroid abnormalities. *Clinical Practice and Epidemiology in Mental Health, 2*(23). doi:10.1186/1745-0179-2-23.

Bould, H., Panicker, V., Kessler, D., Durant, C., Lewis, G., Dayan, C., & Evans, J. (2012). Investigation of thyroid dysfunction is more likely in patients with high psychological morbidity. *Family Practice, 29*(2), 163–167.

Bunevičius, R., Kažanavičius, G., Žalinkevičius, R., & Prange, A. J. Jr. (1999). Effects of thyroxine as compared with thyroxine plus triiodothyronine in patients with hypothyroidism. *New England Journal of Medicine, 340*, 424–429.

Chopra, I. J., Solomon, D. H., & Huang, T. S. (1990). Serum thyrotropin in hospitalized psychiatric patients: evidence for hyperthyrotropinemia as measured by an ultrasensitive thyrotropin assay. *Metabolism, 39*(5), 538–543.

Cooper-Kazaz, R., Apter, J. T., Cohen, R., Karagichev, L., Muhammed-Moussa, S., Grupper, D., . . . Lerer, B. (2007). Combined treatment with sertraline and liothyronine in major depression: a randomized, double-blind, placebo-controlled trial. *Archives of General Psychiatry, 64*(6), 679–688.

Escobar-Morreale, H. F., Botella-Carretero, J. I. & Morreale de Escobar, G. (2015). Treatment of hypothyroidism with levothyroxine or a combination of levothyroxine plus L-triiodothyronine. *Best Practice & Research Clinical Endocrinology & Metabolism, 29*(1), 57–75.

Fava, M., Labbate, L. A., Abraham, M. E., & Rosenbaum, J. F. (1995). Hypothyroidism and hyperthyroidism in major depression revisited. *Journal of Clinical Psychiatry, 56*(5), 186–192.

Fontes, R., Coeli, C. R., Aguiar, F., & Vaisman, M. (2013). Reference interval of thyroid stimulating hormone and free thyroxine in a reference population over 60 years old and in very old subjects (over 80 years): comparison to young subjects. *Thyroid Research, 6*(1), 13.

Garber, J. R., Cobin, R. H., Gharib, H., Hennessey, J. V., Klein, I., Mechanick, J. I., . . . Kenneth, A. (2012). Clinical practice guidelines for hypothyroidism in adults: cosponsored by the American Association of Clinical Endocrinologists and the American Thyroid Association. *Thyroid, 22*(12), 1200–1235.

Grozinsky-Glasberg, S., Fraser, A., Nahshoni, E., Weizman, A., & Leibovici, L. (2006). Thyroxine-triiodothyronine combination therapy versus thyroxine monotherapy for clinical hypothyroidism: meta-analysis of randomized controlled trials. *Journal of Clinical Endocrinology and Metabolism, 91*(7), 2592–2599.

Gussekloo, J., van Exel, E., de Craen, A. J., Meinders, A. E., Frölich, M., & Westendorp, R. G. (2004). Thyroid status, disability and cognitive function, and survival in old age. *JAMA, 292*(21), 2591–2599.

Hein, M. D., & Jackson, I. M. D. (1990). Thyroid function in psychiatric illness. *General Hospital Psychiatry, 12*, 232–244.

Hennessey, J. V., & Jackson, I. M. D. (1996). The interface between thyroid hormones and psychiatry. *Endocrinologist, 6*, 214–223.

Hennessey, J. V., & Espaillat, R. (2015). Diagnosis and management of subclinical hypothyroidism in elderly adults: a review of the literature. *Journal of American Geriatrics Society, 63*(8), 1663–1673.

Hennessey, J. V., & Espaillat, R. (2018). Current evidence for the treatment of hypothyroidism with levothyroxine/levotriiodothyronine combination therapy versus levothyroxine monotherapy. *International Journal of Clinical Practice, 72*(2). doi:10.1111/ijcp.13062.

Hennessey, J. V., & Espaillat, R. (2018). Current evidence for the treatment of hypothyroidism with levothyroxine/levotriiodothyronine combination therapy versus levothyroxine monotherapy. *International Journal of Clinical Practice, 72*, e13062.

Jackson, I. M. D., & Whybrow, P. C. (1995). The relationship between psychiatric disorders and thyroid function. *Thyroid Update, 9*, 1–7.

Jackson, I. M. D. (1998). The thyroid axis and depression. *Thyroid, 8*(10), 951–956.

Joffe, R. T., Brimacombe, M., Levitt, A. J., & Stagnaro-Green, A. (2007). Treatment of clinical hypothyroidism with thyroxine and triiodothyronine: a literature review and metaanalysis. *Psychosomatics, 48*(5), 379–384.

Joffe, R. T. (2006). Is the thyroid still important in major depression? *Journal of Psychiatry & Neuroscience, 31*(6), 367–368.

Jorde, R., Waterloo, K., Storhaug, H., Nyrnes, A., Sundsfjord, J., & Jenssen, T. G. (2006). Neuropsychological function and symptoms in subjects with subclinical hypothyroidism and the effect of thyroxine treatment. *Journal of Clinical Endocrinology and Metabolism, 91*(1), 145–153.

Jorgensen, P., Langhammer, A., Krokstad, S., & Forsmo, S. (2015). Diagnostic labelling influences self-rated health. A prospective cohort study: the HUNT Study, Norway. *Family Practice, 32*(5), 492–499.

Kim, J. S., Zhang, Y., Chang, Y., Ryu, S., Guallar, E., Shin, Y. C., . . . Cho, J. (2018). Subclinical hypothyroidism and incident depression in young and middle-age adults. *Journal of Clinical Endocrinology and Metabolism, 103*(5), 1827–1833.

Lindholm, J., & Laurberg, P. (2011). Hypothyroidism and thyroid substitution: historical aspects. *Journal of Thyroid Research, 2011*, 809341.

Nelson, J. C. (2000). Augmentation stategies in depression 2000. *Journal of Clinical Psychiatry, 61*(Suppl 1), 13–19.

Ott, J., et al. (2011). Hashimoto's thyroiditis affects symptom load and quality of life unrelated to hypothyroidism: a prospective case-control study in women undergoing thyroidectomy for benign goiter. *Thyroid, 21*(2), 161–167.

Panicker, V., Evans, J., Bjøro, T., Asvold, B. O., Dayan, C. M., & Bjerkeset, O. (2009). A paradoxical difference in relationship between anxiety, depression and thyroid function in subjects on and not on T4: findings from the HUNT study. *Clinical Endocrinology, 71*(4), 574–580.

Panicker, V., Saravanan, P., Vaidya, B., Evans, J., Hattersley, A. T., Frayling, T. M., & Dayan, C. M. (2009). Common variation in the DIO2 gene predicts baseline psychological well-being and response to combination thyroxine plus triiodothyronine therapy in hypothyroid patients. *Journal of Clinical Endocrinology and Metabolism, 94*(5), 1623–1629.

Pardridge, W. M. (1979). Carrier medicated transport of thyroid hormones through the rat blood-brain barrier: primary role of albumin bound hormone. *Endocrinology, 105*, 605–612.

Parle, J., Roberts, L., Wilson, S., Pattison, H., Roalfe, A., Haque, M. S., . . . Hobbs, F. D. (2010). A randomized controlled trial of the effect of thyroxine replacement on cognitive function in community-living elderly subjects with subclinical hypothyroidism: the Birmingham Elderly Thyroid study. *Journal of Clinical Endocrinology and Metabolism, 95*(8), 3623–3632.

Pollock, M. A., Sturrock, A., Marshall, K., Davidson, K. M., Kelly, C. J., McMahon, A. D., & McLaren, E. H. (2001). Thyroxine treatment in patients with symptoms of hypothyroidism but thyroid function tests within the reference range: randomized double blind placebo controlled crossover trial. *British Medical Journal, 323*(7318), 891–895.

Samuels, M. H., Kaimal, R., Waring, A., Fink, H. A., Yaffe, K., Hoffman, A. R., . . . Bauer, D. (2016). Thyroid function variations within the reference range do not affect quality of life, mood, or cognitive function in community-dwelling older men. *Thyroid, 26*(9), 1185–1194.

Samuels, M. H., Kolobova, I., Niederhausen, M., Janowsky, J. S., & Schuff, K. G. (2018). Effects of altering levothyroxine (L-T4) doses on quality of life, mood, and cognition in L-T4 treated subjects. *Journal of Clinical Endocrinology and Metabolism, 103*(5), 1997–2008.

Sarne, D., & DeGroot, L. J. (2002). Effects of the environment, chemicals and drugs on thyroid function. *Endocrine Education.* www.thyroidmanager.org.

Sawka, A. M., Gerstein, H. C., Marriott, M. J., MacQueen, G. M., & Joffe, R. T. (2003). Does a combination regimen of thyroxine (T4) and 3,5,3'-triiodothyronine improve depressive symptoms better T4 alone in patients with hypothyroidism? Results of a double-blind, randomized, controlled trial. *Journal of Clinical Endocrinology and Metabolism, 88*(10), 4551–4555.

Stott, D. J., Rodondi, N., & Bauer, D. C. (2017). Thyroid hormone therapy for older adults with subclinical hypothyroidism. *New England Journal of Medicine, 377*(14), e20.

Surks, M. I., & Hollowell, J. G. (2007). Age-specific distribution of serum thyrotropin and antithyroid antibodies in the US population: implications for the prevalence of subclinical hypothyroidism. *Journal of Clinical Endocrinology and Metabolism, 92*(12), 4575–4582.

Taylor, P. N., Iqbal, A., Minassian, C., Sayers, A., Draman, M. S., Greenwood, R., . . . Dayan, C. (2014). Falling threshold for treatment of borderline elevated thyrotropin levels-balancing benefits and risks: evidence from a large community-based study. *JAMA Internal Medicine, 174*(1), 32–39.

Tremont, G., & RA, S. (1997). Use of thyroid hormone to diminish the cognitive side effects of psychiatric treatment. *Psychopharmacol Bulletin, 33*(2), 273–280.

Walsh, J. P., Shiels, L., Lim, E. M., Bhagat, C. I., Ward, L. C., Stuckey, B. G., . . . Cussons, A. J. (2003). Combined thyroxine/liothyronine treatment does not improve well-being, quality of life, or cognitive function compared to thyroxine alone: a randomized controlled trial in patients with primary hypothyroidism. *Journal of Clinical Endocrinology and Metabolism, 88*(10), 4543–4550.

Walsh, J. P., Ward, L. C., Burke, V., Bhagat, C. I., Shiels, L., Henley, D., . . . Stuckey, B. G. (2006). Small changes in thyroxine dosage do not produce measurable changes in hypothyroid symptoms, well-being, or quality of life: results of a double-blind, randomized clinical trial. *Journal of Clinical Endocrinology and Metabolism, 91*(7), 2624–2630.

Watt, T., Hegedüs, L., Bjorner, J. B., Groenvold, M., Bonnema, S. J., Rasmussen, A. K., Feldt-& Rasmussen, U. (2012). Is thyroid autoimmunity per se a determinant of quality of life in patients with autoimmune hypothyroidism? *European Thyroid Journal, 1*(3), 186–192.

Whybrow, P. C. (1994). The therapeutic use of triiodothyronine and high dose thyroxine in psychiatric disorders. *Acta Medica Austriaca, 21,* 47–52.

Williams, M. D., Harris, R., Dayan, C. M., Evans, J., Gallacher, J., & Ben-Shlomo, Y. (2009). Thyroid function and the natural history of depression: findings from the Caerphilly Prospective Study (CaPS) and a meta-analysis. *Clinical Endocrinology, 70*(3), 484–492.

Wirth, C. D., Blum, M. R., da Costa, B. R., Baumgartner, C., Collet, T. H., Medici, M., . . . Rodondi, N. (2014). Subclinical thyroid dysfunction and the risk for fractures: a systematic review and meta-analysis. *Annals of Internal Medicine, 161*(3), 189–199.

Wouters, H. J., van Loon, H. C., van der Klauw, M. M., Elderson, M. F., Slagter, S. N., Kobold, A. M., . . . Wolffenbuttel, B. H. (2017). No effect of the Thr92Ala polymorphism of deiodinase-2 on thyroid hormone parameters, health-related quality of life, and cognitive functioning in a large population-based cohort study. *Thyroid, 27*(2), 147–155.

VI

REPRODUCTIVE ENDOCRINOLOGY

CHAPTER 48

DIFFERENCES (DISORDERS) OF SEXUAL DIFFERENTIATION

Richard O. Roberts, III and Robert H. Slover

1. Describe the first level of sexual differentiation.

   The first level of sexual differentiation is the establishment of chromosomal sex. The vast majority of infants are either 46XX females or 46XY males because chromosomal sex typically determines gonadal sex. Gonadal structures differentiate from the bipotential, or primordial, gonadal ridge. The Y chromosome contains an area known as the sex-determining region, or SRY. The *SRY* gene product initiates the differentiation of the bipotential gonad into a testis. In its absence, the gonad becomes an ovary under the influence of other genes.

2. What is the next level of sex determination?

   The next level of sex determination involves the differentiation of the structures of the genital ducts. The genital duct structures are initially identical and bipotential in the embryonic male and female, and can give rise to differentiated male or female genitalia. In the normal male, testicular Leydig cells produce testosterone, which is necessary to maintain ipsilateral Wolffian duct structures (e.g., vas deferens, epididymis, seminal vesicles). The Sertoli cells of the testis produce anti-Müllerian hormone (AMH), which acts ipsilaterally to cause regression of Müllerian duct structures (Fallopian tubes, uterus, upper third of the vagina). In the absence of testosterone, Wolffian duct structures regress, while in the absence of AMH, Müllerian duct structures are preserved.

3. Discuss the development of the external genitalia.

   Male and female external genitalia arise from the same embryologic structures. In the absence of androgen stimulation, these structures differentiate into the female pattern, whereas the presence of androgens causes male differentiation (virilization). For complete virilization, testosterone must be converted to dihydrotestosterone (DHT) by the enzyme 5-alpha reductase, and androgen receptors must be functional. Excessive androgens virilize a female. Inadequate androgen production, inability to convert testosterone to DHT, or inability to respond to androgens, as in androgen receptor defects, result in undervirilization of a genetic XY male.

4. What is testis-determining factor?

   The testis-determining factor (TDF) promotes differentiation of the bipotential gonad into a testis; SRY was eventually characterized as TDF. SRY belongs to a family of deoxyribonucleic acid (DNA)–binding proteins. Specific manipulations have shown that the introduction of SRY results in sex reversal of XX mice, and site-directed mutagenesis of the *SRY* gene in XY mice yields an XY female. The activation of *SRY* is influenced by the Wilms tumor suppressor gene, *WT1*, which is instrumental in the differentiation of the bipotential gonad into a testis. Other genes that play a role downstream of *SRY* include *SOX9, SF-1, FGF-9, DAX 1, WNT4, DMRT1, ATRX, DHH, FOXL2*, and *GATA4*, among others.

5. Describe the Lyon hypothesis. In which cells are two X chromosomes necessary for normal development?

   Dr. Mary Lyon addressed the question of the extra X chromosomal material in females. Simply put, if two X chromosomes are necessary in each cell, how can males be developmentally normal? Lyon suggested that in each cell, one of the two X chromosomes is inactive and that in any given cell line, which X is active is randomly determined. In fact, the inactive X may be identified in many cells as a clump of chromatin at the nuclear membrane (Barr body). The important exception is in the ovary, where two functional X chromosomes are necessary for normal sustained ovarian development. Without two X chromosomes per cell (as in 45 XO Turner syndrome), the ovary involutes and leaves only fibrous tissue, termed a *streak gonad*.

6. Describe normal male sexual differentiation.

   Prior to the initiation of sexual differentiation, the fetus is sexually bipotential. Fig. 48.1 shows schematically how male development is accomplished. The undifferentiated gonad is derived from coelomic epithelium, mesenchyme, and yolk sac–derived germ cells, which, in the presence of SRY, give rise to Leydig cells, Sertoli cells, seminiferous tubules, and spermatogonia. Testes are formed at 7 weeks. Testicular production of testosterone by Leydig cells leads to Wolffian duct development, and concomitant production of AMH by Sertoli cells leads to Müllerian duct regression. Masculinization of the external genitalia is mediated by DHT, which is produced from testosterone by the action of the enzyme 5-alpha reductase.

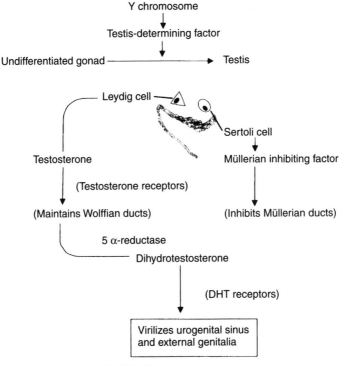

Fig. 48.1. Normal male development.

7. Describe normal female sexual differentiation.
In the absence of *SRY*, and under the influence of proovarian genetic factors, the undifferentiated gonad gives rise to follicles, granulosa cells, theca cells, and ova. Ovarian development occurs in the 13th to 16th week of gestation. Lack of testosterone and AMH allows regression of the Wolffian ducts and maintenance of the Müllerian ducts, respectively. Lack of DHT results in the maintenance of female external genitalia.

8. How is external genital development determined?
The external genitalia arise from the urogenital tubercle, urogenital swelling, and urogenital folds. In females, these become the clitoris, labia majora, and labia minora, respectively. In males, under the influence of DHT, the genital tubercle becomes the glans of the penis, the urogenital folds elongate and fuse to form the shaft of the penis, and the genital swellings fuse to form the scrotum. Fusion is completed by 70 days of gestation and penile growth continues to birth under the effects of both testosterone and growth hormone.

External female differentiation does not require ovaries or hormonal influence, whereas normal development of male genitalia requires normal testosterone synthesis, conversion to DHT by 5-alpha reductase, and normal androgen receptors. See Fig. 48.2.

KEY POINTS: DIFFERENCES (DISORDERS) OF SEXUAL DIFFERENTIATION

- Sexual ambiguity in a newborn must be seen as a medical, social, and psychological emergency requiring a multidisciplinary team approach to discuss the implications of the newborn's specific ambiguity and guide the parents' decision on sex of rearing. Members of the team include the pediatric endocrinologist, urologist, geneticist, pediatrician, appropriate counselors, and an ethicist.
- Evaluation of ambiguity must consider the five major categories of children presenting with this problem; namely, virilized 46,XX females, under-virilized 46,XY males, disorders of gonadal differentiation, including chromosomal abnormalities, and unclassified forms (cryptorchidism, hypospadias, developmental anomalies).
- The most common cause of sexual ambiguity in newborns is congenital adrenal hyperplasia due to 21-hydroxylase deficiency, accounting for > 50% of all diagnosed genital ambiguity and up to as much as 90% of genital ambiguity in individuals with an XX karyotype.

There are three large categories of ambiguity (Table 48.1):
1. Sex chromosome DSD
2. 46,XY DSD
3. 46,XX DSD

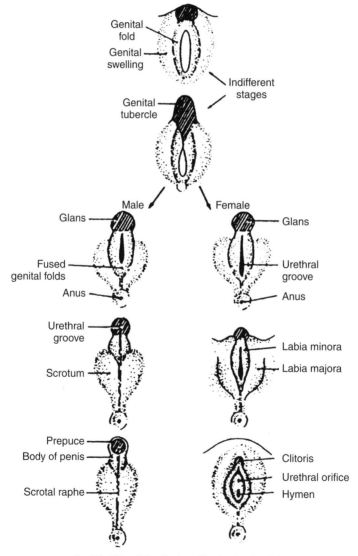

Fig. 48.2. Differentiation of male and female external genitalia.

Table 48.1. New Classification of DSD (Chicago Consensus).

Sex chromosome DSD	45,X (Turner's syndrome and variants) 47,XXY (Klinefelter's syndrome and variants) 45,X/46,XY (mixed gonadal dysgenesis, ovotesticular DSD) 46,XX/46,XY (chimeric, ovotesticular DSD)
46,XY DSD	Disorders of testicular development (complete and partial gonadal dysgenesis, gonadal regression, and ovotesticular DSD) Disorders of androgen biosynthesis, complete and partial androgen insensitivity, disorders of anti-Müllerian hormone [AMH]/AMH receptor, LH receptor defects Other (severe hypospadias, cloacal exstrophy)
46,XX DSD	Disorders of ovarian development (ovotesticular DSD, gonadal dysgenesis) Androgen excess (fetal [21 hydroxylase and 11-hydroxylase deficiency], fetoplacental [aromatase deficiency, POR], maternal [exogenous, luteoma]) Other (vaginal atresia, cloacal exstrophy)

Revised Nomenclature:	
New	**Old**
DSD	Intersex
46, XY DSD	Male pseudohermaphrodite, undervirilization of an XY male, and undermasculinization of an XY male
46, XX DSD	Female pseudohermaphrodite, overvirilization of an XX female, and masculinization of an XX female
Ovotesticular DSD	True hermaphrodite
46, XX testicular DSD	XX male or XX sex reversal
46, XY complete gonadal dysgenesis	XY sex reversal

AMH, Anti-Müllerian hormone; *DSD,* disorders of sexual differentiation; *LH,* luteinizing hormone; *POR,* P450 oxidoreductase.

10. What is a virilized female?

A virilized female (previously called *female pseudohermaphroditism*) is characterized by a 46 XX karyotype, ovaries, normal Müllerian duct structures, absent Wolffian duct structures, and virilized genitalia due to exposure to androgens during the first trimester. See Table 48.2.

11. What is the most common cause of a virilized female?

The most common cause is congenital adrenal hyperplasia (CAH) resulting from 21-hydroxylase deficiency. In fact, this disorder is the single most common cause of sexual ambiguity. In this condition, the gene responsible for encoding the 21-hydroxylase enzyme is mutated, causing deficient enzymatic activity in the fetal adrenal gland. This enzyme blockage occurs along the steroidogenic pathway to cortisol and aldosterone. Because of low or absent levels of cortisol, the feedback mechanism of the hypothalamic–pituitary–adrenal (HPA) axis produces increased adrenocorticotropic hormone (ACTH), which drives the pathway further and results in accumulation of precursor hormones, the measurement of which is useful for making a diagnosis. The increased ACTH level also drives the production of excess adrenal androgens, which result in virilization. Virilization may also be caused by maternal exposure to androgens or synthetic progesterones during the first trimester of pregnancy.

Table 48.2. Prader's Classification: Degree of Virilization of External Genitalia.

Type 1	Clitoral hypertrophy
Type 2	Clitoral hypertrophy, urethral, and vaginal orifices present, but very near in proximity
Type 3	Clitoral hypertrophy, single urogenital orifice, posterior fusion of the labia majora
Type 4	Penile clitoris, perineoscrotal hypospadias, complete fusion of the labia majora
Type 5	Complete masculinization (normal-looking male genitalia) but no palpable testes

12. How do virilized female infants present?

Of importance, affected infants may present with a wide spectrum of ambiguity, ranging from clitoromegaly alone to complete fusion of the labial swellings to form a scrotum and large phallus, mimicking a normal male phenotype with bilateral cryptorchidism. However, even in the most virilized girls, a penile urethra is rare, although possible.

13. What is an undervirilized male?

An undervirilized male (previously called *male pseudohermaphroditism*) refers to a 46 XY male who has ambiguous or female external genitalia. The abnormality may range from hypospadias to a completely female phenotype. Such disorders result from deficient androgen stimulation of genital development and most often are caused by Leydig cell agenesis, testosterone biosynthetic defects, 5-alpha-reductase deficiency, and partial or total androgen resistance (androgen receptor defects).

14. Which boys with hypospadias should be evaluated for sexual ambiguity?

Glandular or distal (first or second degree) hypospadias as the sole presenting genital abnormality has no apparent endocrine basis and need not be evaluated. The incidence of this anomaly is 1 to 8 in 1000 births. In contrast, proximal (third-degree) hypospadias is a feature of many etiologies of sexual ambiguity, and a child with this finding should be fully evaluated as ambiguous.

15. What is gonadal dysgenesis?

Patients with Y-related chromosomal or genetic disorders that cause maldevelopment of one or both testes are said to have gonadal dysgenesis. They present with ambiguous genitalia and may have hypoplasia of Wolffian duct structures and inadequate virilization. AMH may be absent, allowing Müllerian duct structures to persist. Duct asymmetry is, therefore, common. The Y-containing dysgenetic testes are at risk for developing gonadoblastomas and must be removed.

16. An infant is born with ambiguous genitalia, and the sex of the infant is uncertain. How does the health care provider proceed?

Honesty and diplomacy are essential. Explain that the genitalia are not phenotypically male or female and that further testing is necessary to determine the infant's sex. Reference to more commonly understood birth defects may be useful. Explain that it may take several days to complete the testing and that a team will participate to make an accurate diagnosis and a considered recommendation.

17. What history is necessary to evaluate the infant?

Maternal history is particularly important and should include illnesses, drug ingestion, alcohol intake, and use of supplemental hormones during pregnancy. Was progestational therapy used for threatened abortion or androgens for endometriosis? Does the mother have signs of excessive androgen exposure? Explore family history for occurrence of ambiguity, neonatal deaths, consanguinity, or infertility.

18. How should a health care provider direct the physical examination?

The diagnosis of the etiology of sexual ambiguity can rarely be made by examination alone, but physical findings can help direct further evaluation. Look for the following:
1. Are gonads present? Are they normal in size, consistency, and position? Because gonadal descent is tied to Müllerian duct regression, a palpable gonad implies AMH action on that side.
2. What is the phallic length? Measure along the dorsum of the phallus from the pubic ramus to the tip of the glans. At term, a stretched phallic length of 2.5 cm is 2.5 standard deviations (SDs) below the mean. Assess phallic width and development.
3. Note the position of the urethral meatus and look for evidence of hypospadias and chordee (ventral curvature secondary to shortened urethra).
4. What is the degree of fusion of the labioscrotal folds? The folds may range from normal labia majora to a fully fused scrotum. In subtle cases, the ratio of the distance from the posterior fourchette to the anus is compared with the total distance from the urethral meatus.
5. Is there an apparent vaginal orifice?

19. What other areas should be evaluated?

Certain forms of congenital adrenal hyperplasia may cause dehydration, hypo- or hypertension, or areolar or genital hyperpigmentation. Turner's stigmata may be present, including webbed neck, low hairline, and edema of hands and feet. Other associated congenital anomalies may indicate a complex that includes ambiguity.

20. Explain which radiographic studies are necessary.

Structural studies are needed to address the presence of gonads and Müllerian structures. Pelvic ultrasonography should be performed by qualified and experienced personnel as soon as possible to identify Mullerian structures or crypthorchid testes. If necessary, genitography may be performed by inserting contrast material into the urogenital orifice (or vaginal orifice) to define vaginal size, presence of a cervix, and any fistulae. Additionally, cystourethros-copy by an experienced urologist can allow for direct visualization of the internal anatomy.

21. Explain the role of karyotyping.
A karyotype is essential and must be obtained expeditiously. Buccal smears are absolutely contraindicated because they are inaccurate. In many laboratories, a karyotype can be completed within 48 to 72 hours. Some laboratories can also do rapid fluorescence in situ hybridization analysis for the presence of the *SRY* gene and the X centromere to determine chromosomal sex.

22. What single laboratory test is very helpful in almost all cases?
Because 21-hydroxylase deficiency is a common cause of sexual ambiguity, the level of 17-hydroxyprogesterone (17-OHP) is assessed in all such infants who do not have palpable gonads.

23. How is further evaluation directed?
Further evaluation must be directed by information provided through the history, examination, and initial studies. Determining the presence or absence of palpable gonads (presumably testes), the presence or absence of a uterus, the karyotype, and any other concomitant congenital anomalies allows for classification of the infant as a virilized female, an undervirilized male, having a disorder of gonadal differentiation, or having one of the unclassified forms.

24. The infant has no palpable gonads and has fused labioscrotal folds and a prominent phallus. Ultrasonography reveals a uterus and tubes with possible ovaries. The karyotype is 46 XX. How should the health care provider proceed now?
The infant is a virilized female. If there is no history of maternal androgen exposure or virilization, the infant has one of three forms of CAH. Of these, 21-hydroxylase deficiency is most common and is confirmed by finding an elevated serum level of 17-OHP. In 11-beta-hydroxylase deficiency, 11-deoxycortisol is elevated, whereas 17-hydroxypregnenolone and dehydroepiandrosterone (DHEA) are elevated in 3-beta-hydroxysteroid dehydroge-nase deficiency. The baseline levels are usually diagnostic but can be confirmed by using an ACTH stimulation test, if necessary. The electrolyte disturbances seen with such disorders do not usually occur until 8 to 14 days of life; however, plasma renin activity will be elevated earlier and should be measured as a marker of salt wasting caused by aldosterone deficiency. Screening of newborns for CAH with measurement of a 17-OHP level is now mandated in all 50 states in the United States and in many countries throughout the world.

25. An undervirilized male represents a more complex diagnostic dilemma. In an infant with palpable gonads, no Müllerian structures, and a 46 XY karyotype, how should the health care provider proceed?
Defects in testosterone synthesis include three enzyme blocks common to the adrenal and testicular pathways (steroidogenic acute regulatory protein [StAR] defect, 3-beta-hydroxysteroid dehydrogenase deficiency, and 17-alpha-hydroxylase deficiency). Enzyme blocks are diagnosed with ACTH stimulation testing and measurement of steroid precursors. Those with StAR defects have no measurable precursors but show high levels of ACTH and a low cortisol response. Infants with 3-beta-hydroxysteroid dehydrogenase deficiency have elevated levels of 17-hydroxypregnenolone and DHEA. Patients with 17-alpha-hydroxylase deficiency have elevated levels of progesterone, desoxycorticosterone, and corticosterone, with associated hypertension. See Fig. 48.3.

26. Discuss the two remaining defects that involve deficiencies of testicular, but not adrenal, enzymes.
The two remaining defects in testosterone synthesis involve deficiencies of specific testicular rather than adrenal enzymes: 17,20-lyase and 17-beta-hydroxysteroid dehydrogenase. Thus, they are not associated with elevations of ACTH or electrolyte disturbances. Both deficiencies are diagnosed by measuring the precursor response to ad-ministration of human chorionic gonadotropin (hCG). Infants with 17,20-lyase deficiency have elevated levels of 17-hydroxypregnenolone and 17-OHP, whereas infants with 17-beta-hydroxysteroid dehydrogenase deficiency have elevated levels of DHEA and androstenedione.

27. What other possibilities should be investigated?
- Infants with Leydig cell hypoplasia have low levels of testosterone before and after hCG stimulation but have normal adrenal function. Testicular biopsy reveals normal seminiferous tubules and Sertoli cells but absent or few Leydig cells.
- Stimulation with hCG also allows measurement of the testosterone-to-dihydrotestosterone ratio. If the ratio is elevated, 5-alpha-reductase deficiency should be suspected and may be confirmed by cultures of genital skin fibroblasts.
- Finally, normal-to-high testosterone levels with no abnormalities in ACTH and hCG testing lead to the diag-nosis of partial androgen insensitivity (androgen receptor defects). The diagnosis is made by demonstrating abnormal androgen binding in cultures of genital skin fibroblasts in a research laboratory, or by molecular analysis.

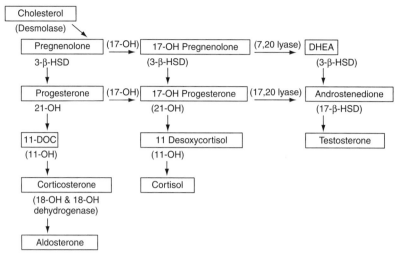

Fig. 48.3. Testosterone synthesis pathway.

28. What is complete androgen insensitivity?

The androgen receptor, encoded on the X chromosome, binds testosterone and, more avidly, binds dihydrotestosterone. Androgen insensitivity results from abnormalities of the androgen receptor. Complete androgen resistance occurs with a frequency of 1 in 20,000 to 1 in 64,000 XY individuals.

29. How do infants with complete androgen insensitivity present?

Complete androgen insensitivity (testicular feminization) rarely presents as ambiguity in the newborn period or early childhood. Unless the testes have descended and are palpable in the labia majora, affected infants appear as phenotypically normal females.

　　Affected children grow as normal females until puberty. They feminize with normal breast development at puberty because high levels of testosterone are aromatized to estrogen, but they have little to no pubic or axillary hair and no menses. Because they produce AMH, they lack Müllerian duct structures. Wolffian duct structures are also rudimentary or absent because they lack normal testosterone receptors. Gender identity is usually female. Patients come to medical attention because of primary amenorrhea in their teenage years. The diagnosis is, therefore, frequently made when patients are in their mid- to late teens.

　　Androgen insensitivity may also be partial and may present with varying degrees of ambiguity in the newborn period. Patients however still lack Mullerian duct structures given normal AMH production. Gender identity may be variable.

30. When should intraabdominal testicular tissue be removed?

The intraabdominal testes of patients with androgen insensitivity or XY gonadal dysgenesis are at risk for malignancy (up to 30% in some series), particularly after the onset of puberty. Timing of gonadectomy is still being debated. Because the risk of malignancy is low until puberty, some prefer to leave the gonads intact until spontaneous pubertal development; however, because carcinoma in situ has been found in prepubertal patients, others recommend early removal. Gonadectomy is controversial and the risks and benefits should be discussed on an individual basis with each patient. If the testes are removed before puberty, estrogen therapy is necessary for normal pubertal progression. If gonads are left in place, they should be monitored closely for the development of malignancy. Because the upper section of the vagina is Müllerian in origin, affected individuals may have shortened vaginas and require plastic surgical repair.

31. Summarize the physiologic results of 5-alpha-reductase deficiency.

Deficiency of 5-alpha-reductase impairs the conversion of testosterone to DHT, leading to incomplete virilization and differentiation of the external genitalia, which are dependent on the action of DHT. The disorder is particularly well documented in large kindred in the Dominican Republic and Gaza, in whom it is inherited as an autosomal recessive condition.

32. Describe the clinical picture in children with 5-alpha-reductase deficiency.

Male infants with 5-alpha-reductase deficiency are born with sexual ambiguity. External genitalia range from a penis with simple hypospadias to a blind vaginal pouch and clitoris-like phallus. The most common presentation is a urogenital sinus with a blind vaginal pouch. During puberty, affected boys undergo virilization because levels of testosterone are higher and alternative isoenzymes mediate conversion of testosterone to DHT; affected females are normal.

Historically, infants with 5-alpha-reductase deficiency were raised as females until puberty, then continued life as males and, in some cases, achieved fertility. Recently, however, the condition has been recognized early in life, and affected males are now raised from infancy as boys.

33. **What is ovotesticular DSD?**

Ovotesticular DSD (previously known as *true hermaphroditism*) is a disorder of gonadal differentiation in which individuals have both ovarian and testicular elements. Affected children may have bilateral ovotestes, an ovary or testis on one side with an ovotestis on the other, or an ovary on one side and testis on the other. Because the effects of AMH and testosterone on duct structures are ipsilateral and localized, internal duct development is often asymmetric. Thus, a Fallopian tube and unicornuate uterus, with absent or vestigial male duct structures, may develop on the side without testicular elements, whereas an epididymis, vas deferens, and seminal vesicles without Müllerian structures may develop on the side with testicular elements. The external genitalia may be male, female, or ambiguous, depending on the amount of functioning testicular tissue.

34. **Why is a multidisciplinary team necessary for the management of an infant with sexual ambiguity?**

Sexual ambiguity is a complex issue in many respects. An accurate diagnosis is essential and may take some time. Sex assignment should be discussed in detail with the family and should be based not only on the underlying diagnosis and karyotype but also on probable adult gender identity, psychosocial factors, anticipated adult sexual function, potential for fertility, psychological health, and minimization of physical/surgical risks. For these reasons, input from several specialties, including endocrinology, genetics, neonatology, psychology, and urology, as well as an ethicist, is important. All members of the team must communicate adequately with each other. The goal of the multidisciplinary team is to provide parents with a clear understanding of the degree of ambiguity and offer guidance in the determination of sex assignment. Additionally, the team should delineate the expected future medical care and support the family through development with attention to the child's wishes and developing gender identity.

35. **How is the decision about sex assignment made?**

Exogenous and endogenous hormones are clearly important, as is the appearance of the genitalia. The decision about sex assignment must be carefully made, taking into consideration each "level" of sex determination. Sex assignment also depends on fetal sex hormone exposure, potential for adult sexual function, and psychological and cultural considerations. It is vital that parents completely understand this process is not perfect and assigned sex may not match gender identity in the future. Flexibility and support of the child, as well as age-appropriate discussions of the diagnosis throughout development, are critical to allow the child to participate in his or her care.

36. **After the etiology of sexual ambiguity has been determined in an infant, what factors should be considered in assigning a sex of rearing?**

Arriving at a precise diagnosis provides the treating team an understanding of potential risks and benefits of either sex assignment. For example, in poorly virilized males, the difference in outcomes among children with defects in Leydig cell development, testosterone synthesis, 5-alpha-reductase activity, and incomplete or complete androgen sensitivity is enormous. A child with Leydig cell agenesis or defective enzyme-related testosterone synthesis may be raised as a male or a female, depending on other factors; a child with complete androgen insensitivity should be raised as a female; and a boy with 5-alpha-reductase deficiency usually is raised as a male. Yet children affected by any of the three conditions have 46 XY karyotypes.

37. **What other factors must be considered?**

- What is the potential for unambiguous genital appearance?
- What is the potential for normal sexual function?
- Is there a potential for fertility?
- What was the in utero hormone exposure, with particular reference to exposure of the developing brain to excess androgens?
- What are the factors likely to affect gender identity and psychological health?
- Phallic size, urethral position, vaginal anatomy, and presence or absence of Müllerian or Wolffian duct structures, and gonadal characteristics and karyotype must all be considered.
- Parental backgrounds and expectations, broader family dynamics, social factors, and ethnic or cultural influences also must be considered.

38. **To which gender are virilized females usually assigned?**

Virilized females are usually assigned a female gender. They have normal ovaries as well as Müllerian structures and, with potential for surgical correction if desired by the patient and steroid replacement, can have normal sexual function and achieve fertility. Approximately 95% of XX individuals with virilizing CAH have a female gender identity and, therefore, should generally be assigned female sex. In severely virilized females with more phenotypically male external genitalia, male sex assignment may be considered in conjunction with input from the family and consideration of the additional factors listed above.

39. How is sex assignment determined in undervirilized males?

Undervirilized males are often infertile and sex assignment has usually been based on phallic size. Because a stretched penile length of 2.5 cm is 2.5 SD below the mean, an infant with a phallus < 2.5 cm may have been assigned female sex of rearing historically. However, phallic size (penis or clitoris) has been challenged as a major factor in decisions regarding gender assignment. Adult social and fulfilling sexual function should be the primary goals of gender assignment. If male sex assignment is contemplated, a trial of depot testosterone (50 mg every 3–4 weeks) for 1 to 3 months indicates whether phallic growth is possible.

40. Summarize the factors that determine sex assignment in patients with gonadal dysgenesis.

In patients with gonadal dysgenesis and Y chromosomal material, gonadectomy should be considered because of the risk of malignant transformation. Potential for fertility should be considered, although, typically, fertility is not possible. Internal duct structures are also frequently deranged. Degree of virilization is often weighed in the determination of sexual assignment, although a multifactorial approach again is of the utmost importance.

41. How is sex assignment determined in ovotesticular DSD?

Individuals with ovotesticular differences in sexual differentiation who have a unilateral ovary and Müllerian structures may have spontaneous puberty and normal fertility and may be raised as females. External genital size and structure may allow male assignment, but more commonly external genitalia are poorly virilized and affected infants are assigned female sex.

42. What principles should be kept in mind when sex assignments are made?

We have much to learn about gender identity and must consider which decisions might be made later than previously thought (e.g., surgery). Some surgical interventions are cosmetic or affect future fertility, and some affected patients have expressed the wish that they should make the decisions in adolescence or adulthood. This field challenges many of the perceptions of sex and gender and the role of physicians. Although the infant with genital ambiguity presents a medical and social emergency, decisions should be made carefully, cautiously, and with all necessary biochemical and anatomic information available. Most importantly, the multidisciplinary team approach must involve the parents in an open and honest discussion of the options. In the end, it is the parents, in the best interests of their child, who come first in decision making on sex assignment.

BIBLIOGRAPHY

Brown, J., & Warne, G. (2005). Practical management of the intersex infant. *Journal of Pediatric Endocrinology & Metabolism, 18,* 3–23.
Douglas, G., Axelrad, M. E., Brandt, M. L. Crabtree, E., Dietrich, J. E., French, S., … Reid Sutton, V. (2012). Guidelines for evaluating and managing children born with disorders of sexual development. *Pediatric Annals, 41,* 4.
Eugenides, J. (2003). *Middlesex* [novel]. New York: Picador.
Goodall, J. (1991). Helping a child to understand her own testicular feminization. *Lancet, 337,* 33–35.
Houk, C. P., & Lee, P. A. (2005). Intersexed states: diagnosis and management. *Endocrinology and Metabolism Clinics of North America, 34,* 791–810.
Houk, C. P., & Lee, P. A. (2010). Approach to assigning gender in 46,XX congenital adrenal hyperplasia with male external genitalia: replacing dogmatism with pragmatism. *Journal of Clinical Endocrinology and Metabolism, 95*(10), 4501–4508.
Jasso, N., Boussin, L., Knebelmann, B., Nihoul-Fékété, C., & Picard, J. Y. (1991). Anti-Müllerian hormone and intersex states. *Trends in Endocrinology and Metabolism, 2,* 227–233.
Joseph A. A., Kulshreshtha B., Mehta M., Ammini A. C. Sex of rearing seems to exert a powerful influence on gender identity in the absence of strong hormonal influence: report of two siblings with PAIS assigned different sex of rearing. *J Pediatr Endocrinol Metab.* 2011;24(11–12):1071–5.
Kaplan, S. (1990). *Clinical Pediatric Endocrinology.* Philadelphia: W.B. Saunders.
Kim, K. S., & Kim, J. (2012). Disorders of sex development. *Korean Journal of Urology, 53*(1), 1–8.
Lee, P. A., Houk, C. P., Ahmed, S. F., & Hughes, I. A. (2006). Consensus statement on management of intersex disorders. *Pediatrics, 118,* e488–e500.
Liu, A. X., Shi, H. Y., Cai, Z. J., Liu, A., Zhang, D., Huang, H. F., & Jin, H. M. (2014). Increased risk of gonadal malignancy and prophylactic gonadectomy: a study of 102 phenotypic female patients with Y chromosome or Y-derived sequences. *Human Reproduction, 29*(7), 1413–1419.
Low, Y., & Hutson, J. M. (2003). Rules for clinical diagnosis in babies with ambiguous genitalia. *Journal of Paediatrics and Child Health, 39,* 406–413.
McGillivray, B. C. (1992). The newborn with ambiguous genitalia. *Seminars in Perinatology, 16,* 365–368.
Meyers-Seifer, C. H., & Charest, N. J. (1992). Diagnosis and management of patients with ambiguous genitalia. *Seminars in Perinatology, 16,* 332–339.

Mieszczak, J., Houk, C. P., & Lee, P. A. (2009). Assignment of the sex of rearing in the neonate with a disorder of sex development. *Current Opinion in Pediatrics, 21,* 541–547.

Mulaikal, R. M. Migeon, C. J. & Rock, J. A. (1987). Fertility rates in female patients with congenital adrenal hyperplasia due to 21-hydroxylase deficiency. *New England Journal of Medicine, 316,* 178–182.

Ogilvy-Stuart, A. L., & Brain, C. E. (2004). Early assessment of ambiguous genitalia. *Archives of Disease in Childhood,* 89, 401–407.

Pagona, R. A. (1987). Diagnostic approach to the newborn with ambiguous genitalia. *Pediatric Clinics of North America, 34,* 1019–1031.

Penny, R. (1990). Ambiguous genitalia. *American Journal of Diseases of Children, 144,* 753.

Rangecroft, L. (2003). British association of paediatric surgeons working party on the surgical management of children born with ambiguous genitalia: surgical management of ambiguous genitalia. *Archives of Disease in Childhood, 88,* 799–801.

Thigpen, A. E., Davis, D. L., Gautier, T., Imperato-McGinley, J., & Russell, D. W. (1992). Brief report: the molecular basis of steroid 5 alpha-reductase deficiency in a large Dominican kindred. *New England Journal of Medicine, 327,* 1216–1219.

Thyen, U., Lanz, K., Holterhus, P. M., & Hiort, O. (2006). Epidemiology and initial management of ambiguous genitalia at birth in Germany. *Hormone Research, 66*(4), 195–203.

Warne, G. L., & Kanumakala, S. (2002) Molecular endocrinology of sex differentiation. *Seminars in Reproductive Medicine, 20,* 169–180.

Woodhouse, C. R. J. (2004). Hypospadias Surgery: an Illustrated Guide. *European Journal of Plastic Surgery, 27*(4), 213.

Zucker, K. J., Bradley, S. J., Oliver, G., Blake, J., Fleming, S., & Hood, J. (1996). Psychosexual development of women with congenital adrenal hyperplasia. *Hormones and Behavior, 30*:300–318.

CHAPTER 49

DISORDERS OF PUBERTY

Shanlee M. Davis and Sharon H. Travers

1. What physiologic events initiate puberty?

   The hypothalamic–pituitary–gonadal (HPG) axis is activated twice in postnatal life: in infancy and again at the time of true puberty. Mature gonadotropin-releasing hormone (GnRH) neurons in the hypothalamus secrete GnRH in pulses. GnRH pulses stimulate the pituitary gland to secrete pulses of gonadotropins, luteinizing hormone (LH), and follicle-stimulating hormone (FSH), with a relatively greater rise in LH. In response to the increased secretion of gonadotropins, there is increased production and secretion of gonadal hormones, leading to the progressive development of secondary sexual characteristics and gametogenesis. *Central puberty* refers to reactivation of the HPG axis, which is regulated by kisspeptin and several other neuropeptides that stimulate GnRH neurons. In both sexes, normal progression through puberty requires maturation of gonadal function via the HPG axis as well as increased secretion of adrenal androgens.

2. What are the first signs of puberty?

   The first physical sign of HPG activation in males is *gonadarche,* or testicular enlargement to a testicular volume of $\geq$ 4 mL or length $\geq$ 2.5 cm. In females, we cannot easily measure ovarian size; therefore, the first physical sign of HPG activation is *thelarche,* or breast buds, indicating estrogen production.

3. How is pubertal development measured?

   Sexual maturity is determined by physical examination and is described in a scale devised by John Tanner in 1969 (Table 49.1). Breast development in females and pubic hair in both sexes progress from Tanner stage I (prepubertal) to Tanner stage V (complete maturation). Testicular volume in males can be measured using an orchidometer, with < 4 mL representing prepubertal volumes and $\geq$ 4 mL representing pubertal volumes. In addition to the physical examination, the tools to assess pubertal development include determination of skeletal maturation with radiography of the left hand (bone age), growth velocity, growth pattern, and specific endocrine laboratory studies.

4. What is adrenarche?

   Adrenarche refers to the time during puberty when the adrenal glands increase their production and secretion of adrenal androgens: dehydroepiandrosterone (DHEA), DHEA-sulfate (DHEA-S), and androstenedione. In typically developing children, signs of adrenarche, such as pubic hair, axillary hair, acne, and body odor, occur at a time similar to that of central puberty. The control of adrenal androgen secretion is not clearly understood, but it appears to be separate from the HPG axis.

5. What is the normal pattern of puberty in boys?

   The mean age of gonadarche is 11.8 years, with a range of 9 to 14 years. There are racial differences in pubertal onset, with black boys starting puberty as early as 8 years of age. Pubic hair and penile enlargement typically occur after gonadarche but occasionally occur earlier because of production of adrenal androgens. It is not until midpuberty when testosterone levels are rising that boys experience voice change, axillary hair, facial hair, and the peak growth spurt. Spermatogenesis is mature at a mean age of 13.3 years.

6. What is the normal pattern of puberty in girls?

   Girls normally begin puberty between ages 8 and 13 years (mean age: 10.4 years for white girls; 9.8 years for Hispanic girls; and 9.5 years for black girls). The initial pubertal event is thelarche, the appearance of breast buds, although a small percentage of girls will develop pubic hair first. In an even smaller percentage of girls, menstrual cycling may appear first. Initial breast development often occurs asymmetrically and should not be of concern. Breast development is primarily under the control of estrogens secreted by the ovaries, whereas pubic hair and axillary hair growth result mainly from production of adrenal androgens. Unlike in boys, the pubertal growth spurt in girls occurs at the onset of puberty. Menarche usually occurs 18 to 24 months after the onset of breast development (mean age: 12.5 years). Although most girls have reached about 97.5% of their maximum height potential at menarche, this can vary considerably. Consequently, age of menarche is not necessarily a good predictor of final adult height.

Table 49.1. Tanner Stages of Pubertal Development.

STAGE CHARACTERISTICS	STAGE CHARACTERISTICS
Girls: Breast Development	Girls: Pubic Hair Development
I. Prepubertal; elevation of papilla only II. Breast buds are noted or palpable; enlargement of areola III. Further enlargement of breast and areola, with no separation of their contours IV. Projection of areola and papilla to form secondary mound above level of breast V. Adult contour breast with projection of papilla only	I. Prepubertal; no pubic hair II. Sparse growth of long, straight, or slightly curly, minimally pigmented hair, mainly of labia III. Considerably darker and coarser hair spreading over mons pubis IV. Thick, adult-type hair that does not yet spread to medial surface of thighs V. Hair adult in type and distributed in classic inverse triangle
Boys: Genital Development	Boys: Pubic Hair Development
I. Prepubertal; testicular length < 2.5 cm II. Testes > 2.5 cm in longest diameter, scrotum thinning and reddening III. Growth of penis in width and length and further growth of testes IV. Penis further larger, with enlarged testes; darker scrotal skin color V. Genitalia adult in size and shape	I. Prepubertal; no pubic hair II. Sparse growth of slightly pigmented, slightly curly pubic hair, mainly at base of penis III. Thicker, curlier hair, spread to mons pubis IV. Adult-type hair that does not yet spread to medial surface of thighs V. Adult-type hair spread to medial thighs

Data from Marshall, W. E., & Tanner, J. M. (1969) Variations in the pattern of pubertal changes in girls. *Archives of Disease in Childhood, 44,* 291–303; Marshall, W. E., & Tanner, J. M. (1970). Variations in the pattern of pubertal changes in boys. *Archives of Disease in Childhood, 45,* 13–23.

7. What controls the pubertal growth spurt?

In both boys and girls, the pubertal growth spurt is primarily controlled by the gonadal steroid estrogen. In both sexes, gonadal (and adrenal) androgens are aromatized to estrogens. Estrogens augment growth hormone (GH) and insulin-like growth factor-1 (IGF-1) secretion. Estrogens also suppress osteoclast activity and prolong the life span of osteoblasts and osteocytes. Androgens have a small independent role in linear growth and maintenance of adequate bone mineral density. At the end of puberty, linear growth is nearly complete because of the effects of gonadal steroids on skeletal maturation and epiphyseal fusion.

8. What is precocious puberty?

Precocious puberty is defined as pubertal development occurring below the limits of age set for normal onset of puberty. In girls, this is pubertal signs before age 8 years in white girls, age 6.6 years in black girls, and age 6.8 years in Hispanic girls. For boys, precocious puberty is pubertal signs occurring before age 9 years in white and Hispanic boys, and age 8 years in black boys.

9. Why does precocious puberty matter?

The most important reason to evaluate early pubertal signs is to rule out an underlying pathologic etiology that would need treatment, such as a tumor or genetic condition. Precocious puberty can also lead to short adult height because of premature epiphyseal fusion and psychosocial stress. If there is no concerning etiology and predicted height is not concerning, precocious puberty may not require extensive evaluation or treatment.

10. How is precocious puberty evaluated?

Evaluation of precocious puberty begins with a thorough history, including timing of onset of pubertal signs, rate of progression, exposure to exogenous steroids or estrogen receptor agonists (E.g., lavender or tea tree oil), presence or history of central nervous system (CNS) abnormalities, and pubertal history of other family members. A physical examination should be performed, with a focus on Tanner staging, proportions, and neurologic signs. Height measurements should be plotted on a growth chart to determine growth pattern, and linear growth velocity should be calculated. Radiography of the left hand and wrist is helpful to determine skeletal maturity (bone age) and skeletal advancement. Depending on this initial assessment, laboratory testing and/or imaging may be needed. Fig. 49.1 provides a simplified flow diagram that can be useful when evaluating a child with precocious puberty.

11. What is GnRH-dependent (central) precocious puberty, and how is it diagnosed?

Central precocious puberty (CPP) involves activation of the GnRH pulse generator, an increase in gonadotropin secretion, gonadarche, and a resultant increase in the production of sex steroids. Consequently, the sequence of

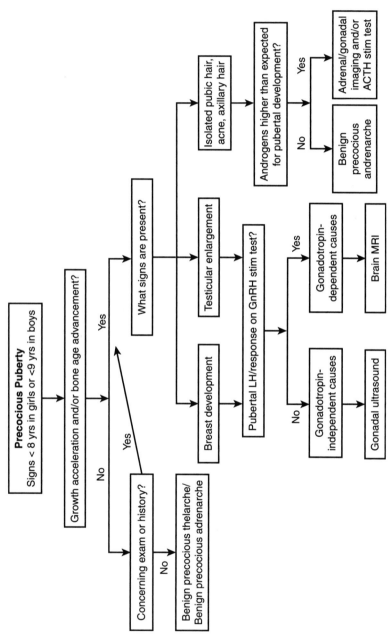

Fig. 49.1. Evaluation of precocious puberty. *ACTH*, Adrenocorticotropic hormone; *GnRH*, gonadotropin–releasing hormone; *MRI*, magnetic resonance imaging; *stim*, stimulation.

hormonal and physical events in CPP is identical to the progression of normal puberty. CPP is much more common in girls than in boys. The GnRH stimulation test is the single most important test to diagnose CPP. A child with CPP will have a predominant LH response to a single dose of a GnRH agonist (leuprolide). Measurement of random gonadotropins may not be helpful because of overlap between prepubertal and early pubertal values. If non-stimulated gonadotropins are obtained, an early-morning sample measured on a third-generation assay will be more likely to identify early pubertal LH concentrations.

12. What causes CPP?

In the large majority of cases, CPP is idiopathic, especially in girls. CPP can also be caused by any CNS disturbance that disrupts the balance regulating the GnRH pulse generator. This includes structural disruptions, such as brain tumors and pre-existing malformations. Often, there will be other signs of a CNS lesion, but occasionally precocious puberty can be the presenting sign. Certain genetic conditions or inherited single-gene mutations can also cause CPP.

13. When is brain imaging indicated?

Girls younger than 6 years of age and boys of any age who are diagnosed with CPP should undergo a magnetic resonance imaging (MRI) study of the brain to evaluate for CNS lesions. It is much less likely that an abnormality will be found in girls between ages 6 and 8 years, so the need for an MRI in this age group should be assessed on an individual basis.

14. How is CPP treated?

Children with CPP can be treated with long-acting GnRH agonists, such as leuprolide or histrelin. GnRH agonists disrupt the endogenous pulsatile secretion of GnRH, thus downregulating pituitary GnRH receptors and decreasing gonadotropin secretion. The most important clinical criteria for GnRH agonist therapy is documented progression of pubertal development, which is based on the recognition that many girls with CPP, especially those between ages 6 and 8 years, have a slowly progressive form and reach normal adult height without any intervention. With GnRH agonist treatment, physical changes of puberty regress or cease to progress, linear growth reverts to the prepubertal rate, and skeletal maturation slows. Projected final adult height often increases because of the slowing of skeletal maturation. GnRH agonists can be given as monthly or every 3-month depot intramuscular injections, or by placement of a small hydrogel implant under the skin that releases a GnRH agonist (histrelin) continuously. Children on GnRH agonists should be monitored every 4 to 6 months to evaluate for pubertal regression or treatment failure. After discontinuation of therapy, pubertal progression resumes, and normal rates of fertility are expected.

15. What is GnRH-independent (peripheral) precocious puberty, and how is it diagnosed?

Peripheral precocious puberty occurs independent of gonadotropin secretion. Early autonomous production of sex steroids from the adrenal glands or gonads can result in peripheral precocious puberty. Basal serum FSH and LH are low (often suppressed), and the LH response to GnRH stimulation is not in a pubertal range. There are numerous etiologies of peripheral precocious puberty (Table 49.2), but these conditions are much less common than CPP. Evaluation for a specific diagnosis will depend on whether signs of androgens or estrogens are present.

16. How is peripheral precocious puberty evaluated?

In girls with signs of estrogen production without CPP, a pelvic ultrasonography can be performed to evaluate for an ovarian cyst or tumor, as well as the size of the uterus and endometrial stripe (particularly if vaginal bleeding is present).

In boys or girls with signs of adrenarche (without testicular enlargement in boys), evaluation should include laboratory studies for nonclassic congenital adrenal hyperplasia (CAH) and adrenal tumors. Serum 17-hydrodroxyprogesterone, testosterone, DHEA-S, and androstenedione levels should be obtained, and, depending on the situation, possibly adrenocorticotropic hormone (ACTH)–stimulated steroid intermediates (e.g., 17-hydroxyprogesterone, 17-hydroxypregnenolone, 11-deoxycortisol). With elevated adrenal androgen levels suggestive of a tumor, imaging of the adrenal glands should be pursued. Genetic testing for CAH may be helpful, particularly if the biochemical testing is nondiagnostic.

In boys with testicular enlargement but a prepubertal response to a GnRH stimulation test, human chorionic gonadotropin (hCG) and testosterone should be measured. Asymmetric or unilateral enlargement of the testes suggests a Leydig cell tumor, and testicular ultrasonography should be performed.

17. What is McCune-Albright syndrome, and how is it treated?

McCune-Albright syndrome is a triad consisting of GnRH-independent precocious puberty, irregular (coast of Maine) café-au-lait lesions on the skin, and polyostotic fibrous dysplasia, but only two of these are necessary to make the diagnosis. It can affect both sexes but is seen infrequently in boys. In girls, breast development and vaginal bleeding occur with sporadic increases in estradiol from autonomously functioning ovarian cysts. Serum gonadotropin levels are low, and GnRH testing elicits a prepubertal response. With time, however, increased estradiol may cause maturation of the hypothalamus, thus leading to true central GnRH-dependent precocity. The syndrome can

Table 49.2. Clinical Findings in Girls with Turner's Syndrome.

PHYSICAL FEATURES	FREQUENCY (%)
Short stature	95–100
Increased upper-to-lower segment ratio	97
Short neck	40
Webbed neck	25
Low posterior hairline	40
Micrognathia	60
High arched palate	35
Epicanthal folds	10
Strabismus	15
Ptosis	10
Cubitus valgus	50–80
Short fourth metacarpals	35
Madelung deformity	5
Edema of hands and feet	25
Fingernail dysplasia/hypoplasia	5
Scoliosis	12
Genu valgum	35–86
Multiple pigmented nevi	25
Congenital Anomalies	
Bicuspid aortic valve	14–34
Coarctation of the aorta	7–14
Renal aplasia	3
Horseshoe kidney	10
Abnormal position or duplication of the renal pelvis/collecting system	15
Physiologic Features	
Otitis media	60
Delayed puberty (no thelarche)	70
Primary amenorrhea	90
Infertility	95
Hypertension	50
Thyroiditis and hypothyroidism	15–30
Alopecia	5
Vitiligo	5
Celiac disease	8
Glucose intolerance	15–50
Type 2 diabetes	10

Data from Gravholt, C. H., Andersen, N. H., Conway, G. S., Dekkers, O. M., Geffner, M. E., Klein, K. O., ... Backeljauw, P. F. (2017). Clinical practice guidelines for the care of girls and women with Turner syndrome: proceedings from the 2016 Cincinnati International Turner Syndrome Meeting. *European Journal of Endocrinology, 177*(3): G1–G70.

be associated with other endocrine dysfunctions, including hyperthyroidism, growth hormone excess, and hyper-cortisolism. In affected tissues, there is an activating mutation in the gene that encodes the alpha-subunit of Gs, the G-protein that stimulates adenylate cyclase. Endocrine cells with this mutation have autonomous hyperfunc-tion and secrete excess amounts of their respective hormones.

Girls with McCune-Albright syndrome are generally treated with an aromatase inhibitor, such as letrozole or anastrozole, which inhibits the conversion of testosterone to estrogen. Trials using tamoxifen, an estrogen receptor antagonist, have also been performed. In boys, treatment consists of either inhibiting androgen production with ketoconazole or use of a combination of an aromatase inhibitor and an antiandrogen. For both sexes, if central puberty has been induced, GnRH agonists may also be part of the treatment plan. Because of other manifestations that can occur in this condition, routine screening is required throughout childhood.

18. What is testotoxicosis, and how is it treated?
Familial testotoxicosis is a male-limited autosomal dominant, gonadotropin-independent form of male precocious puberty. Boys with this condition begin to develop true precocity with bilateral testicular and phallic enlargement and growth acceleration by age 4 years. Serum testosterone concentrations are high, but serum gonadotropins are low and GnRH stimulation shows a prepubertal response. By mid-adolescence to adulthood, GnRH stimulation demonstrates a more typical LH-predominant pubertal response. This condition is caused by an activating muta-tion in the gene encoding the LH receptor. The mutant LH receptors in the testes are constitutively overactive and do not require LH binding for their activity, resulting in autonomous testosterone production. Because Leydig cells are a minority of cells in the testes, testicular size is only modestly enlarged. Treatment options are the same as for boys with McCune-Albright syndrome. If CPP has been induced, GnRH agonists may also be part of the treat-ment plan.

19. What is nonclassic CAH, and how is it treated?
CAH is usually caused by genetic mutations in the *CYP21A2* gene, resulting in 21-hydroxylase deficiency, which prevents the normal production of glucocorticoids by the adrenal glands. Because of the underproduction of these hormones, ACTH is elevated, driving adrenal production of androgens. In classic CAH, there is no functional enzyme, so the presentation is more severe with virilization of female fetuses and salt-losing crises within the first weeks of life in both sexes. In nonclassic CAH, there is partial function of the enzyme so the presentation is milder, often without signs of adrenal insufficiency. These children may present with premature adrenarche, tall stature, and skeletal advancement. Unstimulated 17-hydroxyprogesterone levels may or may not be elevated; therefore, an ACTH stimulation test may be needed to diagnose nonclassic CAH. Genetic testing can be consid-ered, particularly if it would change management.

Nonclassic CAH can be treated with glucocorticoids to reduce pituitary ACTH secretion and thereby decrease the overproduction of adrenal hormones. However, this treatment causes iatrogenic adrenal insufficiency, and therefore the risks and benefits of this treatment need to be weighed on an individual basis.

20. What is the association between hypothyroidism and precocity?
Rarely, severe primary hypothyroidism may cause breast development in girls and increased testicular size in boys. This is often called *Van Wyk and Grumbach syndrome*. The exact mechanism is unclear but one theory is that thyroid-stimulating hormone (TSH), which is elevated in primary hypothyroidism, can stimulate the FSH receptor on the gonads. These children generally present with growth deceleration, as typically seen in hypothyroid-ism, rather than growth acceleration, as typically seen in precocious puberty. Bone age is usually delayed. Thyroid hormone replacement results in regression of pubertal changes, and no other therapy is necessary.

21. When can early puberty signs be benign?
Isolated thelarche or adrenarche that occur early but fail to progress through all pubertal stages can be variants of normal puberty. In these benign conditions, pubertal development is usually isolated (i.e., just thelarche or just adrenarche) and often does not progress beyond Tanner stage II–III. There is usually no significant growth acceleration or bone age advancement. Testicular enlargement is not seen in benign variants. An assessment needs to reasonably exclude pathologic and progressive forms of precocious puberty before determining the pattern is consistent with a benign process.

22. What is benign premature thelarche, and how is it managed?
Benign premature thelarche is defined as isolated breast development in girls without other signs of puberty. Benign premature thelarche is most common in girls who are either under 2 years or between ages 6 and 8 years. Girls with benign premature thelarche may have a history of slowly progressing breast development or waxing and waning of breast size. GnRH stimulation may provoke an FSH-predominant response, as opposed to the typical LH-predominant response seen in true central puberty.

The natural course of benign premature thelarche is for the breast tissue to regress or fail to progress. Be-cause of its benign nature, treatment is not necessary except for reassurance and follow-up. Follow-up is critical because premature thelarche occasionally is the first sign of what later becomes apparent as CPP. Measurement of breast tissue diameter during the clinic visit can be helpful for comparison at a later visit.

23. What is benign premature adrenarche, and how is it treated?

Benign premature adrenarche, which occurs in both sexes, is defined as the early development of pubic hair with or without axillary hair, body odor, and acne (isolated adrenarche). There are no signs of gonadarche—girls have no breast development and boys have no testicular enlargement. Benign premature adrenarche is caused by early secretion of the adrenal androgens, primarily DHEA and DHEA-S, and measurement of these hormones correspond to the Tanner stage of development (usually Tanner stage II–III).

The natural course of benign premature adrenarche is a slow progression of the signs of adrenarche, with no effect on the timing of true puberty. Because pubic hair development may be the first sign of puberty, follow-up is necessary to evaluate for evidence of gonadarche. Girls with benign premature adrenarche are at an increased risk of developing polycystic ovarian syndrome as adolescents or adults.

24. What is physiologic gynecomastia in puberty? When and how should it be treated?

Typically developing boys often have either unilateral or bilateral breast enlargement during puberty. Breast development generally starts midpuberty and resolves within 2 years, likely as a result of a transient imbalance of estradiol and testosterone. Pubertal gynecomastia is common and benign and usually only requires reassurance. However, a thorough history and physical examination should be done to evaluate for pathologic causes of gynecomastia, including hypogonadism, rare malignancies, medications, drug abuse, and exposure to lavender or tea tree oils.

Pharmacologic treatment with antiestrogens (tamoxifen) or aromatase inhibitors have been used to treat gynecomastia with mixed results. If resolution of gynecomastia does not occur or if the breast enlargement is excessive, surgery may be warranted. Surgery should be avoided until puberty is complete to avoid recurrence of gynecomastia.

25. What is delayed puberty?

Delayed puberty is absence of pubertal signs by age 13 years in girls or age 14 years in boys. An abnormality in the pubertal axis may also present as lack of normal pubertal progression, which is defined as $\geq$ 4 years between the first signs of puberty and menarche in girls or $\geq$ 5 years for completion of genital growth in boys. Failure to achieve menarche by age 16 years or within 4 years after thelarche is primary amenorrhea.

26. What features are present in the history of an adolescent with pubertal delay?

The history should include questions regarding the presence of chronic illnesses, autoimmune disorders, nutritional disorders, exercise history, galactorrhea, sense of smell, medications, family history of infertility, and timing of puberty in parents and siblings. Weight gain or loss should also be noted.

27. What features are seen in the physical examination of an adolescent with pubertal delay?

Physical examination should include measurement of arm span and upper-to-lower segment ratio. Signs of any chronic illness, malnutrition, anorexia, hypothyroidism, glucocorticoid excess, or features of Turner's syndrome (in girls) or Klinefelter's syndrome (in boys) should be noted. A careful examination should be made for any signs of puberty, such as pubic hair, axillary hair, acne, testicular size (boys), penile length (boys), or breast development (girls). Pubic hair may represent only adrenal androgen production. Testicular volume $\geq$ 4 mL (length $\geq$ 2.5 cm) indicates gonadotropin stimulation. Breast development and vaginal maturity are indicators of estrogen exposure. In addition, visual fields and olfaction should be evaluated. The growth chart should be analyzed to evaluate for short or tall stature relative to parental heights and to determine if linear growth has been normal.

28. How are radiographic studies and gonadotropin levels helpful in the diagnosis of pubertal delay?

Assessment of bone age is critical in determining biological age and the time of expected pubertal development. If linear growth is normal and bone age is less than the normal age for pubertal onset, the diagnosis is likely to be constitutional growth delay. If linear growth is impaired and bone age is delayed, it may be necessary to evaluate growth hormone or thyroid function. If bone age has advanced beyond the age for normal puberty, gonadotropin levels are helpful to distinguish between gonadotropin deficiency and primary gonadal failure.

29. What other laboratory tests may be needed?

Additional laboratory studies may include a chemistry panel, complete blood count (CBC), celiac testing, thyroid function tests, estradiol (girls), testosterone (boys), and prolactin levels. If gonadotropins are elevated, chromosome analysis is indicated for both sexes. In the case of low gonadotropins, olfactory testing and cranial MRI with views of the pituitary gland and olfactory sulci and bulbs are recommended.

30. What is constitutional growth delay, and how does it affect puberty?

Constitutional growth delay is the most common cause of delayed puberty. Children with this growth pattern generally have slower linear growth velocity within the first 2 years of life. After this, growth returns to normal, but along a lower growth trajectory than would be expected for parental heights. Skeletal maturation is also delayed, and the onset of puberty is commensurate with bone age rather than chronologic age. For example, a 14-year-old boy with a bone age of 11 years will start puberty when his bone age is closer to 11.5 to 12 years. This delay in puberty postpones the pubertal growth spurt and closure of growth plates, so that the child continues to grow after his or her peers have reached their final adult height. A key feature of this growth pattern is normal linear growth after 2 years of age. There is often a family history of "late bloomers."

31. When is hypogonadism diagnosed?

Functional or permanent hypogonadism should be considered when there are no signs of puberty and bone age has advanced to beyond the normal ages for puberty to start. A eunuchoid body habitus is often evident in children with abnormally delayed puberty—a decreased upper-to-lower body ratio and long arm span characterize this habitus. As a rule, serum gonadotropin levels are measured first to determine whether there is hypogonadotropic hypogonadism (gonadotropin deficiency) or hypergonadotropic hypogonadism (primary gonadal failure). If a child's bone age is below the normal age for puberty to start, gonadotropin levels are not necessarily a reliable means of making this diagnosis.

32. What are the causes of hypogonadotropic hypogonadism?

Normal or suppressed gonadotropins indicate that there is failure of the pituitary to stimulate gonadal steroid production. Chronic illness, excessive exercise, malnutrition, anorexia, and depression can cause a functional deficiency of gonadotropins; however, it is reversed when the underlying condition improves. Hyperprolactinemia can cause hypogonadotropic hypogonadism, and only in 50% of cases there is a history of galactorrhea. Other endocrinopathies, such as diabetes mellitus, glucocorticoid excess, and hypothyroidism, can cause hypogonadotropic hypogonadism when these conditions are uncontrolled. Drug abuse, particularly of heroin or methadone, has been associated with hypogonadotropic hypogonadism. Permanent gonadotropin deficiency is suspected if these conditions are ruled out and gonadotropin levels are low. Gonadotropin deficiency may be associated with other pituitary deficiencies from such conditions as septo-optic dysplasia; tumors, such as craniopharyngioma; trauma; empty sella syndrome; pituitary dysgenesis; Rathke's pouch cysts; or cranial irradiation. Various syndromes, such as Kallmann's syndrome, Laurence-Moon-Bardet-Biedl syndrome, and Prader-Willi syndrome, are also associated with gonadotropin deficiency, so genetic testing may be considered, depending on the phenotype. Isolated gonadotropin deficiency (i.e., occurring without another pituitary deficiency) is often difficult to diagnose because hormonal tests do not distinguish with certainty whether a child can produce enough gonadotropins or whether he or she simply has very delayed puberty. If gonadotropin deficiency cannot be clearly distinguished from delayed puberty, a short course of sex steroids can be given. Patients with constitutional delay often enter puberty after such an intervention. If spontaneous puberty does not occur, the diagnosis of gonadotropin deficiency may be made.

33. What is Kallmann's syndrome?

Kallmann's syndrome is a specific cause of idiopathic hypogonadotropic hypogonadism with reduced sense of smell (hyposmia or anosmia). Genetic defects lead to abnormal development and/or migration of the GnRH and olfactory neurons. On MRI, this can be appreciated through the presence of hypoplastic or aplastic olfactory bulbs. Undescended testes, micropenis, and gynecomastia are common in boys with Kallmann's syndrome. Other features than can be seen in Kallmann's syndrome include cleft lip/cleft palate, congenital deafness, color blindness, renal anomalies, and certain neurologic differences.

34. What are the causes of hypergonadotropic hypogonadism?

Elevated gonadotropin levels indicate that there is a failure of the gonads to produce enough sex steroids to suppress the hypothalamic–pituitary axis. These elevated levels are diagnostic for gonadal failure at two periods: (1) before age 6 months in boys and before age 2 to 3 years in girls; and (2) after bone age is at or beyond the normal age for puberty to start. If hypergonadotropic hypogonadism is diagnosed, a karyotype should be performed. Potential etiologies include:

- Variants of ovarian or testicular dysgenesis—Turner's syndrome, Klinefelter's syndrome, pure XX or XY gonadal dysgenesis
- Gonadal toxins—chemotherapy (particularly alkylating agents), radiation treatment
- Androgen enzymatic defects—17-alpha-hydroxylase deficiency in the genetic male or female, 17-ketosteroid reductase deficiency in the genetic male
- Complete or partial androgen insensitivity syndrome (mutation in the androgen receptor gene) in genetic males
- Galactosemia; fragile X premutation (in girls only)
- Other miscellaneous disorders—infections, gonadal autoimmunity, vanishing testes, trauma, torsion

35. What is Klinefelter's syndrome?

Klinefelter's syndrome is the most common cause of testicular failure and results from at least one extra X chromosome. The most common karyotype, 47,XXY, occurs in ~1:650 male births. Associated physical features include tall stature, long extremities, small testes, and gynecomastia. Developmental delays and learning disabilities are common. Boys with Klinefelter's syndrome will have spontaneous pubertal onset but may fail to progress completely through puberty. Gonadotropins rise out of the normal range within a couple years of pubertal onset and testosterone often plateaus or even declines, rather than sustaining adult concentrations. Testosterone supplementation is indicated in many boys over time to support normal secondary sex characteristics, metabolism,

---

Box 49.1. Causes of Precocious Puberty.

Central (GnRH Dependent)
- Idiopathic true precocious puberty
- CNS tumors (hamartomas, hypothalamic tumors)
- CNS disorders (meningitis, encephalitis, hydrocephalus, trauma, abscesses, cysts, granulomas, radiation therapy)

Peripheral (GnRH Independent)
Males
- hCG-secreting tumors (CNS, liver)
- CAH (21-hydroxylase, 3-beta-hydroxysteroid dehydrogenase, or 11-hydroxylase deficiency)
- Adrenal tumors
- Leydig cell testicular tumors
- Familial gonadotropin-independent Leydig cell maturation (testotoxicosis)
- McCune-Albright syndrome (polyostotic fibrous dysplasia)

Females
- Follicular cysts
- Ovarian tumors
- Adrenal tumors
- CAH (21-hydroxylase, 3-beta-hydroxysteroid dehydrogenase, or 11-hydroxylase deficiency)
- Exogenous estrogen
- McCune-Albright syndrome (polyostotic fibrous dysplasia)

CAH, Congenital adrenal hyperplasia; *CNS,* central nervous system; *GnRH,* gonadotropin-releasing hormone; *hCG,* human chorionic gonadotropin.

---

and bone health. Germ cells are decreased in number from birth; Sertoli and Leydig cells are affected to a lesser degree. Men with Klinefelter's syndrome are usually azoospermic and infertile; however, advanced reproductive techniques can now help achieve successful sperm extraction in about half of young men with Klinefelter's syndrome.

36. What is Turner's syndrome?
   Any consideration of pubertal delay and/or amenorrhea in girls must include the possibility of Turner's syndrome. Turner's syndrome is characterized by an absent or structurally abnormal second X chromosome. Turner's syndrome occurs in approximately 1:2000 live female births. Girls with Turner's syndrome often have short stature and dysmorphic features, and are at a higher risk of congenital and acquired heart disease, renal anomalies, frequent otitis media and hearing loss, autoimmunity, and math learning disability. See Box 49.1 for additional clinical findings associated with Turner's syndrome.
      In the absence of a second functional X chromosome, oocyte degeneration is accelerated, often leaving fibrotic streaks in place of normal ovaries. Because of primary gonadal failure, serum gonadotropin levels rise and are elevated in infancy and again after reactivation of the HPG axis. Approximately 10% to 20% of girls with Turner's syndrome have some ovarian function at puberty that promotes spontaneous breast development. A small percentage of this group will have normal periods, and an even smaller percentage (< 1% of girls with Turner's syndrome) are actually fertile.

37. How is Turner's syndrome treated?
   Most girls with Turner's syndrome require exogenous estrogen replacement. Low-dose unopposed estradiol, followed by estrogen and progestin, allows development of secondary sexual characteristics. The timing for initiation of estrogen therapy is critical and should be decided by an endocrinologist through discussions with each patient and her family. This decision depends on several factors, including height and psychosocial factors. In girls with Turner's syndrome, short stature can be treated with growth hormone, with taller final adult height outcomes achieved when growth hormone treatment is started at a younger age. Turner's syndrome is ideally managed by an interdisciplinary care team to address the many medical and neurodevelopmental differences that girls with Turner's syndrome may experience.

38. How is delayed puberty managed?
   The treatment of delayed puberty depends on the underlying cause. If the delayed pubertal development is secondary to anorexia, excessive exercise, hypothyroidism, or illness, treatment of these underlying conditions results in spontaneous onset of puberty. Puberty also begins spontaneously, albeit late, in constitutional growth delay so that reassurance alone to the patient and family may be sufficient. In some patients with constitutional growth delay, treatment to induce puberty may be appropriate. For boys, a 4- to 6-month course of low-dose

depot testosterone (50–100 mg intramuscularly every 4 weeks) can be offered if the bone age is at least 11 to 12 years. This treatment results in some virilization without adversely affecting final adult height. Spontaneous puberty often begins, as evident by testicular enlargement, 3 to 6 months after the end of the testosterone course. For girls, a 3-month course of low-dose estradiol (0.25-0.5 mg orally every day) can be offered if the bone age is at least 10 to 11 years. Therapy is then stopped and physical changes are evaluated. Withdrawal bleeding is unusual after one course of estrogen therapy but may occur with subsequent courses.

39. What is the treatment of hypogonadism in boys?

In boys with hypogonadotropic hypogonadism for whom fertility is not an immediate issue and in all boys with primary hypogonadism, long-term testosterone therapy is required. While the patient is growing, careful attention must be paid to growth velocity and bone age. Most commonly, depot testosterone esters (enanthate or cypionate) are given intramuscularly in 50-mg doses every 3 to 4 weeks for pubertal initiation. The dose is gradually raised to mimic the rise in testosterone during normal puberty over several years. The adult maintenance dose is around 400 mg per month, usually divided into weekly or every-2-week injections. Alternatively, a transdermal testosterone gel or patch may be used.

40. What is the treatment for hypogonadism in girls?

Estrogen replacement therapy in hypogonadal girls is begun with very low-dose unopposed estrogen treatment for 12 to 18 months. Estrogen can be given via an oral tablet or via a transdermal patch, the latter of which is felt to be more physiologic. The dosage used varies, depending on height projections and individual response. After this period of unopposed estrogen, cyclic or daily progesterone is added. Progesterone therapy is necessary to counteract the effects of estrogen on the uterus; unopposed estrogen can cause endometrial hyperplasia and increase the risk of carcinoma. Replacement of gonadal steroids in both sexes is also necessary for normal bone mineralization and to prevent osteoporosis.

41. How do you evaluate a girl with primary amenorrhea?

To sort out the many causes of amenorrhea, it is helpful to distinguish girls who produce sufficient estrogen from those who do not by performing a progesterone challenge. Girls who are producing estrogen will have a withdrawal bleed after 5 to 10 days of oral progesterone, whereas those who are estrogen deficient will have very little or no bleeding. Those who do not have bleeding should be evaluated for hypogonadism, as described previously. There are, however, two situations in which girls who have sufficient estrogen will not have a withdrawal bleed: obstruction of the cervix or absence of the cervix or the uterus. In Rokitansky's syndrome, maldevelopment of the Müllerian structures leads to an absent or hypoplastic uterus or cervix (or both). Complete androgen insensitivity syndrome (testicular feminization) in a genetic male results in a phenotypic female who has normal breast development due to the aromatization of testosterone to estrogen. The production of anti-Müllerian hormone in patients with androgen insensitivity syndrome leads to regression of the Müllerian structures, and thus the absence of a uterus. The absence of a cervix is found in both Rokitansky's syndrome and complete androgen insensitivity syndrome. Consequently, a pelvic examination should be considered in all girls who present with primary amenorrhea. (See also Chapter 53.)

KEY POINTS: DISORDERS OF PUBERTY

- Central precocious puberty occurs more frequently in girls than boys. Boys with central precocity, however, have a much higher incidence of underlying central nervous system pathology.
- Precocious puberty must be distinguished from normal variants of early development, such as benign premature thelarche and benign premature adrenarche.
- The most useful diagnostic test to evaluate precocious puberty is a gonadotropin-releasing hormone stimulation test.
- Children with delayed puberty and normal linear growth will most likely have constitutional growth delay.
- Bone age assessment is the first step in evaluating a child with delayed puberty.
- After it has been determined that a child has abnormally delayed puberty, gonadotropins should be measured. If gonadotropins are elevated, a chromosome analysis is generally the next step.

BIBLIOGRAPHY

Carel, J. C., Eugster, E. A., Rogol, A., Ghizzoni, L., Palmert, M. R., Antoniazzi, F., … Berenbaum, S. (2009). Consensus statement on the use of gonadotropin-releasing hormone analogs in children. *Pediatrics, 123*(4), e752–762.

Carretto, F., Salinas-Vert, I., Granada-Yvern, M. L., Murillo-Vallés, M., Gómez-Gómez, C., Puig-Domingo, M., & Bel, J. (2014). The usefulness of the leuprolide stimulation test as a diagnostic method of idiopathic central precocious puberty in girls. *Hormone and Metabolic Research, 46*(13), 959–963.

Cortes, M. E., Carrera, B., Rioseco, H., Pablo del Río, J., & Vigil, P. (2015). The role of kisspeptin in the onset of puberty and in the ovulatory mechanism: a mini-review. *Journal of Pediatric and Adolescent Gynecology, 28*(5), 286–291.

Davis, S., Howell, S., Wilson, R., Tanda, T., Ross, J., Zeitler, P., & Tartaglia, N. (2016). Advances in the interdisciplinary care of children with Klinefelter syndrome. *Advances in Pediatrics, 63*(1), 15–46.

Durbin, K. L., Diaz-Montes, T., & Loveless, M. B. (2011). Van wyk and grumbach syndrome: an unusual case and review of the literature. *Journal of Pediatric and Adolescent Gynecology, 24*(4), e93–96.

Eugster, E. A., Clarke, W., Kletter, G. B., Lee, P. A., Neely, E. K., Reiter, E. O., … Tierney, D. (2007). Efficacy and safety of histrelin subdermal implant in children with central precocious puberty: a multicenter trial. *Journal of Clinical Endocrinology and Metabolism, 92*(5), 1697–1704.

Fuqua, J. S. (2013). Treatment and outcomes of precocious puberty: an update. *Journal of Clinical Endocrinology and Metabolism, 98*(6), 2198–2207.

Gravholt, C. H., Andersen, N. H., Conway, G. S., Dekkers, O. M., Geffner, M. E., Klein, K. O., … Backeljauw, P. F. (2017). Clinical practice guidelines for the care of girls and women with Turner syndrome: proceedings from the 2016 Cincinnati International Turner Syndrome Meeting. *European Journal of Endocrinology, 177*(3), G1–G70.

Herman-Giddens, M. E., Slora, E. J., Wasserman, R. C., Bourdony, C. J., Bhapkar, M. V., Koch, G. G., & Hasemeier, C. M. (1997). Secondary sexual characteristics and menses in young girls seen in office practice: a study from the Pediatric Research in Office Settings network. *Pediatrics, 99*(4), 505–512.

Kang, E., Cho, J. H., Choi, J. H., & Yoo, H. W. (2016). Etiology and therapeutic outcomes of children with gonadotropin-independent precocious puberty. *Annals of Pediatric Endocrinology & Metabolism, 21*(3), 136–142.

Latronico, A. C., Brito V. N., & Carel, J. C. (2016). Causes, diagnosis, and treatment of central precocious puberty. *Lancet Diabetes & Endocrinology, 4*(3), 265–274.

Layman, L. C. (2007). Hypogonadotropic hypogonadism. *Endocrinology and Metabolism Clinics of North America, 36*(2), 283–296.

Macedo, D. B., Silveira, L. F., Bessa, D. S., Brito, V. N., & Latronico, A. C. (2016). Sexual precocity—genetic bases of central precocious puberty and autonomous gonadal activation. *Endocrine Development, 29*, 50–71.

Magiakou, M. A., Manousaki, D., Papadaki, M., Hadjidakis, D., Levidou, G., Vakaki, M., … Dacou-Voutetakis, C. (2010). The efficacy and safety of gonadotropin-releasing hormone analog treatment in childhood and adolescence: a single center, long-term follow-up study. *Journal of Clinical Endocrinology and Metabolism, 95*(1), 109–117.

Maione, L., Dwyer, A. A., Francou, B., Guiochon-Mantel, A., Binart, N., Bouligand, J., & Young, J. (2018). Genetics in endocrinology: genetic counseling for congenital hypogonadotropic hypogonadism and Kallmann syndrome: new challenges in the era of oligogenism and next-generation sequencing. *European Journal of Endocrinology, 178*(3), R55–R80.

Marsh, C. A. & Grimstad, F. W. (2014). Primary amenorrhea: diagnosis and management. *Obstetrical & Gynecological Survey, 69*(10), 603–612.

Marshall, W. A. & Tanner, J. M. (1969). Variations in pattern of pubertal changes in girls. *Archives of Disease in Childhood, 44*(235), 291–303.

Marshall, W. A. & Tanner, J. M. (1970). Variations in the pattern of pubertal changes in boys. *Archives of Disease in Childhood, 45*(239), 13–23.

Novello, L. & Speiser, P. W. (2018). Premature adrenarche. *Pediatric Annals, 47*(1), e7–e11.

Pasquino, A. M., Pucarelli, I., Accardo, F., Demiraj, V., Segni, M., & Di Nardo, R. (2008). Long-term observation of 87 girls with idiopathic central precocious puberty treated with gonadotropin-releasing hormone analogs: impact on adult height, body mass index, bone mineral content, and reproductive function. *Journal of Clinical Endocrinology and Metabolism, 93*(1), 190–195.

Rosenfield, R. L., Lipton, R. B., & Drum, M. L. (2009). Thelarche, pubarche, and menarche attainment in children with normal and elevated body mass index. *Pediatrics, 123*(1), 84–88.

Schoelwer, M. & Eugster, E. A. (2016). Treatment of peripheral precocious puberty. *Endocrine Development, 29*, 230–239.

Wu, T., Mendola, P., & Buck, G. M. (2002). Ethnic differences in the presence of secondary sex characteristics and menarche among US girls: the Third National Health and Nutrition Examination Survey, 1988–1994. *Pediatrics, 110*(4), 752–757.

MALE HYPOGONADISM

Katherine N. Vu, Vinh Q. Mai, and Robert A. Vigersky

CHAPTER 50

1. **What is male hypogonadism?**

   Male hypogonadism is the clinical and biochemical/laboratory abnormality resulting from failure of proper functioning of the hypothalamic–pituitary–gonadal (HPG) axis. Normal testes have two functions: (1) synthesis and secretion of testosterone from Leydig cells and (2) production of sperm from the seminiferous tubules. Testicular disorders causing deficiency of one and/or both functions lead to primary hypogonadism and/or infertility. When a disorder affects the hypothalamus/pituitary, it can result in secondary or central hypogonadism resulting from lack of appropriate stimulation of gonadotropins (follicle-stimulating hormone/luteinizing hormone [FSH/LH]) on the testes. Depending on the stage of development, hypogonadism may have varied manifestations.

2. **What are the manifestations of in utero hypogonadism?**

   In utero androgen deficiency leads to a female phenotype or ambiguous genitalia (male pseudohermaphroditism), most commonly caused by a block in the production of testosterone as a result of congenital testosterone biosynthetic enzyme defects. Rarely, peripheral tissues cannot respond normally to testosterone, resulting in the androgen insensitivity syndromes of testicular feminization (complete) and Reifenstein's syndrome (incomplete). Other manifestations include micropenis, hypospadias, and cryptorchidism.

3. **What are the manifestations of peripubertal hypogonadism?**

   Childhood androgen deficiency results in delayed, incomplete, or absent pubertal development. Common manifestations include:
   - Eunuchoid proportions (ratio of pubis-to-vertex/pubis-to-floor is < 0.9 and/or arm span is > 5 cm compared with height. This phenotype is caused by the delayed closure of the epiphyses.
   - Small testes (< 20 ml or < 4.5 cm $\times$ 3.0 cm)
   - Decreased body hair
   - Gynecomastia
   - Reduced peak bone mass
   - Reduced male musculature
   - Persistently higher-pitched voice

4. **What are the manifestations of hypogonadism in early adulthood?**

   In early adulthood, a decrease in sperm output (azoospermia/oligospermia) without deficient production of testosterone is common and results in male infertility; thus, infertility is a form of male hypogonadism. A decrease in testosterone production in adulthood is usually accompanied by a decline in production of sperm. When it is not, the term "fertile eunuch" is used (eunuchoid proportions, low levels of LH, low levels of testosterone, normal levels of FSH, and spermatogenesis). Libido and/or potency may be diminished in the "fertile eunuch."

5. **What are the manifestations of hypogonadism in mid-to-late adulthood?**

   The most frequent circumstance in which adult hypogonadism occurs is in the middle-aged or senescent man with decreased libido or potency. Semen analysis is rarely performed in these men because these individuals are usually not concerned about fertility. Other findings may include osteoporosis, diminished androgen production, and small prostate. If the onset of hypogonadism is acute, the patient may experience hot flashes and sweats.

6. **How is production of testosterone normally regulated?**

   LH is episodically secreted from the anterior pituitary in response to pulses of gonadotropin-releasing hormone (GnRH) from the hypothalamus, thus stimulating the production of testosterone by Leydig cells. Once testosterone is secreted into the bloodstream, it is bound by sex hormone-binding globulin (SHBG) and albumin. The non–SHBG-bound (or "free") testosterone provides negative feedback to the hypothalamic–pituitary unit and thus inhibits output of LH. This classic endocrine negative feedback loop serves to maintain serum testosterone at a predetermined level; if serum testosterone falls below the set point, the pituitary is stimulated to secrete LH, which, in turn, stimulates testicular output of testosterone until serum levels return to the set point. Conversely, if serum testosterone rises above the set point, decreased output of LH results in decreased testicular output of testosterone until serum levels have declined back to the set point.

7. How are serum testosterone levels measured?

Although most automated total testosterone assays are reliable and generally are able to distinguish hypogonadism from eugonadism in men, abnormalities in the SHBG level may give falsely low or high total testosterone levels. Equilibrium dialysis is the gold standard for measuring free testosterone levels, but it is not commonly available and should only be ordered to be done in a reliable reference laboratory. Liquid chromatography/mass spectrometry or gas chromatography/mass spectrometry is being used by some reference laboratories to measure testosterone. This is a very accurate but expensive methodology. Analog methods for determining free testosterone are more widely available but are not accurate in the low ranges.

8. What are some conditions associated with decreased or increased serum SHBG levels?

Increased SHBG Levels → High Total Serum Testosterone Levels	*Decreased SHBG Levels → Low Total Serum Testosterone Levels*
• Aging	• Moderate obesity
• Anticonvulsant use	• Nephrotic syndrome
• Estrogen (oral contraceptive pill [OCP]) use in (male-to-female) transgender persons or herbal preparations for "prostate health" that contain plant-derived estrogens	• Hypothyroidism
	• Medications (notably glucocorticoids and androgenic steroids)
	- Diabetes Mellitus
• Hepatic cirrhosis	- Acromegaly
• Human immunodeficiency virus (HIV) infection	
• Hyperthyroidism	

9. How is sperm production normally regulated?

The regulation of sperm production is complex and less clearly understood than regulation of testosterone production. Both hormonal and nonhormonal factors are important. Sertoli cells within the seminiferous tubules seem to play an important coordinating role. Sertoli cells respond to FSH by producing inhibin (secreted into the blood) and androgen-binding protein, transferrin, and other proteins (secreted into the seminiferous tubular lumen). Inhibin inhibits the output of FSH from the pituitary gland, thus completing a feedback loop. In theory, if spermatogenesis declines, production of inhibin also should decline; thus, the negative feedback effect on the pituitary would be reduced, leading to an increased output of FSH, which would then stimulate spermatogenesis. However, not all aspects of this feedback loop (FSH–inhibin–spermatogenesis) have been verified experimentally. Moreover, spermatogenesis depends on intratesticular production of testosterone mediated by androgen receptors within Sertoli cells. Initiation of spermatogenesis during puberty requires both LH and FSH. However, reinitiation of the process is disrupted by exogenous factors (see the following) and requires only LH (or human chorionic gonadotropin [hCG]), although FSH may be needed to produce a normal number of sperm.

10. What is the difference between primary hypogonadism and secondary hypogonadism?

Failure of testicular function may result from a defect either at the testes or the hypothalamic–pituitary level. Testicular disorders leading to hypogonadism are termed *primary hypogonadism* (Fig. 50.1), whereas disorders of hypothalamic–pituitary function leading to hypogonadism are termed *secondary (central) hypogonadism* (Fig. 50.2). This distinction has therapeutic implications. In men with secondary (central) hypogonadism, fertility can generally be restored with appropriate hormonal treatment. Men with primary hypogonadism have fewer options and more limited success with improvement in fertility. In addition, the evaluation of secondary hypogonadism can reveal a pituitary mass or systemic illness as the underlying cause. Primary hypogonadism is also referred to as *hypergonadotropic hypogonadism,* and secondary hypogonadism is also termed *hypogonadotropic hypogonadism.*

11. What is the initial laboratory workup for hypogonadism?

Primary hypogonadism resulting from a testicular disorder leads to a decline in production of testosterone and sperm, a consequent decrease in the negative feedback effects on the pituitary, and a corresponding increase in serum levels of LH and FSH. Conversely, in secondary or central hypogonadism caused by a hypothalamic–pituitary disorder, serum LH and FSH may be subnormal or "inappropriately" normal (explainable, in part, by decreased bioactivity) despite a low serum testosterone level. A subnormal sperm count and a normal testosterone level with normal LH and elevated FSH levels suggest primary hypogonadism with dysfunction of the seminiferous tubules and sperm production but intact Leydig cell function.

An algorithm for the evaluation of hypogonadism is shown in Fig. 50.3.

12. List the congenital causes of primary hypogonadism
- Klinefelter's syndrome (47XXY and mosaics)
- Microdeletions of azoospermia factor (AZF) regions of Yp telomere (15% of men with nonobstructive azoospermia; 5%–10% of those with oligospermia)

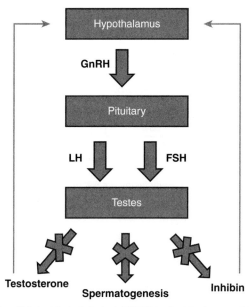

Fig. 50.1. Primary hypogonadism – Defects at the testicular level. *FSH*, Follicle-stimulating hormone; *GnRH*, gonadotropin-releasing hormone; *LH*, luteinizing hormone.

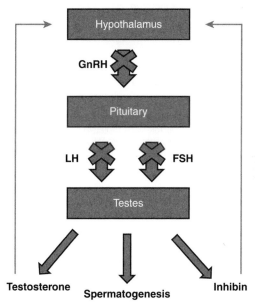

Fig. 50.2. Secondary hypogonadism – Defects in the pituitary or hypothalamus leading to low testosterone levels. *FSH*, Follicle-stimulating hormone; *GnRH*, gonadotropin-releasing hormone; *LH*, luteinizing hormone.

- Cryptorchidism
- Myotonic dystrophy
- Congenital adrenal hyperplasia (3-beta-hydroxysteroid dehydrogenase, 17-alpha-hydroxylase or 17-beta-hydroxysteroid dehydrogenase deficiency)
- Androgen receptor gene mutation (qualitative or quantitative)
- LH receptor mutations (male phenotype, if mild; female phenotype, if severe)

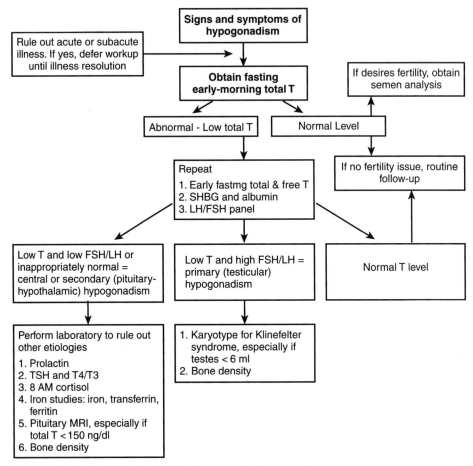

Fig. 50.3. Algorithm for the evaluation of hypogonadism. *FSH*, follicle-stimulating hormone; *LH*, luteinizing hormone; *MRI*, magnetic resonance imaging; *SHBG*, sex hormone-binding globulin; *T*, testosterone; *TSH*, thyroid-stimulating hormone.

13. List the acquired causes of primary hypogonadism
    - Cancer therapy: chemotherapy (alkylating agents > cisplatin and carboplatin) and radiation therapy (may be permanent with external radiation; usually transient with radioactive iodine)
    - Drugs (e.g., ketoconazole, 5-alpha-reductase inhibitors)
    - Testicular injury
    - Hyperthyroidism
    - Infiltrative disease (e.g., hemochromatosis)
    - Infections (e.g., HIV [may be multifactorial], mumps orchitis)
    - Systemic illness (e.g., uremia, cirrhosis): may be multifactorial

14. Is normal aging associated with primary hypogonadism?
    Symptomatic hypogonadism, defined by at least three symptoms and/or signs of testosterone deficiency and an unequivocally consistently low serum total testosterone level (< 320 ng/dL) and/or low free testosterone (< 64 pg/mL), are present in about 2% of men aged 40 to 79 years. Using only biochemical criteria, the prevalence is higher (2%–6%) in that age range and even higher (18%–30%) in men age > 70 years. Not all hypogonadism is symptomatic. A number of cross-sectional studies have noted that older men have mildly reduced levels of serum total testosterone but significantly reduced levels of free testosterone (because of a rise in SHBG with age) compared with younger men. This decline is associated with a rise in LH and FSH, suggesting it results from a primary gonadal cause. Studies have demonstrated an average 1% to 2% decline in serum total testosterone and an even greater reduction in free testosterone (because of elevations in SHBG) per year associated with normal aging. Further complicating the situation is the observation that there has been a population-level decrease in serum testosterone levels in American men over the last 20 years.

15. What are the causes of secondary hypogonadism?

Any disease that affects the hypothalamic–pituitary axis can cause secondary hypogonadism. Involvement of the hypothalamus or pituitary stalk interferes with the secretion of GnRH or the ability of GnRH to communicate with the pituitary. Various anatomic lesions of the pituitary cause secondary hypogonadism by interfering with the production and release of LH and FSH. Such lesions include benign tumors and cysts, malignant tumors (both primary central nervous system [CNS] tumors and metastatic tumors from distant sources), vascular aneurysms, infiltrative diseases (e.g., hemochromatosis), pituitary hemorrhage, and pituitary trauma. Certain inflammatory diseases (e.g., sarcoidosis and histiocytosis) can also affect the hypothalamus and pituitary and decrease testosterone production. Congenital disorders in which output of LH and FSH is impaired, such as Kallmann's syndrome (see below), also lead to secondary hypogonadism. Hyperprolactinemia, obesity, sleep apnea, depression, and human immunodeficiency virus/acquired immunodeficiency syndrome (HIV/AIDS) are associated with secondary hypogonadism as well. Drugs commonly used in the treatment of benign prostatic hypertrophy, the 5-alpha-reductase inhibitors, finasteride and dutasteride, are among the iatrogenic causes of hypogonadism. Others include narcotic analgesics, glucocorticoids, androgen-deprivation therapy with GnRH agonists, or the abuse of anabolic steroids by athletes.

16. What assessment for congenital hypogonadotropic hypogonadism (CHH) should be done?

Kallmann's syndrome is a congenital condition characterized by hypogonadotropic hypogonadism affecting puberty (delayed or impaired) and an impaired sense of smell. The sense of smell in the patient (and his relatives) should be assessed by direct questioning. A quantitative or semiquantitative method is olfactometry. In addition, magnetic resonance imaging (MRI) can be performed to assess the olfactory bulb. If the sense of smell is normal and there does not appear to be a syndromic form of CHH (i.e., Kallmann's syndrome), then the most common gene abnormalities are those of *GNRHR, KISS1R, GnRH1, TAC3*, and *TACR3*. If the sense of smell is decreased or absent in a man with CHH, then the diagnosis is Kallmann's syndrome. *KAL1* mutations cause Kallmann's syndrome, especially in men with mirror movements (bimanual synkinesis), renal agenesis, and an X-linked pattern of inheritance. *FGFR1* mutations occur more often in patients with Kallmann's syndrome and midline abnormalities (e.g., cleft lip/palate, short metacarpals, and/or metatarsals) but can occur in normosmic CHH. *FGF8, PROK2*, or *PROKR2* mutations are more common in Kallmann's syndrome but can also occur in normosmic CHH.

17. What is the most common pituitary tumor in adults?

The most common pituitary tumor found in adults is a prolactin-secreting adenoma. These tumors primarily cause hypogonadism as a result of local destruction and compressive effect against normal pituitary tissue, inhibiting the production and release of LH and FSH. Elevated prolactin levels can also interrupt secretion of GnRH, although this is usually of much less significance in men compared with the mass effect.

18. How do other pituitary adenomas cause hypogonadism?

Pituitary adenomas that produce growth hormone (acromegaly) or adrenocorticotropic hormone (Cushing's disease) and nonfunctioning pituitary tumors may similarly cause secondary hypogonadism by their mass effects.

19. What clinical symptoms are seen in male hypogonadism?

- Loss of the sperm-producing function of the testes leads to infertility, usually defined as failure of a normal female partner to conceive after 12 months of unprotected intercourse.
- Loss of testosterone production by the testis may lead to loss of libido and erectile dysfunction, as well as diminution of secondary sexual characteristics, such as facial and pubic hair, and decrease in testicular volume.
- Decreased production of testosterone also may cause more generalized symptoms, such as decreased muscle mass and strength, malaise, and fatigue. In boys who develop hypogonadism before sexual maturation, delay or absence of the onset of puberty is typical.
- Tender gynecomastia is frequently seen in hypogonadism.
- Numerous nonspecific symptoms are also commonly associated with hypogonadism, such as poor concentration, depressed mood, and increased body fat and body mass index.
- A normochromic, normocytic anemia is also a feature of hypogonadism.

20. What questions are most helpful in determining if a man may have hypogonadism?

When associated with low total and/or free testosterone levels, the following questions are useful in establishing a diagnosis of clinical hypogonadism:

a. How frequently have you awakened with a full erection in the past month?

b. Are you able to get and maintain an erection sufficient for sexual intercourse?

c. How often do you think about sex?

21. How does hypogonadism affect bone architecture?

Osteoporosis is now a well-recognized result of both primary hypogonadism and secondary hypogonadism. Trabecular architecture (as well as bone strength) is even more severely disturbed than bone density in men with hypogonadism. Thus, it is not surprising that hypogonadism is found in up to 30% of men with vertebral fractures.

Estradiol that is aromatized from testosterone may be the most important factor in preserving bone architecture and density in both men and women. However, androgen receptors are also found in bone and may explain the sexual dimorphism of bone density.

22. What laboratory tests help confirm a suspected diagnosis of male hypogonadism?
    The main functions of the testes, production of sperm and production of testosterone, are readily assessed by semen analysis and measurement of serum testosterone, respectively.
    A. Normal semen analysis values in men following 2 to 3 days of abstinence are: 20 million sperm per milliliter and > 60% motility of the sperm. Because sperm density is highly variable from day to day in all men, accurate assessment usually involves several semen analyses done with the same abstinence period each time.
    B. The best initial test for testosterone production is measurement of the fasting morning serum total testosterone level. Serum testosterone also varies considerably from moment to moment, fasting versus nonfasting state as glucose and food intake suppress testosterone levels, and from morning to night in response to LH secretion because of diurnal variation; again, several samples may be needed to establish an accurate measurement. In addition, most testosterone in serum is bound to plasma proteins, particularly SHBG; thus, in patients who have increased or decreased SHBG levels (see above), and in those men in whom plasma protein levels may be disrupted, measurement of the physiologically active "free" testosterone may prove informative.
    C. Bone density measurement using dual energy x-ray absorptiometry (DXA) may provide helpful baseline information and assist in deciding whether to provide androgen replacement therapy and to screen for bone loss/osteoporosis (especially in patients with chronic hypogonadism).

23. What other diagnostic tests are useful in defining the cause of male hypogonadism?
    Additional diagnostic testing should be based on clinical suspicion and the results of preliminary testing. For example, in cases of secondary hypogonadism, measurement of serum prolactin and pituitary imaging, preferably MRI with gadolinium, should be done. Computed tomography (CT) of the sella turcica usually detects macroadenomas (> 1 cm) but will miss many clinically significant microadenomas and is, therefore, less preferable than MRI. Plain skull or sella turcica films are not adequate for diagnosis. Measurement of other pituitary hormones also may be appropriate to assess either possible tumoral hypersecretion (e.g., Cushing's disease, acromegaly) or tumor-related hypopituitarism. Visual field testing is indicated if a macroadenoma is present or there is suprasellar extension. Likewise, the initial findings in primary hypogonadism may suggest additional tests. For example, small firm testes, gynecomastia, azoospermia, modestly reduced serum testosterone, and high levels of serum LH and FSH in a young man should lead to chromosome analysis to confirm a presumptive diagnosis of Klinefelter's syndrome. Measurement of serum estradiol levels may be helpful when feminization is prominent clinically, as with secondary hypogonadism related to production of estrogen by testicular or adrenal tumors or surreptitious use by transgender persons. If infertility is the primary issue and no hormonal abnormality is found, genetic causes should be investigated. This includes testing for Y chromosome microdeletion syndromes. Testis biopsy rarely provides information that is useful in establishing a specific diagnosis, prognosis, or treatment. In addition, if an infiltrative process is suspected, ferritin and an iron panel should be ordered to screen for possible hemochromatosis.

24. Define the term *hermaphrodite.*
    Hermaphrodite refers to someone who has both ovarian and testicular elements in the body. These individuals usually have a 46XX or 46XX/46XY karyotype. They may have an ovary and a testis or an ovotestis. They most often have ambiguous genitalia.

25. Define the term *pseudohermaphrodite.*
    Pseudohermaphrodite refers to someone whose external genitalia are not consistent with his or her gonadal sex. A male pseudohermaphrodite, for example, has a 46XY karyotype and testes but has either ambiguous genitalia or a complete female phenotype. Most often, this results from genetic disorders of testosterone biosynthetic enzymes, the androgen receptor, or the 5-alpha-reductase enzyme; the severity of the phenotype depends on the severity of the genetic defect. A female pseudohermaphrodite, in contrast, has a 46XX karyotype and ovaries but has ambiguous external genitalia. The most common cause of this is congenital adrenal hyperplasia, which results in virilization of the female fetus in utero.

26. How do you treat hypogonadism?
    Deficiency of testosterone is easily treated with testosterone replacement therapy (TRT) (Table 50.1). An alternative approach to therapy is oral clomiphene citrate, which blocks the feedback of estrogen on the hypothalamic–pituitary axis, thereby causing an increase in LH and FSH and a resultant increase in testosterone production. In general, the treatment goal for all TRT is normalization of the serum total testosterone level in the mid-normal range. However, in elderly men, the goal of therapy should be to raise serum testosterone levels to the low-normal range. There is currently considerable controversy over whether or not men with age-associated hypogonadism should be treated with testosterone replacement. Although some short-term studies have demonstrated treatment benefits, long-term large studies are lacking and are needed to clarify the criteria for treatment, as well as the risks and benefits associated with testosterone replacement in this population. A recent study in older men with hypogonadism

Table 50.1. Testosterone Treatment Options in the United States.

FORMULATION	REGIMEN	ADVANTAGES	DISADVANTAGES
Parenteral			
Testosterone enanthate or cypionate in oil	75–100 mg intramuscular (IM) per week or 50–400 mg IM every 2–4 weeks (deep subcutaneous [SC] may be preferable route of administration)	Relatively inexpensive; flexibility of dosing	IM injection resulting in supra-physiologic serum T levels which then decline into the hypogonadal range; "peak" and "trough" fluctuation can cause emotional lability and "let-down" effect
Testosterone undecanoate	Start 750 mgIM, followed by 750 mg 4 weeks later, followed by 750 mg every 10 weeks	Extra-long-acting injection	Injection-associated pulmonary oil microembolism (POEM)
Transdermal/Topical			
Testosterone gel (1%, 1.62%, or 2%)	Apply 20–100 mg daily to clean, dry, intact skin but not to genitals (Dosage depends on formulation)	Good skin tolerability; flexibility of dosing; ease of application	Potential of transfer to others by direct skin-to-skin contact; occasion skin irritation; moderately high dihydro-testosterone (DHT) levels
Testosterone patch	Apply 2–6 mg daily to clean, dry, intact skin but not to genitals	Ease of application	Frequent skin irritation at the application site
Testosterone topical solution	Apply 30 mg to each axilla daily	Good skin tolerability; flexibility of dosing; uses an applicator	Potential of transfer to others by direct skin-to-skin contact; occasion skin irritation
Other			
Testosterone implant pellets	150–450 mg subcutaneous implant every 3–6 months	Ensures compliance	Requires surgical incision for insertions; pellets may extrude spontaneously
Buccal testosterone	Apply 30 mg every 12 hours to gums above the incisor teeth		Gum-related adverse events in 16%
Nasal testosterone gel	11 mg two or three times daily	Rapid absorption and avoid hepatic first-pass metabolism	Local nasal irritation/side effects, not good with nasal disorders, frequent administration
Oral			
Not available in the United States			

and impaired mobility was stopped early because of an increase in cardiovascular events. It should be recognized that some older men with testosterone deficiency are unconcerned about sexual function and may not desire testosterone replacement. In testosterone-deficient men of any age, TRT may be considered to improve osteoporosis and/or reduced hematopoiesis, even in the absence of decreased libido or erectile dysfunction; however, osteoporosis is more effectively and safely treated with osteoporosis medication approved by the U.S. Food and Drug Administration (FDA). Testosterone preparations are presently designated as schedule III drugs by the *Anabolic Steroid Control Act* because of their potential for abuse by athletes and others.

27. What are the potential adverse effects of testosterone treatment?
    Gynecomastia and acne may occur in the first few months after initiating testosterone treatment; these side effects may resolve with continued treatment, although temporary dose reduction may be helpful. Abnormalities in liver function tests are uncommon with currently used injectable and transdermal preparations but can be seen with seldom-used oral preparations. A testosterone-induced increase in hematocrit is common, especially when testosterone injections are used, although clinically significant polycythemia is quite rare unless the drug is being abused. Testosterone treatment may also precipitate or worsen sleep apnea; marked increases in hematocrit may

be a clue to this side effect. Skin reactions are commonly seen in patients using the transdermal patch and are occasionally, but much less frequently, seen with the use of gels. In boys who have not yet gone through puberty, the rapid increase in serum testosterone after initial treatment may lead to considerable psychological difficulties and physically aggressive behavior; initiating treatment with smaller doses may be helpful. TRT, when titrated to the recommended targets, has no adverse effect on lipid profiles compared with eugonadal men, but overtreatment can lead to several lipid abnormalities, including decreases in high-density lipoprotein cholesterol levels. There does not appear to be a significant increase in cardiovascular disease associated with physiologic testosterone replacement, and some studies have even suggested a treatment benefit. However, patients with class III or IV heart failure should be given testosterone replacement cautiously. In addition, there is an increase in risk of venous thromboembolism (VTE), especially in the first 6 months after testosterone initiation, as reported in a large population-based case-control study in the United Kingdom.

28. Does testosterone replacement therapy affect the prostate in older men?

In older men the effects of testosterone on the prostate must be considered, including the possibility of precipitating urinary retention due to testosterone-induced enlargement of the prostate. Short-term studies have not shown any adverse histologic or gene expression effects of testosterone replacement. However, prostate volume, which is often low in men with hypogonadism, increases with long-term testosterone therapy to a level comparable with that in eugonadal men, usually without any significant associated changes in symptoms, urine flow rates, or residual volumes. Nonetheless, individual men may experience voiding symptoms associated with this enlargement, and they should be advised to monitor this. Testosterone therapy with a scrotal patch or gel (but not nonscrotal products) increases levels of dihydrotestosterone more than testosterone, and it is the former that stimulates prostate enlargement. It is advisable to perform a digital rectal examination (DRE) of the prostate and to monitor prostate-specific antigen (PSA) in middle-aged and older men before initiating therapy and annually while they are receiving any TRT. Although no compelling evidence indicates that testosterone treatment causes prostate carcinoma, the potential for testosterone stimulation of occult prostate carcinoma exists. Men with an elevated PSA level or an abnormal result on DRE should be evaluated further, potentially including a prostate biopsy, prior to initiation of testosterone therapy.

29. How does one treat the deficiency of sperm production in primary hypogonadism?

In men with primary hypogonadism, as manifested by elevated levels of serum FSH, there seems to be no effective pharmacologic treatment for increasing the sperm count. Anatomic lesions, such as varicoceles and ejaculatory duct obstructions, can be corrected surgically, but improvement in spermatogenesis may not result. If one plans to use a medication known to cause hypogonadism (e.g., cancer chemotherapeutic agents), it may be desirable to cryopreserve semen specimens before treatment, provided that treatment is not unduly delayed

30. How does one treat deficient sperm production in secondary hypogonadism?

The outlook is more optimistic with secondary hypogonadism, particularly if the condition developed after puberty. Treatment with gonadotropins (hCG with or without FSH) may be successful in restoring production of sperm, as well as testosterone. The pretreatment size of the testes is often a clue to prognosis; a larger testis size is associated with a better outcome. Production of testosterone and sperm in men with secondary hypogonadism also may be enhanced with pulsatile administration of GnRH via a portable infusion pump, provided that the pituitary retains the capability to make gonadotropins. Treatment with gonadotropins or GnRH tends to be both costly and prolonged.

31. What alternative is available to men with hypogonadism who do not respond to therapy with an increase in spermatogenesis?

In men with primary or secondary hypogonadism who have not responded to specific therapy when appropriate and who have preservation of some germ cells in either ejaculate or testes, intracytoplasmic sperm injection (ICSI) may offer some hope, although at a high financial cost. The prognosis for successful ICSI is dependent on the site and extent of microdeletions on the Y chromosome. If microdeletions are found, the patient should be counseled about the possibility of passing this on to his male child. Microsurgical testicular sperm extraction (micro-TESE) is a surgical method for harvesting sperm. Fertility options that should be discussed also include donor sperm and adoption.

32. What are the advantages and disadvantages of the various forms of androgen replacement therapy?

The available forms of testosterone (T) treatment in the United States are shown in Table 50.1.

33. What parameters should be monitored in men on testosterone therapy?

The following should be determined at baseline and at 3 months after initiation of therapy and then monitored at least yearly, once the patient's condition is stabilized:
- Hematocrit and hemoglobin
- Prostate size by digital rectal examination

- Serum PSA
- Liver function tests
- Development of gynecomastia, acne, or edema
- Serum testosterone levels in all forms of treatment
- Serum dihydrotestosterone levels in those receiving scrotal patches or gel
- Development of or worsening of sleep apnea
- Bone mineral density at baseline and at 1- to 2-yearly intervals should be performed

34. In what conditions is testosterone therapy absolutely or relatively contraindicated?
    Absolute contraindications are as follows:
    - Carcinoma of the prostate
    - Uncontrolled obstructive sleep apnea
    - Polycythemia vera
    - Symptomatic and/or severe benign prostatic hypertrophy
    - Breast carcinoma

    Relative contraindications are as follows:
    - Prostate nodule that has not been biopsied
    - Elevated serum PSA level
    - Class III or IV congestive heart failure
    - Myocardial infarction or stroke within the last 6 months
    - Thrombophilia
    - Severe lower urinary tract symptoms (LUTS)

KEY POINTS: MALE HYPOGONADISM

- The manifestations of hypogonadism vary, depending on the patient's stage of development when the hypogonadism occurs.
- A reduction in testicular volume < 20 mL is the most common manifestation of hypogonadism and is seen in nearly all cases of longstanding hypogonadism.
- Classify hypogonadism as primary (a disorder at the level of the testes) or secondary (a disorder at the level of the hypothalamus or pituitary).
- Therapeutic goals are generally to correct testosterone to the mid-normal range topically or by injection.
- Monitor patients on testosterone replacement for polycythemia, sleep apnea, gynecomastia, psychological difficulties, prostate size, prostate symptoms, and increases in prostate-specific antigen (PSA) levels.

⊕ WEBSITES

1. https://academic.oup.com/jcem/advance-article/doi/10.1210/jc.2018-00229/4939465
2. https://www.aace.com/files/hypo-gonadism.pdf
3. http://www.nlm.nih.gov/medlineplus/ency/article/000390.htm
4. https://www.hormone.org/diseases-and-conditions/mens-health/low-testosterone
5. https://www.hormone.org/diseases-and-conditions/mens-health/klinefelter
6. http://www.mayoclinic.com/health/male-hypogonadism/DS00300

ACKNOWLEDGMENTS

The views expressed in this manuscript are those of the authors and do not reflect the official policy of the Department of the Army, Navy, the Department of Defense, the National Institutes of Health, or the United States Government. Dr. Vu and Dr. Mai are military service members. This work was prepared as part of our official duties. Title 17 U.S.C. 105 provides the "Copyright protection under this title is not available for any work of the United States Government." Title 17 U.S.C. 101 defines a U.S. Government work as a work prepared by a military service member or employee of the U.S. Government as part of that person's official duties. We certify that all individuals who qualify as authors have been listed; each has participated in the conception and design of this work, the analysis of data (when applicable), the writing of the document, and/or the approval of the submission of this version; that the document represents valid work; that if we used information derived from another source, we obtained all necessary approvals to use it and made appropriate acknowledgements in the document; and that each takes public responsibility for it.

BIBLIOGRAPHY

Adamopoulos, D. A., Lawrence, D. M., Vassilopoulos, P., Contoyiannis, P. A., Swyer, G. I. (1978). Pituitary–testicular relationships in mumps orchitis and other viral infections. *British Medical Journal, 1*, 1177.

Armory, J. K., Wang, C., Swerdloff, R. S., Anawalt, B. D., Matsumoto, A. M., Bremner, W. J., . . . Clark, R. V. (2007). The effect of 5 reductase inhibition with dutasteride and finasteride on semen parameters and serum hormones in healthy men. *Journal of Clinical Endocrinology and Metabolism, 92*, 1659–1665.

Araujo, A. B., Esche, G. R., Kupelian, V., O'Donnell, A. B., Travison, T. G., Williams, R. E., . . . McKinlay, J. B. (2007). Prevalence of symptomatic androgen deficiency in men. *Journal of Clinical Endocrinology and Metabolism, 92*(11), 4241–4247.

Bagatell, C. J., & Bremner, W. J. (1996). Androgens in men—uses and abuses. *New England Journal of Medicine, 334*, 707–714.

Baker, H. W. G., Burger, H. F., de Kretser, D. M., Hudson, B., O'Connor, S., Wang, C., . . . Rennie, G. C. (1976). Changes in the pituitary–testicular system with age. *Clinical Endocrinology, 5*, 349.

Basaria, S., Coviello, A. D., Travison, T. G., Storer, T. W., Farwell, W. R., Jette, A. M., . . . Bhasin, S. (2010). Adverse events associated with testosterone administration. *N Engl J Med, 363*, 109–122.

Bannister, P., Handley, T., Chapman, C., & Losowsky, M. S. (1986). Hypogonadism in chronic liver disease: impaired release of luteinising hormone. *British Medical Journal, 293*, 1191.

Bhasin, S., Brito, J. P., Cunningham, G. R., Hayes, F. J., Hodis, H. N., Matsumoto, A. M., . . . Yialamas, M. A. (2018). Testosterone therapy in men with hypogonadism: an Endocrine Society Clinical Practice Guideline. *Journal of Clinical Endocrinology and Metabolism, 103*(5), 1–30.

Bhasin, S. (2007). Approach to the infertile man. *Journal of Clinical Endocrinology and Metabolism, 92*, 1995–2004.

Byrne, M., & Nieschlag, E. (2003). Testosterone replacement therapy in male hypogonadism. *Journal of Endocrinological Investigation, 26*(5), 481–489.

Brambilla, D. J., Matsumoto, A. M., Araujo, A. B., & McKinlay, J. B. (2009). The effect of diurnal variation on clinical measurement of serum testosterone and other sex hormone levels in men. *Journal of Clinical Endocrinology and Metabolism, 94*(3), 907–913.

Caronia, L. M., Dwyer, A. A., Hayden, D., Amati, F., Pitteloud, N., & Hayes, F. J. (2013). Abrupt decrease in serum testosterone levels after an oral glucose load in men: implications for screening for hypogonadism. *Clinical Endocrinology, 78*(2), 291–296.

Castro-Magana, M., Bronsther, B., & Angulo, M. A. (1990). Genetic forms of male hypogonadism. *Urology, 35*, 195.

Dada, R., Gupta, N. P., & Kucheria, K. (2003). Molecular screening for Yq microdeletion in men with idiopathic oligospermia and azoospermia. *Journal of Biosciences, 28*, 163–168.

Gambineri, A., Pelusi, C., Vicennati, V., Pagotto, U., & Pasquali, R. (2001). Testosterone in ageing men. *Expert Opinion on Investigational Drugs, 10*(3), 477–492.

Griffin, J. L., & Wilson, J. D. (1980). The syndromes of androgen resistance. *New England Journal of Medicine, 302*, 198.

Gromoll, J., Eiholzer, U., Nieschlag, E., & Simoni, M. (2000). Male hypogonadism caused by homozygous deletion of exon 10 of the luteinizing hormone (LH) receptor: differential action of human chorionic gonadotropin and LH. *Journal of Clinical Endocrinology and Metabolism, 85*, 2281–2286.

Guo, C. Y., Jones, T. H., & Eastell, R. (1997). Treatment of isolated hypogonadotropic hypogonadism effect on bone mineral density and bone turnover. *Journal of Clinical Endocrinology and Metabolism, 82*, 658–665.

Harman, S. M., Metter, E. J., Tobin, J. D., Pearson, J., & Blackman, M. R. (2001). Longitudinal effects of aging on serum total and free testosterone levels in healthy men. Baltimore Longitudinal Study of Aging. *Journal of Clinical Endocrinology and Metabolism, 86*, 724–731.

Hayes, F. J., Seminara, S. B., & Crowley, W. F. (1998). Hypogonadotropic hypogonadism. *Endocrinology and Metabolism Clinics of North America, 27*(4), 739–763.

Hopps, C. V., Mielnik, A., Goldstein, M., Palermo, G. D., Rosenwaks, Z., & Schlegel, P. N. (2003). Detection of sperm in men with Y chromosome microdeletions on the AZFa, AZFb and AZFc regions. *Human Reproduction, 18*, 1660–1665.

Hsueh, W. A., Hsu, T. H., & Federman, D. D. (1978). Endocrine features of Klinefelter's syndrome. *Medicine, 57*, 447.

Kalyani, R. R., Gavini, S., & Dobs, A. S. (2007). Male hypogonadism in systemic disease. *Endocrinology and Metabolism Clinics of North America, 36*(2), 333–348.

Kidd, G. S., Glass, A. R., & Vigersky, R. A. (1979). The hypothalamic-pituitary-testicular axis in thyrotoxicosis. *Journal of Clinical Endocrinology and Metabolism, 48*, 798–802.

Layman, L. C. (2007). Hypogonadotropic hypogonadism. *Endocrinology and Metabolism Clinics of North America, 36*(2), 283–296.

Lee, P. A., & O'Dea, L. S. (1990). Primary and secondary testicular insufficiency. *Pediatric Clinics of North America, 37*, 1359.

Lehtihet, M., Arver, S., Bartuseviciene, I., & Pousette, A. (2012). S-testosterone decrease after a mixed meal in healthy men independent of SHBG and gonadotropin levels. *Andrologia, 44*(6), 405–410.

Lieblich, J. M., Rogol, A. D., White, B. J., & Rosen, S. W. (1982). Syndrome of anosmia with hypogonadotropic hypogonadism (Kallman syndrome): clinical and laboratory studies in 23 cases. *American Journal of Medicine, 73*, 506.

Marks, L. S., Mazer, N. A., Mostaghel, E., Hess, D. L., Dorey, F. J., Epstein, J. I., . . . Nelson, P. S. (2006). Effect of testosterone replacement therapy on prostate tissue in men with late-onset hypogonadism. *Journal of American Medical Association, 296*, 2351–2361.

Martinez, C., Suissa, S., Rietbrock, S., Katholing, A., Freedman, B., Cohen, A. T., & Handelsman, D. J. (2016). Testosterone treatment and risk of venous thromboembolism: population based case-control study. *British Medical Journal, 355*, i5968.

Matsumoto, A. M., & Bremner, W. J. (1987). Endocrinology of the hypothalamic–pituitary–testicular axis with particular reference to the hormonal control of spermatogenesis. *Bailliere's Clinical Endocrinology and Metabolism, 1*, 71.

Mirone, V., Debruyne, F., Dohle, G., Salonia, A., Sofikitis, N., Verze, P., . . . Chapple, C. (2017). European Association of Urology Position Statement on the Role of the Urologist in the Management of Male Hypogonadism and Testosterone Therapy. *European Urology, 72*, 164–167.

Rhoden, E. L., & Morgentaler, A. (2004). Risks of testosterone-replacement therapy and recommendations for monitoring. *New England Journal of Medicine, 350*(5), 482–492.

Schwartz, I. D., & Root, A. W. (1991). The Klinefelter syndrome of testicular dysgenesis. *Endocrinology and Metabolism Clinics of North America, 20*, 153.

Seminara, S. B., Hayes, F. J., & Crowley, W. F. Jr. (1998). Gonadotropin-releasing hormone deficiency in the human (idiopathic hypogonadotropic hypogonadism and Kallmann's syndrome): pathophysiological and genetic considerations. *Endocrine Reviews, 19*, 521.

Silveira, L. F., MacColl, G. S., & Bouloux, P. M. (2002). Hypogonadotropic hypogonadism. *Seminars in Reproductive Medicine, 20*(4), 327–338.

Snyder, P. J., Peachey, H., Berlin, J. A., Hannoush, P., Haddad, G., Dlewati, A., . . . Strom, B. L. (2000). Effects of testosterone replacement in hypogonadal men. *Journal of Clinical Endocrinology and Metabolism, 85,* 2670–2677.

Swerdloff, R. S., Wang, C., Cunningham, G., Dobs, A., Iranmanesh, A., Matsumoto, A. M., . . . Berman, N. (2000). Long-term pharmacokinetics of transdermal testosterone gel in hypogonadal men. *Journal of Clinical Endocrinology and Metabolism, 85,* 4500–4510.

Szulc, P., Munoz, F., Claustrat, B., Garnero, P., Marchand, F., Duboeuf, F., & Delmas, P. D. (2001). Bioavailable estradiol may be an important determinant of osteoporosis in men: the MINOS study. *Journal of Clinical Endocrinology and Metabolism, 86,* 192.

Tenover, J. L. (1998). Male hormone replacement therapy including "andropause." *Endocrinology and Metabolism Clinics of North America, 27*(4), 969–987.

Whitcomb, R. W., & Crowley, W. F. (1993). Male hypogonadotropic hypogonadism. *Endocrinology and Metabolism Clinics of North America, 22,* 125.

Wu, F. C. W., Tajar, A., Beynon, J. M., Pye, S. R., Silman, A. J., Finn, J. D., . . . Huhtaniemi, I. T. (2010). Identification of late-onset hypogonadism in middle-aged and elderly men. *New England Journal of Medicine, 363*(2), 123–135.

Young, J. (2012). Approach to the male patient with congenital hypogonadotropic hypogonadism. *Journal of Clinical Endocrinology and Metabolism, 97,* 707–718.

Vita, R., Settineri, S., Liotta, M., Benvenga, S., & Trimarchi, F. (2018). Changes in hormonal and metabolic parameters in transgender subjects on cross-sex hormone therapy: a cohort study. *Maturitas, 107,* 92–96.

CHAPTER 51

ERECTILE DYSFUNCTION

Mark M. Cruz, Thanh D. Hoang, and Robert A. Vigersky

1. **What is impotence?**
   A more descriptive term for impotence is *erectile dysfunction (ED)*. Classically, ED has been defined as the inability to attain and maintain an erection of sufficient rigidity for sexual intercourse in ≥ 50% attempts over a period of at least 3 months. This definition is important to consider because any normal male can experience occasional ED, and treating men with only occasional symptoms is not without risk.

2. **Do men with ED have disturbances in other sexual functions?**
   Most men with ED are able to ejaculate. Premature ejaculation may precede the development of ED and is sometimes associated with drug therapy. Sexual desire (libido) is also usually preserved; loss of libido is suggestive of hypogonadism or severe systemic or psychiatric illness.

3. **Is impotence common?**
   At least 10 million American men, perhaps as many as 30 million, are impotent. Another 10 million may suffer from partial ED. The prevalence of impotence increases with age; about 2% of 40-year-old, 20% of 55-year-old, and 50% to 75% of 80-year-old men are impotent. Of interest, there is a libido–potency gap, in that many elderly men continue to have active libidos, but only 15% of them engage in sexual activity.

4. **How does normal erection occur?**
   Erection is primarily a vascular event that results from the complex interplay of the hormonal, vascular, and the peripheral and central nervous systems. There is considerable psychiatric interplay in that underlying psychiatric conditions or medications can cause decreased erectile function. Conversely, undesired sexual symptoms can also adversely affect mood and self-perception.

5. **Explain the role of the nervous system in achieving erection.**
   Erection is usually initiated by various psychological and/or physiologic stimuli in the cerebral cortex. The stimuli are modulated in the limbic system and other areas of the brain, integrated in the hypothalamus, transmitted down the spinal cord, and carried to the penis via both autonomic and sacral spinal nerves ("nervi erigentes" derived from the Latin *erigo, erigere, erexi, erectus*). Sensory nerves from the glans of the penis enhance the message and help maintain erection during sexual activity via a reflex arc.

6. **Explain the hormonal aspects of erection.**
   Nervous system stimuli release neurotransmitters that reverse the tonic smooth muscle constriction maintained by norepinephrine, endothelin, and other vasoconstrictive factors. The most important of these are the potent vasodilators, nitric oxide (NO) and prostaglandin E1 (PGE1). In addition to neural sources, NO is derived from endothelial cells, which may explain why endothelial integrity may be necessary for the maintenance of erection. NO works by increasing cyclic guanosine monophosphate (cGMP) and causing a decrease in intracellular calcium. This results in relaxation of vascular smooth muscle cells as a result of the dissociation of actin–myosin. The role of testosterone in erectile function remains complex and controversial. Testosterone has a critical role in stabilizing intracavernosal NO synthase, and for fully satisfactory sexual function, a "normal" quotient of testosterone must be present. Testosterone is also the main hormonal mediator of a male's libido, which means that deficiency can have a psychologic impact on erectile function. Regardless, some men with testosterone levels below the reference limit still can achieve normal erection. Testosterone replacement is, therefore, not guaranteed to cure ED in men with hypogonadism, nor is it indicated in men with normal testosterone levels but impaired sexual function.

7. **What vascular changes in the penis result in erection?**
   Within the two spongy corpora cavernosa of the penis are millions of tiny spaces called *lacunae*, each lined by a wall of trabecular smooth muscle. As neurotransmitters dilate cavernosal and helicine arteries to the penis and relax the trabecular smooth muscle, the lacunar spaces in the penis become engorged with blood. This results in entrapment of outflow vessels between the expanding trabecular walls and the rigid tunica albuginea that surrounds the corpora cavernosa, thereby greatly reducing venous outflow from the penis. This veno-occlusive mechanism accounts for both rigidity and tumescence. Failure of venous occlusion (venous leak) is one of the intractable causes of impotence.

8. What types of nerves and neurotransmitters play a role in penile erection?
At least three neuroeffector systems play a role in penile erection. Adrenergic nerves generally inhibit erection; cholinergic nerves and nonadrenergic, noncholinergic (NANC) substances enhance erection as follows:
- Sympathetic nerves (via beta-adrenergic receptors): constrict cavernosal and helicine arteries, contract trabecular smooth muscle.
- Parasympathetic nerves (via cholinergic receptors): inhibit adrenergic fibers, stimulate NANC fibers.
- NANC messengers (NO, vasoactive intestinal polypeptide, and PGs or other endothelium-derived factors): dilate cavernosal and helicine arteries, relax trabecular smooth muscle.

9. How does detumescence occur?
Phosphodiesterase 5 (PD5), by causing a decrease in cGMP, allows for reversal of the process; that is, detumescence, making PD5 inhibitors, such as sildenafil, vardenafil, tadalafil, and avanafil, important therapeutic agents for the treatment of impotence (see the following).

10. What are the common causes of impotence?
The frequency of the various causes of impotence is difficult to assess because of the large number of patients who do not report the problem, confusion regarding the diagnosis, and variability in the sophistication of the initial evaluation. Primary causes of impotence in men presenting to a medical outpatient clinic are estimated as follows:
- Endocrine factors (hyper- and hypothyroidism, hypogonadism, hyperprolactinemia, hyper/hypocortisolism): 30%
- Diabetes mellitus and metabolic syndrome: 15%
- Medications (antihypertensives, antidepressants, antipsychotics, antiandrogens, recreational drugs, etc.): 20%
- Systemic disease and alcoholism: 10%
- Primary vascular causes: 5% (Alterations of blood flow are thought to play a role in many causes of impotence, but specific lesions amenable to therapy are relatively rare.)
- Primary neurologic causes (multiple sclerosis, Parkinson's disease, myotonic dystrophy, spinal cord diseases, stroke, central nervous system tumors, etc.): 5%
- Psychogenic or unknown causes: 15%

11. What lifestyles are associated with impotence?
- Low levels of physical activity
- Overeating/obesity
- Smoking
- Excessive TV viewing
- Alcohol consumption

12. Besides diabetes mellitus, what are the three most common endocrine causes of impotence?
- Primary (hypergonadotropic) hypogonadism (increased luteinizing hormone [LH] and decreased testosterone)
- Secondary (hypogonadotropic) hypogonadism ("inappropriately" normal or actually decreased LH combined with decreased testosterone)
- Hyperprolactinemia
- Less common causes include hyperthyroidism, hypothyroidism, adrenal insufficiency, and Cushing's syndrome

13. Describe the most common drugs known to induce impotence.
Nonprescription drugs, such as alcohol (as the porter says to Macduff in Act II, Scene 3, in *Macbeth,* "It provokes the desire but takes away the performance"), and illicit drugs, such as cocaine, methadone, and heroin, can cause impotence. The prescription drugs most commonly associated with impotence include the following:
- Antihypertensive agents, especially methyldopa, clonidine, beta blockers, vasodilators (e.g., hydralazine), thiazide diuretics, and spironolactone
- Antipsychotic medications (neuroleptics, etc.)
- Antidepressants and tranquilizers (selective serotonin reuptake inhibitors [SSRIs], tricyclic antidepressants [TCAs], etc.)
- Others (especially cimetidine, digoxin, phenytoin, carbamazepine, ketoconazole, metoclopramide, and megestrol)

14. Which antihypertensive agents should be used in patients with impotence?
Virtually every blood pressure medication has been associated with impotence. Although there is little overall difference in the rate of erectile problems among the commonly prescribed antihypertensive agents, angiotensin-converting enzyme (ACE) inhibitors, angiotensin receptor blockers (ARBs), and calcium channel blockers are the agents least likely to affect erectile ability. When beta blockade is required, selective beta antagonists, such as atenolol or acebutolol, are preferred as they have minimal impact on sexual function.

15. What is "stuttering" impotence? What is its significance?
Impotence alternating with periods of entirely normal sexual function is termed *stuttering impotence.* Multiple sclerosis (MS) is the most significant organic cause of stuttering impotence. It may be the initial manifestation of MS and may be present in up to 50% of men with the disease.

Table 51.1. Organic Impotence Versus Psychogenic Impotence.

	ORGANIC	PSYCHOGENIC
Was onset abrupt?	No	Yes
Is impotence stress dependent?	No	Yes
Is libido preserved?[a]	Yes	No
Do you have morning erections?	No	Yes
Do you have orgasms?	Yes	No
Can you masturbate?	No	Yes
Does impotence occur with all partners?	Yes	No

[a]There is a general relationship between libido and hypogonadal levels of testosterone in populations, but on an individual basis, libido may not be a reliable discriminator.

16. **What information in patient history helps separate organic impotence from psychogenic impotence?**
True psychogenic impotence is uncommon and should be a diagnosis of exclusion. Questions that may help to separate psychogenic from organic impotence are listed in Table 51.1. A detailed history assessing for contributing physical/psychiatric conditions can also help with this distinction. These include obesity, hypertension, hyperlipidemia, atherosclerosis, diabetes mellitus or other endocrinopathy, neurologic disease, prior pelvic surgery or irradiation, trauma, Peyronie's disease, substance abuse, depression, or the aforementioned medications. A detailed social history is also important and includes assessment of stressors and the patient's coping mechanisms; concomitant psychosexual problems, such as premature ejaculation; and relationship dynamics with partner(s).

17. **Name the essential components of a physical examination in a man with a complaint of impotence.**
    - Secondary sexual characteristics, such as muscle development, hair pattern, and presence of breast tissue.
    - Vascular examination, especially of the femoral and lower extremity pulses and the presence of bruits.
    - Focused neurologic examination, including assessing the presence of peripheral neuropathy with vibratory and light touch sensation, and of autonomic neuropathy by using the cremasteric reflex, anal sphincter tone, and/or the bulbocavernosus reflex, evaluation for postural hypotension with standing and supine blood pressure measurement, and measurement of the heart rate response to deep breathing and Valsalva maneuver (diabetics rarely have autonomic neuropathy as a cause of impotence in the absence of peripheral neuropathy).
    - Examination of the genitalia to determine penile size, shape, presence of plaque or fibrous tissue (Peyronie's disease); size and consistency of the testes; prostate examination (prostatic enlargement or irregularity/nodularity). The normal testis size is more than 5×3 cm or 20 mL (by orchidometer).
    - Thyroid-relevant examination including size, the presence of nodularity, and abnormal reflexes.

18. **What is the appropriate laboratory assessment for men with impotence?**
Laboratory assessment should be based on history and physical examination findings. It can discover previously unknown disease in 6% of men. Generally, it should include the following:
    - Complete blood count
    - Urinalysis
    - Fasting plasma glucose and (in known diabetics) hemoglobin A_{1c} (HbA_{1c})
    - Fasting serum lipid profile
    - Serum creatinine
    - Serum free thyroxine and thyrotropin
    - Serum testosterone (fasting, morning sample), LH, and follicle-stimulating hormone (FSH)

19. **Should prolactin levels be measured in all men with impotence?**
Whether serum prolactin should be measured in all men with impotence is somewhat controversial. In general, patients with normal levels of testosterone and LH and a normal result on neurologic examination do not require measurement of prolactin. However, if testosterone is low and associated with low or low-normal LH, or if history or examination suggests a pituitary lesion, prolactin should be measured. Because prolactin interferes with the action of testosterone, prolactin status should be assessed in hypogonadal men unresponsive to testosterone replacement therapy. Hypothyroidism and renal failure also may elevate prolactin.

20. **What is a penile brachial index?**
Comparison of the penile and brachial systolic blood pressures allows for a general assessment of the vascular integrity of the penis. This technique is not highly sensitive, but it is noninvasive and easy to perform and may help to identify men who require more extensive vascular studies. Penile systolic blood pressure obtained with

Doppler ultrasonography should be the same as brachial systolic pressure (i.e., ratio approximately = 1.0). An index < 0.7 is highly suggestive of vasculogenic impotence. Diagnostic yield is increased if the penile brachial index is repeated after exercising the lower extremities for several minutes. This maneuver may uncover pelvic steal syndrome (loss of erection caused by pelvic thrusting) that is characterized by a difference of > 0.15 between the resting and exercise ratios.

21. What is nocturnal penile tumescence monitoring?
Most men experience 3 to 6 erections during the night that are entrained to rapid eye movement (REM) sleep. By monitoring such events, one can assess the frequency, duration, and, with some instruments, even the rigidity of erection. This procedure helps distinguish organic impotence from psychogenic impotence. This can be done at home either semiquantitatively (by using a Snap-Gauge) or more quantitatively (by using the RigiScan). The nocturnal penile tumescence and rigidity evaluation should be done on at least 2 nights, with a functional erectile mechanism indicated by an erectile event of at least 60% rigidity recorded at the penile tip that lasts for > 10 minutes.

22. What are the therapeutic options for impotence?
Once drugs with a high likelihood of causing impotence are discontinued and/or other underlying conditions are aggressively treated (e.g., diabetes mellitus, hypercholesterolemia), broad categories of medical and surgical therapy are available; these are summarized in Table 51.2. Important adjuncts include:
- Medical treatment, in addition to lifestyle modifications and/or weight reduction
- External mechanical aids and vacuum/suction devices
- Psychological therapy (especially in the absence of an obvious organic cause)

23. What options are available for medical treatment?
- Testosterone replacement in men with hypogonadism, with the goal of achieving a mid-normal level of serum testosterone (see chapter 50 on hypogonadism)
- Dopamine agonists (bromocriptine or cabergoline) to reduce hyperprolactinemia in men with hypogonadism who are unresponsive to testosterone treatment
- PD5 inhibitors, such as sildenafil citrate (Viagra), vardenafil (Levitra), tadalafil (Cialis), or avanafil (Stendra) (Table 51.3)
- Adrenergic receptor blockers (e.g., yohimbine, 6.5 mg three times daily)
- Herbal remedies (e.g., Korean red ginseng, 90 mg three times daily)
- SSRI for premature ejaculation

24. Summarize the role of intracavernosal injections.
Intracavernosal injection of vasoactive substances (PGE, papaverine, and phentolamine) individually or in combination (Trimix) may be effective in men when PD5 inhibitors have failed or are contraindicated.

25. List the surgical procedures used to treat impotence.
- Revascularization procedures
- Obliteration of venous shunts
- Penile venous stripping surgery
- Venous ligation surgery
- Surgical penile implants

26. How effective are PD5 inhibitors?
The introduction of the selective PD5 inhibitors (sildenafil citrate [Viagra], vardenafil [Levitra], tadalafil [Cialis], and avanafil [Stendra]) has produced a paradigm shift in the approach to the treatment of impotence by reducing the relevance of finding a specific cause of the problem. There appears to be no tachyphylaxis to their effect for at least 5 years. When taken 1 hour before anticipated sexual activity (and, for sildenafil, vardenafil, and avanafil, avoiding a fatty meal, which inhibits absorption), they are successful in up to 80% of men with organic impotence (although in only about 50%–70% of men with diabetes and 50% of elderly men). Tadalafil can also be prescribed at lower doses for continuous daily use. Unfortunately, well-performed comparisons of the available treatments for ED are not available. The literature on PD5 inhibitors, in particular, is limited by inconsistent study designs, inclusion/exclusion criteria, dosages, treatment durations, randomization, and crossover. When assessing "success" of ED therapy, it is important to consider more than the quality of erection or frequency of penetration, because effective but invasive interventions (i.e., intracavernosal injections) are not uniformly preferred by patients. In terms of PD5 inhibitors, maximum doses are generally preferred to submaximal doses, and longer treatment durations are generally preferred to shorter durations. Younger men with ED of psychogenic origin tend to prefer tadalafil for its greater duration of action, whereas older men with moderate or severe organic ED tend to prefer sildenafil and vardenafil for their better efficacy and side effect profiles. Switching from one PD5 inhibitor to another is sometimes beneficial for nonresponders. There may also be a place for testosterone "rescue" in patients who do not respond to PD5 inhibitors and who also have low testosterone levels.

Table 51.2. Treatment Options for Impotence.

	ORAL PD5 INHIBITORS	INTRAURETHRAL ALPROSTADIL	INTRACAVERNOUS INJECTIONS (ALPROSTADIL, PAPAVERINE, PHENTOLAMINE)	PENILE PROSTHESIS IMPLANTATION
Pharmacology	Inhibit PD5, potentiate vasodilation by nitric oxide-generated cGMP Metabolized by CYP450, require hepatic dosing	Synthetic vasodilator identical to PGE1 Relaxes arterial smooth muscle Inhibits platelet aggregation	Agent specific Relax smooth muscle	Available in inflatable and noninflatable versions
Contraindications	Nitrate use within 24 hours (48 hours for tadalafil) Prolonged QT (vardenafil) Caution if using alpha blockers Caution if penile deformity Caution if liver/kidney disease	Sickle cell anemia Multiple myeloma Leukemia Penile deformities Penile implants	Sickle cell anemia Multiple myeloma Leukemia Penile deformity Penile implant	Active systemic, cutaneous, or urinary infection
Side effects	Flushing Nasal congestion Headache Hearing loss Dyspepsia Visual side effects (sildenafil, avanafil, and vardenafil) Back pain Mild QT prolongation (vardenafil) Hypotension Syncope MI, angina Stroke	Hypotension Syncope Priapism GU pain	Priapism Penile fibrosis Hypotension Hematoma Ecchymosis Penile pain Bleeding Angulation/Peyronie's disease	Infection Erosion Mechanical failure (6%–16% at 5 years) Penile shortening Reduced efficacy of medical therapy if prosthesis fails Autoinflation
Monitoring parameters	Creatinine at baseline	Initial dose under supervision (risk of syncope)	Initial dose under supervision, train for management of priapism	Physical examination

cGMP, Cyclic guanosine monophosphate; *GU,* genitourinary; *MI,* myocardial infarction; *PD5,* phosphodiesterase 5; *PGE1,* prostaglandin E1.

Table 51.3. Comparison of PD5 Inhibitors.[a]

	SILDENAFIL (VIAGRA)	VARDENAFIL (LEVITRA)	TADALAFIL (CIALIS)	AVANAFIL (STENDRA)
Onset	20 minutes	10 minutes	20 minutes	15 minutes (100-mg/ 200-mg doses 30 minutes (50-mg dose)
T_{max}	1 hour	45 minutes	2 hours	30–45 minutes
T½	3–5 hours	4–5 hours	17.5 hours	5 hours
Initial dose	50 mg (25mg if age $\geq$ 65 years)	10mg (5 mg if age $\geq$ 65 years)	2.5 mg or 10 mg	50 mg
Max dose	100 mg	20 mg	20 mg	200 mg
Notes	Original PD5 inhibitor. It has the most data on safety and efficacy. Avoid high-fat meals when dosing	Avoid high-fat meals when dosing	Comparable efficacy and safety when 2.5–5 mg taken daily for men having intercourse $>$ 2 times per week. No dietary restriction needed Also approved for daily use at 2.5–5 mg/day	Avoid high-fat meals when dosing

[a]Comparative efficacy data are lacking for the four available agents. Failure of one agent is not a contraindication to trial of a different PD5 inhibitor.
PD5, Phosphodiesterase 5; *T½,* half-life; *T_{max},* time to maximum plasma concentration.

27. Discuss the side effects of PD5 inhibitors.
    The few immediate side effects associated with PD5 inhibitors (headache, flushing, dyspepsia, hearing loss, nasal congestion, and a blue haze in vision) rarely cause discontinuation of their use. Vardenafil, tadalafil, and avanafil cause less crossover inhibition of retinal PD6 and, therefore, are associated with fewer visual side effects. Since PD5 inhibitors cause vasodilatation similar to that of nitrates, they are contraindicated in men taking any form of nitrates. The long half-life of tadalafil (the so-called "weekend pill") may prove to be particularly troublesome if a patient develops angina within 72 to 96 hours of taking it. Priapism (persistent and painful erection of the penis) may occur as a result of using PD5 inhibitors. Some studies have reported a small increased risk of malignant melanoma associated with PD5 inhibitors.

28. What drug interactions are associated with PD5 inhibitors?
    Because PD5 inhibitors are metabolized via CYP3A4, any drugs that block that enzyme (e.g., erythromycin and other macrolide antibiotics; ketoconazole and other antifungal drugs; human immunodeficiency virus [HIV] protease inhibitors, such as saquinavir and ritonavir; and cimetidine) increase the plasma concentrations of PD5 inhibitors. In such cases, PD5 inhibitors should be started at one fourth to one half of the usual dose. Because PD5 inhibitors may potentiate the hypotensive effect of alpha-adrenergic blocking agents, they should be given in lower doses (sildenafil) or not at all (vardenafil) in men on alpha blockers for control of blood pressure or for benign prostatic hypertrophy. Grapefruit and grapefruit juice should be avoided within 24 hours of PD5 inhibitor use.

29. When are intracavernosal or intraurethral injections recommended?
    Injection of vasodilatory substances directly into the corpora cavernosa of the penis should be reserved for men in whom PD5 inhibitors are ineffective, contraindicated, or limited by intolerable adverse effects. Such "PD5 salvage" therapy results in erections satisfactory for intercourse in some men with ED. PGE1 (Caverject), papaverine, and phentolamine may be used alone or in combination (Trimix).

30. Discuss the side effects of intracavernosal and intraurethral injections.
    Side effects, which depend on the type and quantity of substances injected, include hypotension, elevation of liver enzymes, headache, penile pain, and bleeding. Local complications include hematoma, swelling, inadvertent injection into the urethra, and local fibrosis with long-term use. The most serious local complication is priapism

for > 4 hours, which may necessitate injection of alpha-adrenergic agonists or corpora cavernosal aspiration. PGE1 is also available as an intraurethral suppository (medicated urethral system for erection [MUSE]) and, because it is less invasive and easier to use, may be a more appropriate second-line agent than intracavernosal injection. No controlled studies have evaluated the success of either approach in PD5 inhibitor failures.

31. **Does the onset of ED have other health implications?**
The development of impotence is associated with a 45% increased risk of cardiovascular events. This is in the same range of other well-known risk factors, such as current smoking and a family history of a myocardial infarction (MI). This has implications on management because treatment of ED carries a 2.5-fold risk of nonfatal MI. This is comparable with having had a prior MI, where the risk of a subsequent MI is increased 2.9-fold. The risk increase in ED treatment is probably a result of the increased level of exertion (approximately 3–4 metabolic equivalent tasks [METs]) associated with intercourse. Despite these observations, the absolute risk of MI while on ED treatment is still extremely low (20 cases per million per hour of use in patients with prior MI), and therefore known cardiac disease is not a strict contraindication to treatment. High-risk patients, however, should be stabilized prior to treatment of ED:
    - Unstable or refractory angina
    - Uncontrolled hypertension
    - Congestive heart failure
    - MI or stroke in the last 2 weeks
    - High-risk arrhythmias
    - Hypertrophic or other cardiomyopathy
    - Moderate-to-severe valvular disease

32. **What other modalities are available to treat men with impotence?**
Vacuum erection devices provide a noninvasive, mechanical solution for impotence. They are somewhat cumbersome to use and require the placement of an occlusive ring at the base of the penis to prevent venous outflow. They may be particularly effective in those men who have a "venous leak" as the etiology of their impotence. The constrictive ring prevents antegrade ejaculation because of the urethral constriction. Surgical revascularization has a limited place in the treatment of impotence because of its invasiveness and limited success rate. Similarly, penile prosthesis insertion is rarely done because of the availability of several effective and noninvasive alternatives. In men in whom premature ejaculation is the major problem, intermittent use of topical anesthetic agents, tramadol, and/or SSRIs has been efficacious in delaying time to ejaculation.

33. **What future treatments may be forthcoming?**
A novel therapy using intracavernous injection of adipose-derived stem cells to treat erectile dysfunction is currently under investigation. Taking another approach is the use of centrally acting melanocortin receptor agonists. These can be administered by nasal spray and are in clinical trials. They appear to be effective alone or in combination with PD5 inhibitors. Another emerging technology is low-intensity shock therapy (LIST) to stimulate angiogenesis and neovascularization in the penile tissue, enhance blood flow/endothelial function, and convert PDE5 inhibitor nonresponders to responders. Finally, a novel use of metformin as an adjunct to sildenafil may alleviate ED in patients without diabetes but who have insulin resistance.

KEY POINTS: ERECTILE DYSFUNCTION

- Erections are mediated by neural and endothelial nitric oxide (NO) release, which induces vasodilation.
- The specific cause can be diagnosed in 85% of men with impotence.
- Besides diabetes mellitus, the three most common endocrine causes of impotence are primary hypogonadism, secondary hypogonadism, and hyperprolactinemia.
- The antihypertensives that are least likely to cause impotence are angiotensin-converting enzyme (ACE) inhibitors, angiotensin receptor blockers (ARBs), and calcium channel blockers.
- The roles of risk factors, lifestyle modification, and psychological counseling should be considered in all patients with impotence.
- Serum prolactin level should be measured in patients with secondary hypogonadism or with results suggesting a pituitary lesion.
- Consider possibility of concomitant cardiovascular disease in patients with impotence and treat unstable cardiac conditions prior to initiation of therapy of erectile dysfunction (ED).
- PD5 inhibitors (sildenafil, vardenafil, tadalafil, and avanafil) are the most effective drugs in treating nonhormonal impotence. Avoid a fatty meal which can inhibit absorption when taking sildenafil, vardenafil and avanafil.
- PD5 inhibitors are contraindicated in men taking any form of nitrates because PD5 inhibitors can cause vasodilatation similar to that of nitrates.

🌐 WEBSITES

1. https://academic.oup.com/jcem/article/95/6/2536/2597900
2. https://www.niddk.nih.gov/health-information/urologic-diseases/erectile-dysfunction/all-content
3. https://www.hormone.org/diseases-and-conditions/mens-health/erectile-dysfunction
4. http://auanet.org/guidelines

ACKNOWLEDGEMENTS

The views expressed in this manuscript are those of the authors and do not reflect the official policy of the Department of the Army, Navy, the Department of Defense, the National Institutes of Health, or the United States Government. Dr. Cruz and Dr. Hoang are military service members. This work was prepared as part of our official duties. Title 17 U.S.C. 105 provides the "Copyright protection under this title is not available for any work of the United States Government." Title 17 U.S.C. 101 defines a U.S. Government work as a work prepared by a military service member or employee of the U.S. Government as part of that person's official duties. We certify that all individuals who qualify as authors have been listed; each has participated in the conception and design of this work, the analysis of data (when applicable), the writing of the document, and/or the approval of the submission of this version; that the document represents valid work; that if we used information derived from another source, we obtained all necessary approvals to use it and made appropriate acknowledgements in the document; and that each takes public responsibility for it.

BIBLIOGRAPHY

Adams, M. A., Banting, B. D., Maurice, D. H., Morales, A., & Heaton, J. P. (1997). Vascular control mechanisms in penile erection: phylogeny and the inevitability of multiple and overlapping systems. *International Journal of Impotence Research, 9*, 85–95.

Andersson, K. E. (2003). Erectile physiological and pathophysiological pathways involved in erectile dysfunction. *Journal of Urology, 170*, S6–S14.

Bagatell, C. J., & Bremner, W. J. (1997). Androgens in men—uses and abuses. *New England Journal of Medicine, 334*, 707–714.

Bhasin, S., Cunningham, G. R., Hayes, F. J., Matsumoto, A. M., Snyder, P. J., Swerdloff, R. S., & Montori, V. M. (2006). Testosterone therapy in adult men with androgen deficiency syndromes: an Endocrine Society Clinical Practice Guideline. *Journal of Clinical Endocrinology and Metabolism, 91*, 1995–2010.

Cohan, P., & Korenman, S. G. (2001). Erectile dysfunction. *Journal of Clinical Endocrinology & Metabolism*, 86, 2391–2394.

Cookson, M. S., & Nadig, P. W. (1993). Long-term results with vacuum constriction device. *Journal of Urology*, 149, 290–294.

Esposito, K., Giugliano, F., Di Palo, C., Giugliano, G., Marfella, R., D'Andrea, F., . . . Giugliano, D. (2004). Effect of lifestyle changes on erectile dysfunction in obese men: a randomized controlled trial. *Journal of the American Medical Association, 291*, 2978–2984.

Esposito, K., Giugliano, F., Martedi, E., Feola, G., Marfella, R., D'Armiento, M., & Giugliano, D. (2005). High proportions of erectile dysfunction in men with the metabolic syndrome. *Diabetes Care, 28*, 1201–1203.

Feldman, H. A., Goldstein, I., Hatzichristou, D. G., Krane, R. J., & McKinlay, J. B. (1994). Impotence and its medical and psychosocial correlates: results of the Massachusetts male aging study. *Journal of Urology, 151*, 54–61.

Goldstein, I., Lue, T. F., Padma-Nathan, H., Rosen, R. C., Steers, W. D., & Wicker, P. A. (1998). Oral sildenafil in the treatment of erectile dysfunction. *New England Journal of Medicine*, 338, 1397–1404.

Goldstein, I., Young, J. M., Fischer, J., Bangerter, K., Segerson, T., & Taylor, T. (2003). Vardenafil, a new phosphodiesterase type 5 inhibitor, in the treatment of erectile dysfunction in men with diabetes: a multicenter double-blind placebo-controlled fixed-dose study. *Diabetes Care, 26*, 777–783.

Grimm, R. H., Jr., Grandits, G. A., Prineas, R. J., McDonald, R. H., Lewis, C. E., Flack, J. M., . . . Elmer, P. J. (1997). Long-term effects on sexual function of five antihypertensive drugs and nutritional hygienic treatment in hypertensive men and women. Treatment of Mild Hypertension Study (TOMHS). *Hypertension, 29*, 8–14.

Guay, A., Spark, R. F., Bansal, S., Cunningham, G. R., Goodman, N. F., Nankin, H. R., . . . Perez, J. B. (2003). American Association of Clinical Endocrinologists medical guidelines for clinical practice for the evaluation and treatment of male sexual dysfunction: a couple's problem – 2003 update. *Endocrine Practice, 9*, 77–95.

Hanash, K. A. (1997). Comparative oriented therapy for erectile dysfunction. *Journal of Urology, 157*, 2135–2139.

Herrmann, H. C., Chang, G., Klugherz, B. D., & Mahoney, P. D. (2000). Hemodynamic effects of sildenafil in men with severe coronary artery disease. *New England Journal of Medicine, 342*, 1622–1626.

Hong, B., Ji, Y. H., Hong, J. H., Nam, K. Y., & Ahn, T. Y. (2002). A double-blind crossover study evaluating the efficacy of Korean red ginseng in patients with erectile dysfunction: a preliminary report. *Journal of Urology, 168*, 2070–2073.

Khera, M., Albersen, M., & Mulhall, J. P. (2015). Mesenchymal stem cell therapy for the treatment of erectile dysfunction. *The Journal of Sexual Medicine, 12*(5), 1105–1106.

Krane, R. J., Goldstein, I., & DeTejada, J. S. (1989). Impotence. *N Engl J Med, 321*, 1648–1659.

Krassas, G. E., Tziomalos, K., Papadopoulou, I., Pontikides, N., & Perros, P. (2008). Erectile dysfunction in patients with hyper- and hypothyroidism: how common and should we treat? *Journal of Clinical Endocrinology and Metabolism, 93*, 1815–1819.

Lerner, S. F., Melman, A., & Christ, G. J. (1993). A review of erectile dysfunction: new insights and more questions. *Journal of Urology, 149*(5 pt 2), 1246–1252.

Linet, O. I., & Ogrinc, F. G. (1996). Efficacy and safety of intracavernosal prostaglandin in men with erectile dysfunction. *New England Journal of Medicine, 334*, 873–878.

McMahon, C. (2005). Comparison of the safety, efficacy, and tolerability of on-demand tadalafil and daily dosed tadalafil for the treatment of erectile dysfunction. *Journal of Sexual Medicine, 2*, 415–427.

McMahon, C. G., & Touma, K. (1999). Treatment of premature ejaculation with paroxetine hydrochloride as needed: two single-blind placebo controlled crossover studies. *Journal of Urology, 161*, 1826–1830.

McNamara, E. R., & Donatucci, C. F. (2011). Newer phosphodiesterase inhibitors: comparison with established agents. *Urologic Clinics of North America, 38*, 155–163.

Melman, A. (2007). Gene therapy for male erectile dysfunction. *Urologic Clinics of North America, 34*, 619–630.

Molodysky, E., Liu, S. P., Huang, S. J., & Hsu, G. L. (2013). Penile vascular surgery for treating erectile dysfunction: current role and future direction. *Arab Journal of Urology, 11*(3), 254–266.

Montague, D. K., Jarow, J. P., Broderick, G. A., Dmochowski, R. R., Heaton, J. P., Lue, T. F., . . . Sharlip, I. D. (2005). The management of erectile dysfunction: an AUA update. *Journal of Urology, 174*, 230–239.

Morley, J. E., & Kaiser, F. E. (1993). Impotence: the internists' approach to diagnosis and treatment. *Advances in Internal Medicine, 38*:151-168.

Mulhall, J. P., & Montorsi, F. (2006). Evaluating preference trials of oral phosphodiesterase 5 inhibitors for erectile dysfunction. *European Urology, 49*, 30–37.

Meisler, A. W., & Carey, N. P. (1990). A critical reevaluation of nocturnal penile tumescence monitoring in the diagnosis of erectile dysfunction. *J Nerv Ment Dis, 178*, 78–79.

NIH Consensus Conference: Impotence. (1993). *JAMA, 270*, 83–90.

Nunes, K. P., Labazi, H., & Webb, R. C. (2012). New insights into hypertension-associated erectile dysfunction. *Current Opinion in Nephrology and Hypertension, 21*(2), 163–170.

Padma-Nathan, H., Hellstrom, W. J., Kaiser, F. E., Labasky, R. F., Lue, T. F., Nolten, W. E., . . . Gesundheit, N. (1997). Treatment of men with erectile dysfunction with transurethral alprostadil. Medicated Urethral System for Erection (MUSE) Study Group. *New England Journal of Medicine, 336*, 1–7.

Park, K., Ku, J. H., Kim, S. W., & Paick, J. S. (2005). Risk factors in predicting a poor response to sildenafil citrate in elderly men with erectile dysfunction. *BJU International, 95*, 366–370.

Porst, H., Padma-Nathan, H., Giuliano, F., Anglin, G., Varanese, L., & Rosen, R. (2003). Efficacy of tadalafil for the treatment of erectile dysfunction at 24 and 36 hours after dosing: a randomized controlled trial. *Urology, 62*, 121–125.

Rajfer, J., Aronson, W. J., Bush, P. A., Dorey, F. J., & Ignarro, L. J. (1992). Nitric oxide as a mediator of relaxation of the corpus cavernosum in response to nonadrenergic, noncholinergic neurotransmission. *New England Journal of Medicine, 326*, 90–94.

Rendell, M. S., Rajfer, J., Wicker, P. A., & Smith, M. D. (1999). Sildenafil for treatment of erectile dysfunction in men with diabetes. A randomized controlled trial. *JAMA, 281*, 421–426.

Rey Valzacchi, G. J., Costanzo, P. R., Finger, L. A., Layus, A. O., Gueglio, G. M., Litwak, L. E., & Knoblovits, P. (2012). Addition of metformin to sildenafil treatment for erectile dysfunction in eugonadal non-diabetic men with insulin resistance. A prospective, randomized, double blind pilot study. *Journal of Andrology, 33*, 608–614.

Rosenthal, B. D., May, N. R., Metro, M. J., Harkaway, R. C., & Ginsberg, P. C. (2006). Adjunctive use of Androgel (testosterone gel) with sildenafil to treat erectile dysfunction in men with acquired androgen deficiency syndrome after failure using sildenafil alone. *Urology, 67*, 571–574.

Sidi, A. A. (1988). Vasoactive intracavernous pharmacotherapy. *Urologic Clinics of North America, 15*, 95–101.

Thompason, I. M., Tangen, C. M., Goodman, P. J., Probstfield, J. L., Moinpour, C. M., & Coltman, C. A. (2005). Erectile dysfunction and subsequent cardiovascular disease. *Journal of the American Medical Association, 294*, 2996–3002.

Witherington, R. (1989). Mechanical aids for treatment of impotence. *Clinical Diabetes, 7*, 1–22.

CHAPTER 52

GYNECOMASTIA

Mark Bridenstine, Brenda K. Bell, and Micol S. Rothman

1. Define gynecomastia.

   Gynecomastia is defined as the presence of palpable breast tissue in a male. True gynecomastia resulting from enlargement of glandular breast tissue should be distinguished from excess adipose accumulation (i.e., pseudogynecomastia).

2. How does gynecomastia present clinically?

   Gynecomastia usually presents as a palpable discrete button of tissue arising concentrically beneath the nipple and areola. Gynecomastia feels firm, mobile, and "gritty" compared with surrounding adipose tissue. Fatty tissue, unlike gynecomastia, will not cause resistance until the nipple is reached. If any doubt remains, soap and water on the breast can facilitate the examination by decreasing skin friction.

3. What is the significance of painful gynecomastia?

   Gynecomastia is frequently asymptomatic and incidentally discovered. Pain or tenderness implies recent, rapid growth of breast tissue. This may indicate a pathologic cause for the gynecomastia and should prompt further evaluation.

4. Is gynecomastia always bilateral?

   The involvement tends to be bilateral, but asymmetry is common. Unilateral enlargement is present in 5% to 25% of patients and may be a preliminary stage in the development of bilateral disease. In autopsy studies, unilateral enlargement is often found to be bilateral gynecomastia histologically.

5. Summarize the pathophysiology of gynecomastia.

   Gynecomastia results from an imbalance between the stimulatory effect of estrogen on ductal proliferation and the inhibitory effect of androgen on breast development. The imbalance is most commonly caused by increased production of estrogens, decreased production of testosterone, or increased conversion of androgens to estrogens in peripheral tissue. Disorders of sex hormone–binding globulin (SHBG) or androgen receptor binding and function can also result in gynecomastia.

6. Where are estrogens produced in the male?

   Direct testicular production of estrogens accounts for < 15% of male estrogen production. The majority of estrogens come from the conversion of adrenal and testicular androgens to estrogens by aromatase enzymes in peripheral tissues, particularly adipose tissue and the liver.

7. What is the most common cause of gynecomastia?

   Asymptomatic palpable breast tissue is common in normal males, particularly in the neonate (60%–90%), at puberty (60%–70%, ages 12 and 15 years), and with increasing age (20%–65%, age > 50 years). Prevalence of histopathologically confirmed gynecomastia is up to 40% in autopsy series. Because of this high prevalence, gynecomastia is considered a relatively normal finding during these periods of life. Gynecomastia is often described as *physiologic* or *idiopathic* at these ages.

8. Why does gynecomastia occur so commonly during these stages of life?

   Neonatal gynecomastia is caused by placental transfer of estrogens. During early puberty, production of estrogens begins sooner compared with testosterone production, causing a temporary imbalance in the ratio of estrogens to androgens. With aging, testosterone production decreases, and conversion of peripheral androgen to estrogen often increases because of an age-related increase in adipose tissue. There may also be a higher prevalence of offending medications and medical conditions in the elderly population.

9. What are the other causes of gynecomastia?

   Patients with idiopathic or pubertal gynecomastia make up the majority of cases. Drugs account for 10% to 20% of cases and hypogonadism for another 10%. Adrenal or testicular tumors account for < 3% of cases; gynecomastia may even precede the identification of the testicular tumor. Other causes combined account for < 10% of cases and include androgen-resistance disorders, malnutrition, cirrhosis, alcohol abuse, renal disease, congenital adrenal hyperplasia, extragonadal tumors, refeeding gynecomastia, and hyperthyroidism. Case reports of atypical infectious etiologies (e.g., tuberculosis and filariasis) and topical exposure to essential oils (e.g., lavender and tea tree) have been described.

10. What drugs cause gynecomastia?

Many drugs have been implicated, some with well-characterized steroid effects, others noted in case reports and without a clearly elucidated mechanism (Table 52.1).

11. How do testicular tumors cause gynecomastia?

Germ cell tumors can produce human chorionic gonadotropin (hCG). Like luteinizing hormone (LH), hCG increases testicular estradiol production. Leydig cell tumors, in contrast, may directly secrete estradiol.

12. What extragonadal tumors cause gynecomastia?

Pancreatic, gastric, and pulmonary tumors, transitional cell bladder carcinoma, and renal cell carcinoma have been associated with hCG production. Hepatomas may have increased aromatase activity that results in excess conversion of androgens to estrogens.

13. Who should undergo evaluation for gynecomastia?

History and physical examination are indicated in all cases and will determine the cause in 30% to 40% of patients. Gynecomastia, however, is so common that many experts are cautious about attaching importance to the detection of a small amount of breast tissue in an otherwise asymptomatic male. In adolescents, there is no reason to consider endocrine testing unless the enlargement is massive or the gynecomastia persists for > 2 years. Acute development of enlargement and tenderness in males age > 20 years warrants additional evaluation, as do eccentric, hard masses and lesions > 4 cm in size.

14. What information is significant in the history?

See Box 52.1.

Table 52.1. Causes and Mechanisms of Gynecomastia Development.

PROPOSED MECHANISM	REPORTED AGENTS
Altered Estrogen/Androgen Ratio	
Estrogen excess (exogenous)	Androgens and anabolic steroids (via aromatization of androgens to estrogens), estrogen creams and systemic formulations, human chorionic gonadotropin (hCG), digitoxin (estrogen-like activity), lavender and tea tree essential oils
Androgen deficiency/inhibition of androgen synthesis	Finasteride, dutasteride, ketoconazole, metronidazole, methotrexate, various chemotherapeutic agents, gonadotropin-releasing hormone (GnRH) agonists (e.g., leuprolide, goserelin)
Decreased androgen action	Spironolactone, cimetidine, ranitidine, antiandrogen prostate cancer therapies (e.g., bicalutamide, enzalutamide, flutamide), marijuana, cyproterone acetate
Increased Prolactin	
Antidopaminergic agent	Haloperidol, risperidone, metoclopramide, domperidone, phenothiazines
Mechanism Unknown	
ACE inhibitors	Captopril, enalapril
Calcium channel blockers	Nifedipine, amlodipine, diltiazem, verapamil
Alpha-receptor blockers	Doxazosin, prazosin
Centrally acting agents	Clonidine, methyldopa, reserpine, diethylpropion, amphetamines
Statins (? inhibition of adrenal/gonadal steroid synthesis)	Rosuvastatin, lovastatin, pravastatin, simvastatin
Immunomodulatory agents	Thalidomide, imatinib, dasatinib
Antidepressants	Tricyclic antidepressants, duloxetine, fluoxetine
Antiepileptics	Phenytoin, diazepam, gabapentin
Antituberculosis agents	Isoniazid, ethionamide
Supplements	Melatonin, dong quai, hCG diet
Other	Amiodarone, protease inhibitors, proton pump inhibitors, growth hormone, fenofibrate, heroin, methadone, alcohol, minocycline, penicillamine, etretinate, theophylline, auranofin, sulindac

Box 52.1. Significant Information to Ascertain in Patients with Gynecomastia.

Age	Family history of gynecomastia or breast cancer
Thyroid symptoms	Other illnesses
Duration of enlargement	Congenital abnormalities
Drugs, herbs, supplements	Nutritional status and recent changes in weight
Breast symptoms (tenderness, discharge)	Pubertal progression
Alcohol and illicit drug use	Impotence and libido

15. What should be noted on the physical examination?

    Important features include characteristics of the breast tissue (size, irregular, firm, eccentric, nipple discharge), overlying skin changes (ulceration, nipple retraction), testes (size, asymmetry), abdomen (liver enlargement, ascites, spider angiomas), secondary sexual characteristics, thyroid status (goiter, tremor, reflexes), and signs of excessive cortisol (buffalo hump, central obesity, hypertension, purple striae, moon facies), body mass index (BMI)/ body habitus (bodybuilder physique, obesity).

KEY POINTS: GENERAL APPROACH TO GYNECOMASTIA

- The most important differentiation is between gynecomastia and breast cancer. If doubt remains after physical examination, mammography should be performed.
- Most cases are bilateral, asymptomatic, and incidentally discovered. History, physical examination, and reevaluation in 3 to 6 months are appropriate for such men.
- Rapid enlargement, size > 4 cm, pain, and age < 10 years or between 20 and 50 years correlate with a systemic illness/pathologic cause for the gynecomastia. Such men should be evaluated thoroughly if the cause is not apparent after history and physical examination.
- Malignant tumors can cause gynecomastia, although rarely. Consider testicular, pulmonary, and abdominal (pancreatic, adrenal, gastric, renal/bladder) tumors.

16. Should laboratory tests be ordered?

    Some believe that hormonal testing is not cost effective and favor the use of testicular ultrasonography alone to rule out the 3% incidence of feminizing tumors. Most, however, favor measuring liver enzymes, blood urea nitrogen, creatinine, thyrotropin (thyroid-stimulating hormone [TSH]), and testosterone (total and free). Estradiol, human chorionic gonadotropin (hCG), prolactin, luteinizing hormone (LH), and follicle-stimulating hormone (FSH) may follow the initial screen. If the hCG or estradiol level is elevated, testicular ultrasonography is indicated. If this is negative, chest radiography and abdominal computed tomography (CT) should follow. For prepubertal patients, adrenal CT would precede testicular ultrasonography.

17. What findings raise the suspicion of breast cancer?

    Breast cancer is rare in men (0.2%). The risk is increased in Klinefelter's syndrome (3%–6%) and in male relatives of young women with breast cancer. Carcinoma is usually unilateral, painless, and nontender. Bloody discharge, ulceration, firmness, fixation to the underlying tissue, eccentric location, and adenopathy are suspicious findings. If any doubt remains, mammography or biopsy should be considered. The sensitivity and specificity of mammography for the diagnosis of male breast cancer approaches 90%. The diagnostic accuracy of fine-needle aspiration cytology is > 90%. Excisional biopsy or mastectomy would be recommended for malignant or suspicious cytology or mammographic appearance.

18. Will gynecomastia spontaneously regress?

    Gynecomastia of recent onset and < 3 cm in size will regress in 85% of patients. It may take 18 to 36 months for gynecomastia to resolve during puberty, but resolution will occur in > 90% of pubertal boys. Persistence is uncommon after age 17 years. Gynecomastia caused by a medication or underlying disease should also resolve after discontinuing the inciting agent or treating the underlying disease. This should be emphasized if anabolic steroid use is suspected as an etiology. Persistent tissue becomes more fibrous with time, however, and is less likely to remit spontaneously if it has been present for > 12 months. More highly developed breast tissue (Tanner stages III, IV, and V) is also less likely to regress.

19. What is the treatment when gynecomastia does not regress?

Hormonal therapy can be attempted. Tamoxifen, clomiphene, danazol, dihydrotestosterone, testolactone, and anastrozole have all been used. Although studies are small, and this is an off-label use, tamoxifen has the fewest side effects and the highest response rate for both improvement in tenderness and decrease in mass size. Partial regression can be seen in approximately 80% of patients and complete regression in about 60%. Tamoxifen is given at a dosage of 10 mg twice daily with follow-up in 3 months to assess response. Diarrhea, constipation, and hot flashes are commonly reported adverse events. Aromatase inhibitors, which decrease estradiol levels via blocking aromatization of testosterone, appear less efficacious and have potential adverse associations with bone mass, body fat accumulation, and sexual function in men. Medication is more likely to work if gynecomastia has been present for < 4 months and the size of the tissue is < 3 cm. For recurrent or persistent gynecomastia > 3 cm, surgery is the recommended therapy. Liposuction/ultrasound-guided liposuction, excision, or both may be used. Prophylactic low-dose bilateral breast irradiation and tamoxifen have also been studied in trials to prevent the development of gynecomastia caused by estrogens and antiandrogens used in the treatment of prostate cancer.

KEY POINTS: TREATMENT OF GYNECOMASTIA

- Most cases resolve spontaneously or after removal of the offending medication or treatment of the underlying disease.
- Medical management with tamoxifen can be attempted for 3 to 6 months, if desired.
- The longer the tissue has been present and the larger the amount of tissue, the less likely is the response to tamoxifen. Surgery is indicated in these cases.

BIBLIOGRAPHY

Braunstein, G. D. (2007). Clinical practice. Gynecomastia. *New England Journal of Medicine, 357,* 1229–1237.

Braunstein, G. (2003). Pathogenesis and diagnosis of gynecomastia. *Up to Date in Endocrinology and Diabetes, 11*(2), 1–11.

Braunstein, G. (2003). Prevention and treatment of gynecomastia. *Up to Date in Endocrinology and Diabetes, 11*(3), 1–9.

Bowers, S. P., Pearlman, N. W., McIntyre, R. C., Jr., Finlayson, C. A., & Huerd, S. (1998). Cost-effective management of gynecomastia. *American Journal of Surgery, 176,* 638–641.

Carlson, H. E. (2011). Approach to the patient with gynecomastia. *Journal of Clinical Endocrinology and Metabolism, 96,* 15–21.

Ersöz, H. Ö., Onde, M. E., Terekeci, H., Kurtoglu, S., & Tor, H. (2002). Causes of gynaecomastia in young adult males and factors associated with idiopathic gynaecomastia. *International Journal of Andrology, 25,* 312–316.

Evans, G. F., Anthony, T., Turnage, R. H., Schumpert, T. D., Levy, K. R., Amirkhan, R. H., … Appelbaum, A. H. (2001). The diagnostic accuracy of mammography in the evaluation of male breast disease. *American Journal of Surgery, 181,* 96–100.

Fruhstorfer, B. H., & Malata, C. M. (2003). A systematic approach to the surgical treatment of gynaecomastia. *British Journal of Plastic Surgery, 56,* 237–246.

Gruntmanis, U., & Braunstein, G. (2001). Treatment of gynecomastia. *Current Opinion in Investigational Drugs, 2,* 643–649.

Henley, D. V., Lipson, N., Korach, K. S., & Block, C. A. (2007). Prepubertal gynecomastia linked to lavender and tea tree oils. *New England Journal of Medicine, 356,* 479–485.

Ismail, A. A., & Barth, J. H. (2001). Endocrinology of gynecomastia. *Annals of Clinical Biochemistry, 38,* 596–607.

Khan, H. N., & Blarney, R. W. (2003). Endocrine treatment of physiological gynaecomastia. *British Medical Journal, 327,* 301–302.

Kolhi, K., & Jain, S. (2012). Filariasis presenting as gynecomastia. *The Breast Journal, 18,* 83–84.

Koh, J., & Tee, A. (2009). Images in clinical medicine: tuberculous abscess manifesting as unilateral gynecomastia. *New England Journal of Medicine, 361,* 2270.

Narula, H. S., & Carlson, H. E. (2007). Gynecomastia. *Endocrinology and Metabolism Clinics of North America, 36,* 497–519.

Widmark, A., Fossa, S. D., Lundmo, P., Damber, J. E., Vaage, S., Damber, L., ,… Klepp, O. (2003). Does prophylactic breast irradiation prevent antiandrogen induced gynecomastia? Evaluation of 253 patients in the randomized Scandinavian trial SPCG-7/SFUO-3. *Urology, 61,* 145–151.

William, M. J. (1963). Gynecomastia: its incidence, recognition and host characterization in 447 autopsy studies. *American Journal of Medicine, 34,* 103–112.

Yaturu, S., Harrara, E., Nopajaroonsri, C., Singal, R., & Gill, S. (2003). Gynecomastia attributable to HCG secreting giant cell carcinoma of the lung. *Endocrine Practice, 9,* 233–235.

Finkelstein, J. S., Lee, H., Burnett-Bowie, S. A., Pallais, J. C., Yu, E. W., Borges, L. F., , … &… Leder, B. Z. (2013). Gonadal steroids and body composition, strength, and sexual function in men. *New England Journal of Medicine, 369,* 1011–1022.

CHAPTER 53

AMENORRHEA

Micol S. Rothman and Margaret E. Wierman

1. Define amenorrhea.

   Amenorrhea is the absence of menstrual periods. *Primary amenorrhea* is the failure to ever begin menses; *secondary amenorrhea* refers to cessation of menstrual periods after cyclic menses have been established. *Oligomenorrhea* refers to lighter and irregular menses.

2. Describe the normal timing of puberty.

   Puberty usually begins after age 8 years in girls and is heralded by the initiation of breast development. The average age for girls in the United States to begin menses is 12 years. This event generally signals the end of the pubertal process, occurring after the growth spurt and most somatic changes are completed. National Health and Nutrition Examination Survey (NHANES) data have noted the average age of menarche to be decreasing slightly, and African American girls have a mean earlier age of breast development onset compared with Caucasian girls (8.9 years versus 10 years).

3. Summarize the underlying process of pubertal development.

   The process is triggered by Kisspeptin activation of gonadotropin-releasing hormone (GnRH)–induced episodic secretion of luteinizing hormone (LH) and follicle-stimulating hormone (FSH) from the pituitary gland. The pulsatile release of gonadotropins activates the ovaries, causing maturation of follicles and production of estrogen and, later, progesterone. These gonadal steroids give feedback at the level of the hypothalamus and pituitary to regulate GnRH and gonadotropin secretion. A final maturation event is the development of positive feedback by estradiol to induce the midcycle LH surge that stimulates ovulation. In many adolescents, menstrual cycles are anovulatory, and thus irregular, for the first 12 to 18 months. As the hypothalamic–pituitary–gonadal (HPG) axis matures, ovulatory cycles become more frequent. In normal adult women, all but one or two cycles per year are ovulatory.

4. What types of disorders cause primary amenorrhea?

   Primary amenorrhea is defined as lack of menses by age 16 years or lack of secondary sexual characteristics by age 14 years. It usually results from abnormal anatomical development of the female reproductive organs or from a hormonal disorder involving the hypothalamus, pituitary gland, or ovaries (Table 53.1). The presence of normal secondary sexual characteristics in such patients suggests an anatomic problem, such as obstruction or failure of development of the uterus or vagina. In contrast, a lack of secondary sexual characteristics indicates a probable hormonal cause.

5. What are the hypothalamic and pituitary causes of primary amenorrhea?

   Idiopathic hypogonadotropic hypogonadism (IHH) can be caused by maturational arrest of GnRH-producing neurons during embryonic development (also called Kallmann's syndrome when associated with anosmia) or failure of GnRH secretion at the time of puberty. The Kisspeptin/Kiss receptor system has recently been shown to regulate GnRH secretion at puberty. Mutations in this pathway, as well as the GnRH receptor in the pituitary, may also cause failure of or impaired sexual maturation. Pituitary tumors, craniopharyngiomas, and Rathke's pouch cysts, can cause impaired LH and FSH secretion in adolescence, disrupting sexual maturation.

6. Summarize the ovarian causes of primary amenorrhea.

   Ovarian function may be impaired because of gonadal dysgenesis caused by Turner's syndrome (45XO karyotype) or destruction by chemotherapy or radiation before the completion of sexual maturation. The presence of ambiguous genitalia or palpable gonads in the labia or inguinal area may indicate a disorder of sexual differentiation, such as congenital adrenal hyperplasia (CAH) (21-hydroxylase deficiency) or an androgen resistance syndrome (testicular feminization) resulting from mutations in the androgen receptor.

7. What disorders cause secondary amenorrhea?

   Secondary amenorrhea, which is much more common than primary amenorrhea, occurs in the postpubertal period. The causes are outlined in Table 53.2. Pregnancy should be excluded in all women with amenorrhea. Onset of irregular menses after prior regular menses with associated hot flashes should suggest premature ovarian insufficiency (POI; i.e., premature menopause). Hypothalamic amenorrhea occurs in 3% to 5% of women and is caused by abnormal GnRH-induced gonadotropin secretion, often as a result of stress or eating disorders, but is a diagnosis of exclusion. Hyperprolactinemia caused by medications or tumors occurs in 10% of women with amenorrhea. Pituitary tumors can also result in secondary amenorrhea. Hyperandrogenic anovulatory disorders,

Table 53.1. Causes of Primary Amenorrhea.

- Anatomic
  - Congenital absence of ovaries, uterus, or vagina
  - Cervical stenosis
  - Imperforate hymen
- Hormonal
  - Hypothalamic
  - GnRH deficiency
  - Hypothalamic tumor (craniopharyngioma)
- Pituitary
  - Prolactinoma
  - Rathke's cleft cyst
  - Panhypopituitarism from a genetic mutation
- Ovarian
  - Gonadal dysgenesis (XO)
  - Chemotherapy or radiation damage of the ovaries
  - Androgen resistance syndromes (XY)
- Other: congenital adrenal hyperplasia

Table 53.2. Causes of Secondary Amenorrhea.

- Pregnancy
- Hypogonadotropic hypogonadism
- Hyperprolactinemia (resulting from drugs or prolactinoma)
- Pituitary tumor inhibiting gonadotropin production
- Hypothalamic amenorrhea
- Hypergonadotropic hypogonadism
- Premature ovarian insufficiency (surgical or autoimmune)
- Gonadotropin producing pituitary tumors
- Hyperandrogenic anovulation

such as polycystic ovary syndrome (PCOS), CAH, and, rarely, gonadal or adrenal tumors, are usually associated with oligomenorrhea, rather than amenorrhea, and signs and symptoms of excess androgens, such as hirsutism and acne.

8. How do you evaluate a patient with amenorrhea?
   One must determine whether the disorder is anatomic or hormonal, congenital or acquired, and where the defect is located. A complete history and physical examination provide the first essential clues. Pregnancy testing should always be ordered. Timed measurement of serum gonadotropin levels (LH and FSH) should be done within the first 5 days after the onset of a spontaneous or induced menses. However, it should be noted that patients who have been on birth control pills or other forms of hormonal contraceptives may need to wait a cycle to ensure accurate results. Patients with low or normal levels of LH and FSH (hypogonadotropic hypogonadism) have a disorder at the level of the hypothalamus or pituitary gland. In contrast, patients with high LH and/or FSH levels (hypergonadotropic hypogonadism) may have a defect at the level of either the ovary or hypothalamic-pituitary unit (e.g., PCOS, in which the hypothalamic GnRH pulse generator is abnormally accelerated or a gonadotrope pituitary tumor that secretes the gonadotropins, FSH, and/or LH).

   Other laboratory examinations to consider include measurement of prolactin level to exclude hyperprolactinemia and thyroid function tests to exclude thyroid disorders. In a patient with signs of excess androgens, dehydroepiandrosterone sulfate (DHEAS) and testosterone should be obtained. In the appropriate patient, Cushing's syndrome should be excluded with a 24-hour urine free cortisol, 1 mg dexamethasone suppression test, or late-night salivary cortisol testing. Exclusion may require more than one test.

9. Discuss the major congenital causes of hypogonadotropic hypogonadism.
   Idiopathic hypogonadotropic hypogonadism (IHH) is caused by GnRH deficiency. Female patients present with primary amenorrhea and lack of secondary sex characteristics. When associated with anosmia, the disorder is termed *Kallmann's syndrome*. GnRH deficiency occurs in 1 in 8000 males and 1 in 40,000 females and may be X-linked, autosomal dominant, autosomal recessive, or sporadic. The X-linked form is associated with a mutation in the *KAL-1* gene, which encodes anosmin, a neural cell adhesion protein thought to be important in providing the scaffolding for GnRH neurons in their migration from the olfactory placode to the hypothalamus during embryonic development. Similarly, mutations in FGF8 or its receptor FGFR1 also disrupt neuronal and olfactory nerve migration.

Thus, GnRH neurons fail to reach their target in the hypothalamus. All other hypothalamic–pituitary function is normal. Recently, investigators have found that mutations in the Kisspeptin/KissR system that mediates GnRH secretion at puberty can also cause IHH. In these young women, estrogen administration is used to initiate the development of secondary sexual characteristics, and fertility can be attained using pulsatile GnRH or gonadotropin therapy.

10. What are the most frequent acquired forms of amenorrhea caused by hypogonadotropic hypogonadism?
   • Hyperprolactinemia
   • Hypothalamic amenorrhea

11. How does hyperprolactinemia cause amenorrhea?
   Elevated prolactin levels may be caused by prolactinomas, hypothyroidism, medications (usually psychotropic drugs), or pregnancy. Hyperprolactinemia impairs the normal function of the HPG axis at multiple levels, but the major site of inhibition is the hypothalamic GnRH pulse generator. As prolactin levels rise, luteal phase defects develop, ovulation ceases, and menstrual cycles become shorter and irregular. Higher levels of prolactin are associated with amenorrhea. Treatment of the underlying cause of the elevated prolactin level usually normalizes menstrual cycles.

12. What is hypothalamic amenorrhea?
   Hypothalamic amenorrhea refers to amenorrhea resulting from acquired disorders of the GnRH pulse generator. Excessive stress, exercise, and weight loss have been shown to act centrally to disrupt the GnRH-induced pulsatile gonadotropin secretory pattern. In men, GnRH-induced LH pulses normally occur every 2 hours. In contrast, the LH pulse pattern in women must change across the menstrual cycle, accelerating from every 90 to 60 minutes across the follicular phase to every 30 minutes at ovulation and then slowing from every hour to every 4 to 8 hours across the luteal phase. Disruption of this precisely timed pattern results in anovulation, irregular menses, and, eventually, amenorrhea.

13. What types of GnRH pulse generator defects cause hypothalamic amenorrhea?
   Hypothalamic amenorrhea may result from several types of gonadotropin secretory disorders. Some women with anorexia nervosa have absent GnRH-induced LH pulsations (prepubertal pattern), some have pulsations only at night (early pubertal pattern), and still others have LH pulses throughout the 24-hour period, but they are significantly reduced in amplitude or frequency.

14. How do you make a diagnosis of hypothalamic amenorrhea?
   The diagnosis depends on excluding other causes of amenorrhea and then relies heavily on a history of weight loss, high levels of exercise or stress, or a combination of these. Supportive findings on physical examination include evidence of decreased estrogen effects and absence of other major illnesses. Laboratory testing usually reveals low serum estradiol and low or low-normal serum LH and FSH levels; the test for beta-hCG is negative, and the prolactin level is normal. Elevated FSH levels with low estradiol levels, in contrast, indicate probable POI.

15. What are the consequences of estrogen deficiency?
   Short-term consequences of estrogen deficiency may include painful intercourse, hot flashes, and sleep disturbances. Among the more important long-term consequences are osteoporosis and premature coronary artery disease.

16. What treatment options are available for hypothalamic amenorrhea?
   Interventions to reduce stress and balance nutritional intake with degree of exercise should be attempted initially. If these interventions are unsuccessful, estrogen replacement therapy can be instituted. However, data are mixed as to the protective effect of estrogen on bone health in women with anorexia nervosa. Recent Endocrine Society guidelines suggest avoiding ethinyl estradiol and treating with transdermal estrogen and cyclic progesterone. It should be noted that this does not provide contraception and may be associated with irregular bleeding in older women with more mild defects. Fertility, if desired, may be achieved by ovulation induction with clomiphene in mild cases or with human menopausal gonadotropins or pulsatile GnRH administration if the disorder is more severe.

17. What disorders cause amenorrhea with hypergonadotropic hypogonadism?
   • Premature ovarian insufficiency (high FSH, later high LH and low estrogen)
   • PCOS (low FSH, high LH, and normal estrogen)
   • Gonadotropin-secreting pituitary tumors (high FSH and/or LH, often in postmenopausal women low estrogen)

18. How do you make a diagnosis of POI?
   POI, which is defined as menopause before age 40 years, may be caused by surgical removal or autoimmune destruction of the ovaries. Autoimmune destruction of the ovaries is characterized by a history of normal puberty and regular menses followed by the early onset of hot flashes, irregular menses, and eventual amenorrhea. Elevated serum FSH levels are the laboratory hallmark of gonadal failure resulting from loss of inhibin. To avoid

misdiagnosis, blood for FSH and estradiol should be drawn in the early follicular phase (day 1–5 after onset of a spontaneous or induced menses) because FSH levels rise along with LH at midcycle in normally ovulating women. Turner's syndrome mosaics (XO/XX) may have several menses before they undergo menopause; therefore, a karyotype may be helpful if ovarian failure occurs in adolescence or the early 20s. Measurement of anti-Müllerian hormone (AMH) may predict the age of menopause and assess for premature ovarian insufficiency. AMH is produced by granulosa cells in the ovary and decreases over time with eventual absence at the time of menopause.

19. What other disorders may coexist with POI?
    Both patients and family members are at risk for other autoimmune disorders, including primary adrenal insufficiency (Addison's disease), autoimmune thyroid disorders (Graves' disease, Hashimoto's thyroiditis), type 1 diabetes mellitus, pernicious anemia (vitamin B_{12} deficiency), celiac sprue (often with vitamin D and iron deficiencies), and/or rheumatologic disorders.

20. What are the treatment options for women with POI?
    Estrogen therapy, in combination with progesterone, is used to decrease postmenopausal bone loss and premature coronary artery disease. Options for fertility in women with POI include incubation of donor eggs with the partner's sperm with in vitro fertilization protocols, along with sex hormonal preparation of the patient to enable her to carry the fetus in her uterus.

21. What is hyperandrogenic anovulation?
    Hyperandrogenic anovulation refers to the cluster of disorders that present with irregular menses or amenorrhea and signs of androgen excess, such as hirsutism and acne. The disorders in this group include PCOS, androgen-secreting tumors of the ovaries or adrenal glands, Cushing's syndrome, CAH (classic or attenuated form), and obesity-induced irregular menses. PCOS is the most common disorder of this type, described in 6% to 10% of reproductive-age women. This is described in more detail in Chapter 54.

22. How do tumors cause hyperandrogenic anovulation?
    Androgen-producing ovarian and adrenal tumors are suggested by a rapid progression of hirsutism and virilization (temporal hair recession, clitoris enlargement, and breast atrophy), as well as high serum androgen levels (testosterone or DHEAS). They are usually associated with serum testosterone levels > 200 ng/dL or DHEAS levels > 1000 ng/mL. However, there is no level of testosterone or DHEAS that absolutely confirms or excludes the diagnosis. The diagnosis of these tumors depends on accurate imaging studies.

23. What clinical and biochemical features suggest a patient with hirsutism has CAH?
    CAH (most commonly caused by 21-hydroxylase deficiency) presents in infancy with ambiguous genitalia in girls and occasionally with salt-wasting syndromes. Milder forms present in adolescence with early pubarche and irregular menses. Family history and ethnicity (Ashkenazi Jews, Italians, Hispanics, Inuit) increase the suspicion for CAH. CAH is diagnosed by high basal (> 2–3 ng/mL) or adrenocorticotropic hormone (ACTH)–stimulated (> 10 ng/mL) levels of 17-hydroxyprogesterone, with the test performed in the follicular phase. See Chapter 37.

24. When should you suspect obesity-induced hyperandrogenic anovulation?
    Obesity-induced hyperandrogenic anovulation is suggested by a history of normal puberty and menses until progressive weight gain triggers the development of hirsutism, acne, oligomenorrhea, and, later, amenorrhea. Affected women have low serum levels of FSH and LH in the follicular phase in contrast to women with PCOS (see subsequent discussion).

25. Describe the pathophysiology of obesity-induced hyperandrogenic anovulation.
    Fat tissue contains aromatase and 5-alpha-reductase enzymes. Aromatase converts androgens to estrogens; when aromatase is present in increased amounts, as in obesity, constant (rather than fluctuating) serum estrogen levels are produced, inhibiting LH and FSH secretion and thereby impairing normal ovulation. Increased activity of 5-alpha-reductase, which converts testosterone to dihydrotestosterone (DHT), results in excessive DHT production, promoting the development of hirsutism and acne. Primary treatment with weight loss often results in restoration of normal reproductive function.

KEY POINTS: AMENORRHEA

- Amenorrhea with estrogen deficiency can result in osteoporosis and premature cardiovascular disease.
- Hyperprolactinemia and hypothalamic amenorrhea are the most common causes of acquired amenorrhea with low estrogen and low follicle-stimulating hormone (FSH) levels.
- Premature ovarian insufficiency (POI) is an autoimmune disease; affected females are at risk for other autoimmune disorders, such as adrenal and thyroid disease, pernicious anemia, celiac sprue, and rheumatologic disorders.

KEY POINTS: AMENORRHEA—cont'd

- *Hyperandrogenic anovulation* refers to amenorrhea with hirsutism and acne.
- Polycystic ovarian syndrome (PCOS) is the most common type of hyperandrogenic amenorrhea, associated with risks of infertility, endometrial cancer, the metabolic syndrome, and type 2 diabetes.

BIBLIOGRAPHY

Berga, S. L. (1996). Functional hypothalamic chronic anovulation. In W. Y. Adashi, J. A. Rock, & Z. Rosenwaks (Eds.), *Reproductive Endocrinology, Surgery, and Technology* (pp. 1061–1075). Philadelphia: Lippincott-Raven.

Broer, S. L., Eijkemans, M. J., Scheffer, G. J., van Rooij, I. A., de Vet, A., Themmen, A. P., ... Broekmans, F. J. (2011). Anti-Mullerian hormone predicts menopause: a long-term follow-up study in normoovulatory women. *Journal of Clinical Endocrinology and Metabolism, 96*(8), 2532–2539.

Cumming, D. C. (1996). Exercise-associated amenorrhea, low bone density, and estrogen replacement therapy. *Archives of Internal Medicine, 156*, 2193–2195.

Gordon, C. M., Ackerman, K. E., Berga, S. L., Kaplan, J. R., Mastorakos, G., Misra, M., ... Warren, M. P. (2017). Functional hypothalamic amenorrhea: an Endocrine Society Clinical Practice guideline. *Journal of Clinical Endocrinology and Metabolism, 102*, 1413–1439.

Legro, R. S. (2007). A 27-year-old woman with a diagnosis of polycystic ovary syndrome. *Journal of the American Medical Association, 297*, 509–519.

Legro, R. S., Barnhart, H. X., Schlaff, W. D., Carr, B. R., Diamond, M. P., Carson, S. A., ... Myers, E. R. (2007). Clomiphene, metformin, or both for infertility in the polycystic ovary syndrome. *New England Journal of Medicine, 356*, 551–566.

Norman, R. J., Dewailly, D., Legro, R. S., & Hickey, T. E. (2007). Polycystic ovary syndrome. *Lancet, 370*(9588), 685–697.

Rothman, M. S., & Wierman, M. E. (2008). Female hypogonadism: evaluation of the hypothalamic-pituitary-ovarian axis. *Pituitary, 11*, 163–169.

Pralong, F. P., & Crowley, W. F., Jr. (1997). Gonadotropins: normal physiology. In M. E. Wierman (Ed.), *Diseases of the Pituitary: Diagnosis and Treatment* (pp. 203–219). Totowa: Humana Press.

Santoro, N. (2011). Update in hyper- and hypogonadotropic amenorrhea. *Journal of Clinical Endocrinology and Metabolism, 96*(11), 3281–3288.

Schlechte, J. A. (1997). Differential diagnosis and management of hyperprolactinemia. In M. E. Wierman (Ed.), *Diseases of the Pituitary: Diagnosis and Treatment* (pp. 71–77). Totowa: Humana Press.

Taylor, A. E., Adams, J. M., Mulder, J. E., Martin, K. A., Sluss, P. M., & Crowley, W. F. Jr. (1996). A randomized, controlled trial of estradiol replacement therapy in women with hypergonadotropic amenorrhea. *Journal of Clinical Endocrinology and Metabolism, 81*, 3615–3621.

Warren, M. P. (1997). Anorexia, bulimia, and exercise-induced amenorrhea: medical approach. *Current Therapy in Endocrinology and Metabolism, 6*, 13–17.

Welt, C. K., & Hall, J. E. (1997). Gonadotropin deficiency: differential diagnosis and treatment. In M. E. Wierman (Ed.), *Diseases of the Pituitary: Diagnosis and Treatment* (pp. 221–246). Totowa: Humana Press.

Wierman, M. E. (1996). Gonadotropin releasing hormone. In W. Y. Adashi, J. A. Rock, & Z. Rosenwaks (Eds.), *Reproductive Endocrinology, Surgery, and Technology* (pp. 665–681). Philadelphia: Lippincott-Raven.

CHAPTER 54

POLYCYSTIC OVARIAN SYNDROME

Melanie Cree-Green and Anne-Marie Carreau

1. How does the patient with polycystic ovarian syndrome (PCOS) present clinically?

   Most women with PCOS have symptoms in adolescence with a history of early adrenarche ($<$ 8 years) and menarche ($<$ 10 years), and persistently irregular menses, although many women do not present to care until adulthood when they experience difficulty with conception. Hirsutism and acne can present in adolescence, are common features of the disorder, and are often a reason for primary presentation. Approximately 60% of women with PCOS become overweight, and therefore, persistent weight gain and difficulty with weight loss are additional common presenting complaints. Women with PCOS also have other dermatologic findings, including acanthosis nigricans (a velvety, hyperpigmented cutaneous lesion on the neck and in the axillae), excess skin tags, hidradenitis, pilonidal cysts, and androgenic alopecia. Rarely, PCOS can be diagnosed at the time of presentation for endometrial hyperplasia or carcinoma.

2. Describe the pathogenesis of PCOS.

   The intrinsic primary disorder causing PCOS is still debated among experts. There are three prevailing theories for the primary cause of hyperandrogenism: (1) primary ovarian dysfunction; (2) insulin resistance and hyperinsulinism-induced thecal cell hypertrophy; and (3) hypothalamic/pituitary dysfunction causing increased luteinizing hormone (LH) production. All these pathways appear to contribute to the pathophysiology and clinical manifestations of PCOS.

   Several studies have shown an insulin-mediated mechanism contributing to hyperandrogenism, anovulation, and other metabolic manifestations of the syndrome. At least 40% to 70% of women with PCOS, regardless of body mass index (BMI), are insulin resistant and display compensatory hyperinsulinemia. Ovarian androgen production seems to be partly dependent on insulin and may be hyperresponsive to insulin, even in lean and normo-insulinemic women.

   Ovarian and adrenal hyper-responsiveness to LH and to adrenocorticotropin (ACTH) are also important features of PCOS. Women with PCOS often have increased secretory ratios of LH to follicle-stimulating hormone (FSH), resulting in recruitment of multiple ovarian follicles without dominant follicle development and inability to trigger a gonadotropin-releasing hormone (GnRH)–induced LH surge. This results in anovulation and the appearance of multiple subcapsular cysts. The abnormal GnRH pattern triggers constant estrogen and enhanced androgen production by the ovaries. Additionally, excess anti-Müllerian hormone (AMH), which is released by excess follicles, may inhibit GnRH secretion.

   Genome-wide association studies (GWAS) have demonstrated an underlying genetic predisposition to the ovarian dysfunction and insulin resistance, although no specific gene has been identified. Women with PCOS often have a family history of PCOS or type 2 diabetes. Additionally, PCOS development may also be related to intrauterine factors, such as maternal obesity, poor fetal growth, and prenatal environment, including maternal androgen and AMH concentrations.

3. What are the criteria for diagnosis of PCOS in adults?

   There are three primary guidelines for the diagnosis of PCOS in adult women; these vary slightly and are summarized below. The National Institutes of Health (NIH) criteria are the most stringent and more likely to identify women with metabolic disease. Other causes for irregular menses or signs of hyperandrogenism must be excluded.

Measurement	*NIH, 1990*	*Rotterdam, 2003*	*Androgen Excess Society, 2006*
Oligomenorrhea ($\leq$ 8 menses a year)	+	+/−	+/−
Hyperandrogenism (clinical or biochemical, testosterone)	+	+/−	+
Polycystic ovaries on ultrasound ($>$ 10 mL size and $>$ 12 follicles)	+/−	+/−	+/−
To meet criteria for PCOS	**Must have first 2**	**Need 2 of 3**	**Need androgens + one other**

4. What are the criteria for diagnosis of PCOS in adolescents?

Adolescents must meet three criteria to be given a diagnosis of PCOS:

1. Menstrual abnormalities defined as (a) oligomenorrhea with < 9 menses a year at least 2 years after menarche; or (b) at least 90 days between menses at least 1 year post-menarche or (c) primary amenorrhea after age 15 years.
2. Clinical (acne/hirsutism/androgenic alopecia) and/or biochemical evidence of hyperandrogenism
3. No other cause for irregular menses or signs of hyperandrogenism

There is no role for ovarian ultrasonography in girls for confirming the diagnosis of PCOS because normative data for follicle count and ovarian size are not well established for this age. The original Rotterdam ovarian criteria were developed on the basis of data from women at a mean age of 28 years; because follicle count peaks in early adolescence, these criteria cannot be applied to adolescents. Furthermore, many girls will not tolerate vaginal ultrasonography, and abdominal ultrasonography is not as accurate, especially in girls who are obese. Ultrasonography can be useful to investigate anatomic causes of primary amenorrhea, thickness of the endometrial lining in case of failure to have a withdrawal bleed after a progesterone challenge, or ovarian pain with a suspected large cyst or torsion.

5. What are the long-term consequences of PCOS?

Long-term consequences of PCOS include infertility, endometrial cancer, metabolic syndrome (hypertension, central adiposity, dyslipidemia, hyperglycemia), and type 2 diabetes mellitus.

The relative risk of developing type 2 diabetes is almost four times higher in women with PCOS compared with controls after adjustment for age and 2.4 times higher after further adjustment for BMI. Epidemiologic studies have not yet defined a clear increase in long-term cardiovascular events, but the risk factors for cardiovascular disease, early atherosclerosis deposition, and endothelial dysfunction are clearly present in women with PCOS.

6. How is hyperandrogenism defined, and what can affect the measurements of testosterone?

Hyperandrogenism is defined as having serum testosterone values in excess of the laboratory-defined normative data. Many women will also have mildly elevated dehydroepiandrosterone sulfate (DHEAS) levels. Testosterone has a strong diurnal rhythm, so laboratory examination must be done in the morning to catch the peak value, ideally before 10 AM. Testosterone can rise during ovulation and, thus, is best checked in the first 5 days of the cycle in women who are having cycles. Sex hormone–binding globulin (SHBG) can be decreased in obesity, and thus, measuring serum free testosterone level is ideal in women who are obese. Testosterone assays have been problematic in the past. It is currently recommended that total testosterone be measured with tandem liquid chromatography/mass spectroscopy and free testosterone with equilibrium dialysis.

7. What is the differential diagnosis for suspected PCOS?

PCOS is a diagnosis of exclusion. Other etiologies for hirsutism and amenorrhea need to be excluded.

Condition	Laboratory Testing	Other Signs
Prolactinoma	↑Prolactin	Galactorrhea; breast enlargement/ tenderness; visual field defects
Hypothyroidism	↑Thyroid-stimulating hormone and normal or ↓thyroxine	Constipation; dry skin; fatigue
Primary ovarian insufficiency	↑Luteinizing hormone, ↑follicle-stimulating hormone, ↓estradiol	Hot flashes; vaginal dryness
Hypothalamic amenorrhea	↓Luteinizing hormone, ↓follicle-stimulating hormone, ↓estradiol	Excess exercise; body mass index (BMI) extremes—high or low
Congenital adrenal hypoplasia	↑Morning 17-hydroxyprogesterone	Premature adrenarche; short stature for family; family history
Androgen-secreting tumors	↑DHEAS, ↑androstenedione	
Cushing's syndrome	↑Bedtime salivary cortisol, ↑24-hour urine cortisol, ↑AM cortisol after 1 mg dexamethasone suppression test	Central obesity; rapid-onset symptoms; thick, violaceous striae; proximal muscle weakness
Exogenous androgens	History	

8. What is the role of obesity in PCOS?

Overall, it appears that the risk of developing PCOS is the same in women who are not obese as in women who are. However, obesity is associated with exacerbation of the clinical manifestations of PCOS because it increases insulin resistance and, thus, hyperandrogenism. Women who are obese may be more prone to consult for PCOS because of more severe symptoms that may incite them to seek medical advice.

9. What metabolic screening needs to be done in PCOS?

Women with PCOS are at increased risk for metabolic diseases, including insulin resistance, prediabetes, type 2 diabetes, hyperlipidemia, nonalcoholic fatty liver disease, and, potentially, cardiovascular disease. Women with

PCOS should have a 2-hour 75-g oral glucose tolerance test at diagnosis and then every 1 to 3 years, regardless of their body weight. Measurement of hemoglobin A_{1c}, although less accurate, is also an acceptable test for hyperglycemia. A fasting lipid panel should be performed annually, and blood pressure measurement taken at every visit. All modifiable cardiovascular disease risk factors should be identified. There is currently no accurate laboratory screening test for nonalcoholic fatty liver disease, but this will likely change in the next 10 years. Liver ultrasonography with transient elastography may be a noninvasive way to diagnose fatty liver disease when suspected.

10. What other conditions need to be screened for in women with PCOS?

Psychiatric disease: Women with PCOS have higher rates of psychiatric disease, especially depression and anxiety. These tend to be worse in women with more extreme dermatologic manifestations and in those undergoing infertility treatments.

Obstructive sleep apnea: Women with PCOS have > 2-fold increased risk for obstructive sleep apnea compared with weight-matched controls. Untreated sleep apnea can contribute to metabolic disorders, mood alterations, increased appetite, and fatigue. All women should be screened by using questionnaires on quality of sleep and polysomnography ordered in those who have symptoms suggestive of obstructive sleep apnea. Obstructive sleep apnea should be treated in those with a confirmed diagnosis.

Endometrial cancer: Women presenting later in life with a longer history of irregular menses are at increased risk for endometrial cancer. Screening is discussed below.

11. Which patients need counseling on lifestyle modification?

Healthy lifestyle recommendations should be given to all women with PCOS regardless of their body weight. Diet and exercise may have less effect in normal-weight women with PCOS in terms of normalization of menses, but a healthy lifestyle will still modulate their risk for associated metabolic diseases. Among women who are obese, up to 60% can have normalization of menses and decreases in serum testosterone if they achieve an 8% to 10% loss in body weight.

12. What is the most effective lifestyle modification for women with PCOS?

According to the literature on obesity, the most effective lifestyle intervention is one that the patient can maintain, and every effort should be made to develop a personalized approach to ensure optimal patient outcome. Overall dietary recommendations should focus on caloric restriction; to date, there are no specific recommendations regarding macronutrients for patients with PCOS per se, although diets low in concentrated sugar and fructose are beneficial for those with glucose intolerance, hypertriglyceridemia, and nonalcoholic fatty liver disease. The first approach to exercise should be an increase baseline activity, as women who are obese may have significant deconditioning. This should later be increased to aerobic-type exercises 3 to 5 days a week. There is no conclusive evidence supporting a role for any nutritional supplementation in PCOS. Weight loss medications should be considered as adjunctive therapy if needed.

13. What are the pregnancy complications found in women with PCOS?

Women with PCOS are at increased risk of pregnancy-induced hypertension and preeclampsia (around 3–4 times higher than normal). They are also at a three times higher risk for gestational diabetes. Those disorders are also exacerbated by obesity. Therefore, a thorough baseline assessment and management of obesity and weight gain are of paramount importance. Pregnant women with PCOS are also at increased risk of preterm delivery. It is still debated if PCOS confers an increased risk of early pregnancy miscarriage.

14. Does PCOS affect menopause?

The diagnosis of PCOS in perimenopause and menopause is challenging, and needs to be made on the basis of past history of irregular menses and hyperandrogenism symptoms. Usually, symptoms of PCOS tend to attenuate around menopause, with a natural decline of androgen production and ovarian follicle attrition. However, because the risk of metabolic complications will still be present, it is important to consider diagnosis, prevention, and treatment of these complications. It has been shown that women with PCOS may have a slightly later menopause.

15. What are the treatment options for patients with PCOS not desiring pregnancy?

The initial therapy goals should be personalized to address what the patient identifies as her primary complaints. For menstrual regulation, this would include combined oral contraceptives, estrogen patches, vaginal rings, or cyclic progesterone. Those not desiring regular menses and who do not have significant hirsutism can benefit from long-acting contraceptives, such as a progesterone intrauterine device or a slow-release progesterone implant. Women who are primarily concerned about metabolic diseases or weight gain may wish to initiate therapy with metformin and/or a weight-loss medication. Treatment for dermatologic manifestations is discussed below.

16. What are the options for treating dermatologic manifestations?

For dermatologic manifestations related to the increased androgens (acne, hirsutism, and androgenic alopecia), the best therapy is to restore a normal estrogen-to-testosterone ratio with estrogen therapy by using combined oral contraceptives, estrogen patches, or vaginal rings. Androgen receptor blockers, such a spironolactone, may be of benefit, and topical therapy with eflornithine can be helpful, although these therapies do not cause long-term changes in hair follicles. More definitive therapies, such as electrolysis and laser hair reduction, can be recommended. Minoxidil topical therapy is helpful in women experiencing androgenic alopecia.

Standard over-the-counter acne therapies with salicylic acid or benzoyl peroxide are the first-line treatment. Severe acne may necessitate consultation with a dermatologist for courses of antibiotics, topical retinoids, or oral isotretinoin in cases of severe cystic acne. Many of these therapies can be teratogenic and cannot be used in women desiring fertility.

For women with hidradenitis or folliculitis, wearing properly fitting clothes and undergarments made of absorptive material, such as cotton, is critical. Topical cleaning with chlorhexidine can be combined with application of topical antibiotics and/or oral antibiotics in cases of abscesses or more severe infections.

17. What are the risks and benefits of combined oral contraceptives in women with PCOS?

Combined oral contraceptives are highly effective for regulating menses and treating the dermatologic manifestations of PCOS. Women with PCOS are thought to have a slightly higher thrombotic risk, and thus, standard screening for thrombotic risk factors, such as a personal or family history of venous thromboembolic disease, strokes, and complex migraines with aura, are critical. The role of long-term estrogen therapy in altering cardiovascular disease risk in PCOS is not clear. Overall population studies have indicated that combined oral contraceptives do not cause weight gain, but each case is unique; some women will gain weight, whereas other women may lose weight. Oral contraceptives may worsen insulin resistance, and this should be considered in women with obesity and signs of insulin resistance or hyperglycemia. Mood disorders may sometimes be exacerbated by estrogen, and this should be monitored in women with preexisting psychiatric disease.

18. Is there a role for insulin sensitizers in the treatment of women with PCOS?

Reducing insulin resistance and serum insulin levels with metformin or other insulin sensitizers results in improvement in serum androgen levels, decreased blood pressure, improved lipids, improvement in menstrual regularity, and better glucose tolerance. However, it takes time for metformin therapy to reach its full impact on hyperandrogenism symptoms and can take up to 6 months to improve menstrual cyclicity. Metformin is recommended for the treatment of PCOS in women with impaired glucose tolerance or diabetes, which may represent > 20% to 40% of women with PCOS.

The thiazolidinedione class of insulin sensitizers has been shown to be essentially equivalent to metformin for improving metabolic and hyperandrogenism symptoms in PCOS, but weight gain, cardiovascular concerns, and risk of osteoporosis have limited their use.

Recent small trials have investigated glucagon-like peptide-1 (GLP-1) agonist therapy in PCOS; study results so far have suggested that these agents may have the potential to decrease serum testosterone levels and improve ovulation and menstrual cycle regularity after 3 to 6 months of treatment.

19. What are the treatment options for maintaining endometrial health?

Because chronic anovulation leads to an increased risk of endometrial hyperplasia and cancer, it is important to ensure cyclicity of endometrial proliferation and/or daily progestin exposure. There are several options available to cause cyclic shedding: combined oral contraceptives, estrogen patches or vaginal rings, or intermittent progesterone. Combination contraceptives have the advantage of reducing hyperandrogenism and thereby improving acne and hirsutism. Intermittent progesterone for 10 to 14 days per month or two will also provide endometrial protection but has side effects that may limit utilization in these patients. Furthermore, this does not provide contraception. Long-acting progestins, provided by progesterone intrauterine devices or slow-release progesterone implants, cause endometrial thinning and are also thought to be effective in the prevention of endometrial hyperplasia over the long term. Metformin may increase cyclicity and ovulation and will provide endometrial protection but may take 3 to 6 months to be effective.

20. What are the indications for endometrial biopsy in women with PCOS?

Women with PCOS are at threefold increased risk for the development of endometrial cancer. Risk factors other than anovulation include nulliparity, hypertension, BMI > 30 kg/m^2, and family history of endometrial cancer. As dysfunctional uterine bleeding is also a symptom of endometrial cancer, it is recommended that women with increased risk for endometrial cancer and compatible symptomatology should be considered for endometrial biopsy. This is particularly important for women age > 45 years, as the risk increases with age. Abnormal uterine bleeding not corrected after treatment should always be assessed for endometrial cancer.

21. What are the fertility treatment options for patients with PCOS desiring pregnancy?

Natural pregnancy is definitely possible in women with PCOS because most of these women still have ovulatory cycles. In women who are overweight or obese, lifestyle modifications and weight loss may be beneficial for the reestablishment of ovulatory cycles, increased fertility treatment efficiency, and better pregnancy outcomes. However, many women will need ovulation induction; treatment options include clomiphene citrate, letrozole, metformin, and gonadotropins.

Clomiphene citrate (selective estrogen receptor modulator) and letrozole (aromatase inhibitor) both act by decreasing the feedback from estrogens at the hypothalamic level and thereby promote FSH secretion and subsequent ovulation. Both agents have been proven to increase the rate of pregnancy and live births in comparison with placebo and are considered first-line therapies in women with PCOS and anovulatory infertility. However, it is unclear if one is superior to the other. They both increase the risk of multiple pregnancies (around 5%), and this risk is dose dependent.

Metformin has been suggested as an alternative therapy because it does not increase the risk of multiple pregnancies. The results from randomized controlled trials with metformin monotherapy have failed to show an increased pregnancy rate and demonstrated lower efficacy compared with clomiphene citrate. Metformin may be useful as an adjuvant therapy to other ovulation induction strategies, particularly in women who are obese, but the literature supporting this is still limited.

Gonadotropins are a second-line therapy and must be managed by fertility specialists because they confer a risk of ovarian hyperstimulation syndrome and multiple pregnancies.

KEY POINTS

- Clinical signs and symptoms of polycystic ovarian syndrome (PCOS) include infrequent or irregular menses, infertility, hirsutism, acne, alopecia, and weight gain.
- PCOS is a diagnosis of exclusion, and other causes of irregular menses and hirsutism/acne need to be ruled out.
- PCOS is associated with many other conditions including type 2 diabetes, nonalcoholic fatty liver disease, hypertension, obstructive sleep apnea, and depression.
- All women with PCOS should be encouraged to make healthy lifestyle choices, regardless of weight.
- Pharmacotherapy can include estrogen therapy and/or insulin sensitizers, as well as specific treatments for associated conditions, and should be personalized to achieve patient-specific treatment goals.

BIBLIOGRAPHY

Balen, A. H., Franks, S., Legro, R. S., Wijeyaratne, C. N., Stener-Victorin, E., Misso, M., . . . Teede, H. (2016). The management of anovulatory infertility in women with polycystic ovary syndrome: an analysis of the evidence to support the development of global WHO guidance. *Human Reproduction Update, 22*(6), 687–708.

Committee on Practice Bulletins—Gynecology. (2012). Practice bulletin no. 128: Diagnosis of abnormal uterine bleeding in reproductive-aged women. *Obstetrics and Gynecology, 120*(1), 197–206.

Goodman, N. F., Cobin, R. H., Futterweit, W., Glueck, J. S., Legro, R. S., & Carmina, E. (2015). American Association of Clinical Endocrinologists, American College of Endocrinology, and Androgen Excess and PCOS Society disease state clinical review: guide to the best practices in the evaluation and treatment of polycystic ovary syndrome—Part 1. *Endocrine Practice, 21*(11), 1291–1300.

Goodman, N. F., Cobin, R. H., Futterweit, W., Glueck, J. S., Legro, R. S., & Carmina, E. . . . (2015). American Association of Clinical Endocrinologists, American College of Endocrinology, and Androgen Excess and PCOS Society disease state clinical review: guide to the best practices in the evaluation and treatment of polycystic ovary syndrome—Part 2. *Endocrine Practice, 21*(12), 1415–1426.

Grover, A., & Yialamas, M. A. (2011). Metformin or thiazolidinedione therapy in PCOS? *Nature Reviews. Endocrinology, 7*(3), 128–129.

Legro, R. S., Arslanian, S. A., Ehrmann, D. A., Hoeger, K. M., Murad, M. H., Pasquali, R., & Welt, C. K.; (2013). Diagnosis and treatment of polycystic ovary syndrome: an Endocrine Society clinical practice guideline. *Journal of Clinical Endocrinology and Metabolism, 98*(12), 4565–4592.

Legro, R. S. (2016). Ovulation induction in polycystic ovary syndrome: current options. *Best Practice & Research. Clinical Obstetrics & Gynaecology, 37*, 152–159.

Martin, K. A., Anderson, R. R., Chang, R. J., Ehrmann, D. A., Lobo, R. A., Murad, M. H., ... Rosenfield, R. L. (2018). Evaluation and treatment of hirsutism in premenopausal women: an Endocrine Society clinical practice guideline. *Journal of Clinical Endocrinology and Metabolism, 103*(4), 1233–1257.

Niafar, M., Pourafkari, L., Porhomayon, J., & Nader, N. (2016). A systematic review of GLP-1 agonists on the metabolic syndrome in women with polycystic ovaries. *Archives of Gynecology and Obstetrics, 293*(3), 509–515.

Rosenfield, R. L., & Ehrmann, D. A. (2016). The pathogenesis of polycystic ovary syndrome (PCOS): the hypothesis of PCOS as functional ovarian hyperandrogenism revisited. *Endocrine Reviews, 37*(5), 467–520.

Teede, H. J., Misso, M. L., Costello, M. F., Dokras, A., Laven, J., Moran, L., . . . Norman, R. J. (2018). Recommendations from the international evidence-based guideline for the assessment and management of polycystic ovary syndrome. *Clinical Endocrinology, 89*(3), 251–268.

Witchel, S. F., Oberfield, S., Rosenfield, R. L., Codner, E., Bonny, A., Ibáñez, L., Pena, A., . . . Lee, P. A. (2015). The diagnosis of polycystic ovary syndrome during adolescence. *Hormone Research in Paediatrics 83*:376–389.

CHAPTER 55

HIRSUTISM AND VIRILIZATION

Tamis M. Bright and Aziz Ur Rehman

1. Define hirsutism.

   Hirsutism is the excessive growth of terminal hair in androgen-dependent areas: upper lip, chin, sideburns, earlobes, tip of the nose, back, chest, areolae, axillae, lower abdomen, pubic triangle, and anterior thighs. Hirsutism affects 5% to 10% of females and is frequently associated with irregular menses and acne. Hirsutism should be distinguished from hypertrichosis, which is a non–androgen-dependent increase in vellus hair. Hirsutism can be quantified by using the modified Ferriman-Gallwey scoring system, which assigns a score for the amount of terminal hair growth in each of the nine androgen-dependent areas.

2. Define virilization.

   Virilization refers to hirsutism, acne, and irregular menses, along with signs of masculinization—which are deepening of the voice, increased muscle mass, temporal balding, clitoromegaly, and increased libido. Virilization results from high circulating levels of androgens, close to or in the male range, and is usually caused by an androgen-secreting tumor.

3. Where are androgens produced?

   Twenty-five percent of testosterone in women comes from the ovaries, 25% from the adrenal glands, and 50% from peripheral conversion of androstenedione, which is produced by both the ovaries and adrenals. Testosterone is converted into dihydrotestosterone (DHT) by the enzyme 5-alpha-reductase, which is present in hair follicles, or to estradiol by the aromatase enzyme present in adipose tissue (Fig. 55.1). DHT binds to androgen receptors and is responsible for the transformation of vellus into terminal hair. Hair follicles also contain the enzymes that convert dehydroepiandrosterone (DHEA), which is produced by the adrenals, and androstenedione into testosterone.

4. What causes hirsutism?

   Hirsutism is caused by hyperandrogenism. Androgens transform the fine, downy, minimally pigmented vellus hair in androgen-sensitive areas into coarse, pigmented, terminal hair. An increase in any of the androgenic steroids may cause high levels of DHT in the hair follicle and result in hirsutism.

   Low levels of sex hormone–binding globulin (SHBG), which is produced by the liver, may promote hirsutism. Decreases in SHBG increase the free fraction of hormone available to androgen-sensitive hair. Hyperinsulinemia from insulin resistance, androgen excess, and hypothyroidism can decrease SHBG.

   Increased activity of 5-alpha-reductase in the hair follicle, even with normal circulating androgen levels, also may cause hirsutism by the excessive conversion of testosterone into DHT and is referred to as *idiopathic hirsutism*.

5. List the conditions that result in hirsutism.
   - Polycystic ovary syndrome (PCOS)
   - Idiopathic or familial hirsutism
   - Congenital adrenal hyperplasia (CAH)
   - Cushing's syndrome
   - Prolactinoma
   - Hypothyroidism
   - Acromegaly
   - Medications

6. Describe the pathophysiology of PCOS.

   The exact cause of PCOS is unknown, but affected individuals have been shown to have an accelerated rate of pulsatile gonadotropin-releasing hormone (GnRH) secretion from the hypothalamus. The gonadotropin secretory profile is highly dependent on the rate of GnRH pulsatility. Rapid GnRH pulses stimulate the secretion of luteinizing hormone (LH), but not follicle-stimulating hormone (FSH), from the pituitary gland. The increased LH/FSH secretory ratio results in arrested ovarian follicle development with cyst formation and hypertrophy of theca cells (hyperthecosis). This leads to constant estrogen and increased androgen production with chronic anovulation. Genome-wide association studies (GWAS) have now identified a number of genetic targets linked to PCOS.

7. How does PCOS manifest?

   PCOS affects 5% to 10% of premenopausal women and manifests with symptoms of hyperandrogenism and anovulation. PCOS is the most common cause of hirsutism, resulting in about 70% to 80% of cases. The hirsutism

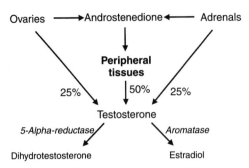

Fig. 55.1. Testosterone production and metabolism.

is gradually progressive, usually beginning at puberty, and most patients have irregular menses from the onset of menarche. However, in a study of patients with hirsutism and regular menses, 50% had polycystic ovaries. Patients with PCOS also frequently have insulin resistance and hyperinsulinemia. Because insulin decreases SHBG and increases the ovarian androgen response to LH stimulation, the hyperinsulinemia contributes to the elevated free androgen levels in PCOS. Thus, PCOS presents as a spectrum: Some patients have minimal findings, whereas others have the entire constellation of hirsutism, acne, obesity, infertility, amenorrhea or oligomenorrhea, male-pattern alopecia, acanthosis nigricans, hyperinsulinemia, and hyperlipidemia.

8. Describe the pathophysiology of idiopathic and familial hirsutism.
   Idiopathic hirsutism is believed to be caused by increased cutaneous activity of 5-alpha-reductase or enhanced skin sensitivity to androgens. Familial hirsutism is an ethnic tendency to have a higher density of hair follicles per unit area of skin. Mediterranean populations and Hispanics have increased hair density, whereas Asians have lower density. Patients with idiopathic or familial hirsutism usually have the onset of hirsutism shortly after puberty with a slow subsequent progression. They have a normal hormonal profile, including androgen levels, as well as normal menses and fertility.

9. Describe the pathophysiology of the hyperandrogenism in congenital adrenal hyperplasia (CAH).
   CAH results from a deficiency of one of the key enzymes in the cortisol biosynthesis pathway. Ninety percent of CAH is due to 21-hydroxylase deficiency, which causes a defect in the conversion of 17-hydroxyprogesterone (17-OHP) to 11-deoxycortisol and of progesterone to deoxycorticosterone (DOC). The resulting low cortisol production rate leads to hypersecretion of pituitary adrenocorticotropic hormone (ACTH), which stimulates overproduction of 17-OHP and progesterone, as well as adrenal androgens, particularly androstenedione (Fig. 55.2). In its classic form, CAH causes adrenal insufficiency at birth and ambiguous genitalia in females. Women with CAH may develop hirsutism if they are inadequately treated or noncompliant with steroids. The late-onset or nonclassic type of CAH

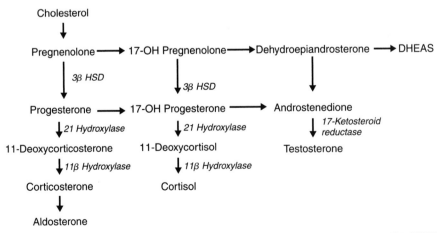

Fig. 55.2. Adrenal steroid biosynthesis. 3-beta-hydroxysteroid dehydrogenase (3β HSD) dehydroepiandrosterone-sulfate (DHEAS).

(NCCAH) results from milder deficiencies of the same enzyme, manifests later, and may cause childhood or post-pubertal hirsutism in women.

10. Do any other causes of NCCAH result in hirsutism?

Other enzyme deficiencies besides 21-hydroxylase deficiency are extremely rare causes of NCCAH. Deficiency of 11-beta-hydroxylase decreases the conversion of 11-deoxycortisol to cortisol and of DOC to corticosterone. This stimulates hypersecretion of ACTH, with consequent overproduction of 11-deoxycortisol, DOC, and androstene-dione. Patients also frequently develop hypertension from the mineralocorticoid DOC.

Deficiency of 3-beta-hydroxysteroid dehydrogenase (3-beta-HSD) decreases the conversion of pregnenolone to progesterone and 17-hydroxypregnenolone to 17-OHP. This defect increases pregnenolone, 17-hydroxypregnenolone, and the androgens DHEA, DHEA sulfate (DHEAS), and androstenediol, which promote the development of hirsutism (see Fig. 55.2).

11. How do Cushing's syndrome, prolactinomas, hypothyroidism, and acromegaly cause hirsutism?

All causes of Cushing's syndrome may result in hypertrichosis because of increased vellus hair on the face, forehead, limbs, and trunk secondary to cortisol hypersecretion. Cushing's syndrome resulting from an adrenal tumor also may produce hirsutism and virilization from increased secretion of androgens with the cortisol.

Hyperprolactinemia suppresses GnRH activity, which diminishes pulsatile LH secretion from the pituitary gland and results in decreased ovarian estrogen production and amenorrhea. Prolactin also increases the adrenal androgens, DHEA and DHEAS. The combination of low estrogen and increased androgens leads to hirsutism.

Hypothyroidism decreases SHBG and thereby leads to an increase in free testosterone. Acromegaly is frequently associated with PCOS, and the hirsutism may result from the PCOS in conjunction with excessive insulin-like growth factor-I (IGF-I), growth hormone, and insulin resistance.

12. Which medications can cause hirsutism?

Danazol, testosterone, glucocorticoids, metyrapone, phenothiazines, anabolic steroids, and valproic acid can cause hirsutism. Transference via skin contact of topical androgens used by a partner can cause hirsutism. Phenytoin, cyclosporine, diazoxide, minoxidil, glucocorticoids, streptomycin, penicillamine, and psoralens can cause hypertrichosis.

13. What conditions cause virilization?

Ovarian Tumors	*Adrenal Disorders*
Thecoma	Congenital adrenal hyperplasia
Fibrothecoma	Adenoma
Granulosa and granulosa-theca cell tumors	Carcinoma
Arrhenoblastoma (Sertoli-Leydig cell tumors)	
Hilus cell tumors	
Adrenal rest tumors of the ovary	Other: anabolic steroids
Luteoma of pregnancy	

KEY POINTS: HIRSUTISM

- Hirsutism is the excessive growth of terminal hair and is frequently associated with irregular menses.
- Virilization consists of hirsutism and irregular menses associated with signs of masculinization.
- Hirsutism and virilization usually result from excess androgens.
- The common causes of hirsutism are polycystic ovary syndrome, nonclassic congenital adrenal hyperplasia (NCCAH), idiopathic or familial hirsutism, and medications.
- The common causes of virilization are ovarian tumors, adrenal tumors, and congenital adrenal hyperplasia (CAH).

14. When should a patient be evaluated for hirsutism?

Any patient with moderate-to-severe hirsutism or an increased Ferriman-Gallwey score, rapid development of hirsutism, or coexistence of amenorrhea, irregular menses, infertility, acanthosis, or virilization should be evaluated. A patient with regular menses who shows significant distress over her hirsutism also may warrant a workup.

15. What information is important in the history?

- Age at onset, progression, and extent of hair growth
- Current measures of hair removal and frequency of use

- Age at menarche, regularity of menses, and fertility
- Family history of hirsutism
- Change in libido or change in voice
- Symptoms of Cushing's syndrome, prolactinoma, acromegaly, or hypothyroidism
- Medications, anabolic steroid use, partner's use of topical androgens

16. What findings are important on physical examination?
   - Distribution and degree of hirsutism
   - Increased muscle mass, temporal balding, clitoromegaly, or acne
   - Obesity
   - Acanthosis nigricans
   - Visual field defects
   - Moon facies, plethora, buffalo hump, supraclavicular fat pads, striae, or thin skin
   - Galactorrhea
   - Goiter, loss of lateral eyebrows, periorbital edema, dry skin, or delayed reflexes
   - Acromegalic features
   - Abdominal or pelvic masses

17. What laboratory tests should be ordered for a patient with hirsutism?
   Laboratory testing should be guided by the results of the history and physical examination. Most authors advocate against testing in patients with regular menses and only gradual progression of mild hirsutism. Serum levels of total and free testosterone, SHBG, DHEAS, and 17-OHP can be useful tests, depending on the individual patient. Some authors screen with all the tests at once, but recent guidelines recommend initial screening with total testosterone followed by a free testosterone level, if the total testosterone is normal. DHEAS and 17-OHP are measured only in those patients with high total or free testosterone to determine the etiology of the hyperandrogenism. If a patient is from a high-risk ethnic group for NCCAH, then a 17-OHP can be obtained even with normal androgen levels. Patients with signs or symptoms of hypothyroidism, hyperprolactinemia, acromegaly, or Cushing's syndrome also should be evaluated with serum thyroid-stimulating hormone (TSH), prolactin, insulin-like growth factor-I (IGF-I), or Cushing's screening (24-hour urine cortisol, late-night salivary cortisol, or a 1-mg overnight dexamethasone test), respectively. Otherwise, these tests need not be obtained in every patient.

18. How are the results of these laboratory tests interpreted?
   For a patient without signs of virilization, it is important to differentiate idiopathic hirsutism, PCOS, and NCCAH, because each is treated differently. Idiopathic hirsutism has normal levels of both total and free testosterone. PCOS has high-normal or increased total and/or free testosterone, normal or slightly increased DHEAS, and normal 17-OHP. NCCAH has elevated testosterone and DHEAS, and mild-to-marked elevation of 17-OHP. An early-morning follicular phase level (random morning if amenorrheic) of 17-OHP > 1000 ng/dL confirms NCCAH. A level of 200 to 1000 ng/dL is strongly suggestive of NCCAH and should be confirmed with an ACTH stimulation test. NCCAH is confirmed if the 60-minute 17-OHP value after 250 mcg of ACTH is > 1000 ng/dL. (See Chapter 37 on Congenital Adrenal Hyperplasia for additional discussion on this issue.)

19. What laboratory tests should be ordered in a patient with virilization?
   After excluding anabolic steroid abuse as an etiology, a patient with virilization should be evaluated to determine whether she has an ovarian tumor, an adrenal tumor, or NCCAH. Tests should include serum total testosterone, DHEAS, and 17-OHP. A markedly increased testosterone level, usually in the adult male range, with normal values on the other tests points to an ovarian tumor. High levels of DHEAS (> 700 ng/mL) with or without high testosterone levels suggest an adrenal tumor. Increased levels of 17-OHP with modest elevations of DHEAS and testosterone are more consistent with NCCAH and can be confirmed, as above, with an ACTH stimulation test. Laboratory values suggesting tumors should be followed with a transvaginal ultrasonography of the ovaries or computed tomography (CT) of the adrenals or ovaries. If no mass is found, 18F fluorodeoxyglucose (18F-FDG) positron emission tomography (PET) or venous sampling of the ovarian or adrenal veins can be performed for localization before surgical removal.

20. How is hirsutism treated?
   For patients not desiring pregnancy, the most common treatment is oral contraceptive pills (OCPs). Antiandrogens can also be prescribed in addition to OCPs or alone, if another form of reliable contraception is utilized. Multiple different cosmetic measures are effective and are often used in conjunction with OCPs and antiandrogens. For patients who desire fertility, only cosmetic measures are safe.

   For patients with PCOS, weight reduction should be encouraged; this usually improves SHBG levels, may help regulate menses, and may resolve anovulation. GnRH agonists have been tried in severe cases when other modalities have not been effective. Patients with PCOS should also be evaluated for glucose intolerance, diabetes, and hyperlipidemia because of their high prevalence in this disorder. These problems should be addressed separately because they are not resolved by treating the hyperandrogenism alone.

If patients with NCCAH do not have improvement of their hirsutism with the above measures, prednisone 4 to 6 mg or dexamethasone 0.25 to 0.5 mg at night will frequently decrease androgen levels to normal. The medication can then be tapered to the lowest effective dose, and the patient should be monitored for any adverse effects of the glucocorticoid therapy.

21. Describe how OCPs are used for the treatment of hirsutism.
OCPs are the most commonly used therapy for hirsutism. The progestin decreases LH and thereby decreases androgen production, and the estrogens increase SHBG, which decreases free testosterone levels. OCPs also decrease the risk of endometrial hyperplasia in women with amenorrhea or oligomenorrhea. Monophasic and triphasic preparations work equally well. Studies with preparations containing the more androgenic progestin levonorgestrel had similar effects on hirsutism as the less androgenic progestins. Low-dose estrogen (20 mcg) OCPs also were shown to have the same effect as higher dose estrogen.

Potential side effects include weight gain, bloating, nausea, emotional lability, breast pain, and venous thromboembolism (VTE). Low-dose estrogen OCPs have less risk of VTE. OCPs containing levonorgestrel, norgestimate, or norethindrone have a lower risk of VTE compared with those containing other progestins.

22. Describe how antiandrogens are used for the treatment of hirsutism.
Spironolactone is an androgen receptor blocker that also inhibits 5-alpha-reductase. Side effects include diuresis, fatigue, hyperkalemia, and dysfunctional uterine bleeding. Doses are 50 to 100 mg twice daily. Finasteride, a 5-alpha-reductase inhibitor, effectively decreases hirsutism at dosages of 2.5 to 7.5 mg/day. Side effects are minimal. Flutamide, another androgen receptor blocker, has similar effectiveness as the other antiandrogens but has been associated with rare fatal hepatotoxicity and, therefore, is not recommended. The antiandrogens are usually used in combination with OCPs for additive effects and to give adequate birth control because antiandrogens can feminize a male fetus. If the patient is not on OCPs, then another form of reliable birth control needs to be utilized.

23. Describe how GnRH agonists are used for the treatment of hirsutism.
By providing constant rather than pulsatile GnRH levels to the pituitary, GnRH agonists reduce gonadotropin secretion and thereby decrease ovarian production of both estrogen and androgen. Estrogen replacement must be given to avoid hot flashes, vaginal dryness, and bone density loss. Leuprolide (3.75 mg per month intramuscularly), nafarelin nasal spray, and goserelin subcutaneous implants have been utilized. Some studies demonstrated an increased effect over OCPs alone, whereas others showed similar effects. The preparations are expensive and, thus, are usually reserved for patients with severe PCOS unresponsive to other therapies.

KEY POINTS: DIAGNOSIS AND TREATMENT OF HIRSUTISM AND VIRILIZATION

- Appropriate laboratory testing includes at least a serum total testosterone, followed by a free testosterone, dehydroepiandrosterone sulfate, and 17-hydroxyprogesterone in select patients.
- Treatment of hirsutism is usually with a combination of oral contraceptive pills, an antiandrogen, eflornithine, and cosmetic measures.
- Treatment of virilization is surgical removal of the tumor or steroid treatment for congenital adrenal hyperplasia.

24. What topical agent is approved for the treatment of hirsutism?
Eflornithine hydrochloride 13.9% cream applied twice daily is used for the treatment of facial hirsutism. Eflornithine irreversibly inhibits ornithine decarboxylase, an enzyme necessary for hair follicle cell division. Inhibition of ornithine decarboxylase results in a decreased rate of hair growth; improvement in hirsutism can be seen by 6 to 8 weeks of use. The most common side effects are pseudofolliculitis barbae, burning, tingling, erythema, dry skin, or rash over the applied area. Generally, side effects resolve without treatment and rarely require discontinuation of the medication. The hirsutism will return to baseline by 8 weeks after discontinuation of the medication.

25. What cosmetic measures can be used for the treatment of hirsutism?
Shaving, plucking, waxing, and chemical depilating are effective measures that can be used to temporarily remove terminal hair. Bleaching can also make hair less apparent. These measures can be used alone or in combination while the patient waits for medications to decrease new growth and rate of transformation into terminal hair. Electrolysis, either through thermolysis or direct current, is a permanent method of hair removal but can be painful.

Photoepilation using ruby, alexandrite, diode, or yttrium aluminum garnet lasers, or intense pulsed light therapy, is an effective treatment for hirsutism. At least three to six treatments about 4 to 6 weeks apart are required. The techniques result in removal of hair through thermal injury to the hair follicle with a period of usually 6 months before regrowth of hair, which is then thinner and lighter. Patients with light skin and dark hair have the best results with the fewest side effects. The side effects include minimal discomfort, local edema and erythema lasting 24 to 48 hours, burns, and infrequent hypo- or hyperpigmentation. A very rare side effect of laser treatment is paradoxical hirsutism, which is increased hair growth instead of removal.

26. How do you choose the appropriate therapy for the patient's hirsutism?

Most patients are given a trial of OCPs for 6 months and are advised to use cosmetic measures while waiting for the medication to work. If needed, an antiandrogen can then be added. Topical eflornithine may be used alone or in combination with the other measures. Because of their more serious side effects and/or higher cost, the other medications are reserved for the most severe cases where OCPs and antiandrogens fail. No matter what therapy is chosen, the patient must be made aware that results will not be seen for at least 3 to 6 months. Although many medications have been used, only topical eflornithine is currently approved by the U.S. Food and Drug Administration (FDA) for the treatment of hirsutism. Unfortunately, most patients have a relapse of hirsutism approximately 12 months after discontinuation of medical therapy.

⊕ WEBSITES

1. Hirsutism: https://www.endocrine.org/guidelines-and-clinical-practice/clinical-practice-guidelines/hirsutism: Endocrine Society

BIBLIOGRAPHY

Barrionuevo, P., Nabhan, M., Altayar, O., Wang, Z., Erwin, P. J., Asi, N., . . . Murad, M. H. (2018). Treatment options for hirsutism: a systematic review and network meta-analysis. *The Journal of Clinical Endocrinology and Metabolism, 103*(4), 1258–1264.

Ferriman, D., & Gallwey, J. D. (1961). Clinical assessment of body hair growth in women. *The Journal of Clinical Endocrinology and Metabolism, 21*(11), 1440–1447.

Goodman, N. F., Cobin, R. H., Futterweit, W., Glueck, J. S., Legro, R. S., & Carmina, E. (2015). American Association of Clinical Endocrinologists, American College of Endocrinology, and Androgen Excess and PCOS Society disease state clinical review: Guide to the best practices in the evaluation and treatment of polycystic ovary syndrome—Part 1. *Endocrine Practice, 21*(11), 1291–1300.

Lapidoth, M., Dierickx, C., Lanigan, S., Paasch, U., Campo-Voegeli, A., Dahan, S., . . . Adatto, M. (2010). Best practice options for hair removal in patients with unwanted facial hair using combination therapy with laser: guidelines drawn up by an expert working group. *Dermatology, 221*, 34–42.

Legro, R. S., Arslanian, S. A., Ehrmann, D. A., Hoeger, K. M., Murad, M. H., Pasquali, R., & Welt, C. K.; Endocrine Society. (2013). Diagnosis and treatment of polycystic ovary syndrome: an Endocrine Society clinical practice guideline. *The Journal of Clinical Endocrinology and Metabolism, 98*(12), 4565–4592.

Martin, K. A., Anderson, R. R., Chang, R. J., Ehrmann, D. A., Lobo, R. A., Murad, M. H., . . . Rosenfield, R. L.(2018). Evaluation and treatment of hirsutism in premenopausal women: an Endocrine Society clinical practice guideline. *The Journal of Clinical Endocrinology and Metabolism, 103*(4), 1233–1257.

Practice Committee of the American Society for Reproductive Medicine. (2006). The evaluation and treatment of androgen excess. *Fertility and Sterility, 86*, S241–S247.

Rosenfield, R., & Ehrmann, D. (2016). The pathogenesis of polycystic ovary syndrome (PCOS): the hypothesis of PCOS as functional ovarian hyperandrogenism revisited. *Endocrine Reviews, 37*(5), 467–520.

Rothman, M. S., & Wierman, M. E. (2011). How should postmenopausal androgen excess be evaluated? *Clinical Endocrinology, 75*, 160–164.

Vinogradova, Y., Coupland, C., & Hippisley-Cox, J. (2015). Use of combined oral contraceptives and risk of venous thromboembolism: Nested case-control studies using the QResearch and CPRD databases. *British Medical Journal, 350*, h2135.

Wolf, J. E., Jr., Shander, D., Huber, F., Jackson, J., Lin, C. S., Mathes, B. M., & Schrode, K.; Eflornithine HCl Study Group. (2007). Randomized, double-blind clinical evaluation of the efficacy and safety of topical eflornithine HCl 13.9% cream in the treatment of women with facial hair. *International Journal of Dermatology, 46*, 94–98.

Zimmerman, Y., Eijkemans, M. J., Coelingh Bennink, H. J., Blankenstein, M. A., & Fauser, B. C. (2014). The effect of combined oral contraception on testosterone levels in healthy women: a systematic review and meta-analysis. *Human Reproduction Update, 20*(1), 76–105.

CHAPTER 56

MENOPAUSE

Wesley Nuffer

1. Define menopause.

   The formal definition of *menopause* is clinically defined as the permanent cessation of menses 12 months after a woman's last menstrual period. It marks the end of a woman's normal ovarian function.

2. When does menopause usually occur?

   The median age for the last menses is 51.4 years. There is large variability in the exact age for menopause to occur. There appears to be a genetic component involved, as women often will experience menopause around the same time as their mother or sister, but there are numerous examples of circumstances when this does not hold true. It also appears that women in Asia may experience menopause at an earlier age.

3. How is menopause diagnosed clinically?

   In a woman age > 45 years, 12 months of secondary amenorrhea is sufficient for the diagnosis of menopause. Although a pelvic examination may reflect some atrophy of the vaginal mucosa, this is not always remarkable. There are usually elevations in both follicle-stimulating hormone (FSH), which rises significantly (approximately 10- to 20-fold), and luteinizing hormone (LH), which has a more modest rise (approximately threefold). It is generally considered that an FSH level above 40 IU/L indicates ovarian failure, but these levels are not reliable for diagnosis because, in some circumstances, these hormones may be elevated prior to menopause.

4. What is perimenopause?

   Menopause should not be thought of as occurring suddenly but, rather, as a transitional process over time. Perimenopause (also called *menopause transition*) describes the transition toward menopause, when cycles can vary in frequency and severity. Menopause symptoms often begin to appear during this time.

5. What determines the timing of physiologic menopause?

   The absence of ovarian oocytes signals the cessation of menstruation in women. Oocyte numbers decline throughout a woman's life, actually peaking in number in utero and declining quite rapidly before birth, when approximately 80% of oocytes have been lost. Eventual exhaustion of most or all oocytes causes menses to cease.

6. What is premature ovarian insufficiency?

   Ovarian insufficiency is considered premature when it occurs in women age < 40 years. Symptoms are very similar to those experienced by women entering menopause at the usual time. There can be several causes of this condition, including autoimmune disorders, chromosomal defects, chemotherapy treatment, and some unknown causes. The incidence of premature ovarian insufficiency is estimated to be 0.3% within the United States.

7. What are the symptoms of menopause?

   The hallmark symptom of menopause, which often occurs during the perimenopause transition, is recurrent hot flashes. These are episodes that last seconds to minutes during which a woman experiences a tremendous warming of her body, often with accompanying redness of the skin and sweat production. Women going through menopause often describe this variable temperature control as occurring at night, thus the term "night sweats." Other symptoms that are less prevalent can include insomnia, short-term memory loss or "mental fogginess," vaginal dryness, and loss of "youthfulness" of the skin, hair, and nails.

8. Will all women experience menopause symptoms?

   It is estimated that the majority of women (approximately 85%) will experience some type of vasomotor symptoms with menopause. This can vary greatly in severity, with the most severe symptoms usually occurring in women who have had their ovaries surgically removed, thereby transitioning to what has been called "instant menopause."

9. Do menopausal symptoms last indefinitely?

   Generally, menopausal symptoms are most prominent during perimenopause or the first few years after menopause. Most women are able to tolerate these symptoms better after approximately 3 to 5 years. Some women, however, continue to suffer from hot flashes and other menopause symptoms even 10 years or longer after menopause occurs, at almost the same severity as when they first appeared.

10. **What other physiologic changes accompany menopause?**
Loss of bone mineral and protein matrix, increased rates of coronary artery disease, skin and vaginal atrophy, hot flashes, and alterations in the lipid profile (increased triglycerides and low-density lipoprotein cholesterol, and decreased high-density lipoprotein cholesterol) all occur through and after menopause.

11. **What estrogen(s) are present in a woman's body?**
Women naturally have three distinct estrogens present in varying amounts—estrone (E1), estradiol (E2), and estriol (E3). E2 is the most potent of these; it binds equally to both the alpha- and beta-estrogen receptors, and converts freely back and forth with E1 in the body. There is some evidence to suggest that E1 has a higher carcinogenic risk compared with the other estrogens, possibly because of its higher affinity for the alpha-estrogen receptor (alpha/beta ratio approximately 5:1). E3 is a metabolite of E2 and E1 and will not convert back to E1 or E2 once formed but, rather, is excreted through urine. It has a higher selective binding to the beta-estrogen receptor (beta/alpha ratio 3:1).

12. **What is the predominant circulating estrogen during and after menopause?**
E2 is the most abundant estrogen in women during the reproductive years, being produced by the ovaries. During menopause, E2 production wanes and then stops, and E1 becomes the dominant estrogen. E1 is formed by the aromatase enzyme in adipose tissue from androstenedione, which is secreted from the adrenal glands.

13. **There was a major shift in managing women at menopause after the Women's Health Initiative (WHI) trial. Why did this occur?**
The WHI trial, a landmark study from the National Institutes of Health (NIH), enrolled over 27,000 women 50 to 79 years of age. Those women with no previous hysterectomy received combined conjugated equine estrogen (CEE) plus medroxyprogesterone acetate (MPA) or placebo (16,608 women), and those women with a previous hysterectomy received either CEE or placebo (10,739 women). The primary outcome for this trial was coronary heart disease events. Much media attention was directed toward this trial when the combined arm of CEE and MPA was stopped early in July 2002, after investigators found that the associated health risks outweighed the potential benefits of therapy. Data showed an increased risk of invasive breast cancer, along with increased incidences of coronary heart disease, pulmonary embolism, and stroke. Positive outcomes included a reduction in colon cancer and lower incidence of hip fractures. The estrogen-alone arm also showed increased risk of stroke and blood clots without preventing heart disease (Fig. 56.1).

14. **What are some of the limitations of the WHI trial data?**
One of the largest recognized limitations to these data is the age of women at enrollment; it is widely believed that a woman's greatest benefit derived from hormone replacement occurs in the years just after menopause, or in the age range of 50 to 60 years. Enrolling women 50 to 79 years of age included a large number of women age > 60 years, and this may have impacted the results of the trial. The other major limitation was that only one hormone regimen (CEE 0.625 mg/day and MPA 2.5 mg/day) was used in women who had an intact uterus, and only CEE 0.625 mg/day was given to women who had previously had hysterectomies; therefore, the rationale behind extrapolating these results to conclude that all hormone products (oral and transdermal estradiol and progesterone preparations) carry the same risk is questionable.

15. **What do national organizations say regarding hormone replacement in menopausal women?**
Overall, there is a strong consensus across major organizations regarding the role of hormone replacement therapy (HRT) in menopause. Both the American College of Obstetrics and Gynecology (ACOG) and the North American

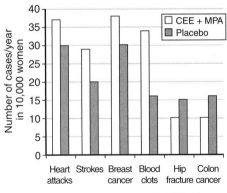

WHI Trial Disease Rates For Women

Fig. 56.1. The Women's Health Initiative (WHI) trial.

Menopause Society (NAMS) recommend estrogen and possible progestogen therapy only for symptomatic relief. They further recommend that women should be on the lowest dose possible for the shortest amount of time. Similarly, the American Association of Clinical Endocrinologists (AACE) clinical guidelines recommend against long-term HRT and that it not be used for cardiovascular disease prevention. Estrogen is indicated for osteoporosis prevention, but the risks of long-term use are considered to outweigh the benefits; therefore, this indication is generally reserved for women age < 60 years, and each individual should be carefully evaluated on the basis of her risk and possible use of other osteoporosis medications. Although HRT should not be used for cardiovascular protection, current evidence suggests that the use of HRT in women during early menopause does not increase heart disease risk. Because the greatest benefits of HRT are seen in women age < 60 years, it is generally recommended that any HRT use should occur between ages 50 and 60 years, and that attempts be made to taper the therapy to discontinuation every 3 to 5 years. The ultimate decision on whether a woman should be treated with HRT for severe symptoms should be an individualized one, made on the basis of shared decision making between the patient and the provider. Perceived risks based on the WHI trial data and the accompanying literature should be presented and weighed against the severity of symptoms and the woman's health-related quality of life.

16. Does the route of administration matter when it comes to HRT?

Administering hormones transdermally (through the skin) produces different effects from taking the same hormones orally because it avoids the "first pass effect," whereby the liver is exposed to much higher concentrations of hormones compared with the rest of the body and metabolizes them to some partially active or inactive metabolites. The AACE guidelines recognize that transdermal estrogen may theoretically have lower risks of thromboembolic disease. Likewise, oral progesterone is metabolized extensively, and some of its byproducts can be extremely sedating; therefore, administering progesterone by the transdermal route can allow for lower doses with less sedation side effects. Topical administration is also beneficial for alleviating some symptoms, such as vaginal dryness, where local symptom relief is achieved with less systemic absorption. Generally, topical formulations of hormones contain lower doses compared with their oral counterparts.

17. What is a bioidentical hormone?

The term *bioidentical* was coined to describe hormones that are identical to what the body naturally produces. Although bioidentical hormones are often promoted by compounding pharmacies, many of the prescription hormone products approved by the U.S. Food and Drug Administration (FDA), such as estradiol and progesterone, are also bioidentical. This term has been used to contrast these from other hormone products, most notably CEE, which originates from pregnant mare urine, and MPA, a synthetic progestogen compound.

18. Are bioidentical hormones safer for supplementation?

There has been a tremendous amount of publicity for and promotion of bioidentical hormones after the WHI trial because of women seeking other options for controlling severe menopausal symptoms. Currently, the majority of the evidence suggests that all estrogen products are similar in nature and effects, regardless of the source. Proponents of bioidentical hormones argue that the physiologic similarity of these molecules yields benefits that are not seen with other estrogen and progestogen hormones. Some compounded hormones include E3, which is not FDA approved for use in the United States, although it is used in Europe and other countries. There are limited data to support the efficacy of E3; the FDA took a strong stance in 2008 in response to a petition from Wyeth Ayerst to prohibit the use of E3, citing lack of evidence of its safety and efficacy. With regard to progesterone, there are some data to support different physiologic activities in comparison with MPA, and evidence from obser-vational trials and controlled primate trials suggest a better safety profile in comparison with that of MPA, but large, randomized, placebo-controlled trials to confirm this potential benefit have yet to be conducted.

KEY POINTS: MENOPAUSE

- Menopause is the cessation of menses, comprising approximately the last third of a woman's life.
- Menopausal symptoms are most severe early during perimenopause and menopause, with the hallmark symptom being hot flashes.
- Hormone replacement therapy should be reserved primarily for symptomatic relief, targeting women 50 to 60 years of age, using the lowest doses for the shortest interval of time.
- The term *bioidentical* refers to any hormone identical to what is found in the body and includes both prescription hormones (i.e., estradiol, progesterone) as well as compounded products.
- Hormone therapy should be based on symptom control, not based on blood or saliva hormone levels.

19. If a woman is on HRT, should dosing be based on serum or saliva hormone levels?

According to the AACE guidelines, HRT should be based on a woman's symptoms and not on specific hormone levels. Among proponents of hormone level monitoring, there is debate as to whether serum or saliva is a better source for measuring hormone levels. Saliva test supporters cite that sex hormones are generally lipophilic and protein bound and that active hormones are, therefore, not reliably measured in blood, whereas saliva levels more closely represent circulating free and intracellular hormone levels. Saliva levels, however, are documented to vary substantially, depending on the time of day when they are collected, and have not been established as a reliable indicator of therapeutic response. Their assays are not FDA approved and generally are not considered to correlate with serum hormone levels. It is also often difficult for women to obtain coverage of payment for saliva levels through their medical benefits, and the cost can be significant. Finally, because there are no clearly established therapeutic ranges for serum or salivary estrogens or progestogens in postmenopausal women, current recommendations are to base therapy on the lowest possible doses that will adequately control menopausal symptoms.

20. **What is the role of progestagen supplementation?**
Progestogens, most notably MPA, are used in conjunction with estrogen treatment to protect women from developing endometrial cancer. They are given to women who have not had a hysterectomy. There is a suggestion, based on small studies, that progesterone supplementation may yield additional benefits, even in women who have had a hysterectomy, but it is not routinely recommended for use beyond endometrial protection.

21. **Do women need androgen supplementation?**
This is a controversial topic. The Endocrine Society's consensus statement recommends against diagnosing androgen deficiency in women, citing lack of data documenting what the "normal" androgen levels in women across their life span are. There is evidence that in some women, supplementing low doses of testosterone (often starting with 1% testosterone creams) may help treat symptoms of fatigue, low energy, and decreased libido. When supplemented, dosing is often limited by unwanted side effects (oily skin and acne, hirsutism, voice lowering).

22. **Are there other therapies available for managing menopausal symptoms?**
Based on the nature and severity of a woman's symptoms, various other approaches are available for management without HRT. Antidepressant drugs, such as fluoxetine, paroxetine, and venlafaxine, have documented evidence for benefit in managing hot flash symptoms; clonidine has also been used successfully for this, particularly at night, although side effects (hypotension and dry mouth) limit its use. A new class of medications, called neurokinin B (NKB) antagonists, are currently being evaluated for the treatment of hot flashes and other menopausal symptoms. These drugs block NKB, a chemical that has been linked to causing hot flashes. There are herbal products, such as soy derivatives and black cohosh, for which some success has been documented by virtue of relatively weak phytoestrogen activity. These typically do not have the potency to control severe menopausal symptoms but may adequately manage mild-to-moderate symptoms. Behavioral and complementary interventions, including acupuncture, meditation, and yoga, have been evaluated and shown to have some benefits in the control of mild-to-moderate symptoms.

23. **Are compounded hormones superior to other hormone treatment?**
Currently, there is no evidence that compounded hormones outperform other forms of HRT. Concerns have been raised by some national organizations, such as the ACOG, regarding compounded hormone therapy. They cite lack of evidence, concerns about the variable purity and potency of the products, and the lack of safety and efficacy data. The quality of compounded medications depends on a reliable source, so women who seek compounded hormones should identify a pharmacy that performs its own quality assurance on products, follows proper protocols, and has reliable equipment to provide consistent, accurate products. Some data suggest that compounded progesterone creams may not yield sufficiently high systemic levels to provide adequate endometrial protection.

24. **Does male menopause exist?**
Androgen levels decline with age in men, and there are indications for supplementation in some circumstances. This is not considered "male menopause," primarily because it does not appear to be a physiologically programmed event.

25. **What are some good menopause/HRT references?**
The chapter *The post-menopausal woman* by McAvey and Santoro on Endotext.com is a good general reference on the topic. Reviews of the literature on bioidentical hormones are provided in Cirigliano, M. (2007). Bioidentical hormone therapy: A review of the evidence. *Journal of Women's Health (Larchmt), 16*(5), 600–631; and Holtorf, K. (2009). The bioidentical hormone debate: are bioidentical hormones (estradiol, estriol, and progesterone) safer or more efficacious than commonly used synthetic versions in hormone replacement therapy? *Postgraduate Medicine, 121*(1), 73–85.

KEY POINTS

- It appears that women in Asia may experience menopause 5 to 10 years earlier compared with American and European women.
- Prescription products with estradiol and progesterone are considered to be "bioidentical."
- Although the WHI trial had an excellent study design, its results may not accurately translate to all menopausal women because of the wide age range of enrollment up through age 79 years.

🌐 WEBSITES

1. American College of Obstetrics and Gynecology: www.acog.org
2. Menopause: www.menopause.org
3. American Association of Clinical Endocrinologists: https://www.aace.com/files/menopause.pdf

BIBLIOGRAPHY

Anderson, G. L., Limacher, M., Assaf, A. R., Bassford, T., Beresford, S. A., Black, H., . . . Wassertheil-Smoller, S.; (2004). Effects of conjugated equine estrogen in postmenopausal women with hysterectomy: The Women's Health Initiative randomized controlled trial. *Journal of the American Medical Association, 291*(14), 1701–1712.

Bachmann, G., & Rojas, V. (2016). Menopausal hormonal therapy: more good news for women. *Journal of Women's Health, 25*(5), 419.

Cirigliano, M. (2007). Bioidentical hormone therapy: a review of the evidence. *Journal of Women's Health (2002), 16*(5), 600–631.

Goodwin, T. M. (2010). *Management of common problems in obstetrics and gynecology* (5th ed.). Chichester, West Sussex; Hoboken, NJ: Wiley-Blackwell.

Grady, D. (2006). Clinical practice. Management of menopausal symptoms. *New England Journal of Medicine, 355*(22), 2338–2347.

Holtorf, K. (2009). The bioidentical hormone debate: are bioidentical hormones (estradiol, estriol, and progesterone) safer or more efficacious than commonly used synthetic versions in hormone replacement therapy? *Postgraduate Medicine, 121*(1), 73–85.

Kohrt, W. M., & Wierman, M. E. (2017). Preventing fat gain by blocking follicle-stimulating hormone. *New England Journal of Medicine, 377*, 293–295.

Mahmud, K. (2010). Natural hormone therapy for menopause. *Gynecological Endocrinology, 26*(2), 81–85.

Nelson, H. D. (2004). Commonly used types of postmenopausal estrogen for treatment of hot flashes: scientific review. *Journal of the American Medical Association, 291*(13), 1610–1620.

The NAMS 2017 Hormone Therapy Position Statement Advisory Panel. (2017). The 2017 hormone therapy position statement of the North American Menopause Society. *Menopause (New York, N.Y.), 24*(7), 728–753.

Rossouw, J. E., Anderson, G. L., Prentice, R. L., LaCroix, A. Z., Kooperberg, C., Stefanick, M. L., ,. . ., . . . Ockene, J.; (2002). Risks and benefits of estrogen plus progestin in healthy postmenopausal women: principal results from the Women's Health Initiative randomized controlled trial. *Journal of the American Medical Association, 288*(3), 321–333.

Santoro, N., Braunstein, G. D., Butts, C. L., Martin, K. A., McDermott, M., & Pinkerton, J. V. (2016). Compounded bioidentical hormones in endocrinology practice: an Endocrine Society Scientific statement. *Journal of Clinical Endocrinology and Metabolism, 101*, 1318–1343.

Shepherd-Banigan, M., Goldstein, K. M., Coeytaux, R. R., McDuffie, J. R., Goode, A. P., Kosinski, A. S., ,. . . . . . & Williams, J. W., Jr. (2017). Improving vasomotor symptoms; psychological symptoms; and health-related quality of life in peri- or post-menopausal women through yoga: an umbrella systematic review and meta-analysis. *Complementary Therapies in Medicine, 34*, 156–164.

Stuenkel, C. A., Davis, S. R., Gompel, A., Lumsden, M. A., Murad, M. H., Pinkerton, J. V., & Santen, R. J. (2015). Treatment of symptoms of the menopause: an Endocrine Society clinical practice guideline. *Journal of Clinical Endocrinology and Metabolism, 100*, 3975–4011.

Weinstein, M., & O'Connor, K. (2010). *Reproductive aging.* Boston, MA: Blackwell Publishing on behalf of the New York Academy of Sciences.

CHAPTER 57

GENDER-AFFIRMING TREATMENT FOR ADULTS WITH GENDER INCONGRUENCE AND GENDER DYSPHORIA

Micol S. Rothman and Sean J. Iwamoto

1. **What is gender identity?**

   Gender identity refers to a person's innate, self-identified gender (e.g., as man, woman, or other) that may or may not align with that person's external genitalia or sex assigned at birth. Gender identity is not visible to other people.

2. **What is the difference between gender incongruence and gender dysphoria?**

   Gender incongruence is defined as a person's gender identity and/or gender expression differing from that person's sex assigned at birth or what is typically associated with the designated gender. Not everyone with gender incongruence has gender dysphoria or seeks treatment.

   Gender dysphoria refers to the distress and unease associated with gender incongruence. The phrase "gender identity disorder" is no longer used, particularly after the 2013 American Psychiatric Association's *Diagnostic and Statistical Manual,* 5th edition (DSM-5) replaced it with "gender dysphoria." See Table 57.1 for other terminology.

   Society and the medical literature are continually evolving when it comes to *transgender* (trans) and gender incongruent/dysphoric terminology. Although the above-mentioned list is not exhaustive, it represents some of the current terms used in practice. There has been a shift away from using "male-to-female" (MTF) to represent trans women and "female-to-male" (FTM) to represent trans men, although one may still see or hear these terms.

   It is important to be aware that biological sex or sex assigned at birth, gender identity, and gender expression are not identical. Knowing someone's gender identity, which may or may not fall into the traditional gender binary of male or female, does not tell you the person's sexual orientation, sexual behavior, or sexual attraction. Make no assumptions, and always ask patients for the name, gender, and pronouns they use.

3. **What is the prevalence of gender dysphoria among adults in the United States?**

   It has historically been difficult to assess the prevalence of gender dysphoria because it requires self-identification. However, with the greater awareness and acceptance of *gender nonconforming/gender nonbinary* people, more recent estimates are higher compared with previous ones. A 2016 Williams Institute study estimated there were 1.4 million adults who identified themselves as "transgender" (approximately 0.6% of the population). Limitations remain in relation to self-reporting and the terminology used, as noted above. The Williams Institute study did not include transgender youth, who are also increasingly seeking care at younger ages. Other studies have suggested a higher prevalence of gender dysphoria among the U.S. veteran population compared to the general population.

4. **Why is it important for endocrinologists to be trained in transgender medicine?**

   Although the awareness of gender dysphoria has improved substantially in the last decade, barriers continue to exist in health care for transgender individuals. In the 2015 U.S. Transgender Survey, with 27,715 respondents from all 50 states, 33% of individuals reported a negative experience with a health care provider, and 23% stated they did not seek care because of fears of mistreatment. Creating a welcoming environment for patients includes, but is not limited to, provider and staff education, identifying and using patients' chosen names and pronouns, being mindful of protected health information on paper and electronic forms, and establishing gender-neutral facilities.

   With their detailed knowledge of hormone physiology and treatment, endocrinologists are uniquely positioned to provide gender-affirming hormone therapy. A 2017 Mayo Clinic and Endocrine Society (ES) Web-based anonymous survey of endocrinology fellowship program directors, with just over a 50% response rate, found that 72% of respondents provided teaching on transgender health topics, but 94% indicated that fellowship training in transgender health is important. Of the practicing U.S. medical doctor ES members who responded to the same survey (only 6% response rate), 80% had treated a transgender patient, but 81% had never received training in transgender management. There was also low confidence in the nonhormone aspects of care among endocrine providers. These results indicated that confidence and competence among endocrinologists needs to increase, especially as the number of patients being referred to endocrinologists rises.

Table 57.1. Terminology.

TERM/PHRASE	DEFINITION
Cisgender, Cis	Those whose gender identity and gender expression align with their sex assigned at birth (i.e., not transgender; e.g., cis women, cis men). Avoid using the term, "normal," when referring to cisgender people.
Cross-dresser	One who wears clothing, jewelry, and/or makeup that is not traditionally associated with their anatomic sex; generally do not intend or desire to change their anatomic sex; more often associated with men; more often occasional; does not necessarily reflect sexual orientation or gender identity. *Note:* The term "transvestite" has significant negative connotation and should be avoided.
Gender expression	The external manifestations of a person's gender. May or may conform to the socially defined behaviors and external characteristics that are historically referred to as *masculine* or *feminine* (e.g., clothing, haircut, jewelry, social interactions, speech patterns)
Gender nonbinary, gender fluid, pangender, polygender	Those who may identify and present themselves as both or alternatively male and female, as neither male nor female, or as a gender outside the male/female binary.
Gender nonconforming	Having a gender expression that is neither masculine nor feminine, or is different from traditional or stereotypic expectations of how a man or woman should appear or behave.
Intersex	A rare group of conditions involving anomalies of the sex chromosomes, gonads, reproductive ducts, and/or genitalia (e.g., born with both male and female genitalia, or having ambiguous genitalia). The term "hermaphrodite" has a negative connotation and should not be used.
Sex assigned at birth	Refers to sex assigned at birth typically based on genitalia (e.g., male, female, or intersex).
Sexual orientation	The physical, romantic, emotional, and/or spiritual attraction a person has for another person (e.g., lesbian, gay, heterosexual, bisexual, pansexual, polysexual, or asexual)
Transgender, Trans	Encompasses those whose gender identity and/or gender expression differs from their sex assigned at birth; independent of the decision whether to use gender-affirming hormones or undergo surgery. The term "transgendered" should not be used.
Trans man/Trans male/ Transmasculine	Generally refers to a person who was assigned female at birth but whose gender identity and/or gender expression is male/masculine.
Trans woman/Trans female/ Transfeminine	Generally refers to a person who was assigned male at birth but whose gender identity and/or gender expression is female/feminine.
Two spirit, Two-spirited	Those who display characteristics of both male and female genders; has been referred to as a third gender or the male-female gender; derived from the traditions of some indigenous North American cultures.

5. **What medical and psychiatric health disparities are seen in transgender patients?**

Medical and psychiatric health disparities do exist between transgender and *cisgender* (cis, denoting or relating to a person whose sense of personal identity and gender corresponds with their sex assigned at birth) people. One case-control study utilizing International Statistical Classification of Diseases and Related Health Problems–Clinical Modification (ICD-9–CM) codes for transgender identification of U.S. veterans between 1996 and 2013 revealed statistically significant disparities with regard to depression, suicidality, posttraumatic stress disorder (PTSD), eating disorders, and other mental health conditions compared with cisgender veterans. Transgender veterans were more likely to have been homeless, to have reported sexual trauma while on active duty, and to have been incarcerated. Human immunodeficiency virus (HIV) infection was the medical diagnosis with the largest disparity (adjusted odds ratio [OR] 4.98; 95% confidence interval [CI] 3.70–6.69), although others, such as cardiac arrest, cerebral vascular disease, congestive heart failure, diabetes, hypercholesterolemia, hypertension, ischemic heart disease, and obesity, were also documented to have increased ORs.

Data from 22 states that participated in gender identity questions in the 2015 U.S. Behavioral Risk Factor Surveillance Survey revealed that trans men were 2.5 times more likely than cis men and almost four times more likely than cis women to lack health care coverage. Trans men had no difference in self-reported overweight or obesity, hypertension, myocardial infarction (MI), angina or coronary heart disease, stroke, or diabetes. In contrast, trans women were over two times more likely to self-report binge drinking compared with cis women. Of the above cardiometabolic diseases, trans women were about three times more likely than cis women to report a history of MI; there was no significant difference in MI between cis women and cis men.

6. What type of evaluation should be done prior to initiating gender-affirming hormone therapy?

There have been varying recommendations regarding real-life experiences, meaning how much time the patient has spent living full-time in the desired gender, prior to hormone therapy. Previous iterations of the ES Clinical Practice Guidelines and the World Professional Association for Transgender Health (WPATH) Standards of Care (SOC) have required real-life experience, but more recent guidelines do not state this as a requirement for initiating gender-affirming hormone therapy. Both the ES and the WPATH do specify a need for persistent gender dysphoria, age of majority, and capacity to consent and recommend that mental health and medical concerns, if present, be reasonably well controlled prior to the initiation of hormone therapy. Of note, studies have shown decreases in anxiety and depression in patients after initiation of gender-affirming hormone therapy and that these conditions are certainly not considered contraindications to hormonal treatment.

The role of the mental health provider has also been a topic of controversy in recent guidelines. Although previously it was required that patients seek a diagnostic evaluation and a letter from a mental health professional prior to the initiation of hormone therapy, the ES guidelines specify that any adult with expertise can make this diagnosis. There are other models, known as "informed consent" models, wherein the medical provider makes the assessment and diagnosis and then assesses the capacity for the patient to provide consent for treatment. Some providers and clinics require a signed informed consent form, whereas others document their informed discussions and patient understanding in the chart.

In our integrated transgender health clinic, we require a diagnosis of gender dysphoria to be confirmed by a mental health professional prior to hormone initiation. Although it is important not to pathologize gender incongruence or gender dysphoria, we have seen the diagnosis being confused with other mental health concerns (e.g., body dysmorphic disorder) that the hormone provider may not be as well-versed in diagnosing. There are also stressors that occur related to gender transition, as in any life change, and the mental health provider on the team plays a valuable role in providing support during this time. We do not see this as a hoop that patients must jump through but, rather, as a way to provide a holistic approach to patient care.

7. What are the options for gender-affirming hormone therapy in trans women?

For patients with gender incongruence/gender dysphoria wishing to pursue feminizing therapy, estrogen is the main hormonal therapy. It can be administered via the oral, transdermal, or intramuscular routes. Although not listed in the guidelines as a route of administration and there are no studies to provide an evidence base in this population, some trans women take oral estradiol sublingually, with varied effects on hormone levels. Antiandrogens can be used in conjunction with estrogen. In the United States, spironolactone is the most widely available antiandrogen. (*Note:* Cyproterone acetate is not available in the United States.) Gonadotrophin-releasing hormone (GnRH) agonists are also utilized at times to block the production of testosterone; these must be given as an injection and can be costly. 5-alpha reductase inhibitors are mentioned in some guidelines as being helpful in treating scalp hair loss and skin changes, although action (blocking the conversion of testosterone to the more active 5-alpha-dihydrotestosterone) may be limited in those already with significant androgen blockade. References for the ES, WPATH, and UCSF guidelines are provided at the end of this chapter.

8. When can physical changes be expected to occur with estrogen and antiandrogen therapy?

Patients should be counseled that physical changes occur slowly, just as in biological puberty, although the feminizing effects are widely variable from person to person. There are no data to suggest that larger doses lead to more rapid changes; in fact, there can be increased adverse events with larger doses. Typical changes seen over the course of the first year are fewer erections, skin changes, fat redistribution, and breast development. Changes in libido are an expected outcome and should be discussed with patients in advance. It is important to educate patients that maximum changes can take more than 3 years to achieve and may be less evident in adults who start gender-affirming hormone therapy at an older age. For trans women who went through male puberty, voice pitch does not go higher with estrogen alone and voice training with a speech pathologist is most effective.

9. What changes in laboratory values can be seen with estrogen and antiandrogen therapy, and how should they be monitored?

Estradiol levels are expected to increase when using estradiol-based preparations. However, estradiol levels will not reflect the use of conjugated estrogens or ethinyl estradiol. These preparations are no longer recommended for routine use in gender-affirming hormone therapy. It is also expected that testosterone levels will decline on all types of estrogen therapy but may not suppress completely, hence the often needed antiandrogen medication. The ES guidelines suggest that goal serum estradiol levels not exceed a peak of 100 to 200 pg/mL and that testosterone levels be suppressed to < 50 ng/dL. They also suggest that patients be evaluated every 3 months for the first year with measurements of serum estradiol and testosterone, with the addition of electrolytes if on spironolactone. Thereafter, assessments and laboratory testing can be done once or twice a year, if the values are stable.

Serum triglycerides may increase on oral estrogen therapy but this can be mitigated with the use of transdermal preparations. Estrogens also typically increase high-density lipoprotein cholesterol levels. Prolactin elevations have been reported as well.

10. What are contraindications to initiating estrogen therapy?

Although there are no absolute contraindications to initiating estrogen therapy, there are conditions considered to pose higher risks for adverse outcomes, according to the ES guidelines. The highest risk is that of venous thromboembolism (VTE). Other moderate risk conditions include cardiovascular or cerebrovascular disease, breast cancer, macroprolactinoma, hypertriglyceridemia, and cholelithiasis. Questions have been raised about migraine with aura because this is a known contraindication to combined oral contraceptive pills, which contain ethinyl estradiol, in cis women. There are no data to answer this question yet in the setting of the specific types of estradiol used in gender-affirming hormone therapy, but some guidelines suggest using oral or transdermal estrogen (as opposed to intramuscular estrogen) to maintain more consistent levels. The risks and benefits of estrogen therapy should be discussed with each patient. At times, we have found consultation with colleagues in other specialties, such as neurology or hematology, to be useful regarding risk factors and management of thromboembolic disease.

11. Is there a role for progesterone in trans women?

There are no data to support the routine use of progesterone for breast growth in trans women. One study that evaluated different hormone protocols (with and without progesterone) did not find a difference in rates of requests for breast augmentation among the various protocols. In Turner's syndrome patients, there are concerns that early administration of progesterone can cause less breast growth overall. In addition, concerns have been raised regarding the role of progesterone in the development of breast cancer. In the Women's Health Initiative (WHI), conjugated equine estrogens plus medroxyprogesterone given to older cis women was associated with increased risk of breast cancer compared with that in the estrogen-only arm of the study. Medroxyprogesterone may also have unfavorable effects on lipid profiles, weight, and mood. Some providers consider micronized progesterone only after some time on estradiol in patients who are adamant on trying it but, again, there are no data to support routine use of progesterone in trans women. We have also seen the use of depot medroxyprogesterone for testosterone suppression though data are also lacking for its routine use.

12. Is the risk of blood clots increased for trans women on estrogen therapy?

Some studies have also suggested an increased risk for VTE in trans women. These include a review of mostly European transgender cohorts showing that trans women were at increased risk of VTE but mostly with the use of ethinyl estradiol, which is no longer recommended. Another recent meta-analysis of mostly uncontrolled and observational studies (including similar cohorts as above) concluded that data regarding the risk of VTE, MI, stroke, and mortality were insufficient to draw conclusions (i.e., too few events reported); however, events were reported more often in trans women than in trans men. More recently, the Study of Transition, Outcomes and Gender (STRONG) cohort, consisting of 6456 Kaiser Permanente members, reported a higher incidence of VTE among the transfeminine cohort compared with reference females and males. Trans women in the study had a higher incidence of VTE, with 2- and 8-year risk differences of 4.1 (95% CI: 1.6–6.7) and 16.7 (95% CI: 6.4–27.5) per 1000 persons relative to cis men, and 3.4 (95% CI: 1.1–5.6) and 13.7 (95% CI: 4.1–22.7) relative to cis women, though absolute rates remained very low.

13. What are some of the other long-term health concerns for trans women on estrogen?

This is an area of active research. The longest study, to date, had a median hormone use duration of 18.5 years in a cohort of 966 trans women. Their average age was 31 years at the initiation of hormone therapy and 20% of subjects were > 40 years of age. There was a significant increase in the standard mortality ratio compared with natal men. In trans women aged 25 to 40 years, the increased mortality risk was mainly attributable to acquired immunodeficiency syndrome (AIDS), suicide, and drug-related deaths, whereas there were increased risks of mortality related to suicide and cardiovascular disease (CVD) in those aged 40 to 64 years. Long-term ethinyl estradiol use was independently associated with a threefold higher risk of death resulting from a cardiovascular cause. This is also a reminder that, although gender dysphoria can be alleviated with hormone therapy, it is important to provide appropriate treatment to gender-nonconforming individuals who have depression. Trans women have higher rates of HIV infection compared with the general population, with even higher rates among sex workers. HIV screening for high-risk patients and referral to a preexposure prophylaxis (PrEP) clinic should be considered, when appropriate.

14. What are the options for gender-affirming hormone therapy in trans men?

For patients with gender incongruence/gender dysphoria who want to pursue masculinizing therapy, testosterone is the mainstay of therapy. It is typically given via subcutaneous or intramuscular injection with weekly or every-other-week dosing of testosterone enanthate or cypionate. Testosterone undecanoate every 3 months is also available. Testosterone can also be administered via transdermal gel or patch, depending on patient preference, compliance, insurance coverage, and cost. A GnRH agonist or progestins have been used when menses persist beyond the first 6 to 12 months of therapy. References for the ES, WPATH, and University of California San Francisco (UCSF) guidelines are provided at the end of the chapter.

15. What are the contraindications to initiating testosterone therapy?

Although there are no absolute contraindications for gender-affirming hormone therapy with testosterone, the condition with the highest risk per the ES guidelines is erythrocytosis with a hematocrit > 50%. Other conditions, listed as moderate risk, include hypertension, liver function abnormalities, coronary or cerebrovascular disease, breast or uterine cancer, and hypertension. In cis men with hypogonadism, there are concerns that testosterone can exacerbate obstructive sleep apnea. More recently, there have been case reports of breast cancer in testosterone-treated trans men both prior to and after mastectomy.

16. When can physical changes be expected to occur with testosterone therapy?

As noted above, patients should be counseled that physical changes occur slowly, just as in puberty, although person-to-person masculinizing effects are widely variable. There are no data to suggest that larger testosterone doses cause more rapid changes, and in fact, there can be increased adverse events with larger doses. The typical changes begin within 3 months and include facial/body hair growth, voice changes, clitoral enlargement, and body fat redistribution with increased muscle mass, but maximal changes can take up to 5 years or more.

17. What changes in laboratory values can be seen with testosterone therapy, and how should they be monitored?

As serum testosterone levels rise, estradiol levels and gonadotropin levels will become suppressed. The ES guidelines suggest aiming for a testosterone level midway between injections of 400 to 700 ng/mL. The guidelines advise monitoring levels every 3 months for the first year and then once or twice yearly going forward. The recommendation for routine monitoring of estradiol levels was removed from the 2017 ES guidelines.

Hematocrit will frequently increase on testosterone therapy and may necessitate a dose reduction or use of a different testosterone formulation/route of administration. Other etiologies of an elevated hematocrit, such as obstructive sleep apnea and tobacco use, should be investigated in addition to family history. Changes in the lipid profile with increases in serum triglycerides and low-density lipoprotein cholesterol with concomitant decreases in HDL cholesterol have been observed. The ES guidelines suggest checking hemoglobin and hematocrit at baseline, every 3 months for the first year of testosterone therapy, and then once or twice yearly. They suggest measuring weight, blood pressure, and lipids at "regular" intervals.

18. What are some of the long-term health concerns for trans men on testosterone?

Again, this is an area of active research, with the longest study to date spanning 18.5 years in 365 trans men. The standard mortality ratio was not significantly increased compared with natal females. It should be noted that the average age in this study was 26 years, with the majority of patients age between 15 and 24 years at the start of the study. Cis women with polycystic ovary syndrome, which could represent a model of biological females with elevated serum testosterone levels, have some concerning changes in cardiovascular parameters, but there are no definitive data as yet to indicate that these individuals develop CVD at a higher rate or at a younger age.

19. What considerations need to be made in elderly transgender patients who wish to start or continue gender-affirming hormone therapy?

As the general population ages, so do transgender patients. Questions arise over the safety of gender-affirming hormone therapy in the elderly transgender population, where aging-related comorbidities are present. There have been no randomized controlled trials investigating the safety of starting or continuing various hormone formulations or routes of administration in older transgender patients, especially with regard to CVD and mortality. Experts have suggested that initiation of gender-affirming hormone therapy has no disproportionate risks and that older age itself should not be a contraindication to initiating hormones. Other areas in need of investigation include dose reductions or even hormone discontinuation after a certain age (although the risk of bone density loss may outweigh any unforeseen benefits). Several institutions consider a change to transdermal estrogens (from oral) in older trans women aged $\geq$45–50 years. A discussion of the risks and benefits, past medical and family histories, current comorbidities, and any modifiable behaviors that may increase risks while on gender-affirming hormone therapy should be conducted with older transgender patients as with younger individuals. Additional topics that have been suggested for future studies among the aging transgender population include palliative care and end-of-life issues.

20. When is gender-affirming surgery indicated?

There are many forms of gender-affirming surgery but surgical transition should not be required of transgender patients. Depending on laws for a given area, surgical transition may still be required for patients to change their legal name, gender marker, or birth certificate. Many trans men will seek a bilateral mastectomy or "top surgery," which does not require a specific duration of testosterone prior to surgery. Breast implants and orchiectomy are often requested by trans women. Some trans women will also seek facial feminization surgery. Gender-affirming genital surgery can be done with creation of a neo-vagina or phalloplasty. Metoidioplasty, wherein the clitoris is brought forward to assist with urinating from a standing position, is also an option for trans men. The ES guidelines and the WPATH recommend at least 1 year of gender-affirming hormone therapy, unless contraindicated, as well as living full-time in the new gender role prior to genital reconstructive surgery. Although breast augmentation surgery can be performed sooner, one reason to postpone surgery is to maximize breast growth on hormones to optimize surgical (aesthetic) results. In the United States, although more insurance companies are covering gender-affirming surgical procedures, persistent barriers include access to a trained surgeon, lack of insurance, and cost. After gonadectomy, hormonal medications can generally be decreased to reflect physiologic dosing because there is no further need for hormonal suppression of the endogenous hormones, and spironolactone can be discontinued in trans women.

21. How common is gonadectomy in transgender patients, and why is that important?

We do not yet fully understand if there are differences in health outcomes (and implications for dosing changes) among transgender patients on gender-affirming hormone therapy who have or have not had gonadectomy. Most published longitudinal data (e.g., CVD risk, body composition, bone density, mental health, quality of life, etc.) have come from the European Network for the Investigation of Gender Incongruence (ENIGI) and an Amsterdam cohort. Additionally, most systematic reviews and meta-analyses have analyzed data that come from the ENIGI cohort. Because of the differences in access to surgery, the ENIGI patient population has had much higher rates of gender-affirming surgery (in particular, gonadectomy); a Dutch cohort, with 86.7% trans women and 94% trans men, has had gonadectomy, and a Belgian cohort, with 64.8% trans women and 85.5% trans men, has had gonadectomy.

In contrast, the 2015 U.S. Transgender Survey reported that only 25% of respondents had undergone *some form* of transition-related surgery, with only 14% of trans men having had hysterectomy—with the status of the ovaries not specified—and only 11% of trans women having had orchiectomy. In that survey, 55% of those who sought coverage for transition-related surgery in the past were denied. Lower rates of hysterectomy with or without oophorectomy (11%) in trans men and a much lower rate of orchiectomy (1.5%) in trans women were seen in the STRONG cohort from Kaiser Permanente, as described above.

22. How should patients be counseled about fertility preservation?

Ideally, patients should be advised about fertility preservation options prior to initiation of hormone therapy due to decreased fertility/sexual function after starting and while taking gender-affirming hormone therapy. Sperm and oocyte banking are available but can be expensive and not covered by insurance. The risks of permanent infertility with long-term hormone therapy are not known at this time. If fertility is desired after the initiation of therapy, typically, hormones are discontinued for some period, with the aim of allowing natal gonadal function to resume. There have been cases of trans men getting pregnant while taking and after stopping testosterone with good outcomes.

It is also important to counsel patients that while gender-affirming hormone therapy may lead to infertility, it is not a reliable contraceptive. Providers should take a thorough sexual history and counsel patients regarding contraception, as appropriate.

23. What are recommendations for osteoporosis screening?

Generally, if patients continue gender-affirming hormone therapy, sex steroids assist in the maintenance of bone density. Testosterone is converted to estradiol, which is considered a key component of bone in cis men. However, if patients do stop therapy after gonadectomy, bone loss can be considerable. There are no fracture data to date, nor is there consensus on bone density interpretation and use of natal gender in bone density reports. There are some concerning data to suggest that a large proportion of trans women have lower bone mineral density prior to starting estrogen, which may be multifactorial and include social and behavioral disparities compared to their peers. The ES guidelines recommend that a baseline bone density be considered in all trans women, with screening of low-risk patients to begin at age 60 years or if hormone use stops. For trans men, they suggest screening if testosterone use stops or other risks arise.

24. What are the recommendations for cancer screening?

Screening for cancers should be done on the basis of existing tissues. For example, both trans women and trans men may have breasts. A trans man with breasts should be screened with mammography or other imaging modality, as deemed appropriate by age and family history; the UCSF Center of Excellence suggests yearly or every-other-year mammography once a trans woman is past 50 years of age and has been on estrogen therapy for > 5 to 10 years. The ES guidelines suggest breast cancer screening for trans women be the same as for cis women per national guidelines.

Cervical cancer screening with Papanicolaou ("Pap") testing is recommended to begin at age 21 years for trans men as it is for cis women. Because this can be an uncomfortable procedure and there are reports of a higher incidence of unsatisfactory results in trans men on testosterone therapy, it is particularly important that this testing be done by an experienced provider. In addition, it is our personal experience that performing Pap testing in a gender-neutral space can improve compliance rates and ease patient distress.

Prostate cancer screening should also be done as appropriate for age and other risk factors. There have been case reports of prostate cancer in trans women.

All other vaccinations and preventive cancer screening should be done as appropriate for age and family history.

25. How do I counsel patients regarding smoking cessation?

Recent studies have shown smoking to be a major risk factor for VTE in patients on hormone therapy, regardless of gender identity. A 2017 retrospective study of 156 transgender patients found that those patients (64% of trans women and 25% of trans men) were more likely to quit smoking after tobacco cessation counseling compared with the general population of adult smokers (6% in a given year). Some guidelines suggest a strong preference to use transdermal estrogen in patients who smoke, although current smoking status is not an absolute contraindication to starting gender-affirming hormone therapy. The same counseling strategies for smoking cessation should be applied to patients regardless of gender identity.

26. What are the benefits of a multidisciplinary approach to transgender care?

Several academic and community hospital–based multidisciplinary approaches to transgender care have been established in recent years (both for adult and pediatric patients). These team models, including our integrated transgender health clinic, utilize experts in a variety of fields (e.g., endocrinology, internal medicine, psychiatry, gynecology, plastic and reconstructive surgery, pediatric endocrinology, urology, infectious diseases, reproductive medicine, dermatology, ENT [ear, nose, and throat], and speech therapy) to provide sensitive and comprehensive care to transgender patients to reduce barriers to access discussed above. There is also interest in learning more about the best approach to transitioning gender-related care from pediatric to adult endocrinology providers.

27. How can providers assist with legal issues?

There will be variation across states and countries as to requirements for document changes. Local Department of Motor Vehicle (DMV) and the federal websites for passports and birth certificates can provide up-to-date information. Often, a letter from a physician is required stating that the patient is receiving medical care and that the gender transition is complete.

KEY POINTS

- Gender incongruence can lead to gender dysphoria, which is the distress and unease that may occur when a person's gender identity and/or gender expression differs from the sex assigned at birth.
- Gender-affirming hormone therapy is associated with many benefits for patients. Hormone preparations that allow for monitoring of serum levels are preferred, with dose adjustments made to keep estradiol and testosterone levels within the laboratory goal ranges and to balance risks, benefits and expectations.
- There appears to be an increased risk of thromboembolic events in trans women and concerns about possible increased risks for cardiovascular disease and mortality, which demonstrate the need for additional high-quality, prospective research.
- There are many questions yet to be answered regarding the long-term effects of gender-affirming hormone therapy, especially among the growing elderly and diverse transgender populations in the United States and around the world.
- Endocrinologists should be familiar with the hormonal management of gender dysphoria and utilize a multi-disciplinary approach with primary care and other specialists to provide comprehensive care. Informed discussion with patients is a key part of making treatment decisions.

BIBLIOGRAPHY

Asscheman, H., Giltay, E. J., Megens, J. A., de Ronde, W. P., van Trotsenburg, M. A., & Gooren L. J. (2011). A long-term follow-up study of mortality in transsexuals receiving treatment with cross-sex hormones. *European Journal of Endocrinology, 164*(4), 635–642.

Baral, S. D., Poteat, T., Strömdahl, S., Wirtz, A. L., Guadamuz, T. E., & Beyrer, C. (2013). Worldwide burden of HIV in transgender women: a systematic review and meta-analysis. *Lancet. Infectious Diseases, 13*, 214–222.

Brown, G. R., & Jones, K. T. (2016). Mental health and medical health disparities in 5135 transgender veterans receiving healthcare in the Veterans Health Administration: a case-control study. *LGBT Health, 3*(2), 122–131.

Center of Excellence for Transgender Health, Department of Family & Community Medicine, University of California, San Francisco, Editor: Deutsch MB. (2016). *Guidelines for the primary and gender-affirming care of transgender and gender nonbinary people* (2nd ed.). Retrieved from http://transhealth.ucsf.edu/pdf/Transgender-PGACG-6-17-16.pdf. Accessed June 8, 2018.

Coleman, E., Bockting, W., Botzer, M., Cohen-Kettenis, P., DeCuypere, G., Feldman, J., Fraser, L., Green, J., Knudson, G., Meyer, W. J., Monstrey, S., Adler, R. K., Brown, G. R., Devor, A. H., Ehrbar, R., Ettner, R., Eyler, E., Garofalo, R., Karasic, D. H., Lev, A. I., Mayer, G., Meyer-Bahlburg, H., Hall, B. P., Pfaefflin, F., Rachlin, K., Robinson, B., Schechter, L. S., Tangpricha, V., van Trotsenburg, M., Vitale, A., Winter, S., Whittle, S., Wylie, K. R., & Zucker, K. (2011). Standards of Care for the health of transsexual, transgender, and gender-nonconforming people, version 7. *International Journal of Transgenderism, 13*(4), 165-232. Also available at: https://www.wpath.org/media/cms/Documents/SOC%20v7/Standards%20of%20Care_V7%20Full%20Book_English.pdf. Accessed 3/18/19.

Davidge-Pitts, C., Nippoldt, T. B., Danoff, A., Radziejewski, L., & Natt, N. (2017). Transgender health in endocrinology: current status of endocrinology fellowship programs and practicing clinicians. *Journal of Clinical Endocrinology and Metabolism, 102*(4), 1286–1290.

Dekker, M. J. H. J., Wierckx, K., Van Caenegem, E., Klaver, M., Kreukels, B. P., Elaut, E., . . . T'Sjoen, G . (2016). A European Network for the Investigation of Gender Incongruence: endocrine part. *Journal of Sexual Medicine, 13*(6), 994–999.

Fenway Health. (2010). *Glossary of gender and transgender terms.* Retrieved from http://fenwayhealth.org/documents/the-fenway-institute/handouts/Handout_7-C_Glossary_of_Gender_and_Transgender_Terms__fi.pdf. Accessed June 8, 2018.

Getahun, D., Nash, R., Flanders, W. D., Baird, T. C., Becerra-Culqui, T. A., Cromwell, L., . . . Goodman, M. (2018). Cross-sex hormones and acute cardiovascular events in transgender persons: a cohort study. *Annals of Internal Medicine, 169*(4), 205–213.

Gooren, L. J., & T'Sjoen, G. (2018). Endocrine treatment of aging transgender people. *Reviews in Endocrine & Metabolic Disorders, 19*(3), 253–262.

Gooren, L. J., Wierckx, K., & Giltay, E. J. (2014). Cardiovascular disease in transsexual persons treated with cross-sex hormones: reversal of the traditional sex difference in cardiovascular disease pattern. *European Journal of Endocrinology, 170*(6), 809–819.

Grant, J. M., Mottet, L. A., Tanis, J., Harrison, J., Herman, J. L., & Keisling, M. (2011). Injustice at every turn: a report of the National Transgender Discrimination Survey. Washington: National Center for Transgender Equality and National Gay and Lesbian Task Force.

Hembree, W. C., Cohen-Kettenis, P. T., Gooren, L., Hannema, S. E., Meyer, W. J., Murad, M. H., . . . T'Sjoen, G. G. (2017). Endocrine treatment of gender-dysphoric/gender-incongruent persons: an Endocrine Society Clinical Practice guideline. *Journal of Clinical Endocrinology and Metabolism. 102*(11), 1–35.

Irwig, M. S. (2017). Testosterone therapy for transgender men. *Lancet. Diabetes & Endocrinology, 5*(4), 301–311.

Kreukels, B. P. C., Haraldsen, I. R., De Cuypere, G., Richter-Appelt, H., Gijs, L., & Cohen-Kettenis, P. T. (2012). A European network for the investigation of gender incongruence: the ENIGI initiative. *European Psychiatry, 27*(6), 445–450.

Maraka, S., Singh Ospina, N., Rodriguez-Gutierrez, R., Davidge-Pitts, C. J., Nippoldt, T. B., Prokop, L. J., & Murad, M. H. (2017). Sex steroids and cardiovascular outcomes in transgender individuals: a systematic review and meta-analysis. *Journal of Clinical Endocrinology and Metabolism, 102*(11), 3914–3923.

Meyers, S. C., & Safer, D. J. (2017). Increased rates of smoking cessation observed among transgender women receiving hormone treatment. *Endocrine Practice, 23*(1), 32–36.

Nokoff, N. J., Scarbro, S., Juarez-Colunga, E., Moreau, K. L., & Kempe, A. Health and cardiometabolic disease in transgender adults in the United States: Behavioral Risk Factor Surveillance System 2015. *Journal of the Endocrine Society, 2*(4), 349–360.

Quinn, V. P., Nash, R., Hunkeler, E., Contreras, R., Cromwell, L., Becerra-Culqui, T. A., . . . Goodman, M. (2017). Cohort profile: Study of Transition, Outcomes and Gender (STRONG) to assess health status of transgender people. *BMJ Open, 7*, e018121.

Streed, C. G., Jr., Harfouch, O., Marvel, F., Blumenthal, R. S., Martin, S. S., & Mukherjee, M. (2017). Cardiovascular disease among transgender adults receiving hormone therapy: a narrative review. *Annals of Internal Medicine, 167*(4), 256–267.

Tangpricha, V., & den Heijer, M. (2017). Oestrogen and anti-androgen therapy for transgender women. *Lancet Diabetes & Endocrinology, 5*(4), 291–300.

James, S. E., Herman, J. L., Rankin, S., Keisling, M., Mottet, L., & Anafi, M. (2016). The Report of the 2015 U.S. Transgender Survey. Washington, DC: National Center for Transgender Equality. http://www.ustranssurvey.org/reports/ Accessed 8/6/18.

Wierckx, K., Gooren, L., & T'Sjoen, G. (2014). Clinical review: Breast development in trans women receiving cross-sex hormones *Journal of Sexual Medicine, 11*(5), 1240–1247.

Wierckx, K., Elaut, E., Declercq, E., Heylens, G., De Cuypere, G., Taes, Y., . . . T'Sjoen, G. (2013). Prevalence of cardiovascular disease and cancer during cross-sex hormone therapy in a large cohort of trans persons: a case-control study. *European Journal of Endocrinology, 169*(4), 471–478.

Williams Institute. (2016). *How many adults identify as transgender in the United States*. Retrieved from https://williamsinstitute.law.ucla.edu/wp-content/uploads/How-Many-Adults-Identify-as-Transgender-in-the-United-States.pdf. Accessed June 8, 2018.

CHAPTER 58

USE AND ABUSE OF ANABOLIC–ANDROGENIC STEROIDS AND ANDROGEN PRECURSORS

Carlos A. Torres and Homer J. LeMar, Jr.

1. **What are anabolic–androgenic steroids?**

   Anabolic–androgenic steroids (AASs) are a group of steroid hormones derived from chemical modification of testosterone. The precursor to testosterone is cholesterol; endogenous synthesis is limited by cholesterol delivery to mitochondria for modification. After synthesis and secretion, testosterone is further converted to strong androgens to include dihydrotestosterone (DHT) via 5-alpha-reductase, and weak androgens to include dehydroepiandrosterone (DHEA) and androstenedione. Testosterone is also converted via aromatase to estradiol, an active metabolite, although not an AAS. The terms *anabolic* and *androgenic* derive from their ability to promote positive nitrogen balance and accretion of lean body mass as well as masculinization.

2. **Where are AASs made?**

   In males, testosterone is made in the Leydig cells of the testes. In females, testosterone is made by the theca cells of the ovary. Testosterone is then peripherally converted to DHT in the skin, prostate, and external genitalia. DHEA, one of the most important weak androgens, is primarily made by the adrenal cortex.

3. **Summarize the biological effects of AASs.**

   Endogenous AASs have diverse effects with three distinct physiologic surges. The first occurs during the fetal period at weeks 6 through 8 of gestation, when they promote the development of male genitalia. The second surge occurs during the neonatal period, when they are involved in the growth of the phallus to normal size, in testicular descent, and spermatogonia development. The final surge assists in the development of secondary sexual characteristics during puberty, including growth and development of the prostate, seminal vesicles, penis, and scrotum. Pubertal changes in hair growth and sebaceous glands result in the male pattern of hair growth on the chin, pubic area, chest, and axillary regions, as well as acne provocation via increased sebum production. Vocal cords begin to thicken, along with enlargement of the larynx, resulting in voice deepening.

   Data indicating decreased urinary nitrogen levels support AAS effects on protein anabolism, resulting in an increase in lean body mass, specifically in the upper girdle, and alterations of fat distribution. Further structural changes occur with increases in bone mineral density and long bone growth, and with closure of the epiphyses. Neurologic changes include increased libido and spontaneous erections. Other effects include promotion of wound healing; stimulation of liver release of clotting factors and erythropoietin with a secondary increase in hematocrit; and suppression of high-density lipoprotein (HDL) synthesis (Table 58.1).

4. **How does testosterone mediate its effects via estradiol?**

   During puberty, when testosterone levels surge to stimulate bone growth, peripheral androgen conversion via aromatase also peaks. Newly synthesized estradiol promotes epiphyseal closure during puberty, counteracting the effects of testosterone. In patients with aromatase deficiency or estradiol receptor dysfunction, long bones continue to grow, but osteoporosis develops because estradiol is the most important regulator of bone mass accretion. Of note, this mechanism is different from estrogen's effect on osteoclasts and osteoblasts associated with osteoporosis in postmenopausal women.

5. **What is the correlation between AAS and age, and how is this important?**

   Total, free, and bioavailable testosterone levels decrease with age. This contributes to the decrease in muscle mass, increase in fat, decreased libido, increased fatigue, and the minor decreases in cognitive function seen in the elderly.

6. **How do AASs exert their effects?**

   Approximately 50% of circulating testosterone is strongly bound to sex hormone–binding globulin (SHBG); 40% is weakly bound to albumin; and 2% is unbound or free. The albumin-bound and unbound forms constitute the "bioavailable" and, thus, active forms of testosterone. AASs act by binding to specific intracellular androgen receptors located throughout the body; this interaction mediates the androgenic and anabolic effects of androgens. Dihydrotestosterone, being a strong androgen, has very high affinity for androgen receptors. Estradiol, formed by aromatase conversion of testosterone, exerts its effects by binding to estrogen receptors throughout the body.

Table 58.1. Physiologic Effects of Androgens.

Fetal Period
- Internal and external male genitalia development

Neonatal Period
- Phallus size development
- Testicular descent
- Spermatogonia development

Puberty
- Growth and development of prostate and seminal vesicles
- Increased size and width of penis
- Increased scrotal size
- Increased male pattern hair growth
- Increased skin thickness
- Increased sebaceous gland production, resulting in oily skin and development of acne
- Deepening of voice via vocal cord thickening and enlargement of larynx
- Increase in lean body mass
- Altered fat distribution
- Increased bone mineral density
- Long bone growth and closure of epiphyses
- Increased libido, sexual desire, and spontaneous erections
- Fibroblast stimulation promoting wound healing
- Liver synthesis of clotting factors and erythropoiesis
- Suppression of high-density lipoprotein cholesterol formation

Adult
- Maintenance of testosterone tissue effects

7. How are androgens metabolized, and why is it necessary to modify testosterone for administration?
   AASs are rapidly metabolized by the first-pass effect through the gut and the liver, making oral testosterone supplements highly ineffective in the absence of modification. Alkylation of testosterone confers resistance to hepatic metabolism and results in AASs that can be administered orally. Esterification of testosterone emulsifies testosterone for intramuscular injection. Addition of carbon chains to the ring structure of testosterone increases fat solubility and extends the duration of action.

8. What are the signs and symptoms of low or high androgen levels?
   Patients with low androgen levels may complain of fatigue, hypoactive sexual desire, erectile dysfunction, diminished pubic and/or facial hair, and testicular atrophy. Other findings include diminished prostate size, abnormal sperm morphology, absent motility of sperm, and a hypoproliferative normochromic anemia. Patients with elevated levels may complain of resistant acne or sudden-onset acne. Women especially will develop hirsutism and irregular menses.

9. What are the indications for AAS therapy?
   AASs are indicated for use in male hypogonadism and constitutional delay of growth and puberty. Use for stimulation of growth is cautioned because it may concomitantly accelerate epiphyseal closure and thereby limit ultimate height achievement. Androgens are also used as prophylaxis in hereditary angioneurotic edema and as second-line therapies for osteoporosis and aplastic or hypoplastic anemias. Gynecologic uses include treatment of endometriosis with weak androgens; reduction of postpartum breast engorgement in conjunction with estrogen; and elimination of estrogen-mediated menstrual bleeding for postmenopausal women undergoing hormone replacement. In oncology, androgens can be used to suppress some breast tumors in premenopausal women.

10. Are there any other potential uses for AASs?
    AASs may help elderly men by increasing body weight and muscle mass, preventing bone loss (vertebral but not femoral bone density), and improving hematocrit; however, AASs are not without side effects. There is also ongoing research on using androgens as male contraceptives, in chronic obstructive pulmonary disease, and in other hypogonadal wasting syndromes, such as muscle wasting in human immunodeficiency virus (HIV) infection and glucocorticoid-induced muscle and bone wasting. All of these uses are still under investigation.

11. What are the uses for androgen antagonists and/or inhibitors?
    5-alpha-reductase inhibitors are used to diminish testosterone conversion to DHT in peripheral tissues, most importantly in the prostate gland and in hair follicles. They have U.S. Food and Drug Administration (FDA) approval for treatment of benign prostatic hyperplasia and to combat early male-pattern baldness. Androgen receptor antagonists are also used to treat metastatic prostate cancer and female hirsutism.

12. **How common is abuse of AASs?**
First noted in the 1950s, AAS abuse was mostly limited to bodybuilders, other muscle-building enthusiasts, and various professional athletes. It is now known that AAS abuse is far more widespread. According to the results of one study, 3.3% of high school students reported anabolic steroid use; in another study, the use of products to improve appearance, muscle mass, or strength was reported by both girls and boys at rates of 8% and 12%, respectively. The National Institute of Drug Abuse (NIDA) report in 2007 noted use in 2.3% of boys versus 0.6% of girls. The NIDA recently estimated that over half a million grade 8 through grade 10 students are abusing AASs. Another study found that 1,084,000 Americans, or 0.5% of the adult population, have admitted to using AAS.

13. **Who is at risk for using illegal AASs?**
In the world of competitive athletics, bodybuilders are the biggest offenders with regard to AAS abuse. Because AASs increase hematocrit through enhanced erythropoietin production, they may also be used by athletes participating in endurance-oriented sports. Nonathletes may use AASs solely to improve appearance. Surveys have shown that the percentage of students who reported lifetime AAS use has increased from 2.7% to 6.1% in the past decade. Most users are men, although up to 2% may be women. Other risk factors include involvement in school sports and the use of other illicit drugs, alcohol, or tobacco.

14. **Do AASs truly help athletes?**
Both athletes and coaches are likely to answer with an unequivocal yes. AASs used in conjunction with adequate protein, carbohydrate intake, and proper training in experienced athletes seem to induce greater and more rapid gains. A study comparing supraphysiologic doses of testosterone enanthate with placebo in eugonadal men found clear increases in muscle size and strength, with or without weight-training exercise. Studies of AAS in athletes have shown an increase of body weight and lean body mass, but no significant decrease in the percentage of body fat. Not only do muscle fibers gain in cross-sectional diameter with anabolic steroid use, but new muscle fibers are also formed. The upper regions of the body show the most prominent gains in muscle mass as a result of AAS use because of the relatively larger number of androgen receptors in these areas.

15. **What doses of AASs are used in attempts to enhance sports performance and appearance?**
Doses used for illicit purposes are markedly higher ($\geq$ 10-fold) than physiologic and therapeutic doses. Furthermore, multiple agents are often used in so-called stacking regimens or arrays, in which multiple steroids at increasing doses are used to derive further effects. The drugs are often taken in 6- to 12-week cycles, with variable periods off the drugs, but some athletes may use them for as long as $\geq$ 1 year. Human chorionic gonadotropin may be used at the end of a cycle to prevent inhibition of gonadal function. Little is known about precise doses or stacking regimens; however, some anecdotal information is available.

16. **What are the potential adverse effects of AAS use?**
The most common side effects are hepatic dysfunction to include cholestatic jaundice and development of hepatic neoplasms; most worrisome is peliosis hepatis, which can rupture causing death. Other common side effects include gynecomastia, acne, male-pattern baldness, increased aggression, and alterations in the cholesterol profile to include an increase in low-density lipoprotein (LDL) and decrease in high-density lipoprotein (HDL). Fortunately, most side effects are temporary and reversible with cessation of AAS (Table 58.2). Long-term use is associated with a reduction in the production of natural sex hormones; this, however, is usually reversible but may take over a year to resolve. There is also an increase in cardiovascular disease as a result of fluid retention, exacerbation of hypertension and dyslipidemia, increased liver synthesis of clotting factors, development of polycythemia, and vasospasm induction via effects on vascular nitric oxide. Males may be at increased risk for development of prostate problems in previously benign or local disease, impotence, and testicular atrophy resulting in infertility. Women may experience menstrual irregularities, such as oligomenorrhea or amenorrhea, and virilizing effects, such as hirsutism, clitoromegaly, and deepening of the voice. In adolescents, there is a risk of premature epiphyseal closure leading to a reduction in final adult height and psychological dysfunction caused by androgen effects on brain development.

17. **What are the neuropsychiatric implications of AAS use?**
Major mood disorders and aggressive or even criminal behavior have been previously reported in the literature. One study performed in 1994 compared neuropsychiatric behavior in men actively taking AASs and those not taking AASs. One hundred and sixty men recruited from gyms responded to a questionnaire about androgen use and psychiatric symptoms. Psychiatric symptoms, including major mood disorders and aggressive behavior, were more common in men who had taken androgens than in those who had never taken androgens; among the former, the symptoms were more common while they were taking androgens. Several studies have also described an association between nonmedical use of androgens and risky or even criminal behavior. In mail surveys of approximately 10,000 to 15,000 college students from 1993 to 2001, nonmedical use of androgens was associated with cigarette smoking, other illicit drug use, drinking and driving, and alcohol use disorder.

18. **What screening tests are used to detect AAS use in athletes?**
Urine samples can be evaluated via mass spectroscopy and gas chromatography, where direct confirmation comes from measurement of protein kinase C (PKC). PCK reflects an exogenous synthetic origin, ruling in or out a potential

Table 58.2. Potential Adverse Effects of Anabolic–Androgenic Steroid (AAS) Use and Abuse.

SYSTEM/ ORGAN	ADVERSE EFFECTS	SYSTEM/ ORGAN	ADVERSE EFFECTS
Liver	• Cholestatic hepatitis • Peliosis hepatis (hemorrhagic liver cysts) • Liver tumors—benign and malignant (oral agents)	Hematologic	• Platelet count and aggregation increased • Polycythemia
Cardiovascular	• Stroke and myocardial infarction incidence increased • High-density lipoprotein (HDL) cholesterol reduced and low-density lipoprotein (LDL) cholesterol increased • Left ventricular enlargement (cardiac androgen receptors) • Increased vasomotor tone and vasospasm (effects on vascular nitric oxide)	Psychological	• Aggressive behavior • Psychotic symptoms • Dependence/Withdrawal • Depression
		Skin	• Sebum production and acne increased • Male-pattern baldness • Hirsutism (women)
Reproductive	• Testicular atrophy • Oligospermia/azoospermia • Priapism • Gynecomastia/breast tenderness • Natural sex hormone production diminished • Prostate disease worsening (benign/local disease) • Clitoral hypertrophy • Menstrual irregularity, amenorrhea and infertility	Other	• Fluid retention resulting in peripheral edema and exacerbation of hypertension and/or congestive heart failure • Deepening of voice • Stunted growth (for adolescents) • Epiphyseal closure with decreased final adult height

physiologic anomaly. The World Anti-Doping Agency (WADA) is currently using two main methods for the detection of AAS use. An increased ratio of urine testosterone to epitestosterone ($> 4{:}1$) is confirmatory of AAS use. The biggest pitfall of this diagnostic study is that positive results can be masked by taking gonadotropins or epitestosterone. The second is the ratio of carbon 13 (C13) to carbon 12 (C12). This test is performed by using isotope mass spectrometry to measure the urinary ratio of testosterone metabolites (C13 and C12). This is currently used as a confirmatory test for people who test positive on testosterone/epitestosterone (T/E) ratio assessment. Exogenous testosterone is manufactured from plant sterols, which have a lower C13/C12 ratio, compared with their animal counterparts. The biggest advantage of C13/C12 over T/E ratio is that the results are not masked by the use of gonadotropins or epitestosterone. Furthermore, urine samples with a high ratio of testosterone to luteinizing hormone (LH) > 30 suggests AAS abuse because LH secretion is suppressed in subjects using testosterone. Detection of derivatives of testosterone can be done via gas chromatography and mass spectrometry as long as the athlete is actively taking AASs at the time of the test. Derivatives of testosterone will also lead to an increase in the T/E ratio.

19. What are some methods currently being used by professional athletes and recreational users to avoid detection of AAS?

Several methods to avoid detection have been previously described both in the literature and in anecdotal sources. The most common one is to discontinue the medication prior to laboratory testing. Urine dilution by drastically increasing fluid intake and using diuretics prior to testing are other frequent methods used. Isolated cases where substances have been directly placed in the urethra to confound test results have also been previously reported. Other methods include to simply refuse to provide urine or blood samples, and more recently, the use of designer steroids has also been reported. In 2003, the Olympic Analytical Laboratory at the University of California, Los Angeles (UCLA) discovered the first designer steroid, tetrahydrogestrinone (THG), which was manufactured by a private laboratory. The drug was could not be detected by using standard testing methods and was only confirmed by using liquid chromatography with tandem mass spectrometry.

20. What are the so-called androgen precursors, or prohormones?

These are products/supplements advertised to be metabolized to testosterone or other active metabolites. In 2004, the U.S. Congress passed the *Anabolic Steroid Control Act*, banning prohormones indefinitely. Data from the past decade are mixed, showing that acute oral ingestion of ≥ 200 mg daily of androstenedione or androstenediol modestly increases serum testosterone and circulating estrogen concentrations in men and women; however, doses < 300 mg taken for up to 12 weeks have shown no effect on body composition or physical performance.

21. What are SARMs, and are they really effective?

Selective androgen receptor modulators (SARMs) are specific nonsteroidal orally active molecules designed to bind to androgen receptors in certain tissues, such as muscle and bone. In the last decade, they have become popular as performance-enhancing drugs. None is approved for human use, and no research is available to back up their efficacy. Many of these SARMs are sold online, and the majority has inaccurate labeling. In a study of 44 SARM products purchased from the Internet and analyzed by using procedures approved by the WADA, only 18 had accurate labeling (e.g., the label showed the correct SARM and dosage). Four products contained no active compounds at all, and the remainder were inaccurately labeled (most of these products had at least one additional unapproved drug or substance [e.g., growth hormone secretagogues and/or androgens]).

22. Have androgen precursors been shown to be anabolic in men or women?

Yes, recent literature has suggested that use of suprapharmacologic doses can be anabolic in certain situations; however, the situations and mechanism of action are unclear and side effects similar to AAS apply.

23. Is AAS becoming a global public health problem?

In 2013, the Centers for Disease Control and Prevention (CDC) reported an astonishing rate of 3.2% use of AASs among high school students in the United States. The prevalence rate increased from 1991 to 2001 (2.7%–5%) and then decreased between 2001 and 2013 (5%–3.2%). The lifetime prevalence of use in high school girls and boys was 2.2% and 4%, respectively. Globally, a meta-analysis of 187 studies demonstrated that the overall global lifetime prevalence rate was 3.3% but was higher among men (6.4%) than among women (1.6%). The rate was higher among recreational athletes than among professional athletes (18.4% versus 13.3%) and varied by region (highest in the Middle East [22%] compared with other regions of the world [2%–5%]).

BIBLIOGRAPHY

108th U.S. Congress. Anabolic Steroid Control Act of 2004.

Althobiti, S. D., Alqurashi, N. M., Alotaibi, A. S., Alharthi, T. F., & Alswat, K. A. (2018). Prevalence, attitude, knowledge, and practice of anabolic androgenic steroid (AAS) use among gym participants. *Materia Socio-Medica, 30*(1), 49–52.

Ayotte, C. (2010). Detecting the administration of endogenous anabolic androgenic steroids. *Handbook of Experimental Pharmacology*, 77–98.

Basaria, S. (2010). Androgen abuse in athletes: detection and consequences. *Journal of Clinical Endocrinology and Metabolism, 95*(4), 1533–1543.

Bhasin, S., & Jameson, J. L. (2012). Disorders of the testes and male reproductive System. Harrison's Online Featuring the Complete Contents of Harrison's Principles of Internal Medicine. 18th ed. New York: McGraw-Hill, Medical Pub. Division, 2012.**

Bonci, L. (2009). DeLee J., Drez D. (eds.) Nutrition, pharmacology, and psychology in sports. In *DeLee & Drez's Orthopaedic Sports Medicine: Principles and Practice* (3rd ed., pp. 399–461). Philadelphia: Saunders.

Buckman, J. F., Farris, S. G., & Yusko, D. A. (2013). A national study of substance use behaviors among NCAA male athletes who use banned performance enhancing substances. *Drug and Alcohol Dependence, 131*(1–2), 50–55.

Chrousos, G. P. (2012). Katzung B. G., Masters S. B., Trevor A. J. (eds.) The gonadal hormones & inhibitors. In *Basic & Clinical Pharmacology* (12th ed.). New York: McGraw-Hill Medical.

Fink, J., Schoenfeld, B. J., & Nakazato, K. (2018). The role of hormone in muscle hypertrophy. *Physician and Sportsmedicine, 46*, 129–134.

Kann, L., Kinchen, S., Shanklin, S. L., Flint, K. H., Kawkins, J., Harris, W. A., . . . Zaza, S. (2014). Youth risk behavior surveillance—United States, 2013. *MMWR Supplements, 63*(4), 1.

Leder, B. Z., Leblanc, K. M., Longcope, C., Lee, H., Catlin, D. H., & Finkelstein, J. S. (2002). Effects of oral androstenedione administration on serum testosterone and estradiol levels in postmenopausal women. *Journal of Clinical Endocrinology & Metabolism, 87*(12), 5449–5454.

Matsumoto, A. M., & Bremner, W. J. (2011). Melmed S, Polonsky K., Larsen P. R., Kronenberg H. M. (eds.) Testicular disorders. In *Williams Textbook of Endocrinology* (12th ed., pp. 688–777). Philadelphia: Saunders.

Morales, A. (2012). Androgen deficiency in the aging male. In *Campbell-Walsh Urology* (10th ed., pp. 810–822). Philadelphia, PA: Elsevier/Saunders.

Nelson, J. B. (2012). Wein A. J., Kavoussi L. R., Novick A. C., Partin A. W., Peters C. A. (eds.) Hormone therapy for prostate cancer. In *Campbell-Walsh Urology* (10th ed., pp. 2934–2953). Philadelphia, PA: Elsevier/Saunders.

Parr, M. K., Laudenbach-Leschowsky, U., Höfer, N., Schänzer, W., & Diel, P. (2009). Anabolic and andogenic activity of 19-norandrostenedione after oral and subcutaneous administration – analysis of side effects and metabolism. *Toxicology Letters, 188*(2), 137–141.

Pope, H. G., Jr., & Katz, D. L. (1994). Psychiatric and medical effects of anabolic-androgenic steroid use. A controlled study of 160 athletes. *Archives of General Psychiatry, 51*(5), 375.

Sagoe, D., Molde, H., Andreassen, C. S., Torsheim, T., & Pallesen, S. (2014). The global epidemiology of anabolic-androgenic steroid use: a meta-analysis and meta-regression analysis. *Annals of Epidemiology, 24*(5), 383–398.

Steroids (Anabolic-Androgenic): Drug Facts. (2018 January). National Institute on Drug Abuse. N.p., n.d. Web. Retrieved from http://www.drugabuse.gov/publications/drugfacts/anabolic-steroids.

Tenover, J. L. (2009). Halter J. B., Ouslander J. G., Tinetti M., Studenski S., High K. P., Asthana S. (eds.) Sexuality, sexual function, androgen therapy, and the aging male. In *Hazzard's Geriatric Medicine and Gerontology* (6th ed.). New York: McGraw-Hill Medical.

Van Wagoner, R. M., Eichner, A., Bhasin, S., Deuster, P. A., & Eichner, D. (2017). Chemical composition and labeling of substances marketed as selective androgen receptor modulators and sold via the internet. *JAMA, 318*(20), 2004.

Weil, P. A. (2012). Murray R. K., Bender D. A., Botham K. M., Kennelly P. J., Rodwell V. W., Weill P. A. (eds.) The diversity of the endocrine system. In *Harper's Illustrated Biochemistry* (29th ed.). New York: McGraw-Hill Medical.

Ziegenfuss, T. N., Berardi, J. M., Lowery, L. M., & Antonio, J. (2002). Effects of prohormone supplementation in humans: a review. *Canadian Journal of Applied Physiology, 27*(6), 628–645.

VII
MISCELLANEOUS TOPICS

CHAPTER 59

AUTOIMMUNE POLYGLANDULAR SYNDROMES

Richard Millstein

1. What are autoimmune polyglandular syndromes?

   Autoimmune polyglandular syndromes (APSs) are a group of disorders characterized by the presence of ≥ 2 glandular autoimmune-mediated diseases. There are two main forms of APS: type 1 and type 2. These two syndromes share the component of autoimmune adrenal disease but differ in the immunologic processes that lead to the resulting conditions. There is also a more recently described type 3 APS.

2. What are the autoimmune endocrinopathies associated with APS 1?

   This condition is characterized by hypoparathyroidism (80%–85%), chronic mucocutaneous candidiasis (70%–80%), primary adrenal insufficiency (60%–70%), type 1 diabetes mellitus (< 20%), hypogonadism (12%), autoimmune thyroid disease (10%), and hypopituitarism (0%–2%). Candidiasis tends to be the presenting condition, and the most common accompanying conditions are hypoparathyroidism and adrenal insufficiency.

3. Are there nonendocrine autoimmune disorders associated with APS 1?

   Yes. Vitiligo, alopecia areata, autoimmune gastritis, pernicious anemia, autoimmune hepatitis, celiac disease, Sjögren's syndrome, rheumatoid arthritis, and myasthenia gravis can all be associated with APS 1.

4. At what age does APS 1 occur?

   Components of APS 1 tend to manifest within the first 20 years of life, most commonly in infancy or childhood (ages 3–5 years). APS 1 has also been called juvenile autoimmune polyglandular polyendocrinopathy or auto-immune polyendocrinopathy candidiasis–ectodermal dystrophy (APECED). The incidence of APS 1 is < 1:100,000.

5. Is there a genetic basis for APS 1?

   Yes. APS 1 is caused by mutations of the *AIRE* (Auto-Immune Regulator) gene. This gene codes for a transcription regulator that promotes central immunologic tolerance, thereby preventing the body from attacking itself. The *AIRE* gene is expressed in the thymus, lymph nodes, and peripheral blood cells.

6. What are the autoimmune endocrinopathies associated with APS 2?

   APS 2 is characterized by autoimmune thyroid disease (70%–75%), type 1 diabetes mellitus (50%–60%), primary adrenal insufficiency (40%), hypoparathyroidism (3%), and hypopituitarism (0%–2%). Mucocutaneous candidiasis is not associated with APS 2.

7. Are there nonendocrine autoimmune disorders associated with APS 2?

   Yes. These include vitiligo, alopecia areata, autoimmune gastritis, and pernicious anemia.

8. At what age does APS 2 occur?

   APS 2 will usually manifest in the third to fourth decade of life. Childhood disease is extremely rare. The appearance of more than one autoimmune disease can take years to decades to manifest.

9. Are there genetic causes of APS 2?

   Yes. APS 2 is a human leukocyte antigen (HLA)–related disorder associated with specific haplotypes within the major histocompatibility loci on chromosome 6.

10. What are Schmidt's and Carpenter's syndromes?

    Schmidt's syndrome is a combination of primary adrenal insufficiency and Hashimoto's thyroiditis, and Carpenter's syndrome is a combination of primary adrenal insufficiency and type 1 diabetes mellitus.

11. Are family members of patients with APS 2 at risk of acquiring autoimmune disorders?

    Yes. The exact risk is difficult to assess but roughly 10% of affected patients can have a family member with at least one autoimmune disease.

Table 59.1 Suggested Auto antibodies and Laboratory Testing for Autoimmune Diseases

AUTOIMMUNE DISEASE	ANTIBODY	LABORATORY
Type 1 diabetes	• Antiglutamic acid decarboxylase (GAD) antibody • Islet cell antibody • Insulin autoantibodies (IAA) • Insulinoma antigen 2 (IA-2)	Elevated blood glucose and low C-peptide level
Hypothyroidism	• Thyroid peroxidase antibody (TPO) • Antithyroglobulin antibody (TgAb)	Elevated TSH and low thyroid hormones (T_4 and/or T_3)
Graves' disease	• TSH receptor antibody (TRAB) • Thyroid-stimulating immunoglobulin (TSI)	Suppressed TSH and elevated thyroid hormones (T_4 and/or T_3)
Primary adrenal insufficiency	• 21 hydroxylase antibody	Low cortisol and elevated ACTH. Consider an ACTH stimulation test.
Hypoparathyroidism	Unknown	Low serum calcium, parathyroid hormone, and 1,25 dihydroxy vitamin D
Hypogonadism	17-alpha-hydroxylase antibody	Low estrogen/testosterone with elevated FSH/LH (postpubertal age)

ACTH, Adrenocorticotropic hormone; *FSH,* follicle-stimulating hormone; *LH,* luteinizing hormone; T_3, triiodothyronine; T_4, thyroxin; *TSH,* thyroid-stimulating hormone.

12. What is autoimmune polyglandular syndrome type 3?

Type 3 APS is defined by multiple autoimmune disorders with the exclusion of autoimmune adrenal disease.

13. What thyroid diseases are associated with all of the APSs?

Autoimmune thyroiditis (Hashimoto's thyroiditis) and/or Graves' disease are the autoimmune thyroid diseases that can be present in all of the APSs.

14. How is APS diagnosed?

Screening can be accomplished on the basis of current guidelines for the various components of APSs, discussed in separate chapters in this book. In young patients with type 1 diabetes or autoimmune adrenal failure, screening for other autoimmune diseases should be performed. In those with autoimmune adrenal disease, antibodies for type 1 diabetes mellitus, and autoimmune hypothyroidism should be assessed every 2 to 3 years. If clinical disease is present, then antibodies should be assessed (Table 59.1).

15. Is the treatment of the hormone disorders in patients with APSs different from treatment of these conditions in patients without APS?

No, but with some exceptions. Each endocrine deficiency is treated by the same medications discussed in the individual chapters devoted to those disorders in this book. However, the provider must always keep in mind that one of the other conditions in their patient's APS might not yet be diagnosed and that its appearance may affect the treatment of the other components. A few examples are worth noting.

A patient with type 1 diabetes who begins having more frequent or more severe hypoglycemic episodes without a clear explanation may have developed adrenal insufficiency. Similarly, the development of unexplained hypoglycemia or hyperglycemia in a patient with type 1 diabetes may signal the presence of hypothyroidism or hyperthyroidism, respectively. Finally, initiating levothyroxine therapy in a patient with coexisting but unrecognized adrenal insufficiency can precipitate an adrenal crisis because thyroid hormone increases the metabolic clearance rate of cortisol; if the drop in serum cortisol cannot be compensated for by increased adrenal cortisol production, an adrenal crisis can occur.

16. How do you treat mucocutaneous candidiasis?

The treatment of choice for mucocutaneous candidiasis is oral fluconazole 100 to 200 mg daily for 7 to 14 days. Response may be initially delayed if extensive skin/nail involvement is present. Fluconazole 100 mg three times weekly can be used as suppressive therapy, and itraconazole or posaconazole can be used for fluconazole-refractive disease.

KEY POINTS: AUTOIMMUNE POLYGLANDULAR SYNDROMES

- Autoimmune polyglandular syndrome type 1 (APS 1) consists of mucocutaneous candidiasis, hypoparathyroidism, and adrenal insufficiency, as well as other autoimmune conditions.
- APS 2 consists of adrenal insufficiency, type 1 diabetes mellitus, and thyroid disorders, as well as other autoimmune conditions.
- APS 1 and 2 can have nonendocrine components.
- The cause of APS type 1 involves the *AIRE* gene, whereas APS type 2 is a polygenic human leukocyte antigen (HLA)–associated disorder.

BIBLIOGRAPHY

American Diabetes Association. (2018). Pharmacologic approaches to glycemic treatment: standards of medical care in diabetes. *Diabetes Care, 41*(Suppl. 1), S73–S85.

Bahn Chair, R. S., Burch, H. B., Cooper, D. S., Garber, J. R., Greenlee, M. C., Klein, I., Laurberg P . . . Stan, M. N. (2011). Hyperthyroidism and other causes of thyrotoxicosis: management guidelines of the American Thyroid Association and American Association of Clinical Endocrinologists, *Thyroid, 21*(6), 593–646.

Betterle, C., Lazzarotto, F., & Presotto, F. (2004). Autoimmune polyglandular syndrome type 2: the tip of an iceberg. *Clinical & Experimental Immunology, 137*(2), 225–233.

Boelaert, K., Newby, P. R., Simmonds, M. J., Holder, R. L., Carr-Smith, J. D., Heward, J. M., . . . & Franklyn, J. A. (2010). Prevalence and relative risk of other autoimmune diseases in subjects with autoimmune thyroid disease. *American Journal of Medicine, 123*(2), 183.

Borstein, S. R., Allolio, B., Arlt, W., Don-Wauchope, A., Hammer, G. D., Husebye, E. S., . . . Torpy, J. J. (2016). Diagnosis and treatment of primary adrenal insufficiency: an Endocrine Society clinical practice guideline. *Journal of Clinical Endocrinology and Metabolism, 101*(2), 364–389.

Brandi, M. L., Bilzikian, J. P., Shoback, D., Bouillon, R., Clarke, B. L., Thakker, R. V., Khan AA, . . . Potts, J. T., Jr. (2016). Management of hypoparathyroidism: summary statement and guidelines. *Journal of Clinical Endocrinology and Metabolism, 101*(6), 2273–2283.

Caja, S., Mäki, M., Kaukinen, K., & Lindfors, K. (2011). Antibodies in celiac disease: implications beyond diagnostics. *Cellular & Molecular Immunology, 8*(2), 103–109.

De Martino, L., Capalbo, D., Improda, N., Lorello, P., Ungaro, C., Di Mase, R., . . . Salerno, M. (2016). Novel findings into AIRE genetics and functioning: clinical implications. *Frontiers in Pediatrics, 4*, 86.

Dittmar, M., & Kahaly, G. J. (2003). Polyglandular autoimmune syndromes: immunogenetics and long term follow-up. *Journal of Clinical Endocrinology and Metabolism, 88*(7), 2983–2992.

Erichsen, M. M., Løvås, K., Skinningsrud, B., Wolff, A. B., Undlien, D. E., Svartberg, J., . . . Husebye, E. S. (2009). Clinical, immunological, and genetic features of autoimmune primary adrenal insufficiency: observations from a Norwegian registry. *Journal of Clinical Endocrinology and Metabolism, 94*(12), 4882–4890.

Jonklass, J., Bianco, A. C., Bauer, A., Burman, K. D., Cappola, A. R., Celi, F. S., . . . Sawka, A. M. (2014). Guidelines for the treatment of hypothyroidism: prepared by the American Thyroid Association Task Force on Thyroid Hormone Replacement. *Thyroid, 24*(12), 1670–1751.

Kahaly, G. J. (2009). Polyglandular autoimmune syndromes. *European Journal of Endocrinology, 161*, 11–20.

Owen, C., & Cheetham, T. (2009). Diagnosis and management of autoimmune polyglandular syndromes. *Endocrinology and Metabolism Clinics of North America, 38*(2), 419–436.

Pappas, P. G., Kauffman, C. A., Andes, D. R., Clancy, C. J., Marr, K. A., Ostrosky-Zeichner, L., . . . Sobel, J. D. (2016). Clinical practice guidelines for the management of candidiasis: 2016 update by the Infectious Disease Society of America. *Clinical Infectious Diseases, 62*(4), e1–e50.

CHAPTER 60

MULTIPLE ENDOCRINE NEOPLASIA SYNDROMES

John J. Orrego

1. What are multiple endocrine neoplasia (MEN) syndromes?

    There are three well-defined and one recently described inherited disorders that are characterized by the occurrence of tumors involving ≥ two endocrine glands. All of these disorders are genetically transmitted in an autosomal dominant fashion. These syndromes are called MEN type 1 (MEN 1), MEN type 2A (MEN 2A), MEN type 2B (MEN 2B), and MEN type 4 (MEN 4).

2. Define MEN 1.

    MEN 1, also known as *Wermer's syndrome*, and which was first described in 1954, consists of hyperplasia or neoplastic transformation of the parathyroid glands (primary hyperparathyroidism), pancreatic islets (pancreatic neuroendocrine tumors [NETs]), and anterior pituitary gland (pituitary adenomas).

3. Define MEN 2A.

    MEN 2A, also known as *Sipple's syndrome*, first described in 1961, consists of hyperplasia or neoplastic transformation of the thyroid parafollicular cells (medullary thyroid carcinoma [MTC]), parathyroid glands (primary hyperparathyroidism), and adrenal medulla (pheochromocytoma).

4. Define MEN 2B.

    MEN 2B consists of hyperplasia or neoplastic transformation of the thyroid parafollicular cells (MTC) and adrenal medulla (pheochromocytoma) in the setting of marfanoid habitus, ocular abnormalities (enlarged corneal nerves and conjunctivitis sicca), and ganglioneuromatosis of the gastrointestinal tract.

5. Define MEN 4.

    MEN 4 describes a small subgroup of MEN 1 patients who do not harbor MEN 1 mutations but, instead, have mutations of the *CDKN1B* gene.

6. How is the diagnosis of MEN 1 made?

    The diagnosis of MEN 1 can be established by one of three criteria:
    1. *Clinical*—two or more primary MEN 1–associated endocrine tumors (parathyroid adenoma, enteropancreatic NET, and pituitary adenoma)
    2. *Familial*—one of the MEN 1–associated tumors in a first-degree relative of a patient with a clinical diagnosis of MEN 1
    3. *Genetic*—identification of a germline *MEN1* mutation in an individual, who may be asymptomatic and free of biochemical or radiologic abnormalities (mutant gene carrier)

7. How common is MEN 1?

    MEN 1 is the most common form of MEN. Its incidence is 1 in 30,000 individuals, and its prevalence is 2 to 3 per 100,000. The incidence of MEN 1 in patients with primary hyperparathyroidism, gastrinomas, and pituitary adenomas ranges from 1% to 18%, 16% to 38%, and < 3%, respectively. The syndrome is characterized by a high degree of penetrance. By age 50 years, 80% and 98% of patients with MEN 1 have developed clinical and biochemical manifestations of the disorder, respectively.

8. What are the similarities and differences between primary hyperparathyroidism in MEN 1 and its sporadic counterpart?

    Primary hyperparathyroidism associated with MEN 1 results from hyperplasia of all four glands, whereas the sporadic version is usually characterized by adenomatous change in a single gland (80%–85% of cases). Primary hyperparathyroidism is the most common and earliest manifestation of MEN 1, occurring in approximately 90% of patients. The typical age at onset in MEN 1 patients is 20 to 25 years, which contrasts with an age at onset of 50 to 60 years in sporadic cases. The former is equally common in men and women; the latter is three times more frequent in women.

    In both conditions, malignant transformation of the affected parathyroid glands is very rare. The complications resulting from primary hyperparathyroidism (bone loss, fractures, nephrolithiasis, and reduced glomerular filtration rate) are similar in both groups of patients.

9. What causes the hyperplasia of parathyroid glands affected by MEN 1?

Hyperplasia of parathyroid glands affected by MEN 1 results from expansion of multiple-cell clones, whereas sporadic parathyroid adenomas result from activation of a single-cell clone. A mitogenic factor, similar to basic fibroblast growth factor, has been found in MEN 1. It has been postulated that this factor may originate from pituitary tumors and specifically stimulate angiogenesis of parathyroid cells.

10. Summarize the therapy for hyperplastic parathyroid glands.

Therapy of both sporadic adenomas and MEN 1–associated hyperplastic glands depends on surgical resection. In sporadic primary hyperparathyroidism, removal of the solitary adenoma, when clinically indicated, is curative in 95% of cases. In MEN 1–associated hyperplasia, either subtotal parathyroidectomy (at least 3.5 glands) or total parathyroidectomy, with or without autologous parathyroid tissue graft in the forearm, is recommended to restore normocalcemia. Concurrent transcervical thymectomy is also suggested at the time of surgery. Despite this approach, persistent or recurrent hypercalcemia within 10 years is evident in 20% to 60% of patients with MEN 1, as opposed to 4% in patients without MEN 1. This recurrence rate dictates that surgery be delayed until complications of hypercalcemia are imminent or gastrin levels are elevated.

11. How common is neoplastic transformation of pancreatic islet cells in MEN 1?

Neoplastic transformation of the pancreatic islet cells is the second most common manifestation of MEN 1, occurring in approximately 40% to 70% of cases. Pancreatic NETs are commonly referred to as PNETs. These PNETs are usually multicentric and are often capable of elaborating several peptides and biogenic amines. They are classified on the basis of the clinical syndrome produced by the predominant secretory product. This group of tumors characteristically progresses from hyperplasia to malignancy, and many patients have regional lymphadenopathy and liver metastases at diagnosis, making curative resection unlikely. PNETs may arise from normal islet cells (eutopic) or cells that are not normal constituents of the adult pancreas (ectopic).

12. What are the most common enteropancreatic tumors in MEN 1?

Gastrinomas, which cause Zollinger-Ellison syndrome, are the most common functional PNETs in MEN 1 (40%–50% of cases). Excessive gastrin secretion from a gastrinoma results in high gastric acid output caused by stimulation of parietal cells and histamine-secreting enterochromaffin-like cells. In addition, gastrin-mediated histamine release also stimulates the parietal cells. Approximately 70% to 80% of gastrinomas are sporadic, but 20% to 30% occur in association with MEN 1. Compared with the former, most of the MEN 1–associated gastrinomas arise in the duodenum ($>$ 70%) and are multiple, submucosal, small ($<$ 5 mm), and less likely to have metastasized to the liver at diagnosis.

Nonfunctioning PNETs affect 20% to 55% of patients with MEN 1. Although they may synthetize peptides and hormones (i.e., pancreatic polypeptide), they do not usually cause any specific symptoms related to them. These tumors can also be malignant and metastasize to the liver.

Insulinomas are the second most common functional PNET in MEN 1 syndrome (10%–30% of cases) and the most common eutopic type. Persistent or disordered insulin secretion causes severe hypoglycemia; inappropriately elevated concentrations of insulin, proinsulin, and C-peptide are present in the serum. Insulinomas associated with MEN 1 syndrome are more frequently multicentric and malignant than are the sporadic tumors. Approximately 1% to 5% of all patients with an insulinoma are eventually discovered to have MEN 1.

Less than 1% of patients with MEN 1 harbor glucagonomas, somatostatinomas, and vasoactive intestinal peptide (VIP)omas.

13. How do patients with MEN 1–associated gastrinomas present?

Excessive gastrin secretion by these tumors causes prolific production of gastric acid with resultant multiple or refractory duodenal and jejunal ulcers, enlarged gastric folds, and diarrhea. The diagnosis is established by demonstrating hypergastrinemia in association with increased basal gastric acid secretion (gastric pH $<$ 2). Basal fasting serum gastrin levels usually exceed 300 pg/mL. A secretin stimulation test may aid in the differentiation of gastrinomas from other hypergastrinemic states; serum gastrin levels in patients with gastrinomas increase by at least 200 pg/mL after the intravenous (IV) administration of secretin.

14. What other conditions may cause hypergastrinemia?

Hypergastrinemia may result from any condition that stimulates normal gastrin secretion (hypercalcemia) or that interferes with normal gastric acid production and feedback to the G cells (achlorhydria, gastric outlet obstruction, retained antrum with a Billroth II procedure, vagotomy, and the use of histamine-2 [H_2] blockers and proton pump inhibitors [PPIs]). Primary hyperparathyroidism can, therefore, elevate serum gastrin levels in patients without gastrinomas.

15. How are gastrinomas treated?

Given that most gastrinomas in patients with MEN 1 are small, multiple, and duodenal, surgical cure is difficult. Fortunately, symptoms of hypergastrinemia can be pharmacologically controlled with administration of a PPI.

These patients usually need higher doses, and some may need the addition of an H_2 blocker. In patients with pancreatic gastrinomas > 2 cm, surgery is recommended. The rationale for this approach is that 50% to 70% of patients with tumors 2 to 3 cm in size and 25% to 40% of those with tumors > 4 cm develop lymph node and liver metastases, respectively. Gastrinomas express surface receptors for somatostatin, potentiating the use of somatostatin receptor scintigraphy in combination with annual magnetic resonance imaging (MRI)/computed tomography (CT) surveillance to monitor tumor progression.

16. Summarize the approach to treatment of hypoglycemia associated with insulinomas.
Insulinomas produce devastating hypoglycemia, which is difficult to counteract medically. Without effective long-term pharmacotherapy, surgical resection of the tumor(s) is required in most patients. Fortunately, when the largest tumor is excised, many of the patient's symptoms are alleviated. Localization is accomplished preoperatively with endoscopic ultrasonography, MRI/CT, or by comparison of insulin levels in the right hepatic vein after selective infusion of the intra-pancreatic arteries with calcium gluconate. Intraoperative ultrasonography may also assist precise localization at the time of surgery. Alternatively, discreet lesions can sometimes be effectively treated with endoscopic alcohol ablation.

17. How do pituitary tumors originate in MEN 1?
Pituitary tumors occur in 20% to 50% of cases of MEN 1. Although they usually result from neoplastic transformation of anterior pituitary cells with clonal expansion to a tumor, they can also originate from excessive stimulation of the pituitary by ectopically produced hypothalamic-releasing factors elaborated by carcinoids or pancreatic islet cells. Fortunately, despite the larger size, more aggressive behavior, and decreased response to therapy, the prevalence of pituitary carcinoma is not increased in these patients.

18. What pituitary adenomas are most commonly associated with MEN 1?
Prolactinomas are the most common pituitary tumors associated with MEN 1, constituting 60% of the total. The symptoms of hyperprolactinemia result from functional impairment of the hypothalamic–pituitary gonadal axis. Thus, women present with galactorrhea, oligorrhea/amenorrhea, and infertility; and men with decreased libido and other typical symptoms of hypogonadism. The tumors are typically multicentric and > 1 cm (macroadenomas) but respond to dopamine agonists, such as cabergoline or bromocriptine. In 15% of patients with MEN 1, a prolactinoma may be the first manifestation of this syndrome.

    The second most commonly encountered pituitary tumor type is the growth hormone (GH)–producing tumor, which is reported in 15% to 25% of patients. Overproduction of GH results in gigantism in children and acromegaly in adults. These patients have high circulating levels of GH and insulin-like growth factor-1 (IGF-1).

    Less common pituitary tumors include nonfunctioning pituitary adenomas and corticotropin (ACTH)–producing tumors that cause Cushing's syndrome.

19. Describe other endocrine tumors associated with MEN 1.
About 10% of patients with MEN 1 also have foregut carcinoids. These may be bronchopulmonary, thymic, or gastric in origin. Unlike bronchial carcinoids, which are four times more common in women, thymic carcinoids occur predominantly in men (ratio 20:1). Foregut NETs cause 50% of deaths in MEN 1. Given that most patients with bronchial and thymic carcinoids are asymptomatic and that these tumors do not usually synthetize substances that can be used as tumor markers, the screening is dependent on radiologic imaging. Type II gastric enterochromaffin-like (ECL) cell carcinoids (ECLomas) are associated with MEN 1, and gastrinoma and may be detected incidentally at the time of upper endoscopy.

    Adrenocortical tumors are present in 40% of patients with MEN 1. These are usually nonfunctioning, bilateral, and benign.

20. Are there any nonendocrine tumors associated with MEN 1?
Yes. Facial angiofibromas (40%–88%) and collagenomas (0%–72%), subcutaneous or visceral lipomas (34%), and meningiomas (8%) are tumors that are frequently found in patients with MEN 1.

21. What is a phenocopy?
Between 5% and 25% of patients with MEN 1 have no mutations of the *MEN1* gene. Although part of this variability in detecting *MEN1* mutations could be attributed to differences in methods used to identify the mutations or to phenotype ascertainment, some of these patients may represent phenocopies or have mutations involving other genes. Phenocopy is the development of typical disease manifestations associated with mutations of a specific gene, but results from another etiology.

22. What causes MEN 1?
The *MEN1* gene is located on the long arm of chromosome 11 (11q13) and consists of 10 exons that encode a 610 amino acid protein known as *menin*, which has been shown to interact with a number of proteins that are involved in genome stability, cell division and proliferation, and transcriptional regulation. Most of the *MEN1* mutations are inactivating and are consistent with those expected in a tumor-suppressor gene. To date, 1133 germline mutations have been discovered, rendering genetic screening extremely challenging. The proband

inherits an allele predisposing to MEN 1 from the affected parent, whereas a normal allele is passed down from the unaffected parent. The gene for this tumor suppressor is unusually susceptible to mutation. If a somatic mutation later inactivates the normal allele, suppressor function is lost, permitting hyperplasia of the gland to occur (Knudson's "two-hit" hypothesis).

23. At what age should screening begin?

Asymptomatic carriers of the *MEN1* mutation should be screened for biochemical and anatomic evidence of tumors. Manifestations of MEN 1 syndrome have been reported as early as 5 years of age; therefore, patients at risk should consider starting endocrine screening at that time. Nearly all people at risk develop the disorder by age 40 years; screening may be unnecessary in members older than 50 years of age who are proven to be disease free.

24. Summarize the tests used for screening of individuals with MEN 1.

In known mutant gene carriers, annual fasting testing for serum calcium, parathyroid hormone (PTH), prolactin, IGF-1, gastrin, glucose, insulin, glucagon, VIP, pancreatic polypeptide, and chromogranin A levels is recommended. CT or MRI of the abdomen annually, CT or MRI of the chest every 1 to 2 years, and MRI of the pituitary gland every 3 years, are recommended.

KEY POINTS: MEN 1

- Multiple endocrine neoplasia type 1 (MEN 1) consists of neoplastic transformation in at least two of these three glands: parathyroid glands, pancreas, and anterior pituitary.
- MEN 1 results from a mutation inactivating the menin tumor suppressor on chromosome 11. Routine clinical testing for the mutation is currently available.
- Therapy for MEN 1 includes surgical resection of hyperplastic parathyroid tissue and pituitary adenomas; surgical cure for the associated enteropancreatic tumors, which are multiple and frequently malignant, is not usually possible.
- Although patients with MEN 1 have decreased life expectancy, presymptomatic tumor detection may improve the prognosis for these patients.

---

25. How is MEN 2 subclassified?

All clinical subtypes of MEN 2 are characterized by the presence of MTC.
1. MEN 2A—this is a heritable predisposition to MTC, pheochromocytoma, and primary hyperparathyroidism. Within MEN 2A, there are four variants:
   a. Classic MEN 2A
   b. MEN 2A with cutaneous lichen amyloidosis
   c. MEN 2A with Hirschsprung's disease
   d. Familial MTC
2. MEN 2B—this is a heritable predisposition to MTC, pheochromocytoma, marfanoid habitus, mucosal neuromas, and intestinal ganglioneuromas.

26. How common is MEN 2?

All these forms of inherited MTC affect 1 in 30,000 individuals. MEN 2A accounts for 80% of hereditary MTC syndromes, compared with familial MTC and MEN 2B, which account for 15% and 5% of these patients, respectively.

27. Is the form of MTC associated with MEN 2A similar to the sporadic form of MTC?

No. MTC results from malignant transformation of the parafollicular cells (or C cells) that normally elaborate calcitonin and are scattered throughout the thyroid gland. MTC accounts for 4% to 5% of all thyroid malignancies. The sporadic form of MTC is more common (75% of all cases), occurs in a solitary form (> 80% of cases), and metastasizes to local lymphatics, lung, bone, and liver early in the course of disease. Sporadic MTC occurs more commonly in an older population (peak age 40–60 years) and is usually located in the upper two thirds of the gland.

Parafollicular cells in patients with MEN 2A characteristically progress through a state of C-cell hyperplasia to nodular hyperplasia to malignant degeneration over a variable period. MTC associated with MEN 2A is multicentric (90% at the time of diagnosis), occurs at a younger age compared with sporadic MTC (as young as 2 years), and generally has a better prognosis than the sporadic form. MTC occurs in virtually all cases of MEN 2A and is usually the first tumor to appear.

28. What are the symptoms of MTC?

In the index case, the clinical presentations and manifestations of MEN 2–associated MTC are similar to those of sporadic MTC. Most patients present with one or more palpable thyroid nodules or thyroid incidentalomas and/or clinically detectable cervical lymphadenopathy.

Systemic symptoms may be caused by hormonal secretion by the tumor. Calcitonin, calcitonin gene–related peptide, or other substances elaborated by the tumor may cause diarrhea or facial flushing. The diarrhea is secretory and affects 4% to 7% of patients at the time of diagnosis but develops in 25% to 30% during the course of the disease.

About 3% of patients with MTC develop Cushing's syndrome as a result of ectopic ACTH secretion by the tumor.

29. How is MEN 2A-associated MTC treated?

It is imperative that patients at risk be diagnosed while still in the C-cell hyperplasia stage. Total thyroidectomy precludes malignant degeneration and metastases; bilateral central neck dissection is also usually recommended at the time of the initial surgery. If frank MTC has already developed, a total thyroidectomy and bilateral central neck node dissection are the treatment of choice.

30. Is C-cell hyperplasia pathognomonic of MEN 2?

No. Patients with hereditary MTC also initially develop primary C-cell hyperplasia, which soon progresses to early invasive medullary microcarcinoma and eventually develops into grossly invasive macroscopic disease. Furthermore, secondary C-cell hyperplasia, which is not a premalignant lesion, occurs with aging, hypergastrinemia, hyperparathyroidism, and Hashimoto's thyroiditis.

Detection of primary C-cell hyperplasia with a pentagastrin or calcium stimulation test has been essentially replaced by *RET* protooncogene testing.

31. What is the second most common neoplasm associated with MEN 2A?

Pheochromocytomas develop in up to 50% of patients with MEN 2A and are bilateral in up to two thirds of the patients. They are usually benign and rarely extraadrenal. Compared with the sporadic form, pheochromocytomas associated with MEN 2A secrete greater amounts of epinephrine. Hypertension is, therefore, less common (30% of cases). Given that 5% of apparently sporadic MTC are associated with *RET* mutations, screening for coexistent pheochromocytoma is mandatory before thyroidectomy in these patients.

32. Summarize the treatment of pheochromocytomas associated with MEN 2A.

Laparoscopic surgical resection is indicated, but controversy surrounds the need for prophylactic resection of contralateral uninvolved adrenals, 50% of which develop pheochromocytomas within 10 years of the original surgery.

33. Is hyperparathyroidism associated with MEN 2A similar to that found in MEN 1?

Yes, but it is encountered much less commonly, involving only up to 30% of cases.

34. What is the genetic basis for the MEN 2A syndrome?

MEN 2A is caused by an activating mutation of the *RET* (REarranged during Transfection) protooncogene, which is located on the long arm of chromosome 10q11.2 and comprises 21 exons. The RET protein is a single-pass transmembrane receptor tyrosine kinase that transduces growth and differentiation signals in several developing tissues, including those derived from the neural crest. This protein is activated by the binding of one of its four ligands, glial cell line–derived neurotrophic factor (GDNF), neurturin, artemin, or persephin, which require their specific coreceptors. Interaction of these molecules results in dimerization of the RET protein, autophosphorylation, and phosphorylation of intracellular substrates. Thus, mutation of the *RET* protooncogene to an oncogene results in constitutive activation of the RET protein, causing unregulated phosphorylation of other critical proteins expressed in the thyroid C cells, adrenal medulla, and other tissues. Inheritance of one *RET* oncogene from one affected parent is sufficient to cause MEN 2A syndrome in the offspring. Five distinct mutations involving exons 10 and 11 have been described in 98% of 203 kindred with the disorder.

35. How should a kindred be screened after the proband with MEN 2A is identified?

Screening initially entails the differentiation of gene carriers from uninvolved family members and the subsequent delineation of organ involvement in the affected members. Direct deoxyribonucleic acid (DNA) sequencing of the *RET* protooncogene causing MEN 2A is clinically available. With appropriate repeat analysis of positive and negative test results, the assay offers near 100% accuracy in identification of affected individuals. Genetic analysis of the kindred should be performed to identify the specific *RET* oncogene mutation; characterization of the familial oncogene precludes the need for repetitive biochemical screening of noncarriers in subsequent generations.

36. How is MEN 2A treated?

Because C-cell hyperplasia has been described in gene carriers as young as 2 years of age, total thyroidectomy is suggested in affected individuals before age 5 years. The American Thyroid Association created a categorization system to guide the timing of prophylactic thyroidectomy, which is based on the specific *RET* mutation and its risk for aggressive MTC. An alternative to preemptive thyroidectomy is to perform annual pentagastrin or calcium stimulation tests and withhold surgery until a positive result is obtained.

Screening for MEN 2A-associated pheochromocytoma should be performed annually by measuring plasma or urinary fractionated metanephrines. This screening should commence by age 8 years in carriers of *RET* mutations in codons 630 and 634, and by age 20 years in carriers of other MEN 2A *RET* mutations.

Serum levels of albumin-corrected calcium or ionized calcium should be assessed every year. After the presence of the syndrome has been established, screening for adrenal and parathyroid involvement should continue through life.

37. **What comprises the MEN 2B syndrome?**
MEN 2B syndrome is the association of MTC and pheochromocytoma with multiple mucosal neuromas. Primary hyperparathyroidism is not associated with MEN 2B. This syndrome is less common than MEN 2A and is more commonly sporadic than familial, but if inherited, it is transmitted in an autosomal dominant fashion.

38. **What findings raise the suspicion of MEN 2B syndrome?**
The occurrence of multiple mucosal neuromas on the distal tongue, lips, eyelids, and along the gastrointestinal tract should always raise the possibility of MEN 2B. Other manifestations of MEN 2B include a marfanoid habitus (without ectopia lentis or aortic aneurysms), hypertrophic corneal nerves, and slipped femoral epiphysis.

39. **How should MEN 2B be treated?**
The MTC associated with this syndrome is more aggressive than other forms; metastatic lesions have been described in infancy. Because of the propensity toward early metastasis, many experts recommend that children with the syndrome should undergo total thyroidectomy as soon as surgery can be tolerated. Pheochromocytomas occur in nearly half of all patients and follow a clinical course similar to those in the MEN 2A syndrome.

40. **What is the overall mortality rate associated with MEN 2B?**
Overall mortality in MEN 2B is much higher; the average age of death among patients with MEN 2A is 60 years, whereas in patients with MEN 2B, the average age of death is 30 years.

41. **Summarize the screening recommendations for MEN 2B.**
Screening of family members with pentagastrin or calcium stimulation tests for MTC should begin at birth and continue through life if thyroidectomy is deferred. Screening for pheochromocytoma should begin at age 8 years and continue for life.

42. **What causes MEN 2B?**
More than 95% of the kindred with MEN 2B have been found to carry a mutation of the *RET* protooncogene at codon 918 (exon 16). This oncogene codes for a methionine-to-threonine substitution, resulting in activation of the innermost tyrosine kinase moiety of the same receptor associated with MEN 2A.

43. **Have the clinical presentations and prognoses of MEN syndromes changed since the time of their original descriptions?**
Yes. When MEN syndromes were initially described, most patients presented with involvement of all of the afore-mentioned organ systems because diagnostic capabilities were limited. At present, early diagnosis of the proband and aggressive screening of the kindred may permit detection of hyperplasia and prompt prophylactic surgery or medical therapy that limits morbidity and mortality.

KEY POINTS: MEN 2A AND MEN 2B

- Multiple endocrine neoplasia type 2A (MEN 2A) consists of neoplastic transformation of parathyroid glands, thyroid parafollicular C cells, and adrenal medulla.
- MEN 2B consists of neoplastic transformation of thyroid parafollicular C cells and adrenal medulla, with mucosal neuromas and marfanoid habitus.
- Genetic testing for the *RET* mutation should be offered to any patient diagnosed with medullary thyroid carcinoma.

44. **Describe MEN 4.**
MEN 4 is found in a small subgroup of patients with MEN 1 who do not harbor *MEN1* mutations but, instead, have mutations of the *CDKN1B* gene, which is located on chromosome 12p13.1 and encodes the 198 amino acid cyclin-dependent kinase inhibitor (CK1), which regulates cell motility and apoptosis. About 3% of patients with MEN 1-associated tumors, such as parathyroid adenomas, pancreatic NETs, and pituitary adenomas, meet this definition. These patients also have thyroid, adrenal, renal, and gonadal tumors. To date, eight different heterozygous loss-of-function mutations in the *CDNK1B* gene have been identified in these patients.

BIBLIOGRAPHY

Chandrasekharappa, S. C. V., Guru, S. C., Manickam, P., Olufemi, S. E., Collins, F. S., Emmert-Buck, M. R., . . . Marx, S. J. (1997) Positional cloning of the gene for multiple endocrine neoplasia type 1. *Science, 276*, 404–407.

Eng, C. (1996). The RET proto-oncogene in multiple endocrine neoplasia type 2 and Hirschsprung's disease. *New England Journal of Medicine, 335*, 943–951.

Eng, C., Clayton, D., Schuffenecker, I., Lenoir, G., Cote, G., Gagel, R. F., . . . Mulligan, L. M. (1996). The relationship between specific RET proto-oncogene mutations and disease phenotype in multiple endocrine neoplasia type 2. *JAMA, 276*, 1575–1579.

Grauer, A., Raue, F., & Gagel, R. F. (1990). Changing concepts in the management of hereditary and sporadic medullary thyroid carcinoma. *Endocrinology and Metabolism Clinics of North America, 19*, 613–635.

Hu, M. I., & Gagel, R. F. (2012). Multiple endocrine neoplasia type 2. *Translational Endocrinology & Metabolism, 2*, 45–76.

Joseph, S., Wang, Y. Z., Philip Boudreaux, J., Anthony, L. B., Campeau, R., Raines, D., . . . Woltering, E. A. (2011). Neuroendocrine tumors: current recommendations for diagnosis and surgical management. *Endocrinology and Metabolism Clinics of North America, 40*, 205–231.

Kloos, R. T., Eng, C., Evans, D. B., Francis, G. L., Gagel, R. F., Gharib, H., . . . Wells, S. A., Jr. (2009). Medullary thyroid cancer: management guidelines of the American Thyroid Association. *Thyroid, 19*, 565–612.

Lemos, M. C., & Thakker, R. V. (2008). Multiple endocrine neoplasia type 1 (MEN1): analysis of 1336 mutations reported in the first decade following identification of the gene. *Human Mutation, 29*, 22–32.

Lenders, J. W. M., Duh, Q. Y., Eisenhofer, G., Gimenez-Roqueplo, A. P., Grebe, S. K., Murad, M. H., . . . Young, W. F., Jr. (2014). Pheochromocytoma and paraganglioma: an Endocrine Society clinical practice guideline. *Journal of Clinical Endocrinology and Metabolism, 99*, 1915–1942.

Marx, S. J. (2018). Recent topics around multiple endocrine neoplasia type 1. *Journal of Clinical Endocrinology and Metabolism, 103*, 1296–1301.

Phay, J. E., Moley, J. F., & Lairmore, T. L. (2000). Multiple endocrine neoplasias. *Seminars in Surgical Oncology, 18*, 324–332.

Romei, C., Pardi, E., Cetani, F., & Elisei, R. (2012). Genetic and clinical features of multiple endocrine neoplasia types 1 and 2. *Journal of Oncology, 15*, 1–15.

Santoro, M., Carlomagno, F., Romano, A., Bottaro, D. P., Dathan, N. A., Grieco, M., . . . Kraus, M. H. (1995). Activation of RET as a dominant transforming gene by germline mutations of MEN-IIa and MEN-IIb. *Science, 267*, 381–383.

Thakker, R. V. (2012). Multiple endocrine neoplasia type 1. *Translational Endocrinology & Metabolism, 2*, 13–44.

Thakker, R. V., Newey, P. J., Walls, G. V., Bilezikian, J., Dralle, H., Ebeling, P. R., . . . Brandi, M. L. (2012). Clinical practice guidelines for multiple endocrine neoplasia type 1 (MEN1). *Journal of Clinical Endocrinology and Metabolism, 97*, 2990–3011.

Thakker, R. V. (2014). Multiple endocrine neoplasia type 1 (MEN1) and type 4 (MEN4). *Molecular and Cellular Endocrinolology, 386*, 2–15.

Tham, E., Grandell, U, Lindgren, E., Toss, G., Skogseid, B., & Nordenskjöld, M. (2007). Clinical testing for mutations in the MEN-I gene in Sweden: a report of 200 unrelated cases. *Journal of Clinical Endocrinology and Metabolism, 92*, 3389–3395.

Vinik, A. I., & Gonzales, M. R. (2011). New and emerging syndromes due to neuroendocrine tumors. *Endocrinology and Metabolism Clinics of North America, 40*, 19–63.

Wells, S. A., Jr., Pacini, F., Robinson, B. G., & Santoro, M. (2013). Multiple endocrine neoplasia type 2 and familial medullary thyroid carcinoma: an update. *Journal of Clinical Endocrinology and Metabolism, 98*, 3149–3164.

Wells, S. A., Jr., Asa, S. L., Dralle, H., Elisei, R., Evans, D. B., Gagel, R. F., . . . Waguespack, S. G. (2015). Revised American Thyroid Association Guidelines for the Management of Medullary Thyroid Carcinoma. *Thyroid, 25*, 567–610.

CHAPTER 61

PANCREATIC NEUROENDOCRINE TUMORS

Michael T. McDermott

1. **What are the pancreatic neuroendocrine tumors?**

   Pancreatic neuroendocrine tumors (PNETs) are neuroendocrine tumors that arise in the pancreas, most commonly in the islets of Langerhans. Most PNETs (50%–75%) are nonfunctioning—that is, they either do not produce any hormones or do not produce hormones that result in a clinical syndrome. Functioning PNETs are generally named for the hormones they secrete. These include insulinomas, gastrinomas, glucagonomas, somatostatinomas, and vasoactive intestinal polypeptide tumors (VIPomas). PNETs can also occasionally secrete adrenocorticotropic hormone (ACTH), corticotropin-releasing factor (CRF), and growth hormone–releasing factor (GRF) (Fig. 61.1).

2. **Are pancreatic neuroendocrine tumors usually benign or malignant?**

   Insulinomas are usually benign (80%–90%); other pancreatic endocrine tumors are frequently malignant and metastatic at presentation (50%–80%).

3. **Are pancreatic neuroendocrine tumors associated with other endocrine disorders?**

   PNETs are usually sporadic tumors but can also be part of inherited endocrine tumor syndromes, such as multiple endocrine neoplasia type 1 (MEN 1), Von Hippel–Lindau (VHL) syndrome, and neurofibromatosis type 1 (NF-1). PNETs occur in ~80% to 100% of patients with MEN 1, in ~20% of patients with VHL, and in ~10% of those with NF-1. PNETs also occur in ~1% of patients with tuberous sclerosis.

4. **What are insulinomas?**

   Insulinomas are insulin-producing tumors within the pancreas. They belong to a larger group of hyperinsulinemic pancreatic beta-cell disorders that include solitary and multiple insulinomas, islet cell hyperplasia, and nesidio-blastosis (neoproliferation of beta cells along the pancreatic ducts).

5. **What is Whipple's triad?**
   - Hypoglycemia
   - Symptoms during hypoglycemia
   - Relief of symptoms with correction of hypoglycemia

6. **What glucose levels indicate hypoglycemia?**

   Glucose levels < 55 mg/dL commonly indicate hypoglycemia, but the best criteria for hypoglycemia continue to be controversial.

7. **What are the symptoms of hypoglycemia?**

   Hypoglycemia symptoms are classified by type and timing in relation to meals. Neuroglycopenia symptoms (confusion, slurred speech, blurred vision, seizures, coma) result from inadequate glucose delivery to the brain. Adrenergia symptoms (tremors, sweating, palpitations, nausea) result from catecholamine discharges. Symptoms that occur within 4 to 5 hours after a meal are considered "postprandial"; those occurring > 5 hours after meals are considered "fasting." Neuroglycopenia symptoms are characteristic of insulinomas, but adrenergic symptoms may also occur. Insulinomas most commonly cause fasting hypoglycemia (73%), but both fasting and postprandial hypoglycemia (21%) and pure postprandial hypoglycemia (6%) may be seen.

8. **What evaluation should be done to test for insulinoma?**

   Blood samples obtained during an episode of witnessed hypoglycemia are very helpful, but more often, the conditions that provoke the hypoglycemia must be replicated. This is most commonly done with a prolonged fast (supervised 72-hour fast or screening outpatient 12- to 18-hour fast). For this procedure, patients are allowed to drink calorie-free, caffeine-free beverages only. Blood is drawn every 6 hours until the glucose is < 60 mg/dL and then every 1 to 2 hours. Sufficient blood is obtained for measurement of glucose, insulin, C-peptide, proinsulin, and beta-hydroxybutyrate; glucose is measured immediately on all samples, and the other tests are run only on samples for which the glucose is < 55 mg/dL. Insulin antibodies are ordered on one sample, and a serum or urine sample is sent for sulfonylureas and meglitinides. The test is stopped when the patient has typical symptoms, when the glucose level is < 55 mg/dL (if Whipple's triad was previously demonstrated) or < 45 mg/dL

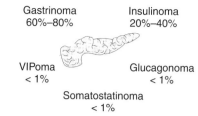

Gastrinoma
60%–80%

Insulinoma
20%–40%

VIPoma
< 1%

Glucagonoma
< 1%

Somatostatinoma
< 1%

Fig. 61.1 Pancreatic islet cell tumors. *VIPoma,* vasoactive intestinal polypeptide tumors.

Table 61.1. Diagnostic Criteria for Insulinoma: Demonstration of Hypoglycemia with Endogenous Hyperinsulinemia.

TEST	THRESHOLD	SENSITIVITY	SPECIFICITY[a]
Glucose	< 55 mg/dL		
Insulin	≥ 3 uU/mL	93%	95%
C-peptide	≥ 0.6 ng/mL	100%	60%
Proinsulin	≥ 5 pmol/L	100%	68%
Beta-hydroxybutyrate	≤ 2.7 mmol/L	100%	100%
Glucose rise after glucagon	≥ 25 mg/dL	91%	95%
Insulin antibodies	Negative		
Sulfonylurea screen	Negative		
Meglitinide screen	Negative		

[a]Compared with normal controls who developed glucose < 60 mg/dL during a 72-hour fast.

(if Whipple's triad was not previously demonstrated), or at the end of 72 hours. At the end of the test, glucagon 1 mg is given intravenously, and glucose is measured 10, 20, and 30 minutes later.

9. What are the diagnostic criteria for insulinomas?
   Hypoglycemia with endogenous hyperinsulinemia must be demonstrated to diagnose insulinoma. Diagnostic criteria are shown in Table 61.1.

10. How can insulinomas be localized?
    Cross-sectional imaging of the pancreas with computed tomography (CT) or magnetic resonance imaging (MRI) is usually the first localization procedure; reported sensitivities of these techniques vary from 15% to 90%. Endoscopic ultrasonography of the pancreas has higher sensitivity (56%–93%) and can detect tumors as small as 2 to 3 mm in size. Intraarterial pancreatic calcium infusion, with measurement of insulin changes in the right hepatic vein, yields similar or superior results but is more invasive. Intraoperative ultrasonography is highly accurate and useful for finding small tumors that could not be localized preoperatively. Cross-sectional imaging also provides the best results in finding metastatic disease because metastatic spread from malignant insulinomas is usually to the liver and regional lymph nodes.

11. What is the treatment for insulinomas?
    Surgery is the treatment of choice. When surgery is not desired or feasible, symptom relief can sometimes be achieved with dietary management (multiple small meals per day) and medical therapy to inhibit insulin secretion with diazoxide, somatostatin analogues (octreotide LAR, lanreotide, and possibly pasireotide), or calcium channel blockers. Malignant insulinomas can show partial responses to cytotoxic chemotherapy (streptozotocin with doxorubicin or 5-fluorouracil). Other considerations may include everolimus, an inhibitor of mammalian target of rapamycin (mTOR), sunitinib, and other inhibitors of vascular endothelial growth factor receptor (VEGF-R), and peptide receptor radioligand therapy with radiolabeled somatostatin analogues, such as 177-Lu DOTATATE, 90-Y edotreotide, or 90-Y DOTA tyr3-octreotide.

12. What are the clinical manifestations of gastrinomas?
    Gastrinomas secrete excessive gastrin, which stimulates prolific gastric acid secretion. Patients develop severe peptic ulcer disease, often associated with secretory diarrhea. This disorder is also known as *Zollinger-Ellison syndrome.*

13. Do gastrinomas always arise from pancreatic islet cells?

Gastrinomas may arise from the pancreatic islets (25%) but more commonly occur in the duodenum (70%).

14. How is the diagnosis of gastrinomas made?

Gastrinomas are diagnosed by demonstrating a fasting serum gastrin level > 1000 pg/mL associated with high gastric acidity (pH ≦ 4.0). For moderately elevated serum gastrin levels (110–1000 pg/mL), a secretin test should be conducted. A gastrin increment of ≧ 200 pg/mL 15 minutes after intravenous (IV) secretin administration is also diagnostic of this condition. Patients should be off proton pump inhibitor therapy for 1 week prior to testing for gastrinomas.

15. What is the best way to localize gastrinomas?

Localization of gastrinomas may be pursued with various techniques, including CT, MRI, endoscopic ultrasonography, somatostatin receptor–based functional imaging (68-Ga DOTATATE or In-111 pentetreotide), transhepatic portal venous sampling, and selective arterial secretin infusions with right hepatic vein gastrin measurements.

16. How are gastrinomas managed?

Most benign and some malignant gastrinomas can be cured with surgery. Otherwise, attention should be directed toward reducing gastric acid overproduction and secretory diarrhea. Proton pump inhibitors, in high doses, are the medications of choice for this purpose. Somatostatin analogues (octreotide LAR, lanreotide) are also effective agents. High-dose histamine-2 blockers may be useful but are rarely adequate by themselves. Patients with refractory disease may require total gastrectomy and vagotomy for symptom relief.

17. How do you treat malignant gastrinomas?

Gastrinomas are usually malignant, and therefore, antitumor therapy is often necessary. Because liver metastases are common, hepatic-directed therapies, such as partial resection, hepatic artery embolization, and liver transplantation, may be considered. Streptozotocin–doxorubicin combination therapy is the most commonly used cytotoxic regimen for malignant pancreatic endocrine tumors. Other potential approaches that have shown some success include everolimus, an inhibitor of mTOR, sunitinib, and other VEGF-R inhibitors, and peptide receptor radioligand therapy using radiolabeled somatostatin analogues such as 177-Lu DOTATATE, 90-Y edotreotide, or 90-Y DOTA tyr3-octreotide.

18. What are the characteristics of glucagonomas?

Glucagon antagonizes insulin action in the liver by stimulating both glycogenolysis and gluconeogenesis. Glucagonomas secrete excessive glucagon, causing diabetes mellitus, weight loss, anemia, and necrolytic migratory erythema, which is a characteristic skin rash. Affected individuals also have an increased risk of thromboembolic events. The diagnosis of a glucagonoma is made by finding a significantly elevated level of serum glucagon (> 500 pg/mL); however, some glucagonomas show only modest hyperglucagonemia. In these cases, other causes of mild-to-moderate glucagon elevations, such as fasting, hypoglycemia, renal failure, liver failure, pancreatitis, sepsis, and trauma, must be ruled out. Techniques similar to those used for gastrinomas are useful for localization.

19. How are glucagonomas treated?

Treatment options include surgery for localized disease, somatostatin analogues (octreotide LAR, lanreotide) to reduce glucagon secretion, hepatic-directed therapies, chemotherapy regimens, and peptide receptor radioligand agents similar to those used for treating gastrinomas. Chronic anticoagulation to reduce the risk of thromboembolic events should also be considered. Finally, zinc supplements and intermittent amino acid infusions may help reduce the skin rash (necrolytic migratory erythema) and to improve the patient's overall sense of well-being.

20. What are the characteristics of somatostatinomas?

Among its multiple systemic effects, somatostatin inhibits secretion of insulin and pancreatic enzymes, production of gastric acid, and gallbladder contraction. Somatostatinomas secrete excess somatostatin, causing diabetes mellitus, weight loss, steatorrhea, hypochlorhydria, and cholelithiasis. The diagnosis is made by finding a significantly elevated serum somatostatin level.

KEY POINTS: PANCREATIC ENDOCRINE TUMORS

1. Insulinomas most often cause fasting hypoglycemia with neuroglycopenic symptoms but sometimes cause mainly postprandial symptoms.
2. Suspected insulinomas are investigated by measuring serum glucose, insulin, C-peptide, proinsulin, beta-hydroxybutyrate, and a sulfonylurea screen during a symptomatic episode or a supervised fast.
3. Insulinomas are treated by surgical resection, when possible, or multiple frequent feedings or medications, such as diazoxide, somatostatin analogues, or calcium channel blockers.
4. Gastrinomas (Zollinger-Ellison syndrome) cause aggressive peptic ulcer disease, which is sometimes associated with secretory diarrhea.

KEY POINTS: PANCREATIC ENDOCRINE TUMORS—cont'd

5. Gastrinomas are diagnosed by finding a markedly elevated serum gastrin or a prominent increase in gastrin after intravenous secretin administration in a patient with significant gastric acidity.
6. Gastrinomas are treated by surgical resection, if possible, or reduction of gastric acid production by high-dose proton pump inhibitors, somatostatin analogs, or a gastrectomy, if necessary.

21. What is the treatment for somatostatinomas?

Surgery is the treatment of choice. When surgery is not possible, the same general treatment options as discussed above for gastrinomas should be considered. However, somatostatin analogue therapy (octreotide LAR, lanreotide) should be avoided.

22. What are the characteristics of VIPomas?

VIPomas cause watery diarrhea, hypokalemia, and achlorhydria (WDHA) syndrome. The diagnosis is made by finding a significantly elevated serum VIP level. This is also known as *Verner-Morrison syndrome* or *pancreatic cholera*.

23. How are VIPomas treated?

Surgery is the treatment of choice. Somatostatin analogues effectively reduce diarrhea in most patients. Radiation therapy and chemotherapy also may effectively reduce diarrhea and tumor size.

24. Briefly discuss other types of pancreatic neuroendocrine tumors.

Other types of pancreatic neuroendocrine tumors are rare. ACTH- and CRF-secreting tumors lead to the development of Cushing's syndrome, and GRF-secreting tumors cause acromegaly. Localization procedures and treatments are similar to those described earlier for other pancreatic neuroendocrine tumors.

BIBLIOGRAPHY

Auernhammer, C. J., Spitzweg, C., Angele, M. K., Boeck, S., Grossman, A., Nölting, S., . . . Bartenstein, P. (2018). Advanced neuroendocrine tumours of the small intestine and pancreas: clinical developments, controversies, and future strategies. *Lancet Diabetes & Endocrinology, 6,* 404–415.

Bainbridge, H. E., Larbi, E., & Middleton, G. (2015). Symptomatic control of neuroendocrine tumours with everolimus. *Hormones & Cancer, 6,* 254–259.

Bousquet, C., Lasfargues, C., Chalabi, M., Billah, S. M., Susini, C., Vezzosi, D., . . . Pyronnet, S. (2012). Clinical review: current scientific rationale for the use of somatostatin analogs and mTOR inhibitors in neuroendocrine tumor therapy. *Journal of Clinical Endocrinology and Metabolism, 97,* 727–737.

Caplin, M. E., Pavel, M., Ćwikła, J. B., Phan, A. T., Raderer, M., Sedláčková, E., . . . Ruszniewski, P. (2014). Lanreotide in metastatic enteropancreatic neuroendocrine tumors. *New England Journal of Medicine, 371,* 224–233.

Cho, J. H., Ryu, J. K., Song, S. Y., Hwang, J. H., Lee, D. K., Woo, S. M., . . . Lee, W. J. (2016). Prognostic validity of the American Joint Committee on Cancer and the European Neuroendocrine Tumors Staging Classifications for Pancreatic Neuroendocrine Tumors: a retrospective nationwide multicenter study in South Korea. *Pancreas, 45,* 941–946.

Cryer, P. E., Axelrod, L., Grossman, A. B., Heller, S. R., Montori, V. M., Seaquist, E. R., & Service, F. J. (2009). Evaluation and management of adult hypoglycemic disorders: an Endocrine Society Clinical Practice Guideline. *Journal of Clinical Endocrinology and Metabolism, 94,* 709–728.

Dasari, A., Shen, C., Halperin, D., Zhao, B., Zhou, S., Xu, Y., . . . Yao, J. C. (2017). Trends in the incidence, prevalence, and survival outcomes in patients with neuroendocrine tumors in the United States. *JAMA Oncology, 3,* 1335–1342.

Deppen, S. A., Liu, E., Blume, J. D., Clanton, J., Shi, C., Jones-Jackson, L. B., . . . Walker, R. C. (2016). Safety and efficacy of 68Ga-DOTATATE PET/CT for diagnosis, staging, and treatment management of neuroendocrine tumors. *Journal of Nuclear Medicine, 57,* 708–714.

Garske-Román, U., Sandström, M., Fröss Baron, K., Lundin, L., Hellman, P., Welin, S., . . . Granberg, D. (2018). Prospective observational study of ^{177}Lu DOTA-octreotate therapy in 200 patients with advanced metastasized neuroendocrine tumours (NETs): feasibility and impact of a dosimetry-guided study protocol on outcome and toxicity. *European Journal of Nuclear Medicine and Molecular Imaging, 45,* 970–988.

Guettier, J. M., Kam, A., Chang, R., Skarulis, M. C., Cochran, C., Alexander, H. R., . . . Gorden, P. (2009). Localization of insulinomas to regions of the pancreas by intraarterial calcium stimulation: the NIH Experience. *Journal of Clinical Endocrinology and Metabolism, 94,* 1074–1080.

Hicks, R. J., Kwekkeboom, D. J., Krenning, E., Bodei, L., Grozinsky-Glasberg, S., Arnold, R., . . . Ramage, J. (2017). ENETS Consensus guidelines for the standards of care in neuroendocrine neoplasia: peptide receptor radionuclide therapy with radiolabeled somatostatin analogues. *Neuroendocrinology, 105*(3), 295–309.

James, P. D., Tsolakis, A. V., Zhang, M., Belletrutti, P. J., Mohamed, R., Roberts, D. J., & Heitman, S. J. (2015). Incremental benefit of preoperative EUS for the detection of pancreatic neuroendocrine tumors: a meta-analysis. *Gastrointestinal Endoscopy, 81,* 848–856.e1.

Kaltsas, G., Caplin, M., Davies, P., Ferone, D., Garcia-Carbonero, R., Grozinsky-Glasberg, S., . . . de Herder, W. W. (2017). ENETS Consensus guidelines for the standards of care in neuroendocrine tumors: pre- and perioperative therapy in patients with neuroendocrine tumors. *Neuroendocrinology, 105*(3), 245–254.

Kasumova, G. G., Tabatabaie, O., Eskander, M. F., Tadikonda, A., Ng, S. C., & Tseng, J. F. (2017). National rise of primary pancreatic carcinoid tumors: comparison to functional and nonfunctional pancreatic neuroendocrine tumors. *Journal of the American College of Surgeons, 224,* 1057–1064.

Kiesewetter, B., & Raderer, M. (2013). Ondansetron for diarrhea associated with neuroendocrine tumors. *New England Journal of Medicine, 368*, 1947–1948.

Knigge, U., Capdevila, J., Bartsch, D. K., Baudin, E., Falkerby, J., Kianmanesh, R., . . . Vullierme, M. P. (2017). ENETS consensus recommendations for the standards of care in neuroendocrine neoplasms: follow-up and documentation. *Neuroendocrinology, 105*(3), 310–319.

Krejs, G. J., Orci, L., Conlon, M., Ravazzola, M., Davis, G. R., Raskin, P., . . . Unger, R. H. (1979). Somatostatinoma syndrome: biochemical, morphologic and clinical features. *New England Journal of Medicine, 301*, 283–292.

Leichter, S. B. (1980). Clinical and metabolic aspects of glucagonoma. *Medicine, 59*, 100–113.

Leoncini, E., Carioli, G., La Vecchia, C., Boccia, S., & Rindi, G. (2016). Risk factors for neuroendocrine neoplasms: a systematic review and meta-analysis. *Annals of Oncology, 27*, 68–81.

Luo, G., Javed, A., Strosberg, J. R., Jin, K., Zhang, Y., Liu, C., . . . Yu, X. (2017). Modified staging classification for pancreatic neuroendocrine tumors on the basis of the American Joint Committee on Cancer and European Neuroendocrine Tumor Society Systems. *Journal of Clinical Oncology, 35*, 274–280.

Oberg, K., Couvelard, A., Delle Fave, G., Gross, D., Grossman, A., Jensen, R. T., . . . Ferone, D. (2017). ENETS consensus guidelines for standard of care in neuroendocrine tumours: biochemical markers. *Neuroendocrinology, 105*(3), 201–211.

Partelli, S., Bartsch, D. K., Capdevila, J., Chen, J., Knigge, U., Niederle, B., . . . Falconi, M. (2017). ENETS consensus guidelines for standard of care in neuroendocrine tumours: surgery for small intestinal and pancreatic neuroendocrine tumours. *Neuroendocrinology, 105*(3), 255–265.

Placzkowski, K. A., Vella, A., Thompson, G. B., Grant, C. S., Reading, C. C., Charboneau, J. W., . . . Service, F. J. (2009). Secular trends in the presentation and management of functioning insulinoma at the Mayo Clinic, 1987–2007. *Journal of Clinical Endocrinology and Metabolism, 94*, 1069–1073.

Sadowski, S. M., Neychev, V., Millo, C., Shih, J., Nilubol, N., Herscovitch, P., . . . Kebebew, E. (2016). Prospective study of ^{68}Ga-DOTATATE positron emission tomography/computed tomography for detecting gastro-entero-pancreatic neuroendocrine tumors and unknown primary sites. *Journal of Clinical Oncology, 34*, 588–596.

Sbardella, E., & Grossman, A. (2016). New developments in the treatment of neuroendocrine tumours – RADIANT-4, NETTER-1 and telotristat etiprate. *European Endocrinology, 12*, 44–46.

Sundin, A., Arnold, R., Baudin, E., Cwikla, J. B., Eriksson, B., Fanti, S., . . . Vullierme, M. P. (2017). ENETS consensus guidelines for the standards of care in neuroendocrine tumors: radiological, nuclear medicine & hybrid imaging. *Neuroendocrinology, 105*(3), 212–244.

van Schaik, E., van Vliet, E. I., Feelders, R. A., Krenning, E. P., Khan, S., Kamp, K., . . . de Herder, W. W. (2011). Improved control of severe hypoglycemia in patients with malignant insulinomas by peptide receptor radionuclide therapy. *Journal of Clinical Endocrinology and Metabolism, 96*, 3381–3389.

Wermers, R. A., Fatourechi, V., Wynne, A. G., Kvols, L. K., & Lloyd, R. V. (1996). The glucagonoma syndrome. Clinical and pathologic features in 21 patients. *Medicine, 75*, 53–63.

Yao, J. C., Shah, M. H., Ito, T., Bohas, C. L., Wolin, E. M., Van Cutsem, E., . . . Öberg, K. (2011). Everolimus for advanced pancreatic neuroendocrine tumors. *New England Journal of Medicine, 364*, 514–523.

Zhang, J., Wang, H., Jacobson, O., Cheng, Y., Niu, G., Li, F., . . . Chen, X. (2018). Safety, pharmacokinetics, and dosimetry of a long-acting radiolabeled somatostatin analog ^{177}Lu-DOTA-EB-TATE in patients with advanced metastatic neuroendocrine tumors. *Journal of Nuclear Medicine, 59*, 1699–1705.

CHAPTER 62

CARCINOID SYNDROME

Michael T. McDermott

1. What are carcinoid tumors, and how are they classified?

Carcinoid tumors are neoplasms that arise from enterochromaffin cells. Today, a more common term for these tumors is *neuroendocrine tumors (NETs).* They are classified according to their site of origin, as foregut carcinoids (bronchus, stomach, duodenum, bile ducts, pancreas), midgut carcinoids (jejunum, ileum, appendix, cecum, ascending colon), or hindgut carcinoids (transverse and descending colon, rectum). Pulmonary NETs are still commonly referred to as *carcinoids,* but when they occur elsewhere, the term *NET*, as proposed by the World Health Organization (WHO) is preferred. Less commonly, NETs can develop in the ovaries, testes, prostate, kidney, breast, thymus, or skin. Approximately 55% of NETs occur in the gastrointestinal (GI) tract, and 30% are found in the bronchopulmonary system. Malignant NETs are referred to as *neuroendocrine carcinomas.*

2. Define carcinoid syndrome.

Carcinoid syndrome refers to a group of symptoms that occur when NETs secrete large amounts of various humoral substances into the systemic circulation. The most common features are cutaneous flushing (85%–90%), secretory diarrhea (75%–80%), bronchospasm (10%–20%), and fibrotic growths involving the endocardium and right heart valves (33%) and sometimes pleural, peritoneal, or retroperitoneal fibrosis. Carcinoid syndrome does not cause hypertension but may cause hypotension, especially during prolonged flushing spells. Carcinoid syndrome most often results from midgut NETs (jejunum, ileum, appendix, cecum, ascending colon) that have metastasized to the liver. Carcinoid syndrome is only rarely associated with foregut and hindgut NETs.

3. Describe the flushing that occurs in carcinoid syndrome.

The classic carcinoid flush that occurs with midgut NETS is characterized by sudden episodes of reddish-to-purplish flushing of the face, neck, and chest associated with cutaneous burning, lasting anywhere from 30 seconds to 30 minutes. More severe or prolonged flushing episodes may be associated with hypotension and tachycardia. Telangiectasias eventually develop on the malar areas, nose, and upper lip as a result of prolonged vasodilation in the cutaneous vasculature.

  Gastric NET flushing is more often patchy, serpiginous, bright red, and intensely pruritic. Pulmonary NET flushing can be prolonged (hours to days) and more severe, and may be associated with hypotension, tachycardia, anxiety, disorientation, periorbital edema, lacrimation, salivation, dyspnea, wheezing, and diarrhea.

4. What are the biochemical mediators of carcinoid syndrome?

Carcinoid syndrome results from humoral mediators secreted by NETs that reach the systemic circulation. Carcinoid syndrome does not usually occur with midgut NETs unless there are extensive liver metastases that impair mediator metabolism in the liver or that secrete mediators directly into the circulation via the hepatic vein. Extraintestinal carcinoids may cause carcinoid syndrome without liver metastases because mediators from these tumors are not secreted into the portal veins.

  Serotonin, histamine, kallikrein, bradykinin, tachykinins, and prostaglandins are considered the most important humoral mediators (Fig. 62.1). Histamine is the main mediator of flushing; kallikrein, bradykinin, and tachykinins may contribute in some cases. Serotonin is the primary mediator of diarrhea and fibrous tissue formation in the heart, serosal tissues (pleural, peritoneal), and retroperitoneal spaces; kinins and prostaglandins may also contribute to the secretory diarrhea. The formation and metabolism of serotonin are shown in Fig. 62.2.

5. Why does niacin deficiency and pellagra often accompany carcinoid syndrome?

Niacin deficiency occurs in carcinoid syndrome because large amounts of tryptophan are diverted from niacin synthesis to produce serotonin (see Fig. 62.2). This can result in the classic features of pellagra—glossitis, angular stomatitis, rough scaly skin, mental confusion, and hypoproteinemia.

6. Do carcinoid tumors cause any other humoral syndromes?

Carcinoids may also secrete corticotropin-releasing factor (CRF) or corticotropin (adrenocorticotropin [ACTH]), causing Cushing's syndrome, or growth hormone–releasing factor (GRF), causing acromegaly. These syndromes have been reported mainly with bronchial and pancreatic carcinoid tumors.

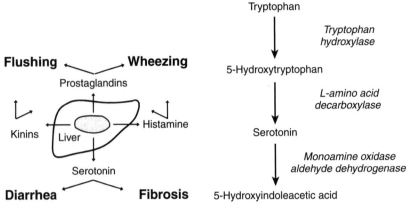

Fig. 62.1. Carcinoid syndrome.

Fig. 62.2. Serotonin metabolism.

KEY POINTS: CARCINOID SYNDROME

- Carcinoid syndrome results from metastatic neuroendocrine tumors (NETs), which produce multiple humoral mediators that cause flushing, diarrhea, bronchospasm, and fibrosis of the endocardium, heart valves, pleura, peritoneum, and retroperitoneal spaces.
- Most patients with carcinoid syndrome have extensive liver metastases that impair the metabolic clearance of mediators secreted by the primary tumor or that secrete the mediators directly into the systemic circulation via the hepatic vein.
- Carcinoid syndrome is usually diagnosed by demonstrating markedly increased urinary excretion of 5-hydroxyindoleacetic acid (5-HIAA).
- Cross-sectional imaging with computed tomography (CT) or magnetic resonance imaging (MRI) is the best way to localize tumors that cause carcinoid syndrome with complementary use of somatostatin receptor-based functional imaging for tumors that cannot be localized with CT or MRI.
- The treatment for carcinoid syndrome is surgical removal of the primary tumor, when possible, or palliation of symptoms by giving medications that reduce secretion of the humoral mediators or antagonize their effects.
- Carcinoid crisis can be precipitated when a patient with carcinoid syndrome or a secreting carcinoid tumor has a procedure of or other manipulation of the carcinoid tumor, or is given an adrenergic or sympathomimetic medication or a monoamine oxidase inhibitor (MAOI).
- Carcinoid crisis is best treated with intravenous octreotide and hydrocortisone, but the use of adrenergic and sympathomimetic agents for the hypotension should be avoided.

---

7. How is the diagnosis of carcinoid syndrome usually made?

Carcinoid syndrome caused by midgut NETs (jejunum, ileum, appendix, cecum, ascending colon) is diagnosed by demonstrating markedly elevated 24-hour urinary 5-HIAA excretion; 5-HIAA is a breakdown product of serotonin (see Fig. 62.2). Normal urinary 5-HIAA excretion is < 8 mg/24 hr. Other causes of mild-to-moderate 5-HIAA elevations are shown in Table 62.1; excretion of 5-HIAA is usually < 30 mg/24 hr in these situations. Carcinoid syndrome is most often associated with urinary 5-HIAA excretion > 100 mg/24 hr, although only mild or normal values may be seen in some patients. Patients should avoid foods that are rich in tryptophan and/or serotonin and medications, which can produce false positive or false negative 5-HIAA results, for 3 days prior to and on the day of collection of the 24-hour urine specimen (Table 62.1).

Table 62.1. Causes of Abnormal 5-Hydroxyindoleacetic Acid (5-HIAA) Excretion Other than Carcinoid Syndrome.

Diseases—malabsorption disorders

Food (tryptophan rich)—bananas, pineapples, kiwi, plums, avocados, eggplant, pecans, walnuts, hickory nuts

Medications that increase 5-HIAA—acetaminophen, ephedrine, guaifenesin, mephenesin, methocarbamol, phenacetin, caffeine, nicotine, methamphetamine, phenobarbital, acetanilid, reserpine, phentolamine, phenmetrazine, coumaric acid, melphalan, fluorouracil

8. How is carcinoid syndrome diagnosed if urinary 5-HIAA is normal?

Foregut carcinoid tumors usually lack the enzyme L-amino acid decarboxylase and, therefore, do not convert 5-hydroxytryptophan to serotonin; serotonin and 5-HIAA values are, therefore, usually normal (see Fig. 62.2). Assays for 5-hydroxytryptophan are not available. Whole-blood serotonin, platelet-rich plasma serotonin, and urinary serotonin assays are available, but their performance characteristics have not yet been established. Accordingly, they are not recommended as routine screening tools; nonetheless, these measurements may be useful in select patients. Similarly, a plasma 5-HIAA assay has been developed, but its usefulness for diagnosing carcinoid syndrome has not been well evaluated, and the test itself is not widely available.

Chromogranins A, B, and C are secreted by multiple types of NETs. Chromogranin A is often significantly elevated in carcinoid syndrome, but there are numerous other conditions and medications (especially proton pump inhibitors) that can elevate serum chromogranin A levels. Because elevations are nonspecific, serum chromogranin A is not recommended as a routine screening test for carcinoid syndrome. Proceeding directly to imaging of the abdomen, pelvis, and chest is often the best option.

9. What procedures are the best to localize the source of carcinoid syndrome?

Cross-sectional imaging with multiphasic contrast-enhanced CT scanning of the areas of suspected tumor location (usually starting with the abdomen and pelvis) is the best initial imaging study. Some authorities prefer MRI because of its superior detection of hepatic metastases. Somatostatin-based functional imaging with 68-Ga DOTATATE or In-111 pentetreotide (octreoscan) is an imaging technique that is particularly useful when a tumor is not detected with cross-sectional imaging. When available, 68-Ga DOTATATE is the preferred functional imaging agent because of demonstrated superior performance.

10. What is the treatment for carcinoid syndrome?

Surgery can be curative when carcinoid syndrome results from a carcinoid tumor that has not metastasized. However, approximately 90% of patients with carcinoid syndrome have extensive metastases at the time of diagnosis. The goal of therapy, therefore, is most often to provide palliation and to prolong survival.

11. How are carcinoid syndrome symptoms controlled?

The most troublesome symptoms patients with carcinoid syndrome experience are intense flushing and secretory diarrhea. Long-acting somatostatin analogues (octreotide, lanreotide) are the most effective available medications for controlling these carcinoid symptoms because approximately 80% of NETs express somatostatin receptors. Recommended starting doses are intramuscular octreotide LAR 20 to 30 mg every 4 weeks (with eventual dose escalation up to 60 mg every 4 weeks) or lanreotide 60 to 120 mg every 4 weeks. Short-acting octreotide can be used to treat intermittent breakthrough symptoms at doses of 100 to 500 mcg, as needed, every 8 hours. Positive somatostatin receptor–based functional imaging (see above) predicts a good response to these somatostatin analogues, but the necessity for positive imaging before starting these agents has not been established. In addition to symptom control, there is evidence that somatostatin analogues may have direct effects to inhibit tumor growth.

12. What medications may be effective when somatostatin analogues do not adequately control carcinoid symptoms?

Telotristat is an orally administered inhibitor of tryptophan hydroxylase, the rate-limiting step in serotonin synthesis. Telotristat used in combination with somatostatin analogues has been shown to significantly reduce both 5-HIAA excretion and diarrhea. This agent may also be effective in preventing or reducing progression of carcinoid heart disease. Other antiflushing and antidiarrheal strategies can be added if symptom control is inadequate. Table 62.2 lists various medication options for relief of refractory symptoms.

13. Are chemotherapy regimens effective in the treatment of carcinoid tumors?

Cytotoxic chemotherapy has yielded disappointing results in patients with carcinoid syndrome. Etoposide–cisplatin combination therapy is the most commonly used regimen for poorly differentiated carcinoid tumors. Everolimus, an antagonist of mammalian target of rapamycin (mTOR), and vascular endothelial growth factor receptor (VEGF-R) antagonists, such as vatalanib, sunitinib, sorafenib, and bevazuzimab, are also under investigation. Other agents that have shown limited benefit include streptozotocin, 5-fluorouracil, lomustine, doxorubicin, and dacarbazine.

14. What other treatments may be effective for palliation or prolongation of survival in patients with carcinoid syndrome?

Hepatic resection is an option in patients with focal liver metastases. Other approaches include hepatic artery embolization, chemoembolization, 90-Y microsphere radioembolization, and peptide receptor radioligand therapy.

15. What is peptide receptor radioligand therapy?

Peptide receptor radioligand therapy takes advantage of the presence of somatostatin receptors on NETs to deliver radiopharmaceuticals directly to these tumors. NETs that show significant tracer uptake on somatostatin receptor–based functional imaging (68-Ga DOTATATE or In-111 pentetreotide) can subsequently be treated with one of several labeled analogues, such as 177-Lu DOTATATE, 90-Y edotreotide, or 90-Y DOTA tyr3-octreotide. Promising results in terms of symptom control have been reported in clinical trials.

Table 62.2. Medications for Relief of Symptoms Related to Carcinoid Syndrome.

Medications to Control Carcinoid Flushing

Octreotide (Sandostatin)	50–150 mcg 2 or 3 times/day subcutaneously
Octreotide, long acting (Sandostatin LAR)	20–30 mg every month intragluteally
Lanreotide (Somatuline)	60–120 mg every month subcutaneously
Phentolamine (Regitine)	25–50 mg 1–3 times/day
Phenoxybenzamine (Dibenzyline)	30 mg/day
Cyproheptadine (Periactin)	2–4 mg 3 or 4 times/day
Methysergide (Sansert)	2 mg 3 times/day
Prochlorperazine (Compazine)	5–10 mg every 4–6 hours
Chlorpromazine (Thorazine)	10–25 mg every 4–6 hours
Clonidine (Catapres)	0.1–0.2 mg 2 times/day
Methyldopa (Aldomet)	250 mg 3 times/day
Cimetidine (Tagamet), plus:	300 mg 3 times/day
• Diphenhydramine (Benadryl)	50 mg 4 times/day
• Glucocorticoids	

Medications to Control Carcinoid Diarrhea

Standard antidiarrheal measures, plus:

Octreotide (Sandostatin)	50–150 mcg 2 or 3 times/day subcutaneously
Octreotide, long acting (Sandostatin LAR)	20–30 mg every month intragluteally
Lanreotide (Somatuline)	60–120 mg every month subcutaneously
Telotristat (Xermelo)	250–500 mg 3 times/day
Clonidine (Catapres)	0.1–0.2 mg 2 times/day
Cyproheptadine (Periactin)	2–4 mg 3 or 4 times/day
Methysergide (Sansert)	2 mg 3 times/day
Ondansetron (Zofran)	8 mg 3 times/day

16. What is carcinoid crisis?

Carcinoid crisis is a life-threatening episode of hypotension, flushing, and bronchospasm that is triggered most often by tumor manipulation or anesthesia and less commonly by chemotherapy, hepatic artery embolization, or radionuclide therapy. It can also be provoked by the administration of adrenergic agents, such as epinephrine and sympathomimetic amines, or monoamine oxidase inhibitors (MAOIs) in patients with underlying carcinoid tumors.

17. How can carcinoid crisis be prevented?

When patients with carcinoid syndrome undergo surgery or hepatic artery embolization for their tumor or metastases, they should be pretreated with octreotide (300–500 mcg) subcutaneously or intravenously 30 to 60 minutes before the procedure. Repeat dosing during the surgery or procedure may be needed to prevent hypotension. Despite these measures, carcinoid crisis can still occur. Anesthesiologists should be specifically notified that the patient has carcinoid syndrome. Epinephrine, sympathomimetic amines, and MAOIs should be avoided in patients with carcinoid syndrome.

18. Which patients should receive prophylaxis to prevent carcinoid crisis?

All patients with symptomatic carcinoid syndrome, even if symptoms are well controlled with the above measures, should receive octreotide prophylaxis for surgery or procedures that can precipitate carcinoid crisis. Patients who have metastatic NETs, even in the absence of carcinoid syndrome symptoms, should have measurement of 24-hour urinary 5-HIAA excretion; octreotide prophylaxis, as described above, should be used in those with elevated urinary 5-HIIA levels.

19. Describe the management of carcinoid crisis.

Effective treatment for carcinoid crisis consists of IV administration of octreotide and glucocorticoids. If this does not abort the episode, additional options include methotrimeprazine (an antiserotonin agent), methoxamine (a direct vasoconstrictor), phentolamine (an alpha-adrenergic blocker), ondansetron (a serotonin receptor antagonist), and glucagon. It is critical to avoid the use of adrenergic and sympathomimetic agents in patients with suspected carcinoid crisis because these drugs can significantly worsen the condition. Effective medication dose regimens for this condition are listed in Table 62.3.

Table 62.3. Management of Carcinoid Crisis.

MEDICATION	DOSE REGIMEN
Octreotide (Sandostatin)	50 mcg IV over 1 min, then 50 mg IV over 15 min
Hydrocortisone (Solu-Cortef)	100 mg IV over 15 min
Methotrimeprazine (Levoprome)	2.5–5.0 mg slow IV push
Methoxamine (Vasoxyl)	3–5 mg slow IV push, followed by an infusion
Phentolamine (Regitine)	5 mg slow IV push
Ondansetron (Zofran)	20 mg IV over 15 min
Glucagon	0.5–1.5 mg slow IV push

IV, Intravenous.
From Warner, R. R. P. (1997). Gut neuroendocrine tumors. In C.W. Bardin (Ed.), *Current therapy in endocrinology and metabolism* (6th ed., pp. 606–614). St. Louis, MO: Mosby

BIBLIOGRAPHY

Auernhammer, C. J., Spitzweg, C., Angele, M. K., Boeck, S., Grossman, A., Nölting, S., . . . Bartenstein, P. (2018). Advanced neuroendocrine tumours of the small intestine and pancreas: clinical developments, controversies, and future strategies. *Lancet Diabetes & Endocrinology, 6*, 404–415.

Bainbridge, H. E., Larbi, E., & Middleton, G. (2015). Symptomatic control of neuroendocrine tumours with everolimus. *Hormones & Cancer, 6*, 254–259.

Caplin, M. E., Pavel, M., Ćwikła, J. B., Phan, A. T., Raderer, M., Sedláčková, E., . . . Ruszniewski, P. (2014). Lanreotide in metastatic enteropancreatic neuroendocrine tumors. *New England Journal of Medicine, 371*, 224–233.

Condron, M. E., Pommier, S. J., & Pommier, R. F. (2016). Continuous infusion of octreotide combined with perioperative octreotide bolus does not prevent intraoperative carcinoid crisis. *Surgery, 159*, 358–365.

Davar, J., Connolly, H. M., Caplin, M. E., Pavel, M., Zacks, J., Bhattacharyya, S., . . . Toumpanakis, C. (2017). Diagnosing and managing carcinoid heart disease in patients with neuroendocrine tumors: an expert statement. *Journal of the American College of Cardiology, 69*, 1288–1304.

Fisher, G. A., Wolin, E. M., Liyanage, N., Lowenthal, S. P., Mirakhur, B., Pommier, R. F., . . . Vinik, A. I. (2018). Lanreotide therapy in carcinoid syndrome: prospective analysis of patient-reported symptoms in patients responsive to prior octreotide therapy and patients naïve to somatostatin analogue therapy in the ELECT phase 3 study. *Endocrine Practice, 24*, 243–255.

Garske-Román, U., Sandström, M., Fröss Baron, K., Lundin, L., Hellman, P., Welin, S., . . . Granberg, D. (2018). Prospective observational study of ^{177}Lu-DOTA-octreotate therapy in 200 patients with advanced metastasized neuroendocrine tumours (NETs): feasibility and impact of a dosimetry-guided study protocol on outcome and toxicity. *European Journal of Nuclear Medicine and Molecular Imaging, 45*, 970–988.

Hicks, R. J., Kwekkeboom, D. J., Krenning, E., Bodei, L., Grozinsky-Glasberg, S., Arnold, R., . . . Ramage, J. (2017). ENETS consensus guidelines for the standards of care in neuroendocrine neoplasia: peptide receptor radionuclide therapy with radiolabeled somatostatin analogues. *Neuroendocrinology, 105*(3), 295–309.

Kaltsas, G., Caplin, M., Davies, P., Ferone, D., Garcia-Carbonero, R., Grozinsky-Glasberg, S., . . . de Herder, W. W. (2017). ENETS consensus guidelines for the standards of care in neuroendocrine tumors: pre- and perioperative therapy in patients with neuroendocrine tumors. *Neuroendocrinology, 105*(3), 245–254.

Kiesewetter, B., & Raderer, M. (2013). Ondansetron for diarrhea associated with neuroendocrine tumors. *New England Journal of Medicine, 368*, 1947–1948.

Knigge, U., Capdevila, J., Bartsch, D. K., Baudin, E., Falkerby, J., Kianmanesh, R., . . . Vullierme, M. P. (2017). ENETS consensus recommendations for the standards of care in neuroendocrine neoplasms: follow-up and documentation. *Neuroendocrinology, 105*(3), 310–319.

Kulke, M. H., Hörsch, D., Caplin, M. E., Anthony, L. B., Bergsland, E., Öberg, K., . . . Pavel, M. (2017). Telotristat ethyl, a tryptophan hydroxylase inhibitor for the treatment of carcinoid syndrome. *Journal of Clinical Oncology, 35*, 14–23.

Oberg, K., Couvelard, A., Delle Fave, G., Gross, D., Grossman, A., Jensen, R. T., . . . Ferone, D. (2017). ENETS consensus guidelines for standard of care in neuroendocrine tumours: biochemical markers. *Neuroendocrinology, 105*(3), 201–211.

Partelli, S., Bartsch, D. K., Capdevila, J., Chen, J., Knigge, U., Niederle, B., . . . Falconi, M. (2017). ENETS consensus guidelines for standard of care in neuroendocrine tumours: surgery for small intestinal and pancreatic neuroendocrine tumours. *Neuroendocrinology, 105*(3), 255–265.

Pavel, M., Hörsch, D., Caplin, M., Ramage, J., Seufferlein, T., Valle, J., . . . Wiedenmann, B. (2015). Telotristat etiprate for carcinoid syndrome: a single-arm, multicenter trial. *Journal of Clinical Endocrinology and Metabolism, 100*, 1511–1519.

Rinke, A., Müller, H. H., Schade-Brittinger, C., Klose, K. J., Barth, P., Wied, M., . . . Arnold, R. (2009). Placebo-controlled, double-blind, prospective, randomized study on the effect of octreotide LAR in the control of tumor growth in patients with metastatic neuroendocrine midgut tumors: a report from the PROMID Study Group. *Journal of Clinical Oncology, 27*, 4656–4663.

Sbardella, E., & Grossman, A. (2016). New developments in the treatment of neuroendocrine tumours – RADIANT-4, NETTER-1 and telotristat etiprate. *European Endocrinology, 12*, 44–46.

Strosberg, J., Weber, J., Feldman, M., Goldman, J., Almhanna, K., & Kvols, L. (2013). Above-label doses of octreotide-LAR in patients with metastatic small intestinal carcinoid tumors. *Gastrointestinal Cancer Research, 6*, 81–85.

Strosberg, J. R., Benson, A. B., Huynh, L., Duh, M. S., Goldman, J., Sahai, V., . . . Kulke, M. H. (2014). Clinical benefits of above-standard dose of octreotide LAR in patients with neuroendocrine tumors for control of carcinoid syndrome symptoms: a multicenter retrospective chart review study. *Oncologist, 19*, 930–936.

Sundin, A., Arnold, R., Baudin, E., Cwikla, J. B., Eriksson, B., Fanti, S., . . . Vullierme, M. P. (2017). ENETS consensus guidelines for the standards of care in neuroendocrine tumors: radiological, nuclear medicine & hybrid Imaging. *Neuroendocrinology, 105*(3), 212–244.

Vinik, A. I., Wolin, E. M., Liyanage, N., Gomez-Panzani, E., & Fisher, G. A. (2016). Evaluation of lanreotide depot/autogel efficacy and safety as a carcinoid syndrome treatment (ELECT): a randomized, double-blind, placebo-controlled trial. *Endocrine Practice, 22*, 1068–1080.

Zhang, J., Wang, H., Jacobson, O., Cheng, Y., Niu, G., Li, F., . . . Chen, X. (2018). Safety, pharmacokinetics, and dosimetry of a long-acting radiolabeled somatostatin analog ^{177}Lu-DOTA-EB-TATE in patients with advanced metastatic neuroendocrine tumors. *Journal of Nuclear Medicine, 59*, 1699–1705.

CHAPTER 63

AGING AND ENDOCRINOLOGY

Kerrie L. Moreau, Sean J. Iwamoto, and Shauna Runchey

1. What effect does aging have on body weight?

   Aging is associated with changes in body composition that may be influenced by the endocrine milieu and can have important endocrine/metabolic consequences (Table 63.1). In general, body weight increases with advancing age until about age 60 years; thereafter, it stabilizes and then declines after age 65 to 70 years. This may be attributed to improved survival of adults without obesity and/or a "die off" effect in the heaviest individuals during middle age. However, the reduction in body weight in older adults, whether intentional or unintentional, appears to be associated with an increase in mortality, morbidity, and disability. Indeed, there is a well-described obesity paradox in older adults, wherein higher body mass index (BMI) is associated with lower overall mortality, and weight loss is associated with greater mortality compared with weight stability. The causes for this are not clear, but it is possible that any sustained weight loss may, in fact, be unintentional, as intentional weight loss is difficult to maintain. Weight loss, in the face of illness or disease raises cytokine levels and may predispose to a disproportionate loss of weight as lean mass (muscle mass). This weight loss exacerbates age-related sarcopenia (loss of muscle mass and strength) and leads to a catabolic state. It is also possible that the apparent obesity paradox of aging is related to the time of onset of obesity in older adults, with obesity beginning at a young age or in middle-age being associated with untoward consequences, and obesity beginning at an older age being less dangerous. Interventions in these two potentially heterogeneous groups might also be expected to produce different health-related outcomes, but these have not yet been studied.

2. What changes in lean body mass occur with aging?

   There is an inevitable loss of lean body mass, mostly skeletal muscle, with aging. Cross-sectional studies demonstrate that starting at age 30 years, 1% to 2% of muscle mass is lost per year, such that a 20% to 30% loss of lean mass is observed by age 80. The mechanisms underlying the loss of muscle mass with aging include declines in sex hormones, myocyte apoptosis and mitochondrial dysfunction. Secondary causes of sarcopenia include disuse resulting from immobility and a sedentary lifestyle, inadequate nutrition, and disease-related muscle loss (e.g., endocrine and inflammatory diseases). The age-related loss of muscle mass has been blamed for much, but not all, of the age-related decline in muscle strength and power. Longitudinal studies have shown that the decline in strength outpaces the loss of lean mass with up to a 60% loss in strength from age 30 to 80 years. Furthermore, the loss of strength and power is not as linear as the loss of muscle mass and seems to accelerate at older ages. A 25% decline in strength has been detected between ages 70 and 75 years. Power (work per unit time) may decline at double the rate of strength. These changes in lean mass, muscle mass, strength and power are complex but have important functional consequences for older people. For example, testosterone supplementation is consistently associated with increases in lean mass but is less consistently associated with improvements in strength or function.

   The term *sarcopenic obesity* refers to the age-associated loss of muscle mass and/or muscle function (i.e., strength) coupled with increased adiposity. Consensus on diagnostic tools for or the definition of sarcopenic obesity is lacking, and therefore, prevalence, clinical relevance, and optimal treatment have not been fully established. Prospective studies show that older men with sarcopenia and obesity have the highest risk of all-cause mortality even after adjustment for lifestyle factors (e.g., smoking, alcohol intake, physical activity, and occupation), cardiovascular disease (CVD), inflammation, and weight loss. These data support the importance of implementing weight-loss programs that maintain lean mass in older adults. One contributing factor to the development of sarcopenic obesity could be weight cycling with loss of both lean and fat mass followed by regain of fat mass only. This may have a greater effect in older patients who are less anabolic and generally less active. The loss of lean mass with aging can have a profound effect on resting metabolic rate and thus predispose to further accretion of fat mass if caloric intake is not reduced.

3. What changes in bone health occur with aging?

   Prospective data indicate that peak bone mass occurs during late teenage years in women and about a decade later in men. Because of intimate structural and functional links between muscle and bone, the occurrence of peak bone mass likely corresponds with peak skeletal muscle development. It is generally thought that bone mass is maintained, or decreases slowly ($< 0.2\%$ per year), at least through age 40 years in women and age 50 years in men. Intuitively, a decline in physical activity during middle age might be expected to induce an even faster rate

Table 63.1. Body Composition Changes with Aging.	
	CHANGE
Fat mass	↑
Lean mass	↓
Muscle mass	↓
Bone mass	↓

of bone loss. However, the increase in body weight that typically also occurs during middle age may counter this to a large extent by increasing mechanical loading forces acting on the skeleton during weight-bearing activity. There is an inevitable loss of bone mass in older age that increases the risk for osteoporosis in elderly men and augments the risk for osteoporosis in postmenopausal women. In elderly women and men, the decrease in bone mineral density (BMD) at the hip appears to be accelerated (~1% per year) relative to changes at the spine. In fact, spine BMD may seem to *increase* in advanced age, when vertebral compression fractures and the development of extravertebral osteophytes lead to an apparent increase in BMD that does not actually reflect increased vertebral bone strength. The utility of measuring spine BMD for the diagnosis of osteoporosis in the elderly can, therefore, be compromised.

In addition to bone density, bone quality is an important component of overall bone strength and changes in bone quality can also increase the risk for an osteoporotic fracture. Bone quality properties include porosity, architecture and geometry, turnover, damage, and mineral content. Higher resolution imaging techniques suggest that overall bone quality declines with age because of factors such as increased cortical and trabecular porosity and decreased volumetric BMD. These changes are not captured by standard dual-energy x-ray absorptiometry (DXA) screening.

4. Does menopause have an independent effect on bone health?
The decline in BMD accelerates in the late perimenopausal and early postmenopausal periods in women. What remains somewhat controversial is whether the menopause-induced increase in bone resorption diminishes after a few years or persists into old age. In this regard, observational studies of women aged 65 years and older indicate that the rate of bone loss continues to increase with age, particularly in the hip region. This is corroborated by observations that serum markers of bone turnover increase at menopause and remain elevated into older age. Recent studies in animals implicate both the decrease in estrogens and the increase in follicle-stimulating hormone (FSH) as mechanisms underlying bone loss with the menopausal transition. Inhibition of FSH activity prevented ovariectomy-induced bone loss in these animal models. However, whether the increase in FSH with menopause contributes to the decline in bone mass in women remains unclear.

5. Can weight-bearing exercise prevent the menopause-related loss of bone mineral density in women?
It is unlikely that even vigorous weight-bearing exercise can completely mitigate the deleterious effects of estrogen deficiency on BMD. Older female athletes not on hormone replacement therapy have lower BMD compared with premenopausal athletes. Additionally, young female athletes with menstrual cycle dysfunction can have BMD levels in the osteopenic (1.0–2.4 standard deviation [SD] below the average peak BMD) and even osteoporotic range (≥ 2.5 SD below the average peak BMD) despite their participation in sports that involve high levels of mechanical loading (e.g., gymnastics, distance running). Moreover, in premenopausal women undergoing ovarian hormone suppression, concurrent resistance exercise training only mitigated some of the BMD decline in the proximal femur and did not prevent the BMD decline at the lumbar spine.

6. Do sex hormones influence the skeletal response to exercise?
In animal models, the effects of mechanical stress in the presence of estrogens (in females) or androgens (in males) on the bone proliferative response have been found to be either additive or synergistic (i.e., more than additive). There is also evidence for additive or synergistic effects of exercise and estrogens on BMD in women. In postmenopausal women, hormone therapy concurrent with exercise training had a greater beneficial effect on hip and spine BMD compared with exercise alone. There is some evidence that in postmenopausal women treated with hormone therapy, mixed loading exercise protocols, such as high-impact weight-bearing activities (e.g., jumping), combined with progressive-resistance training may have a greater benefit on BMD compared with single-mode exercise.

The responses of bone cells to mechanical stress involve activation of estrogen receptor alpha. Recent studies of laboratory animals suggest that estrogen receptor alpha may facilitate the effects of mechanical loading on bone whereas estrogen receptor beta may inhibit such effects. Additionally, the mechanical loading effects facilitated by estrogen receptor alpha signaling may be impaired in postmenopausal women because of reduced estrogen levels. However, the effects of age-related sex hormone deficiency on receptor density and/or function in bone remain unknown.

7. What criteria are used to determine who should be treated for low bone density?

DXA is the best test for monitoring changes in BMD in the elderly population. Clinical practice guidelines recommend bone density screening to identify osteoporosis in all women aged $\geq$ 65 years and in men aged $\geq$ 70 years. Earlier bone density screening and/or vertebral imaging is recommended for adults at age 50 years with clinical risk factors for fracture (see below). T-scores between -1.0 and $+1.0$ indicate normal bone density, whereas T-scores between -1.0 and -2.5 indicate low bone mass or osteopenia. T-scores of ≤ -2.5 indicate osteoporosis. Pharmacotherapy for low BMD is not only reserved for those with osteoporosis by DXA criteria. In 2008, the University of Sheffield launched the FRAX tool, which can be used to evaluate the fracture risk in individuals aged 40 to 90 years. The FRAX algorithm calculates an individual's 10-year probability of major osteoporotic and hip fractures, and can identify those patients who could benefit from treatment. The FRAX tool may be used with or without a screening BMD measurement and takes into account several criteria, including race/ethnicity, age, gender, personal history (and family history) of fracture, current smoking, alcohol use, glucocorticoid use, and having a disorder or chronic disease associated with osteoporosis. A U.S. Food and Drug Administration (FDA)–approved medical therapy should be considered in postmenopausal women and men aged $\geq$ 50 years if they have (1) a hip or vertebral (clinical or morphometric) fracture; (2) a T-score ≤ -2.5 at the femoral neck or spine (excluding secondary causes); and/or (3) a T-score < -1.0 but > -2.5 at the femoral neck or spine *and* a 10-year probability of $\geq$ 20% for a major osteoporosis-related fracture or $\geq$ 3% for a hip fracture. Additionally, clinical judgment and/or patient preference should be considered for patients with T-scores or 10-year fracture probabilities outside of these values.

8. What pharmacologic agents are available for use in elderly patients with low bone density?

In addition to lifestyle recommendations for all patients (adequate intake of calcium and vitamin D through the diet or supplements), several FDA-approved agents are available for management of osteoporosis and osteopenia in individuals at high risk for fractures. Bisphosphonates, antiresorptive agents that act by inhibiting osteoclast attachment to bone matrix and enhancing osteoclast apoptosis, are the first-line drug class for the improvement of bone density and fracture prevention at all major sites. For patients aged >80 years, risedronate and zoledronic acid are the only bisphosphonates to show significant reductions in new vertebral, hip, and nonvertebral fractures during a 3-year period. Possible side effects of oral bisphosphonates include dysphagia and esophagitis. Oral and intravenous bisphosphonates may impair renal function and are, thus, contraindicated in patients with an estimated glomerular filtration rate (eGFR) < 35 mL/min. There have been reports of rare but serious side effects, such as avascular necrosis, osteonecrosis of the jaw, and low-trauma atypical subtrochanteric and diaphyseal femur fractures, associated with long-term bisphosphonate use (> 3–5 years). Recommendations are to periodically reevaluate indications for continued bisphosphonate therapy, particularly in patients who have been treated for over 5 years, and to always ask about such symptoms as new thigh or groin pain.

Commonly prescribed alternatives to oral or intravenous bisphosphonates include denosumab, selective estrogen receptor modulators (SERMs), and anabolic agents.

Denosumab is a human monoclonal antibody that binds receptor activator of nuclear factor kappa-B ligand (RANKL) to prevent RANKL–RANK interaction and thereby reduces osteoclast formation and function. As an antiresorptive osteoporosis agent, it has the net effect of increasing BMD in women and men and reducing the risk of fractures (better data for fracture reduction in women). Use of denosumab could be considered in patients who have failed or are intolerant of bisphosphonates and in patients for whom bisphosphonates are contraindicated for impaired renal function. No dose adjustment is necessary in patients with renal impairment because denosumab is not renally cleared, although patients with renal disease and those with poor calcium absorption are at higher risk for hypocalcemia. Additionally, because RANKL functions within the immune system, long-term monitoring is needed to assess for an increased risk for serious infections and neoplasms. Denosumab, administered once every 6 months by subcutaneous injection, is dosed continuously without a drug holiday. Subsequent therapy with another agent is necessary if denosumab is stopped because patients are at increased risk for vertebral fractures after discontinuation of denosumab.

FDA-approved anabolic drugs include teriparatide, which is recombinant human parathyroid hormone (PTH [1-34]); and abaloparatide, which has 41% homology to PTH (1-34) and 76% homology to parathyroid hormone–related peptide (PTHrP [1-34]). These agents improve BMD and prevent fractures by stimulating osteoblast function through intermittent interaction with the PTH/PTHrP-1 receptor. They are administered via daily subcutaneous injections; this is important to consider in elderly patients who may not have the functional capacity or appropriate assistance to do so. Cumulative anabolic therapy should not exceed 2 years so it is important to evaluate the need for subsequent antiresorptive therapy.

9. Does fat mass increase and/or get redistributed with aging?

The loss of lean mass with aging is accompanied by an increase in overall fat mass. Specifically, there is an increase in total adiposity and a shift from lower body subcutaneous fat to more abdominal visceral fat depots with advancing age. An increase in central adiposity begins in young men who gain excess fat, but this does not appear to occur in women until around the time of the menopausal transition. Aging is also associated with an increase in fat deposition in other ectopic depots, including cardiac and skeletal muscle tissues. Although the loss of lean mass was once thought to be the primary determinant of physical disability in old age, recent studies indicate that increased adiposity is an independent, and perhaps stronger, predictor of disability in older individuals. The infiltration of fat in skeletal muscle is associated with reduced lower leg strength and power, and impaired physical function. This, combined with an increase in visceral adiposity, may play a role in age-associated insulin resistance.

10. Does the menopause trigger an increase in abdominal obesity in women?

Evidence supports an increase in abdominal adiposity with the menopausal transition in women. Cross-sectional comparisons of women across menopausal stages show greater waist size across stages. Prospective cohort studies indicate an increase in total fat mass and a disproportionate increase in abdominal fat that are related to both chronologic and ovarian age, with the most rapid increases in abdominal fat occurring in perimenopausal women. Women who had an oophorectomy before age 40 years had greater waist size compared with women who did not have an oophorectomy. Studies treating premenopausal women with gonadotropin-releasing hormone agonists to suppress sex hormones show fat mass gains of 1 to 2 kg in 4 to 6 months, with a disproportionate increase in central body regions. Finally, several randomized controlled trials (RCTs) have shown that postmenopausal women treated with estrogens with or without progestins gain less weight and have less increase in waist size compared with placebo-treated women. The effects seem to be slightly larger with unopposed estrogens. Recent studies in animals suggest a possible role for an increase in FSH as a mechanism for the increase in adiposity. Animals treated with an FSH antibody had a marked reduction in adiposity that was more pronounced in the abdominal visceral region. It has not yet been determined whether estrogens and/or blocking the increase in FSH specifically prevent or attenuate intraabdominal fat accumulation.

11. What are the results of prospective studies of intentional weight loss (through lifestyle, weight loss medications, or weight loss surgery) in the elderly?

Obesity in older adults is a mounting public health concern given its increasing incidence and association with loss of functional independence and frailty. Hypocaloric diets have been effective in reducing total and visceral fat and improving glucose tolerance, insulin sensitivity, blood pressure, and pulmonary function. Elderly adults with obesity are capable of participating in and adhering to rigorous interventions with diet, exercise, or diet plus exercise. Such studies have found that diet alone and exercise alone both reduce frailty, but the combination of diet and exercise generates the greatest objective functional and subjective benefits.

Intentional weight loss typically results in a loss of lean mass (muscle and bone), which may exacerbate sarcopenia and risk for osteoporosis. This could have adverse effects in elderly adults who are already at risk for osteoporosis. Thus, it has been suggested that exercise training should be added to diet interventions to mitigate the loss of lean mass. Using this approach, the addition of exercise training to diet in older adults with obesity prevented the weight loss–induced increase in bone turnover and attenuated, but did not prevent, the decline in bone mineral density.

Some prospective observational studies have suggested that weight loss in older adults may be associated with increased mortality despite a decrease in comorbidities, such as CVD and type 2 diabetes. However, in randomized controlled weight loss interventions, weight loss did not increase mortality in older adults over a follow-up period of 8 to 12 years. In fact, secondary analyses from one trial suggested that intentional weight loss might reduce the mortality risk in this population. Additional trials of intentional weight loss in older adults are needed to confirm whether it does, indeed, reduce mortality risk and whether the risk-to-benefit profile is similar in older adults who develop obesity earlier versus later in life.

Several weight loss medications can be prescribed with diet and/or exercise in individuals with obesity. However, data are lacking regarding efficacy and safety of antiobesity pharmacotherapy in the geriatric population. Recent clinical trials investigating the antiobesity effects of the combination medication bupropion (antidepressant) and naltrexone (opioid antagonist) as well as lorcaserin (serotonin receptor [5-HT_{2C}] activator) included only ~2% of adults aged $\geq$ 65 years. Moreover, there were not enough older patients in these studies to determine whether response rates differed between geriatric and younger patients. About 7% of participants in the phentermine/topiramate and liraglutide trials were aged $\geq$ 65 years, and there were no differences in safety or effectiveness between geriatric and younger patients. Bupropion/naltrexone, lorcaserin, and phentermine/topiramate have warnings and dose adjustments for worsening renal impairment, which is more common in elderly patients and needs to be considered. Orlistat, which prevents some dietary fat from being absorbed, does not appear to have age-related dosing risks.

Weight loss surgery is effective at reducing weight and medical comorbidities in the elderly, though at higher perioperative risk. A recent systematic review of 26 studies of 8,149 patients aged $\geq$ 60 years revealed a pooled 30-day postoperative mortality rate of 0.01% and overall complication rate of ~15%. After 1 year, pooled mean excess weight loss was 54%, and the resolution rates of diabetes, hypertension, and lipid disorders were 55%, 43%, and 41%, respectively. These improvements are comparable with those seen in younger patients and appear to be independent of bariatric surgery procedure type. There also does not appear to be an increased mortality in elderly patients who underwent Roux-en-Y gastric bypass compared with nonsurgical elderly controls.

12. Why is vitamin D status important in older adults?

Vitamin D supplementation has been found to reduce the incidence of osteoporotic fractures in the elderly. This may occur via increased bone mineralization and/or improved muscle function and reduction in falls. According to the Institute of Medicine, vitamin D deficiency is defined as a serum 25-hydroxyvitamin D (25[OH]D) level < 20 ng/mL (50 nmol/L). National and international groups have suggested that a 25(OH)D level $\geq$ 30 ng/mL

(75 nmol/L) is needed to minimize fracture and fall risk. There are insufficient data to recommend a safe upper limit of 25(OH)D.

It has been estimated that > 40% of community-dwelling older women and men in the United States are vitamin D deficient, and the prevalence is even higher in nursing home residents. There are multiple causes of vitamin D deficiency in older adults, including decreased sun exposure; decreased skin synthesis; decreased intake; impaired absorption, transport, or liver hydroxylation of oral vitamin D; medications altering vitamin D metabolism (e.g., drugs that induce p450 enzymatic activity leading to decreased circulating levels of 25[OH]D); chronic illnesses associated with malabsorption; and liver and kidney diseases.

Bone mineral density is adversely affected when serum 25(OH)D levels are < 30 ng/mL. Although vitamin D_3 supplementation has been found to raise serum 25(OH)D levels above 30 ng/mL, recent meta-analyses did not find that vitamin D_3 (alone or in combination with calcium) supplementation reduced fracture risk among community-dwelling older adults without known vitamin D_3 deficiency, osteoporosis or prior fracture. There is currently no evidence for antifracture efficacy of vitamin D_2 supplementation.

Vitamin D deficiency also causes muscle weakness. Proximal muscle strength is linearly related to serum 25(OH)D when levels are < 30 ng/mL. Vitamin D supplementation has been associated with a 22% reduction in falls. Nursing home residents randomized to receive 800 IU/day of vitamin D_2 plus calcium had a 72% reduction in falls.

In addition to its important role in muscle and bone metabolism, vitamin D deficiency is postulated to influence immune function, cancer risk, parathyroid hormone and renin production, and insulin secretion. Epidemiological studies demonstrate higher mortality in patients with insufficient or deficient levels of 25(OH)D.

13. What are the recommendations for vitamin D supplementation in older adults?

The 2010 Institute of Medicine recommendations for vitamin D supplementation are set at 600 IU/day for men and women aged 51 to 70 years and 800 IU/day for older individuals.

In 2010, the National Osteoporosis Foundation (NOF) recommended that older adults aged ≥ 65 years should have a serum 25(OH)D level of ≥ 30 ng/mL (75 nmol/L) to reduce risk for falls and fractures. Supplementation doses up to 800 to 1000 IU/day were recommended because of the lack of evidence for efficacy of higher doses. These recommendations are also supported by the International Osteoporosis Foundation (IOF) and the American Geriatrics Society (AGS).

The 2011 Endocrine Society clinical practice guidelines suggested maintaining a serum 25(OH)D level of ≥ 30 ng/mL (75 nmol/L) with vitamin D_2 or D_3 1500 to 2000 IU/day.

In 2012, the United States Preventive Services Task Force (USPSTF) reported that supplementation of 400 IU/day of vitamin D in combination with 1000 mg/day of calcium does not reduce fracture risk in noninstitutionalized, community-dwelling, asymptomatic adults without a previous history of fractures. It was further noted that there is a lack of evidence regarding the effectiveness of higher doses of vitamin D and calcium on incident fractures.

14. What interventions have been associated with increased longevity and have they been shown to work in humans?

Studies of yeast, worms, flies, rodents, and mammals have demonstrated that caloric restriction (CR; 30%–40% reduction in daily energy intake) increases mean (i.e., average life expectancy) and maximal life span. Interestingly, generating a negative energy balance in rodents through increased energy expenditure (exercise) results in similar improvements in mean life span as CR but does not increase maximal life span. Studies in humans have suggested that CR produces physiologic, metabolic, and hormonal effects that parallel many of the positive effects found in other species. CR intervention trials with durations of 6 months to 2 years in healthy adults found that CR led to improvements in cardiometabolic risk and did not adversely affect quality of life.

Dietary composition also plays a role in longevity. A large meta-analysis of data from the Consortium on Health and Ageing: Network of Cohorts in Europe and the United States (CHANCES), including 400,000 elderly participants, found that adherence to a healthy diet (limited saturated fats, mono- and disaccharides, and cholesterol; 6%–10% of energy intake from polyunsaturated fatty acids [PUFAs] and 10%–15% from protein; and intake of > 25 g/day of fiber and > 400 g/day of fruits and vegetables), was associated with increased life expectancy. Although prolonged dietary intervention trials for longevity typically study biomarkers of longevity rather than actual lifespan, most of the evidence shows that prolonged adherence to similar diets (e.g., Mediterranean) with or without caloric restriction have led to improved indices of insulin sensitivity, oxidative stress, and other CVD risk factors. A 5-year primary prevention trial in older adults at high CVD risk showed that consumption of Mediterranean-style diets led to a decrease in incident CVD, type 2 diabetes, peripheral artery disease and atrial fibrillation in men and women.

It is estimated that one quarter to one third of the variance in life expectancy in humans is explained by genetic factors. Large-scale collaborations are studying different populations to define biomarkers or genes associated with longevity in humans. Variants of two genes, *APOE* (apolipoprotein E) and *FOXO3A* (forkhead box O3A), have been consistently shown to be associated with longevity. APOE is a major carrier of cholesterol and aids in lipid transport and injury repair in the brain. The *FOXO3A* gene is involved in the insulin/insulin-like growth factor-1 (IGF-1) signaling pathway and may influence longevity via its effects on oxidative stress and insulin sensitivity.

15. What happens to testosterone and estradiol levels with aging in men?

Serum total testosterone represents the unbound and protein-bound testosterone in the circulation. Most testosterone is bound to sex hormone binding globulin (SHBG) and albumin; only 2% to 4% of circulating testosterone

Table 63.2. Hormonal Changes with Aging.

	WOMEN	MEN
Estradiol	↓	↓
Testosterone	↓	↓
Growth hormone	↓	↓
Insulin-like growth factor-1 (IGF-1)	↓	↓
Dehydroepiandrosterone sulfate (DHEA/S)	↓	↓
Thyroid-stimulating hormone (TSH)	↑	↑
Cortisol	↑	↑

is unbound or free. In general, serum total testosterone levels decline gradually with advancing age (Table 63.2). Additionally, SHBG levels increase with age, resulting in an even greater relative reduction in calculated bioavailable and free testosterone with age (declines of −14.5% for total testosterone versus −27% free testosterone [FT] per decade of aging).

Although testosterone is converted to estradiol via aromatase, total serum estradiol levels in adult men do not change significantly with age. In fact, serum total estradiol levels of elderly males may be two- to fourfold higher than postmenopausal women of the same age. However, bioavailable and free estradiol levels decrease as a result of the increase in SHBG with aging (estradiol binds to SHBG with half the affinity of testosterone).

16. What is the cause of decreases in male testosterone levels with aging?

The decline in serum testosterone levels with aging in men is quite variable, and changes in health and lifestyle factors can contribute to this variability. For example, obesity and comorbid disease, including diabetes, are associated with greater rates of decline in serum testosterone. In fact, the decline in total testosterone associated with becoming obese (−12%) is comparable to that associated with 10 years of aging among men who are weight stable (−13%). Acute and chronic illness, some medications (e.g., narcotics, glucocorticoids), nutritional deficiency, sleep disorders (e.g., obstructive sleep apnea), stress, and loss of a spouse can also reduce serum testosterone concentrations.

17. What is the prevalence of hypogonadism in older men?

The prevalence of male hypogonadism is not completely known because of the lack of consensus on the definition of hypogonadism with aging. When using a biochemical definition of hypogonadism of serum total testosterone concentrations < 325 ng/dL, the Baltimore Longitudinal Study of Aging reported increased hypogonadism prevalence rates with advancing age of 12%, 19%, 28%, and 49% of men in their 50s, 60s, 70s, and 80s, respectively. However, the prevalence of symptomatic hypogonadism in this study was not reported. When hypogonadism was defined as total testosterone < 300 ng/dL and free testosterone < 5 ng/dL, almost 50% of men aged > 50 years with hypogonadism were asymptomatic, whereas 65% of men with symptoms had normal testosterone levels. The prevalence of symptomatic androgen deficiency is estimated to be at least 5% in men aged 50 to 70 years and 18% in older men. In 2018, the Endocrine Society published updated testosterone therapy guidelines and recommended that hypogonadism be diagnosed in men with signs and symptoms of testosterone deficiency (e.g., low libido, loss of body hair, hot flushes, decreased energy) and unequivocally and consistently low morning serum testosterone concentrations. It is important to note that defining hypogonadism can be challenging because symptoms can be variable, nonspecific, and influenced by age and other factors (e.g., obesity). Additionally, it is important to confirm low testosterone concentrations because of large day-to-day variability in serum levels. Indeed, 30% of men with an initial testosterone value in the hypogonadal range have a normal serum testosterone level on repeat measures. Serum testosterone has diurnal variation and can be influenced by food and exercise; thus, serum measures should occur in the morning after an overnight fast and abstinence from exercise.

18. Are there benefits of testosterone supplementation for older men with low normal testosterone levels?

Of the RCTs that have been conducted in otherwise healthy, older hypogonadal men, most found an increase or maintenance of fat-free mass (bone and muscle) and a decrease in fat mass (including abdominal visceral and intermuscular fat) with testosterone therapy. Whether such physiologic effects translate into strength or functional improvements remains uncertain. Anemia caused by androgen insufficiency improves with testosterone therapy. Improvements in sexual function and sense of well-being have been inconsistent.

The lack of consistent findings among trials of testosterone supplementation is likely related to variability in study cohorts (e.g., baseline testosterone levels, symptoms, body composition, comorbidities, physical function), the type of testosterone supplementation therapy (e.g. oral, transdermal, intramuscular, dose, and average testosterone concentration achieved), and duration of intervention (e.g. months versus years). A placebo-controlled, randomized trial of testosterone gel (1%) applied daily for 3 years in 308 older men (age ≥ 60 years) that included men with *low-normal* testosterone levels showed no improvement in insulin sensitivity, atherosclerosis progression, sexual function, or health-related quality of life. These results differ from those of the Testosterone Trials (seven coordinated placebo-controlled trials) in 788 older men with low testosterone levels that showed normalization of testosterone levels in older men with low testosterone led to improved sexual and physical function, mood, and bone mineral density, but also showed evidence of atherosclerosis progression. Longer term studies will be necessary to assess cardiovascular outcome risks.

19. Is there evidence for adverse effects of testosterone supplementation in men with low or low-normal testosterone levels?

Common adverse events reported with testosterone supplementation include acne, oily skin, and breast tenderness. Small decreases in high-density lipoprotein cholesterol (HDL-C) may also occur with testosterone therapy. A rise in hematocrit and frank erythrocytosis are dose-related, more common in older than younger men and are exacerbated in the setting of sleep apnea. Worsening of benign prostatic hyperplasia is also relatively common. There is a consistent lack of evidence of increased prostate cancer risk in studies of men on testosterone therapy, but there is evidence that testosterone administration is associated with an increased risk of detecting subclinical prostate cancer in older men; this is likely a result of increased surveillance and testosterone-induced increases in PSA levels that may lead to an increased likelihood of a prostate biopsy.

Although observational studies have consistently reported an association between low testosterone and increased cardiovascular risk and mortality, recent studies have suggested possible cardiovascular harm in older men receiving testosterone therapy. This has led to cautions against testosterone use in older men. In 2010, researchers from the Testosterone in Older Men with Mobility Limitations (TOM) trial published data on adverse events associated with testosterone administration, which led to early termination of the study. The original purpose of the study was to determine the effects of testosterone administration on lower extremity strength and physical function in older men with significant mobility limitations and low serum levels of either total or free testosterone. The participants were men aged $\geq$ 65 years with limitations in mobility and a high prevalence of chronic disease (e.g., diabetes, hypertension, obesity). During the 6-month intervention, men who were randomized to testosterone gel therapy with a goal of attaining a serum total testosterone level > 500 ng/dL unexpectedly had a higher prevalence of cardiovascular, respiratory, and dermatologic adverse events, even after adjustment for baseline risk factors. The increased frequency of cardiovascular events led to trial termination. However, this has not been confirmed in other studies or in meta-analyses of testosterone intervention trials. Furthermore, a recently completed study demonstrated a reduction in cardiovascular adverse events in a testosterone-supplemented group versus a placebo-supplemented group of generally healthy older men with low-normal serum total testosterone levels at baseline. Taken together, there have been no large, long-term, randomized, placebo-controlled trials of testosterone therapy evaluating cardiovascular outcomes to provide any definitive conclusions about cardiovascular risk with testosterone.

20. What are the recommendations for testosterone replacement therapy in older men with androgen deficiency?

The most recent guidelines from the Endocrine Society published in 2018 recommend against routinely prescribing testosterone to all men age $\geq$ 65 years with low serum testosterone concentrations. The Endocrine Society recommends screening for and diagnosing androgen deficiency in older men only when they have consistent signs and symptoms of low androgen levels. They recommend the use of a high-quality assay to measure morning fasted serum total testosterone concentrations and confirming a low result with a repeat morning fasted total testosterone level and/or free or bioavailable testosterone level if SHBG is altered or if total testosterone is borderline. Even if low testosterone levels are confirmed, only men with clinically significant and symptomatic androgen deficiency and no contraindications (i.e., planning fertility, presence of an obstructing urinary tract or prostate condition, elevated hematocrit or thrombophilia, untreated obstructive sleep apnea, or neuro- or cardiovascular event within the preceding 6 months) should be considered for treatment. Men with low testosterone levels should always be evaluated for the cause of androgen deficiency. If therapy is initiated, the clinician should ensure that the patient understands the uncertainty of the risks and benefits of testosterone therapy. The choice of supplementation should be at the discretion of both the clinician and the patient. Although the Endocrine Society advises a target total testosterone level in the mid-normal range when prescribing testosterone therapy, many clinicians aim for total testosterone levels in the low-normal range to avoid potential cardiovascular or respiratory side effects despite lack of evidence supporting this practice. Monitoring patients during the first year of therapy should include evaluations for hematocrit and prostate cancer risk.

At this time, testosterone replacement should continue to be reserved for the minority of older men who have frankly low serum testosterone levels and clear clinical signs and symptoms of hypogonadism, who do not have an existing clear contraindication for androgen therapy.

21. Should estrogen therapy be given to postmenopausal women?

This has been an area of controversy since the completion of the Women's Health Initiative (WHI) trials almost 15 years ago. Similar to debates about testosterone supplementation, there is ongoing controversy regarding criteria for who should be treated (e.g., age, years menopausal, symptomatic), by what formulation (e.g., conjugated estrogens versus estradiol, progesterone versus medroxyprogesterone acetate [MPA], continuous versus intermittent progestins), at what dose (e.g., fixed dose versus targeted serum estradiol levels), by what route (i.e., oral, transdermal, transvaginal), and for what length of time. The WHI trials generated important results but raised equally important questions. The risks of oral conjugated estrogens vary, depending on whether they are used with or without MPA, with a more favorable risk profile when estrogen is used alone. The WHI trials appear to support the "timing hypothesis," that cardiovascular benefits may occur when therapy is initiated near the time of menopause, whereas initiating hormone treatment after 10 or more years of estrogen deficiency may increase risk for cardiovascular events.

The loss of estrogen with menopause appears to be linked with deleterious changes in body composition, including increased central fat accumulation and decreased bone mineral density, which translate long term into increased risk for CVD and fractures. Additionally, the loss of estrogen is associated with hot flashes, decreased sleep quality, vaginal dryness, and worsening of mood disturbances, the sum of which equals decreased quality of life for many women.

In the North American Menopause Society (NAMS) 2017 hormone therapy position statement, hormone therapy is indicated (and approved by the FDA) as first-line therapy for relief of vasomotor symptoms (VMSs) and genitourinary syndrome of menopause (e.g., vaginal atrophy). Hormone therapy is also indicated and FDA approved for use in women with elevated risk for bone loss and fractures, and in those with hypoestrogenism caused by hypogonadism, surgical menopause, or primary ovarian insufficiency. The risks of hormone therapy may differ depending on type, dose, route of administration, duration of use, timing of initiation, and whether a progestin is used. For example, transdermal estradiol appears to be associated with fewer thromboembolic events than oral estrogens. Because the use of continuous conjugated estrogens plus MPA was associated with an increased incidence of invasive breast cancer in the WHI trial (whereas use of conjugated estrogens alone was not), intermittent progesterone may be a better alternative for endometrial protection. The NAMS recommends hormone therapy be individualized with respect to appropriate treatment type and duration to maximize benefits and minimize risks, with periodic reevaluation of the benefits and risks of therapy. Discontinuation of systemic hormone therapy in women age $\geq$ 65 years for safety reasons is not supported by evidence. Decisions to continue hormone therapy use in older women should be judged on an individual basis for quality of life, persistent VMSs, and/or prevention of bone loss and fractures, with appropriate evaluation of risks. Ultimately, a discussion of whether or not to use hormone therapy should be incorporated into recommendations for lifestyle modifications to manage menopausal symptoms and risk for age-associated chronic diseases.

22. How does the serum dehydroepiandrosterone (DHEA) concentration change with aging?

DHEA is the most abundant steroid hormone in humans, with approximately 95% coming from the adrenal glands. DHEA sulfate (DHEAS) is the predominate circulating form of DHEA and is thought to be one of the best biological markers of human aging. Peak serum DHEAS levels are reached early in the third decade and then decline steadily. By age 70 years, circulating DHEAS levels are only about 20% of peak levels. The decrease in DHEA with aging does not represent a general decline in adrenal function, as similar changes in other adrenal hormones do not occur.

23. What are the biologic effects of DHEA?

The actions of DHEA are thought to be mediated primarily through conversion to androgens and/or estrogens, and thus it may function as a large storage pool of prehormone. DHEA is the precursor for 30% to 50% of androgens in older men and > 70% of androgens in older women and is a major source of estrogens in men and postmenopausal women. Tissues that can be targeted by DHEA include muscle, bone, adipose, blood vessels, heart, and liver. As such, the decline in DHEA with aging may contribute to physiologic changes that occur as a result of sex hormone deficiency (e.g., the loss of bone and muscle mass). Other biological effects of DHEA may include increased IGF-1 levels, antiglucocorticoid effects, and antiinflammatory effects via PPAR-alpha agonism.

24. What are the hormonal effects of DHEA supplementation?

In the United States, DHEA is considered a dietary supplement, and therefore, it is not an FDA-regulated drug. Hence, over-the-counter products vary greatly in the amounts of bioactive hormone they contain (if any) and may have quite different pharmacokinetic profiles. Even lot-to-lot variability within a brand can be large. Despite being labeled a "dietary supplement," DHEA has measurable effects on concentrations of hormones. In older adults, 50 mg of bioactive DHEA per day results in a 300% to 600% increase in plasma DHEAS concentration in both men and women; a 100% increase in plasma testosterone in women with nonsignificant changes in men; a 70% to 300% rise in plasma estradiol in women and a 30% to 200% increase in men; and increases in IGF-1 of 25% to 30% in women and 5% to 10% in men. However, the physiologic effects of DHEA supplementation in humans appear quite variable.

25. Summarize the controlled studies of DHEA administration in older adults.

In recent randomized, placebo-controlled trials of 1 to 2 years' duration, DHEA replacement alone in older men and postmenopausal women did not result in significant changes in fat or muscle mass, lipid profiles, glucose levels, mood, or cognitive performance. Studies of DHEA combined with an exercise stimulus (e.g., endurance, resistance, or both) have shown mixed effects. In postmenopausal women, 12 weeks of DHEA was not more effective compared with placebo at potentiating the effects of endurance and resistance exercise on body composition, glucose levels, or lipid metabolism. In contrast, 16 weeks of DHEA improved muscle volume and strength compared with placebo when combined with high-intensity resistance exercise in older women and men.

RCTs on the effects of long-term (i.e., 1–2 years) DHEA (50 mg/day) on BMD in older adults have shown trends for BMD increases at the hip, but improvements at other sites appear to be more study specific and gender specific. Increases in BMD in response to short-term DHEA therapy have generally been small (1%–2%). One study evaluated the effects of DHEA therapy or placebo combined with vitamin D and calcium on BMD in older patients. Compared with placebo, spine BMD increased by 1.7% after 1 year and by 3.6% after 2 years in DHEA-treated older women; there was no effect on hip BMD in postmenopausal women or on spine or hip BMD in older men. The 2-year increment of 3.6% in the spine observed in women was comparable with that seen with bisphosphonate treatment. There have been no RCTs assessing the effect of DHEA on fracture risk.

In general, DHEA replacement trials have not shown significant adverse events (e.g., increases in prostate-specific antigen [PSA]), but much larger trials would be needed to establish safety and efficacy. The most common reported adverse effects have been dermatologic or androgenic symptoms in postmenopausal women.

26. Describe the changes in the growth hormone (GH)–IGF-1 axis with aging.

Aging is associated with a significant decline in the GH area under the curve, as well as the number and amplitude of night-time GH peaks. These changes in GH secretion (approximately 15% decline for every decade after age 30 years) are also associated with a steady decline in IGF-1 production. By age 65 years, most individuals have a serum IGF-1 concentration that is near or below the lower limit of normal for young healthy individuals. The observed decline in the GH–IGF-1 axis appears to occur above the level of the pituitary because chronic treatment with growth hormone–releasing hormone (GHRH) and/or other GH secretagogues (GHS) mitigates much of the decline. The cause of the fall-off in GH–IGF-1 axis activity is not clear but could be explained by age-related decreases in GHRH or ghrelin secretion, increased inhibition by somatostatin, increased sensitivity of somatotrophs to negative feedback inhibition by IGF-1, and/or a decline in pituitary responsiveness to GHRH or ghrelin. Ghrelin appears to be the natural ligand for the GHS receptor. Although there is a close physiologic relationship between GH secretion and slow-wave sleep, it is unclear if the altered GH–IGF-1 axis is the consequence or cause of profound age-related changes in sleep architecture.

27. Is the decline in the GH–IGF-1 axis associated with age-related changes in body composition and function?

Many of the body composition changes and differences in physical and psychological function that occur with aging seem consistent with a GH-IGF-1–deficient state. Indeed, the decrease in GH observed with aging (though milder) is associated with many of the same physiologic abnormalities seen in younger adults with GH deficiency, including:

- Reduced lean body and muscle mass
- Reduced strength and aerobic capacity
- Increased total, central, and intraabdominal (visceral) fat
- High incidence of metabolic syndrome
- Reduced bone mass and density
- Reduced or absent slow-wave (deep) sleep
- High incidence of mood disturbance (depression)
- Deterioration of memory and cognitive function

Despite the association of these changes to both aging in the elderly and GH deficiency in younger adults, causality is still unknown.

28. Is GH replacement recommended for the healthy elderly?

Although GH therapy in younger GH-deficient patients improves body composition, bone mineral density, exercise capacity, cardiac function, cholesterol levels, and quality of life, and may decrease mortality, the efficacy and safety of therapy for the otherwise "healthy" elderly is controversial. A 2007 systematic review of clinical trials of GH in the healthy elderly concluded that GH therapy does increase serum IGF-1 concentrations, although women may require higher doses of GH for longer periods compared with men to achieve physiologic replacement levels. Despite higher GH doses per kilogram of body weight, women do not consistently demonstrate the increase in lean body mass or decrease in fat mass that occur in men. Furthermore, translation into clinically significant changes in strength, function, bone mineral density, and improved metabolic parameters has been difficult to demonstrate in either gender. GH treatment is associated with several important adverse events, such as a significantly increased incidence compared with placebo of soft tissue edema (42%), carpal tunnel syndrome (18%), arthralgias (16%), gynecomastia (6%), impaired glucose tolerance (13%), and new-onset diabetes (4%).

The scant clinical experience with GH treatment for the healthy elderly suggests that although GH may minimally improve body composition, it does not improve other clinically relevant outcomes, such as strength or function, and it is associated with high rates of adverse events. Furthermore, studies in invertebrate and rodent models have suggested that lower GH axis activity may be protective for longevity. On the basis of available evidence, GH cannot be recommended for routine use in the healthy elderly. Large RCTs would be needed to determine the safety and efficacy of GH combined with exercise, sex hormones, and other replacement strategies, such as GHRH, IGF-1, and ghrelin-mimetic GHS.

29. Does GHRH supplementation affect GH secretion, cognition, mood, and sleep?

Elderly individuals often experience lack of sleep at night and feel tired during the day. This may be attributed to the near total loss of slow-wave sleep (stage N3 or "deep sleep"). Of interest, the periods of slow-wave sleep in younger individuals coincide exactly with the nighttime peaks of GH secretion. Indeed, animal and some human data have suggested that appropriately timed GHRH supplementation may restart pulsatile GH secretion and stimulate slow-wave sleep. Also, limited evidence suggests that chronic GHRH supplementation may improve cognitive function, specifically psychomotor and perceptual processing speed, as well as fluid memory. One small randomized, double-blind, placebo-controlled trial of older adults (mean age of 68 years) examined the effects of 20 weeks of daily subcutaneous injections of tesamorelin (a GHRH analogue currently only FDA approved for the treatment of human immunodeficiency virus–associated lipodystrophy) on cognition, mood, and sleep in those with mild cognitive impairment (MCI) versus healthy controls. Intention-to-treat and more complete analyses revealed the favorable effects of GHRH on cognition in both healthy older adults and in those with MCI; the beneficial effect was particularly noteworthy for executive function, with a trend toward benefit on verbal memory, but there was no difference in visual memory. GHRH did not affect mood or sleep quality in healthy older adults or in those with MCI. Larger studies of longer duration are needed to further establish the role for GHRH therapy in promoting cognition, mood, and sleep in the elderly with normal or pathologic aging.

30. What happens to the hypothalamic–pituitary–adrenal (HPA) axis with aging?

The HPA axis activity changes with aging and is different between the genders. The cortisol response to pharmacologic and psychological stressors is augmented with aging in both men and women. Interestingly, women have a more exaggerated response compared with men, suggesting that the loss of female sex hormones may contribute to alterations in HPA axis activity. However, distinguishing among the independent effects of age, declines in sex hormones, and body composition-related changes in the HPA axis is challenging. For example, morning cortisol levels tend to be lower, and stress-induced HPA axis responsiveness tends to be greater in older adults compared with younger adults, but such findings are also associated with central obesity (commonly found with aging; see above). Additionally, dynamic HPA axis responses to various stressors have been reported to be exaggerated in postmenopausal women compared with premenopausal women, with estradiol treatment attenuating the responses in postmenopausal women. However, several characteristics appear to be unique to aging per se. First, there is evidence for a phase advance characterized by an earlier morning cortisol peak. Second, the evening cortisol nadir appears to be higher in older persons, resulting in a compression of the diurnal amplitude. Third, glucocorticoid-mediated negative feedback is decreased. In total, mean 24-hour serum cortisol concentrations are 20% to 50% higher in both older women and older men, likely reflecting alterations in glucocorticoid clearance, HPA axis responsiveness to stress, and central glucocorticoid-mediated negative feedback. Finally, suppression of ovarian hormones for 20 weeks with leuprolide did not alter basal or dynamic HPA axis activity in premenopausal women, but estrogen add-back treatment reduced dynamic HPA axis activity compared with preintervention levels, suggesting that aging, as opposed to the decline in ovarian hormones, is the predominant contributing factor to increased HPA axis activity in older women. However, further research is needed to tease out the complex interaction between sex hormone changes and aging effects on the HPA axis in both women and men.

A recent meta-analysis of four large United Kingdom–based cohort studies of older adults followed up for 8 years showed no association of morning cortisol levels or diurnal cortisol slope with mental well-being. Whether an increase in the exposure to systemic and/or local tissue (via 11-beta hydroxysteroid dehydrogenase-1) glucocorticoids in the elderly contributes to such age-related changes as central obesity, insulin resistance, decreased lean body mass, increased risk for fractures, decreased sleep quality, and poor memory (all common symptoms of cortisol excess) are areas of ongoing investigation.

31. What do thyroid function profiles look like in older adults?

Interpreting data from studies done in elderly subjects regarding thyroid function is difficult because evaluation is often complicated by the increased prevalence of chronic diseases and medication use. Nevertheless, serum TSH concentrations and distributions appear to increase with age, independent of the presence of antithyroid antibodies. This has been hypothesized to be caused by an age-related decline in thyroid function or to recalibration of the baseline TSH setpoint; however serum free thyroxine (fT_4) levels tend to remain stable with age. Older individuals with higher fT_4 levels have been reported to have a lower physical function status and an increase in overall 4-year mortality. Total triiodothyronine (T_3) levels have been shown to be inversely related to physical performance and lean body mass. Serum reverse T_3 (rT3) levels appear to increase with age, presence of disease, and lower physical function status. These trends in thyroid hormone levels may indicate that it is beneficial to have lower activity of the thyroid hormone axis in older age.

Establishment and widespread use of age-specific reference ranges have been proposed and would have important implications for defining subclinical hypothyroidism in the elderly and treatment targets for thyroid hormone replacement.

32. What thyroid conditions are more prevalent with aging?

Thyroid nodules increase with age, with an estimated prevalence of 37% to 57% in the elderly population. The risk of malignancy in a nodule also increases with age, however the prevalence of thyroid cancer is not necessarily higher in adults over age 60 depending on the population studied.

The most frequent cause of hyperthyroidism in older adults is toxic multinodular goiter rather than Graves' disease. Presenting symptoms of hyperthyroidism may be more atypical, with apathetic symptoms being more common in older adults.

Hypothyroidism increases significantly with age as a result of multiple conditions, including autoimmune thyroid disorders and the use of medications that can impair thyroid function. The incidence of myxedema coma is also higher in older adults compared with younger adults.

Subclinical hypothyroidism is defined as having a mildly elevated serum TSH level associated with fT_4 values that are still within the reference range. This condition clearly increases with age, but the actual incidence depends on the definition of the upper normal limit (UNL) for serum TSH. For example, using the common current UNL of 4.5 mIU/L, 15% of disease-free Americans older than 80 years of age have subclinical hypothyroidism. However, if the UNL of the TSH reference range were to change to 2.5 mIU/L, the incidence of subclinical hypothyroidism would be as high as 40%.

33. Should subclinical hypothyroidism or subclinical hyperthyroidism be treated in the elderly?
Subclinical hypothyroidism in individuals < 65 years of age is associated with increased ischemic heart disease and cardiovascular mortality; however, in several meta-analyses of studies in elderly patients, these risk associations were not found. In addition to the diagnostic dilemma posed by the absence of appropriate age-specific TSH ranges, a large proportion (> 40%) of elderly patients with mildly elevated serum TSH levels may revert to euthyroidism after 4 years of follow-up without treatment. Some data suggest that levothyroxine treatment should be considered in older patients with serum TSH levels > 10 mIU/L and who have positive antithyroid antibodies or are symptomatic, to reduce the risk of progression to overt hypothyroidism, decrease the risk of cardiovascular events, and improve quality of life. This begs the question of what the appropriate TSH target level should be for patients being treated for overt hypothyroidism. The goal should be to avoid subclinical and overt hyperthyroidism and, based on epidemiologic studies, a TSH level of 4 to 6 mIU/L is a reasonable target in the elderly. Further guidance on treatment of the elderly with subclinical hypothyroidism should be generated by RCTs.

Recent studies have shown that a large proportion of older patients with subclinical hyperthyroidism (~40%–50%) will also revert to euthyroidism with observation (within 2–7 years), whereas < 10% of patients progress to overt hyperthyroidism. Elderly patients with subclinical hyperthyroidism have been shown to have an increased risk for the development of atrial fibrillation and osteoporotic fractures. Some studies in high-risk elderly patients with persistent subclinical hyperthyroidism have shown increased risk for heart failure hospitalizations, nonfatal CVD and dysrhythmias, whereas other studies have not shown an association with CVD mortality. Work-up for the cause of subclinical hyperthyroidism in older patients is the same as that for younger patients. Whether and how to treat subclinical hyperthyroidism in older adults should be based on the risks and benefits of treatment vs. no treatment.

34. What factors should be considered when determining the management of glycemia in older patients with type 2 diabetes?
Among U.S. residents aged ≥ 65 years, 12 million (25%) were known to have diabetes in 2015. When managing diabetes in the elderly, treatment decisions should be individualized and should consider medical, psychological, functional, and social conditions for each geriatric patient. Duration of diabetes and existing comorbidities, such as heart disease or renal insufficiency, as well as polypharmacy and cost, are other important considerations. The 2018 American Diabetes Association (ADA) recommendations suggest that healthy older individuals with intact cognition and normal functional status should have lower hemoglobin A_{1c} (HbA_{1c}) goals (< 7.5% without hypoglycemia), whereas individuals with chronic illnesses, poor cognition, or functional dependence should have higher HbA_{1c} targets (< 8.0%–8.5%) without hypoglycemia. Elderly patients have increased susceptibility to cognitive decline related to hypoglycemia and are at risk for overtreatment of diabetes. A glycemic target of < 8% may be more prudent in managing diabetes in patients with long-term diabetes, established CVD, limited life expectancy, and increased susceptibility to severe hypoglycemia. The 2018 American College of Physicians (ACP) Guidance Statement recommends that clinicians treat octogenarians with type 2 diabetes or those with life expectancy of ≤ 10 years to minimize symptoms of hyperglycemia and not to reach a specific glycemic target. Large multicenter studies that aimed for intense glycemic control of HbA_{1c} < 6% to 6.5% in older individuals showed no significant reduction in their primary combined cardiovascular endpoints but reported significantly higher rates of hypoglycemia in those patients with intensive blood glucose management. Thus, risks of intensive control likely outweigh the benefits in an elderly population. Given the increasing complexity of glucose management in type 2 diabetes as new medications and drug classes are developed, a patient-centered treatment plan is necessary to reconcile glycemic management and optimize patient outcomes.

35. What medications should be considered for the treatment of type 2 diabetes in older adults?
Special care is required in prescribing and monitoring drug therapy for older patients with diabetes. Metformin has traditionally been considered contraindicated when the eGFR is < 60 mL/min; however, recent studies have shown that metformin can be used safely in patients with an eGFR of 30 to 60 mL/min (with a suggested dose reduction by half when the eGFR is 30–45 mL/min). Because serum creatinine levels alone are often not an adequate reflection of the GFR in older patients, it is important to assess the eGFR that also accounts for age and body weight. Metformin is still contraindicated for those with acute illness, hospitalization, severe renal impairment (eGFR < 30 mL/min), and significantly impaired hepatic function because of the potential risk of lactic acidosis.

Thiazolidinedione use in the elderly is generally not recommended for those at increased risk for congestive heart failure (CHF) or fractures (e.g., elderly postmenopausal females). Furthermore, there is a modest cumulative dose-related increased risk of bladder cancer in patients taking pioglitazone. Long-acting insulin secretagogues, especially the sulfonylurea, glyburide, can cause hypoglycemia in the elderly and are contraindicated. Even the shorter-acting insulin secretagogues (glipizide and glimepiride) should be used with caution because elderly adults are particularly predisposed to hypoglycemia, especially those who skip meals.

Glucagon-like peptide-1 (GLP-1)–based therapies act in a glucose-dependent manner and are associated with much less hypoglycemia. The advantages of Dipeptidyl peptidase-4 (DPP-4) inhibitors are that they can be used (with dose adjustments) in those with renal impairment and are orally dosed once daily. There is concern about an increased risk of CHF hospitalizations in patients using certain DPP-4 inhibitors (saxagliptin). Although the DPP-4 inhibitors are considered weight neutral, GLP-1 receptor agonist therapy tends to cause weight loss. Although dosed once daily to once weekly, GLP-1 injections require good visual and motor skills for proper injection technique.

Insulin injections may be problematic for the patient with visual impairment and require that the patient or = caregiver have sufficient ability to follow a prescribed regimen. Overtreatment with or a mistimed dose of insulin can easily cause hypoglycemia. In the elderly, hypoglycemia may be particularly hard to identify, and recurrent hypoglycemic episodes may be incorrectly diagnosed as irreversible cognitive impairment. Management of diabetes with insulin therapy can be improved in elderly patients with visual impairment through the use of assistive devices, such as glucometers with large easier-to-read screens, audio glucometers, magnifying glasses and preloaded insulin pens.

The newest antidiabetes agents are the sodium–glucose cotransporter-2 (SGLT-2) inhibitors. Meta-analyses of studies have shown that these agents can be used safely in elderly patients with beneficial effects of lowering HbA_{1c}, possible lowering of systolic blood pressure, and reduced body weight. However, SGLT-2 inhibitors have been associated with increased frequency of genital and urinary tract infections and euglycemic ketoacidosis, and thus longer term safety data are needed.

KEY POINTS: HORMONES AND AGING

- Most hormonal axes are associated with a gradual age related changes over time, beginning at about age 30 years, with the exception of a relatively rapid decline in estradiol during the menopause transition in women.
- Serum total testosterone concentrations decrease gradually with age in men, but numerous other factors could be contributing to the decline, including age-related chronic disease and lifestyle.
- By age 70 years, dehydroepiandrosterone, a precursor for androgens and estrogens, is ~20% of peak levels observed in the third decade of life.
- The decline in growth hormone (GH) with aging is accompanied by changes in body composition; however, whether GH declines contribute to age-related metabolic changes, sleep disturbances and visceral adiposity or vice versa is unknown.
- Age-specific reference ranges for thyroid-stimulating hormone may be appropriate and have important implications in defining subclinical hypothyroidism in older adults.

Take Home Messages: No Magic Hormonal Fountain of Youth

1. Estrogen therapy is controversial but is indicated as first-line therapy for relief of postmenopausal vasomotor and genitourinary symptoms, and may be considered as a primary therapy in women with an elevated risk for bone loss and fractures, as well as those with hypoestrogenism caused by hypogonadism, surgical menopause, or premature ovarian insufficiency. There is also be cardiovascular benefits if therapy is initiated early (near time of menopause).
2. Testosterone therapy for older symptomatic hypogonadal men is associated with consistent improvements in body composition (decreased fat and increased fat-free mass), but instituting therapy requires close patient monitoring, especially in regard to cardiovascular status. Consistent evidence for improvement in strength or function is not available. Testosterone therapy is indicated for men with signs and symptoms of androgen deficiency and confirmed low morning serum testosterone levels.
3. DHEA replacement therapy increases levels of estradiol, testosterone (women only), insulin-like growth factor-1 (IGF-1) and bone mineral density, but does not appear to be associated with clear improvements in metabolism or body composition in older humans.
4. Growth hormone supplementation appears to be more effective at increasing lean body mass in older men than in older women. These body compositional changes are not necessarily associated with functional improvements and treatment has been associated with risk of adverse events.
5. Physical activity and long-term caloric restriction have the best evidence for alleviating age-related increases in adiposity, reductions in lean body mass, and cardiovascular risk factors.
6. Weight loss in the obese elderly is associated with improvements in cardiovascular risk factors, but exercise may be needed to attenuate loss of muscle and bone mass during weight loss, and to mitigate against frailty.
7. Adequate calcium and vitamin D intake are essential for fall and fracture prevention and maintenance of bone mineral density.

8. Clinicians caring for older adults with type 2 diabetes must take into consideration the clinical and functional heterogeneity of their patients when setting and prioritizing an individual's treatment goals and drug regimens. Occult hypoglycemia may be much more common in older patients, especially those treated with insulin, and the consequences of this on central nervous system and cardiovascular function must be carefully considered.

Acknowledgements

Dr. Sandra Sobel, Dr. Heather Brooks, Dr. Robert Schwartz, and Dr. Wendy Kohrt wrote this chapter in the 6th edition. Some material from that chapter has been retained in this edition. The authors also acknowledge Dr. Sara Wherry, who provided advice on the bone density sections of this chapter.

BIBLIOGRAPHY

American Diabetes Association. (2018). Older adults: standards of medical care in diabetes-2018. *Diabetes Care, 41*(Suppl. 1), S119–S125.

Araujo, A. B., Esche, G. R., Kupelian, V., O'Donnell, A. B., Travison, T. G., Williams, R. E., ... McKinlay, J. B. (2007). Prevalence of symptomatic androgen deficiency in men. *Journal of Clinical Endocrinology and Metabolism, 92*, 4241–4247.

Atkins, J. L., Whincup, P. H., Morris, R. W., Lennon, L. T., Papacosta, O., & Wannamethee, S. G. (2014). Sarcopenic obesity and risk of cardiovascular disease and mortality: population-based cohort study of older men. *Journal of the American Geriatrics Society, 62*(2), 253–260.

Atzmon, G., Barzilai, N., Hollowell, J. G., Surks, M. I., & Gabriely, I. (2009). Extreme longevity is associated with increased serum thyrotropin. *Journal of Clinical Endocrinology and Metabolism, 94*(4), 1251–1254.

Baker, L. D., Barsness, S. M., Borson, S., Friedman, S. D., Craft, S., & Vitiello, M. V. (2012). Effects of growth hormone-releasing hormone on cognitive function in adults with mild cognitive impairment and healthy older adults: results of a controlled trial. *Archives of Neurology, 69*, 1420–1429.

Basaria, S., Coviello, A. D., Travison, T. G., Storer, T. W., Farwell W. R., Jette A. M., ... Bhasin S. (2010). Adverse events associated with testosterone administration. *New England Journal of Medicine, 363*, 109–122.

Basaria, S., Harman, S. M., Travison, T. G., Hodis, H., Tsitouras, P., Budoff, M., ... Bhasin, S. (2015). Effects of testosterone administration for 3 years on subclinical atherosclerosis progression in older men with low or low-normal testosterone levels: a randomized clinical trial. *JAMA, 314*(6), 570–581.

Bhasin, S., Brito, J. P., Cunningham, G. R., Hayes, F. J., Hodis, H. N., Matsumoto, A. M., ... Yialamas, M. A. (2018). Testosterone therapy in men with hypogonadism: an Endocrine Society Clinical Practice Guideline. *Journal of Clinical Endocrinology and Metabolism,103*(5), 1715.

Centers for Disease Control and Prevention. (2017). *National diabetes statistics report* [Internet]. Retrieved from: https://www.cdc.gov/diabetes/pdfs/data/statistics/national-diabetes-statistics-report.pdf.

Cosman, F., de Beur, S. J., LeBoff, M. S., Lewiecki, E. M., Tanner, B., Randall, S., & Lindsay, R. (2014). Clinician's guide to prevention and treatment of osteoporosis. (Guide developed by expert committee of the National Osteoporosis Foundation). *Osteoporosis International, 25*(10), 2359–2381. doi:10.1007/s00198-014-2794-2.

Cruz-Jentoft, A. J., Baeyens, J. P., Bauer, J. M., Boirie, Y., Cederholm, T., Landi, F., ... Zamboni, M. (2010). European Working Group on Sarcopenia in Older People. Sarcopenia: European consensus on definition and diagnosis: report of the European Working Group on Sarcopenia in Older People. *Age Ageing, 39*(4), 412–423.

Dawson-Hughes, B., Mithal, A., Bonjour, J. P., Boonen, S., Burckhardt, P., Fuleihan, G. E., ... Yoshimura, N. (2010). IOF position statement: vitamin D recommendations for older adults. *Osteoporosis International, 21*(7), 1151–1154.

Ekstrom, N., Scholer, L., Svensson, A. M., Eeg-Olofsson, K., Miao Jonasson, J., Zethelius, B., ... Gudbjörnsdottir, S (2012). Effectiveness and safety of metformin in 51,675 patients with type 2 diabetes and different levels of renal function: a cohort study from the Swedish National Diabetes Register. *BMJ Open, 2*(4), e001076.

Elmore, L. K., Baggett, S., Kyle, J. A., Skelley, J. W. (2014). A review of the efficacy and safety of canagliflozin in elderly patients with type 2 diabetes. *Consultant Pharmacist, 29*(5), 335–346.

Gavin, K. M., Shea, K. L., Gibbons, E., Wolfe, P., Schwartz, R. S., Wierman, M. E., & Kohrt, W. M. (2018). Gonadotropin releasing hormone agonist in premenopausal women does not alter hypothalamic-pituitary-adrenal axis response to corticotropin-releasing hormone. *American Journal of Physiology-Endocrinology and Metabolism. 315*(2), E316–E325.

Giordano, S., & Victorzon, M. (2015). Bariatric surgery in elderly patients: a systematic review. *Clinical Interventions in Aging, 10*, 1627–1635.

Gourlay, M. L., Overman, R. A., & Ensrud, K. E. (2015). Bone density screening and re-screening in postmenopausal women and older men. *Current Osteoporosis Reports, 13*(6), 390–398.

Gozansky, W. S., Van Pelt, R. E., Jankowski, C. M., Schwartz, R. S., & Kohrt, W. M. (2005). Protection of bone mass by estrogens and raloxifene during exercise-induced weight Loss. *Journal of Clinical Endocrinology and Metabolism, 90*, 52–59.

Hennessey, J. V., & Espaillat, R. (2015). Diagnosis and management of subclinical hypothyroidism in elderly adults: a review of the literature. *Journal of the American Geriatrics Society, 63*(8), 1663–1673.

Heilbronn, L. K., de Jonge, L., Frisard, M. I., DeLany, J. P., Larson-Meyer, D. E., Rood, J., ... Ravussin, E. (2006). Effect of 6-mo. calorie restriction on biomarkers of longevity, metabolic adaptation and oxidative stress in overweight subjects. *JAMA, 295*(13), 1539–1548.

Holick, M. F. (2007). Vitamin D deficiency. *New England Journal of Medicine, 357*, 266–281.

Huang, G., Pencina, K. M., Li, Z., Basaria, S., Bhasin, S., Travison T. G., ... Tsitouras, P. (2018). Long-term testosterone administration on insulin sensitivity in older men with low or low-normal testosterone levels. *Journal of Clinical Endocrinology and Metabolism, 103*(4), 1678–1685.

Inzucchi, S. E., Bergenstal, R. M., Buse, J. B., Diamant, M., Ferrannini, E., Nauck, M., ... Matthews, D. R. (2012). Management of hyperglycemia in type 2 diabetes: a patient-centered approach. *Diabetes Care, 35*, 1364–1379.

Jankovic, N., Geelen, A., Streppel, M. T., de Groot, L. C., Orfanos, P., van den Hooven, E. H., ... Feskens, E. J. (2014). Adherence to a healthy diet according to the world health organization guidelines and all-cause mortality in elderly adults from Europe and the United States. *American Journal of Epidemiology, 180*(10), 978–988.

Jankowski, C. M., Gozansky, W. S., Schwartz, R. S., Dahl, D. J., Kittelson, J. M., Scott, S. M., ... Kohrt, W. M. (2006). Effects of dehydroepiandrosterone replacement therapy on bone mineral density in older adults: a randomized, controlled trial. *Journal of Clinical Endocrinology and Metabolism, 91,* 2986–2993.

Jonklass, J., Bianco, A. C., Bauer, A. J., Burman, K. D., Cappola, A. R., Celi, F. S., ... Sawka, A. M. (2014). Guidelines for treatment of hypothyroidism: prepared by the American Thyroid Association Task Force on Thyroid Hormone Replacement. *Thyroid, 24*(12), 1670–1751.

Kahwati, L. C., Weber, R. P., Pan, H., Gourlay, M., LeBlanc, E., Coker-Schwimmer, M., & Viswanathan, M. (2018). Vitamin D, calcium, or combined supplementation for the primary prevention of fractures in community-dwelling adults: evidence report and systematic review for the US Preventive Services Task Force. *JAMA, 319*(15), 1600–1612.

Kaufman, J. M., & Vermeulen, A. (2005). The decline of androgen levels in elderly men and its clinical and therapeutic implications. *Endocrine Reviews, 26,* 833–876.

Kennedy, B. K., Steffen, K. K., & Kaeberlein, M. (2007). Ruminations on dietary restriction and aging. *Cellular and Molecular Life Sciences, 64,* 1323–1328.

Laron, Z. (2005). Do deficiencies in growth hormone and insulin-like growth factor-1 (IGF-1) shorten or prolong longevity? *Mechanisms of Ageing and Development, 126,* 305–307.

Li, J., Li, S., Deng, K., Liu, J., Vandvik, P. O., Zhao, P., ... Sun, X. (2016). Dipeptidyl peptidase-4 inhibitors and risk of heart failure in type 2 diabetes: systematic review and meta-analysis of randomized and observational studies. *British Medical Journal, 352,* i610.

Lipska, K. J., Bailey, C. J., & Inzucchi, S. (2011). Use of metformin in the setting of mild-to-moderate renal insufficiency. *Diabetes Care, 34,* 1431–1437.

Liu, H., Bravata, D. M., Olkin, I., Nayak, S., Roberts, B., Garber, A. M., & Hoffman, A. R. (2007). Systematic review: the safety and efficacy of growth hormone in the healthy elderly. *Annals of Internal Medicine, 146,* 104–115.

Martínez-González, M. A., Salas-Salvadó, J., Estruch, R., Corella, D., Fitó, M., & Ros, E. (2015). Benefits of the Mediterranean diet: insights from the PREDIMED Study. *Progress in Cardiovascular Diseases, 58*(1), 50–60.

Miner, M. M., & Seftel, A. D. (2007). Testosterone and ageing: what have we learned since the Institute of Medicine report and what lies ahead? *International Journal of Clinical Practice, 61,* 622–632.

Qaseem, A., Wilt, T. J., Kansagara, D., Horwitch, C., Barry, M. J., Forciea, M. A. (2018). Hemoglobin A1c targets for glycemic control with pharmacologic therapy for nonpregnant adults with type 2 diabetes mellitus: a guidance statement update from the American College of Physicians. *Annals of Internal Medicine, 168*(8), 569–576.

Ravussin, E., Redman, L. M., Rochon, J., Das, S. K., Fontana, L., Kraus, W. E., ... Roberts, S. B. (2015). A 2-year randomized controlled trial of human caloric restriction: feasibility and effects on predictors of health span and longevity. *The Journals of Gerontology Series A, Biological Sciences and Medical Sciences, 70*(9), 1097–1104.

Shea, K. L. (2015). Body composition and BMD after ovarian hormone suppression. *Menopause, 22,* 1045–1052.

Sherlock, M., & Toogood, A. A. (2007). Aging and the growth hormone/insulin like growth factor-I axis. *Pituitary, 10,* 189–203.

Sirola, J., Kroger, H., Honkanen, R., Jurvelin, J. S., Sandini, L., Tuppurainen, M. T., & Saarikoski, S. (2003). Factors affecting bone loss around menopause in women without HRT: a prospective study. *Maturitas, 45,* 159–167.

Snyder, P. J., Bhasin, S., Cunningham, G. R., Matsumoto, A. M., Stephens-Shields, A. J., Cauley, J. A., ... Ellenberg, S. S. (2018). Lessons from the testosterone trials. *Endocrine Reviews, 39*(3), 369–386.

Sowers, M., Zheng, H., Tomey, K., Karvonen-Gutierrez, C., Jannausch, M., Li, X., ... Symons, J. (2007). Changes in body composition in women over six years at midlife: ovarian and chronological aging. *Journal of Clinical Endocrinology and Metabolism, 92,* 895–901.

Stafford, M., Ben-Shlomo, Y., Cooper, C., Gale, C., Gardner, M. P., Geoffroy, M. C., ... Cooper, R. (2017). Diurnal cortisol and mental well-being in middle and older age: evidence from four cohort studies. *BMJ Open, 7*(10), e016085.

Stott, D. J., Rodondi, N., Kearney, P. M., Ford, I., Westendorp, R. G. J., Mooijaart, S. P., ... Gussekloo, J. (2017). Thyroid hormone therapy for older adults with subclinical hypothyroidism. *New England Journal of Medicine, 376,* 2534–2544.

Surks, M. I., & Hollowell, J. G. (2007). Age-specific distribution of serum thyrotropin and antithyroid antibodies in the U.S. population: implications for the prevalence of subclinical hypothyroidism. *Journal of Clinical Endocrinology and Metabolism, 92,* 4575–4582.

Travison, T. G., Araujo, A. B., Kupelian, V., O'Donnell, A. B., & McKinlay, J. B. (2007). The relative contributions of aging, health, and lifestyle factors to serum testosterone decline in men. *Journal of Clinical Endocrinology and Metabolism, 92,* 549–555.

Turner, R. M., Kwok, C. S., Chen-Turner, C., Maduakor, C. A., Singh, S., & Loke, Y. K. (2014). Thiazolidinediones and associated risk of bladder cancer: a systematic review and meta-analysis. *British Journal of Clinical Pharmacology, 78*(2), 258–273.

US Preventive Services Task Force. (2018). Vitamin D, calcium, or combined supplementation for the primary prevention of fractures in community-dwelling adults. US Preventive Services Task Force Recommendation Statement. *JAMA, 319*(15), 1592–1599.

Van den Beld, A. W., Visser, T. J., Feelders, R. A. Grobbee, D. E., & Lamberts, S. W. (2005). Thyroid hormone concentrations, disease, physical function, and mortality in elderly men. *Journal of Clinical Endocrinology and Metabolism, 90*(12), 6403–6409.

Vanderschueren, D., Venken, K., Ophoff, J., Bouillon, R., & Boonen, S. (2006). Clinical review: sex steroids and the periosteum - reconsidering the roles of androgens and estrogens in periosteal expansion. *Journal of Clinical Endocrinology and Metabolism, 91,* 378–382.

Villareal, D. T., Banks, M., Sinacore, D. R., Siener, C., & Klien, S. (2006). Effect of weight loss and exercise on frailty in obese older adults. *Archives of Internal Medicine, 166,* 860–866.

Villareal, D. T., Miller, B. V. III., Banks, M., Sinacore, D. R., & Klein, S. (2006). Effect of lifestyle intervention on metabolic coronary heart disease risk factors in obese older adults. *American Journal of Clinical Nutrition, 84,* 1317–1323.

Villareal, D. T. & Holloszy, J. O. (2006). DHEA enhances effects of weight training on muscle mass and strength in elderly women and men. *American Journal of Physiology Endocrinology and Metabolism, 291,* E1003–E1008.

Villareal, D. T., Chode, S., Parimi, N., Sinacore, D. R., Hilton, T., Armamento-Villareal, R., ... Shah, K. (2011). Weight loss, exercise, or both and physical function in obese older adults. *New England Journal of Medicine, 364,* 1218–1229.

Weiss, E. P., Shah, K., Fontana, L., Lambert, C. P., Holloszy, J. O., & Villareal, D. T. (2009). Dehydroepiandrosterone replacement therapy in older adults: 1- and 2-y effects on bone. *American Journal of Clinical Nutrition, 89,* 1459–1467.

Wierman, M. E. & Kohrt, W. M. (2007). Vascular and metabolic effects of sex steroids: new insights into clinical trials. *Reproductive Science, 14,* 300–314.

Zhao, J. G., Zeng, X. T., Wang, J., & Liu, L. (2017). Association between calcium or vitamin D supplementation and fracture incidence in community-dwelling older adults: a systematic review and meta-analysis. *JAMA, 318*(24), 2466–2482.

ENDOCRINOPATHIES CAUSED BY IMMUNE CHECKPOINT INHIBITORS

David Saxon and Thomas Jensen

1. How are immune checkpoint inhibitors (ICPIs) classified? Explain their mechanisms of action.

   ICPIs have been developed targeting cytotoxic T lymphocyte–associated-protein 4 (CTLA-4), programmed cell death protein 1 (PD-1) and programmed cell death ligand 1 (PD-L1). These proteins play an important role in the development of peripheral immune self-tolerance and prevention of autoimmunity. Antigen presenting cells (APCs) activate T cells through the binding of antigens (either foreign antigens from infections or mutated self-antigens from cancer cells) on major histocompatibility complexes with T-cell receptors but require additional stimulation. CTLA-4 and PD-L1 receptors on T cells are part of a complex system of checkpoints that promote peripheral immune self-tolerance. CTLA-4 is the primary receptor that prevents activation of naïve T cells in lymph nodes and competes with its homolog receptor on T cells, cluster of differentiation 28 (CD28), for binding of CD80/CD86 on APCs. Binding of CD28 promotes T-cell activation and proliferation, whereas binding of CTLA-4 leads to anergy and reduced T-cell survival. PD-1 regulates previously activated T cells in the periphery and interacts with receptors for PD-L1 or programmed cell death ligand 2 (PD-L2) on peripheral cells to further promote self-tolerance through reduced T-cell activation and survival. Cancer cells have found ways to take advantage of this peripheral tolerance system to evade the immune system. ICPIs block these normal protein interactions, thereby removing the "brakes" on the immune system and resulting in enhanced T cell–mediated death of cancer cells (Fig. 64.1), as well as the adverse endocrinopathies addressed below.

2. What ICPIs are available in the United States? What are the indications for use of these various medications?

   Several ICPIs are currently approved by the U.S. Food and Drug Administration (FDA). Ipilimumab, a CTLA-4 inhibitor, was the first agent approved for use in patients with advanced melanoma. Available PD-1 inhibitors are nivolumab and pembrolizumab. Nivolumab is approved for patients with metastatic melanoma, previously treated metastatic non–small cell lung cancer (NSCLC), recurrent or metastatic squamous cell carcinoma of the head and neck, advanced renal cell carcinoma (often in combination with ipilimumab), hepatocellular carcinoma (previously treated with sorafenib), relapsed or progressive classical Hodgkin's lymphoma (after autologous hematopoietic stem cell transplantation), and certain cases of metastatic colon carcinoma. Pembrolizumab is approved for advanced melanoma, advanced NSCLC, head and neck squamous cell cancer, classical Hodgkin's lymphoma, advanced urothelial cancer, tumors that have microsatellite instability-high (MSI-H) or are mismatch repair deficient, and advanced gastric adenocarcinoma. Available PD-L1 inhibitors are atezolizumab (approved for urothelial cancers and NSCLC), durvalumab (approved for urothelial cancers), and avelumab (approved for Merkel cell carcinoma and urothelial carcinoma). Indications for use of these therapies are rapidly changing and multiple drug combinations are being tested in a variety of cancers.

3. What is the spectrum of immune-related adverse events seen with ICPIs?

   Immune-related adverse events (IRAEs) affect multiple organs and systems, including the skin, gastrointestinal (GI) tract, heart, lungs, kidneys, eyes, musculoskeletal system, nervous system, hematologic system and the endocrine system (Table 64.1).

4. What specific endocrine disorders are seen with ICPIs?

   The most common endocrinopathies associated with ICPIs are acute hypophysitis (with accompanying central adrenal insufficiency, central hypothyroidism, and hypogonadotropic hypogonadism), and thyroid dysfunction. Additional endocrinopathies can include primary adrenal insufficiency, type 1 diabetes mellitus, and hypoparathyroidism, although these are much less common. The risk for development of these endocrinopathies is related to the type of ICPI, the dose, and whether combination ICPI therapy is used.

5. How are organ-specific toxicities caused by immunotherapies graded?

   The National Cancer Institute (NCI) Common Terminology Criteria for Adverse Events (CTCAE) is a descriptive terminology used for adverse event (AE) reporting. A grade refers to the severity of an AE and a general guideline is used to grade AEs on a scale of 1 through 5. Grade 1 AEs are defined as mild or no symptoms and can be clinically monitored without intervention. Grade 2 AEs are moderate and limit age-appropriate activities of daily living (ADLs); minimal, local, or noninvasive intervention is indicated. Grade 3 AEs are severe, but not immediately life-threatening; they limit self-care ADLs, and hospitalization is generally needed. Grade 4 AEs have life-threatening consequences, and urgent intervention is needed. A Grade 5 AE is one that leads to a patient's death.

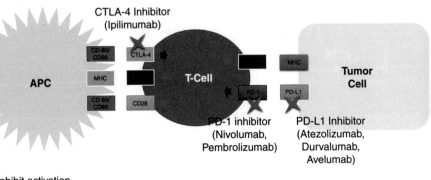

Fig. 64.1 Mechanism of immune checkpoint therapy in cancer treatment.

Table 64.1		
ADVERSE EVENT	**ONSET**	**DURATION**
Pruritis, Rash	3–4 weeks	7–8 weeks
Colitis, Diarrhea	4–6 weeks	5–6 weeks
Hepatic Toxicity	6–8 weeks	7–8 weeks
Hypophysitis	6–8 weeks	Permanent (usually)

6. What is the overall incidence of clinically significant endocrinopathies in patients treated with ICPIs?
   According to a recent systematic review and meta-analysis that included 7551 patients in 38 randomized trials, the overall incidence of endocrinopathies with ICPIs was approximately 10%.

7. What are the rates of various endocrine IRAEs?
   Table 64.2 highlights the overall incidence of various endocrinopathies caused by ICPIs. Differences in AE rates are dependent on whether a CTLA-4 or PD-1 inhibitor or combination therapy is used. Other diseases, such as primary adrenal insufficiency, type 1 diabetes mellitus, and hypoparathyroidism, are rare and will be addressed in detail below.

Table 64.2 Rates of More Common Endocrinopathies Caused by Immune Checkpoint Inhibitors When Used Alone or in Combination				
DRUG	**HYPOPHYSITIS**	**HYPOTHYROIDISM**	**HYPERTHYROIDISM**	**THYROIDITIS**
Ipilimumab	0.5%–18%	0.7%–15% Subclinical hypothyroidism 6% in one study	1%–2.3%, 16% experienced subclinical hyperthyroidism in one study	2% in one study
Nivolumab	0%–0.9%	8.6%	4.2%	NA
Pembrolizumab	0%–2.2%	6.9%–9.3%	1.8%–4.8%	NA
Ipilimumab and Nivolumab	7.7%–12%	13%–22%, 5% Subclinical Hypothyroidism 5%	4.3%–9.9%, 22% subclinical hyperthyroidism in one study	9% in one study
Nivolumab and Pembrolizumab	NA	13%	13% developed subclinical hyperthyroidism	NA

8. How does management of grade 4 endocrine toxicities differ from grade 4 nonendocrine toxicities?

When grade 4 nonendocrine toxicities develop, the offending agent should be permanently discontinued. In contrast, grade 4 endocrine toxicities are usually managed with specific hormone replacements and in many cases the medications can eventually be discontinued.

9. What previously rare pituitary problem is seen with ICPIs? Which medication is it most commonly associated with? How does it present clinically?

Hypophysitis or inflammation of the pituitary gland and stalk leading to pituitary dysfunction is seen relatively frequently with certain ICPIs. Common symptoms of hypophysitis include headache, weakness, and fatigue. Imaging often shows pituitary enlargement, which may be subtle and only evident if pretreatment imaging is available for comparison. The most commonly seen hormonal disorder is central hypothyroidism, followed by central adrenal insufficiency and hypogonadotropic hypogonadism. Prolactin levels are also often low but growth hormone (GH) secretion is relatively spared. Hypophysitis develops most commonly with ipilimumab by itself or in combination with nivolumab, occurring on average in 3.2% and 6.4% of treated patients, respectively; it usually appears 8 to 12 weeks after initiation of the medication. This is thought to be caused, in part, by pituitary cells having a higher level of CTLA-4, which leads to complement activation. The incidence appears to be less with PD-1 and PD-L1 inhibitors as noted in Table 64.2.

10. What is the management for ICPI-related hypophysitis?

There is some controversy regarding the optimal management of ICPI-related hypophysitis. Patients with central adrenal insufficiency should be treated with corticosteroids promptly and prior to other replacement hormones, especially thyroid hormone because initial treatment with thyroid hormone may precipitate an adrenal crisis in patients with coexisting impairment of the hypothalamic–pituitary–adrenal (HPA) axis. There has also been debate about whether to treat with high-dose corticosteroids (prednisone 1 mg/kg/day) or physiologic corticosteroid dosing. Recent studies have shown that high-dose steroids fail to promote resolution of pituitary enlargement and pituitary insufficiency and may cause central adrenal insufficiency (if not present before). High-dose steroids could be considered for patients with severe pituitary enlargement, especially if there is a risk for optic nerve compression. Stress dose steroids should be given initially if a patient presents with an adrenal crisis. Patients who have central hypothyroidism (determined by a low serum free thyroxine (T_4) level with or without a low total triiodothyronine [T_3]) may be placed on thyroid hormone replacement once their adrenal status has been determined to be normal or after corticosteroid replacement has begun. Treatment goals for central hypothyroidism are to maintain serum free T_4 levels in the middle or upper end of the reference range of the particular laboratory assay. Appropriate sex hormone replacement in hypogonadotropic hypogonadism patients (males with testosterone and premenopausal females with estrogen and progesterone as needed) can be considered as well.

It should be noted that in one long-term follow up study (median 33 months), central hypothyroidism resolved in 85% of patients, and hypogonadism resolved in 84% of patients, but corticotroph deficiency was rarely corrected. Therefore, patients with thyroid or gonadal dysfunction should be monitored for recovery if they are asymptomatic or, if started on medication, should later be tapered down or off to see if the respective axes have recovered. Patients with central adrenal insufficiency on physiologic replacement could be rechecked by withholding their steroid dose for 1 or 2 days, followed by measurement of baseline adrenal laboratory values and performance of a cosyntropin stimulation test; however, in most cases, lifelong corticosteroid replacement therapy will be necessary.

11. What thyroid disorders are associated with the use of ICPIs? How are they differentiated, and how are they managed?

A recent study reported that approximately 30% of patients on ICPIs had new-onset of thyroid function abnormalities, and an additional 70% with preexisting thyroid disorders had exacerbations appear on laboratory testing at a median time point of 33 to 46 days after starting ICPI treatment. Because of variation in the definitions of hypothyroidism, hyperthyroidism, and thyrotoxicosis, it can be hard to delineate the true incidence of these conditions in clinical trials and practice. A recent review found a 5.6% incidence of ipilimumab-related hypothyroidism and a 3.2% incidence of thyroiditis. With PD-1 inhibitors, the rates of hypothyroidism and hyperthyroidism were 5.9% and 3.3%, respectively, and with PD-L1 inhibitors the hypothyroidism incidence was 4.3%. The overall incidence of ICPI-related thyroid disease with combination therapy jumps to 13.9% for hypothyroidism, 8% for hyperthyroidism and 16.9% for other thyroid disorders, including destructive thyroiditis.

12. What is the differential diagnosis for an elevated serum thyroid-stimulating hormone (TSH) and a normal or low serum free T_4 in the setting of ICPI therapy?

Primary hypothyroidism should be suspected in the setting of an elevated serum TSH level with a normal or low serum free T_4 value; however, this thyroid test pattern can also be seen in the hypothyroid phase of destructive thyroiditis. An enlarged thyroid gland and positive thyroid antibodies (thyroid peroxidase and thyroglobulin antibodies) suggests autoimmune hypothyroidism, whereas a normal gland size and negative antibodies would favor thyroiditis. When findings are equivocal, follow-up laboratory examinations in 3 to 4 weeks may help determine if a recovering thyroiditis is present.

13. **What thyroid disorders should be considered when TSH is suppressed and thyroid hormone levels are normal or elevated in the setting of ICPI therapy?**

Suppressed serum TSH levels with normal or elevated thyroid hormone values would suggest autoimmune hyperthyroidism (Graves' disease) or the hyperthyroid phase of destructive thyroiditis. Patients with autoimmune hyperthyroidism often have a diffusely enlarged thyroid gland, elevated thyroid-stimulating immunoglobulins (TSIs), or positive thyrotropin receptor antibodies (TRABs) and increased homogenous uptake on an iodine-123 (^{123}I; radioactive iodine [RAI]) scan, whereas patients with destructive thyroiditis usually have a normal-size thyroid gland, normal TSI or TRAB levels, and decreased uptake on an ^{123}I scan. The clinician should also be alert for other underlying causes of thyroid dysfunction, such as medications (amiodarone or lithium) or recent iodinated contrast administration, which may exacerbate underlying thyroid disease and limit the utility of RAI. In addition, central hypothyroidism, characterized by low serum free T_4 levels and low or inappropriately normal serum TSH levels, can occur especially in the setting of CTLA-4 inhibitor use.

14. **How should hypothyroidism be monitored and managed in the setting of ICPI therapy?**

Monitoring for and treatment of these toxicities is critically important. The American Society of Clinical Oncology (ASCO) recommends measuring serum TSH and free T_4 levels every 4 to 6 weeks as part of routine clinical monitoring or for case detection in symptomatic patients on therapy. For primary hypothyroidism, grade 1 toxicity is a serum TSH level that becomes mildly elevated but is < 10 mIU/L in an asymptomatic patient; in this situation, it is recommended that ICPI therapy be continued, with close monitoring of both TSH and free T_4. Grade 2 toxicity is when the serum TSH level is persistently > 10 mIU/L and moderate symptoms are present but the patient can still perform ADLs. In this scenario, thyroid hormone replacement should be prescribed, and ICPI therapy may need to be held temporarily until symptoms improve; TSH should be monitored every 6 to 8 weeks while titrating hormone replacement (alternatively, free T_4 can be checked up to every 2 weeks to titrate hormone replacement if the free T_4 was initially low). Grade 3 or 4 toxicity is defined as severe hypothyroid symptoms with medically significant or life-threatening consequences that prevent a patient from performing ADLs. ICPI therapy should be withheld in such cases until symptoms resolve with thyroid hormone replacement; the patient should be admitted to the hospital and given intravenous (IV) thyroid hormone replacement if signs of myxedema coma (decompensated hypothyroidism) are present (i.e., hypothermia, bradycardia). Prior to initiation of thyroid medication, all patients should have their adrenal axis evaluated to rule out the presence of adrenal insufficiency that maybe exacerbated if untreated prior to the initiation of thyroid hormone therapy.

15. **How should hyperthyroidism be managed in the setting of ICPI therapy?**

Patients with destructive thyroiditis who are asymptomatic can be monitored, and those with significant symptoms (palpitations, tremors) can be treated with beta-blockers and, if necessary, steroids. If and when patients convert to a hypothyroid phase, asymptomatic patients can be monitored with serial thyroid laboratory evaluations every 4 to 6 weeks, and symptomatic patients can be placed on thyroid hormone replacement with dose titration until the serum TSH is within the reference range. After 4 to 8 months, patients can be taken off medication to determine if they still require treatment. Patients with clinical autoimmune hyperthyroidism can be treated with antithyroid medications, such as methimazole (MMI) or propylthiouracil (PTU), and with beta-blockers, as necessary. If a patient is experiencing grade 3 or 4 toxicity, ICPIs should be withheld and the patient hospitalized, as necessary, until stabilized. In addition, avoidance of interventions that may exacerbate thyroid disease, such as iodinated contrast administration, is recommended until the patient is placed on medications that will control the thyroid disease. Treatment with RAI (^{131}I) or thyroidectomy can also be considered.

16. **What other thyroid abnormalities can be seen in patients on ICPIs?**

Finally, normal or mildly low serum TSH levels along with normal or low free T_4 and frankly low total T_3 values suggest the nonthyroidal illness syndrome (euthyroid sick syndrome). These patients should not be given thyroid supplementation but, rather, should have their thyroid laboratory values monitored.

17. **What other endocrinopathies have been seen with ICPIs?**

Primary adrenal insufficiency, type 1 diabetes mellitus, and hypoparathyroidism have been occasionally seen with use of ICPIs. Primary adrenal insufficiency should be suspected in the setting of typical symptoms of adrenal insufficiency (fatigue, light headedness, weight loss, abdominal pain, nausea, vomiting), with an elevated plasma adrenocorticotropic hormone (ACTH) level and a low serum cortisol level (especially < 3 mcg/dL) or a failure to stimulate cortisol to 18 mcg/dL or greater during a cosyntropin stimulation test. Patients with primary adrenal insufficiency need both glucocorticoid and mineralocorticoid supplementation, whereas those with central adrenal insufficiency only require glucocorticoid replacement. Type 1 diabetes can be suspected in patients with sudden-onset diabetes, especially if they present with diabetic ketoacidosis. Antibodies for type 1 diabetes along with C-peptide and insulin levels can help differentiate type 1 diabetes from type 2 diabetes. Hypoparathyroidism presents with symptoms of hypocalcemia (numbness, tingling, tetany), low serum calcium and high serum phosphorus levels, and low or low-normal serum parathyroid hormone (PTH) levels. This condition can be treated with a combination of calcium, calcitriol, and, as necessary, a thiazide diuretic and PTH (Natpara) replacement. Knowledge of the natural history of these disorders is limited because of their rare occurrences at this time.

18. **What is the most frequently reported adverse event with PD-1 and PD-L1 inhibitors?**
Fatigue is the most commonly reported AE with these agents, and the pathogenesis is poorly understood. Individual drug studies report fatigue in 16% to 37% of patients on PD-1 inhibitors and 12% to 24% of patients on PD-L1 inhibitors. Of the patients who report fatigue with these agents, only a minority will have hypothyroidism as a cause. Regardless, patients with even subtle changes in their energy level should have adrenal and thyroid laboratory values assessed to evaluate for potential endocrinopathies.

19. **How much more likely are patients to develop thyroid dysfunction when taking a combination of ipilimumab (CTLA-4 inhibitor) and a PD-1 inhibitor than when taking ipilimumab alone?**
Patients taking combination therapy are approximately 3.8 times more likely to develop hypothyroidism and 4.2 times more likely to develop hyperthyroidism compared with those given ipilimumab alone.

20. **How relatively likely are other endocrinopathies when comparing different classes of ICPIs?**
Patients on PD-1 inhibitors are about twice as likely to develop hypothyroidism as patients on ipilimumab. PD-1 inhibitor therapy is about five times more likely to cause hyperthyroidism compared with PD-L1 inhibitor therapy, but hypothyroidism rates are similar. Patients on ipilimumab are about five times more likely to develop hypophysitis compared with those on PD-1 inhibitor therapy alone, but those who are on a combination of these drugs are more than twice as likely to develop hypophysitis compared with those on ipilimumab alone.

21. **Does development of IRAEs suggest improved cancer treatment outcomes compared with nondevelopment of IRAEs?**
Some data suggest that the occurrence of an IRAE predicts a better cancer response to ICPI treatment. The hypothesis is that the occurrence of an IRAE reflects better activation of the immune system. A meta-analysis with nivolumab in the treatment of melanoma showed a slightly better response rate (44%) in those who required immune-modulating agents to treat IRAEs compared with those who did not receive immune-modulating agents (36%). Another study with ipilimumab in patients with melanoma showed that an early IRAE predicted a better probability of an objective antitumor response; furthermore, all patients who achieved a complete response had more severe IRAEs. In patients treated with pembrolizumab for melanoma, the occurrence of vitiligo was also a predictor of an objective response. Patients who developed early IRAEs while being treated for NSCLC with nivolumab also showed a better objective response (37% versus 17%) and had longer progression-free survival (6.4 months versus 1.5 months). Further studies looking at the exact nature and mechanism of this relationship are needed.

22. **Are any ICPIs being investigated for the treatment of thyroid cancer?**
Small, ongoing clinical trials testing CTLA-4, PD-1, and PD-L1 inhibitors are underway in combination with other treatment modalities in patients with anaplastic, poorly differentiated, and recurrent differentiated thyroid cancers. In a recent case report, a patient with anaplastic thyroid cancer showing BRAF and PD-L1 positivity had complete clinical and radiographic remission 20 months after treatment with emurafenib and nivolumab.

KEY POINTS

- The use of immune checkpoint inhibitors (ICPIs) to treat advanced cancers is growing, and these agents have the potential to cause a variety of endocrinopathies. Available medications fall into three classes: cytotoxic T lymphocyte–associated-protein-4 (CTLA-4), programmed cell death protein 1 (PD-1), and programmed cell death ligand 1 (PD-L1) inhibitors.
- The most common endocrinopathies associated with ICPIs are acute hypophysitis (with accompanying central adrenal insufficiency, central hypothyroidism, and hypogonadotropic hypogonadism) and thyroid dysfunction.
- The overall incidence of endocrinopathies with ICPIs is approximately 10%.
- Hypophysitis, or inflammation of the pituitary gland and stalk leading to pituitary dysfunction, is a previously rare pituitary problem that is seen relatively frequently with ICPIs (most commonly with ipilimumab). Single or multiple hormonal deficiencies can be seen with hypophysitis.
- Thyroid abnormalities that may be encountered when taking care of patients on ICPIs include primary hypothyroidism, Graves' disease, thyroiditis, and euthyroid sick syndrome.

BIBLIOGRAPHY

Barroso-Sousa, R., Barry, W. T., Garrido-Castro, A., Hodi, F. S, Min, L., Krop, I. E., & Tolaney, S. M. (2018). Incidence of endocrine dysfunction following the use of different immune checkpoint inhibitor regimens: A systematic review and meta-analysis. *Journal of the American Medical Association Oncology, 4*(2), 173–182.

Brahmer, J. R., Lacchetti, C., Schneider, B. J., Atkins, M. B., Brassil, K. J., Caterino, J. M., Chau I, ... & Thompson, J. A.; National Comprehensive Cancer Network. (2018). Management of immune-related adverse events in patients treated with immune check-point inhibitor therapy: American Society of Clinical Oncology clinical practice guideline. *Journal of Clinical Oncology, 36*(17), 1714–1768.

Corsello, S. M., Barnabei, A., Marchetti, P., De Vecchis, L., Salvatori, R., & Torino, F. (2013). Endocrine side effects induced by immune checkpoint inhibitors. *Journal of Clinical Endocrinology and Metabolism, 98*(4), 1361–1375.

Downey, S. G., Klapper, J. A., Smith, F. O., Yang, J. C., Sherry, R. M., Royal, R. E., . . . Rosenberg, S. A. (2007). Prognostic factors related to clinical response in patients with metastatic melanoma treated by CTL-associated antigen-4 blockade. *Clinics in Cancer Research, 13*(22 Pt 1), 6681–6688.

Haanen, J. B. A. G., Carbonnel, F., Robert, C., Kerr, K. M., Peters, S., Larkin, J., & Jordan, K.; ESMO Guidelines Committee. (2017). Management of toxicities from immunotherapy: ESMO clinical practice guidelines for diagnosis, treatment and follow-up. *Annals of Oncology, 28*(Suppl. 4), iv119–iv142.

Faje, A. (2016). Immunotherapy and hypophysitis: Clinical presentation, treatment, and biologic insights. *Pituitary, 19*(1), 82–92.

Hua, C., Boussemart, L., Mateus, C., Routier, E., Boutros, C., Cazenave, H., . . . Robert, C. (2016). Association of vitiligo with tumor response in patients with metastatic melanoma treated with pembrolizumab. *Journal of the American Medical Association Dermatology, 152*(1), 45–51.

Illouz, F., Briet, C., Cloix, L., Le Corre, Y., Baize, N., Urban, T., . . . Rodien, P. (2017). Endocrine toxicity of immune checkpoint inhibitors: Essential crosstalk between endocrinologists and oncologists. *Cancer Medicine, 6*(8), 1923–1929.

Joshi, M. N., Whitelaw, B. C., Palomar, M. T., Wu, Y., & Carroll, P. V. (2016). Immune checkpoint inhibitor-related hypophysitis and endocrine dysfunction: Clinical review. *Clinical Endocrinology (Oxford), 85*(3), 331–339.

Kollipara, R., Schneider, B., Radovich, M., Babu, S., & Kiel, P. J. (2017). Exceptional response with immunotherapy in a patient with anaplastic thyroid cancer. *Oncologist, 22*(10), 1149–1151.

Konda, B., Nabhan, F., & Shah, M. H. (2017). Endocrine dysfunction following immune checkpoint inhibitor therapy. *Current Opinions in Endocrinology, Diabetes and Obesity, 24*(5), 337–347.

Patel, N. S., Oury, A., Daniels, G. A., Bazhenova, L., & Patel, S. P. (2018). Incidence of thyroid function test abnormalities in patients receiving immune-checkpoint inhibitors for cancer treatment. *Oncologist, 23*(10), 1236–1241.

Teraoka, S., Fujimoto, D., Morimoto, T., Kawachi, H., Ito, M., Sato, Y., . . . Tomii, K. (2017). Early immune-related adverse events and association with outcome in advanced non-small cell lung cancer patients treated with nivolumab: A prospective cohort study. *Journal of Thoracic Oncology, 12*(12), 1798–1805.

Weber, J. S., Hodi, F. S., Wolchok, J. D., Topalian, S. L., Schadendorf, D., Larkin, J., Sznol M, . . . & . . . Robert, C. (2017). Safety profile of nivolumab monotherapy: A pooled analysis of patients with advanced melanoma. *Journal of Clinical Oncology, 35*(7), 785–792.

CHAPTER 65

SLEEP AND ENDOCRINOLOGY

Roger A. Piepenbrink

"Our 24/7 society has led humans to be the only animal species that routinely ignores its biological clock as we are often awake when the clock is telling us to be asleep. Both chronic disruption of circadian organization and chronic insufficient sleep [quality and quantity] have been associated with a wide range of mental and physical disorders. Modern medicine is only beginning to recognize that the treatment of many disorders of human health may need to take into account circadian medicine to improve overall 24-hour temporal organization between and within the central nervous system and peripheral tissues."

—(Turek, 2017)

In the 1300s, depending on location, between 30% and 60% of the European population was killed by the plague. Because there was no treatment, symptoms developed rapidly, and the patients died. A different type of plaque is working its way through the United States; it starts insidiously in patients, sometimes in their youth, and kills more slowly. Such is the behavior of the plague of obesity, pre–diabetes mellitus (pre-DM), and type 2 diabetes mellitus (T2DM). It is estimated that over 30% of the U.S. adult population age > 20 years already has pre-DM, and by age ≥ 65 years, nearly 60% of the population has contracted this plague. With time, 70% of people with pre-DM will progress to T2DM, the prevalence increasing in parallel with obesity. The epidemic nature and multifactorial mechanisms contributing to the scourges of obesity, pre-DM, and T2DM are challenging clinicians. This chapter explores the endocrine and sleep literature to highlight the metabolic contributions of sleep to select endocrine diseases; we will describe the roles of sleep quality, quantity, and even circadian disruption of sleep, with particular attention to those processes regulated through the hypothalamus. And is it any wonder there is significant homeostatic interaction between sleep and endocrine function, given that the major controllers for these two processes are collocated in the hypothalamus? Here, the 7-mm^3 hypothalamus is the integrative genius, with the pituitary largely following its commands. As will be reviewed, anatomic proximity of neuroendocrine centers and sleep–wake centers in the hypothalamus foster functional integration to accomplish and protect homeostasis. This chapter will also cover normal sleep stages, the controllers for sleep and wake, human hormonal profiles as influenced by sleep–wake cycling, sleep deprivation, and obstructive sleep apnea (OSA) with attention to governing neuroendocrine mechanisms. It will also review the health consequence in the endocrine system of disrupted sleep and the improvements that result from successfully treating sleep abnormalities. Finally, some basics on how to obtain selected history and physical examination data germane to sleep disease will be discussed.

1. Why should endocrinologists concern themselves with sleep–wake cycles and circadian rhythmicity?

   The 24-hour profile of nearly all pituitary hormones is related to the presence and quality of sleep. Stereotypical changes in nearly all hormonal and metabolic variables are observed surrounding sleep cycling and sleep–wake transitions. The absence of sleep, or the interruption of sleep, has potent influences on hormonal ebb and flow. This adds another layer of control to hormone release on top of the well-known feedback loops. Understanding these reproducible changes in view of sleep wake–cycling is fundamental to recognizing normal and *early abnormal* endocrine processes. For example, appreciation of normal hormone changes during the day and night provides insight into a patient's laboratory values drawn at varied times through a 24-hour period.

2. Do sleep disorders cause endocrine disease or does endocrine disease cause sleep disorders?

   Both are true. Sleep experts have dubbed sleep symptoms as the "canary in the mine" for serious medical and psychological diseases. Sleep quality evaluation can be a tool for assessment of disease. Additionally, sleep disorders are common in many endocrine diseases. For example, patients with acromegaly are at risk for sleep apnea (see question 27). Excessive androgens can worsen OSA, as can hypothyroidism. Thyrotoxicosis can contribute to debilitating insomnia, with profound daytime fatigue accompanying other presenting complaints. Disruptive sleep is now known to be associated with increased risk for diabetes and shortened sleep is associated with obesity. Assessment of the sleep habits of patients is often omitted in the pursuit of human pathophysiology. But sleep quality and quantity (i.e., sleep architecture) can be vital to anticipating components of disease.

3. What are the stages of human sleep?

   Normal adult sleep is organized into rapid eye movement (REM) sleep (Table 65.1) and non–rapid eye movement (NREM) sleep, which is further divided into stages N1, N2, and N3. This final NREM stage is also called slow-wave sleep (SWS). In classic teaching, NREM was organized into four stages, but in 2007, stages N3 and N4 were combined. Each of these stages has specific electroencephalography (EEG) characteristics. Typically, adults enter sleep through stage N1. It usually takes 90 to 100 minutes for the first NREM sleep cycle to finish, but once completed, it heralds the first REM period. The hallmark of REM sleep is rapid movement of the eyes compared with the slow

493

Table 65.1. Comparison of Sleep Stages.

CHARACTERISTICS	NREM	REM
Responsiveness to stimuli	Reduced	Reduced to absent
Sympathetic activity	Reduced	Reduced or variable
Parasympathetic activity	Increased	Markedly increased
Eye movements	SEMs	REMs
Heart rate	Bradycardia	Tachycardia/bradycardia
Respiratory rate	Decreased	Variable; apneas can occur
Muscle tone	Reduced	Markedly decreased
Upper airway muscle tone	Reduced	Moderately decreased to absent
Cerebral blood flow	Reduced	Markedly increased
Other characteristics	Sleep walk	Dreams
	Night terrors	

REMs, Rapid eye movements; *SEMs,* slow eye movements.
Modified from: Chokroverty, S. (2006). Disorders of sleep. In *Neurology* (Chapter XIII). American College of Physicians Medicine, WebMD Inc.

eye movements (SEM) seen on electrooculography in stage N1 sleep. Also defining REM is muscle atonia, which manifests as absence of chin muscle movement and attendant low electromyography tone. The only somatic muscles working in REM are the extraocular muscles and the diaphragm! Curiously, we will see that REM predominant OSA, which is OSA predominant in REM, is associated with occult hyperglycemia.

4. What is the progression of sleep stages in a usual night of sleep?
In the adult, NREM and REM sleep typically alternate in 90- to 120-minute cycles (Fig. 65.1). Four to five cycles occur during a normal sleep period, depending on the length of sleep. Each cycle is identifiable with sleep onset initiating in stage N1, progressing to stage N2, then to SWS (N3), back through N2, and into REM. Once the individual achieves sleep, there is not a significant return to stage N1. Sleep cycling can also be thought of as alternating between REM and SWS, with N2 serving as a conduit between these two stages. In a typical night of adult sleep, stage N1 will comprise up to 5% of total sleep, stage N2 up to 50%, SWS up to 20%, and REM up to 25%. SWS is predominately experienced in the first third of a night of normal sleep and REM in the last half of sleep. Not achieving SWS or not achieving REM sleep has neuroendocrine significance. And for the individual, it is not just REM sleep or just achieving SWS that confers a rested feeling, but the full complement of > 7 hours of four to five cycles with normal architecture that is critical to restorative sleep.

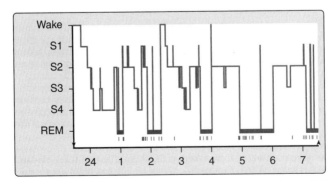

Fig. 65.1. The progression of sleep stages across a single night in a normal young adult volunteer is illustrated in this sleep histogram. The text describes the ideal or average pattern. This histogram was drawn on the basis of continuous overnight recordings on electroencephalography, electrooculography, and electromyography in a normal 19-year-old man. The records were assessed in 30-second epochs for the various sleep stages. *REM,* Rapid eye movement. (Carskadon, M. A., & Dement, W. C. (2017). Normal human sleep: An overview. In M. Kryger, T. Roth, W. C. Dement (Eds.). *Principles and Practice of Sleep Medicine.* (6th ed.). St. Louis, MO: Elsevier.)

5. **How do the sleep stages change during one's life span?**

As we age, total sleep time decreases and sleep begins to fragment (Fig. 65.2). The time in sleep declines with age from 16 to 18 hours a day in a newborn to 9 to 10 hours in a 10-year-old, to 7.5 to 8 hours in the average adult, and eventually to 6 hours in an 80-year-old. A newborn's sleep is up to 50% REM sleep, and this declines to 25% of sleep by adulthood. There is also a progressive decrease in SWS with aging. This change in sleep architecture also has endocrine repercussions because specific anterior pituitary hormone release is associated with particular sleep stages (see question 15).

6. **What are the fundamental changes in the nervous system in NREM versus REM sleep, and what other differences are noted between the phases of NREM and REM?**

Cortical deactivation and autonomic nervous system (ANS) changes typify sleep (see Table 65.1). While awake, we interact with our environment, but when asleep we are largely unresponsive to sensory input and do not generate motor output. During NREM, the cortex is deactivated, EEG activity is slower and of higher voltage than when awake, and blood flow is decreased. During REM sleep, the cortex is activated, EEG readings during sleep are similar to those when awake, and blood flow is increased. There are also changes in the ANS during sleep, with parasympathetic nervous system (PNS) predominance in NREM and even more so in REM. Sympathetic nervous system (SNS)

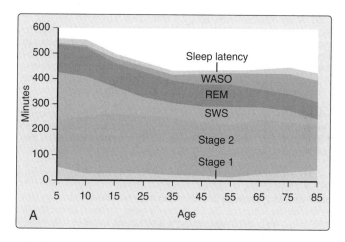

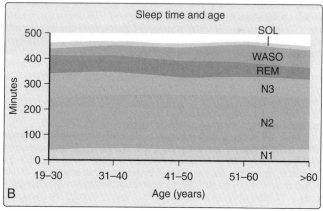

Fig. 65.2. Changes in sleep with age. A, Time (in minutes) for sleep latency and waking after sleep onset (WASO) and for rapid eye movement (REM) sleep and non-REM (NREM) sleep stages 1, 2, and slow-wave sleep (SWS). Summary values are given for ages 5 to 85 years. B, Changes in sleep in adults using the current American Academy of Sleep Medicine (AASM) scoring standards. Time (in minutes) for sleep latency and WASO and for REM sleep and NREM sleep stages N1, N2, and N3. Values are medians. (A, From Ohayon, M., Carskadon, M. A., Guilleminault, C., & Vitiello, M. V. (2004). Meta-analysis of quantitative sleep parameters from childhood to old age in healthy individuals: developing normative sleep values across the human lifespan. *Sleep, 27,* 1255–1273; B, Data from Mitterling, T., Högl, B., Schönwald, S. V., Hackner, H., Gabelia, D., Biermayr, M., & Frauscher, B. (2015). Sleep and respiration in 100 healthy Caucasian sleepers—a polysomnographic study according to American Academy of Sleep Medicine standards. *Sleep, 38,* 867–875.) (Figure from: Carskadon, M. A., & Dement, W. C. (2017). Normal human sleep: An overview. In M. Kryger, T. Roth, W. C. Dement (Eds.). *Principles and practice of sleep medicine.* (6th ed.). St. Louis, MO: Elsevier.)

tone decreases in NREM and usually in REM, but PNS tone and SNS tone can be variable during REM. In NREM, there are decreases in respiratory rate (RR), heart rate (HR), blood pressure (BP), and cardiac output. Normal REM is characterized by fluctuations in BP, HR, and RR. Dreaming and somatic muscle hypotonia to atonia (which includes reduced to absent upper airway muscle tone) are also characteristic REM events. REM may have a few periods of decreased or absent breathing. Cerebral metabolic rates for glucose and oxygen decrease during NREM, but *increase to above waking levels* in REM. As mentioned, REM-predominant OSA is associated with pre-DM and T2DM.

7. What are the systems and neurotransmitters responsible for wakefulness and for the sleep state?
Our contemporary understanding of the endocrine system includes much more neuroendocrinology. The discussion in this chapter highlights the interactions among the cortex, brain stem, hypothalamus, and pituitary. Central nervous system (CNS) accomplishment of sleep–wake changes can be best modeled as flip switches, where neural networks responsible for either state are mutually inhibitory—that is, when one is active, there is inhibition of the other. If the sleep network is active, then the wakefulness network is inhibited. Importantly, sleep is accomplished through the inhibitory influence of primarily one neurotransmitter on the arousal centers, whereas wakefulness is promoted by an arousal system of several nuclei making several neurotransmitters. Transition to sleep is accomplished through wake-inhibiting neurons primarily localized to ventrolateral preoptic (VLPO) nuclei neurotransmitter gamma-aminobutyric acid (GABA). Thus, the transition from wake to sleep is mediated through the release of GABA from VLPO nuclei, inhibiting the arousal system and its thalamocortical projection. If this arousal system, the so-called *reticular activating system* (RAS), is inhibited, sleep is promoted. Conceptually, sleep control is subdivided into sleep switches, with NREM switches governing NREM sleep and REM switches governing REM sleep. During NREM sleep, forebrain NREM-on neurons are firing; during REM sleep, REM-on neurons are firing. In turn, when transitioning from sleep to wakefulness, the RAS inhibits the VLPO nuclei. As mentioned, RAS contains a series of activating nuclei making different neurotransmitters: dopamine, acetylcholine, serotonin, histamine, orexin, norepinephrine. A good mnemonic for the wake-promoting neurotransmitters is, 'DASH ON'. Dorsal and ventral routes of the RAS have been identified. The dorsal route is composed of ascending projections through the thalamus to the cortex; the ventral route projects to the posterior hypothalamus and basal forebrain (BF). This ventral route receives inputs from the melanin-hypocretin (orexin) concentrating neurons in the lateral hypothalamus or cholinergic neurons of the BF. There are also RAS projections down the spinal cord for muscular tone and postural control. Even though these tiny tufts of neurons with their respective neurotransmitters are known as *specific nuclei*, their visualization evades current clinical imaging techniques.

8. What are the two basic processes controlling sleep timing and sleep quality and, therefore, contributing to anterior pituitary hormone cycling in a 24-hour period?
The following should serve as a framework for understating these two time-honored processes. For more in-depth rendering, please see selected references. The first process is called *process-C*, for circadian process (*circadian* from Latin "approximately a day"), and is regulated by the hypothalamic suprachiasmatic nuclei (SCN). This nucleus receives input from environmental cues, the strongest of which is light. Process-C is the broader of the two processes and transmits circadian output to coordinate behavioral, physiologic, and genetic rhythms. The second process is sleep–wake homeostasis (SWH), also known as *process-S*. SWH is dependent on process-C but the circadian process is not dependent on SWH. SWH is presently conceptualized as a process relating the amount and intensity of sleep to the duration of prior wakefulness; however, the actual basis of SWH and its anatomic location remain elusive. So, if one has 24 hours with no sleep, there is increased pressure to sleep. The pressure to sleep is least when a person is most rested. This pressure increases during the day and peaks just before midnight. The continuous interaction between these two processes, process-C and process-S, influences the hypothalamic generators to release or inhibit hormones from the anterior pituitary, which, in turn, contributes to the 24-hour hormone profile.

9. Discuss the basic mechanisms of Process-C (reference Fig. 65.3 in questions 9–13).
Research has uncovered *core molecular clock* machinery responsive to process-C in most tissues! The bilateral or paired SCN of the hypothalamus are regarded as *the sole* master 24-hour pacemaker. Research has shown the circadian process to be a *hierarchy* of oscillations starting with oscillations from the SCN centrally emanating to the periphery—that is, downstream oscillations within the brain and then to peripheral tissues. Interactions between several hypothalamic nuclei are also involved in process-C. Importantly, SCN timing is genetically determined to be slightly > 24 hours and must be modified or reset (synchronized) to the 24-hour day–night cycle by environmental stimuli (*zeitgebers*, German for "time givers" or "time cues"). The brain is employing these mechanisms to adjust to and optimize systematic function according to the location of the body.

10. How is the circadian system organized?
Using engineering parlance, the organization of the circadian system consists of three parts: (1) input system, (2) oscillator network, and (3) output system. The *input system* is represented by the retinal hypothalamic tract (RHT). The *oscillatory network*, itself with three parts, is represented by SCN, entrainment and tissue oscillators. The *output system* is represented by tissue-specific peripheral circadian outputs. For example, circadian outputs of muscle could be glucose uptake and oxidation; in the liver, they could be glucose uptake and production; in adipose tissue, the circadian outputs are lipolysis and lipogenesis; and in the pancreas, they are insulin and

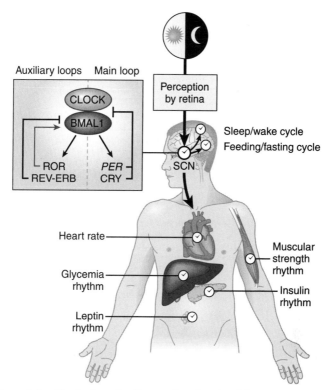

Fig. 65.3. Hierarchic organization of the circadian system. The suprachiasmatic nucleus (SCN) synchronizes a network of brain and peripheral clocks, leading to circadian rhythms of physiologic, metabolic, and hormonal patterns. The molecular clockwork relies on transcriptional – translational feedback loops. The main loop involves CLOCK–BMAL1 stimulating the transcription of Per and Cry genes, which in turn inhibit the transcriptional activity of CLOCK-BMAL1. In the auxiliary loops, after stimulation of their transcription by CLOCK-BMAL1, ROR and REV-ERB stimulate and inhibit the transcription of BMAL1, respectively. The auxiliary loops help stabilize the 24-hour oscillations of the clock proteins. BMAL1, brain-muscle-art – like protein; CLOCK, circadian locomotor output cycles kaput; Cry, Cryptochrome; Per, Period; REV-ERB, reverse viral erythroplastic oncogene products; ROR, retinoic acid receptor–related orphan nuclear receptor. (From: Chapter 38. Grosbellet, M, E Challet. Central and peripheral circadian clocks. In Kryger M, T Roth, WC Dement (eds) *Principles and Practice of Sleep Medicine*, 2017, 6th edition.)

glucagon secretion. In fact, through different experimental sources, epidemiologic, clinical, and, especially, mammalian genetic study techniques, recent work has demonstrated exciting links of circadian disruption with T2DM pathophysiology and its treatment.

11. How does the circadian input system (i.e., the RHT) work?
    Photic information is transmitted from the retina directly to the oscillator network in the SCN via the RHT. However, the photic information is not communicated by retinal rod and cone cells. *Within the retina* there are non-rod, non-cone cells, the so-called *retina ganglion cells* (RGCs). These cells contain a photopigment, melanopsin, which is preferentially excited by the short wavelengths, especially blue light. The RGC/RHT system then can be thought of as a transducer and tract, respectively, for communication of light–dark (LD) information to the SCN. Normally, the SCN is most active during the day and most inactive at night. SCN activity inhibits the tonic activity of the paraventricular hypothalamic (PVH) nuclei, which normally is a stimulus for melatonin synthesis from the pineal. So, by SCN inhibition of the PVH, daytime melatonin production decreases. In the absence of light, the PVH stimulates the pineal gland to allow melatonin secretion. It would be easier to understand if the RHT went directly to the pineal gland. But this would omit levels of integration which are associated with this melanopsin–RHT signal. This chemical LD signal is not just destined for the pineal gland; it also reaches non-SCN circadian centers as well as sleep–wake centers.

12. Since the circadian oscillatory network has three components (SCN, entrainment, and tissue oscillators), what is the basic SCN organization and the basic molecular mechanisms of the circadian clock systems?
    The SCN cytoarchitecture reveals functional organization. In mammals, the SCN comprises some 100,000 neurons and is divided into a primarily light-sensitive *SCN core*, which receives the unique nonimage retinal signaling RGC/RHT,

and a *SCN shell*, which is capable of generating rhythms. As will now be discussed, these central and peripheral circadian oscillations have very similar genetic processes. The nuclear mechanisms controlling these circadian rhythms will now be discussed. Modern laboratory techniques in tissue cultures and genetics are allowing for real-time monitoring of circadian rhythms. The transcriptional and translational processes interact in feedback loop relationships, constantly running in nearly every cell of the body, and are regulated to a 24-hour cycle with periods

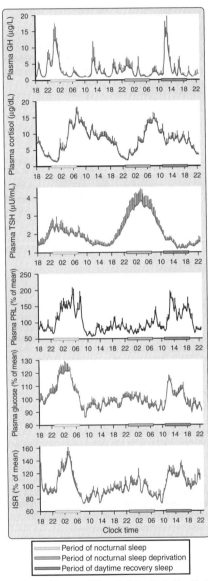

Fig. 65.4. Mean 24-hour profiles of plasma growth hormone (GH), cortisol, thyrotropin (thyroid-stimulating hormone [TSH]), prolactin (PRL), glucose, and insulin secretion rates in a group of eight healthy young men (age 20–27 years) studied during a 53-hour period including 8 hours of nocturnal sleep, 28 hours of sleep deprivation, and 8 hours of daytime sleep. The vertical bars on the tracings represent the standard error of the mean (SEM) at each time point. The horizontal bars are the following periods: light gray is nighttime sleep, medium gray is nocturnal sleep deprivation, and darkest gray is daytime recovery sleep. Caloric intake was exclusively under the form of a constant glucose infusion and the subjects remained recumbent throughout the study period. Shifted sleep was associated with an immediate shift of GH and PRL release. In contrast, the secretory profiles of cortisol and TSH remained synchronized to circadian time. Both sleep-dependent and circadian inputs can be recognized in the profiles of glucose and Insulin Secretion Rate. *(From Van Cauter, E., & E. Tasali. Chapter 20. Endocrine physiology and relationship to sleep and sleep disturbances. In Kryger M., T. Roth, W. C. Dement (Eds.), 2017 Principles and Practice of Sleep Medicine. (6th ed.). Philadelphia: Elsevier Saunders.)*

of activity and quiescence. Importantly, if SCN cells are removed from the body or are placed in complete darkness, they are still capable of maintaining a 24-hour period of activity despite the absence of an external LD cue. This molecular clockwork, as the experts call it, has two primary positive loop genes, *circadian locomotor output cycles kaput (CLOCK)* and *brain and muscle aryl hydrocarbon receptor nuclear translocator-like protein-1 (BMAL1)*. Usually, at the start of the day, these two proteins, CLOCK and BMAL1, will noncovalently join (heterodimerize) and, through a complicated series of events, this heterodimer will activate transcription of negative feedback signals. These negative loop components typically are *periodic circadian protein* (PER1 and PER2) and *cryptochrome* (CRY1 and CRY2). The PER and CRY proteins, in turn, heterodimerize and repress BMAL1–CLOCK activity. The nuclear receptors *Rev-erb alpha/beta* and *ROR alpha/beta* are also involved in control and stabilization of this system because they act as transcriptional repressors and activators, respectively, of BMAL1. Up to 10–50% of all genes expressed in a given tissue use this same genetic method of regulation; specifically included are the regulation of transcription, translation, and messenger ribonucleic acid (mRNA) processing (formation, degradation, micro-turnover, and splicing). The oscillations are independent of retinal input, and destruction of the SCN abolishes oscillations with significant downstream influence (e.g. certain behaviors, such as drinking and movement; and hormonal rhythms, such as cortisol).

13. **On the basis of the description of the circadian system, elaborate on its second part, "entrainment," and how is it related to "synchronization" of circadian rhythms.**
    Circadian rhythms are synchronized to the 24-hour day through the process of entrainment. As outlined above, the SCN is the master autonomous pacemaker for biologic rhythms, but is set at > 24 hours. The synchronization of genetic oscillating systems by a time giver (zeitgeber) is called entrainment. This anchors the internal autonomous clock to external environment. Light is the dominant correcting factor or time cue, capable of inducing sleep phase or wake phase changes. Besides photic stimuli, there are other nonphotic time cues, such as exercise, social interaction, temperature variation, and even feeding; all are capable of shifting circadian rhythms. The interaction between photic and nonphotic clues is complex and the magnitude of contributions to the human system remains to be determined. At this point, it can be said that stable entrainment likely reflects integration of both central and peripheral parameters.

14. **How is melatonin involved in regulation of circadian rhythms, and are there any other hormones that contribute to circadian rhythm regulation?**
    Melatonin communicates a chemical message of LD cycling peripherally, that is, to the remainder of the body. Melatonin levels are involved in synchronization of circadian rhythms through a circuitous neural communication to the SCN and periphery. As mentioned, the intrinsic circadian rhythm from neuronal activity in the SCN is slightly > 24 hours; therefore, the SCN clock must be reset daily by extrinsic time cues, most importantly the LD cycle. The SCN projects into PVH, mediating melatonin synthesis. Melatonin levels in the pineal gland are inhibited by light and increase at sundown, peaking at mid-darkness. This makes the neurohormone, melatonin, the chemical message communicating photoperiod "fine tuning" to the autonomous master clock in the SCN. This communication occurs through specific melatonin receptors. The MT1 and MT2 melatonin receptors are G-protein coupled with characteristic seven transmembrane domains. These two melatonin-receptor families are distributed throughout the brain (including the SCN itself) and in peripheral tissues, such as adipocytes, macrophages, platelets, gastrointestinal tract, liver, heart, kidneys, and adrenal glands. The melatonin receptors are only receptive at the LD transitions, and thus, exogenous administration of melatonin is most effective at these transitions. Therefore, pineal circadian melatonin production results from direct neuronal input from the SCN and can be regarded as hormonal output from the central circadian clock.

    The glucocorticoid (GC) hormone profile joins melatonin as a major modulator of the circadian rhythm, which then confers time-giving properties from central to peripheral clocks. In contrast to other endocrine end-organ hormones (e.g., free thyroxine [fT$_4$], insulin-like growth factor-1 [IGF-1]), which remain generally stable, the blood concentration of GCs oscillates through a 24-hour period (Fig. 65.3) and shorter periods (ultradian) for necessary episodic release. The former provides "gearing up" for the anticipated needs of the body, whereas the latter is episodically called out in rapid response to stressful stimuli. The major external synchronizer for the SCN master clock is ambient light, with melatonin regarded as hormonal output from the central (i.e., SCN) circadian clock. It is the central SCN clock that governs normal CRH secretion, which then governs pituitary ACTH release and the attendant GC secretion from the adrenal cortex. This normal release pathway, CRF→ACTH→GC, ultimately works through the glucocorticoid receptor (GR). However, the master SCN circadian clock does not express GR in significant amounts, and thus, it is not sensitive to the 24-hour CG changes or to episodic CG changes. It follows then that adrenalectomy has little influence on SCN circadian gene expression. Yet, given the ubiquitous somatic distribution of GR, circadian GC release becomes the synchronizer of the central clocks with somatic peripheral clocks. Molecular feedback loops generating central and now peripheral circadian rhythmicity work through the CLOCK and BMAL1 positive feedback loop, which includes the *CRY* and *PER* genes that can inhibit their own CLOCK/BMAL1 translocation, constituting a primary negative feedback loop (see question 12). The key hypothalamic nuclei, including the PVH (stress response, sympathetic tone modulation) and arcuate nucleus (hunger, appetite feeding modulation), have a generous distribution of GR, which allow for synchronization of non-SCN brain clocks with the 24-hour GC profile.

Table 65.2. Primary Influence on 24-Hour Variation.

HORMONE	SLEEP–WAKE HOMEOSTASIS	CIRCADIAN
GH	+++	+
PRL	+++	++
TSH	++	+++
Testosterone	++	++
Cortisol	+	+++

GH, Growth hormone; *PRL,* prolactin; *TSH,* thyroid-stimulating hormone.

15. Name the two hormones that are elevated early in sleep and the two hormones that are elevated late in sleep.
    Recall that SWS predominates during the first third of sleep and REM predominates during the last half of sleep.
    GH and prolactin (PRL) are entrained to SWS (see Fig. 65.4). The increase in GH secretion during sleep is well
    known. Regardless of age and gender, most PRL secretion also occurs when the individual is asleep, with
    nocturnal maximum PRL levels twice that of daytime levels. The nighttime GH and PRL surges are associated
    with the first period of SWS. In fact, the GH surge immediately after sleep onset is the largest of the 24-hour
    period for both genders, although in females the surge is less than in males. Females have two evening GH
    surges; the first is before sleep onset, and a second occurs with SWS. Males have few daytime GH pulses
    compared with females. The surges for PRL and GH are lost during a night of total sleep deprivation and return
    during daytime recovery sleep. It is the onset of sleep and not the time of day that primarily triggers GH and PRL
    release, please note PRL also has the stronger circadian trigger (Table 65.2).
    The hormones that increase later in sleep are testosterone and cortisol. Testosterone rises just after mid-
    night and cortisol begins its rise at 2 AM, peaking at 6 to 9 AM. The timing and amount of REM sleep are related
    to the late-sleep rise of these two hormones in men. But the 24-hour rhythm for both testosterone and cortisol is
    primarily controlled by circadian rhythmicity (process-C) and not sleep–wake homeostasis (process-S). Before we
    leave this subject, it is well known that many drugs increase serum prolactin levels (e.g., narcotics, antiemetics,
    antipsychotics). Added to this list are the benzodiazepine sedatives and imidazopiridine hypnotics, such as
    triazolam and zolpidem. Taking either at bedtime is associated with nocturnal, but not daytime, marked
    increases in serum prolactin.

16. How does gonadotropin release change from youth to adulthood, and is the LH adulthood pattern solely
    responsible for gonadal steroid release?
    a. Regarding changes to maturity: Sexual maturity is geared to enable men and women to achieve daily
       sperm and monthly egg production, respectively. There is a pulsatile release of both luteinizing hormone (LH)
       and follicle-stimulating hormone (FSH) before puberty and increased pulses occur with sleep. Gonadotropin
       secretion during the day is without circadian rhythm, differing from testosterone, which has a significant
       circadian rhythm. The gender-similar gonadotropin patterns diverge with puberty, with the menstrual cycle
       phase exerting unique influences on LH pulses. Indeed, one of the hallmarks of puberty is increased nocturnal
       pulse amplitudes of LH and FSH. Each LH pulse is in direct response to a hypothalamic gonadotropin-
       releasing hormone (GnRH) surge. However, GnRH pulses are not directly related to pituitary FSH secretion.
       With the advent of sexual maturity, the brisk LH and FSH pulses of puberty give way to lower amplitude,
       90-minute interval LH surges without significant diurnal variation. Essentially, the male will continue his
       90-minute interval LH pulses with little FSH pulsatility, whereas the female will show marked increases of
       LH pulse frequency during the follicular phase, with little change to the amplitude in either the follicular or
       luteal phases. There is a nocturnal LH pulse frequency decrease in the early follicular phase but not in the
       luteal phase. This slowing is sleep–wake related and is not circadian (i.e., seen in day-time sleep, but not
       seen in night-time wakefulness). Finally, FSH and LH secretion are increased in men and women as they age,
       with pulse frequency being increased, whereas amplitude is decreased. Additionally, in men age ≥ 30 years,
       there is a progressive decline in total testosterone associated with an increase in sex hormone binding globu-
       lin, resulting in an even greater decline in serum free testosterone levels; for this reason, free or bioavailable
       testosterone measurements may be warranted when evaluating older men for hypogonadism. The serum
       gonadotropin rise and pulse frequency increase are noted in menstruating women age > 40 years. One study
       showed a causal relationship between gonadotropin elevation, vasomotor symptoms (VMSs) and decreases
       in objective and subjective sleep quality. The North American Menopause Society published a 2017 position
       statement regarding the use of menopausal hormone replacement therapy (HRT). There, it is noted that the
       benefit–risk ratios for HRT are most favorable for women age < 60 years or who are within 10 years of the

onset of menopause, and who have no contraindications for HRT treatment of bothersome VMSs and for those at elevated risk for bone loss or fracture.

b. Regarding gonad steroid release: FSH stimulates recruitment and growth of immature ovarian follicles and preservation of growing follicles in females. Once a follicle is in the 8- to 10-mm range, its estradiol secretion markedly increases. Mean monthly estrogen is essentially constant in eumenorrheic females, yet a diurnal free estradiol rhythm exists and consists of two major components: (1) an asymmetrically peaked diurnal cycle; (2) ultradian (shorter than a day) harmonics in the range of 6 to 12 hours. The diurnal and ultradian rhythms are remarkably consistent throughout the menstrual cycle in terms of 24-hour mean level, peak width, and amplitude. In contrast, there is less complicated diurnal variation in males. The early-morning rise in testosterone that started at sleep onset increases to maximum levels during the last half of sleep (REM predominant) and is not associated with corresponding LH surges. The characteristic male night-time LH surges occur later on, during the last half of sleep. Recently, a testosterone surge was observed during adult day-time recovery sleep, and a testosterone decrease followed as the patient remained awake after this day-time recovery sleep. All this suggests that sleep itself, independent of LH bursts, contributes to testosterone release. Therefore, the 24-hour testosterone profile and its response to sleep deprivation and daytime recovery sleep are more like the prolactin profile (see Fig. 65.3).

c. Tying this together by using an example: When a sleep-deprived male resident in internal medicine finally gets some sleep, his testosterone will surge during recovery sleep; remember that during the normal day, and in one who has not slept, testosterone levels are on a decline. So, if low testosterone is found in an individual, it may be from primary hypogonadism, but it may also be sleep deprivation, OSA, or even shift work. For the female shift worker, they will have the typical fragmented and shorter sleep, but the frequently associated menstrual irregularities could be from the altered sleep patterns. But in both genders with normal sleep–wake cycles there is no significant circadian pacemaker for the gonadotropins' diurnal change. It is fair to tell patients to get their testosterone levels drawn first thing in the morning in a rested state, on the basis of the observations that sleep increases testosterone, wakefulness decreases it, and the circadian influence may be less potent than sleep–wake homeostasis.

17. **What are the sleep characteristics associated with rising AM testosterone levels?**
There is accumulating evidence in adult men that the testosterone profile is significantly influenced by NREM–REM cycling. Sleep architecture, characteristics which is associated with a nocturnal rise in AM testosterone, as follows: (1) duration of the first NREM period; (2) daytime recovery sleep; (3) habitual sleep duration. Restriction of sleep to 5 hours/night for just 5 consecutive nights decreases AM serum testosterone levels up to 15% and one night with no sleep or sleeping only 4.5 hours in the first half of the night decreases AM testosterone levels by 20%. These facts argue for assessing sleep habits of patients in the workup for hypogonadism (see last question of the chapter on taking sleep history).

18. **Does penile tumescence have any relation to sleep architecture, and if so what?**
Since the 1970s, it has been known that nocturnal erections are phenomena of REM sleep. Therefore, the classic hypogonadal teaching that decreased morning erections are caused by low testosterone levels may be related to more than one primary problem. The patient with decreased or absent morning erections may have hypogonadism, but the root cause could lie in abnormal sleep architecture (i.e., sleep disease impairing REM density). One recent 12-week randomized trial evaluated the use of continuous positive airway pressure (CPAP) versus vardenafil versus placebo in a two-by-two factorial study design in 61 men (mean age 55 years; body mass index [BMI] 32 kg/m^2) with AM serum total testosterone levels $\leq$ 299.9 ng/dL. The CPAP treatment groups showed improvement in, among other parameters, nocturnal erections. The use of CPAP for 6.2 hours per night resulted in a decrease in respiratory events from a mean apnea–hypopnea index (AHI) of 39 events to 14 events per hour in the per-protocol group. Note that CPAP, in this study, improved OSA from the severe range to the mild range, but not into the normal range (AHI < 5 events/hr). One might speculate that even better results would be seen with normalized breathing (AHI < 5 events/hr) at night. Regardless, the authors conclude "these data may convince some men who highly value erectile function to adhere to CPAP therapy." Other endocrine systems also show a dose–duration response improvement with CPAP. Another inference from these data supports closer historical screening for sleep disease (see question 41) in those patients admitting to decreased or absent morning erections.

19. **Is the testosterone decline observed with aging related to changes associated with the sleep pattern of aging?**
Yes, at least in part, it does. As discussed previously (see Fig. 65.2), aging is associated with less time in overall sleep and less time in SWS. In older men, LH pulses show lower amplitude but increased frequency (see question 16 for a more complete answer). Also, to this author's knowledge, not all the parameters listed in question 17 above have been considered and, therefore, could be confounders to the data associated with testosterone changes in aging. The sleep-related testosterone rise is still seen in older men, although the magnitude is less, and it is no longer associated with duration of the first NREM period.

20. **What factors influence TSH release?**

TSH secretion is primarily related to circadian rhythm, Process-C, though there is SWH, Process-S, influence (see Fig 65.4, third panel from top). TSH secretion in young healthy males shows an early evening circadian elevation before sleep onset, then a decline shortly after sleep onset continuing until it reaches a nadir in the afternoon. The inhibitory influence of sleep on TSH release is thought to occur during SWS. Therefore, clinicians may need to temper therapeutic decisions made on the basis of a sole mid-afternoon TSH value or an evening TSH level ordered in an emergency department. The highest TSH levels in the daytime, when outpatient laboratories are open, are after a person wakes up. With acute sleep loss, TSH takes its usual early-evening upturn at approximately 6 PM but, instead of the usual TSH downturn at sleep onset, with sleep deprivation TSH continues to rise to nearly twice the normal maximum through the middle of the usual sleep period. TSH hits a peak in the middle of the total sleep deprivation period, and from there, it begins a downward trajectory, eventually normalizing in the sleep-deprived individual's day-time recovery sleep. Thus, a TSH value obtained at 7 AM in such a patient reflects the influence of lack of sleep and probably does not reflect the need for thyroid hormone initiation or adjustment. The loss of an inhibitory effect of sleep on the circadian TSH elevation may contribute to elevated TSH values seen in acutely ill hospitalized patients.

21. **TSH and cortisol secretion profiles are circadian, so why are their levels not parallel through the night and day?**

The difference in these two hormone profiles is attributable to the extent that each is influenced by either process-C or process-S (Table 65.2). However, this question is not straightforward. The difference demonstrates nicely the primary process-C contribution to cortisol secretion versus the influence of a combination of process-S plus process-C on TSH secretion. In general, the day-to-night pattern for both hormones is not parallel, but they are similar (see Fig. 65.3). The patterns of both reveal the highest hormone levels during sleep and the lowest levels during the day, but the 24-hour highest level for TSH occurs as a person goes to sleep, whereas the cortisol peak occurs as the person wakes up. The cortisol profile is nearly all circadian governed (process-C), so it does not show significant variation with acute sleep deprivation. In contrast, nocturnal TSH will *increase* with acute sleep loss and *decrease* with daytime-recovery sleep. Thus, the evening TSH increase before sleep onset reveals process-C influence, whereas the decrease of TSH during sleep reflects an influence of process-S. To continue a description of the excursion of these hormones during a normal 24-hour cycle, TSH fluctuations precede those of cortisol, with TSH starting its rise before sleep onset and before the cortisol rise and starting its descent also before the cortisol descent. Cortisol peaks in the last third of the night, and, as mentioned, TSH begins to rise before sleep onset. Then, with sleep achieved, TSH hits its peak between 10 PM and midnight followed by a slow during-the-day TSH decline with a nadir by mid-afternoon. Given that corticotrophin (ACTH) release is primarily influenced by the time of day (process-C), the normal 24-hour cortisol profile does not have a significant change in shape with total sleep deprivation or during daytime recovery sleep. Cortisol will hit its 24-hour nadir after the transition to sleep, between 10 PM and midnight; then, as though someone rattles its cage, cortisol rises abruptly after midnight and peaks at 6 to 9 AM (by the second third of sleep, the cortisol rise is underway regardless of sleep–wake state). Normal awakening is the herald of the cortisol decline, progressing over the entire waking period with a nadir after sleep transition in the successive night of sleep. But, as is well known, cortisol is a stress response hormone and will increase with stress (e.g., someone cuts in front in traffic, or there is a morning dental appointment); with such events, this end-of-the-night/start-of-the-day surge of cortisol pattern will change. This stress-sensitive trigger is not seen with TSH. Therefore, a change to one's sleep-wake cycle influences the release of both hormones but to different extents. In a study of healthy young men during nocturnal sleep deprivation from 10 PM to 6 AM, with the lack of TSH suppression by sleep, TSH more than doubled. That is, TSH rose from its afternoon nadir of approximately 1.5 mU/L to a new peak of approximately 3.8 mU/L at 2 AM and, in the follow-on recovery sleep (10 AM–6 PM), TSH returned to a mean of 1.25 mU/L; but there was no effect on cortisol. It is well documented that interruptions to nocturnal sleep are associated with short-term TSH elevations. TSH levels normalize when normal nocturnal sleep is resumed. In contrast to the absence of acute sleep deprivation effects on cortisol, repeated and prolonged nocturnal sleep interruptions do result in cortisol elevations.

22. **Jet lag is not uncommon. How are some of its symptoms attributable to the observed changes in cortisol and TSH?**

Jet lag is a well-known sleep disorder arising from crossing multiple time zones in a short period. However, it probably has underlying endocrine pathophysiology. Essentially, the circadian process becomes misaligned with the destination time zone. This is particularly true when flying east, which moves time zones ahead and puts the individual at risk for insomnia, whereas flying west moves the time zones back, putting the traveler at risk for daytime sleepiness in the new time zone. For example, if a physician departs London on a nonstop 10-hour flight west to Los Angeles, the doctor's circadian clock is set to London although his or her body is now located in Los Angeles. London is 8 hours ahead of Los Angeles. So, if the flight leaves London at 8 AM, he or she will arrive in Los Angeles at 6 PM London time (in his or her circadian clock); but because of the 8-hour time difference, it is 10 AM Pacific Standard Time (PST). He or she clears customs and, by noon, is home exhausted, sleeps 8 hours, and wakes at 8 PM PST. You can see that this person will struggle with unwanted sleepiness and insomnia until his or her clock shifts from London time to PST.

Patients with insomnia, whose total time asleep/total time in bed is < 70% of normal, have significantly higher evening and early sleep cortisol levels. In a study of young adults whose circadian rhythms were perturbed by a flight from Europe to the US, *GH secretory patterns adjusted within a few days to the new sleep–wake cycle, but the cortisol levels remained disassociated for 2 weeks.* This dissociation is thought to contribute to the symptoms of jet lag syndrome. Disruption of the hypothalamic–pituitary–thyroid axis during prolonged flight has also been studied. The usual TSH-suppressive influence of sleep may not be present in prolonged air travel because the traveler remains awake. This translates to an overall TSH elevation, paralleled by a small, temporary increase in serum T_3 levels. The study related the fatigue and discomfort of jet lag syndrome to the prolonged elevation of thyroid hormone as well as to the desynchronization of multiple circadian rhythms.

23. How do circadian and sleep–wake processes influence glucose and insulin levels?

Glucose and insulin levels are influenced by both process-C and SWH. Studies in normal adults have demonstrated a 30% increase in glucose and a 60% increase in insulin levels during nocturnal sleep (Fig. 65.4, bottom two panels). During sleep deprivation, glucose levels and insulin secretion rates increase at the habitual sleep time, although to a much lesser degree, suggesting circadian modulation. In recovery sleep, however, glucose levels and insulin secretion both markedly increase, suggesting modulation by sleep itself.

In a recent review, evidence was presented suggesting that multiple processes within adipose tissue (e.g., inflammatory pathways, lipogenesis, lipolysis, and even insulin sensitivity, etc.) are controlled by the circadian clock; furthermore, with clock disruption, there is enhanced adiposity, insulin resistance, and increased susceptibility to T2DM development. Finally, compelling evidence was presented highlighting how circadian clocks contribute to islet cell function, having a critical role in the regulation of beta-cell and alpha-cell function and turnover. With regard to therapeutic targeting, as mentioned in question 13, melatonin can be regarded as hormonal output from the central circadian clock. Timed melatonin supplementation in rodents has been shown to reduce adiposity while also decreasing skeletal muscle and hepatic insulin resistance. In addition, islet cells from subjects with T2DM isolated in cell culture showed improved glucose-stimulated insulin secretion and beta cell survival in response to melatonin. The highlighted mechanisms included attenuation of induction of oxidative and endoplasmic reticulum stress.

24. How does aging change hormonal release?

Changes to sleep architecture with aging are thought to lead to hormonal changes. Normal aging is associated with loss of SWS and REM, with increased sleep fragmentation (see Fig. 65.2). Recall that GH and PRL rise primarily in relation to the SWS of NREM, whereas TSH, cortisol, and testosterone increases are primarily under circadian control. In younger men, there is a dose-response relationship between SWS and GH secretion. For example, in 16- to 25-year-old males, SWS is nearly 20% of the sleep period and tails off to 5% to 10% at age > 40 years. This is associated with GH secretion during sleep of ~350 mcg in the 16- to 25-year-old, but not > 100 mcg in individuals age > 35 years. Most of the PRL released during a 24-hour period is during sleep regardless of gender; there is nearly a 50% decrement in nocturnal PRL secretion with aging. The extent of circadian changes in cortisol and TSH are less dramatic with aging. Day–night TSH fluctuations also dampen with age.

25. What is the definition of sleep-disordered breathing (SDB), and how does this differ from OSA?

Confusion arises when the terms *sleep-disordered breathing* (SDB) or *sleep-related breathing disorder* (SRBD), and OSA are used interchangeably in the literature and in sleep laboratory reports. SRBD and SDB are disease headings under which other diseases are arranged, much like chronic obstructive pulmonary disease comprises a general reference for other specific pulmonary disease entities. SRBD, on the one hand, contains adult and pediatric central sleep apnea and OSA syndromes. OSA, on the other hand, is a specific adult and pediatric disorder that is diagnosed with polysomnography (PSG). OSA can be suspected on the basis of complaints from the patient or his or her bed partner. Such complaints include unintentional sleep episodes during wakefulness, daytime sleepiness, unrefreshing sleep, fatigue, insomnia, waking from sleep with breath holding, gasping or choking, loud snoring, and breathing interruptions. Rendering the diagnosis of OSA includes ruling out current medical, neurologic, and/or substance abuse disorders. Of note, some prescribed medications can also increase the risk for OSA.

26. What are respiratory events?

Respiratory events are apnea, hypopnea, and respiratory effort–related arousal (RERA). An apneic episode is an airflow decrease of at least 90% from baseline lasting at least 10 seconds (try holding your own breath for 10 seconds!). Hypopnea is defined as 10 seconds of at least a 30% decrease in airflow, resulting in ≥ 4% desaturation on pulse oximetry. RERA criteria should be sought if an observed event does not meet apnea or hypopnea criteria. RERA is defined as a sequence of breaths > 10 seconds in duration associated with increased respiratory effort and results in an arousal from sleep. The American Academy of Sleep Medicine (AASM) directs that apnea, hypopnea, and RERA, if present, be scored in the routine PSG interpretation. The average number of apnea and hypopnea episodes in 1 hour is referred to as the apnea–hypopnea index (AHI). However, if RERA is present, then the average number of apnea, hypopnea, and RERA should be calculated. This is the respiratory disturbance index (RDI). Note that the AHI does not equal the RDI, even though the terms are sometimes used interchangeably; such an interchange could create confusion.

27. **What is the prevalence of OSA?**

    The prevalence is dependent on the definition of OSA. The earliest epidemiologic investigations, primarily of white men, estimated up to 4% had OSA (60%–90% were obese). The prevalence of OSA for adults age 30 to 60 years is currently *24% in men and 9% in women*. Obesity is a major risk factor. In nonobese patients, genetic craniofacial features, such as retrognathia (maxillary insufficiency), are correlated with OSA. As more data on OSA emerge, the prevalence may become unique to populations or ethnicities. For example, in Asian nonobese male office workers, BMI and age were positively correlated, but the correlation with weight was less than in white, non-Asian subjects. Risk factors for OSA other than adiposity, such as pharyngeal narrowing, retrognathia or micrognathia, and pharyngeal collapsibility, are thought to assume greater pathologic significance in Asians.

28. **Define sleep deprivation. How common is it?**

    Sleep deprivation can be acute or chronic. By definition, going without sleep for 24 hours is total acute sleep loss, whereas sleeping < 6 hours a night for ≥ 6 nights is considered chronic sleep deprivation. People in industrialized nations are sleeping less. In the United States, for example, over 30% of adults age < 64 years report sleeping < 6 hours per night, leaving no doubt that many patients are accumulating chronic sleep deprivation.

29. **What are the key features of sleep deprivation versus sleep apnea?**

    In sleep deprivation, the person does not sleep but breathes normally. In sleep apnea, the person sleeps but does not breathe well during sleep. One can objectively measure excessive daytime sleepiness (EDS) with a standardized tool, such as the Epworth Sleepiness Scale (ESS). One must appreciate that this screening tool is specific but not sensitive. An ESS score > 9 to 10 is consistent with EDS, but not necessarily OSA. The greatest clinical use for this scale is serial tracking of patients in response to therapy. It is important to remember that the ESS does not correlate with (1) objective testing for sleepiness; (2) likelihood of OSA on overnight PSG; and (3) the patient's perception of sleep-related problems. Patients with acute or chronic shortening of sleep resist the drive to sleep with no impairment of gas exchange. In OSA, there is a repetitive collapse of the upper airway, which induces apneic and hypopneic episodes despite persistent thoracic and abdominal respiratory effort. This leads to mechanical loading on the upper airway, chest wall, and diaphragm. What follows are hypoxia, hypercarbia, and a marked increase in SNS tone. OSA often leads to disruption or fragmentation of the usual sleep–wake cycle and endocrine responsiveness. Both can contribute to fatigue and daytime sleepiness. In contrast, if EDS is secondary to sleep deprivation, the patient's sleep continuity is normal and is often associated with an increase in SWS.

30. **In view of increased SNS tone in OSA (see question 29), does the comorbidity of OSA interfere with the assessment of metanephrines and catecholamines when screening for pheochromocytoma?**

    Yes. OSA results in an appropriate release of catecholamines in response to physiologic stress or disease, just as myocardial infarctions, cerebral vascular accidents, and acute heart failure are associated with appropriate acute catecholamine increases. If a 24-hour urinary collection is performed in the setting of undiagnosed or poorly treated OSA, it would likely contain elevated metanephrine and catecholamine levels. This may falsely suggest a diagnosis of pheochromocytoma.

31. **What endocrine diseases are associated with OSA?**

    The endocrine diseases commonly associated with OSA are *hypothyroidism, acromegaly*, and *polycystic ovary syndrome* (PCOS), but the most prevalent are *obesity* and *T2DM*. As would be expected, the statistics for these disorders vary, depending on the series. Although it was once thought that all patients with OSA had subclinical hypothyroidism, this has now been shown not to be the case. In general, 11% to 30% of patients with OSA will have subclinical or overt hypothyroidism, and the prevalence of OSA in patients with hypothyroidism is about 30%. OSA is reversible in the majority of such patients once they are treated appropriately with thyroid hormone replacement. In one prospective study of nonobese, middle-age men and women with newly diagnosed symptomatic hypothyroidism, 30% had OSA by PSG at study onset; 84% of those subjects had reversal of OSA with TSH normalization. Finally, insulin levels and measures of glucose tolerance in PCOS are strongly correlated with the risk and severity of OSA. Additionally, among those PCOS women with normal glucose tolerance, insulin levels are significantly higher in those at high versus low OSA risk, independent of BMI. Therefore, it is reasonable to assess measures of sleep habits and behaviors, and restorative sleep in all patients with PCOS. Probably the most alarming statistics are the prevalence of obesity and its partner in crime, T2DM. Using the older OSA diagnostic criteria, the prevalence of moderate-to-severe OSA in obese women and men age < 65 years, was 4% to 7% and 9% to 14%, respectively. More recent studies, using current diagnostic definitions, reported a substantially higher prevalence of moderate-to-severe OSA of 23% in obese women and 49% in obese men.

32. **How is the sleep apnea of GH excess different from the sleep apnea of thyroid hormone deficiency?**

    GH excess is associated with a high proportion of OSA and central sleep apnea, whereas hypothyroidism is almost uniformly associated with OSA. Up to 60% of patients with acromegaly are eventually found to have sleep apnea by PSG studies. In one series, over 30% had central sleep apnea. Endoscopy revealed little occlusive posterior tongue movement during sleep, indicating that this is not from macroglossia. The mechanism for central sleep apnea in patients with acromegaly is not clear.

33. How does sleep deprivation influence glucose tolerance?

In one study, after 1 week of sleeping 4 hours per night, there were increases in post-breakfast insulin resistance. During sleep restriction, glucose tolerance is nearly 40% worse compared with that in a group with sleep extension. Interestingly, it is first-phase insulin release that has been found to be markedly reduced. When sleep-deprived individuals go into recovery sleep (sleeping during the day because of prior sleep deprivation), there are marked elevations of glucose and insulin levels, indicating that sleep also exerts modulatory influences on glucose regulation independent of the circadian rhythm. At this point, it is important to reference a recent meta-analysis of 36 studies incorporating over 1 million patients, which compared the relative contribution of sleep disturbances risk for T2DM development with traditional T2DM risk factor development; the relative risk of T2DM development is given within parenthesis: overweight (2.99) > family history of T2DM (2.33) > personal history of OSA (2.02) > sleep less than 5 hours (1.48) > shift work or sleeping > 9 hours or the independent characteristic of poor sleep quality (1.4) > physical activity (1.2); this demonstrating traditional RF greater relative contribution than sleep characteristics, but sleep characteristics clearly important.

34. What sleep abnormalities are associated with abnormal glucose metabolism?

Snoring, sleep duration, and OSA have all been linked to hyperglycemia and T2DM risk.

a. Interestingly just *snoring*, in nonobese Asians and especially in those who are obese, has been independently associated with abnormal oral glucose tolerance tests and higher hemoglobin A_{1c} (HbA_{1c}) levels.

b. In epidemiologic studies, *sleep duration* has been both negatively and positively correlated with the risk of developing T2DM. Observational studies have shown that patients who report < 6 hours of sleep per night have an increased prevalence of glucose intolerance and T2DM. Very recently, it was found that the duration of sleep (< 6 and > 8 hours per night) was predictive of an increased incidence of T2DM.

c. *OSA*, as diagnosed with PSG, is independently associated with abnormal glucose metabolism. A recent study extends this independent association through rigorous assessment of the potential confounders of overweight/obesity. In this cross-sectional analysis of 2588 patients, it was shown that impaired fasting glucose (IFG), impaired glucose tolerance (IGT), and occult diabetes are associated (but to different degrees) with OSA in both the normal-weight (BMI < 25 kg/m²) and overweight/obese subgroups. This suggests that individuals with OSA are at special risk for T2DM. Importantly, sleep fragmentation and hypoxemia are likely OSA culprits leading to hyperglycemia. A 2009 study comparing subjects without diabetes who had OSA with patients without diabetes who had mild, moderate, and severe OSA showed 27%, 37%, and 44% decreases, respectively, in insulin sensitivity caused by OSA; this contribution to reduced insulin sensitivity was found to be independent of age, gender, ethnicity, and percent body fat. Furthermore, there were no increases in insulin concentrations. Unfortunately, at present the relative contributions of sleep restriction, sleep fragmentation, and hypoxia cannot be ascertained. The risk of hyperglycemia is likely proportional to OSA severity; data from diverse patient populations suggest that OSA severity is a risk for T2DM development. The prevalence of OSA in patients with T2DM is 60% to 80% based on an evaluation of 12 clinic or community-based cohorts from 2003 to 2016. The prevalence of T2DM in patients with OSA is reported to be 15% to 30%.

35. What are the main mechanisms underlying the development abnormal glucose metabolism in patients with OSA?

The hallmark of OSA is airflow reduction, which is typically associated with intermittent hypoxemia, sleep fragmentation, and SNS stimulation. In animal studies, insulin sensitivity has been shown to vary with intermittent hypoxemia, independent of activation of the SNS. Additionally, it has been shown that in overweight to mildly obese males without diabetes, every 4% decrease in oxygen saturation is associated with an odds ratio that approaches 2.0 for IGT. Sleep fragmentation has also been associated with abnormal glucose metabolism. In one study of *healthy* adults, selective suppression of SWS (without decreasing total sleep time) was associated with decreases in insulin sensitivity of nearly 25%! This suggests that the low levels of SWS in the sleep-restricted, the elderly, and obese subjects may contribute to their increased incidence of T2DM. In a study of consecutive adults with T2DM (age 41–77 years; BMI 20–57 kg/m²), mild OSA was associated with a mean HbA_{1c} of 7.22% and severe OSA with a HbA_{1c} of almost 9.42%. After adjustments for age, gender, race, BMI, number of antidiabetes medications, level of exercise, years of diabetes, and total sleep time, the severity of OSA by AHI correlated significantly with higher mean HbA_{1c} values.

36. With respect to causality, does the use of CPAP improve abnormal glucose metabolism parameters?

Yes. This is seen in subjects without diabetes, in nonobese patients with diabetes, and in patients with poorly controlled diabetes. *Caveat:* In this body of work, the reader must discern from the trial whether or not there was a published measure of CPAP compliance and, when subjects were compliant with CPAP treatment, how effective the treatment was in normalizing events. It is likely that the study group that will get maximum benefit is the one with normalized sleep (duration > 7 hours, with residual AHI < 5 events/hr). Trials reporting definitions for CPAP treatment adherence and those demonstrating no change in BMI during the study period do show improvement. A study of patients without diabetes who had moderate-to-severe OSA reported that CPAP significantly improved insulin sensitivity after only 2 days of treatment and that the improvement persisted at the 3-month follow-up with no significant changes seen in body weight. Interestingly, this benefit was most pronounced in nonobese subjects. In contrast, the same research laboratory showed no improvement in insulin sensitivity in obese patients with T2DM. In other trials, postprandial blood glucose levels improved most significantly after CPAP use in patients with T2DM and OSA. Overall OSA treatment in patients with diabetes translated to a mean decrease in HbA_{1c} of 0.4% (from 8.4% to 8%). The CPAP influence was larger in those with higher initial HbA_{1c} values. In one trial of consecutive patients with poorly controlled T2DM ($HbA_{1c} > 8.5\%$) and moderate or severe OSA (undiagnosed/or known but not untreated), normalization of respiratory events translated to a mean decrease in HbA_{1c} of 0.9%. This is respectable T2DM therapy because most current T2DM medications lower HbA_{1c} by roughly 0.5% to 1.5%. Therefore, one can say that for the price of a good night of sleep the patient with diabetes is also likely to achieve glycemic improvement. Naysayers would argue that although this benefit is reported, it is likely offset by weight gain resulting from CPAP therapy. However, in the randomized controlled trials that addressed this question, there was no change in body composition; furthermore, daytime sleepiness improved and physical activity increased over a 3-month period. It is reasonable to conclude that the use of CPAP is at least weight neutral, but this issue remains under investigation. There remain concerns that the decreased work of breathing with CPAP and the improved GH secretion associated with restoration of sleep architecture may increase the tendency to gain weight (see question 38).

37. **How well are providers in diabetes clinics screening their patients for OSA? What are good tools for screening by history and physical examination?**
    A study of patients with diabetes, using a validated questionnaire to quantify OSA risk and sleepiness, revealed that 56% of patients reported snoring, 29% had fatigue upon awakening, and 34% reported feeling tired during wake time. The authors of the study concluded that 56% of those questioned were at high risk for OSA. This finding supports a call for greater vigilance in screening for OSA in patients with diabetes given the high prevalence of SDB found in this patient population. Certain screening tools may be helpful toward this end. BMI is proportional to OSA risk. Neck size > 17 inches is the most sensitive physical finding. Some craniofacial changes, such as retrognathia, also place a patient at high risk. Keep in mind a patient with OSA is often unaware of the neurocognitive changes that have developed slowly over time, and thus, he or she may not volunteer a history consistent with OSA, unless directly queried.

38. **Does the effective use of CPAP in patients with OSA lead to weight loss?**
    Results are not consistent on this matter. Some 30% of patients treated for OSA may have stable or even increased body weight, with two mechanisms having been implicated: (1) Decreased work of breathing with treated OSA translates to conservation of calories during sleep; and (2) improved sleep architecture leads to increased SWS and, therefore, increased GH secretion with attendant weight gain. For those that lose weight, two distinct mechanisms have also been proposed. First, patients treated for OSA usually wake more rested and with a sense of improved vitality or energy; once on treatment, patients with OSA have even been shown to exercise more. Second, treatment of OSA results in normalization of serum leptin (from the Greek word *leptos*, meaning "thin"), the so-called satiety hormone. As will be discussed below, leptin is suppressed during sleep deprivation and in untreated sleep apnea.

39. **What are the effects of sleep deprivation on leptin ("satiety hormone") and ghrelin ("hunger hormone")?**
    With sleep deprivation, leptin decreases and ghrelin (from the original root *ghre* meaning "to grow") increases. In longer than average sleep, leptin increases, and ghrelin decreases. It has been documented that leptin secretion is blunted in sleep-deprived subjects and that over a 6-month period of time sleep deprived subjects gain an average of 10 lb more compared with rested subjects.

40. **How does the testosterone panel change with OSA? Does OSA treatment influence the panel?**
    The androgen changes of OSA are distinct from those seen with aging and obesity (Table 65.3). In OSA, there are decreases in serum total and free testosterone and sex hormone–binding globulin levels without concomitant gonadotropin increases. In fact, one study showed LH pulse disturbances with untreated OSA. Interestingly, testosterone levels improve with OSA treatment, whether by CPAP or with uvulopalatopharyngoplasty. These findings point to a hypothalamic mechanism for low testosterone levels in untreated OSA.

Table 65.3. Androgen Changes in Common Circumstances.

CONDITION	SHBG	TOTAL TESTOSTERONE	FREE TESTOSTERONE
Aging	↑	↓	↓
Obesity	↓	↓	Normal
OSA	↓	↓	↓

OSA, Obstructive sleep apnea; *SHBG*, sex hormone–binding globulin.

41. **How does androgen replacement therapy influence sleep?**

Exogenous testosterone may worsen existing OSA or lead to changes associated with OSA. One randomized controlled trial revealed that high-dose testosterone administration in hypogonadal, otherwise healthy, elderly men shortened total sleep time and worsened coexisting undiagnosed sleep apnea. Although there have been no substantiated reports of decreased cognition and impaired driving ability with hypogonadism, it is incumbent on the prescriber to screen patients for the possibility of undiagnosed OSA before prescribing androgen replacement therapy.

42. **How does one determine the possible primary contribution of a sleep abnormality in a patient with fatigue?**

Some illustrative examples will be useful. A female patient complains of fatigue and believes it must be caused by a thyroid problem; and a male patient has similar complaints and attributes his fatigue to low testosterone. The following is presented to allow the clinician to pick and choose an individualized approach to each specific patient.

1. Differentiate whether there is an element of sleepiness to what a patient means by "fatigue"—that is, seek to differentiate, if possible, fatigue and sleepiness. Fatigue and sleepiness may mean the same thing to some patients. However, fatigue is usually felt after prolonged exertion or hard physical work. Patients may have a sense of not feeling normal, decreased efficiency, loss of power, and even loss of responsiveness to stimulation. If the fatigue has an element of sleepiness, however, this may be historical evidence that the primary complaint is actually sleepiness. Such a patient usually has deficient sleep duration and/or disrupted sleep (insomnia, untreated OSA, or restless leg syndrome), may admit to sleepiness upon awakening despite > 7 hours of apparent sleep time and/or difficulty staying awake in the late morning, afternoon, or with family in evening.

2. Use a basic sleep history to implicate a problem with sleep habits that might provide a clue to sleep pathology. The average adult should be getting at least 7 hours of consolidated sleep with < 20 to 30 minutes to get to sleep and < 20 to 30 minutes of awake time after they initially achieve sleep. Are the time they go to bed, the time they are asleep, and their wake time usually consistent? Do they have the typical features of SDB; for example, do they wake up frequently during the night, often for reasons unknown, sometimes snoring themselves awake? Are there unprovoked sweating episodes, and are there awakenings consistent with hot flushing (which may also happen during the day)? Do they have increased heartburn at night? Is there increased movement or fitful sleeping, such as moving back and forth or finding the bed covers helter-skelter in the morning? Does their partner complain of loud snoring or breath holding? Is there difficulty with leg movement or features of a clinical diagnosis of restless leg syndrome (RLS)? The mnemonic for diagnosing RLS is "URGE," Urge to move legs (can only be ill-defined leg discomfort), worse with Rest, better if the patient Gets up and walks around, and finally worse in Evening – fascinatingly there is this circadian feature to RLS.

3. Use the screening tools for sleepiness and for risk of occult OSA. Remember, the tools are specific and not sensitive. Use the ESS (see question #29) for assessment of daytime sleepiness; a score in the 9 to 10 range warrants further review of the sleep history (though not necessarily a sleep study). Additionally, one can screen for the risk of sleep apnea using the pneumonic **STOPBANG**:

Snoring loudly (louder than usual speech, or heard behind closed doors)
Tired during the day
Observed apneas
Pressure—treated for hypertension
BMI > 35 kg/m^2
Age > 50 years
Neck circumference > 16 inches (40 cm)
Gender male
Each parameter $= 1$ point. The total score is used to predict risk of OSA: low risk $= 0$ to 2; intermediate risk $= 3$ to 4; high risk $= 5$ to 8.

4. Use the physical examination to look for features that may worsen collapsibility of the already malleable adult posterior oropharynx (OP) during sleep. Recall that it is only the airway segment below the jaw angle and above the manubrium that does not have anatomic buttressing and is, therefore, vulnerable to nighttime narrowing. So, look for anything in the OP that can impact this dynamic. For example, examine the overall anterior perspective of the OP for these features: *narrow jaw* (high arched palate, teeth crowding); *septal deviation; insufficiency of the mandible;* so-called *receding chin* with attendant *maxillary overjet.* For example, is there ≥ 3 to 5 mm space between the posterior surface of the maxillary incisors and the anterior surface of the mandibular incisors? If so, this could indicate a narrowed OP. Another related tip is to check for mandibular insufficiency (i.e., protrusion of the maxillary incisors, also known as "buckteeth"). From the profile view of the face, maxillary insufficiency gives the patient a flat-to-concave facial profile; these patients can also have a smaller zygomatic arch. With the mouth open assess tonsil size. Tonsillar enlargement is graded as follows: grade 0 $=$ tonsils are *absent*; grade 1 $=$ tonsils *hidden behind* tonsillar pillars; grade 2 $=$ tonsils *extend to* pillars; grade 3 $=$ tonsils *visible beyond* pillars; and grade 4 $=$ tonsils *enlarged to midline.* With the mouth still open and the patient seated, inspect the OP directly. Ask the person to protrude the tongue. The following assessment is the Mallampati classification. Class I $=$ all of

the following are visible—the soft palate, uvula, tonsillar columns (anterior and posterior), and fauces (the passage from mouth to throat, anterior boundary behind and lateral to uvula); Class II = the uvula, soft palate, and fauces are visible but tonsillar pillars are not visible; Class III = the soft palate, fauces, and only the base of uvula are visible; Class IV = the soft palate is no longer visible, nor are the fauces, uvula, or tonsillar pillars.

KEY POINTS: SLEEP AND ENDOCRINOLOGY

- Sleep–wake regulators and neuroendocrine controllers are colocated in the hypothalamus and are responsible for functional integration to accomplish and protect homeostasis; this likely underlies the overlap of sleep maladies and endocrine disorders.
- The endocrine diseases associated with abnormal sleep include: type 2 diabetes mellitus, obesity, acromegaly, hyperthyroidism, hypothyroidism, and polycystic ovarian syndrome.
- Normal sleep preserves normal 24-hour hypothalamic–pituitary hormone axis cycling for several hormone systems. Sleep deprivation and obstructive sleep apnea (OSA) can impair hormone cycling.
- Mechanisms responsible for 24-hour hypothalamic–pituitary hormone cycling are circadian, sleep–wake homeostatic, or both. These mechanisms are complex, distinct, and superimposed on classic hormonal feedback loop mechanisms.
- The master circadian clock is located in the suprachiasmatic nucleus of the hypothalamus, which relays an intrinsic rhythm to peripheral organ systems using genetic clockwork: two positive loop genes are *CLOCK* and *BMAL1*, and two negative loop components are *PER* and *CRY*.
- Current evidence links the circadian system to diabetes pathophysiology and treatment.
- States of sleep and wake are best conceived as flip-flop switches. Transitioning from sleep to wakefulness is accomplished by the reticular activating system and is composed of a series of cortical activating nuclei with multiple neurotransmitters. The transition from wake to sleep is accomplished by primarily one neurotransmitter, gamma-aminobutyric acid.
- Sleep architecture changes with aging to consist of less total sleep time and less slow-wave sleep (SWS).
- OSA requires polysomnography for diagnosis.
- Acute sleep loss eliminates the normal nocturnal suppression of thyroid-stimulating hormone secretion.
- Sleep deprivation disrupts SWS, resulting in a decrease in levels of the hormones that are entrained to SWS (growth hormone and prolactin).
- Short-term sleep deprivation increases serum cortisol levels, suppresses insulin secretion, and diminishes glucose tolerance. It also decreases serum leptin and increases ghrelin levels such that sleep-deprived subjects gain weight compared with non–sleep-deprived subjects.
- OSA results in less predictable hormone changes depending on the extent of sleep fragmentation, elevation of adrenergic tone, and hypoxia. It is associated with decreased insulin sensitivity and worsened glucose tolerance proportional to the severity of OSA, and inversely proportional to the time amount of continuous positive airway pressure use.
- Effective treatment of OSA improves sleep architecture, normalizes hormone release, and improves abnormal glucose metabolism.

ACKNOWLEDGEMENT

I dedicate this work to my wife, Laurie, and to our daughter, Amy, and our son, Evan. Since the completion of the second edition of this chapter the author completed 2013-2014 Adult and Pediatric Sleep Medicine Fellowship, Walter Reed National Military Medical Center (WRNMMC), Bethesda, Maryland. I also want to thank the WRNMMC staff physicians, Drs C. Lettieri, A. Holly, J. Dombrowski, R. Kramer, A. Kramstov, V. Steiger, and the Sleep Medicine support team. Thank you to the teaching staff D. Lewin, PhD and J.A. Owens, MD MPH at Children's National Hospital, Washington, DC. Thank you to Emerson Wickwire, PhD at the Howard County Center for Lung & Sleep Medicine, Columbia, MD. Finally thank you to Brendan Lucey, M. D. Neurologist & Director Sleep Medicine Center, Washington University, St Louis Missouri for the review of this chapter. Since Sleep Medicine Fellowship graduation, the author has practiced the combination Adult Endocrinology and Sleep Medicine in the USAF.

🌐 WEBSITE

1. Sleep Research Society: http://www.sleepresearchsociety.org/.
2. NIH, NHLBI, National Center on Sleep Disorders Research: http://www.nhlbi.nih.gov/about/ncsdr/index.htm.
3. American Academy of Sleep Medicine: http://www.aasmnet.org.

BIBLIOGRAPHY

Anothaisintawee, T., Reutrakul, S., Van Cauter, E., & Thakkinstian, A. (2016). Sleep disturbances compared to traditional risk factors for diabetes development, systematic review and meta-analysis. *Sleep Medicine Reviews, 30*, 11–24.

Avidan, A. Y. (2014). Chapter 4: Normal sleep in humans. In M. H. Kyrger, A. Y. Avidan, & R. B. Berry (Eds.), *Atlas of clinical sleep medicine* (2nd ed.). Philadelphia PA: Elsevier Saunders.

Aronsohn, R., Whitmore, H., van Cauter, E., & Tasali, E. Impact of untreated obstructive sleep apnea on glucose control in type 2 diabetes. *American Journal of Respiratory and Critical Care Medicine, 181*, 507–513.

Aurora, R. N., & Punjabi, N. M. (2007). Sleep apnea and metabolic dysfunction: cause or correlation? *Sleep Medicine Clinics, 2*, 237–250.

Borbely, A. A., Daan, S., Wirz-Justice, A., & Deboer, T. (2016). The two-process model of sleep regulation: a reappraisal. *Journal of Sleep Research, 25*, 131–143.

Brzezinski, A. (1997). Melatonin in humans. *New England Journal of Medicine, 336*(3), 186–195.

Chokroverty, S. (2006). Disorders of Sleep. In *Neurology* Chapter XIII. American College of Physicians Medicine. WebMD Inc.

Chung, F., Yegneswaran, B., Liao, P., Chung, S. A., Vairavanathan, S., Islam, S., … Shapiro, C. M. (2008). STOP questionnaire: a tool to screen patients with obstructive sleep apnea. *Anesthesiology, 108*(5), 812–821.

Czeiler, C. A. & Buxton, O. M. (2017). The human circadian timing system and sleep wake regulation. In M. H. Kryger, R. Thomas, & W. C. Dement (Eds.), *Principles and practice of sleep medicine* (6th ed., pp. 362–376). Philadelphia PA: Elsevier Saunders.

Guardiola-Lemaitre, B., & Quera-Salva, M. A. (2011). Melatonin and the regulation of sleep and circadian rhythms. In M. H. Kryger, R. Thomas, & W. C. Dement (Eds.), *Principles and practice of sleep medicine* (5th ed., pp. 420–430). Philadelphia PA: Elsevier Saunders.

Gooley, J. J., & Saper, C. B. (2017). Anatomy of the mammalian circadian system. In M. H. Kryger, R. Thomas, & W. C. Dement (Eds.), *Principles and practice of sleep medicine* (6th ed., pp. 343–350). Philadelphia PA: Elsevier Saunders.

Iber, C., et al. (2007). *The American Academy of Sleep Medicine Manual for the scoring of sleep and associated events: rules, terminology and technical specifications* (1st ed.). Westchester, Illinois: American Academy of Sleep Medicine.

Ip, M. S., Lam, B., Lauder, I. J., Tsang, K. W., Chung, K. F., Mok, Y. W., & Lam, W. K. (2001). A community study of sleep disordered breathing in middle-aged Chinese men in Hong Kong. *Chest, 119*, 62–69.

Jha, A., Sharma, S. K., Tandon, N., Lakshmy, R., Kadhiravan, T., Handa, K. K., … Chaturvedi, P. K. (2006). Thyroxine replacement therapy reverses sleep-disordered breathing patients with primary hypothyroidism. *Sleep Medicine, 7*, 55–61.

Javeed, N., & Matveyenko, A. V. (2018). Circadian etiology of type II diabetes mellitus. A review. *Physiology, 33*, 138–150.

Jun, J., & Polotsky, V. Y. (2007). Sleep disordered breathing and metabolic effects: evidence from animal models. *Sleep Medicine Clinics, 2*, 263–277.

Kelly, E., Cullen, G., & McGurk, C. (2008). Are we missing OSAS in the diabetic clinic? *European Journal of Internal Medicine, 19*, e13.

Knutson, K. L., Spiegel, K., Penev, P., & van Cauter, E. (2007). The metabolic consequences of sleep deprivation. *Sleep Medicine Reviews, 11*, 163–178.

Kuehn, B. M. (2017). Resetting the circadian clock might boost metabolic health. *JAMA, 317*(13), 1303–1305.

Lemaire, J. J., Nezzar, H., Sakka, L., Boirie, Y., Fontaine, D., Coste, A., … De Salles, A. (2013). Maps of the adult hypothalamus. *Surgical Neurology International, 4*(Suppl. 3), S156–S163.

Liu, P. Y., Caterson, I. D., Grunstein, R. R, & Handelsman, D. J. (2007). Androgens, obesity and sleep-disordered breathing in men. *Endocrinology and Metabolism Clinics of North America, 36*, 349–363.

Melehan, K. L., Hoyos, C. M., Hamilton, G. S., Wong, K. K., Yee, B. J., McLachlan, R. I., … Liu, P. Y. (2018). Randomized trial of CPAP and vardenafil on erectile and arterial function in men with obstructive sleep apnea and erectile dysfunction. *Journal of Clinical Endocrinology and Metabolism, 103*(4), 1601–1611.

Oster, H., Chalet, E., Ott, V., Arvat, E., de Kloet, E. R., Dijk, D. J., … Van Cauter, E. (2017). The functional and clinical significance of the 24-hour rhythm of circulating glucocorticoids. *Endocrine Reviews, 38*(1), 3–45.

Parish, J. M., Adam, T., & Facchiano, L. (2007). Relationship of metabolic syndrome and obstructive sleep apnea. *Journal of Clinical Sleep Medicine, 3*, 467–472.

Pinkerton, J. V., Sánchez Aguirre, F., Blake, J., Cosman, F., Hodis, H. N., Hoffstetter, S., … Utian, W. H. (2017). The 2017 hormone therapy position statement of the North American Menopause Society. *Menopause, 24*(7), 728–753.

Punjabi, N. M., Sorkin, J. D., Katzel, L. I., Goldberg, A. P., Schwartz, A. R., & Smith, P. L. (2002). Sleep-disordered breathing and insulin resistance in middle-aged and overweight men. *American Journal of Respiratory and Critical Care Medicine, 165*, 677–682.

Reutrakul, S., & Mokhlesi, B. (2017). Obstructive sleep apnea and diabetes mellitus: a state of the art review. *Chest, 152*(5), 1070–1086.

Rosenwassen, A. M., & Turek, F. W. (2017). Physiology of the mammalian circadian system. In M. H. Kryger, R. Thomas, & W. C. Dement (Eds.), *Principles and practice of sleep medicine* (6th ed., pp. 351–361). Philadelphia PA: Elsevier Saunders.

Sack, R. L. (2010). Clinical practice. Jet lag. *New England Journal of Medicine, 362*(5), 440–447.

Seicean, S., Kirchner, H. L., Gottlieb, D. J., Punjabi, N. M., Resnick, H., Sanders., M., … Redline, S. (2008). Sleep disordered breathing and impaired glucose metabolism in normal-weight and overweight/obese individuals: the Sleep Heart Health study. *Diabetes Care, 31*(5), 1001–1006.

Spiegel, K., Leproult, R., L'hermite-Balériaux, M., Copinschi, G., Penev, P. D., & Van Cauter, E. (2004). Leptin levels are dependent on sleep duration: relationships of sympathovagal balance, carbohydrate regulation, cortisol, and thyrotropin. *Journal of Clinical Endocrinology and Metabolism, 89*, 5762–5771.

Spiegel, K., Leproult, R., & Van Cauter, E. (1999). Impact of sleep debt on metabolic and endocrine function. *Lancet, 354*, 1435–1439.

Tasali, E., Mokhlesi, B., & Van Cauter, E. (2008). Obstructive sleep apnea and type 2 diabetes: Interacting epidemics. *Chest, 133*, 496–506.

Tasali, E., Leproult, R., Ehrmann, D. A., & Van Cauter, E. (2008). Slow wave sleep and the risk of type 2 diabetes in humans. *Proceedings of the National Academy of Science USA, 105*(3), 1044–1049.

Tasali, E., Van Cauter, E., & Ehrmann, D. A. (2006). Relationships between sleep disordered breathing in glucose metabolism in polycystic ovarian syndrome. *Journal of Clinical Endocrinology and Metabolism, 91*(1), 36–42.

Tuomilehto, H., Peltonen, M., Partinen, M., Seppä, J., Saaristo, T., Korpi-Hyövälti, E., … Tuomilehto, J. (2008). Sleep duration is associated with an increased risk for prevalence of type 2 diabetes in middle-aged women –The FIN-D2D survey. *Sleep Medicine, 9*, 221–227.

Turek, F. W., & Zee, P. C. (2017). Introduction to Book Section 5: Chronobiology. Chapter 32 introduction: master circadian clock and master circadian rhythm. In M. H. Kyrger, T. Ross, & W. C. Dement (Eds.), *Principles and practice of sleep medicine* (6th ed., pp. 340–342). Elsevier.

Van Cauter, E., & Tasali, E. (2017). Endocrine physiology in relationship to sleep and sleep disturbances. In M. H. Kryger, R. Thomas, & W. C. Dement (Eds.), *Principles and practice of sleep medicine* (6th ed., pp. 202–219). Philadelphia PA: Elsevier Saunders.

Young, W. F. Jr. (2008). Endocrine hypertension. In H. M. Kronenberg, S. Melmed, K. S. Polonsky, & P. R. Larsen (Eds.), *Williams textbook of endocrinology* (11th ed.). Philadelphia PA: Elsevier Saunders.

Zee, P. C., & Manthena, P. (2007). The brain's master circadian clock: implications and opportunity for therapy of sleep disorders. *Sleep Medicine Reviews, 11*, 59–70.

CHAPTER 66

THYROID AND PARATHYROID SURGERY

Logan R. McKenna, Maria B. Albuja-Cruz, Robert C. McIntyre Jr., and Christopher D. Raeburn

THYROID

1. Using the Bethesda System, list the possible results of fine-needle aspiration (FNA) of thyroid nodules and describe the appropriate surgical intervention.
   - *Nondiagnostic:* Repeat FNA with ultrasound guidance. Thyroid lobectomy if still non-diagnostic.
   - *Benign:* Risk of cancer is < 5%. Clinical follow-up is appropriate.
   - *Atypia of undetermined significance (AUS) or follicular lesion of undetermined significance (FLUS):* Risk of cancer 10% to 40%. Options include observation (if determined to be low risk on the basis of ultrasound appearance and other clinical factors), repeat FNA with or without molecular testing, or surgery.
   - *Follicular neoplasm (FN):* Risk of cancer 15% to 35%. Options include repeat FNA for molecular testing or surgery.
   - *Suspicious:* Risk of cancer 60% to 75%. Surgery for either thyroid lobectomy or thyroidectomy.
   - *Malignant:* Risk of cancer > 97%. Surgery for thyroid lobectomy or thyroidectomy is generally recommended; however, active surveillance can be considered in patients with very low risk cancers (<1 cm, no evidence of invasion, metastasis, or aggressive features) or in patients with high surgical risk or short expected remaining life spans because of comorbidities.

2. A patient underwent a thyroid lobectomy for a suspicious thyroid nodule, and the final pathology result revealed carcinoma. How do you decide whether completion thyroidectomy is necessary?
   Patients undergoing lobectomy for an indeterminate/suspicious thyroid nodule should be counseled that a second surgery for completion thyroidectomy may be necessary in some cases. In brief, a completion thyroidectomy would be indicated if a thyroidectomy would have been recommended had the final diagnosis been available prior to the thyroid lobectomy. A lobectomy may be sufficient treatment for low-risk patients who meet the following criteria: unifocal tumor < 4 cm, without invasion, and no regional or distant metastases. For high-risk and some intermediate-risk patients, completion thyroidectomy is indicated to enable radioactive iodine therapy or to facilitate follow-up based on individual patient characteristics and preferences.

3. Why not just do an intraoperative frozen section on indeterminate thyroid nodules to help guide the extent of surgery?
   Unfortunately, the accuracy of frozen section for most thyroid nodules is not much better than FNA and is, therefore, not routinely used. To distinguish a benign from malignant follicular thyroid lesion requires a detailed assessment for capsular and/or vascular invasion, which cannot practically be accomplished intraoperatively. Frozen section can sometimes be useful for definitive diagnosis of cancer in nodules that are in the suspicious category (Bethesda V).

4. What is the role for molecular testing of thyroid nodules?
   About 15% to 30% of thyroid nodules are cytologically indeterminate on FNA (Bethesda III and IV), and the majority (60%–85%) of these nodules are benign. The goal of molecular diagnostic testing of thyroid nodules is to further stratify the risk of malignancy in those with indeterminate cytology to decrease the number of patients who undergo unnecessary surgery for benign disease. There are multiple commercially available tests that analyze for the genetic mutations/alterations and/or gene expression profiles known to occur in thyroid cancer. Although not perfect, some of these tests are now in their second (Afirma GSC) and third (Thyroseq v3.0) generation, and are reported to have excellent negative-predictive (95%) and reasonable positive-predictive (50%-70%) values. When appropriately utilized, these tests can safely and cost-effectively avoid unnecessary surgery in up to 20% of patients with indeterminate thyroid nodules.

5. Differentiate among total, near-total, and subtotal thyroidectomies.
   A total thyroidectomy removes all grossly visible thyroid tissue. A near-total thyroidectomy removes all grossly visible thyroid tissue except for a small amount (< 1 g) adjacent to where the recurrent laryngeal nerve enters the larynx. Total and near-total thyroidectomies have equivalent oncologic outcomes and are often considered synonymous. A subtotal thyroidectomy leaves more than 1 g of thyroid tissue and is not an appropriate cancer operation. It is used occasionally in patients with benign multinodular goiter or hyperthyroidism in an attempt to

leave enough thyroid hormone so that replacement is not required. However, subtotal thyroidectomy for hyperthyroidism significantly increases the risk of recurrent hyperthyroidism (8%) compared with near-total/total thyroidectomy (0%) and is generally not recommended.

6. **What is the appropriate extent of thyroidectomy for differentiated thyroid carcinoma?**
   For differentiated (papillary, follicular, Hürthle cell) cancers, the extent of surgery is determined by tumor size, history of radiation, family history, and clinical evidence of metastases. For low-risk microcarcinomas (< 1 cm, no invasion or evidence of nodal/distant metastasis), active surveillance may be considered; otherwise, a thyroid lobectomy should be performed unless there is a clear indication to remove the contralateral lobe. Until recently, total or near-total thyroidectomy was recommended for all tumors > 1 cm; however, multiple studies have found that in properly selected low- to intermediate-risk patients, thyroid lobectomy and thyroidectomy have equivalent outcomes. Therefore, the most current guidelines state that the initial surgical procedure for unifocal tumors 1 to 4 cm in size without extrathyroidal extension and without nodal/distant metastases can be *either* thyroidectomy *or* thyroid lobectomy. Factors which might lead to thyroidectomy being chosen over lobectomy include older age (> 45 years), contralateral nodules (> 5 mm), history of radiation exposure, family history of thyroid cancer, or potential need for radioactive iodine. For high-risk tumors (> 4 cm, gross invasion, clinically apparent nodal/distant metastases) a thyroidectomy is indicated.

7. **What is the incidence of lymph node metastases in differentiated thyroid cancer (DTC), and when is a neck dissection indicated?**
   DTC (predominantly papillary) involves cervical lymph nodes in 30% to 80% of cases. In the majority of cases, the metastatic nodes are not clinically evident; therefore, all patients should undergo preoperative full-neck ultrasonography to assess for abnormal nodes. Unlike many other malignancies, the presence of *occult* lymph node metastases does not worsen the outcome for most patients with differentiated thyroid cancer, and routine neck dissection does not clearly improve outcomes except for patients in the high-risk group. Moreover, neck dissection may increase the risk of complications. For these reasons, the decision to perform a prophylactic neck dissection for differentiated thyroid cancer is somewhat controversial. The following are some general guidelines:
   - All patients with clinically palpable nodes require a compartment (central and/or lateral) dissection at the same time as thyroidectomy.
   - Any suspicious nodes on preoperative ultrasonography should be subjected to FNA and, if positive, should be removed via formal neck dissection as above.
   - Physical examination, ultrasonography, and intraoperative assessment are not sensitive in detecting nodal metastases in the central neck. It has been debated whether a *prophylactic* central neck dissection at the time of thyroidectomy is indicated for papillary carcinoma. The current American Thyroid Association (ATA) Guidelines Task Force state that prophylactic central neck dissection may be indicated in patients with advanced tumors (> 4 cm and/or grossly invasive) or if there are known lateral nodal or distant metastases. Thyroidectomy alone may be appropriate for noninvasive tumors < 4 cm.

8. **What is a central and modified radical neck dissection?**
   A central neck dissection removes all the perithyroidal and tracheoesophageal groove nodes (level VI) from the hyoid bone superiorly down to the sternal notch. Laterally, the dissection extends from carotid to carotid artery. The lateral spread of disease usually involves the jugular lymph nodes (levels II–IV) and less commonly posterior (level V) nodes. A modified radical neck dissection, sometimes referred to as a *functional dissection*, removes all lymphatic tissue from level II to level IV (and sometimes V) and spares the internal jugular vein, sternocleidomastoid muscle, and spinal accessory nerve because sacrificing these structures (radical neck dissection) does not improve outcomes.

9. **Describe the appropriate surgical management for medullary thyroid carcinoma (MTC).**
   MTC accounts for $< 5\%$ of thyroid cancers but occurs as part of an inherited syndrome in 20% to 25% of cases. Thus, all patients with MTC should be considered for genetic testing. If the patient has multiple endocrine neoplasia type 2 (MEN 2) syndrome, a prophylactic thyroidectomy is indicated, and the specific mutation in the *RET* gene can help determine at what age the surgery should occur. Patients with MEN 2 should also be screened for pheochromocytoma and primary hyperparathyroidism so that these conditions can be surgically corrected prior to or concomitant with the thyroidectomy, respectively. Because medullary thyroid cancer is not sensitive to radioiodine or thyroid-stimulating hormone (TSH) suppression, a total thyroidectomy is indicated. Because of the high incidence of regional lymph node involvement, a central neck dissection is performed at the time of thyroidectomy. Some surgeons also advocate routine prophylactic ipsilateral or bilateral modified radical neck dissection at the initial surgery; however, despite this aggressive approach, biochemical cure (normalization of serum calcitonin) is uncommon in patients with positive nodes. In the latest ATA guidelines, the task force did not achieve consensus. Some recommend that lateral neck dissection should be performed *selectively* based on clinically or ultrasonographically abnormal nodes. Others consider basal serum calcitonin levels, recommending ipsilateral central and lateral neck dissection for levels > 20 pg/mL and bilateral lateral dissection for levels > 200 pg/mL.

10. Discuss the role of surgery in anaplastic carcinoma of the thyroid.

Anaplastic carcinoma of the thyroid accounts for < 1% of thyroid cancers but is one of the most aggressive solid tumors known and is rarely curable. Median survival is about 6 months. At the time of diagnosis, 50% of patients harbor distant metastases, and 95% have local invasion precluding curative resection. Thus, surgery is usually restricted to a diagnostic or palliative role. Incisional biopsy of the thyroid is sometimes necessary to differentiate anaplastic cancer from thyroid lymphoma, poorly differentiated thyroid cancer, or metastasis to the thyroid gland because the treatments and outcomes are very different. Palliative surgical debulking and tracheostomy should be reserved for patients with airway compromise because they do not prolong survival. An attempt at a curative resection should be reserved for younger patients who do not have distant disease and only when all gross cervical and mediastinal disease can be resected without excessive morbidity. In this select subgroup of patients, curative-intent surgery combined with adjuvant external beam radiation and/or chemotherapy has been shown to prolong survival compared with patients treated with adjuvant therapy alone. Recent studies have shown promising results with the use of combined tyrosine kinase inhibitors, dabrafenib, and trametinib.

11. When is surgery indicated for recurrent thyroid cancer?

Suspected recurrent disease in the neck should be evaluated by using FNA. Confirmed nodal recurrence should be treated with a formal dissection of the involved neck compartment. A recurrence in a neck compartment that has already been subjected to formal neck dissection can be challenging because of scarring of the tissue planes, which renders repeat formal neck dissection virtually impossible. In these situations, the risks and benefits of additional surgery must be carefully considered because the risk of complications increases and the likelihood of cure decreases with each subsequent surgery for recurrence. Observation may be the best option for patients with low-risk disease. When indicated, focused resection of nodal recurrences that are palpable can be performed. If not palpable, intraoperative ultrasonography can be used to guide the excision. For patients who are poor surgical candidates or have had multiple neck operations, percutaneous ethanol injection of nodal metastases is an alternative. Radioiodine is the standard therapy for distant metastatic disease, but isolated metastases can occasionally be surgically resected or treated with external beam radiation.

12. How many times should a thyroid cyst be aspirated if it reaccumulates fluid?

Purely cystic nodules are most often benign, and FNA is not indicated for diagnosis. Aspiration may be performed if a cyst is large and symptomatic. If aspirated, the cyst fluid should be sent for cytology. Recurrence of thyroid cysts occurs in > 50%; recent controlled studies have shown that aspiration followed by ethanol injection has a higher success rate compared with aspiration alone. If the cyst recurs after a second aspiration, and it is still symptomatic, surgical excision may be considered

13. List the indications for thyroidectomy in hyperthyroidism.

In the United States, thyroidectomy is not commonly performed for hyperthyroidism unless it is secondary to a single hyperfunctioning adenoma or because of a toxic multinodular goiter associated with compressive symptoms or containing a suspicious nodule. Despite the excellent success, low recurrence rate, safety, and more rapid return to a euthyroid state, < 10% of patients with hyperthyroidism undergo thyroidectomy. Possible indications for thyroidectomy in patients with hyperthyroidism include:

1. Failure of antithyroid medications
2. Large goiter and low radioiodine uptake
3. Compression symptoms, such as dysphagia, stridor, or hoarseness
4. Nodules suspicious for cancer
5. Young children (age < 5 years)
6. Pregnant patient who is difficult to treat medically
7. Young female who wants to become pregnant in the near future (< 6 months)
8. Moderate-to-severe Graves' ophthalmopathy
9. Concomitant primary hyperparathyroidism requiring surgery
10. Cosmetic concerns

14. How should patients with hyperthyroidism be prepared for surgery?

It is important to render patients euthyroid prior to surgery for hyperthyroidism to avoid perioperative thyroid storm. Antithyroid medications administered for 4 weeks prior to surgery are usually adequate. Because recovery of TSH may lag behind thyroid hormone levels, serum thyroxine (T_4) and triiodothyronine (T_3) levels should be used to determine adequacy of antithyroid therapy. It is recommended that patients receive saturated solution of potassium iodide (SSKI; or Lugol's solution, 3–5 drops three times a day) for 10 days prior to surgery to decrease the vascularity of the goiter and reduce the risk of bleeding. Patients who are very symptomatic may benefit from preoperative beta-blockade. For more rapid induction of a euthyroid state, patients may also be given corticosteroids, which can return serum T_4 and T_3 to within the normal range in < 7 days. In cases of severe, refractory hyperthyroidism, plasmapheresis may occasionally be indicated.

15. **What is the effect of thyroidectomy on Graves' ophthalmopathy compared with other treatment modalities?**
Ophthalmopathy occurs in about one third of patients with Graves' disease, with 5% having moderate-to-severe eye disease. For those without ocular involvement or with only mild Graves' eye disease, the outcome of the eye disease is felt to be equivalent among different treatment modalities. For patients with mild Graves' eye disease being treated with radioiodine, concurrent use of glucocorticoids is recommended to decrease the risk of the eye disease worsening. Because of the transient increase in TSH receptor antibody level that occurs following radioiodine therapy and the concern for this exacerbating Graves' ophthalmopathy, thyroidectomy is recommended for patients with active moderate-to-severe Graves' ophthalmopathy.

16. **What are the complications of thyroidectomy?**
Thyroidectomy is a safe procedure that is typically performed either as an outpatient procedure or, more commonly, with a single overnight stay. The incidence rates of specific complications after thyroidectomy include:
1. Cervical hematoma: 1%
2. Permanent/severe hoarseness (i.e., recurrent laryngeal nerve injury): 1%
3. Mild/temporary hoarseness: 10%
4. Temporary hypocalcemia: 10% to 15%
5. Permanent hypoparathyroidism: 1% to 3%
6. Mortality: < 0.1%

17. **What is the significance of a "hot" thyroid nodule incidentally discovered on positron emission tomography (PET)?**
Fluorodeoxyglucose (FDG) whole-body PET scan is commonly used in the evaluation and surveillance of patients with various types of cancer. A focal area of increased FDG uptake within the thyroid is incidentally noted in up to 4% of PET scans. The risk of malignancy in these lesions is about 33%. Thus, thyroid incidentalomas noted on PET scans have a high risk of malignancy and warrant appropriate diagnostic evaluation. Diffuse FDG uptake is usually related to underlying thyroiditis and, in most cases, is not indicative of malignancy.

18. **What is the appropriate therapy for an intrathoracic (substernal) goiter?**
Intrathoracic goiters are typically cervical goiters with mediastinal extension. Although commonly asymptomatic, up to 40% of patients present with compressive symptoms resulting from impingement on the esophagus, airway, vascular structures, or nerves. There is general agreement that medical therapy (thyroid hormone suppression and/or radioiodine) is ineffective for intrathoracic goiters. Controversy exists as to whether there is an increased risk of unexpected malignancy in intrathoracic compared with cervical goiters; however, when cases of incidental microcarcinoma are excluded, there does not appear to be an increased risk of malignancy in intrathoracic goiters. Despite this, the presence of an intrathoracic goiter is considered by many as an indication for thyroidectomy. Because the arterial supply of intrathoracic goiters originates in the neck, the vast majority of these tumors can be resected through a cervical approach. Extension into the posterior mediastinum, malignancy, or compression of the vena cava may necessitate a combined cervical and sternotomy approach, although this is required in < 5% of cases.

19. **When should thyroglossal duct cysts be removed? Describe the operation.**
During the embryologic development of the thyroid, a diverticulum forms from the foramen cecum at the base of the tongue and descends as the thyroglossal duct to the future anatomic position of the thyroid overlying the anterolateral surface of the upper tracheal rings. The thyroglossal duct normally disappears during further development but, in rare cases, will persist as a patent duct or as a thyroglossal duct cyst. Patients may experience infections, pain or compressive symptoms, or may have cosmetic concerns. Because of the risk of infection, thyroglossal duct cysts should be removed; this requires excision of the entire cyst and cyst tract from the origin at the foramen cecum down to the cyst itself. Because the tract nearly always passes through the hyoid bone, the center of the hyoid should be resected to lower the risk of recurrence; this causes no disability and requires no repair.

PARATHYROID

20. **Which patients with primary hyperparathyroidism (HPT) should undergo parathyroidectomy?**
All patients with primary hyperparathyroidism and "classic" symptoms attributable to the disease (e.g., kidney stones, severe bone disease/fragility fractures, overt neuromuscular syndrome) should undergo surgical intervention; however, most patients do not have these classic symptoms. The National Institutes of Health (NIH) established criteria to assist clinicians in determining which patients with "asymptomatic" HPT should undergo surgery. If the patient meets any one of the criteria then surgery is recommended:
- Age < 50 years
- Serum calcium level > 1 mg/dL above normal
- Bone mineral density reduced > 2.5 standard deviations below mean peak adult value (T score)
- Impaired renal function (glomerular filtration rate < 60 mL/minute)

- Severe hypercalciuria (24-hour calcium > 400 mg/24 hr)
- Silent nephrolithiasis on radiography, ultrasonography, or computed tomography (CT)
- Silent vertebral fractures on spine radiography, CT, or magnetic resonance imaging (MRI)
- Patients unwilling or unable to undergo surveillance

    If the patient does not meet any of the criteria, then *either* surgery *or* continued surveillance are reasonable and safe options.

21. **Should subjective symptoms, such as fatigue, irritability, and difficulty concentrating, be considered indications for surgery in primary hyperparathyroidism?**

Although only a minority of patients with primary HPT manifest the *classic* symptoms, as many as 90% of patients experience more subtle, subjective symptoms, such as fatigue, weakness, musculoskeletal pains, abdominal discomfort, depression, anxiety, irritability, or memory/cognitive difficulties. In fact, some have argued that there is no such thing as truly "asymptomatic" primary HPT! Although some studies have shown that patients undergoing parathyroidectomy have improvement in these subjective symptoms, the results are inconsistent, and it is not possible to predict in any one patient whether or not these symptoms will improve after surgery. Similarly, some studies have found primary HPT to be associated with an increased risk of cardiovascular disease and early mortality; however, the results of studies investigating whether parathyroidectomy reduces these risks have been conflicting. In contrast to the NIH guidelines, the American Association of Endocrine Surgeons guidelines include neurocognitive and/or neuropsychiatric symptoms as an indication for surgery, and recommend that a history of cardiovascular disease as well as other nontraditional symptoms be considered in the decision for parathyroidectomy.

22. **When should preoperative parathyroid localization studies be performed?**

An experienced parathyroid surgeon does not require preoperative localization prior to an initial bilateral neck exploration and will have a surgical success rate of > 95%. However, about 85% of patients with primary HPT have a single parathyroid adenoma, and therefore, preoperative imaging is commonly performed. If an adenoma is localized, then a focused parathyroidectomy (also known as *minimally invasive parathyroidectomy*) can be performed. Ultrasonography and 99m technetium sestamibi scanning are the most common modalities utilized, but high-resolution CT with intravenous contrast, commonly referred to as a "4-D CT," is increasingly being used. Advantages of ultrasonography are its low cost, absence of ionizing radiation, and ability to evaluate for concomitant thyroid pathology. Sestamibi scanning and CT are more costly and entail radiation exposure but may have improved sensitivity compared with ultrasonography. Centers vary as to which modality is used preferentially. Patients with a prior history of neck surgery and certainly all patients with persistent or recurrent hyperparathyroidism should undergo preoperative localization studies prior to planned reexploration. Parathyroid venous sampling with or without arteriography may be useful in select situations of persistent or recurrent hyperparathyroidism when other modalities have failed to localize the abnormal gland.

23. **What is the best treatment for a 45-year-old female with primary hyperparathyroidism but negative preoperative localization studies?**

Surgery! Patient age < 50 years warrants parathyroidectomy. Remember, failure to localize an abnormal parathyroid on imaging has nothing to do with whether or not a patient *has* HPT or whether or not the patient should undergo surgery. The sensitivity of preoperative localization studies is not perfect, and they fail to localize an abnormal parathyroid approximately 15% of the time. Although multiglandular disease is more common when preoperative localization studies are negative, most patients with negative localization will still turn out to have a single adenoma as the cause of their HPT. The success rate of surgery, if performed by an experienced surgeon, is still high (> 90%–95%) when preoperative localization is negative.

24. **Define minimally invasive parathyroidectomy.**

A conventional parathyroidectomy entails bilateral neck exploration, identification of all four glands, and removal of the grossly enlarged gland(s). The development of accurate preoperative localization studies and a rapid intra-operative parathyroid hormone (ioPTH) assay has fostered the development of minimally invasive approaches to parathyroidectomy. A focused unilateral approach utilizes preoperative imaging to limit the dissection to one side. The abnormal gland is found and removed and after 10 to 15 minutes a postexcision blood sample is drawn and the PTH level is compared with a preexcision blood sample. A reduction of the PTH to 50% of the preoperative level and into the normal range predicts successful removal of all hyperfunctioning glands, and the surgery is terminated. If the PTH does not drop appropriately, then all four glands must be identified because the patient likely has multiglandular disease.

25. **What is MIRP?**

Minimally invasive radio-guided parathyroidectomy (MIRP) is a second alternative to conventional parathyroidec-tomy and involves 99m technetium sestamibi scanning the morning of the surgery. An incision is made; either a unilateral or a bilateral neck exploration is performed; and abnormal parathyroid(s) are removed. A small, hand-held gamma probe is then used to measure the ex vivo radioactive counts of the excised parathyroid to determine whether the gland is hyperfunctioning. If the radioactive counts of the excised parathyroid are ≥ 20% higher than the counts in the operative bed, then the gland is presumed to be an adenoma. Contrary to common perception, the gamma probe is not typically used to *localize* the abnormal parathyroid. This is because the thyroid gland also takes up sestamibi, so the high radioactive counts of the thyroid obscure the ability to use the probe to discern the location of the parathyroid. Although this technique can be useful in confirming that an excised parathyroid is hyperfunctioning, it does not rule out the possibility of additional hyperfunctioning glands. Either all four parathyroids must be evaluated or an ioPTH assay should be used to exclude the possibility of multiglandular disease (15%).

26. Summarize the advantages of minimally invasive approaches.
Multiple studies have shown the minimally invasive approaches to be as safe and effective as conventional para-thyroidectomy. However, there are also multiple studies showing that a conventional parathyroidectomy (bilateral neck exploration) can similarly be performed through a small incision, on an outpatient basis, and with excellent results. Some studies have found the minimally invasive approaches to be more efficient in terms of time and cost because they limit the amount of dissection required. Because the minimally invasive approach is typically performed through a slightly smaller incision, cosmesis may be improved.

27. How is the ioPTH assay utilized in parathyroid surgery?
The half-life of PTH is 3 to 5 minutes, allowing for a rapid assay for ioPTH to be used intraoperatively to assess the functional success of the operation. This test is performed by drawing a sample of blood before the operation and 10 minutes after the suspected abnormal glands have been removed. A reduction of the ioPTH by 50% pre-dicts successful removal of all hyperfunctioning glands, and the surgery is terminated. The rate of multiglandular disease is approximately 5% to 15% when ioPTH is used to determine the completeness of resection, whereas the rate is 10% to 35% when conventional parathyroidectomy is performed (i.e., bilateral neck exploration and removal of grossly enlarged parathyroids). Therefore, the use of ioPTH may prevent the unnecessary removal of glands that *appear* enlarged but are not hyperfunctional.

28. What is the expected success of surgery for primary hyperparathyroidism?
Parathyroidectomy is highly successful for primary hyperparathyroidism, correcting hypercalcemia in > 95% of patients when performed by an experienced surgeon. Bone density stabilizes or increases in the vast majority of patients. Successful parathyroidectomy significantly decreases the risk of kidney stone recurrence. Following successful surgery, many patients experience improvement in the vague nonspecific symptoms of hyper-parathyroidism.

29. Describe the appropriate management of a "missing" parathyroid.
Despite meticulous operative technique during conventional parathyroidectomy (identification of all four glands), the surgeon occasionally encounters a "missing gland." Up to 20% of parathyroid glands are ectopic, with the most common locations being within the thymus, retroesophageal, and intrathyroidal. A systematic search of the most common ectopic locations is required for successful outcome in these patients. When three normal glands have been identified and the fourth gland is not in a normal position, the most likely ectopic location depends on whether the upper gland or the lower gland is missing.

30. List the likely locations for an ectopic inferior parathyroid gland.
- Thyrothymic ligament
- Thymus
- Mediastinum outside thymus
- Undescended gland

31. List the likely locations for an ectopic superior parathyroid gland.
- Retroesophageal
- Tracheoesophageal groove
- Posterosuperior mediastinum
- Intrathyroidal

32. What if a patient has multiglandular parathyroid disease?
A single adenoma is, by far, the most common cause of primary HPT (85%). Depending on the method used to define multiglandular disease (i.e., ioPTH assay versus gross appearance/size), the reported rates range from 5% to 35%. Multiglandular disease can be caused by either multiple adenomas or four-gland hyperplasia. Hyperplasia may be sporadic or secondary to a genetic predisposition, such as MEN syndrome. When all four glands are hyperplastic, a subtotal parathyroidectomy is required (removal of 3½ glands). It is important that the surgeon be careful to preserve the blood supply to the parathyroid remnant. If after removing half the final parathyroid the remnant appears ischemic, then it should be excised and autotransplanted, either to the brachioradialis muscle in the nondominant forearm or the sternocleidomastoid muscle. Most patients (95%) will have normal calcium and low or normal parathyroid hormone levels; however, permanent hypoparathyroidism occurs in 2% to 3% and recurrent hyperparathyroidism occurs in about 10% of patients.

33. What are the indications for surgery for tertiary hyperparathyroidism?

Although all patients with dialysis-dependent renal failure develop secondary hyperparathyroidism, only a minority of patients develop tertiary hyperparathyroidism, which develops when somatic mutations occur within one or more of the hyperplastic parathyroids resulting in adenomatous transformation. Medical management with phosphate binders, active vitamin D analogues (calcitriol), and calcimimetics (Cinacalcet) will keep the PTH, calcium, and phosphate levels under control in most patients. Most experts agree that parathyroidectomy is indicated in patients who, despite optimal medical management, have refractory hyperparathyroidism (PTH > 800 pg/mL) and significant associated signs and symptoms. The most common signs and symptoms include hypercalcemia with hyperphosphatemia (calcium $\times$ phosphate product = > 50), bone and joint pain and/or fractures, proximal muscle weakness, extraskeletal calcification and/or calciphylaxis, and pruritus. Indications for parathyroidectomy in asymptomatic patients with refractory hyperparathyroidism is more controversial, but some recommend it for patients who have PTH > 1000 pg/mL, who are younger (i.e., age < 65 years), and who do not have other significant comorbidities.

34. Discuss the advantages and disadvantages of subtotal parathyroidectomy (SPTx) versus total parathyroidectomy with autotransplantation (TPTx + AT) for refractory tertiary hyperparathyroidism.

There is no significant difference in persistent/recurrent HPT or the rate of permanent hypoparathyroidism between SPTx and TPTx + AT. The advantage of TPTx + AT is that persistent or recurrent hypercalcemia can be treated by partially or completely removing the grafts (usually placed in a forearm muscle) under local anesthesia, whereas the same complication occurring after SPTx requires repeat neck operation with higher morbidity.

35. List the complications of parathyroidectomy for primary hyperparathyroidism and their prevalence.

- Persistent hyperparathyroidism: < 5%
- Recurrent hyperparathyroidism: 5% to 10%
- Transient hypocalcemia: 10% to 25%
- Permanent hypoparathyroidism: 2% to 5% (< 1% for solitary adenoma)
- Temporary recurrent laryngeal nerve injury: 3%
- Permanent recurrent laryngeal nerve injury: < 1%
- Mortality: < 0.1%

36. Define persistent and recurrent hyperparathyroidism.

Persistent hyperparathyroidism is defined as failure of calcium and PTH levels to normalize or remain normal in the initial 6 months after operation, whereas recurrent hyperparathyroidism is defined as recurrence of hypercalcemia after 6 months.

37. What is the most common cause of an elevated serum PTH with normal serum calcium after parathyroidectomy?

Persistent PTH elevation with normal serum calcium can be observed in up to 30% of patients after parathyroidectomy. This can be disconcerting to the patient and the surgeon, but in the vast majority of cases, it is not caused by persistent or recurrent HPT. The cause of this phenomenon is likely multifactorial, but vitamin D deficiency, rapid bone turnover ("hungry bone syndrome"), and inadequate calcium intake are thought to be the main causes. Postoperative supplementation with calcium and vitamin D decreases this phenomenon. Long-term studies have shown that the PTH level eventually returns to normal in most patients and that the long-term recurrence rate is not increased in this subset of patients.

38. Discuss the approach to patients with persistent or recurrent hyperparathyroidism.

The approach to patients with persistent or recurrent hyperparathyroidism requires confirmation of the diagnosis (exclude familial hypocalciuric hypercalcemia, vitamin D deficiency, etc.), estimation of disease severity to ensure that reoperation is justified, careful review of the operative and pathology reports, and preoperative localization. If undergoing repeat operation, assessing vocal cord function should be considered. Causes of failure include missed adenoma in a normal location, ectopic glands, inadequate resection in multiglandular disease, and supernumerary glands.

39. Discuss the options for treatment of persistent or recurrent hyperparathyroidism.

Although preoperative localization is optional prior to an initial surgery for HPT, it is essential in cases of persistent or recurrent disease because the success rate of the surgery is much higher when the abnormal gland has been accurately localized. Multiple modalities are often utilized with 99m technetium sestamibi scanning, neck ultrasonography, and CT being the most common. Having correlation of the location of the abnormal gland on two different imaging modalities is very reassuring and is used by some surgeons as a criterion for reoperation in persistent HPT. Repeat cervical exploration is successful in normalizing PTH levels in about 85% of patients, and may be aided by intraoperative ultrasonography and ioPTH assay. Mediastinal parathyroid tissue is most often removed via the transcervical approach, but thoracoscopy or median sternotomy may be required 1% to 2% of the time. Angiographic ablation of mediastinal parathyroid tissue using high doses of ionic contrast may be successful in selected patients and prevent sternotomy.

40. How can parathyroid cancer be recognized?

Parathyroid cancer is the rarest of all endocrine tumors, with a reported incidence of < 1% in patients with primary HPT. It is difficult to distinguish parathyroid cancer from the more common benign causes of HPT, and the diagnosis is frequently not suspected preoperatively. Parathyroid cancer should be suspected preoperatively when patients present with rapid-onset, severe, symptomatic hypercalcemia (> 14 mg/dL), very high PTH levels (> 5 times normal), a palpable neck mass, or hoarseness. It should be suspected intraoperatively when the tumor is large, firm, fibrotic, or invasive to the thyroid or other surrounding structures. Successful outcome requires early recognition and complete resection of the tumor and any involved structures.

41. Describe the management of parathyroid cancer.

Surgery is the mainstay of treatment for parathyroid cancer because radiation and chemotherapy have shown little benefit. Local invasion and pathologic nodes should be assumed to represent cancer. Any suspicious parathyroid lesions should be carefully removed without disrupting the parathyroid capsule because this may result in tumor spillage and local recurrence. If a parathyroid gland is obviously abnormal and infiltrating other tissues, those tissues should be resected en bloc with the tumor whenever possible, including the ipsilateral thyroid lobe when necessary. Removal of the central nodes on the side of the tumor is indicated at the initial operation. Any obviously enlarged lateral nodes should be resected by formal neck dissection. Prophylactic neck dissections have shown no benefit. The histopathologic diagnosis of this cancer is also difficult; thus, intraoperative frozen section is rarely useful other than to confirm parathyroid tissue.

42. Give the recurrence and survival rates for parathyroid cancer.

Recurrence rates are high and depend on whether the patient underwent a routine parathyroidectomy for presumed benign disease (> 50% recurrence) or an en bloc resection for suspicion of cancer (10%–33%). Despite this high recurrence rate, prolonged survival is still possible. The National Cancer Database reports 5- and 10-year survival rates of 85.5% and 49.1%, respectively.

KEY POINTS: THYROID AND PARATHYROID SURGERY

- Low-risk thyroid microcarcinomas (< 1 cm, no invasion or evidence of nodal/distant metastasis) can sometimes be managed by active surveillance if both the patient and physician agree; otherwise, a thyroid lobectomy should be performed unless there is a clear indication to remove the contralateral lobe.
- Current guidelines recommend that the initial surgical procedure for unifocal thyroid tumors 1 to 4 cm in size without extrathyroidal extension and without nodal/distant metastases can be *either* thyroidectomy *or* thyroid lobectomy.
- Lymph node involvement in thyroid cancer should be treated with a systematic compartment node dissection.
- Incidental thyroid hot spots discovered on positron emission tomography (PET) scans have a high rate of malignancy and should be evaluated by ultrasound-guided fine-needle aspiration (FNA).
- All patients with primary hyperparathyroidism and "classic" symptoms attributable to the disease (e.g., kidney stones, severe bone disease/fragility fractures, overt neuromuscular syndrome) should undergo surgical intervention.
- Indications for surgery in patients with asymptomatic hyperparathyroidism include high serum calcium (> 1.0 mg/dL above normal), urinary calcium excretion > 400 mg/24 hr, age under 50 years, osteoporosis, and reduced creatinine clearance.
- Surgery for primary hyperparathyroidism results in normalization of serum calcium in > 95% of patients when performed by an experienced parathyroid surgeon.
- Parathyroid cancer is rare but should be suspected in patients with a palpable mass and symptomatic hypercalcemia that is severe and of rapid onset.

BIBLIOGRAPHY

Bilezikian, J. P., Brandi, M. L., Eastell, R., Silverberg, S. J., Udelsman, R., Marcocci, C., . . . J. T., Jr.. (2014). Guidelines for the management of asymptomatic primary hyperparathyroidism: summary statement from the Fourth International Workshop. *Journal of Clinical Endocrinology and Metabolism, 99*(10), 3561–3569.

Bilezikian, J. P. (2018). Primary hyperparathyroidism. *Journal of Clinical Endocrinology and Metabolism, 103*(11), 3993–4004.

Cibas, E. S., & Ali, S. Z. (2017). The 2017 Bethesda system for reporting thyroid cytopathology. *Thyroid, 27*(11), 1341–1346.

Haugen, B. R., Alexander, E. K., Bible, K. C., Doherty, G. M., Mandel, S. J., Nikiforov, Y. E., . . . Wartofsky, L. (2016). 2015 American Thyroid Association Management Guidelines for adult patients with thyroid nodules and differentiated thyroid cancer: the American Thyroid Association Guidelines Task Force on thyroid nodules and differentiated thyroid cancer. *Thyroid, 26*(1): 1–133.

Nixon, I. J., Ganly, I., Patel, S. G., Palmer, F. L., Whitcher, M. M., Tuttle, R. M., . . . Shah, J. P. (2012). Thyroid lobectomy for treatment of well differentiated intrathyroid malignancy. *Surgery, 151,* 571–579.

Wells, S. A., Asa, S. L., Dralle, H., Elisei, R., Evans, D. B., Gagel, R. F., . . . Waguespack, S. G.; American Thyroid Association Guidelines Task Force on medullary thyroid carcinoma. (2015). Revised American Thyroid Association guidelines for the management of medullary thyroid carcinoma. *Thyroid, 25*(6), 567–610.

Wilhelm, S. M., Wang, T. S., Ruan, D. T., Lee, J. A., Asa, S. L., & Duh, Q. Y. (2016). The American Association of Endocrine Surgeons guidelines for definitive management of primary hyperparathyroidism. *Journal of the American Medical Association Surgery,151*(10), 959–968.

CHAPTER 67

ADRENAL SURGERY

Oliver J. Fackelmayer, Chris Raeburn, Robert McIntyre Jr., and Maria Albuja-Cruz

1. Should all incidentally discovered adrenal masses be resected?
   No. Incidentally discovered, clinically occult adrenal masses, referred to as *incidentalomas,* are common (4.4% in modern abdominal computed tomography [CT] series) and increasingly encountered with the ubiquity of abdominal CT. Most incidentally discovered adrenal nodules are nonfunctional and benign (80% are cortical adenomas), requiring only surveillance. Adrenalectomy is indicated for tumors > 4 cm, imaging characteristics concerning for malignancy, and biochemically hyperactive lesions.

2. A patient with right lower quadrant pain underwent CT of the abdomen with intravenous (IV) contrast in the emergency department; a 2-cm left adrenal nodule was noted. What is the next step?
   The patient should be evaluated with a thorough history (query current colonoscopy, mammography, chest radiography [CXR] for smokers; prior malignancy, including skin cancer, especially melanoma) and physical examination. The patient should undergo biochemical testing to assess for tumor functionality. The adrenal nodule should be evaluated with a dedicated adrenal protocol CT. If the biochemical testing is negative and the initial CT was performed with IV contrast and did not have concerning features, it is reasonable to delay dedicated adrenal imaging until the 6-month follow-up. If the condition is stable, annual screening should be pursued with imaging for 1 to 2 years and biochemical testing for 5 years. The risk of an adrenal mass becoming hormonally hyperactive during 1, 2, and 5 years is 17%, 29%, and 47%, respectively.

3. What is the laboratory workup of an adrenal mass?
   Up to 20% of adrenal incidentalomas are found to be biochemically hyperfunctional and should be resected. Therefore, patients should be screened for hypercortisolism, hyperaldosteronism (if hypertensive), and pheochromocytoma with the following tests:
   - 1 mg overnight dexamethasone suppression test (8:00 AM cortisol):
     - ≦1.8 mcg/dL—excludes autonomous cortisol secretion
     - 1.9–4.9 mcg/dL—evidence of possible autonomous cortisol secretion
     - ≧ 5 mcg/dL—evidence of autonomous cortisol secretion
   - Only in patients with concomitant hypertension or unexplained hypokalemia—plasma aldosterone concentration (PAC) to plasma renin activity (PRA) ratio (PAC/PRA)—suggestive of aldosteronoma if PAC > 15 ng/dL and PAC/PRA > 20.
   - 24-hour urine metanephrines and catecholamines or plasma metanephrines and normetanephrines—diagnostic of pheochromocytoma if ≧ 3-fold above upper limit of normal.
     Routine screening for excess androgens or estrogens is not included in the screening algorithm because sex hormone–secreting adrenal tumors are rare and usually clinically apparent.

4. What imaging studies are available for evaluating adrenal pathology?
   There are three main imaging techniques for the differentiation of malignant from benign adrenal tumors: CT, magnetic resonance imaging (MRI), and positron emission tomography with fluorodeoxyglucose (FDG-PET/CT). CT and MRI are mainly techniques to identify benign lesions and exclude adrenal malignancy. FDG-PET/CT is mainly used for detection of malignant disease.
     Abdominal CT is the initial modality of choice. An adrenal protocol CT consists of thin-cut imaging through the adrenal glands first without IV contrast, and then with contrast, followed by delayed (usually 10–15 minutes) images to assess contrast washout.
     MRI is considered essentially equivalent to CT for adrenal tumors and is a reasonable, although more expensive, alternative; MRI should be considered in patients with contrast allergy and in situations where radiation exposure should be limited (pregnancy, children, patients with known germline mutations). MRI is recommended in patients with known or suspected metastatic pheochromocytomas.
     FDG-PET/CT standard uptake value (SUV) has been utilized to differentiate between benign and malignant adrenal lesions.
     Meta-iodo-benzyl-guanidine (MIBG) nuclear medicine scans are best utilized for recurrent, familial, or extraadrenal pheochromocytomas.

5. What findings on CT help distinguish between benign and malignant tumors?
   Adrenal nodule size and imaging characteristics are the two major predictors of malignancy. Adrenocortical carcinoma (ACC) accounts for only 2% of lesions < 4 cm but up to 25% of those > 6 cm. Benign adenomas are

typically < 4 cm, are homogeneous with smooth borders, have a high lipid content (low attenuation—< 10 Hounsfield units [HU] on noncontrast images), and rapid contrast washout (> 50% washout) on delayed images 10 minutes after the contrast bolus. Malignant tumors are typically > 6 cm, heterogeneous with irregular borders, and have increased noncontrast attenuation (> 10 HU) and slower contrast washout.

6. Should all adrenal nodules be evaluated with percutaneous biopsy?
No. Percutaneous biopsy is reserved for patients who have a history of extraadrenal malignancy with an adrenal mass, and only if the results of the biopsy will alter the treatment plan for the extraadrenal malignancy. Pheochromocytoma must be excluded with biochemical testing prior to biopsy to avoid potentially precipitating a hypertensive crisis. Percutaneous biopsy cannot differentiate an adrenal adenoma from an adrenocortical carcinoma.

7. Is adrenalectomy best performed with an open technique or the laparoscopic technique?
Laparoscopic adrenalectomy is the approach of choice for benign adrenal tumors except when very large (> 8 cm). Laparoscopic adrenalectomy has been associated with shorter hospital stay, less postoperative pain, less blood loss, faster recovery, and overall increased patient satisfaction compared with the open techniques. Open adrenalectomy and conversion from laparoscopic technique to open technique should be undertaken when malignancy is suspected.

8. What are the possible laparoscopic approaches for adrenalectomy?
The most common technique is via an anterolateral laparoscopic transabdominal approach in which the patient is placed in the lateral decubitus position with the side of the lesion up. This provides excellent exposure but does not permit removal of both glands without repositioning the patient. A supine anterior transabdominal approach provides access to both adrenal glands, but exposure is more difficult. A posterior laparoscopic retroperitoneal approach (retroperitoneoscopic) in the prone position avoids entering the peritoneal cavity altogether and affords access to both adrenals without repositioning but is limited by a smaller working space that precludes removal of larger lesions (> 4 cm). The various laparoscopic approaches are felt to be equivalent in terms of safety and recovery, and are selected according to the surgeon's preference and patient/tumor characteristics.

9. What is hyperaldosteronism?
Primary hyperaldosteronism (PA), also known as Conn's disease, is a clinical syndrome of refractory hypertension (requiring > 3 antihypertensive agents) combined with spontaneous hypokalemia (serum potassium < 3.5 mEq/L) or severe (< 3mEq/L) diuretic-induced hypokalemia. In the vast majority of patients, PA is caused by either bilateral adrenal hyperplasia (60%–65%) or an aldosterone-producing adenoma (APA; 30%–40%).

10. What is adrenal vein sampling (AVS), and when is it indicated?
AVS is an interventional radiology procedure in which endovascular catheters are used to selectively cannulate and sample blood from the right and left adrenal veins. There are technical limitations to accurate sampling, and the technique may not be universally available. APAs are typically < 2 cm in diameter, and therefore the sensitivity of CT is only 85%. AVS should be used in most patients with biochemically confirmed PA to exclude bilateral hyperplasia and confirm the correct side in those with an APA, which may be in the "normal" gland in the setting of an incidentaloma. Imaging results can be misleading in up to 20% of patients (bilateral adrenal masses but unilateral APA; unilateral adrenal nodule but small APA detected in contralateral "normal" gland). AVS may be omitted in younger patients (age < 35 years), as they are less likely to have confounding adrenal nodules.

11. Describe the AVS ratios for localization?
Both aldosterone and cortisol are measured in all AVS samples to determine the cortisol-corrected aldosterone values. The criteria used to determine lateralization of aldosterone hypersecretion depend on whether the AVS is done under cosyntropin administration. With cosyntropin administration, a cortisol-corrected aldosterone ratio from high-side to low-side of > 4:1 indicates the presence of a unilateral APA. In the absence of cosyntropin, some investigators consider a cortisol-corrected aldosterone lateralization ratio (high to low side) of > 2:1 as consistent with an APA. Suppression of aldosterone secretion in the contralateral adrenal is also suggestive of an APA.

12. What is the aldosterone resolution score (ARS)?
The ARS accurately identifies individuals at low (ARS ≤ 1) or high (ARS ≤ 4) likelihood of complete resolution of hypertension without further need for lifelong antihypertensive medications after adrenalectomy for aldosteronoma.

	Points	
Predictor	*Present*	*Absent*
No. of antihypertensive medications ≤ 2	2	0
Body mass index ≤ 25	1	0
Years of hypertension ≤ 6	1	0
Female	1	0
Total*	5	0

*Possible score range 0 to 5.

13. Describe the appropriate perioperative management of pheochromocytomas.

Surgical resection is the only chance for cure for patients with pheochromocytomas. All patients with the biochemical diagnosis of a pheochromocytoma should undergo preoperative alpha-adrenergic blockade for 7 to 14 days to prevent unstable intraoperative blood pressure. Phenoxybenzamine is a nonselective long-acting alpha-adrenergic blocker; the starting dose is 10 mg twice daily and the dosage is titrated up to achieve the goals of treatment. Short-acting alpha-adrenergic blockers (prazosin, doxazosin, terazosin) and calcium channel blockers (nicardipine) are alternative options.

Preoperative beta-adrenergic receptor blockade is indicated for tachyarrhythmias only after alpha-adrenergic blockade is established. Propranolol (10–40 mg every 6 to 8 hours) is the most commonly used beta-blocker in this scenario.

The goals of treatment are a blood pressure $< 130/80$ mm Hg seated and > 90 systolic when standing; the heart rate should be 60 to 70 beats per minute seated and 70 to 80 beats per minute standing.

Patients should increase their fluid and salt intake (> 5 g/day) after starting alpha-blockers to attain fluid expansion because they have intravascular volume depletion.

Genetic testing is recommended for all patients with pheochromocytoma because it is now known that up to 40% of cases are hereditary. Also, lifelong annual biochemical testing to assess for recurrent or metastatic disease is recommended because up to 25% of pheochromocytomas are malignant, and the malignant nature of pheochromocytomas (metastases) may not be apparent for many years (up to 40 years) after the initial resection. Patients with mutations encoding succinate dehydrogenase subunit B (SDHB) have a 40% chance of metastatic disease.

Chromogranin A is a nonspecific marker of neuroendocrine tumors and is commonly used as a marker for monitoring disease as it is elevated in 91% of patients with pheochromocytomas and should be checked prior to adrenalectomy.

14. What is cortical-sparing adrenalectomy, and when is it indicated?

Patients with pheochromocytomas associated with a familial syndrome are at increased risk of developing bilateral and/or recurrent pheochromocytomas. These patients may be treated with cortical-sparing (partial) adrenalectomy in an effort to prevent adrenal insufficiency should another pheochromocytoma arise requiring additional adrenal-ectomy. This approach balances the benefit of avoiding the need for lifelong hormone replacement with a low risk of recurrence in the adrenal remnant ($\approx 7\%$).

15. Describe the appropriate perioperative management of a cortisol-producing adrenal adenoma.

Diabetes and hypertension should be adequately treated prior to surgery. Patients with Cushing's syndrome have an increased relative risk for thromboembolic complications; therefore, measures to prevent venous thromboembolism (VTE) should be implemented. Intraoperative replacement of glucocorticoids is controver-sial for patients with Cushing's syndrome. However, patients with Cushing's syndrome have a suppressed hypothalamic–pituitary–adrenal (HPA) axis, leading to atrophy of the contralateral gland. Therefore, after adrenalectomy for cortisol-producing adrenal adenomas, patients generally require glucocorticoid replace-ment to prevent adrenal insufficiency. A cosyntropin stimulation test can be done on postoperative day 1 to determine the need for glucocorticoid replacement after adrenalectomy; basal serum cortisol and plasma adrenocorticotropin (ACTH) levels should be checked, and serum cortisol level should be evaluated 60 minutes after IV administration of cosyntropin 250 mcg. Patients do not need glucocorticoid replacement if the basal serum cortisol level is > 5 mcg/dL, the stimulated cortisol level is > 18 mcg/dL, and there are no clinical symptoms of adrenal insufficiency. However, patients will need glucocorticoid replacement if the basal cortisol is $\leqq 5$ mcg/dL, the stimulated cortisol is $\leqq 18$ mcg/dL, or there are clinical symptoms of adrenal insufficiency.

The time required for the HPA axis to recover after surgery ranges from 6 to 18 months. Cosyntropin stimulation studies can be done every 3 to 6 months to determine when the steroid therapy can be discontinued.

16. Summarize the long-term success of adrenalectomy for functional tumors.

Patients with an APA can expect a $\approx 100\%$ cure of hypokalemia, and $> 90\%$ will show significant improvement in hypertension after adrenalectomy. Approximately 30% to 60% can completely stop antihypertensive therapy. Factors that predict a favorable outcome include young age (< 40 years), shorter duration of hypertension (< 6 years), ≤ 2 antihypertensive agents, a good response to spironolactone, female gender, and less severe hypertension. In older patients with severe, longstanding hypertension associated with renal dysfunction, adrenalec-tomy may not normalize blood pressure but often results in easier control of hypertension with fewer or lower dose medications.

Adrenalectomy for nonfamilial pheochromocytomas is curative in most cases. However, a long-term recurrence rate as high as 25% (metastases indicating that the primary tumor was malignant) has been reported; thus, patients should undergo annual laboratory surveillance for the rest of their lives.

Adrenalectomy in patients with cortisol-producing adrenal adenomas results in excellent improvement in the symptoms of Cushing's syndrome and improves patient quality of life. Hypertension and diabetes resolve in 65% to 80% of patients, and the physical changes of Cushing's syndrome are reversed in 85%. These improvements take 6 to 12 months to occur.

17. Describe the appropriate management of adrenal malignancy.

Adrenocortical carcinoma (ACC) is a rare (1–2 per million) and aggressive cancer with a poor prognosis. At the time of diagnosis, approximately 25% of patients have nodal involvement, and 20% have distant metastases. Roughly 60% of ACCs are functioning tumors, and the mean size of tumors at the time of diagnosis is > 10 cm. The overall 5-year survival rate is around 25% and depends largely on the stage at diagnosis. Patients undergoing complete resection of small tumors (< 5 cm) without local invasion (stage 1) have a 5-year survival of 66%, whereas patients with metastases or invasion into other organs (stage 4) have a median survival of < 12 months. The only chance for cure is surgery, which should be offered to all patients who do not have metastases and who have a reasonable surgical risk. The operation for ACC should be performed with an open approach, and when a malignant tumor is suspected, a minimally invasive approach should be converted to an open approach. Surgery should also be considered for young patients with an isolated, easily resectable metastasis. Despite limited response rates, patients with stage 3 or 4 disease are frequently offered adjuvant therapy with mitotane (+/− cytotoxic chemotherapy) and/or radiotherapy because of the high recurrence rate (up to 85%). Mitotane is an adrenocorticolytic agent indicated for suspected incomplete resection and tumors with a high proliferative rate (Ki67 > 10%).

KEY POINTS: ADRENAL TUMORS

- During the evaluation of an adrenal incidentaloma the following three questions should be answered:
  - Is the tumor hormonally hyperactive?
  - Does it have imaging characteristics concerning for primary adrenal malignancy (adrenocortical carcinoma)?
  - Does the patient have a history of a prior malignancy?
- Biopsy of an adrenal mass is only indicated if a metastatic deposit in the adrenal gland is suspected, and the biopsy results will alter management of the primary malignancy. Pheochromocytoma must be rule out prior adrenal biopsy.
- Alpha blockade for 7 to 14 days is crucial in patients undergoing adrenalectomy for pheochromocytoma.
- Adrenal vein sampling is indicated in most patients with a biochemical diagnosis of primary aldosteronism to distinguish unilateral versus bilateral disease. Adrenalectomy only has a role in unilateral primary aldosteronism.
- Glucocorticoid replacement may be required after adrenalectomy for Cushing's syndrome.
- Open adrenalectomy is the procedure of choice for adrenocortical carcinoma.

BIBLIOGRAPHY

Aronova, A., Gordon, B. L., Finnerty, B. M., Zarnegar, R., & Fahey, T. J. 3rd. (2014). Aldosteronoma resolution score predicts long-term resolution of hypertension. *Surgery, 156,* 1387–1393.

Berruti, A., Fassnacht, M., Baudin, E. (2010). Adjuvant therapy in patients with adrenocortical carcinoma: a position of an international panel. *Journal of Clinical Oncology, 28,* e401.

Bovio, S, Cataldi, A., Reimondo, G., Sperone, P., Novello, S., Berruti, A., . . . Terzolo, M. (2006). Prevalence of adrenal incidentaloma in a contemporary computerized tomography series. *Journal of Endocrinological Investigation, 29*(4), 298.

Carey, R. M. (2012). Primary aldosteronism. *Journal of Surgical Oncology, 106*(5), 575–579.

Fassnacht, M., Arlt, W., Bancos, I., Dralle, H., Newell-Price, J., Sahdev, A., . . . Dekkers, O. M. (2016). Management of adrenal incidentalomas: European Society of Endocrinology Clinical Practice Guideline in collaboration with the European Network for the Study of Adrenal Tumors. *European Journal of Endocrinology, 175*(2), G1–G34.

Funder, J. W., Carey, R. C., Mantero, F., Murad, M. H., Reincke M., Shibata, H., . . . Young, W. F. Jr. (2016). The management of primary aldosteronism: case detection, diagnosis, and treatment: an Endocrine Society clinical practice guideline. *Journal of Clinical Endocrinology & Metabolism, 101*(5), 1889–1916.

Harvey, A. M. (2014). Hyperaldosteronism: diagnosis, lateralization, and treatment. *Surgical Clinics of North America, 94*(3), 643–656.

Icard, P., Goudet, P., Charpenay, C., Andreassian, B., Carnaille, B., Chapuis, Y., . . . Proye, C. (2001). Adrenocortical carcinomas: surgical trends and results of a 253-patient series from the French Association of Endocrine Surgeons study group. *World Journal of Surgery, 25,* 891.

Lee, J., El-Tamer, M., Schifftner, T., Turrentine, F. E., Henderson, W. G., Khuri, S., . . . Inabnet, W. B. 3rd. (2008). Open and laparoscopic adrenalectomy: analysis of the National Surgical Quality Improvement Program. *Journal of the American College of Surgeons, 206,* 953–959.

Lenders, J. W. M., Duh, Q-Y., Eisenhofer, G., Gimenez-Roqueplo, A-P., Grebe, S. K. G., Murad, M. H., . . . Young, W. F. Jr; Endocrine Society. (2014). Pheochromocytoma and paraganglioma: an Endocrine Society clinical practice guideline. *Journal of Clinical Endocrinology & Metabolism, 99*(6), 1915–1942.

Mantero, F., Terzolo, M., Arnaldi, G., Osella, G., Masini, A. M., Alì, A., , . . . Angeli, A. (2000). A survey on adrenal incidentaloma in Italy. Study Group on Adrenal Tumors of the Italian Society of Endocrinology. *Journal of Clinical Endocrinology & Metabolism, 85*(2), 637.

Martucci, V. L., & Pacak, K. (2014). Pheochromocytoma and paraganglioma: diagnosis, genetics, management, and treatment. *Current Problems in Cancer, 38*(1), 7–41.

McKenzie, T. J., Lillegard, J. B., Young, Jr., W. F., & Thompson, G. B. (2009). Aldosteronomas—state of the art. *Surgical Clinics of North America, 89*(5), 1241–1253.

Stewart, P. (2010). Is subclinical Cushing's syndrome an entity or a statistical fallout from diagnostic testing? Consensus surrounding the diagnosis is required before optimal treatment can be defined. *Journal of Clinical Endocrinology & Metabolism, 95*(6), 2618–2620.

Terzolo, M., Angeli, A., Fassnacht, M., Daffara, F., Tauchmanova, L., Conton, P. A., . . . Berruti, A. (2007). Adjuvant mitotane treatment for adrenocortical carcinoma. *New England Journal of Medicine, 356,* 2372.

Zeiger, M., Thompson, G., Duh, QY., Hamrahian, A., Angelos, P., Elaraj, D., Angelos P, . . . Kharlip, J.; American Association of Clinical Endocrinologists; American Association of Endocrine Surgeons. (2009). American Association of Clinical Endocrinologists and American Association of Endocrine Surgeons medical guidelines for the management of adrenal incidentalomas. *Endocrine Practice, 15*(Suppl. 1), 1–20.

Zini, L., Porpiglia, F., & Fassnacht, M. (2011). Contemporary management of adrenocortical carcinoma. *European Journal of Urology, 60,* 1055.

CHAPTER 68

PANCREAS AND OTHER ENDOCRINE TUMOR SURGERY

Stephanie Davis, Maria Albuja-Cruz, Chris Raeburn, and Robert McIntyre, Jr.

1. What are pancreatic neuroendocrine tumors (PNETs)?

   PNETs are a group of epithelial neoplasms originating from the islet cells of the pancreas (also known as *islet cell tumors*). They are categorized as either functional or nonfunctional, depending on the tumor's ability to secrete hormones, such as insulin, gastrin, glucagon, vasoactive intestinal peptide (VIP), or somatostatin. The majority (60%–90%) of PNETs are nonfunctional. Nonfunctional PNETs typically manifest similarly to pancreatic adenocarcinoma, with abdominal pain or biliopancreatic duct obstruction, secondary to mass effect. They are often diagnosed at advanced stages because of their slow growth pattern leading to a delay in onset of symptoms. Nonfunctional PNETs are also increasingly being discovered incidentally with the increasing use of high-quality abdominal imaging. Functional PNETs are often diagnosed on the basis of presenting symptoms caused by over-production of hormones. They can be small and difficult to localize with imaging. PNETs are usually sporadic but can be associated with genetic syndromes about 10% of the time; these include multiple endocrine neoplasia types I and IV (MEN 1 or 4), von Hippel-Lindau (VHL) syndrome, neurofibromatosis-1 (NF-1), and tuberous sclerosis complex (TSC).

2. How common are PNETs?

   PNETs are rare, with an incidence of 0.43 per 100,000 population per year. The incidence in the United States has increased in frequency over the past 30 years because of growing awareness, improvements in diagnostic imaging, and overall increased use of computed tomography (CT) and magnetic resonance imaging (MRI). Autopsy series find a prevalence of 0.8% to 10%. PNETS account for only 1% to 3% of all pancreatic tumors and 7% of all NETs; only gastrointestinal (GI) carcinoids are more common.

3. What are the subtypes and syndromes of functional PNETs?

   Insulinoma is the most common functional PNET and is malignant in < 10% of cases. The most common presenting symptom is hypoglycemia, causing neuroglycopenic or cardiovascular symptoms. These tumors are found in an even distribution through the entire pancreas.

   Gastrinoma is the second most common functional PNET and causes Zollinger-Ellison syndrome (ZES). Approximately 60% to 90% are malignant. The most common presenting symptoms are severe peptic ulcer disease, abdominal pain, and diarrhea. The vast majority (70%–95%) of gastrinomas are located in the first portion of the duodenum and not in the pancreas, as previous studies had suggested.

   Glucagonoma is the next most common functional PNET and 50% to 80% of these tumors are malignant. The most common presenting symptoms are necrolytic migratory erythema, diabetes, deep vein thrombosis, and diarrhea. These tumors are found in an even distribution through the entire pancreas, are often quite large, and usually present with metastases.

   VIP–secreting tumors (VIPomas) are rare, malignant 40% to 70% of the time, and present with watery diarrhea, hypokalemia, and achlorhydria (also known as *Werner-Morrison syndrome*). The most common tumor locations are the body and tail of the pancreas.

   Somatostatinomas are the rarest functional PNETs and are malignant > 70% of the time. The most common presenting symptoms are diabetes, steatorrhea, and cholelithiasis. These tumors are most commonly found in the pancreas (55%) or the proximal small bowel (duodenum/jejunum; 44%).

4. What are the principles of biochemical testing?

   When a hormonally active tumor is suspected, the diagnosis should be confirmed biochemically before any imaging is performed. This is important not only for cost-effectiveness but also because some localization studies are invasive. For most biochemical studies an 8-hour fast is recommended. It is important to recognize that certain medications can affect test results, especially proton pump inhibitors (PPIs), which significantly increase serum gastrin and chromogranin A levels. Patients with suspected insulinoma should undergo a 72-hour fast with serial measurements of glucose, serum insulin, proinsulin, C-peptide, and sulfonylurea screening. Evaluation for possible ZES should include measurements of fasting serum gastrin levels and gastric pH. Those suspected of having a glucagonoma, VIPoma, or somatostatinoma should have measurements of serum glucagon, VIP, and somatostatin levels, respectively. If a familial syndrome is suspected, screening for other syndromic components should be undertaken, and genetic testing should be considered. For example, if MEN 1 is being considered, patients should be evaluated for coexisting hyperparathyroidism and pituitary tumors, and genetic testing for the menin gene mutation is usually appropriate.

5. **How should functional PNETs be imaged?**

Given the small size of many functional PNETs, preoperative localization can be difficult. Multiphasic CT or MRI is often the first imaging modality pursued. Somatostatin receptor scintigraphy (octreotide scan) is highly sensitive (60%–90%) in locating most PNETs and is especially useful in identifying metastatic disease but is less sensitive for insulinomas because of their low level of expression of type 2 somatostatin receptors. An emerging imaging technique is the use of gallium-labeled radioligands (e.g., 68Ga-DOTATATE and 68Ga-DOTATOC), for which uptake is measured with positron emission tomography/CT. This technology has been shown to be superior to standard imaging (CT, MRI, octreotide scanning) in the detection of primary NETs and metastases in multiple studies (sensitivity and specificity of 97% and 92%, respectively). Endoscopic ultrasonography has also emerged as a valuable imaging modality (sensitivity and specificity of 82% and 92%, respectively), particularly for small insulinomas often missed on CT, and has the added advantage of the ability to perform a biopsy and even tattoo lesions to aid in identification during minimally invasive surgical approaches. Provocative arterial stimulation studies (secretin for gastrinomas and calcium for insulinomas) with hepatic venous sampling have higher sensitivity than portal vein sampling and have, therefore, replaced it; however, their invasiveness and ability to only regionalize a tumor make them less desirable options for localization.

6. **What is the appropriate surgical approach for insulinomas?**

Surgical excision of PNETs remains the only curative treatment. The small size of many insulinomas (< 2 cm) and the rarity of malignancy in these tumors allow for pancreatic parenchymal sparing excision by simple enucleation in most cases. It is becoming increasingly common to utilize a laparoscopic approach for simple enucleation. If a patient is not a candidate for enucleation (size, concerning features, proximity to main pancreatic duct), then a formal pancreaticoduodenectomy for tumors in the pancreatic head or a distal pancreatectomy for tumors in the body or tail may be required. When the tumor cannot be localized with preoperative imaging, intraoperative ultrasonography with bimanual palpation has up to 95% sensitivity in localizing the tumor.

7. **Describe the surgical approach to gastrinomas.**

The surgical approach to gastrinomas is more complex because these tumors are more frequently malignant and the majority occur outside the pancreas. Tumors in the pancreatic head can often be enucleated, reserving formal pancreaticoduodenectomy for more invasive tumors or those in close proximity to the pancreatic duct or superior mesenteric vessels. Tumors in the body or tail of the pancreas should be resected by distal pancreatectomy. Upper endoscopy with duodenal transillumination can aid in identification of lateral wall tumors. Duodenotomy should be performed in every operation to reduce the risk of missing a gastrinoma located in the duodenal wall (98% of gastrinomas will be found by doing this). Routine duodenotomy has also been shown to improve the long-term cure rate. Small submucosal lesions can be enucleated, but full-thickness resection of the duodenal wall may be necessary. These tumors have a propensity to metastasize to lymph nodes, and recent studies have shown not only that lymph node status has important prognostic value, but also that resection of lymph nodes improves survival and reduces the risk of persistent disease. Thus, it is recommended that routine lymph node resection be performed in all gastrinoma cases.

8. **Should PNETs occurring in patients with MEN 1 be approached differently from PNETs occurring sporadically?**

Yes. Approximately 70% of patients with MEN 1 develop PNETs, with gastrinoma being the most common. Gastrinomas are commonly multifocal in these patients and, thus, aggressive surgery is often necessary to achieve a biochemical cure; however, this is not routinely recommended. The morbidity and mortality rates of aggressive surgical resection for multifocal gastrinomas combined with the availability of effective medical management of gastric acid hypersecretion sway many clinicians toward avoiding surgical resection unless there is suspicion of malignancy. It is recommended that surgery be avoided for tumors < 2 cm in size because of the low risk of hepatic metastases. For tumors > 2 cm in size, the risk of hepatic metastases is much higher. Enucleation of tumors in the pancreatic head combined with distal pancreatectomy is the recommended procedure. Pancreaticoduodenectomy is recommended in select cases of large tumors in the pancreatic head that are not amenable to enucleation.

9. **Describe the presentation of nonpancreatic GI neuroendocrine tumors (carcinoid tumors).**

Carcinoid tumors can occur in many different organs throughout the body but most commonly occur in the GI tract (approximately 70% of the time). Within the GI tract, the most common locations, listed in descending order, are the small intestine, rectum, appendix, large intestine, and stomach. Neuroendocrine tumors of the small intestine are the most likely to cause carcinoid syndrome, which typically does not occur until the patient has developed metastases to the liver. These tumors frequently result in a desmoplastic (fibrotic) reaction of the adjacent mesentery, causing bowel obstructions. Hindgut carcinoids do not usually produce active hormones and are typically found incidentally during endoscopy performed for other reasons. Gastric carcinoids are also frequently found incidentally on endoscopy but may cause such symptoms as pain or bleeding.

10. Describe carcinoid syndrome.

Carcinoid syndrome results from the production and release of biologically active amines and peptides (e.g., serotonin, histamine, or tachykinins) from neuroendocrine tumors. Approximately 8% to 28% of these tumors result in carcinoid syndrome. The liver metabolizes serotonin to inactive products and, therefore, most patients do not develop carcinoid syndrome until they have significant liver metastases, which permit serotonin to directly enter the systemic circulation. Because serotonin is rapidly metabolized, it cannot be measured. However, 5-hydroxyindoleacetic acid (5-HIAA) is the main serotonin metabolite and can be measured in 24-hour urine samples.

Carcinoid syndrome most commonly results from small bowel primary tumors. Classic symptoms include intermittent flushing, diarrhea, wheezing (from bronchoconstriction), and right-sided heart failure (from valvular fibrosis of the right-sided valves). Carcinoid crisis is a life-threatening exacerbation of carcinoid syndrome, which manifests as profound flushing, bronchospasm, tachycardia, and volatile swings of blood pressure. Patients with foregut or midgut carcinoid tumors (with or without having carcinoid syndrome) are at risk for carcinoid crisis during manipulation, whether that be surgery or radiologic intervention.

11. Once a patient is diagnosed with carcinoid syndrome, what is the next step?

The tumor must be localized. This may be difficult because of the small size of many carcinoid tumors. Multiphasic CT or MRI and somatostatin receptor scintigraphy are generally recommended to localize any carcinoid tumor. Luminal evaluation by endoscopy with consideration for endoscopic ultrasonography is also recommended for ileal, rectal, large intestine, and gastric carcinoids. Echocardiography should be performed if right-sided heart disease is suspected in cases of carcinoid syndrome.

12. Describe the appropriate surgical management for non–PNETs (carcinoid tumors).

Gastric carcinoids are classified into three types. Types I and II account for most gastric carcinoids (> 75%) and are associated with chronic hypergastrinemia resulting from chronic atrophic gastritis (type I) and ZES (type II), respectively. These tumors are most commonly small (< 1 cm) and multifocal and are typically treated by endoscopic resection and surveillance with excellent outcomes. Octreotide or lanreotide therapy can control symptoms in patients with type II gastric carcinoids and ZES. Type III gastric carcinoids occur sporadically and are usually larger, solitary, and invasive. They are treated similarly to gastric adenocarcinoma with formal gastric resection and lymph node dissection. For tumors < 2 cm in size, endoscopic or wedge resection is possible.

Small intestinal carcinoids without metastases should be excised by segmental resection and lymph node dissection. Some studies advocate the use of prophylactic octreotide (preoperative bolus and/or continuous infusion) during surgery for foregut and midgut carcinoids to prevent carcinoid crisis; however, this remains controversial because some studies have shown it to be ineffective. Appendiceal carcinoids are typically incidentally discovered and occur most commonly at the appendiceal tip. Distal lesions < 2 cm are adequately treated with appendectomy. The presence of a carcinoid tumor near the appendiceal base, size > 2 cm, or gross lymph node involvement requires a formal right hemicolectomy. Rectal carcinoids often manifest with bleeding or are incidentally found on endoscopy. Tumors < 1 cm can be subjected to endoscopic resection, tumors 1 to 2 cm to transanal excision, and tumors > 2 cm or with evidence of lymph node metastasis on endoscopic ultrasonography to surgical resection (low anterior resection or abdominoperineal resection).

13. Discuss the role of surgery for liver metastases from neuroendocrine tumors (both pancreatic and nonpancreatic).

Surgical resection is the recommended treatment for patients with liver metastases from intestinal NETs and/or PNETs. These patients experience symptomatic improvement and have prolonged survival (58%–70% versus 25%–30% 5-year survival rates) compared with similar patients who do not undergo hepatic resection. Patients with unresectable liver metastases, those with poor baseline liver function, or those with tumor recurrence (after prior hepatic resections) may benefit from other therapies, such as radiofrequency thermal ablation and/or transarterial chemoembolization. Nonresectable NET liver metastasis resistant to medical treatment and confined to the liver is an accepted indication for liver transplantation; however, most patients eventually develop recurrence.

14. What are the principles of systemic therapy in patients with unresectable or metastatic NETs?

There is no known role for adjuvant systemic therapy. Patients who have metastatic NETs and carcinoid syndrome should be treated with a somatostatin analogue (octreotide or lanreotide). The long-acting release (LAR) preparations are often effective for symptom management; intercurrent symptom flares can be treated by temporarily adding a short-acting somatostatin analogue. Telotristat is orally administered for the inhibition of tryptophan hydroxylase, which is the rate-limiting step in serotonin synthesis. Telotristat can be used in combination with somatostatin analogues and has been shown to significantly reduce both 5-HIAA excretion and diarrhea. There is no consensus on initiation of treatment in the asymptomatic patient with a low tumor burden. The use of octreotide or lanreotide in patients with clinically significant tumor burdens or progressive disease can help control tumor growth. Systemic chemotherapy and hepatic artery embolization have not been very effective in palliative therapy for patients with diffuse hepatic metastases; however, selective hepatic artery chemoembolization, when possible, has been successful in decreasing tumor burden and alleviating symptoms.

For patients with progressive metastatic carcinoid, everolimus (an inhibitor of mechanistic target of rapamycin) can be given with octreotide LAR. Cytotoxic chemotherapy regimens, such as combination capecitabine and oxaplatin, or 5-fluorouracil, streptozotocin, or doxorubicin, have shown only modest response rates. Patients who have failed to respond to somatostatin analogues can be treated with interferon-alpha. There are some reports of benefit from treatment with radiolabeled somatostatin analogues in patients with advanced disease.

KEY POINTS: PANCREAS AND OTHER GASTROINTESTINAL NEUROENDOCRINE TUMORS

- Insulinoma, the most common functional pancreatic neuroendocrine tumor (PNET), is usually benign and, in most cases, can be treated with enucleation.
- Gastrinoma is usually malignant and can occur in the pancreas, duodenum (most common), and lymph nodes.
- Carcinoid tumors are most commonly located in the small intestine, and when metastatic to the liver, it can result in carcinoid syndrome.
- PNETs in patients with multiple endocrine neoplasia type 1 are most commonly gastrinomas, are frequently multifocal, and are usually treated medically. Tumors > 2 cm should be resected.
- Resection of isolated liver metastasis from neuroendocrine tumors improves symptoms and prolongs survival.

BIBLIOGRAPHY

Caplin, M. E., Pavel, M., Cwikla, J. B., Phan, A. T., Raderer, M., Sedláƒäková, E., . . . Ruszniewski, P.; (2014). Lanreotide in metastatic enteropancreatic neuroendocrine tumors. *New England Journal of Medicine, 371*(3), 224–233.

Chan, M. Y., Ma, K.W., & Chan, A. (2018). Surgical management of neuroendocrine tumor-associated liver metastases: a review. *Gland Surgery,* 7(1), 28–35.

Ellison, T. A., Wolfgang, C. L., Shi, C., Cameron, J. L., Murakami, P., Mun, L. J., . . . Edil, B. H. (2014). A single institution's 26-year experience with nonfunctional pancreatic neuroendocrine tumors: a validation of current staging systems and a new prognostic nomogram. *Annals of Surgery, 259*(2), 204–212.

Faggiano, A., Malandrino, P., Modica, R., Agrimi, D., Aversano, M., Bassi, V., . . . Colao, A. (2016). Efficacy and safety of everolimus in extrapancreatic neuroendocrine tumor: a comprehensive review of literature. *Oncologist, 21*(7), 875–886.

Falconi, M., Eriksson, B., Kaltsas, G., Bartsch, D. K., Capdevila, J., Caplin, M., . . . Zheng-Pei, Z. (2016). ENETS consensus guidelines update for the management of patients with functional pancreatic neuroendocrine tumors and non-functional pancreatic neuroendocrine tumors. *Neuroendocrinology, 103*(2), 153–171.

Jensen, R. T., & Norton, J. A. (2017). Treatment of pancreatic neuroendocrine tumors in multiple endocrine neoplasia type 1: Some clarity but continued controversy. *Pancreas, 46*(5), 589–594.

Maxwell, J. E., & Howe, J. R. (2015). Imaging in neuroendocrine tumors: an update for the clinician. *International Journal of Endocrine Oncology, 2*(2), 159–168.

McKenna, L. R., & Edil, B. H. (2014). Update on pancreatic neuroendocrine tumors. *Gland Surgery, 3*(4), 258–275.

Nell, S., Verkooijen, H. M., Pieterman, C. R. C., de Herder, W. W., Hermus, A. R., Dekkers, O. M., . . . Valk, G. D. (2018). Management of MEN1 related nonfunctioning pancreatic NETs: a shifting paradigmresults from the Dutch MEN1 Study Group. *Annals of Surgery, 267*(6), 1155–1160.

Norton, J. A., Krampitz, G., Zemek, A., Longacre, T., & Jensen, R. T. (2015). Better survival but changing causes of death in patients with multiple endocrine neoplasia type 1. *Annals of Surgery, 261*(6), e147–e148.

Strosberg, J. R., Halfdanarson, T. R., Bellizzi, A. M., Chan, J. A., Dillon, J. S., Heaney, A. P., . . . Bergsland, E. K. (2017). The North American Neuroendocrine Tumor Society consensus guidelines for surveillance and medical management of midgut neuroendocrine tumors. *Pancreas, 46*(6), 707–714.

CHAPTER 69

BARIATRIC SURGERY

Jonathan A. Schoen and Kevin B. Rothchild

1. **Define obesity. How common is it?**
   Obesity is simply defined as the excess of body fat. The degree of body fat relative to weight is calculated by the body mass index (BMI; kg/m^2). Overweight is a BMI 25.0 to 29.9 kg/m^2; obesity is a BMI $\geq$ 30 kg/m^2; morbid obesity is a BMI $\geq$ 40 kg/m^2. Increasing BMI correlates with increasing health issues, including diabetes mellitus, hypertension, sleep apnea and Pickwickian syndrome, asthma, coronary artery disease, cardiomyopathy, gastroesophageal reflux disease, degenerative joint disease, hyperlipidemia, fatty liver (hepatic steatosis and nonalcoholic steatohepatitis), gout, urinary incontinence, gallbladder disease, psychological disorders, menstrual irregularities, infertility, and certain cancers (endometrial, colon, breast, and kidney). Most importantly, a BMI > 40 kg/m^2 increases the risk of death from all causes twofold. Approximately 127 million adults (64%) in the United States are considered overweight, and 93 million adults (39.8%) are considered obese. Nearly 18.5% of children and adolescents are obese, with wide variation in certain regions.

2. **In what populations does BMI have limited utility as a precise indicator of obesity?**
   The utility of BMI alone is limited in those with a higher proportion of fat relative to muscle (i.e., the elderly) and in those with an unusually high proportion of muscle (i.e., bodybuilders).

3. **How successful is nonsurgical treatment of obesity?**
   Evidence suggests that nonsurgical treatment (diet/behavior modification, exercise programs, and psychological support) for morbid obesity has a > 90% long-term failure rate. Pharmacologic therapy for morbid obesity, although improving, has been hampered by serious side effects, lack of insurance coverage, and, overall, disappointing results.

4. **What are the indications for obesity surgery?**
   A National Institutes of Health (NIH) Consensus Conference held in 1991 recommended that the following patients be considered for bariatric surgery:
   - BMI $\geq$ 40 kg/m^2
   - BMI of 35 to 40 kg/m^2 if associated with other severe obesity-related medical problems that are likely to improve with weight reduction (i.e., hypertension, diabetes mellitus, obstructive sleep apnea)

5. **Are there other important inclusion criteria for surgery?**
   The initial medical and surgical history and physical examination will determine a person's eligibility for bariatric surgery. The patient must meet the 1991 NIH Consensus Conference weight criteria, as discussed above. The patient must also clear psychological testing and evaluation and preferably have a referral from their primary care provider or internist. Endocrine disorders, such as hypothyroidism and Cushing's disease, should be ruled out, as should any medications causing weight gain. A documented history of failed prior weight loss attempts through dietary, behavioral, lifestyle, and/or medical interventions must be reviewed and verified. Last, but most important, the patient must be motivated and have a basic understanding of the procedure, its risks, benefits, complications, and long-term outcomes prior to any further evaluation for surgery

6. **Have there been any recent updates to the classic surgical indications listed above?**
   - The U.S. Food and Drug Administration in 2011 expanded the use of the Lap Band to include obese individuals who have a BMI of 30 to 34 kg/m^2 and also have an existing obesity-related comorbidity.
   - The International Diabetes Federation in its 2011 position statement, as well as the American Diabetes Association in its recent position statement, stated that surgery should be considered a treatment option in patients who have type 2 diabetes mellitus and a BMI between 30 and 34.9 kg/m^2 if hyperglycemia cannot be adequately controlled by an optimal medical regimen.

7. **List the relative contraindications to bariatric operations.**
   - Endocrine disorders that cause or contribute to morbid obesity
   - Psychological instability
   - Alcohol or drug abuse
   - End-stage organ disease, unless used as a bridge to transplantation
   - Terminal cancer
   - Inability to comprehend or comply with postoperative nutritional and behavioral guidelines

8. Categorize the various surgical options for weight reduction.
   I. Restrictive
   II. Malabsorptive
   III. Combination restrictive/Malabsorptive
   IV. Other

9. List the options for restrictive surgery.
   - *Vertical-banded gastroplasty (historical):* A stapling device is used to divide the stomach vertically along the lesser curve to create a small (20 mL) pouch. A prosthetic device is then wrapped around the outlet of the pouch to prevent it from dilating over time. This operation is no longer performed because of poor long-term success, obstructive symptoms, and reflux.
   - *Gastric banding:* This procedure is performed laparoscopically and involves placement of an adjustable band around the proximal stomach to create a small (15-mL) pouch. The band is connected to a reservoir placed in the subcutaneous tissue that enables band adjustment. Concerns about long-term complications and variable weight loss success have led to a substantial decline in popularity (Fig. 69.1).
   - *Sleeve gastrectomy:* This procedure is gaining in popularity and has now surpassed the gastric bypass as the most common operation done for weight loss. It involves stapling and removing a majority of the gastric body and fundus, leaving the lesser curvature and a small amount of antrum. This amounts to approximately 80% to 85% of the stomach being excised and removed. The pylorus remains intact and the small intestine is unaltered. The short-term complications are essentially the same as for gastric bypass, but the long-term risks and side effects are considerably less than for gastric bypass and biliopancreatic diversion. It is, however, less effective than these operations with regard to weight loss and resolution of diabetes and other comorbidities (Fig. 69.2).

10. What is the option for malabsorptive surgery?
    Biliopancreatic diversion with and without a duodenal switch is a surgical option for malabsorption. A subtotal gastrectomy or sleeve gastrectomy is performed, leaving a gastric remnant of 250 to 500 mL. The small bowel is divided 200 to 300 cm proximal to the ileocecal valve, and the ileum is anastomosed to the stomach or first portion of the duodenum (duodenal switch). The jejunum is connected to the side of the ileum approximately 50 to 100 cm from the ileocecal valve—the "common channel." This procedure results in malabsorption by creating a short common channel for digestion and absorption of food/calories. Chronic diarrhea is common if the patient is not very careful with diet. Similarly, a "distal" gastric bypass involves creating a short common channel, leading to considerable malabsorption. These are the most effective options for weight loss and resolution of comorbidities but carry the highest short-term and long-term risks. The biliopancreatic diversion has been gaining in popularity because of its excellent long-term weight loss results and is now being studied as a single anastomosis operation to decrease the morbidity and make it a more applicable option (Fig. 69.3).

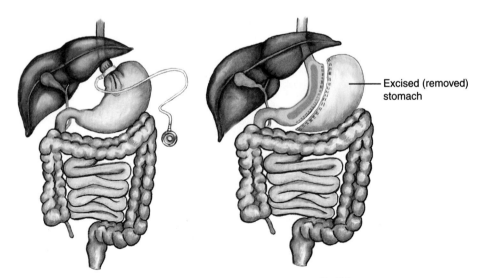

Excised (removed) stomach

Fig. 69.1. Adjustable gastric band "Lap Band" (Kuzmak).   **Fig. 69.2.**

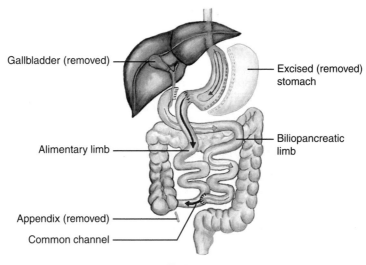

Gallbladder (removed)

Excised (removed) stomach

Alimentary limb

Biliopancreatic limb

Appendix (removed)

Common channel

Fig. 69.3.

11. Explain the combined restrictive/malabsorptive option.

Known as the "proximal" Roux-en-Y gastric bypass, the proximal stomach is stapled to create a small 15- to 30-mL proximal stomach pouch, which is completely separated from the excluded remnant stomach. This small reservoir restricts the amount of food that can be ingested at one time, forcing portion control similar to the purely restrictive surgical options. The proximal jejunum is then divided distal to the ligament of Treitz, and the distal end is anastomosed to the small stomach pouch (the Roux limb). The proximal end of the jejunum (the biliopancreatic limb) is then anastomosed to the side of the Roux limb (the "Y" connection) 75- to 150-cm distal to the gastrojejunostomy. The length of this Roux limb determines to a small degree the amount of calorie malabsorption; it is typically made longer for patients with high BMIs. There is malabsorption of vitamin and minerals from the bypass of the proximal jejunum. The effect of creating the Roux limb leads to dumping syndrome and forced aversion, and avoidance of simple sugars and fatty foods. This operation causes weight loss as a result of portion control (restriction), dumping syndrome, and, to a lesser degree, malabsorption of calories (Fig. 69.4).

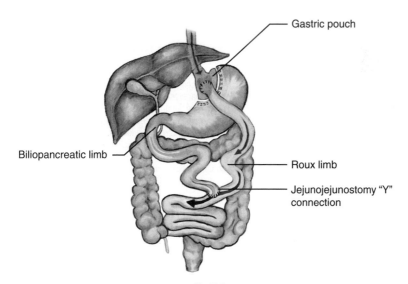

Gastric pouch

Biliopancreatic limb

Roux limb

Jejunojejunostomy "Y" connection

Fig. 69.4.

12. **What options are in the "other" category of procedures?**
    Vagal nerve stimulation, greater curvature plication, intragastric balloons, endoscopic gastric plication, gastrostomy tube placement, and gastric artery embolization are all being studied as viable weight loss options but, as of yet, have not shown long-term results comparable with those of the surgical options already discussed and are generally not covered by insurance.

13. **How much weight do patients lose following bariatric surgery?**
    Success following bariatric surgery is determined by both weight loss and improvement in obesity-related comorbidities. Most surgical studies report outcomes as percentage of excess weight lost (EWL) and consider loss of at least 50% of excess weight as a minimum criterion for success. The lap band typically produces 40% to 60% EWL gradually over 2 to 3 years but has up to a 50% failure and explant rate at 10 years. The gastric bypass typically produces 60% to 80% EWL rapidly over 2 years with fairly low rates of weight regain (approximately 10%–15%) and an estimated 10% overall failure rate. The biliopancreatic diversion is the most effective weight loss procedure and results in loss of 80% of excess weight maintained over the long term. Its popularity is limited by a small percentage of patients who have excessive weight loss or severe vitamin, mineral, and protein deficiencies. The sleeve gastrectomy has shown effective and durable weight loss, with up to 80% of patients achieving 60% EWL at 5 years. Long-term data are still lacking, but the overall failure rate is estimated at 20%.

14. **What are the effects of bariatric surgery on obesity-related comorbidities?**
    Bariatric surgery has been shown to significantly reduce obesity-related comorbidities. Approximately 85% of patients with diabetes, hyperlipidemia, and obesity hypoventilation syndrome will have improvement or effective remission at 2 years after surgery. Glycemic control occurs immediately and dramatically after bariatric surgery, especially after gastric bypass and biliopancreatic diversion, and for reasons which are not entirely clear. This effect is largely caused by dietary changes, adipose reduction with decreased cytokine production, and gastrointestinal (GI) hormonal changes. Hypertension, hyperlipidemia, sleep apnea, pseudotumor cerebri, and non-alcoholic fatty liver disease also improve or resolve in over two thirds of patients after successful weight loss surgery. Salutary effects on other comorbidities, such as asthma, depression, arthritic pain, and even disability are frequently observed after surgery.

15. **Explain the incretin effect in relation to weight loss surgery.**
    Rapid transit of nutrients from the gastric pouch to the distal ileum in those with Roux-en-Y anatomy or the duodenal switch causes increased release of incretins (glucagon-like peptide-1, glucose-dependent insulinotropic polypeptide) with subsequent enhancement of glucose-stimulated insulin secretion and beta-cell sensitivity to oral glucose, especially in patients with type 2 diabetes, in whom this relationship is impaired. Similar effects are seen after the sleeve gastrectomy, although the results are less dramatic and substantial. This may indicate the possible role of ghrelin as an incretin hormone because this hormone level drops immediately after surgery. These early GI hormone changes likely explain much of the initial improvement in blood glucose levels after weight loss surgery. However, long-term data show that glycemic control can wane over time, likely as a result of weight regain or poor diet choices. This may also relate to the existing islet cell mass at the time of surgery because the best and most durable responses occur in patients with diabetes existing for < 5 years and not on insulin therapy.

16. **What are the complications of bariatric surgery?**
    Perioperative (30-day) mortality for bariatric procedures has fallen to approximately 0.1% overall, comparable with that for cholecystectomy or hip replacement. The laparoscopic technique has changed the pattern of perioperative complications. Wound complications and postoperative cardiopulmonary complications are less frequent, whereas anastomotic stenosis, GI bleeding, and bowel obstruction occur more frequently with laparoscopic techniques compared with open techniques. Mean hospital stay after laparoscopic bariatric surgery is 1 to 3 days, which is significantly shorter than after open surgery (5–7 days). Thus, all procedures should be done laparoscopically, if possible. The lap band is usually performed as either an outpatient procedure or requires a 24-hour stay. Each procedure has its own unique risk of complications, the lap band having the lowest number of serious complications but the highest reoperation rate and the biliopancreatic diversion having the highest serious complication rate.

17. **Give the incidence of complications after laparoscopic bariatric procedures in general.**
    - Anastomotic leak (1%)
    - Anastomotic stenosis (5%–10%)
    - Postoperative bowel obstruction (3%)
    - GI bleed (2%)
    - Gallstones (10%)
    - Protein-calorie malnutrition (3%–5%)
    - Anemia (30%)
    - Vitamin deficiency (30%)
    - Wound complications (infection, dehiscence, and hernia) (4%–5%)
    - Band slippage or erosion into stomach (1%–5%)

KEY POINTS: BARIATRIC SURGERY

- Surgery is the only therapy that consistently results in significant, long-term weight loss in morbidly obese patients.
- Laparoscopic sleeve gastrectomy is now the most common bariatric operation performed in the United States, followed by the laparoscopic Roux-en-Y gastric bypass. These procedures typically result in loss of 60% to 80% of excess weight (weight above ideal body weight).
- Surgical weight loss significantly reduces obesity-related comorbidities and is the most effective treatment for diabetes mellitus.

BIBLIOGRAPHY

Adams, T. D., Davidson, L. E., Litwin, S. E., Kim, J., Kolotkin, R. L., Nanjee, M. N., . . . Hunt, S. C. (2017). Weight and metabolic outcomes 12 years after gastric bypass. *New England Journal of Medicine, 377*, 1143–1155.

Biertho, L., Steffen, R., Ricklin, T., Horber, F. F., Pomp, A., Inabnet, W. B., , . . . Gagner, M. (2003). Laparoscopic gastric bypass versus laparoscopic adjustable gastric banding: a comparative study of 1,200 cases. *Journal of the American College of Surgery, 197*(4), 536–544, (discussion 544–545).

Biertho, L., Steffen, R., Ricklin, T., Horber, F. F., Pomp, A., Inabnet, W. B., , . . . Gagner, M. (2003). Laparoscopic gastric bypass versus laparoscopic adjustable gastric banding: a comparative study of 1,200 cases. *Journal of the American College of Surgery, 197*(4), 536–544, (discussion 544–545).

Brolin, R. E. (2002). Bariatric surgery and long-term control of morbid obesity. *Journal of the American Medical Association, 288*, 2793–2796.

Buchwald, H., Avidor, Y., Braunwald, E., Jensen, M. D., Pories, W., Fahrbach, K., & Schoelles, K. (2004 Oct 13). Bariatric surgery: a systematic review and meta-analysis. *Journal of the American Medical Association, 292*(14), 1724–1737.

Laferrére, B. (2016). Bariatric surgery and obesity: Influence on the incretins. *International Journal of Obesity, 6*(suppl 1), S32–S36.

NIH Consensus Conference. (1991). Gastrointestinal surgery for severe obesity. *Annals of Internal Medicine, 115*, 956–961.

Podnos, Y., Jimenez, J. C., Wilson, S. E., Stevens, C. M., & Nguyen, N. T. (2003). Complications after laparoscopic gastric bypass. *Archives of Surgery, 138*, 957–961.

Pories, W., Swanson, M. S., MacDonald, K. G., Long, S. B., Morris, P. G., Brown, B. M., , ... & Dolezal, J. M.. (1995). Who would have thought it? An operation proves to be the most effective therapy for adult-onset diabetes mellitus. *Annals of Surgery, 222*, 339–351.

Schauer, P. R., Burguera, B., Ikramuddin, S., Cottam, D., Gourash, W., Hamad, G., , . . . & . . . Kelley, D. (2003). Effect of laparoscopic Roux-en Y gastric bypass on type 2 diabetes mellitus. *Annals of Surgery, 238*, 467–484, (discussion 84–85).

Schauer, P. R., Bhatt, D. L., Kirwan, J. P., Wolski, K., Aminian, A., Brethauer, S. A., & Navaneethan, S. D. (2017). Bariatric surgery versus intensive medical therapy for diabetes—5-year outcomes. *New England Journal of Medicine, 376*, 641–651.

CHAPTER 70

ENDOCRINOLOGY IN AFRICA

Helen Y. Bitew and Abdurezak A. Abdela

1. How prevalent is diabetes mellitus in Africa?

    Low- and middle-income countries carry the major burden of diabetes mellitus (DM) worldwide. Eighty percent of people with DM live in these countries. The International Diabetes Federation (IDF) Africa region has on record > 15.9 million people with DM, and this number is projected to increase by 162% by 2045. However, North Africa is not an IDF Africa region and, therefore, the actual number of people with DM in the African continent is much higher than the number indicated above. In addition, 70% of DM in Africa is undiagnosed, making it the home of the highest percentage of undiagnosed people with DM in the world. There is, of course, a significant variation across different regions and countries within Africa, ranging from 0.7% in Benin to 18.4% in Re'union. Ethiopia, which has a large population, has the highest number of people with DM (2.65 million) despite a prevalence of 4.8%.

2. What are the peculiarities seen among Africans with Type 1 diabetes mellitus?

    Although it is difficult to make generalizations about an entire continent and its people, a few peculiarities can be observed among Africans. Some studies have suggested that the frequency of antibody positivity among African patients with type 1 DM (T1DM) is lower than that reported in the American and European populations (7%–44% versus 80%–97%). One of the hypotheses for low antibody positivity with T1DM in Africa is the existence of malnutrition-related or modified DM as a cause of insulin-requiring DM. Some epidemiologic peculiarities include average age of onset that is later by about a decade, male predominance, and poor socioeconomic status correlated with higher risk.

3. What is malnutrition-related diabetes mellitus (MRDM)?

    Although it is not in the current classification of diabetes, MRDM is noted in parts of sub-Saharan Africa and Asia. It was listed as a subtype of type 1 DM in the 1985 World Health Organization (WHO) classification but was later removed, with the citation that there was not enough evidence. There are two forms of MRDM: fibrocalcific pancreatic diabetes (FCPD) and protein-deficient pancreatic diabetes (PDPD; also known as the *Jamaica type* or *J-type*). It is reported that insulin requirements of patients with MRDM are higher than for typical patients with T1DM. African patients' insulin requirements tend to be less than those of Indian or Jamaican patients.

4. What are the features of MRDM in Africa?

    The features suggestive of MRDM are onset before age 30 years, body mass index (BMI) < 19 kg/m^2, absence of ketosis on insulin withdrawal, poor socioeconomic status, history of childhood malnutrition, and insulin requirements > 2 U/kg/day (suggesting insulin resistance). FCPD will be diagnosed if, in addition to the above, the patient has a history of recurrent abdominal pain from an early age, pancreatic calculi on plain radiography of the abdomen, and/or typical changes on ultrasonography of the pancreas, in the absence of alcoholism, gallstones, or hyperparathyroidism.

5. Discuss ketosis-prone type 2 diabetes mellitus (T2DM).

    A group of patients with the phenotypic T2DM appearance present with acute, severe hyperglycemia with ketosis. This phenomenon has been described among Africans and African Americans. It is characterized by a strong family history of T2DM, young adult age, male gender (three times more common in men than in women), rare islet autoimmunity, and high human papilloma virus-8 prevalence. Although insulin is required in the short term to control hyperglycemia, unlike classic T2DM, patients with ketosis-prone T2DM may achieve full remission with no need for continuing medical treatment. However, recurrence is possible.

6. How is a hyperglycemic crisis diagnosed and treated in resource-limited settings?

    The diagnosis of diabetic ketoacidosis (DKA) is made on the basis of clinical presentation, blood glucose levels, and urine ketones. Serum ketones, arterial blood gas analysis, and serum electrolytes are not readily available. Most facilities administer regular insulin hourly because of lack of infusion capability and insulin analogues. This leads to increased complications. Missed doses of regular insulin result in patients taking days longer to clear their ketones. The long turnaround time to get results from laboratories adds further difficulty in following the DKA protocol. Finally, it is difficult to confirm resolution of DKA, often resulting in premature discontinuation of hourly insulin administration and subsequent DKA relapses.

7. How prevalent is gestational diabetes in Africa?

There have been few studies done in Africa, with only 11% of the 54 African countries having prevalence data on gestational diabetes mellitus (GDM). The prevalence data reported from one systematic review ranges from 0% in Tanzania to 13.9% in urban Nigeria. This difference could be because of the use of different diagnostic criteria. Many sub-Saharan countries do not have screening and treatment protocols for GDM. In contrast to the standard practice of using insulin for GDM, metformin and glyburide are mainly used to treat these women; however, there have not been increased reported fetal or maternal complications. These oral agents are preferred because they are relatively inexpensive, less invasive, and require minimal self-monitoring of blood glucose.

8. What is the most common cause of hospital admissions for patients with T2DM in Africa?

Diabetic foot disease (ulcer with and/or gangrene) is the leading cause of hospital admission in patients with T2DM in Africa. Neuropathy is not the most common cause of foot ulcer; instead, the cause for the majority of foot ulcers is unidentified. Poorly fitting shoes and blunt trauma contribute to a third of cases. Foot ulcers result in significant morbidity and mortality, accounting for close to 50% of amputations and > 20% of in-hospital mortality.

9. How is diabetes care organized in Africa, and what are the care gaps?

The rate of undiagnosed DM in Africa is high. Patients usually present late, significantly increasing the chances of having chronic complications. In many African countries, care is integrated with other services at the primary care level. However, most centers fail to meet the IDF recommendations for resource-limited settings. The identified care gaps include limited number of health care professionals, patient overload, access to basic laboratories, self-monitoring of blood glucose, diabetes education, and access to and affordability of oral and injectable medications.

10. What options are there to manage diabetes in places where there are few endocrinologists/diabetologists?

A "task shifting/sharing" approach is increasingly being used in the management of chronic illnesses in areas with few specialized human resources for health care. A similar approach is used in the management of diabetes in Africa. Nurses, health care officers/medical officers, general practitioners, and internists are trained to provide comprehensive noncommunicable-disease care. The fact that task sharing requires continuous support and mentorship from specialists has shaped the role of the endocrinologist in Africa.

11. What are the common thyroid disorders in Africa?

The leading cause of thyroid disorders in Africa is iodine deficiency. In addition to the low iodine status of the region, selenium deficiency and thiocyanate toxicity in inadequately cooked cassava contribute to iodine deficiency. Endemic goiter (> 5% of 6- to 12-year-old children with goiter) is prevalent in different regions. The common causes for hyperthyroidism are toxic multinodular goiter, Graves' disease, and toxic adenoma. The common causes for hypothyroidism are thyroidectomy, Hashimoto's thyroiditis, and atrophic thyroiditis.

12. What is the impact of iodine deficiency in Africa?

The WHO recommends iodine intake of 150 mcg/day for the general population, 250 mcg/day during pregnancy, and 290 mcg/day when lactating. Two billion people, including 285 million school-age children, still have iodine deficiency (urinary iodine excretion of < 100 mcg/L). This has substantial effects on growth and development, and is the most common cause of preventable mental impairment worldwide. In areas where the daily iodine intake is below 50 mcg, goiter is usually endemic, and when the daily intake falls below 25 mcg, congenital hypothyroidism is common. Eight percent of newborns from sub-Saharan Africa are afflicted by learning disabilities resulting from iodine deficiency related disorders.

13. What are the challenges of diagnosing thyroid diseases in Africa?

Most diagnostic modalities are not readily available in sub-Saharan Africa. Thyroid function tests are in common use for assessment of functional status. However, radioactive iodine uptake measurements, thyroid scans, and thyroid antibody tests are rarely available. Ultrasonography is being used increasingly to characterize thyroid nodules. Fine-needle aspiration cytology (FNAC) is also available.

14. What are the therapeutic options available for treatment of hyperthyroidism and hypothyroidism in Africa?

Antithyroid drugs (ATDs) and surgery are the mainstays of treatment for hyperthyroidism. Propylthiouracil is the main ATD in use, with limited availability of carbimazole and methimazole. There are centers that perform large volumes of thyroid surgery, with common indications being large goiters, retrosternal goiters, failure to respond to and control hyperthyroidism on ATDs, compressive symptoms, and thyroid malignancies. Radioactive iodine (RAI) therapy is not readily available. Hypothyroidism is treated with levothyroxine (LT_4). The availability of levotriiodothyronine (LT_3) and different dosage formulations of LT_4 is very limited.

15. How do you follow up a patient on an ATD in an African setting?

It takes more than a year for thyroid-stimulating hormone (TSH) levels to reach closer to normal values among African patients. This may be attributable to prolonged suppression of the thyrotropes from long-standing untreated hyperthyroidism, but other significant factors include repeated treatment interruptions caused by erratic availability of medications, the high cost of thyroid function tests forcing less frequent testing and adjustment of doses, and poor patient adherence. Therefore, responses to treatment are followed mainly with free T_4 and T_3.

16. **What are the comparative challenges in providing endocrinologic care other than that for diabetes in Africa?**
Endocrinologic care in Africa is comparatively less developed and organized compared with diabetes care. There are challenges related to diagnosis, including laboratory assays for determining hormone levels, performing stimulation or suppression tests, and imaging (magnetic resonance imaging/computed tomography) of the endocrine glands. In addition, there are challenges for providing appropriate treatment because of lack of medications and less developed endocrine and neurosurgery services. There is lack of a sustainable supply of medications, such as bromocriptine; furthermore, cabergoline, hydrocortisone, fludrocortisone, growth hormone, and RAI treatment are not available at all in most sub-Saharan countries. These challenges have resulted in significant suffering of patients who have treatable endocrine diseases.

17. **What training opportunities in endocrinology are available in Africa?**
There are few specialist and subspecialty training programs in sub-Saharan Africa. Some parts of Africa have more developed endocrinology training programs (e.g., Egypt, Nigeria, and South Africa). However, in most sub-Saharan African countries there are very limited training opportunities. Even when training opportunities are available, the capacity of programs to take large numbers of fellows is limited. In addition, the fact that the pool of medical graduates is small makes it difficult to attract a large number of fellows into programs. In some African countries, such as Kenya, programs are focused only on pediatric endocrinology, whereas in others, such as Ethiopia, programs are open to take candidates from adult and pediatric specialties.

18. **What are the diagnostic challenges of thyroid cancer?**
Most patients with thyroid nodules characteristically present late for care. The high prevalence of goiters has led to the general perception that thyroid nodules are benign conditions. In some places, goiters are even considered a mark of beauty. Even when patients present early, the absence of ultrasound-guided FNAC expertise and lack of availability of tumor genetic marker testing significantly affects diagnostic accuracy. The general lack of a multidisciplinary approach to care further complicates management after diagnosis.

19. **How is thyroid cancer managed?**
Once the diagnosis is made, care is generally directed to surgeons and then radiation oncologists. There is no access to RAI therapy or thyroglobulin tests for follow-up. Most patients are followed-up by surgeons and radiation oncologists, effectively alienating endocrinologists from patients with thyroid cancer. This creates significant barriers to proper patient management and follow-up care with regard to LT_4 dosing required to achieve optimal TSH suppression and investigations needed to detect recurrence.

20. **What are the peculiar roles and responsibilities of an endocrinologist in Africa?**
Endocrinology is a comprehensive subspecialty and, therefore, an endocrinologist in Africa cannot afford to focus on specific endocrine pathology for specialization. In addition, he or she is expected to play more roles than purely that of an endocrinologist, who is also a general practitioner. Endocrinologists in Africa must be leaders, consultants, trainers, coordinators of care team, and advocates.

BIBLIOGRAPHY

Abdulkadir, J., Mengesha, B., Welde Gabriel, Z., Keen, H., Worku, Y., Gebre, P., ... Taddesse, AS. (1990). The clinical and hormonal (C-peptide and glucagon) profile and liability to ketoacidosis during nutritional rehabilitation in Ethiopian patients with malnutrition-related diabetes mellitus. *Diabetologia, 33*, 222–227.

Alemu, S., Dessie, A., Seid, E., Bard, E., Lee, P. T., Trimble, E. R., ... Parry, E. H. O. (2009). Insulin-requiring diabetes in rural Ethiopia: should we reopen the case for malnutrition-related diabetes? *Diabetologia, 52*, 1842–1845.

Atun, R., Davies, J. I., Gale, E. A. M., Bärnighausen, T., Beran, D., Kengne, A. P., ... Werfalli, M. (2017). Diabetes in sub-Saharan Africa: from clinical care to health policy. *The Lancet Diabetes & Endocrinology Commission, 5*(8), 622–667.

Chattopadhyay, P. S., Gupta, S. K., Chattopadhyay, R., Kundu P. K., & Chakraborti, R. (1995). Malnutrition-related diabetes mellitus (MRDM), not diabetes-related malnutrition: a report on genuine MRDM. *Diabetes care, 18*(2), 276–277.

Gill, G. V., Mbanya, J. C., Ramaiya, K. L., & Tesfaye, S. (2009). A sub-Saharan African perspective of diabetes. *Diabetologia, 52*, 8–16.

Gizaw, M., Harries, A. D., Ade, S., Tayler-Smith, K., Ali, E., Firdu, N., & Yifter, H. (2015). Diabetes mellitus in Addis Ababa, Ethiopia: admissions, complications and outcomes in a large referral hospital. *Public Health Action, 5*(1), 74–78.

International Diabetes Federation. (n.d.). *IDF Diabetes Atlas.* (8th ed.). Brussels, Belgium: IDF.

Kebede, D., Abay, Z., & Feleke, Y. (2012). Pattern, clinical presentations and management of thyroid diseases in national endocrine referral clinics, Tikur Anbessa Specialized Hospital, Addis Ababa, Ethiopia. *Ethiopian Medical Journal, 50*(4), 287–295.

Macaulay, S., Dunger, D. B., & Norris, S. A. (2014). Gestational diabetes mellitus in Africa: a systematic review. *PloS One, 9*(6), e97871.

Ogbera, A. O. & Kuku, S. F. (2011). Epidemiology of thyroid diseases in Africa. *Indian Journal of Endocrinology & Metabolism, 15*(Suppl. 2), S82–S88.

Palace, M. R. (2017). Perioperative management of thyroid dysfunction. *Health Services Insights*, 1–5. Retrieved from: https://journals.sagepub.com/doi/10.1177/1178632916689677.

Siraj, E. S., Gupta, M., Scherbaum, W. A., Yifter, H., Ahmed, A., Kebede, T., ... Abdulkadir, J. (2016). Islet-cell associated autoantibody in Ethiopian patients with diabetes. *Journal of Diabetes and Its Complications, 30*(6), 1039–1042.

Vanderpump, M. P. J. (2011). Epidemiology of thyroid disease and swelling. In A. H. John, P. Wass, M. Stewart, S. A. Amiel, & M. J. Davies (Eds.), *Oxford textbook of endocrinology and diabetes* (2nd ed.). Oxford, UK: Oxford University Press.

Wondwossen, A., Reja, A., & Amare, A. (2011). Diabetic foot disease in Ethiopian patients: a hospital based study. *Ethiopian Journal of Health Development, 25*(1), 17–21.

CHAPTER 71

FAMOUS PEOPLE WITH ENDOCRINE DISORDERS

Pratima Kumar, Kenneth J. Simcic,[a] and Michael T. McDermott

1. Name the former college basketball star from Gonzaga University who was diagnosed with type 1 diabetes mellitus (T1DM) at age 14 years.

   Adam Morrison. After his final college season, Morrison shared college basketball's Player of the Year Award with J.J. Redick of Duke University. He was then selected third overall in the 2006 National Basketball Association (NBA) draft by the Charlotte Bobcats.

2. This female track star recovered from Graves' disease and went on to win the title of "fastest woman in the world" at the 1992 Summer Olympics in Barcelona. Who is she?

   Gail Devers. Devers repeated as champion in the women's 100 meters at the 1996 Olympics in Atlanta. She enjoyed remarkable longevity in her sport. In February 2007, at age 40 years, she won the 60-meter hurdles at the Melrose games with a time of 7.86 seconds.

3. Name the dwarf actor who gained fame for his role as Tattoo on the television series Fantasy Island (1977–1984).

   Herve Villechaize (1943–1993). Villechaize's short stature was secondary to achondroplasia. His adult height was only 3 feet, 2 inches.

4. Television and film actress Mary Tyler Moore had what endocrine disorder?

   T1DM. Moore was diagnosed at age 33 years. Her diabetes had been complicated by retinopathy and recurrent foot infections. She died as a result of pneumonia in 2017 at age 80 years. Diabetes was never an obstacle to her success as an actress.

5. George Bush and his wife Barbara were both diagnosed with Graves' disease during his presidency (1989–1993). How did the president's Graves' disease manifest clinically?

   Atrial fibrillation. Mrs. Bush's Graves' disease was also complicated by ophthalmopathy. In addition to radioactive iodine (RAI) for her hyperthyroidism, she also required treatment with glucocorticoids and orbital radiation therapy for her eye disease.

KEY POINTS

- Because many endocrine disorders are common, it is not surprising that famous people have or have had endocrine disorders.
- Most endocrine disorders are either curable or treatable.
- Many famous people have accomplished great things despite their endocrine disorders. The lives of these famous people can serve as sources of encouragement to patients who suffer from similar endocrine conditions.

6. Pulitzer Prize–winning film critic Roger Ebert was diagnosed with what endocrine disorder at age 59 years?

   Papillary thyroid cancer (treated with thyroidectomy and RAI). Ebert had a major risk factor for papillary thyroid cancer. As a child, he was given radiation treatment for an ear infection. He was unable to speak, but he used a computer program to turn text into speech.

7. Name the actor who had acromegalic gigantism and played the character Jaws in the James Bond films *The Spy Who Loved Me* (1977) and *Moonraker* (1979).

   Richard Kiel (Kiel was 7 feet, 2 inches tall).

8. Name the 2-foot, 8-inch, dwarf actor best known for his role as Mini-Me in the film *Austin Powers: The Spy Who Shagged Me* (1999).

   Vern Troyer. Troyer's dwarfism was secondary to chondrodysplasia. He had acting roles in $>$ 15 feature films.

---

[a]Deceased.

9. Name the NFL quarterback who developed T1DM in 2007.
Jay Cutler. He lost 35 pounds at the time of his diagnosis in 2007 but regained his weight and strength on insulin therapy. He performed athletically at the highest level despite having diabetes because of his devotion to good glucose control on and off the field.

10. Ancient Egyptian sculptures and paintings suggest that Tutankhamen (1357–1339 BC) and other pharaohs of the Eighteenth Egyptian Dynasty had what endocrine disorder?
Gynecomastia. Familial aromatase excess syndrome is a possible explanation for this historical finding.

11. What famous male ice skater overcame growth failure related to a childhood illness to win the gold medal at the 1984 Winter Olympics in Sarajevo?
Scott Hamilton. As a child, Hamilton suffered from Shwachman's syndrome, a rare disorder of the pancreas. His adult height is 5 feet, 3 inches. Hamilton was also diagnosed with testicular cancer at age 38 years and with a craniopharyngioma at age 46 years.

12. Name the late professional wrestler (and actor) who was well known for his height and acromegalic facial features.
Andre "The Giant" Rousimoff (1947–1993).

13. Charles Sherwood Stratton (1838–1883) reached an adult height of only 3 feet, 4 inches. What was his circus name?
General Tom Thumb. In 1863, Stratton married fellow diminutive circus performer Lavinia Warren, whose height was only 2 feet, 8 inches.

14. Actress Catherine Bell, who starred as Lt. Col. Sarah "Mac" MacKenzie on the television series JAG (1995–2005), has been treated for what thyroid disorder?
Papillary thyroid cancer.

15. Oscar award–winning actress Halle Berry was diagnosed with what endocrine disorder at age 21 years?
T1DM.

16. After successful treatment for Graves' disease, this professional golfer captained the United States team to the 1999 Ryder Cup in what has been called the greatest comeback in Ryder Cup history. Who is he?
Ben Crenshaw.

17. Vocalist Rod Stewart has had surgery for what endocrine disorder?
Thyroid cancer (most likely papillary). It took 9 months for Stewart to recover his voice after the surgery.

18. Ron Santo won six Golden Glove Awards and played in nine All Star games while playing third base for the Chicago Cubs. He was diagnosed with T1DM at what age?
Eighteen years, just after signing his first contract to play major league baseball. Since his retirement from baseball, Santo has suffered the following macrovascular complications of his diabetes: coronary artery disease, requiring a quadruple coronary artery bypass operation and implantation of an automatic cardiac defibrillator device, and bilateral below-knee amputations for peripheral vascular disease. He died at age 70 years in 2010.

19. Name the 3-foot, 7-inch, 65-pound midget who batted one time for the St. Louis Browns on August 19, 1951.
Eddie Gaedel (1925–1961). Gaedel was walked on four pitches by Detroit Tigers' pitcher Bob Cain.

20. Gheorghe Muresan of the Washington Bullets is the tallest player in the history of the NBA (7 feet, 7 inches). What treatments has he received for his acromegaly and gigantism?
Transsphenoidal pituitary surgery, pituitary radiation, and somatostatin analogue injections. (*Note:* Shaquille O'Neal is 7 feet, 1 inch tall.)

21. In his 6-year NBA career (Washington Bullets 1993–1997; New Jersey Nets 1998–2000), Muresan twice led the league in what category?
Field goal percentage (1995–1996 season: 0.584; 1996–1997 season: 0.604).

22. Regardless of acting ability, it seems that every famous giant gets an acting role in a movie. Gheorghe Muresan starred in what movie with Billy Crystal?
My Giant (1998).

23. The late actor Rondo "The Creeper" Hatton had severe acromegalic facial features. He played the villain in numerous horror films, such as the *Pearl of Death* (1944), *House of Horrors* (1946), and *The Brute Man* (1946). How old was Hatton at the time of his death?

    Hatton died of a myocardial infarction at age 51 years. At the time of his death, he also reportedly suffered from diabetes and loss of vision. All these conditions were probably sequelae of his untreated acromegaly.

24. What endocrine disorder was Nick Jonas diagnosed with in 2005?

    Pop singer Nick Jonas was diagnosed with T1DM in 2005 at the age of 13. He is currently involved in singing, acting, and songwriting.

25. Name the former chief justice of the U.S. Supreme Court who died of anaplastic thyroid cancer at age 80 years.

    William Rehnquist. Rehnquist was diagnosed with anaplastic cancer in October 2004, and he died < 1 year later, in September 2005.

26. Grammy award–winning vocalists Johnny Cash (1932–2003), Ella Fitzgerald (1917–1996), Waylon Jennings (1937–2002), and Luther Vandross (1951–2005) all died of complications of what endocrine disorder?

    Type 2 diabetes mellitus (T2DM).

27. Track star Carl Lewis competed in five consecutive Olympics. He is one of only three athletes who have won nine gold medals in an Olympic career. With what endocrine disorder was he diagnosed at age 35 years?

    Primary hypothyroidism (secondary to Hashimoto's thyroiditis).

28. Name the American swimmer who was diagnosed with T1DM 18 months before he won two gold medals at the 2000 Olympics in Sydney, Australia.

    Gary Hall, Jr.

29. Carla Overbeck, women's soccer star and captain of the 1996 U.S. gold medal Olympic team, was diagnosed with what endocrine disorder at age 32 years?

    Graves' disease.

30. Based on a true story, the film *Lorenzo's Oil* (1992) portrays a family's struggle with what rare adrenal disorder?

    Adrenoleukodystrophy. The film's main character, Lorenzo Odone, was diagnosed with this condition at age 5 years.

31. Despite his T1DM, this former National Hockey League star led the Philadelphia Flyers to back-to-back Stanley Cup championships in 1973 to 1974 and 1974 to 1975.

    Bobby Clarke. Clarke's diabetes was diagnosed at age 13 years.

32. The demanding ironman Triathlon requires a 2.4-mile swim followed by a 112-mile bike ride and a 26.2-mile run. Name the three-time member of the U.S. National Team for Long Course Triathlon who was diagnosed with T1DM at age 24 years.

    Jay Hewitt. Hewitt began competing in the triathlon after his diagnosis of diabetes.

33. Name the Supreme Court justice who has T1DM.

    Justice Sonia Sotomayor was diagnosed with T1DM at age 7 years. She went to Princeton University and earned a law degree from Yale. She became the first Hispanic Supreme Court Justice in 2009 and is still serving her country in that capacity.

34. What Major League Baseball player broke the racial barrier in 1947 and became one of the greatest baseball players of all time despite having diabetes mellitus?

    Jackie Robinson became the first African American athlete to play major league baseball when he joined the Brooklyn Dodgers in 1947. He led the league in stolen bases his first year and was the league's Most Valuable Player in 1949. Despite being diagnosed with T2DM while still in his baseball career, he became a Baseball Hall of Fame player and one of the greatest of all time.

35. What was the most likely reason for President Eisenhower's erratic blood pressure?

    President Eisenhower suffered a heart attack in 1955 and died of ischemic cardiomyopathy 14 years later. His autopsy revealed a 1.5 cm pheochromocytoma in the left adrenal gland. The pheochromocytoma was the most likely cause of his erratic blood pressure.

KEY POINTS

- Although T1DM is a serious disease, athletes with this condition have been able to compete and succeed at a professional level in almost every sport.
- The accomplishments of track star Gail Devers emphasize the excellent prognosis of properly treated Graves' disease.
- Perhaps the most fascinating of all endocrine disorders are the disorders of growth. This explains why dwarfs and giants have been so popular as circus performers and movie actors.
- The curability of most thyroid cancers is illustrated by the lives of Rod Stewart and Catherine Bell.
- The high mortality of untreated acromegaly is illustrated by the short lives of wrestler Andre "The Giant" Rousimoff and actor Rondo Hatton.

BIBLIOGRAPHY

D'Arrigo, T. (2007). Hot shot NBA rookie Adam Morrison scores with control. *Diabetes Forecast, 60,* 42–45.
https://dlife.com/famous-with-diabetes-bobby-clarke/
Drimmer, F. (1991). *Very special people.* New York: Carol Publishing Group.
Falcon, M., & Shoop, S. A. (March 20, 2003). Roger Ebert reviews his thyroid cancer (April 5, 2002). *USA Today.* Retrieved from: www.usatoday.com/news/health/spotlight/2002/03/20-ebert.htm.
https://www.iol.co.za/lifestyle/health/celebrities-who-had-diabetes-17349864
http://www.futureofpersonalhealth.com/advocacy/jay-cutler-inspires-children-to-tackle-diabetes
Lerner, B. H. (2006). *When illness goes public.* Baltimore, MD: Johns Hopkins University Press.
Mandernach, M. (1996). Short hitter, long memory. *Sports Illustrated, 2,* 5.
https://www.webmd.com/diabetes/ss/slideshow-celebrities-with-diabetes
Messerli, F., Loughlin, K. R., Messerli, A. W., & Welch, W. R. (2007). The President and the pheochromocytoma. *American Journal of Cardiology, 99*(9), 1325–1329.
Montville, L. Giant. (1995). *Sports Illustrated, 2,* 50–56.
Paulshock, B. Z. (1980). Tutankhamen and his brothers: familial gynecomastia in the Eighteenth Dynasty. *Journal of the American Medical Association,* 244, 160–164.
https://www.verywellhealth.com/celebrity-thyroid-patients-4020422
USA Today (June 21, 2011). Sotomayor opens up about her diabetes. Retrieved from: http://usatoday30.usatoday.com/news/washington/judicial/supremecourtjustices/2011-06-21-sotomayor-diabetes-court_n.htm.
http://www.endocrineweb.com/conditions/thyroid/celebrities-thyroid-disorders.

CHAPTER 72

INTERESTING ENDOCRINE FACTS AND FIGURES

Michael T. McDermott

1. Who is the tallest man on record?

   The man with the greatest medically documented height was Robert Wadlow of Alton, Illinois. He was 8 feet, 11.1 inches (272 cm) tall and weighed 439 lb (199 kg) when he died in 1940 at age 22 years; he was 7 feet, 8 inches (233.6 cm) at age 15 years. His condition was the result of a growth hormone–secreting pituitary tumor that developed before closure of the skeletal epiphyseal plates (gigantism). The tallest currently living man is Sultan Kosen of Turkey, who stands 8 feet, 2 inches (251 cm) tall.

2. Name the tallest woman on record.

   Zeng Jinlian of Hunan Province, China, is the tallest woman on record. She was 8 feet, 1 inch (246 cm) tall just before her death at age 17 years in 1982 and had been 7 feet, 1.5 inches tall at age 13 years. She also had a growth hormone–secreting tumor that had developed during childhood. The tallest currently living woman is Siddiqa Parveen of India, who is 7 feet 8 inches (233.6 cm) tall; it has been estimated that she may be as tall as 8 feet, 2 inches (249 cm), but her height estimates are inexact because she is unable to stand.

3. How tall was the shortest man on record?

   Chandra Bahadur Dangi of Nepal was measured at 21.49 inches (54.6 cm) tall in 2012. The shortest currently living man is Khagendra Thapa Magar of Nepal, whose height was measured at 2 feet, 2.4 inches (67 cm) in 2010.

4. Who is the shortest woman on record?

   The shortest adult woman on record was Pauline Musters of The Netherlands. She was 23.2 inches (≈61 cm) tall and weighed 9 lb shortly before her death at age 19 years in 1895. Because of her relatively normal proportions, she is believed to have had pituitary growth hormone deficiency, although growth hormone assays were clearly not available in 1895. The shortest currently living woman is Jyoti Amge of India, who stood 2 feet, 0.7 inches (62.8 cm) tall at age 18 years in 2011.

5. Who had the most variable adult stature?

   Adam Rainer of Austria was a 3-feet, 10.45-inch (118 cm) dwarf at age 21 years but rapidly grew into a 7-foot, 1.75-inch (218 cm) giant at age 32 years in 1931. He was 7 feet, 8 inches (234 cm) tall when he died in 1950 at age 51 years.

6. Which is the tallest tribe in Africa?

   The Watusi (or Tutsi) tribe of Sudan, Rwanda, Burundi, and Central African Republic are the tallest in the world. The men average 6 feet, 5 inches, and the women average 5 feet, 10 inches. Their tall stature is believed to be a genetic adaptation.

7. Which is the shortest tribe in Africa?

   The Mbuti pygmies of central Africa have the lowest mean height. The men average 4 feet, 6 inches and the women 4 feet, 5 inches. Their short stature is thought to result from genetic resistance to growth hormone, possibly as a result of deficient growth hormone receptors.

8. Who was the heaviest man on record?

   Jon Brower Minnoch of Bainbridge Island, Washington, was 6 feet, 1 inch tall and weighed approximately 1400 lb when he was admitted to the hospital at age 37 years for congestive heart failure. He remained in the hospital for 2 years on a 1200-calorie diet and was discharged at 476 lb; his weight loss of 924 lb is also a record. He weighed 798 lb when he died at age 42 years in 1983. The heaviest currently living man is Juan Pedro Franco Salas of Mexico, whose peak weight was 1311 lb (597.8 kg); he has been diagnosed with type 2 diabetes, hypertension, and a thyroid disorder.

9. How much did the heaviest woman on record weigh?

   The heaviest woman on record was Rosalie Bradford, who weighed 1199 lb (543.9 kg) in 1987. She also holds the record for weight loss, having shed 917 lb over the subsequent 7 years.

10. What is the greatest rate of weight gain ever recorded?

Arthur Knorr of the United States gained 294 lb (134.7 kg) during the last 6 months of his life; this is an average weight gain of 1.6 lb a day. Since a pound of fat has about 3500 kcal, this represents an excess intake (above caloric expenditures) of 5600 kcal a day. Doris James holds the record for women, having gained 328 lb (148.8 kg) in the last year of her life (3150 kcal/day excess) before she died at age 38 years, weighing 675 lb (306.2 kg).

11. What is the largest recorded waist size?

Walter Hudson of New York, who stood 5 feet, 10 inches (177.8 cm) tall, had a peak weight of 1197 lb (543 kg) and a waist size of 119 inches (302 cm).

12. Who are the heaviest twins on record?

Billy McCrary and Benny McCrary of Hendersonville, North Carolina, weighed 743 and 723 pounds (337 and 330 kg), respectively. Both had 84-inch (213 cm) waists. One brother died in a motorcycle accident, but the other is alive at the time of this printing.

13. What is the longest anyone has ever survived without food or water?

Andreas Mihavecz of Austria was put in jail in 1979. The guards forgot about him and gave him no food or water for 18 days, after which he was found still alive, but barely.

14. What is the greatest known number of children born to one woman in a lifetime?

Valentina Vassilyev, a peasant woman from Shuya, east of Moscow, Russia, gave birth to 69 children from 1725 to 1765. She had 27 pregnancies, producing 16 pairs of twins, 7 sets of triplets, and 4 sets of quadruplets. Sixty-seven of the children survived infancy. Her husband had 18 more children with a second wife.

15. Who is the oldest known woman to give birth?

Adriana Emilia Illiescu of Romania gave birth to a daughter by cesarean section in 2005, at age 66 years, 230 days. Donna Maas of California is the oldest woman to give birth to twins, having delivered twin boys by cesarean section in 2004 at age 57 years, 286 days.

16 What is the highest reported number of multiple births for a single gestation?

Ten births (decaplets) were reported in Brazil (1946), China (1936), and Spain (1924). Nine births (nonuplets) were recorded in Australia (1971), Philadelphia (1972), and Bangladesh (1977). The largest number to survive a multiple gestation is seven (septuplets), which has happened on three occasions; the mothers were Bobby McCaughey of Nebraska (1997), Nikem Chukwu of Texas (1998), and Hasna Mohammed Humair of Saudi Arabia (1998).

17. What is the highest single birth weight ever recorded?

In 1879, Anna Bates, living in Seville, Ohio, gave birth to a 23 pound, 12 ounce (10.8 kg) baby boy, who died 11 hours later. Anna was 7 feet, 5.5 inches (227 cm) tall. Carmelina Fedele of Italy gave birth in 1955 to the largest surviving baby, who weighed 22 pounds, 8 ounces (10.2 kg).

18. What is the oldest age to which a human has been documented to live?

Jeanne Louise Calment of Arles, France, lived to be 122 years, 164 days old. She died on August 4, 1997. The oldest man was Shigechiyo Izumi of Japan, who lived to be 120 years, 237 days old and died in 1986.

19. What is the highest blood glucose level ever reported?

A 12-year-old boy with new-onset diabetes mellitus was still conscious when he was discovered to have a blood glucose level of 2350 mg/dL in 1995.

20. What is the record for most kidney stones produced by one individual?

Don Winfield of Canada passed 3711 kidney stones over a 15-year period (1986–2001).

21. What is the largest tumor ever reported?

A 328-lb ovarian cyst was removed from a woman in Texas in 1905.

22. What is the record for the longest hair?

Hoo Sateow of Thailand had his hair measured at 16 feet, 11 inches in 1997. He had not cut his hair for 70 years.

23. What is the record distance walked by an individual in 24 hours?

The record for men is 142.25 miles, by Jesse Castenda of the United States in 1976. The record for women is 131.27 miles by Annie Van der Meer-Timmerman of The Netherlands in 1986. The 24-hour record for an individual in a wheelchair is 77.58 miles by Nik Nikzaban of Canada in 2000.

24. Did King David of Israel have an endocrine disorder?

"When King David was old and advanced in years, though they spread covers over him, he could not keep warm. His servants therefore said to him, 'Let a young virgin be sought to attend you, lord king, and to nurse you. If she sleeps with your royal majesty, you will be kept warm.' … The maiden, who was very beautiful, nursed the king and cared for him, but the king did not have relations with her." (I Kings 1:1–4) Some speculate that King David was afflicted with hypothyroidism.

25. What endocrine disorder might Goliath of Gath have had?

Goliath of Gath, who was killed by a stone from David's sling (I Samuel 17:1–51), probably stood about 6 feet, 10 inches. His tall stature may have resulted from a growth hormone–secreting pituitary tumor. Others add that the ease with which David's stone became embedded in Goliath's skull may have resulted from hyperparathyroidism, and his bizarre behavior may have resulted from hypoglycemia caused by an insulinoma. He may, thus, be the earliest known case of multiple endocrine neoplasia type 1 syndrome.

26. What endocrine disorder did President John F. Kennedy have?

John Kennedy, the 35th president of the United States (1961–1963), had primary adrenal insufficiency—Addison's disease. This was believed to have developed when he was a Navy PT boat captain in the South Pacific during World War II. He was sustained throughout his adult life and his presidency through therapy with oral glucocorticoids.

27. What US President had a pheochromocytoma?

Dwight D. Eisenhower, the 34th president of the United States (1953–1961), had an acute myocardial infarction in 1955 while playing golf at Fitzsimmons Army Medical Center in Aurora, Colorado, the current site of the University of Colorado Denver School of Medicine and University of Colorado Hospital. Eisenhower died 14 years later of an ischemic cardiomyopathy. At autopsy, a 1.5-cm pheochromocytoma was discovered. It is not known if this tumor was ever symptomatic.

 WEBSITE

http://www.guinnessworldrecords.com

BIBLIOGRAPHY

Baumann, G., Shaw, M. N., & Merimee, T. J. (1989). Low levels of high affinity growth hormone-binding protein in African Pygmies. *New England Journal of Medicine, 320*, 1705–1709.

Farlan, D. (Ed.). (1991). *The Guinness book of world records 1991*. New York: Bantam Books.

Folkard, C. (Ed.). (2003). *The Guinness book of world records 2003*. New York: Bantam Books.

Glenday, C. (Ed.). (2007). *The Guinness book of world records 2007*. New York: Bantam Books.

Padgett, J., Allman, M., & Mansfield, D. (Eds.). (2018). *The Guinness book of world records 2018*. San Diego: Portable Press.

Messerli, F. H., Loughlin, K. R., Messerli, A. W., & Welch, W. R. (2007). The President and the pheochromocytoma. *American Journal of Cardiology, 99*, 1325–1329.

Catholic Publishers. (1971). *The New American Bible*. Camden, NJ: Thomas Nelson, Inc.

CHAPTER 73

ENDOCRINE CASE STUDIES

Michael T. McDermott

1. A 34-year-old woman has new-onset hypertension. Initial blood pressure (BP) was 158/98 mm Hg. Her serum potassium level is 2.7 mEq/L. Initial hormone screening shows a plasma aldosterone (PA) of 55 ng/dL (normal [nl] 1–16) and a plasma renin activity (PRA) of 0.1 ng/mL/hr (nl 0.15–2.33). What is the probable diagnosis, and what is the next step?

   Primary aldosteronism (Conn's syndrome) is strongly suggested by the presence of hypertension and spontaneous hypokalemia. Initial screening confirms this by finding a significantly elevated PA, a suppressed PRA, and a high PA/PRA ratio. Confirmatory testing with a saline infusion or oral salt-loading test to assess suppressibility of PA is often the recommended next step. However, the 2016 Endocrine Society Guideline Committee on Primary Aldosteronism recommended that confirmatory testing is not needed when all three of the following—spontaneous hypokalemia, suppressed PRA, and PA > 20 ng/dL—are present because nothing else really causes this group of results. The next step, therefore, is to establish whether the cause is an aldosterone-producing adenoma or bilateral adrenal hyperplasia; abdominal computed tomography (CT) should be ordered. Her abdominal CT scan showed a 2-cm left adrenal cortical adenoma with < 10 Hounsfield Units (HU). Adrenal vein sampling (AVS) may be needed at this point if an accurate diagnosis is not apparent, but the 2016 guidelines also recommend that AVS is not needed if all three of the following are present: age < 35 years, PA markedly elevated, unilateral cortical adenoma on imaging study. This patient also meets these criteria. The treatment for this aldosterone-producing adrenal adenoma is surgery. Spironolactone and or eplerenone should be given to control BP and to normalize the serum potassium preoperatively (see Chapter 32).

2. A 32-year-old business executive develops amenorrhea. She has not recently lost weight but states that her job is very stressful. Evaluation reveals the following laboratory results: serum estradiol = 14 pg/mL (nl 23–145); luteinizing hormone (LH) = 1.2 mIU/mL (nl 2–15); follicle-stimulating hormone (FSH) = 1.5 mIU/mL (nl 2–20); prolactin = 6.2 ng/mL (nl 2–25); thyroid-stimulating hormone (TSH) = 1.2 mU/L (nl 0.5–5.0); and negative result on serum pregnancy test. Magnetic resonance imaging (MRI) of her pituitary gland shows normal results. What is the probable diagnosis, and what is the best management approach?

   This patient has secondary amenorrhea with low estradiol and gonadotropin levels. These results are most consistent with hypothalamic amenorrhea, which may occur in women who exercise excessively, have very low body weight, or have stressful jobs. The disorder results from reduced gonadotropin-releasing hormone (GnRH) pulse frequency in the hypothalamus. Treatment consists of stress management and, if menses do not resume, estrogen replacement therapy (see Chapter 53).

3. A nulliparous 48-year-old woman presents with symptoms of thyrotoxicosis. She has a modest, nontender goiter and no exophthalmos. She takes no medications or supplements and has had no recent radiology procedures. The following results are found on thyroid evaluation: TSH < 0.1 mU/L; free thyroxine (T_4) = 3.5 ng/dL (nl 0.8–1.8); thyroglobulin = 35 ng/mL (nl 2–20); erythrocyte sedimentation rate (ESR) = 10 mm/hr; and 24-hour radioactive iodine uptake (RAIU) = 1% (nl 20%–35%). What is the likely diagnosis, and what are your management recommendations?

   This 48-year old woman has clinical and biochemical thyrotoxicosis with a low RAIU. The differential diagnosis includes postpartum thyroiditis, silent thyroiditis, subacute thyroiditis, factitious thyrotoxicosis, and iodine-induced thyrotoxicosis. She has never been pregnant and denies medication use and recent iodine exposure. The nontender gland, elevated thyroglobulin, and normal ESR are most consistent with silent thyroiditis. A transient (1–3 months) thyrotoxic phase followed by a transient (2–6 months) hypothyroid phase is expected before the condition resolves; 20% of patients, however, remain hypothyroid. If symptomatic, the thyrotoxic phase is best treated with beta-blockers, and the hypothyroid phase can be managed, if necessary, with temporary levothyroxine replacement (see Chapters 39 and 41).

4. A 38-year-old man has coronary artery disease, xanthomas of the Achilles tendons, and serum lipid profile as follows: cholesterol = 482 mg/dL; triglycerides (TG) = 125 mg/dL; high-density lipoprotein (HDL) cholesterol = 42 mg/dL; and low-density lipoprotein (LDL) cholesterol = 415 mg/dL. What is the probable diagnosis, and what are the management options?

   Significant elevations of total cholesterol and LDL cholesterol, normal TG, tendon xanthomas, and premature coronary artery disease are most consistent with a diagnosis of heterozygous familial hypercholesterolemia. Genetic mutations resulting in deficient or dysfunctional LDL receptors (LDLRs) are the most common cause. Less common monogenic hypercholesterolemia disorders include apolipoprotein B (apo-B) mutations that produce a defective apo-B that cannot bind to LDLRs, proprotein convertase subtilisin-like kexin type 9 (PCSK9) mutations that cause accelerated LDLR degradation, LDLR adaptor protein 1 mutations that prevent normal clustering of LDLR in cell surface clathrin-coated pits, and adenosine triphosphate (ATP)–binding cassette G5 or G8 (ABCG5/8) mutations that cause abnormal cellular transport of cholesterol and plant sterols (sitosterolemia).

The recommended criteria for diagnosing heterozygous familial hypercholesterolemia are the following: LDL > 190 mg/dL (adults) or > 160 mg/dL (children) *plus* premature coronary artery disease, or history of a similarly affected first-degree relative, or the identification of a genetic defect. Aggressive lipid lowering with a combination of statins and PCSK9 inhibitors is often required for satisfactory LDL control; ezetimibe and bile acid resins may be added, if needed. In many cases, LDL apheresis is also indicated (see Chapter 10).

5. A 28-year-old man presents with complaints of infertility. He is found to have small, firm testes and gynecomastia. Laboratory testing shows the following abnormalities: testosterone = 171 ng/dL (nl 300–1000); LH = 88 mIU/mL (nl 2–12); and FSH = 95 mIU/mL (nl 2–12). What is the likely diagnosis, and what is the recommended treatment?
   The patient has hypergonadotropic hypogonadism. The small, firm testes and gynecomastia are most consistent with a diagnosis of Klinefelter's syndrome. These patients usually have a 47XXY karyotype, but mosaic patterns are also common. Androgen replacement therapy is the treatment of choice (see Chapter 50).

6. A 38-year-old nurse presents in a stuporous state; the blood glucose level is 14 mg/dL. Additional blood is drawn, and the patient is quickly resuscitated with intravenous (IV) glucose. Further testing on the saved serum reveals the following: serum insulin = 45 mcU/mL (nl < 22); C-peptide = 4.2 ng/mL (nl 0.5–2.0); and proinsulin = 7 pmol/L (nl < 5). A sulfonylurea screen yields negative results. What is the probable diagnosis, and what are the next steps in management?
   The patient has hyperinsulinemic hypoglycemia. The differential diagnosis includes insulinoma, surreptitious insulin injection, and oral sulfonylurea ingestion. The elevated serum C-peptide and proinsulin levels are most consistent with an insulinoma. After an appropriate localizing procedure, surgical removal·is the treatment of choice (see Chapters 9 and 61).

7. A 28-year-old woman presents with amenorrhea. Her menses started at age 13 years and have been regular since age 16 years. She has type 1 diabetes mellitus (T1DM). Further tests show the following: estradiol = 15 pg/mL (nl 23–145); LH = 78 mIU/mL (nl 2–15); FSH = 92 mIU/mL (nl 2–20); prolactin = 12 ng/mL (nl 2–25); TSH = 1.1 mU/L; the pregnancy test yields negative results. What is the most likely diagnosis, and how would you treat her?
   The patient has secondary amenorrhea, with very low estradiol and elevated gonadotropin levels. In a patient with another autoimmune disease (T1DM), the most likely diagnosis is premature ovarian insufficiency (POI) caused by autoimmune ovarian destruction. Hormone replacement therapy is the treatment of choice (see Chapter 53).

8. A 34-year-old woman presents with a milky breast discharge, amenorrhea, headaches, fatigue, and weight gain. Laboratory evaluation reveals the following: prolactin = 58 ng/mL (nl 2–25); free T_4 = 0.2 ng/dL (nl 0.8–1.8); and TSH > 60 mU/L (nl 0.5–5.0). The pituitary gland is observed to be enlarged on MRI. What is the cause of her elevated prolactin, and what is the most appropriate treatment?
   The patient has moderately increased serum prolactin levels, pituitary enlargement, and severe primary hypothyroidism. Her entire clinical picture is most likely explained solely by the hypothyroidism, which is well known to cause secondary hypersecretion of prolactin and pituitary enlargement resulting from thyrotroph hyperplasia. All abnormalities should resolve after adequate thyroid hormone replacement is established (see Chapters 25 and 40).

9. A 6-year-old girl has developed breast enlargement and some pubic hair. She has not complained of headaches and has had good health otherwise. Her older sister entered puberty at approximately age 8 years. Her height is at the 90th percentile for her age, and her physical examination reveals Tanner's stage III breast development and stage II pubic hair growth. Abdominal and pelvic examinations are normal. Laboratory tests show the following results: LH = 7 mIU/mL (nl 2–15); FSH = 8 mIU/mL (nl 2–20); prolactin = 6 ng/mL (nl 2–25); TSH = 1.9 mU/L (nl 0.5–5.0); and a normal result on pituitary MRI. Her bone age is 1.8 years ahead of the chronologic age. What is the probable diagnosis, and what is the most appropriate management?
   This patient has gonadotropin-dependent true precocious puberty. The etiology includes pituitary and hypothalamic tumors, but in most cases in girls, the condition is idiopathic. The normal pituitary MRI result points to a diagnosis of idiopathic precocious puberty. A long-acting GnRH analogue should successfully arrest her premature development and allow her to enter puberty at a later, more appropriate time (see Chapter 49).

10. A 19-year-old man presents with excessive thirst and urination. Laboratory evaluation shows the following: serum glucose = 88 mg/dL; sodium = 146 mmol/L; osmolality = 298 mOsm/kg; and urine volume = 8800 mL/24 hr. A water deprivation test is performed: it shows a urine osmolality of 90 mOsm/kg, with no response to water deprivation, and an increase in urine osmolality to 180 mOsm/kg after the administration of vasopressin. What is the likely diagnosis, and what are your treatment recommendations?
    The differential diagnosis of polyuria and polydipsia with maximally dilute urine includes central diabetes insipidus, nephrogenic diabetes insipidus, and primary polydipsia. The lack of response to water deprivation and the > 50%

increase in urine osmolality after administration of vasopressin are most consistent with central diabetes insipidus. This may be caused by inflammatory or mass lesions in the hypothalamus but is often idiopathic. MRI of the pituitary–hypothalamic region should be performed. The treatment of choice is intranasal or oral desmopressin (see Chapters 22 and 29).

11. A 45-year-old man has a 4-year history of worsening hypertension, which has not yet been controlled with three antihypertensive medications. Serum potassium had been 3.7 mEq/L when his hypertension was first discovered. There is no family history of hypertension. His medications include the following: lisinopril 40 mg daily; amlodipine 10 mg daily; and hydrochlorothiazide (HCTZ) 25 mg daily. His vitals are as follows: BP 165/95 mm Hg and pulse 72 beats per minute. Physical examination results are normal. Recent laboratory values are as follows: sodium (Na) 144 mEq/L; potassium (K) 2.5 mEq/L; and creatinine 1.1 mg/dL. Morning, seated PA was 24 ng/dL (nl 1–21), and PRA was < 0.6 ng/mL/hr (nl 0.6–4.3). PA after a 2-L saline infusion was 21 ng/dL. What do you recommend next for evaluation and subsequent treatment?

    Primary aldosteronism (Conn's syndrome) is strongly suggested by the presence of resistant hypertension (uncontrolled on a three-drug regimen that includes a thiazide diuretic) and easily induced (thiazide diuretic) hypokalemia. Initial screening confirms this through the following findings: significantly elevated PA, suppressed PRA, and a high PA/PRA ratio. Confirmatory testing with a saline infusion (or oral salt-loading test) to assess suppressibility of PA was indicated according to the 2016 Endocrine Society Guideline Committee on Primary Aldosteronism (confirmatory testing is not needed when all three of the following are present: spontaneous hypokalemia, suppressed PRA and PA > 20 ng/dL); this patient had easily induced but not spontaneous hypokalemia. The next step, therefore, is to establish whether the cause is an aldosterone-producing adenoma or bilateral adrenal hyperplasia with an abdominal CT scan; abdominal CT showed bilateral but asymmetrical adrenal enlargement with the left side being significantly larger than the right.

    The next step should be AVS because he does not meet the criteria for not needing AVS (all three of the following must be present: age < 35 years, PA markedly elevated, and unilateral cortical adenoma on imaging study). AVS did not show significant lateralization, indicating that the most likely underlying disorder in this patient is bilateral adrenal hyperplasia (idiopathic hyperaldosteronism). The management for this condition is the use of an aldosterone receptor antagonist (spironolactone with or without eplerenone) and the use of other antihypertensive medications, as needed, to adequately control his BP. Aldosterone receptor antagonist therapy should be titrated until the serum potassium is normal without a need for potassium supplements and PRA is in the upper end of the reference range (see Chapter 32).

12. A 25-year-old woman presents with a rounded face, prominent supraclavicular adiposity, and purplish striae in the axillae. The results of hormone testing are as follows: 24-hour urine cortisol = 318 mcg (nl 10–50); after 1 mg of dexamethasone at bedtime, morning serum cortisol = 28 mcg/dL (nl 5–25); and baseline morning plasma adrenocorticotropic hormone (ACTH) = 65 pg/mL (nl 10–80). After an 8-mg oral bedtime dose of dexamethasone, the morning serum cortisol is 3 mcg/dL. What is the probable diagnosis, and what are the next steps for evaluation and management?

    Cushingoid features and significantly elevated urinary cortisol excretion confirm the diagnosis of Cushing's syndrome. Endogenous Cushing's syndrome is most often caused by ACTH-secreting pituitary adenomas (65%–80%), ectopic ACTH production by nonpituitary tumors (10%–15%), and cortisol-producing adrenal adenomas (10%–15%). The normal plasma ACTH level, which is inappropriate for the elevated serum cortisol level, and serum cortisol suppression with high-dose dexamethasone are most consistent with a pituitary adenoma (Cushing's disease). This should be confirmed with MRI of the pituitary gland and, unless a pituitary adenoma ≥ 7 mm in size is identified, inferior petrosal sinus sampling should follow. Transsphenoidal surgical removal is the treatment of choice. When surgery does not result in remission, treatment options include repeat surgery, radiation therapy, and medical therapy with ketoconazole, metyrapone, or pasireotide to reduce cortisol production or mifepristone to block cortisol tissue action (see Chapter 27).

13. An 8-year-old boy with known adrenal insufficiency complains of frequent muscle cramps and paresthesias of the lips, hands, and feet. He has positive Chvostek's and Trousseau's signs on examination. Results of blood testing are as follows: calcium (Ca) = 6.2 mg/dL (nl 8.5–10.2); phosphorus (P) = 5.8 mg/dL (nl 2.5–4.5); intact parathyroid hormone (PTH) = 3 pg/mL (nl 10–65); and 25-hydroxy vitamin D = 42 ng/mL (nl 30–100). What is the most likely diagnosis, and what is the best treatment approach?

    Hypocalcemia, hyperphosphatemia, and a low serum PTH level are diagnostic of primary hypoparathyroidism. This disorder, which is often autoimmune in nature, may occur in association with adrenal insufficiency as part of the autoimmune polyendocrine syndrome type I (APS I). Hypoparathyroidism must be treated with both Ca and calcitriol supplementation. Calcitriol is necessary because PTH, the missing hormone, is necessary for normal renal conversion of 25-hydroxy vitamin D into 1,25-dihydroxy vitamin D, the active vitamin D metabolite that is necessary for normal intestinal Ca and P absorption. A thiazide diuretic is also often helpful to further increase serum Ca and to reduce treatment-induced hypercalciuria. For patients with persistent hypocalcemia, hyperphosphatemia, or hypercalciuria despite these measures, treatment with recombinant human PTH 1–84 (Natpara) is available (see Chapters 20 and 59).

14. A 52-year-old man has a personal and family history of early coronary artery disease, minimal alcohol consumption, and no xanthomas on examination. He has the following results on serum testing: cholesterol = 328 mg/dL; TG = 322 mg/dL; HDL = 35 mg/dL; LDL = 229 mg/dL; apo-B = 178 mg/dL (nl 60–130), apo-E phenotype = E3/E3; TSH = 2.1 mU/L (nl 0.1–4.5); and glucose = 85 mg/dL. What is the probable diagnosis, and what are the treatment options?

    This patient has elevations of both serum cholesterol and TG and no detected disorders that cause secondary dyslipidemia. The differential diagnosis is familial combined hyperlipidemia and familial dysbetalipoproteinemia. The elevated apo-B level and the normal apo-E phenotype are most consistent with familial combined hyperlipidemia; an E2/E2 apo-B phenotype is characteristic of familial dysbetalipoproteinemia. The top treatment priority is LDL reduction with use of a statin. After the LDL cholesterol level is brought to the individualized-goal level, persistent TG elevations can be addressed with further dietary medication and weight loss and the possible addition of a fibrate, niacin, or fish oils (see Chapter 10).

15. A 58-year-old man reports recently developed diabetes mellitus, weight loss, and a skin rash that is most prominent on the buttocks; a dermatologist suspects this to be necrolytic migratory erythema and performs biopsy and histopathologic analysis to confirm this. What is the probable underlying diagnosis, and what are the therapeutic options?

    Diabetes mellitus, weight loss, and necrolytic migratory erythema are virtually diagnostic of a glucagon-secreting pancreatic neuroendocrine tumor (glucagonoma). The diagnosis can be confirmed with the finding of a significantly elevated serum glucagon level. After appropriate localizing procedures, treatment options include surgery for localized disease, somatostatin analogues (octreotide LAR, lanreotide) to reduce glucagon secretion, hepatic-directed therapies (partial resection, hepatic artery embolization), chemotherapy (streptozotocin/doxorubicin), everolimus (an inhibitor of mTOR [mechanistic target of rapamycin]), sunitinib, and other vascular endothelial growth factor receptor (VEGF-R) inhibitors, and peptide receptor radioligand therapy with use of radiolabeled somatostatin analogues, such as 177-Lu DOTATATE, 90-Y edotreotide, or 90-Y DOTA tyr3-octreotide. Chronic anti-coagulation to reduce the increased risk of thromboembolic events and supplementation with zinc and amino acid infusions to reduce the skin rash and improve quality of life should also be considered (see Chapter 61).

16. A 29-year-old woman has asymptomatic hypercalcemia. Her mother and one of her sisters also have hypercalcemia and have had failed neck explorations for presumed parathyroid tumors. Further testing results are as follows: serum Ca = 11 mg/dL (nl 8.5–10.2); P = 3 mg/dL (nl 2.4–4.5); creatinine = 0.9 mg/dL; intact PTH = 66 pg/mL (nl 10–65); 25-hydroxyvitamin D = 42 ng/mL (nl 30–100); 24-hour urine Ca = 13 mg (nl 100–300); and creatinine = 1100 mg. What is the probable diagnosis, and what is the recommended management?

    The vast majority of patients with hypercalcemia and a mildly elevated serum PTH level have primary hyperpara-thyroidism. However, in this case, the very low urinary calcium excretion and family history of unsuccessful para-thyroid surgeries point to a suspected diagnosis of familial hypocalciuric hypercalcemia (FHH). The diagnosis is confirmed by finding a Ca/creatinine clearance ratio (urine Ca × serum creatinine/serum calcium × urine creatinine) of < 0.01. This autosomal dominant disorder results from heterozygous inactivating mutations of the calcium sensor receptor gene. The mutant sensor receptors, present in parathyroid and renal tubular cells, have a raised threshold for calcium recognition. The result is a raised physiologic equilibrium, in which hypercalcemia coexists with mild elevations of PTH and low urinary calcium excretion. The disorder causes no morbidity and does not require treatment (see Chapters 17 and 18).

17. A 39-year-old human immunodeficiency virus (HIV)–positive man with *Pneumocystis jiroveci* pneumonia (PJP) has the following serum thyroid hormone values: free T_4 = 0.8 ng/dL (nl 0.8–1.8); total T_3 = 22 ng/dL (nl 90–200); TSH = 0.5 mU/L (nl 0.5–5.0); and T_3 resin uptake = 48% (nl 35%–45%). What is the most likely endocrine diagnosis, and what is the best management approach?

    The very low T_3, low-normal free T_4, low-normal TSH, and elevated T_3 resin uptake are most consistent with the euthyroid sick syndrome (nonthyroidal illness syndrome). This is not a primary thyroid disorder but is, instead, a set of circulating thyroid hormone abnormalities that occur in the presence of nonthyroidal illnesses; it is corrected when the underlying illness resolves. Treatment of the condition with thyroid hormone administration is not currently recommended, although this remains controversial (see Chapter 45).

18. An 18-year-old female has not yet begun menstruating. She has a height of 56 inches, a small uterus, and no breast development. The results of hormone tests are as follows: estradiol = 8 pg/mL (nl 23–145); LH = 105 mIU/mL (nl 2–15); FSH = 120 mIU/mL (nl 2–20); prolactin = 14 ng/mL (nl 2–15); and TSH = 1.8 mU/L (nl 0.5–5.0). What is the probable diagnosis, and what are the management options?

    Primary amenorrhea, short stature, low serum estradiol, and elevated gonadotropins are most consistent with a diagnosis of Turner's syndrome. This disorder, characterized by ovarian dysgenesis, is associated with a 45XO karyotype. These patients should be given hormone replacement therapy with estrogen and progesterone. Growth hormone (GH) therapy should be considered because it improves longitudinal growth and final height (see Chapter 49 and 53).

19. A 62-year-old woman presents for evaluation of recent nephrolithiasis and low back pain. Her estimated calcium intake is 800 mg/day, and she takes no vitamins. Her physical examination is unremarkable. Spinal radiography shows a compression fracture of the second lumbar vertebra (L2). Laboratory evaluation shows the following: serum Ca = 13.0 mg/dL (nl 8.5–10.5); P = 2.3 mg/dL (nl 2.5–4.5); albumin = 4.4 g/dL (nl 3.2–5.5); intact PTH = 72 pg/mL (nl 11–54); and 24-hour urine Ca = 312 mg (nl 100–300). What is the most likely diagnosis? Hypercalcemia, hypophosphatemia, and elevated serum PTH levels are characteristic of primary hyperparathyroidism. Hyperparathyroidism is usually caused by a solitary parathyroid adenoma, but familial cases and those associated with multiple endocrine neoplasia (MEN) syndromes more often have four-gland hyperplasia. Surgical indications include serum calcium levels > 1 mg/dL above the normal range, urinary calcium excretion > 400 mg/24 hr, renal impairment, osteoporosis, age < 50 years, or symptoms related to hyperparathyroidism. Observation alone or bisphosphonate therapy may be appropriate for patients with mild, asymptomatic disease or only mild bone loss. This patient should be referred for parathyroid surgery (see Chapters 18 and 60).

20. A 32-year-old woman presents with recent-onset fatigue, palpitations, profuse sweating, and emotional lability. She gave birth to her second child 8 weeks ago. Her pulse is 100 beats per minute, and she has mild lid retraction, a fine hand tremor, and a slightly enlarged, nontender thyroid gland. She is not breast feeding her child. Laboratory tests are as follows: TSH < 0.03 mU/L (nl 0.5–5.0); free T_4 = 3.8 ng/dL (nl 0.8–1.8); and RAIU < 1% at 4 and 24 hours. What is the probable diagnosis, and what treatment do you recommend for her? Postpartum thyrotoxicosis is most often caused by Graves' disease or postpartum thyroiditis. RAIU will distinguish the two, being high in Graves' disease and low in postpartum thyroiditis. RAIU is contraindicated in patients who are breast feeding; in those cases, measurement of TSH receptor antibodies (TRAbs) is often useful, being positive in Graves' disease and negative in postpartum thyroiditis. This patient has postpartum thyroiditis, a condition caused by lymphocytic inflammation with leakage of thyroid hormone from the inflamed gland. There is often a thyrotoxic phase (lasting 1–3 months) followed by a hypothyroid phase (lasting 2–6 months) and eventual return to euthyroidism, although nearly 20% of patients remain permanently hypothyroid. Treatment consists of beta-blockers, if necessary, for symptom control in the thyrotoxic phase, and levothyroxine, if necessary, for symptom control in the hypothyroid phase and for those who remain permanently hypothyroid (see Chapters 39 and 41).

21. A 70-year-old man presents complaining of a 1-year history of weakness, weight loss, and hand tremors. He has been treated with amiodarone for nearly 3 years for paroxysmal atrial flutter. Laboratory tests show the following: TSH < 0.01 mU/L (nl 0.5–5.0); free T_4 = 3.35 ng/dL (nl 0.8–1.8); and the RAIU was 2.7% at 6 hours and 4.1% at 24 hours. Thyroid scan showed patchy tracer uptake. Color doppler shows increased blood flow. What is the likely diagnosis, and what is the best treatment plan? This man has amiodarone-induced thyrotoxicosis (AIT). The condition occurs in up to 10% of patients using amiodarone, which has a very high iodine content. There are two subtypes: type 1 AIT results from iodine overload, and type 2 AIT results from amiodarone-induced thyroid follicular damage (thyroiditis). It can be very difficult to determine which type is present in a patient, and in fact, there can be mixed cases with features of both types. AIT type 1 usually occurs in patients with underlying goiters or nodules; RAIU is low but may be detectable and color Doppler studies show increased flow. AIT type 2 is more often seen in patients without underlying goiters or nodules; RAIU is very low (often < 1%), and color Doppler studies show decreased flow. Serum interleukin-6, when available, is often elevated in type 2 AIT. Type 1 AIT is best treated with methimazole, although lithium and perchlorate (when available) may also add benefit, whereas type 2 AIT responds better to steroid therapy. Mixed or refractory cases may require both methimazole and steroids, plasmapheresis, or thyroidectomy (see Chapters 39 and 41).

22. A 20-year-old man presents with failure to enter puberty. He has small, soft testes, no gynecomastia, normal visual fields, and decreased sense of smell. Laboratory evaluation is as follows: serum testosterone = 40 ng/dL (nl 300–900); LH = 2.0 mIU/mL (nl 2–12); FSH = 1.6 mIU/mL (nl 2–12); prolactin = 7 ng/mL (nl 2–20); and TSH = 0.9 mU/L (nl 0.5–5.0). MRI of the pituitary gland shows normal results. What is the probable diagnosis, and what is the recommended treatment? This picture is most consistent with idiopathic hypogonadotropic hypogonadism (IHH), also known as *Kallmann's syndrome* when it is accompanied by anosmia. The disorder is caused by deficiency of GnRH and may be X-linked, autosomal dominant, autosomal recessive, or sporadic. The X-linked form results most commonly from mutations of the *Kal-1* gene, which encodes anosmin, a neural cell adhesion protein that is critical for the scaffolding for GnRH neuron migration from the olfactory placode to the hypothalamus during embryonic development. In addition to GnRH deficiency, this mutation causes maldevelopment of the olfactory lobe, resulting in anosmia. Mutations in fibroblast growth factor 8 (FGF8) or its receptor, FGFR1, or in the Kisspeptin/KissR system have also been found to underlie some cases of IHH. Androgen therapy is indicated to promote appropriate masculinization. When desired, these patients can also become fertile by receiving treatment with GnRH or gonadotropin preparations (see Chapters 49 and 50).

23. A 40-year old man is brought to the emergency department with sudden onset of inability to stand. He endorses recent muscle aches and weakness. His past medical history and family history are negative. He is a

naturalized citizen originally from Korea. He takes no medications. His vitals are as follows: BP = 124/68 mm Hg, P = 88; height = 5 feet 6 inches; weight 142 lb. Physical examination findings are as follows: bilateral flaccid leg weakness (0/5); bilateral proximal arm weakness (3/5); reduced reflexes; thyroid: diffuse goiter; eyes: lid lag, no proptosis. Laboratory testing results are as follows: TSH < 0.01 mU/L (nl 0.45–4.5); free T_4 2.52 ng/dL (nl 0.8–1.8). What is his likely diagnosis, and what do you recommend next?

This patient was suspected of having thyrotoxic periodic paralysis (TPP). Serum potassium drawn during the episode was 2.1 mEq/L, confirming the diagnosis. TPP is a potentially fatal complication of hyperthyroidism that occurs as a sporadic (noninherited) disorder predominantly in Asian males. Episodes of mild-to-severe muscle weakness or paralysis associated with severe hypokalemia result from sudden intracellular shifts of potassium caused by thyrotoxicosis-induced increased sensitivity of Na-K-ATPase (adenosine triphosphatase) pump activity. TPP attacks are treated acutely with potassium supplementation (oral or IV) and can be prevented by successful treatment of the hyperthyroidism.

24. A 32-year-old man presents with complaints of impotence and intermittent retroorbital headaches for the past year. He is adopted and does not know his natural family history. He has bitemporal visual field loss, but his examination is otherwise normal. Laboratory tests reveal the following: serum calcium = 11.8 mg/dL (nl 8.5–10.5); P = 2.5 mg/dL (nl 2.5–4.5); albumin = 4.8 g/dL (nl 3.2–5.5); intact PTH = 58 pg/mL (nl 11–54); prolactin = 2650 ng/mL (nl 0–20); testosterone 72 ng/dL; LH 2.1 mIU/mL (nl 2–12); and FSH = 1.1 mIU/mL (nl 2–12). What is the likely diagnosis, and how should this be further evaluated?

This patient has a prolactinoma, manifesting as impotence, headaches, bitemporal hemianopsia, secondary hypogonadism, and a significantly elevated serum prolactin level. Hypercalcemia with an elevated serum PTH level indicates that he also has hyperparathyroidism. MEN 1 syndrome, which consists of hyperparathyroidism, pituitary tumors, and pancreatic endocrine tumors, results from an inherited mutation in the *Menin* gene. This patient should be screened for a gastrinoma by ordering a fasting serum gastrin and for insulinoma by measuring serum glucose, insulin, C-peptide, proinsulin, and beta-hydroxybutyrate after an overnight fast or during a prolonged supervised fast. After pituitary imaging studies, he should be treated with a dopamine agonist, transsphenoidal surgery, or both, and subsequently with parathyroid surgery (see Chapters 25 and 60).

25. A 45-year old man presented to his primary care provider with progressive dyspnea on exertion. Laboratory testing revealed hypercalcemia, prompting a referral to you. Past medical history: hepatitis C. Medications: interferon, ribavirin. Dietary Ca: 600 mg/day. He takes no supplements. He smokes half a pack of cigarettes per day and drinks one to two beers per day. Physical examination results are normal except for diffuse rales in all lung fields. Laboratory testing results are as follows: Ca = 12.4 mg/dL; creatinine = 1.2 mg/dL; carbon dioxide (CO_2) = 23 mEq/L; and P = 5.9 mg/dL. Additional laboratory examinations yielded these results: PTH < 1 pg/mL; PTH-related peptide (PTHrp) < 1 pmol/L; 25-hydroxy vitamin D = 34 ng/mL (nl 30–100); 1,25-dihydroxy vitamin D 186 pg/mL (nl 15–75). What is the most likely cause of his hypercalcemia and what treatment options are available?

Chest radiography showed hilar adenopathy and diffuse interstitial disease; biopsy revealed noncaseating granulomas, consistent with sarcoidosis. Hypercalcemia associated with low serum PTH levels and high 1,25-dihydroxy vitamin D levels is most often caused by granulomatous disorders or lymphomas. In these cases, the granulomatous tissue or lymphoma expresses high levels of 1-alpha-hydroxylase that converts circulating 25-hydroxy vitamin D into 1,25-dihydroxy vitamin D in high concentrations, resulting in 1,25-dihydroxy vitamin D–mediated hypercalcemia. The most common cause of 1,25-dihydroxy vitamin D–mediated hypercalcemia is sarcoidosis (~50% of cases), followed by lymphoma (~17%), granulomatous infections (~8%), other granulomatous diseases (~4%), and idiopathic cases (~3%). Treatment for the hypercalcemia consists of hydration and glucocorticoids; if these measures do not reduce serum calcium sufficiently, ketoconazole or hydroxychloroquine can be added (see Chapters 17 and 19).

26. A 52-year-old woman complains of a 1-year history of progressive fatigue, puffy eyes, dry skin, and mild weight gain. She had acromegaly treated with transsphenoidal surgery and radiation therapy 10 years ago. Physical examination showed normal visual fields, mild periorbital edema, and dry skin. Laboratory testing revealed the following: GH = 1.2 ng/mL (nl < 2.0); insulin-like growth factor-1 (IGF-1) = 258 ng/mL (nl 182–780); TSH = 0.2 mU/L (nl 0.5–5.0); and free T_4 = 0.3 ng/dL (nl 0.8–1.8). What is the most likely cause of this patient's symptoms, and what treatment do you recommend?

She has central hypothyroidism caused by pituitary damage from the combined effects of surgery and radiation treatment of her pituitary tumor 10 years earlier. Such a lengthy delay in the development of this condition is not uncommon. The most common conditions that cause central hypothyroidism are tumors, surgery, radiation, hemorrhage, infections, infiltrative disorders, and trauma affecting the hypothalamus or pituitary gland. Medications that have been shown to suppress thyroid-releasing hormone (TRH) or TSH production include opioids, glucocorticoids, mitotane, and bexarotene; use of these medications may cause central hypothyroidism. Metformin has also been reported to suppress TSH secretion and may interfere with thyroid test interpretation but, as yet, has not been implicated in causing de novo central hypothyroidism.

The diagnosis of central hypothyroidism is based on the presence of symptoms of thyroid hormone deficiency, a low serum free T_4, and a low or low-normal serum TSH. Treatment consists of levothyroxine replacement in doses sufficient to relieve symptoms and to maintain the serum free T_4 level in the mid-normal or upper-normal range. Because TSH secretion is impaired, the serum TSH level cannot be used to monitor this patient's response to therapy. Assessment of her pituitary–adrenal axis with a cosyntropin stimulation test and plasma ACTH level is also indicated (see Chapters 22 and 40).

27. A 32-year-old woman complains of deep pain in both thighs. She was diagnosed as having type 1 diabetes mellitus at age 20 years. She currently has two to three bowel movements each day. Her menses are regular. Her diet is well balanced, with adequate calcium intake, and she takes a multivitamin. Physical examination results are normal. Laboratory studies show the following: serum Ca = 8.2 mg/dL (nl 8.5–10.5); P = 2.3 mg/dL (nl 2.5–4.5); alkaline phosphatase = 312 U/L (nl 25–125); PTH = 155 pg/mL (nl 11–54); and 25-hydroxy vitamin D = 7 ng/mL (nl 30–100). Explain the findings in this patient, and suggest a probable underlying diagnosis and treatment plan.

    Her biochemical profile of hypocalcemia, hypophosphatemia, elevated alkaline phosphatase, and significant secondary hyperparathyroidism suggests vitamin D deficiency, which is confirmed by the low serum 25-hydroxy vitamin D level. The elevated serum alkaline phosphatase suggests that the vitamin D deficiency has been sufficiently severe and prolonged to result in osteomalacia. Lactose intolerance can cause chronic diarrhea but seldom results in vitamin D and calcium malabsorption. Celiac disease (gluten-sensitive enteropathy), which occurs with increased frequency in patients with T1DM, should be suspected. The diagnosis can be confirmed through measurement of tissue transglutaminase antibodies or small bowel biopsy. The treatment is elimination of gluten (wheat, rye, barley, oats) from the diet and supplementation with calcium and vitamin D.

28. A 31-year old woman is referred for abnormal results on thyroid tests that had been ordered to evaluate fatigue, insomnia, and headaches for the past 6 months. Vitals: BP 132/73 mm Hg; P = 72; height = 5 feet 8 inches; weight = 139 lb. Physical examination results are as follows: normal except for a diffuse goiter and warm moist skin; eyes appear normal. Laboratory tests are reviewed and repeated: TSH = 4.74 and 5.04 mU/L (nl 0.45–4.5); and free T_4 2.91 and 2.82 ng/dL (nl 0.8–1.8). What is the differential diagnosis, and what do you recommend next?

    Elevated or normal serum TSH levels in the presence of elevated serum free T_4 levels are clearly inappropriate. The following causes of inappropriate TSH levels should be considered: thyroid hormone resistance syndromes, TSH-producing pituitary tumors, human antimouse antibodies (HAMA), macro-TSH, and high-dose biotin supplements.

    The patient was asked about biotin supplements, and she confirmed that she was not taking them. HAMA testing was negative. The alpha-subunit (ASU) was measured; ASU was elevated at 1.4 ng/mL and the ASU/TSH molar ratio was > 1.0. This prompted MRI evaluation, which showed a 2.4-cm pituitary tumor that abutted, but did not displace, the optic chiasm. Transsphenoidal surgery was performed, and the tumor stained heavily for TSH and ASU. Final diagnosis: TSH-producing pituitary adenoma (see Chapters 28 and 39).

29. A 42-year-old man presents for evaluation of a skin rash that has recently developed. He has a history of T2DM. He drinks two to three alcoholic beverages several nights each week. Physical examination shows eruptive xanthomas (red papules with golden crowns) all over his body, most prominently on the buttocks, thighs, and forearms. Laboratory studies reveal the following: glucose = 310 mg/dL; hemoglobin A_{1c} (HbA_{1C}) = 12.9%; cholesterol = 1082 mg/dL; and TG = 8900 mg/dL. Discuss the cause, risks, and treatment of this lipid disorder.

    This patient has severely elevated serum TGs. This condition usually results from the combination of an inherited TG disorder (familial hypertriglyceridemia or familial combined hyperlipidemia) with a secondary cause of TG elevation (uncontrolled diabetes mellitus, excess alcohol use). His LDL cholesterol cannot be assessed until the serum TG levels are < 400 mg/dL. He is at high risk of developing acute pancreatitis because of the severely elevated TG levels; acute pancreatitis has a 3% to 5% mortality rate in this setting. The priority, therefore, is to quickly lower his serum TG level to < 1000 mg/dL. This goal can be achieved most effectively with a temporary very-low-fat (< 5% fat) diet, blood glucose control, and discontinuation of alcohol. TG levels will fall by about 20% to 25% a day on this regimen. A fibrate or fish oil (or both) should then be added, and he should be advised to follow an American Heart Association diet. Diabetes management must also be improved and further alcohol intake discouraged (see Chapter 10).

    Our practice is to not start TG-lowering medications until the serum TG level is < 1000 mg/dL because, in our experience, patients tend to ignore the acute dietary modification in the belief that the medications will lower the TG level sufficiently. However, TG-lowering medications are ineffective when serum TG levels exceed 1000 mg/dL because the enzyme lipoprotein lipase is saturated at this level. The only currently effective intervention for serum TG levels above 1000 mg/dL is the very-low-fat diet, as described above.

30. A 26-year-old woman requests to be tested for a type of thyroid cancer that has recently been found in her mother and two of five siblings. She notes that she has had intermittent headaches and palpitations for the past year. Her BP is 164/102 mm Hg. She has a 1-cm, left-sided thyroid nodule without associated lymphadenopathy. Laboratory testing shows the following results: serum Ca = 11.2 mg/dL (nl 8.5–10.5); P = 2.4 mg/dL (nl 2.5–4.5); albumin = 4.5 g/dL (nl 3.2–5.5); intact PTH = 55 pg/mL (nl 11–54); calcitonin = 480 pg/mL (nl 0–20); and 24-hour urine metanephrines = 1788 mcg (nl 0–400). Discuss her diagnosis and management.

The thyroid nodule, elevated serum calcitonin, and family history make medullary carcinoma of the thyroid (MCT) likely. Hypertension, headaches, palpitations, and high urinary metanephrines indicate a probable pheochromocytoma. She also has hyperparathyroidism. MEN type 2A (MEN 2A) consists of MCT, pheochromocytoma, and hyperpara-thyroidism. It is an autosomal dominant syndrome that results from a germ-line mutation in the *Ret* gene. After initiation of alpha-blocker therapy and blood pressure control, treatment should consist of removal of the pheochromocytoma(s), followed by removal of the abnormal thyroid and parathyroid glands. Screening at-risk family members for the *Ret/MCT* oncogene should also be performed (see Chapters 43 and 60).

31. A 68-year-old man presents with complaints of a 10-year history of progressive pain in the shins, knees, and left arm. He also notes progressive hearing loss. Physical examination reveals tenderness above the left elbow and enlarged, bowed shins. Bone scan shows intense uptake in both tibias and the left humerus. Skeletal radiography shows enlargement, with multiple focal lytic and sclerotic areas, in the tibias and the distal left humerus. Laboratory evaluation reveals: serum Ca = 9.8 mg/dL (nl 8.5–10.5); and alkaline phosphatase = 966 U/L (nl 25–125). What is the probable diagnosis, and what treatment recommendations would you give?
Bone pain and deformity, reduced hearing, and markedly elevated serum alkaline phosphatase levels suggest a diagnosis of Paget's disease. Intense radioisotope uptake on bone scanning supports this diagnosis, and the characteristic findings on skeletal radiography confirm it. Treatment options include analgesics, IV bisphosphonates (zoledronic acid preferred), subcutaneous denosumab and calcitonin. A single infusion of zoledronic acid, 5 mg intravenously, will likely reduce symptoms and serum alkaline phosphatase levels for an extended period (see Chapter 16).

32. A 19-year-old man has been experiencing fatigue, muscle weakness, and dizziness for the past 3 weeks. This morning he fainted when he went outdoors to exercise. His BP is 95/60 mm Hg, and his pulse is 110 beats per minute. His skin is cool, dry, and tanned. His thyroid feels normal. Laboratory testing shows the following: hematocrit = 36%; glucose = 62 mg/dL; Na = 120 mmol/L; K = 6.7 mmol/L; creatinine = 1.4 mg/dL; and blood urea nitrogen (BUN) = 36 mg/dL. What endocrine disorder should be considered and evaluated?
Hyponatremia with hyperkalemia always suggests primary adrenal insufficiency. Fatigue, weakness, hypotension, tanned skin, anemia, azotemia, and hypoglycemia are also consistent with this diagnosis. The most common cause is autoimmune destruction of the adrenal glands. The diagnosis is made by finding a basal serum cortisol level < 3 mcg/dL or by a cosyntropin stimulation test that shows a low basal serum cortisol level and failure to increase to at least 18 mcg/dL after ACTH administration. During an adrenal crisis, however, there is no time to wait for test results. When this diagnosis is suspected, blood should be drawn for serum cortisol measurement (if a diagnosis of adrenal insufficiency is not already established) and then treatment started with IV fluids and glucocorticoids. The recommended treatment regimen for an adrenal crisis is the following: IV normal saline (1 L over 1 hour, then guided by clinical evaluation) and hydrocortisone (Solu-Cortef) 100 mg IV immediately, then a 200 mg/24-hr infusion for 24 hours, followed by a 100 mg/24 hr infusion for 24 hours. Precipitating conditions should also be actively sought and treated. After that the patient should be transitioned to an oral replacement regimen of glucocorticoids (hydrocortisone or prednisone) and, usually a mineralocorticoid (fludrocortisone) (see Chapter 36).

33. A 72-year old woman is found to have elevated serum calcium on preoperative laboratory examinations before elective surgery, prompting a referral to you. She reports noting recent fatigue and "fuzzy thinking." Past medical history: gastroesophageal reflux disease (GERD), osteopenia. Medications: calcium carbonate 2000 mg four times daily ("maybe more often"). Vitals: BP 139/80 mm Hg; P = 82; height = 5 feet 5 inches; weight = 142 lb. Physical examination results are normal. Further laboratory testing reveals the following: Ca = 14.1 mg/dL; creatinine = 7.1 mg/dL; CO_2 = 37 mEq/L; and P = 2.7 mg/dL. More tests were ordered: PTH < 1 pg/mL (nl 10–65); PTHrp < 1 pmol/L (nl 0–3); 25-hydroxy vitamin D = 35 ng/mL (nl 30–100); and venous pH = 7.54. What is the most likely cause of her hypercalcemia, and what treatment options are available?
Milk alkali syndrome consists of the triad of hypercalcemia, metabolic alkalosis, and renal insufficiency associated with the ingestion of calcium and absorbable alkali, most commonly calcium carbonate. Alkalosis occurs because the calcium-induced diuresis results in volume depletion, which stimulates renal bicarbonate absorption (contraction alkalosis). Milk alkali syndrome is the third most common cause of hypercalcemia after primary hyperparathyroidism and hypercalcemia of malignancy. Treatment is hydration and stopping calcium, alkali, and vitamin D intake until the biochemical abnormalities resolve. Dialysis may be needed in some cases (see Chapters 17 and 19).

34. A 38-year old woman is referred for hyperthyroidism. She has recently been experiencing anxiety, fatigue, insomnia, thinning hair, and brittle nails. Medications: vitamins, multiple supplements. Vitals: BP 122/78 mm Hg; P = 66; height = 5 feet 4 inches; weight = 145 lb. Physical examination results are as follows: thyroid: normal; eyes: normal; hair: normal; and nails: normal. Repeat evaluation: TSH = 0.05 mU/L (nl 0.45–4.5); free T_4 = 3.6 ng/dL (nl 0.8–1.8); TRabs = positive; RAIU = 18%; and scan: homogeneous uptake. What is her likely diagnosis, and what should be done next?
The patient was asked about her intake of vitamins and supplements; her list included a hair-and-nail treatment that contained high amounts of biotin. She was asked to stop the supplements temporarily, and 3 days later, her

thyroid test results were normal. This is a case of biotin interference in hormone assays, with results mimicking Graves' disease. Biotin is a component of the reagents for immunoassays of some hormones, such as TSH, T_4, T_3, TRAb, PTH, cortisol, and others. As a result, patients who take high doses of biotin supplements, a common over-the-counter treatment for hair loss and brittle nails, can cause falsely and significantly elevated serum levels of free T_4, free T_3, PTH, cortisol, estradiol, and dehydroepiandrosterone sulfate (DHEAS) for several hours or longer after biotin ingestion; TSH levels can be low, high, or normal, depending on which assay is used. Measurement of these hormones after at least an 8-hour (preferably 2–3 days) abstinence from biotin corrects the anomaly in this laboratory value (see Chapter 38).

BIBLIOGRAPHY

Beck Peccoz, P., Rodari, G., Giavoli, C., & Lania, A. (2017). Central hypothyroidism – a neglected thyroid disorder. *Nature Reviews Endocrinology, 13,* 588–598

Berglund, L., Brunzell, J. D., Anne, C., Goldberg, A. C., Sacks, F., Murad, M. H., & Stalenhoef, A. F. (2012). Evaluation and treatment of hypertriglyceridemia: an Endocrine Society Clinical Practice Guideline. *Journal of Clinical Endocrinology and Metabolism, 97,* 2969–2989.

Bornstein, S. R., Allolio, B., Arlt, W., Barthel, A., Don-Wauchope, A., Hammer, G. D., . . . Torpy, D. J. (2016). Diagnosis and treatment of primary adrenal insufficiency: an Endocrine Society Clinical Practice Guideline. *Journal of Clinical Endocrinology and Metabolism, 101*(2), 364–389.

Brandi, M. L., Bilezikian, J. P., Shoback, D., Bouillon, R., Clarke B. L., Thakker, R. V., . . . Potts, J. T. Jr. (2016). Management of hypoparathyroidism: summary statement and guidelines. *Journal of Clinical Endocrinology and Metabolism, 101,* 2273–2283.

Chaker, L., Bianco, A. C., Jonklass, J., & Peeters, R. P. (2017). Hypothyroidism. *Lancet, 390,* 3550–3562.

Cryer, P. E., Axelrod, L., Grossman, A. B., Heller, S. R., Montori, V. M., Seaquist, E. R., & Service, F. J. (2009). Evaluation and management of adult hypoglycemic disorders: an Endocrine Society Clinical Practice Guideline. *Journal of Clinical Endocrinology and Metabolism, 94,* 709–728.

Fleseriu, M., Hashim, I. A., Karavitaki, N., Melmed, S., Murad, M. H., Salvatori, R., & Samuels, M. H. (2016). Hormonal replacement in hypopituitarism in adults: an Endocrine Society Clinical Practice Guideline. *Journal of Clinical Endocrinology and Metabolism, 101,* 3888–3921.

Funder, J. W., Carey, R. M., Mantero, F., Murad, M. H., Reincke, M., Shibata, H., . . . Young, W. F. Jr. (2016). The management of primary aldosteronism: case detection, diagnosis, and treatment: an Endocrine Society Clinical Practice Guideline. *Journal of Clinical Endocrinology and Metabolism, 101*(5), 1889–1916.

Elston, M., Shegal, S., Du Toit, S., Yarndley, T., & Conaglen, J. V. (2016). Factitious Graves' disease due to biotin immunoassay interference – a case and review of the literature. *Journal of Clinical Endocrinology and Metabolism, 101,* 3251–3255

Gravholt, C. H., Andersen, N. H., Conway, G. S., Dekkers, O. M., Geffner, M. E., Klein, K. O., . . . Backeljauw, P. F. (2017). Clinical practice guidelines for the care of girls and women with Turner syndrome: proceedings from the 2016 Cincinnati International Turner Syndrome Meeting. *European Journal of Endocrinology, 177*(3), G1–G70.

Grunenwald, S., & Caron, P. (2015). Central hypothyroidism in adults: better understanding for better care. *Pituitary, 18,* 169–175.

Jellinger, P. S., Handelsman, Y., Rosenblit, P. D., Bloomgarden, Z. T., Fonseca, V. A., Garber, A. J., . . . Davidson, M.. (2017). American Association of Clinical Endocrinologists and American College of Endocrinology Guidelines for Management of Dyslipidemia and Prevention of Cardiovascular Disease. *Endocrine Practice, 23*(Suppl. 2), 1–87.

Jonklaas, J., Bianco, A. C., Bauer, A. J., Burman, K. D., Cappola, A. R., Celi, F. S., . . . Sawka, A. M. (2014). Guidelines for the treatment of hypothyroidism prepared by the American Thyroid Association Task Force on Thyroid Hormone Replacement. *Thyroid, 24,* 1670–1751.

Lenders, J. W., Duh, Q. Y., Eisenhofer, G., Gimenez-Roqueplo, A. P., Grebe, S. K., Murad, M. H., . . . Young, W. F. Jr. (2014). Pheochromocytoma and paraganglioma: an Endocrine Society Clinical Practice Guideline. *Journal of Clinical Endocrinology and Metabolism, 99*(6), 1915–1942.

Li, D., Radulescu, A., Shrestha, R. T., Root, M., Karger, A. B., Killeen, A. A., . . . Burmeister, L. A. (2017). Association of biotin ingestion with performance of hormone and non-hormone assays in healthy adults. *JAMA, 318,* 1150–1160.

Machado, M. C., Bruce-Mensah, A., Whitmire, M., & Rizvi, A. A. (2015). Hypercalcemia associated with calcium supplement use: prevalence and characteristics in hospitalized patients. *Journal of Clinical Medicine, 4*(3), 414–424

Nieman, L. K., Biller, B. M., Findling, J. W., Newell-Price, J., Savage, M. O., Stewart, P. M., & Montori, V. M. (2008). The diagnosis of Cushing's syndrome: an Endocrine Society Clinical Practice Guideline. *Journal of Clinical Endocrinology and Metabolism, 93*(5), 1526–1540.

Nieman, L. K., Biller, B. M., Findling, J. W., Murad, M. H., Newell-Price, J., Savage, M. O., & Tabarin, A. (2015). Treatment of Cushing's syndrome: an Endocrine Society Clinical Practice Guideline. *Journal of Clinical Endocrinology and Metabolism, 100*(8), 2807–2831.

Ross, D. S., Burch, H. B., Cooper, D. S., Greenlee, M. C., Laurberg, P., Maia, A. L., . . . Walter, M. A. (2016). 2016 American Thyroid Association guidelines for diagnosis and management of hyperthyroidism and other causes of thyrotoxicosis. *Thyroid, 26,* 1343–1421.

Rossi, G. P., Auchus, R. J., Brown, M., Lenders, J. W., Naruse, M., Plouin, P. F., . . . Young, W. F. Jr. (2014). An expert consensus statement on use of adrenal vein sampling for the subtyping of primary aldosteronism. *Hypertension, 63,* 151–160.

Stone, N. J., Robinson, J. G., Lichtenstein, A. H., Bairey Merz, C. N., Blum, C. B., Eckel, R. H., . . . Tomaselli, G. F. (2014). 2013 ACC/AHA guideline on the treatment of blood cholesterol to reduce atherosclerotic cardiovascular risk in adults: a report of the American College of Cardiology/American Heart Association Task Force on Practice Guidelines. *Circulation, 129,* S1–S45.

Tebben, P. J., Singh, R. J., & Kumar, R. (2016). Vitamin D mediated hypercalcemia: mechanisms, diagnosis and treatment. *Endocrine Reviews, 37*(5), 521–547.

INDEX

A

AACE. *See* American Association of Clinical Endocrinologists
AAS. *See* Anabolic-androgenic steroids
Abaloparatide, 124–125t, 127, 475
ABC. *See* ATP-binding cassette
Abnormal growth
  causes of, 245
  curve, 244
  syndromes associated with, 245
Abnormal intellectual development, 353
Abnormal visual fields, 221
Absorptive hypercalciuria, 170
  phosphorus in, 173
  PTH in, 173
ACE. *See* Angiotensin-converting enzyme
Acquired hypertriglyceridemia, 95
Acromegaly, 205b.*See also* Gigantism
  actor with, 212
  clinical effects of, 209t
  death from, 208
  diagnosis of, 209
  endocrine syndromes in, 209, 210t
  hirsutism and, 429
  IGF-1 and, 209
  medical therapy for, 210
  OSA and, 504
  patient examination in, 208
  radiation therapy for, 211
  sleep apnea and, 208
  symptoms and physical abnormalities improvement, 211
  transsphenoidal surgery for, 211
  treatment of, 210
ACTH. *See* Adrenocorticotropic hormone
Actin-myosin, 404
Action in Diabetes and Vascular Disease: Preterax and Diamicron Modified Release Controlled Evaluation (ADVANCE) study, 20–21, 32
Action to Control Cardiovascular Risk in Diabetes (ACCORD) study, 20–21, 32
Acute thyroiditis, 315
ADA. *See* American Diabetes Association
Adenomas. *See specific types*
Adenosine triphosphate (ATP), 93
ADH. *See* Antidiuretic hormone
Adrenal cancer
  cortisol-producing, 277
  primary aldosteronism and, 262
  types of, 275–279
Adrenal crisis, 284t
  diagnosis of, 283
  management of, 283
Adrenal glands
  cancer in, 275–279
  pathology, imaging for, 518
  surgery, 518–522
Adrenal hyperplasia, 289, 289f
Adrenal incidentalomas, 271–274, 273b
  defined, 271–273
  diagnostic evaluation of, 271
  etiologies of, 271
  excess cortisol secretion by, 271–272
  hormone evaluation for, 272, 272t

Adrenal incidentalomas *(Continued)*
  hormone syndromes caused by, 271
  imaging studies for, 271, 272t
  management of, 273, 273t
  monitoring of, 273
  pheochromocytoma and, 272
  prevalence of, 271
  primary aldosteronism in, 272
Adrenal insufficiency, 281–287
  causes of, 281, 281t
  central, 283
  chronic, 284
    "stress dose" glucocorticoids for, 285–286, 285t
    treatment of, 285
  classification of, 286b
  defined, 281
  DHEA for, 284–285
  diagnosis
    biochemical, 282, 282f
    in critical care setting, 284
  drugs and, 286
  evaluation of, 283, 283f
  glucocorticoids for, 284
  hyperkalemia in, 281–282
  hyponatremia in, 281–282
  hypothyroidism and, 231
  imaging tests for, 283
  laboratory abnormalities in, 281–282
  presentation of, 281
  primary, 282, 283, 549
  symptoms of, 281
  treatment of, 287b
    deficiencies, 284
Adrenal malignancies, 275–280, 278b
  management of, 521
Adrenal mass, 518, 521b
  biopsy for, 273
  CT for, 518
  CT of, 275
  FDG-PET of, 275
  laboratory workup for, 518
  percutaneous biopsy in, 519
Adrenal vein sampling (AVS), 261
  by experienced interventional radiologist, 261
  indications for, 519
  performing, 261
Adrenalectomy
  cortical-sparing, 520
  for functional tumors, long-term success of, 520
  laparoscopic approaches for, 519
  open technique in, 519
Adrenal-producing adenomas, 263
Adrenarche, 382
  benign premature
    diagnosis of, 388
    treatment of, 388
  in puberty, 387
Adrenocortical carcinomas
  adjuvant therapy for, 276
  biopsy for, 275
  clinical presentation of, 275
  distribution of, 276

Adrenocortical carcinomas *(Continued)*
  functioning, 275
  genetic abnormalities causing, 276
  histologic features of, 276
  imaging features of, 275
  initial treatment of, 276
  management of, 521
  nonfunctioning, 277
  prognosis of, 277, 278t
  staging system for, 276
  steroid hormone secreting, 275
Adrenocorticotropic hormone (ACTH), 182
  carcinomas, 223
  Cushing's syndrome and, 214t, 216
  deficiency, 182, 183
    treatment of, 185
  diagnosis of, 216
  stimulation tests, 283
Adrenoleukodystrophy, 537
ADVANCE study. *See* Action in Diabetes and Vascular
    Disease: Preterax and Diamicron Modified Release
    Controlled Evaluation (ADVANCE) study
Africa
  diabetes mellitus in, 532
  endocrinology in, 532–534
    training opportunities in, 534
  gestational diabetes in, 533
  hyperthyroidism in, 533
  hypothyroidism in, 533
  iodine deficiency in, 533
  malnutrition-related diabetes mellitus in, 532
  thyroid disorders in, 533
    diagnosis of, 533
  type 1 diabetes mellitus in, 532
  type 2 diabetes mellitus in, 533
AFTNs. *See* Autonomously functioning thyroid nodules
Aging, 473–486
  anabolic-androgenic steroids and, 446
  body composition changes with, 474t
  body weight and, 473
  bone health in, changes of, 473–474
  DHEA in, 480
  estradiol with, 477–478
  fat mass and, 475–476
  GH-IGF-1 axis with, 481
  growth hormone and, 255–256
  hormonal changes with, 478t
  hormonal release and, 503
  HPA axis with, 482
  hyperparathyroidism and, 153
  lean body mass in, 473
  primary hypogonadism and, 396
  sleep stages and, 495, 495f
  take home messages in, 484–485
  testosterone and, 477–478, 501
  thyroid conditions in, 482–483
Agouti-related peptide (AGRP), 102
Agranulocytosis, 307
AGRP. *See* Agouti-related peptide
AIT. *See* Amiodarone-induced thyrotoxicosis
Albuminuria, DKD and, 18
Aldosterone receptor antagonist therapy, 544
Aldosterone resolution score (ARS), 519
Aldosterone-producing adenoma (APA), 258, 260
  CT of, 260–261
  IHA *versus*, 260
  management of, 262–263
  MRI of, 260–261
  surgery, 262
Aldosterone/renin ratio (ARR), 259
Aldosteronism, primary, 257–264, 263b, 542, 544
  clinical manifestations of, 258

Aldosteronism, primary *(Continued)*
  defined, 258
  detection of, 259
  diagnosis of, 259
    confirmation, 260
  evaluation and management algorithm for, 263, 263f
  forms of, 260, 263
  imaging study for, 260–261
  medications for, 262
  postoperative period of, 262–263
  prevalence of, 258
  screening for, 259
Alendronate, 124–125t
Alpha blockade, 268
5-Alpha reductase, 372
  deficiency
    in children, 378–379
    physiologic results of, 378
Alpha subunit/TSH molar ratio, 220, 220t
Alpha-glucosidase inhibitors, 36, 88–89
17Alpha-hydroxylase, 289
  deficiency of, 291–292
Alpha-melanocortin, 102
Alternate-day fasting, 104
Ambiguous genitalia, 292..*See also* Sexual ambiguity
  patient evaluation for, 376
  physical examination of, 376
  radiographic studies in, 376–377
  surgical correction of, 294
Amenorrhea, 417–421, 420–421b
  defined, 417
  evaluation of, 391
  with hypergonadotropic hypogonadism, 419
  hyperprolactinemia causing, 419
  hypothalamic, 419
    causes of, 419
    diagnosis of, 419
  patient evaluation for, 418
  primary, 391
    causes of, 417, 418t
    ovarian, 417
  secondary, 542, 543
    causes of, 417–418, 418t
American Association of Clinical Endocrinologists (AACE), 434–435
American College of Cardiology/American Heart Association
    (ACC/AHA), 95
American College of Obstetricians and Gynecologists (ACOG),
    69, 434–435
  early screening guidelines, 77
  on GDM, 76
  glucose tolerance test results, 77t
  risk factors, 78t
American Diabetes Association (ADA)
  early screening guidelines, 77
  on GDM, 76–77
  glucose tolerance test results, 77t
  risk factors, 78t
American Thyroid Association (ATA), 304
Amge, Jyoti, 539
Amino acids, 68
Aminoglycosides, 167
Amiodarone-induced thyrotoxicosis (AIT), 318, 319t, 546
Amphetamine, 105, 360t
Anabolic agents, 124, 124–125t
Anabolic Steroid Control Act, 449–450
Anabolic-androgenic steroids (AAS), 446–450
  abuse of, 448
  adverse effects of, 448, 449t
  age and, 446
  athletes using, 448
  avoid detection of, 449
  biological effects of, 446, 447t

Anabolic-androgenic steroids *(Continued)*
defined, 446
doses of, 448
effects of, 446
as health problem, 450
illegal, 448
indications for, 447
metabolism of, 447
neuropsychiatric implications of, 448
potential uses of, 447
production of, 446
screening tests for, 448–449
Anaplastic thyroid cancer (ATC), 331–332, 332b
defined, 331
staging of, 331, 332t
surgery for, 512
treatment of, 331–332
Anastrozole, 416
Androgen
antagonists, 447
changes, 506t
deficiency, 479
dermatologic manifestations related to, 424–425
excess, 251
insensitivity, 378
in menopause, 436
precursors, 446–450
anabolic, 450
production of, 427
replacement therapy, 400, 507
symptoms of low/high levels of, 447
Angiotensin receptor blocker (ARB), for DKD, 18
Angiotensin-converting enzyme (ACE), 18
inhibitors, preconception counseling and, 71
ANP. *See* Atrial natriuretic peptide
Antiandrogen therapy, 440
Antiandrogens, 431
Anticonvulsants, 364t
Antidepressants. *See also specific drugs*
depression and, 365
thyroid function and, 365
thyroid hormone and, 368
Antidiuretic hormone (ADH), 225. *See also* Syndrome of inappropriate secretion of antidiuretic hormone
plasma concentrations of, 235
secretion
conditions influencing, 229
drugs affecting, 230t
physiologic changes affecting, 229
water restriction and values for, 235t
Antihypertensives. *See also specific drugs*
for impotence, 405
Antiobesity medications, 105, 106t
Antipsychotics, 364t
Antiresorptive agents, 124, 124–125t
Antithyroid antibody tests, 301–302
Antithyroid drugs (ATDs), 306
in African setting, 533–534
breast-feeding and, 352
effectiveness of, 307
laboratory tests, in patient taking, 308
pretreatment with, 308
side effects of, 307
APA. *See* Aldosterone-producing adenoma
Apathetic hyperthyroidism, 305
Apnea, 503
Apo A1, 93
Apoprotein(a), 94
Apoproteins, 92
Appropriate growth chart, 244
APS. *See* Autoimmune polyendocrinopathy syndromes
Aquaporins (AQPs), 228–229

ARB. *See* Angiotensin receptor blocker
Areolae, 213–214
Arginine vasopressin, 228–229
ARR. *See* Aldosterone/renin ratio
Arterial thrombosis, 93
Arthropathy, 307
Ascending reticular activating system (ARAS), 496
Aspart, in pregnancy, 74
ATA. *See* American Thyroid Association
ATC. *See* Anaplastic thyroid cancer
ATDs. *See* Antithyroid drugs
Atherosclerotic cardiovascular disease (ASCVD)
prevention of, 20
type 2 diabetes mellitus with, 37
Atherosclerotic plaque, 93
Atorvastatin, 96
ATP. *See* Adenosine triphosphate
ATP-binding cassette (ABC), 94
Atrial natriuretic peptide (ANP), 226
Atypical femoral fractures, 126, 126f
Autoimmune disorders, 167
Autoimmune polyendocrinopathy syndromes (APS), 451–454,
454b
defined, 452
diagnosis of, 453, 453t
thyroid diseases associated with, 453
treatment of, 453
type 1
defined, 452
genetic basis for, 452
nonendocrine autoimmune disorders associated with, 452
occurrence of, 452
type 2
autoimmune disorders and, 452
defined, 452
genetic causes of, 452
nonendocrine autoimmune disorders associated with, 452
occurrence of, 452
type 3, 453
Autoimmune thyroid disease
clinical characteristics of, 316
depression and, 363
Autonomously functioning thyroid nodules (AFTNs), 305
Autonomy, 304
Avanafil, 407
Azoospermia factor (AZF), 394

B
Band keratopathy, 154
Bariatric surgery, 527–531, 531b
classic surgical indications for, 527
combined restrictive/malabsorptive option, 529
complications of, 530
contraindications for, 527
inclusion criteria for, 527
laparoscopic, complications after, 530
on obesity-related comorbidities, 530
weight loss in, 530
Baroreceptors, 226, 227f
Barr body, 372
Basal insulin, 34t, 36
coverage, 22
dose selection of, 62
with MDI, 22
preparations, 23
timing, 24
Basal metabolic rate (BMR), 102
Bates, Anna, 540
Beckwith-Wiedemann syndrome, 251
Bell, Catherine, 536
Benign premature adrenarche, 388
Benign premature thelarche, 387

Berry, Halle, 536
Beta-blockers, 268, 306
  for nursing women, 352
  during pregnancy, 350
11Beta-hydroxylase, 289, 290
  deficiency of, 291
17-Beta-hydroxysteroid dehydrogenase, 377
Bethesda System for Reporting Thyroid Cytopathology, 324
Biguanides, 34t
Bile acid sequestrants, 96t
Biochemical testing, principles of, 523
Biochemical thyrotoxicosis, 542
Bioidentical hormone, 435
  safety of, 435
Biotin, 549–550
  affecting thyroid function laboratory assays, 355
Biotin, in thyroid function, 302
Birth. *See also* Pregnancy
  greatest known number of children, 540
  highest birth weight, 540
  multiple, highest number of, for single gestation, 540
  oldest woman to give, 540
Bisphosphonates, 125
  for low bone density, 475
  mechanism of action, 151t
  ONJ and, 125
Blood glucose (BG)
  correction factor, 50
  correctional insulin, 27
  high, causes of, 26
  highest recorded level, 540
  in hospital setting, 61
  postprandial, 27, 28
  self-monitored, 24, 39
  troubleshooting, 27
Blood pressure, 537–538
Bloodstream
  lipids in, 92–98
  lipoproteins in, 92
BMD. *See* Bone mineral density
BMI. *See* Body mass index
BMR. *See* Basal metabolic rate
BNP. *See* Brain natriuretic peptide
Body mass index (BMI)
  coronary artery disease and, 101f
  hypertension and, 101f
  obesity and, 527
Body weight. *See also* Weight gain; Weight loss
  aging and, 473
  water as, 226t
Bolus insulin
  correctional
    half, 28
    initial, 27
    timing, 28
    usage, 28
  coverage, 22
  with MDI, 22
  preparations, 22–23
  timing, 23–24
Bolus on board (BOB), 50
Bone densitometry
  criteria, 110
  report, 111
Bone density screening test, 116, 117t
Bone disease, 165
Bone mass measurement, 116–122, 121b
  anatomic sites, 116
  L-spine, 117
  in postmenopausal women and men age, 118
  preferred method for, 116

Bone mass measurement *(Continued)*
  techniques, 116
  T-score, 117
  vertebra, 117
  WHO classification in, 117–118
  Z-score, 117
Bone matrix protein, 146
Bone metabolism, 205
Bone mineral density (BMD), 473–474
  absolute, 111
  calcium in, 484
  in children, 120
  cost-effective evaluation of, 112
  defined, 116
  forearm, 117
  importance of, 116
  low
    causes of, 112
    criteria for, 475
    pharmacologic agents for, 475
  L-spine, 118, 119f
  measurement
    with DXA, 111
    indications for, 111
    technique, 111
  monitoring, anatomic sites for, 118
  significant change in, 118
  trend at total hip, 118–119, 120f
  vitamin D in, 484
Bone remodeling, 124, 124f
Bone sialoprotein, 146
Bradford, Rosalie, 539
Brain natriuretic peptide (BNP), 226
Breast cancer, 415
Breastfeeding
  ATDs and, 352
  beta-blockers and, 352
  [131]I ablation and, 308, 352
Buccal testosterone, 399t
Bupropion, 105
Bush, George, 535

C

CAH. *See* Congenital adrenal hyperplasia
Calcimimetic drugs, for hypercalcemia, 150–152
Calcitonin, 124–125t, 151t
  measurement of, 302
  mechanism of action, 151t
Calcitriol-mediated hypercalcemia, 161
Calcium
  for bone mineral density, 484
  dietary intake
    assessment of, 123
    ensuring adequate, 123
  FGF 23 and, 145
  filtered and excreted load, 172
  kidney and, 172
  metabolism, 149f
  phosphate and, 147, 148t
  serum
    correcting levels, 164
    factors controlling, 148t
    hypercalciuria and, 172
    ionized, 164
    low, 164
    serum albumin and, 164
    source of, 144
    vitamin D metabolism and, 164
Calcium acetate, 168t
Calcium carbonate, 168t
Calcium channel blockers, 71

Calcium chloride, 168t
Calcium citrate, 168t
Calcium gluceptate, 168t
Calcium gluconate, 168t
Calcium-sensing receptor (CaSR), 146
Calment, Jeanne Louise, 540
cAMP. *See* Cyclic adenosine monophosphate
Cancer. *See also specific types*
　hypercalcemia with, 149
　hypocalcemia and, 167
　screening, 443
Carbamazepine, 364t
　on thyroid function, 365
Carbohydrate counting, 26, 50–60
　accuracy of, 50
　assessment of, 59
　basics, 51, 51t
Carbohydrate-to-insulin (C:I) ratio, 26
　adjusting, 26, 27f
　basal insulins and, 26
　bolus insulins and, 26
　determining, 26, 50
　usage, 28
Carboxy-terminal PTH (CPTH) fragments, 146
Carcinoid crisis
　defined, 470
　management of, 470, 471t
　prevention of, 470
　prophylaxis for, 470
Carcinoid syndrome, 467–472, 468b
　biochemical mediators of, 467, 468f
　defined, 467
　description of, 525
　diagnosis of, 468, 468t, 525
　flushing in, 467
　5-HIAA and, 469
　localization of, 469
　medications for, 469, 470t
　niacin deficiency and, 467
　pellagra and, 467
　symptoms of, control of, 469
　treatment of, 469
Carcinoid tumors
　chemotherapy for, 469
　classification of, 467
　humoral syndromes from, 467–468
　surgical management for, 525
Carcinoma. *See specific types*
Cardiac autonomic neuropathy, 19
Cardiac septal hypertrophy, 80
Cardiovascular disease, 291
Carney's complex, 210t
Carpenter's syndrome, 452
Cash, Johnny, 537
CaSR. *See* Calcium-sensing receptor
Castenda, Jesse, 540
Catecholamines
　adrenergic receptors and, 266–267
　measurement of, medications causing interference
　　with, 267
　metabolism of, 266
　OSA and, 504
　synthesis of, 266
Catecholamine-secreting tumors, 265–270
　clinical manifestations of, 265
　diagnosis of, 267
　molecular taxonomy of, 269
　nonclassic manifestations of, 266
　prevalence of, 265
C-cell hyperplasia, 459
Celiac antibody, 248

Central hypothyroidism, 547
　euthyroid sick syndrome *versus,* 341–342
Central idiopathic precocious puberty, 390b
Central neck dissection, 511
Central precocious puberty (CPP)
　causes of, 385
　treatment of, 385
Cerebral tetany, 165
Cerebrospinal fluid (CSF) leak, 190
CETP. *See* Cholesterol ester transfer protein
CF. *See* Correctional bolus insulin
CGM. *See* Continuous glucose monitoring
cGMP. *See* Cyclic guanosine monophosphate
Chemotherapy
　for carcinoid tumors, 469
　for pheochromocytoma, 269
CHH. *See* Congenital hypogonadotropic hypogonadism
Childhood hypoglycemia, 89
Cholesterol, 67–68, 92
　lowering therapy, 97
Cholesterol ester transfer protein (CETP), 93, 93t
Chronic adrenal insufficiency
　management of, 284
　"stress dose" glucocorticoids for, 285–286, 285t
　treatment of, 285
Chronic renal failure, 136
Chvostek's sign, 165
Chylomicrons, 92
C:I ratio. *See* Carbohydrate-to-insulin (C:I) ratio
Cinacalcet, 151t
　mechanism of action, 151t
Circadian rhythm
　concerns, 493
　cortisol in, 502
　entrainment in, 499
　glucose levels and, 503
　input system, 497
　insulin levels and, 503
　melatonin in, 498f, 499
　molecular mechanisms of, 497–499
　organization of, 496–497, 497f
　synchronization of, 499
　TSH in, 363, 502
Cirigliano, M., 436
Cisgender, 439t
Citrate toxicity, 165
Clarke, Bobby, 537
Clinical inertia, 40
Clinical thyrotoxicosis, 542
Clomiphene, 416
Clomiphene citrate, 425–426
Clonidine suppression test, 267
Colesevelam, 36
Collagen, 146
Complete androgen insensitivity, 378
Completion thyroidectomy, in thyroid nodule, 510
Compounded hormones, 436
Computed tomography (CT), 111
　of adrenal mass, 275
　for adrenal pathology, 518
　of aldosterone-producing adenoma, 260–261
　of benign and malignant tumors, 518–519
　of idiopathic hyperaldosteronism (IHA), 260–261
　of pheochromocytoma, 268
Congenital adrenal hyperplasia (CAH), 288–298, 296b, 376
　cardiovascular disease and, 291
　causes of, 290
　classic, therapy for, 295
　clinical consequences of, 290–291
　　in females, 291
　　in males, 291

Congenital adrenal hyperplasia *(Continued)*
  clinical features of, 292
  confirmation of, 293
  defined, 288
  diagnosis of, 292
  form of, 290
  genetic defects confirmed in, 293
  hirsutism and, 420, 428–429, 428f
  hydrocortisone for, 294
  21-hydroxylase-deficient, 387
  incidentalomas and, 292
  inherited, 289
  newborn screening, 293
  nonclassic, 292
    diagnosis, 293, 293f
    glucocorticoid treatment in, 295
    predicted adult height and, 295
    pregnancy and, 295
  prevalence of, 288
  rarer forms of, 290
  treatment of, 295t, 387
    in adolescents and adults, 294–295
    in children, 294
    monitoring, 296
    in neonates, 294, 294f
    prenatal, 296
Congenital hypogonadotropic hypogonadism (CHH), 397
Conivaptan, 238
Connective tissue disorders, 251
Conn's syndrome, 542, 544
Constitutional advanced growth, 251
Constitutional growth delay, 388–389
  defined, 245
  diagnosis of, 245
  puberty and, 389
  testosterone therapy for, 245–248
Continuous glucose monitoring (CGM), 25–26, 45, 46f, 47f, 48f, 73–74
  benefits of, 45
  correction dose and, 50–51
  major problems with, 45
Continuous positive airway pressure (CPAP)
  for abnormal glucose metabolism, 505–506
  for OSA, 506
Continuous subcutaneous insulin infusion (CSII) device, 43, 48–49b
  complications of, 44
  components of, 43, 43b
  in inpatient setting, 65
  insulin delivery setting on, 44
Contraceptive agents, 84
Coronary artery disease
  BMI and, 101f
  cholesterol-lowering therapy, 97
  diabetes and, 71
  diabetes mellitus and, 20
  pregnancy and, 71
Correctional bolus insulin (CF)
  half, 28
  initial, 27
  timing, 28
  usage, 28
Cortical-sparing adrenalectomy, 520
Corticotropin-releasing hormone (CRH), 213, 289
  Cushing's syndrome and, 218
Cortisol
  circadian rhythm and, 502
  clinical symptoms of excessive, 213
  jet lag and, 502–503
  normal function of, 213
  presentation of, 213
  regulation of, 213

Cortisol *(Continued)*
  in sleep, 500
  24-hour profiles of, 498f
  urine free, 215
Cortisol-producing adrenal adenomas, perioperative management of, 520
CPAP. *See* Continuous positive airway pressure
CPTH fragments. *See* Carboxy-terminal PTH (CPTH) fragments
Crenshaw, Ben, 536
CRH. *See* Corticotropin-releasing hormone
Cross-dresser, 439t
CSII. *See* Continuous subcutaneous insulin infusion
CT. *See* Computed tomography
Cushing's syndrome, 213–218, 218b, 544
  ACTH and, 214t, 216
  adrenal incidentalomas and, 271
  biochemical testing of, 216
  causes of, 214, 214t
  clinical findings of, 213
  CRH and, 218
  death in, 214
  diagnosis of, 215f
  differential diagnosis of, 215
  hirsutism and, 429
  MRI findings in, 216
  screening tests for, 215
  surgery for, 216
    transsphenoidal, 216
  symptoms and signs of, 214t
Cutler, Jay, 536
Cyclic adenosine monophosphate (cAMP), 228–229, 348–349
Cyclic guanosine monophosphate (cGMP), 404
CYP11B1, 289
CYP17A1 (17alpha-hydroxylase), 289
CYP21A2 (21-hydroxylase), 289
  deficiencies, 290
Cyst fluid, 512

D
Danazol, 416
Dangi, Chandra Bahadur, 539
DCCT. *See* Diabetes Control and Complications Trial
DCT. *See* Distal convoluted tubule
DDP-4 inhibitors. *See* Dipeptidyl peptidase (DPP)-4 inhibitors
Dehydroepiandrosterone (DHEA), 284–285, 418, 423, 484
  aging and, 480
  biologic effects of, 480
  hormonal effects of, 480
  for older adults, 480–481
Dehydroepiandrosterone sulfate (DHEA-S), 272, 284–285
Deiodinase enzymes
  for euthyroid sick syndrome, 343
  function of, 342–343, 342f, 342t
Denosumab, 124–125t, 125, 151t
  for low bone density, 475
  mechanism of action, 151t
  precautions, 125
Depo-Provera, 84
Depression
  antidepressant medication for, 366
  autoimmune thyroid disease and, 363
  diabetes mellitus and, 19
  subclinical, 360
  thyroid axis and, 363
  thyroid hormone and, 366
  TRH and, 363
Destructive thyroiditis, 318
Detemir, pregnancy and, 74
Detumescence, 405
Devers, Gail, 535

DHEA. *See* Dehydroepiandrosterone
DHEA-S. *See* Dehydroepiandrosterone sulfate
Diabetes care, in Africa, 533
Diabetes Control and Complications Trial (DCCT), 21
Diabetes insipidus
  diagnosis of, 237
  management of, 237
  pituitary insufficiency and, 182
  polyuria in, 234–235
Diabetes mellitus, 7–11, 11b, 61–66. *See also* Gestational
    diabetes mellitus; Type 1 diabetes mellitus; Type 2
    diabetes mellitus
  in Africa, 532
  apps available for, 46
  breastfeeding and, 82
  causal factors, 9–10
  classification of, 8–9, 9t
  complications of
    acute, 14–22
    chronic, 14–22
  congenital abnormalities and, 70
  coronary artery disease and, 71
  defined, 8
  depression and, 69
  diagnosis of, 8
  epidemiology of, 8
  in first trimester, 68
  foot problems in, 19
  glycemic control in, 20
  home regimen of, 65
  inpatient management of, 62
  ketosis-prone, 9
  macrosomia and, 70
  malnutrition-related, 532
  management of, 533
  monogenic, 10
  occurrence of, 8
  OSA and, 506
  overt, 77t
  pathophysiology of, 8
  preconception counseling and, 69
  in pregnancy, 67–86, 75–76b
    White classification, 73
  prevention of, 10
  screening for, 10
  in second trimester, 68
  sleep in, 68
  surgery and, 65
  in third trimester, 68
  thyroid disease and, 71
  type 3c, 10
Diabetes Prevention Program (DPP), 10, 40
Diabetes-related distress, 19
Diabetic autonomic neuropathy, 19
Diabetic ketoacidosis (DKA), 20–21b
  causes of, 14
  defined, 14
  diagnosis of, 15, 532
  fetal growth and, 75
  HHS *versus*, 15, 16t
  insulin infusion for, 15
  ketones in, 15
  management of, 15
  mortality rate for, 14
  precipitating factors for, 14
  pregnancy and, 75
    physician remember about, 75–76
  prevalence of, 14
  symptoms and signs of, 14
  type 1 diabetes mellitus and, 14
Diabetic macular edema (DME), 18

Diabetic nephropathy
  preeclampsia and, 72
  pregnancy and, 72
Diabetic neuropathy, 18
Diabetic retinopathy
  management of, 18
  manifestation of, 18
  pregnancy and, 73
  prevalence of, 17
Dialysis, 151t
  mechanism of action, 151t
Diet
  calcium in, 123
  low-calorie, 104
  obesity and, 104
  patient readiness for changing, 103
  postpartum management and, 81
  very-low-calorie, 104
Dietary carbohydrates, 26
Differentiated thyroid cancer (DTC), 327–331, 331b
  lymph node metastases in, 511
  preoperative evaluation of, 328–329
  prognosis of, 330, 330t
  radioactive iodine for, 330, 330t
  recurrence of, 331
  risk factors for, 327
  staging for, 327, 328t
  surgery for, 329
  thyroidectomy for, 511
Dihydrotestosterone, 372, 416
Dipeptidyl peptidase (DPP)-4 inhibitors, 34t, 35–36, 484
Diplopia, 189
Distal convoluted tubule (DCT), 229
Distal symmetric polyneuropathy, 18
DKA. *See* Diabetic ketoacidosis
Dopamine agonists, 205
DPP. *See* Diabetes Prevention Program
DTC. *See* Differentiated thyroid cancer
Dual-energy x-ray absorptiometry (DXA), 475
Duloxetine, for diabetic neuropathy, 18–19
Duration of insulin action (DIA), 50
DXA. *See* Dual-energy x-ray absorptiometry
Dyslipidemias
  bile acid sequestrants for, 96t
  cholesterol absorption inhibitors for, 96t
  ezetimibe for, 96t
  fibrates for, 96t
  medications for, 95, 96t
  niacin for, 96t
  nicotinic acid for, 96t
  omega 3 fatty acids for, 96t
  PCSK9 inhibitors for, 96t
  primary, 94
  secondary, 95, 545
  statins for, 96t
  treatment of, 95

E
EABV. *See* Effective arterial blood volume
Ebert, Roger, 535
ECG. *See* Electrocardiography
ECT. *See* Electroconvulsive therapy
Ectopic inferior parathyroid gland, locations for, 515
Ectopic superior parathyroid gland, locations for, 515
ECV. *See* Effective circulating volume
Effective arterial blood volume (EABV), 226
Effective circulating volume (ECV), 226, 229
  baroreceptors and, 226, 227f
Eisenhower, Dwight D., 541
Electrocardiography (ECG), 71
Electroconvulsive therapy (ECT), 366–367

Electrolyte free water clearance, 240
Empty sella syndrome, 184–185
Endocrine case studies, 542–550
Endocrine disorders
    famous people with, 535–538, 535b
    OSA and, 504
    pancreatic neuroendocrine tumors associated
        with, 462
    sleep disorders and, 493
Endocrine toxicities, grade 4, 489
Endocrine tumors
    associated with MEN 1, 457
    surgery for, 523–526
Endocrinologist, roles and responsibilities of, 534
Endocrinology
    in Africa, 532–534
        training opportunities in, 534
    aging and, 473–486
    sleep and, 493–509, 508b
Endocrinopathies
    caused by immune checkpoint inhibitors, 487–492,
        491b
    rates of, 488t
    overall incidence of, 488
Endometrial cancer, 424
Endometrial health, treatment options for, 425
Energy balance, 103
Energy expenditure
    components of, 102
    obesity and, 102
    physical activity, 102
Enteral nutrition (EN), 64
Enteropancreatic tumors, in MEN 1, 456
Epidermal growth factor receptors, 146
Erb's palsy, 80
Erectile dysfunction, 404–412, 410b
Erection
    detumescence, 405
    disturbances in other sexual functions, 404
    hormonal aspects of, 404
    nervous system in, 404
    neurotransmitters, 405
    nocturnal penile tumescence, 407
    normal, 404
    vascular changes in, 404
Ergogenic aid, 254
Estradiol
    aging and, 477–478
    monitoring, 440
Estrogen
    during and after menopause, 434
    deficiency, 419
    excess, 251
    for female hypogonadism, 391
    in male, 413
    therapy, 124–125t
        contraindications for, 441
        laboratory values in, 440
        physical changes caused by, 440
        for postmenopausal women, 479–480, 484
Etelcalcetide, 150–152
Etomidate, 217, 277
Eunuchoid body habitus, 389
Euthyroid sick syndrome, 341–344, 343b, 490, 545
    as adaptive mechanism, 343
    causes of, 342
    central hypothyroidism *versus,* 341–342
    deiodinase enzymes, 342–343
    deiodinase function in, 343, 343f
    pathophysiology of, 342
    prognostic significance of, 343–344

Excessive growth, 251
    genetic syndromes associated with, 251–252
    hormonal causes of, 251
Exercise
    contraindications, 81
    GDM and, 81
    postpartum management and, 81
    sex hormones and, 474
    weight loss and, 105
    weight-bearing, 474
External genitalia development, 372
    determination, 373–374
    differentiation of, 374f
Extracellular fluid (ECF), 225
Eye disease, 305
Ezetimibe
    for dyslipidemia, 96t
    role of, 98

F
Factitious hypoglycemia, 89
Falls, 112
Familial combined hyperlipidemia (FCH), 94
Familial dysalbuminemic hyperthyroxinemia (FDH),
        219, 301
Familial dysbetalipoproteinemia (FDL), 94
Familial hirsutism, 428
Familial hypercholesterolemia (FH), 94, 542–543
Familial hyperchylomicronemia (FHC), 95
Familial hyperphosphatemic tumoral calcinosis, 113
Familial hypertriglyceridemia (FHT), 95
Familial hypocalciuric hypercalcemia (FHH), 150, 545
    primary hyperparathyroidism *versus,* 154
Familial low HDL, 95
Familial pheochromocytoma, 278, 278t
Familial short stature, 245
    distinguishing, 245, 246f
Fasting hypoglycemia, 87
Fasting plasma glucose levels, 10
Fat distribution, 100
Fat mass, menopause and, 475–476
FCH. *See* Familial combined hyperlipidemia
FDA. *See* Food and Drug Administration
FDH. *See* Familial dysalbuminemic hyperthyroxinemia
Fertility preservation, 443
Fetal acidemia, 80
Fetal growth
    DKA and, 75
    hyperglycemia and, 70
Fetal hypoxia, 80
Fetal surveillance, 80
Fetal thyroid function, 347
Fetal thyroid hormone, 347
Fetal well-being, 69–70, 74–75
FFA. *See* Free fatty acid
^{18}F-FDG PET/CT. *See* Fluorodeoxyglucose positron emission
        tomography/computed tomography
FGF 23. *See* Fibroblast growth factor 23
FH. *See* Familial hypercholesterolemia
FHC. *See* Familial hyperchylomicronemia
FHT. *See* Familial hypertriglyceridemia
Fibrates
    for dyslipidemias, 96t
    pregnancy and, 72
    role of, 98
Fibroblast growth factor 23 (FGF 23), 145
    calcium and, 145
    effects on calcium metabolism, 146–147
    phosphate and, 145
    vitamin D and, 145
Fine-needle aspiration (FNA), of thyroid nodule, 510

First trimester, 67
  diabetes management in, 68
FISH. *See* Fluorescence in situ hybridization
Fitzgerald, Ella, 537
Fludrocortisone, 284
Fluorescence in situ hybridization (FISH), 248
Fluoride, 167
Fluorodeoxyglucose positron emission tomography/computed tomography (^{18}F-FDG PET/CT)
  for adrenal pathology, 518
  for pheochromocytoma, 268
Fluvastatin, 96
FNA. *See* Fine-needle aspiration
Follicle-stimulating hormone (FSH), 500–501
Food and Drug Administration (FDA), 254
Foot ulcers, diabetic, 19
Foscarnet, 167
Fracture, prevention of, 127
Fragility fracture, 110
Franco, Juan Pedro, 539
FRAX risk assessment criteria, 111–113, 475
Free fatty acid (FFA), 67
  GDM and, 79
  macrosomia and, 79
Free water clearance, 239–240
  electrolyte, 240
  osmolar, 240
FSH. *See* Follicle-stimulating hormone (FSH)
Fuel metabolism, 67–76
Functional pancreatic neuroendocrine tumors
  imaging for, 524
  subtypes and syndromes of, 523
Functioning adrenocortical carcinomas, 275, 275f
Functioning prolactinoma, 190
Furosemide, 151t, 167
  mechanism of action, 151t

G

GAD. *See* Glutamic acid decarboxylase
Gaedel, Eddie, 536
Galactorrhea, in prolactin-secreting pituitary tumors, 203
Gamma-aminobutyric acid (GABA), 496
Gastric banding, 530, 528
Gastrinomas, 523
  clinical manifestations of, 463
  diagnosis of, 464
  localization of, 464
  malignant, treatment of, 464
  management of, 464
  in MEN 1, 456
  from pancreatic islet cells, 464
  surgical approach to, 524
Gastrointestinal disorders, 248
Gastrointestinal neuroendocrine tumors, 526b
Gastroparesis, 19
Gender dysphoria, 438–445
  in adults, 438
  gender incongruence and, 438
  transgender medicine and, 438
Gender expression, 439t
Gender identity, 438
Gender incongruence, 438–445
  gender dysphoria and, 438
  transgender medicine and, 438
Gender-affirming treatment, 438–445, 444b
  in elderly transgender, 442
  evaluation prior, 440
  indications for, 442
  legal issues in, 444
  in transmen, 441
  in transwomen, 440

Gender-fluid, 439t
Gender-nonbinary, 439t
Gender-nonconforming, 439t
General Tom Thumb, 536
Gestational diabetes mellitus (GDM)
  ACOG on, 76
  in Africa, 533
  causes of, 78
  complications of, 79
  contraceptive agents and, 84
  defined, 76
  diagnosis of, 76
  diet therapy for, 81
  exercise and, 81
  fetal complications of, 79–80
  fetal growth in, 79
  fetal surveillance in, 80
  FFAs and, 79
  glyburide and, 70–71
  insulin secretion in, 78–79
  insulin treatment of, 82
  lipids in, 79
  long-term sequelae of, 80–81
  medical therapy for, 81–82
  one-step approach to, 76–84
  postpartum management and, 82–83
  risks to the mother with, 79
  sulfonylureas in, 82
  triglycerides and, 79
  two-step approach, 76
Gestational transient thyrotoxicosis (GTT), 347–348
  Graves' disease from, 348
GFR. *See* Glomerular filtration rate
GH. *See* Growth hormone
Ghrelin
  defined, 102
  sleep deprivation on, 506
Giant prolactinoma, 206
Gigantism. *See also* Acromegaly
  diagnosis of, 209
  endocrine syndromes in, 209
  treatment of, 210
Glargine, 74
Glimepiride, 35
Glipizide, 35
Glomerular filtration rate (GFR), 229
  estimating, 158
GLP-1. *See* Glucagon-like peptide 1
Glucagon
  causing hypocalcemia, 167
  for hypoglycemia, 29–30
Glucagon-like peptide 1 (GLP-1), 64, 484
  receptor agonists, 34t, 35
Glucagonomas, 464, 523, 545
Glucagon-secreting pancreatic neuroendocrine tumor, 545
Glucocorticoid-induced osteoporosis, prevention and treatment of, 129
Glucocorticoid-remediable aldosteronism, 258, 262
Glucocorticoids
  for adrenal insufficiency, 284
  causing osteoporosis, 113
  growth pattern and, 251
  mechanism of action, 151t
  monitoring of, 113
  in nonclassic CAH, 295
  potencies of, 284t, 285
  stress dose, 285–286, 285t
Gluconeogenesis, 14
Glucose, 226–227
  for brain metabolism, 88
  circadian rhythm and, 503

Glucose *(Continued)*
  control, 69–70, 73
  hepatic, 78
  intolerance, 77, 250
  metabolism, abnormal
    CPAP for, 505–506
    with OSA, 505
    sleep abnormalities and, 505
  sleep-wake processes and, 503
  tolerance of, sleep deprivation in, 505
  24-hour profiles of, 498f
Glucose tolerance test
  ACOG criteria, 77t
  ADA criteria, 77t
Glutamic acid decarboxylase (GAD), 78
Glyburide
  GDM and, 70–71, 82
  pregnancy and, 70–71
Glycemia, in type 2 diabetes mellitus, 483
Glycemic control
  CSII improving, 43–44
  in diabetes mellitus, 20
    type 2, 31–32
Glycemic targets, 61b
  in critically ill, 61
  determination of, 32
  of non-critically ill patients, 61
  in pregnant patients, 61
Glycerol, 226–227
Glycine, 226–227
Glycoprotein hormones, 219
Glycoprotein-secreting pituitary tumors, 219–224, 222b
  differential diagnosis of, 219–220
  types of, 219
Glycosaminoglycans, 172
GnRH. *See* Gonadotropin-releasing hormone
GnRH-dependent (central) precocious puberty, 383–385
Goiter, 321–326
  defined, 321
  evaluation of, 321
  role of iodine in, 321
  simple nodular, 321
  toxic multinodular, 305
Goliath of Gath, 541
Gonadal dysfunction, 203
Gonadal dysgenesis, 376
  sex assignment in, 380
Gonadal failure, 389
Gonadal toxins, 389
Gonadectomy, in transgender, 443
Gonadotroph adenomas, 221–222
Gonadotropin
  deficiency, 182, 183
    treatment, 185
  for PCOS, 426
  release change from youth to adulthood, 500–501
Gonadotropin-dependent true precocious puberty, 543
Gonadotropinomas
  medical therapy for, 222
  presenting symptoms, 222, 222t
  treatment of, 222
Gonadotropin-releasing hormone (GnRH)
  agonists, 431
  mature, 382
  pulse generator, 419
Granulomatous disorders, in hypercalcemia, 547
Granulomatous hypophysitis, 196
Graves' disease, 453t, 535
  defined, 304
  GTT from, 348
  ¹³¹I ablation and, 308
  in postpartum period, 351

Graves' disease *(Continued)*
  pregnancy and, 348–349
    alternatives to, 351
    fetal risks, 348–349
    natural history of, 351
    treatment of, 349
Graves' ophthalmopathy, 513
Graves' orbitopathy, 308
Growth, 244b
  after pubertal growth spurt, 243
  charts, 246f, 247f, 248f
    appropriate, 244
    errors in, 243
    interpreting, 244
    physical examination and, 244
    radiologic imaging and, 244
  curve, 245
    abnormal, 244
  measurements, 244
  before pubertal growth spurt, 243–252
  variants, 252b
Growth disorders, 243–252
  excessive growth, 251
    genetic syndromes associated with, 251–252
    hormonal causes of, 251
    gastrointestinal disorders and, 248
    glucocorticoids and, 251
Growth hormone (GH), 253–256
  abuse, 255b
    in athletes, 255
    testing for, 255
  actions of, 253, 254t
  administration of, 254
  aging and, 255–256
  carcinomas, 223
  deficiency, 252b
    in adults, 254
    causes of, 249
    conditions associated with, 253
    diagnosis of, 249
    height prognosis and, 250
    idiopathic, 249
    IGF-1 and, 249
    laboratory evaluation for, 249
    signs and symptoms of, 253
    treatment of, 250
  defined, 253–256
  effects of, 253
  as ergogenic aid, 254
  excessive, 253
    characteristics of, 251
    clinical features of
      in adults, 208
      in children, 208
    OSA and, 504
  FDA-approved, 254
  human cadaver-derived, 254
  normal function of, 208
  peripheral tissues and, 208
  potential uses of, 254
  regulation of, 208, 253
  replacement of, for healthy elderly, 481
  secretion of, 253
  in sleep, 500
  supplementation of, 484
  testing, 249
  therapy, 250
    adverse effects of
      in adults, 255
      in athletes, 255
      in children, 255
    indications for, 250

Growth hormone *(Continued)*
   risks of, 250
    side effects of, 250
    for Turner's syndrome, 250
  24-hour profiles of, 498f
  use, 255b
Growth hormone (GH)-IGF-1 axis, with aging, 481
Growth hormone-releasing hormone (GHRH), 482
Growth hormone-secreting pituitary tumors, 208–212
  causes of, 209
  MRI of, 210
  size of, 210
GTT. *See* Gestational transient thyrotoxicosis
Gynecomastia, 413–416, 415b, 416b, 536
  bilateral, 413
  causes of, 413
  defined, 413
  drugs causing, 414, 414t
  evaluation for, 414
  extragonadal tumors and, 414
  hormonal therapy for, 416
  laboratory tests, 415
  painful, 413
  as palpable discrete button, 413
  pathophysiology of, 413
  patient history of, 415b
  physical examination of, 414, 415
  regression of, 415
  significance of, 413
  during stages of life, 413
  testicular tumors causing, 414

H
Hall, Gary, Jr., 537
HAMAs. *See* Heterophile antimouse antibodies
Hamilton, Scott, 536
Hatton, Rondo "The Creeper, " 537
hCG. *See* Human chorionic gonadotropin
HDL. *See* High-density lipoproteins
Headaches, 188
Height. *See also* Short stature
  CAH and, 295
  familial, 245
  GH deficiency and, 250
  measurement of, 243
    children, 243
    infant, 243
    midparental, 244
    recording, 243
Heparin, 167
Hepatic glucose production, 78
Hepatic lipase, 93t
Hepatotoxicity, 307
Hermaphroditism
  defined, 398
  true, 379
Heterophile antimouse antibodies (HAMAs), 302
Heterozygous familial hypercholesterolemia, 542–543
Hewitt, Jay, 537
HHM. *See* Humoral hypercalcemia of malignancy
HHS. *See* Hyperglycemic hyperosmolar state
High-density lipoproteins (HDL), 92
  familial low, 95
  function of, 93
High-oxalate foods, 175t
Hirsutism, 213, 422, 427–432, 429b
  acromegaly and, 429
  antiandrogens and, 431
  CAH and, 420, 428–429, 428f
  causes of, 427
  conditions resulting in, 427
  cosmetic measures for, 431

Hirsutism *(Continued)*
  Cushing's syndrome and, 429
  defined, 427
  diagnosis of, 431b
  evaluation of, 429
  familial, 428
  GnRH agonists for, 431
  history in, 429–430
  hypothyroidism and, 429
  idiopathic, 428
  laboratory tests for, 430
    interpretation of, 430
  medications causing, 429
  oral contraceptive pills and, 431
  PCOS and, 423
  physical examination in, 430
  prolactinomas and, 429
  topical agent for, 431
  treatment of, 430–431
Holtorf, K., 436
Homeostatic Model Assessment of Insulin Resistance (HOMA-IR)
  score, 10
Homocystinuria, 251
Hormone replacement therapy (HRT), 126
  dosing, 435–436
  during menopause, 434–435
  references, 436–437
  route of, 435
HRT. *See* Hormone replacement therapy
Hudson, Walter, 540
Human chorionic gonadotropin (hCG), 345, 377
  beta-subunit of, 345–346
Humoral hypercalcemia of malignancy (HHM), 161–163, 163b
  cancer causing, 161
  diagnostic features of, 161
  differential diagnosis of, 162t
  hypercalcemia and, 156t
  primary hyperparathyroidism *versus*, 156
  prognosis for, 163
  treatment of, 162–163t, 162–163
  types of, 161
Humoral syndromes, 467–468
Hybrid closed-loop insulin delivery system, 45
Hydralazine, 71
Hydrochlorothiazide, 237
Hydrocortisone, 284t, 294
3-hydroxy-3-methyl-glutaryl-coenzyme A reductase, 93t
5-hydroxyindoleacetic acid (5-HIAA), carcinoid syndrome and, 468, 468t, 469
21-hydroxylase, 289, 377
  deficiency, 387
  gene encodes for, 290
  heterozygote carriers of, 290
  phenotype for, 290
Hyperadrenergic spells, differential diagnosis of, 267
Hyperaldosteronism, defined, 519
Hyperandrogenic anovulation, 420
  tumors causing, 420
Hyperandrogenism, 423
Hypercalcemia, 149b, 144–152. *See also* Humoral hypercalcemia of malignancy
  with cancer, 149
  causes of, 148, 149b, 150
  classification of, 144
  defined, 144
  ECG changes in, 162
  familial hypocalciuric, 545
  granulomatous disorders in, 547
  incidence of, 144
  lithium and, 152
  mechanisms and causes of, 147t
  signs and symptoms of, 144

Hypercalcemia *(Continued)*
 therapy for, 150, 151t
  mechanisms of action of, 150, 151t
 of unknown cause, diagnostic approach for, 161, 162f
Hypercalcemic crisis, 161
Hypercalciuria
 absorptive, 170
  phosphorus in, 173
  PTH in, 173
 conditions associated with, 170
 defined, 170
 idiopathic, 170
  etiology of, 172
  forms of, 173, 173t
  pathophysiology of, 172
 renal leak, 173
 serum calcium and, 172
 sodium and, 172
Hypercholesterolemia, 96, 97t
 heterozygous familial, 542–543
Hyperemesis gravidarum, thyrotoxicosis related to, 347–348
Hypergastrinemia, 456
Hyperglycemia, 9–10, 14, 61–66
 causes of, 16
 defined, 64
 diabetes medications associated with, 16
 enteral nutrition for, 64
 fetal growth and, 70
 P_{Na} correction factor, 238
 prevention of, 17
 rebound, 29
 risk factors for, 61
 risk of, 16
 signs and symptoms of, 16
 steroid-induced, 64
 total parenteral nutrition for, 64
 treatment of, 17, 64, 64b
Hyperglycemic crisis, 532
Hyperglycemic hyperosmolar state (HHS), 15
 development of, 15
 diagnosis of, 16
 DKA *versus*, 15, 16t
 insulin therapy for, 16
 symptoms and signs of, 15
 treatment of, 16
Hypergonadotropic hypogonadism, 543
 amenorrhea with, 419
 causes of, 389
Hyperinsulinemia
 pancreatic islet cell, 89
 PCOS and, 427–428
Hyperinsulinemic hypoglycemia, 543
Hyperkalemia, in adrenal insufficiency, 281–282
Hypernatremia
 approach to, 236t
 brain adapting to, 232
 causes of, 236t
 patient with, 235
 symptoms and signs of, 231
Hyperoxaluria
 defined, 173
 nephrolithiasis and, 173–174
Hyperparathyroidism, 153–160, 157b
 associated with MEN 2A, 459
 asymptomatic
  monitoring of, 158
  parathyroidectomy for, 158
  surgical treatment of, 158
 laboratory tests for, 155, 156t
 parathyroid tumor, 157
 persistent, 516

Hyperparathyroidism *(Continued)*
 primary, 153, 546
  age and, 153
  anatomic alterations in, 153
  causes of, 153
  CKD and, 154
  classic radiographic findings in, 154–155
  diagnosis of, 153
  differential diagnosis of, 154, 155
  familial hypocalciuric hypercalcemia *versus,* 154
  in MEN 1, 455
  normocalcemic, 159
  parathyroidectomy for, 513–514
  pathophysiologic changes in, 155
  prevalence of, 153
  surgery for, 514
  symptoms and signs of, 154, 155t
  therapeutic options for, 158–159
  treatment of, 514
 PTH assay for, 157
 recurrent, 516
 secondary, 155–156
 tertiary
  pathophysiologic changes in, 156
  surgery for, indications for, 516
Hyperpigmentation, 213–214
Hyperplastic parathyroid glands, therapy for, 456
Hyperprolactinemia, 419
Hypertension, 101f
Hyperthyroidism, 304–310, 309b
 in Africa, 533
 aging and, 483
 apathetic, 305
 autonomy in, 304
 causes of, 304
  rare, 305
 causing eye disease, 305
 country of residence significant in, 348
 fetal, 349
 ^{123}I scan of, 352
 in immune checkpoint inhibitors, 490
 iodine for, 307, 350
 mood disorders and, 360t
 neonatal, 349
  mortality rate of, 349
 pregnancy and, 347
  diagnostic approach, 348
  risk of, 348
  risk to, 348
  treatment, 349
 subclinical, 349, 360
 surgery for, 306–307
  preparation for, 512
 thyroid antibody testing for, 305–306
 thyroidectomy in, 512
 thyrotoxicosis *versus,* 304
 treatment of, 306, 351
Hypertriglyceridemia, 98
Hyperuricosuria, 174
Hypoalbuminemia, 164
Hypocalcemia, 164–169, 168b
 affecting cardiac function, 165–167
 autoimmune disorders associated with, 167
 cancer and, 167
 causes of, 164–165
 defining, 164
 differential diagnosis of, 166t
 drugs causing, 167
 in intensive care settings, 167
 laboratory tests for, 165
 ophthalmologic findings in, 167

Hypocalcemia *(Continued)*
  physical signs, 165
  radiographic findings of, 165
  symptoms of, 165
  treatment of, 167–168
Hypocalciuric hypercalcemia, familial, 545
Hypoglycemia
  alcohol causing, 90
  artifactual causes of, 88
  autoimmune syndromes and, 90
  causes of, 87
  childhood, 89
  clinical symptoms of, 87
  defined, 87–90
  drugs causing, 90
  evaluation for, 462–463
  factitious, 89
  fasting, 87
  food intake and, 87
  glucagon for, 29–30
  glucose levels in, 462
  hyperinsulinemic, 88, 543
  insulinomas and, 457
  management options for, 89
  postprandial or reactive, 87
  pregnancy and, 70, 74
  rebound hyperglycemia in, 29
  symptoms of, 462
  treatment of, 29
  type 1 diabetes mellitus and, 74
  unawareness, 17
  underlying medical illness, attributed to, 90
Hypoglycemic disorders, 87–91, 90b
Hypogonadism, 453t
  congenital hypogonadotropic, 397
  diagnosis of, 389
  in girls, 391
  hypergonadotropic, 389, 543
  hypogonadotropic, 389
    amenorrhea with, 419
    idiopathic, 418–419, 546
    major congenital causes of, 418–419
  laboratory workup for, 394, 396f
  male, 393–403
    affecting bone architecture, 397–398
    clinical symptoms in, 397
    defined, 393
    determining, 397
    diagnosis of, 398
    prevalence of, 478
    treatment of, 391
  manifestations of
    in early adulthood, 393
    in mid-to-late adulthood, 393
  peripubertal, 393
  pituitary adenomas and, 397
  primary, 222, 394–395
    acquired causes of, 396
    aging and, 396
    congenital causes of, 394–395
    laboratory tests for, 222
    sperm production in, 400
  secondary, 394, 395f
    causes of, 397
    sperm production in, 400
  treatment of, 398–399
  in utero, 393
Hypogonadotropic hypogonadism, 389
  amenorrhea caused, 419
  idiopathic, 418–419, 546
  major congenital causes of, 418–419

Hypokalemia, 258
Hypomagnesemia, 165
Hyponatremia
  adrenal insufficiency and, 231, 281–282
  approach to, 233t
  brain adapting to, 231
  causes of, 233t
  hypothyroidism and, 231
  patients with, 232
  symptoms and signs of, 231
  translocation, 238–239
  vasopressin receptor antagonists for, 238
  volume assessment in, 232
Hypoparathyroidism, 165, 453t
  with immune checkpoint inhibitors, 490
  primary, 544
Hypophosphatasia, 113
Hypophysitis, 184, 196
  angiotensin-converting enzyme (ACE) in, 199
  antipituitary antibody in, 199
  clinical presentation of, 198
  in immune checkpoint inhibitors, 489
  immunoglobulin G4 in, 199
  immunotherapeutic agents causing, 199
  ipilimumab-induced, 199–200, 200f
  pituitary macroadenomas *versus*, 198t
  primary
    autoimmune disorders associated with, 197
    natural history of, 199
    and treatment options for, 199
    types of, 196–197
  secondary, 197, 197t
Hypopituitarism, 182
  diagnosis of, 183
  life expectancy and, 186–187
  magnetic resonance imaging in, 184
  organic, 183t
Hypopnea, 503
Hypospadias, 376
Hypothalamic amenorrhea, 419, 542
  diagnosis of, 419
  treatment options for, 419
Hypothalamic-pituitary-adrenal (HPA) axis, 215
  aging and, 482
Hypothyroidism, 311–314, 312b, 453t, 543
  abnormal intellectual development and, 353
  adrenal insufficiency and, 231
  in Africa, 533
  aging and, 483
  causes of, 311, 311f
  central, 547
  defined, 311
  diagnosis of
    in acutely ill inpatients, 312
    in outpatient setting, 312
  hirsutism and, 429
  hyponatremia and, 231
  in immune checkpoint inhibitors, 489
  laboratory tests during, 312
  levothyroxine and, 361–362
  liothyronine and, 361–362
  LT_4, 313
  mood disorders and, 360t
  myxedema *versus*, 314
  neuropsychiatric symptoms of, 365–366
  OSA and, 504
  overtreatment of, 313
  physical examination in, 311
  precocious puberty and, 387
  pregnancy and, 352
  presentation of, 312

Hypothyroidism *(Continued)*
  prevalence of, 311
  primary, 313
  psychiatric disorders and, 359
  surgery for, 313
    emergent, 313
  symptoms of, 311, 313
  treatment of, 312

I
^{123}I scan, 352
^{131}I ablation
  ATD pretreatment, 308
  Breastfeeding and, 308, 352
  for Graves' disease, 308
  pregnancy and, 308
Ibandronate, 124–125t
ICF. *See* Intracellular fluid
ICSI. *See* Intracytoplasmic sperm injection
Idiopathic hirsutism, 428
Idiopathic hyperaldosteronism (IHA), 258, 260
  APA *versus*, 260
  CT of, 260–261
  management of, 262–263
  MRI of, 260–261
  pharmacologic options, 262
  symptoms of, 258
Idiopathic hypercalciuria (IH), 170
  etiology of, 172
  forms of, 173, 173t
  pathophysiology of, 172
Idiopathic hypogonadotropic hypogonadism (IHH), 417, 546
Idiopathic postprandial syndrome, 87
Idiopathic short stature, 251
IGF-1. *See* Insulin-like growth factor-1
IH. *See* Idiopathic hypercalciuria
IHA. *See* Idiopathic hyperaldosteronism
IHH. *See* Idiopathic hypogonadotropic hypogonadism
Illiescu, Adriana Emilia, 540
IIT. *See* Intensive insulin therapy
I-MIBG ablation, for pheochromocytoma, 269
Immune checkpoint inhibitors (ICPIs)
  classification of, 491
  endocrinopathies caused by, 487–492, 491b
  free T$_4$ in, 489
  hyperthyroidism in, 490
  hypothyroidism in, 490
  immune-related adverse events in, 487
  indications for, 487
  mechanisms of action of, 487, 488f
  pituitary problem in, 489
  specific endocrine disorders with, 487
  thyroid abnormalities in, 490
  for thyroid cancer, 491
  thyroid disorders with, 489, 490
  in United States, 487
Immune-related adverse events (IRAEs)
  in cancer treatment, 491
  endocrine, rates of, 488
  with ICPIs, 487
Impotence
  antihypertensives and, 405
  causes of, 405
  defined, 404
  drugs and, 405
  endocrine causes of, 405
  future treatments, 410–411
  health implications of, 410
  laboratory assessment for, 406
  lifestyle and, 405
  medical treatment, 407

Impotence *(Continued)*
  modalities of, 410
  organic, 406t
  physical examination in, 406
  prevalence of, 404
  prolactin in, 406
  psychogenic, 406t
  "stuttering, " 405
  surgical procedures for, 407
  therapeutic options for, 407
  treatment options for, 408t
In utero hypogonadism, 393
Incidentalomas, 518
  CAH and, 292
Incretin
  mimetics, 35
  in weight loss surgery, 530
Inferior petrosal sinus sampling (IPSS), 216
Inflammatory bowel disease, 248
Insulin, 103
  basal, 34t
    coverage, 22
    dose selection of, 62
    with MDI, 22
    preparations, 23
    timing, 24
  bolus
    coverage, 22
    with MDI, 22
    preparations, 22–23
    timing, 23–24
  circadian rhythm and, 503
  continuous subcutaneous, 65
  correctional, 63t
  in CSII device, 43
  for DKA, 15
  dose adjustment of, 62
  for GDM, 82
  for HHS, 16
  impaired secretion in GDM, 78–79
  initiation of, 37–39
  intensification, 39
  intravenous infusion
    adjusting, 62
    defined, 62
    rate of, 62
    total daily dose, 62
    transitioning off, 62
  nutritional dosing of, 63t
  pharmacodynamics of, 23t
  prandial dose of, 62
  pump, 24, 24t, 48–49b
    benefits of, 25, 25f
    candidate for, 44
    challenges using, 44
    initial basal rate for, 28
    initiation of, 24–25
    limitations of, 25
    nighttime basal rate adjustments, 28–29
    pregnancy and, 74
  rapid-acting, 74
  resistance, 10
  sleep-wake processes and, 503
  sliding-scale for, 62–64
  titration of, 37–39
Insulin pen, 46
Insulin secretion rates (ISR), 24-hour profiles of, 498f
Insulin-like growth factor-1 (IGF-1), 383
  acromegaly and, 209
  GH deficiency and, 249
  serum level of, 249

Insulinomas, 89, 523
  defined, 462
  diagnostic criteria for, 463, 463t
  hypoglycemia associated with, treatment of, 457
  localization of, 463
  in MEN 1, 456
  surgical approach for, 524
  treatment, 463
Intensive insulin therapy (IIT), 30b
  basal insulin coverage *versus* bolus insulin coverage, 22, 22f
  candidates for, 21
  components of, 21
  risks of, 22
  for type 1 diabetes mellitus, 23
Interferons, 146
Interleukins, 146
Intersex, 439t
Interstitial fluid (ISF), 225
Intraabdominal testicular tissue, 378
Intracavernosal injections, 407, 408t
  side effects of, 409–410
Intracellular fluid (ICF), 225
Intracytoplasmic sperm injection (ICSI), 400
Intraoperative parathyroid hormone (ioPTH) assay, in parathyroid
    surgery, 515
Intrathoracic (substernal) goiter, 513
Intraurethral alprostadil, 408t
Intraurethral injections, 409
  side effects of, 409–410
Intravenous insulin infusion
  adjusting, 62
  defined, 62
  rate of, 62
  total daily dose, 62
  transitioning off, 62
Iodine
  deficiency, 533
  in goiters, 321
  for hyperthyroidism, 307
  in pregnancy
    contraindications, 350
    insufficient intake, 346
Ipilimumab-induced hypophysitis, 199–200, 200f
  biopsy in, 200
  natural history of, 200
  treatment of, 200
IPSS. *See* Inferior petrosal sinus sampling
ISF. *See* Interstitial fluid
Islet beta cell hyperfunction, 88
Isoniazid, 167
Izumi, Shigechiyo, 540

J
James, Doris, 540
Jennings, Waylon, 537
Jet lag, 502–503
Jinlian, Zeng, 539
Jod-Basedow phenomenon, 305
Johnson, Nicole, 537
JUPITER trial. *See* Justification for the Use of Statins in Primary
    Prevention: An Intervention Trial Evaluating Rosuvastatin
    (JUPITER) trial
Justification for the Use of Statins in Primary Prevention: An In-
    tervention Trial Evaluating Rosuvastatin (JUPITER) trial, 97

K
Kallmann's syndrome, 389, 546
Karyotype, 248
Karyotyping, 377
Kennedy, John F., 541
Keratinocytes, 146

Ketoacidosis, hyperglycemic hyperosmolar state and, 15
Ketoconazole, 167, 217
Ketones, in DKA, 15
Ketosis-prone diabetes, 9
Ketosis-prone type 2 diabetes mellitus, 532
Kidneys
  calcium and, 172
  CaSR in, 146
  salt and, 229
  water and, 229
Kidney stones
  asymptomatic, 178
  chemical precursors, 171
  composition of, 170
  conditions associated with, 170
  defined, 170
  diagnosis of, 175–176
  formation of, 171
    diet in, 174
    inhibitors, 171
    promoters, 172
  frequency of, 170, 171f
  history in, 175
  hyperuricosuria and, 174
  nephrocalcin and, 172
  pathophysiologic factors influencing, 171
  physical examination in, 175
  radiographic tests of, 177
  risk for, 170
  size 1 to 2 cm, 178
  size 3 cm or larger, 178
  symptomatic, 178
  symptoms and signs of, 174–175
  therapeutic approach to, 176
  urinalysis and, 176
  urinary crystals in, 176–177
  urinary pH and, 174
Kiel, Richard, 535
King David, 541
Klinefelter's syndrome, 251, 543
  defined, 389–390
Knorr, Arthur, 540
Kosen, Sultan, 539
Kussmaul respirations, 14

L
Lactation, maternal thyroid status and, 351
LADA. *See* Latent autoimmune diabetes of adulthood
Laparoscopic adrenalectomy
  for pheochromocytoma, 268
  techniques for, 519
Laparoscopic bariatric procedures, 530
Latent autoimmune diabetes of adulthood (LADA), 9, 78
LCAT. *See* Lecithin cholesterol acyl transferase
LDL. *See* Low-density lipoprotein
Lecithin cholesterol acyl transferase (LCAT), 93, 93t
Leptin
  deficiency, 102
  defined, 102
  sleep deprivation and, 506
Letrozole, for PCOS, 425–426
Levothyroxine (LT₄), 312
  for depression, 367
  for differentiated thyroid cancer, 329
  hypothyroidism and, 361–362
  pharmacologic doses of, 367
  during pregnancy, 354
  symptomatic euthyroid subjects, 362
Leydig cell, 372
  hypoplasia, 377
LH. *See* Luteinizing hormone

Lifestyle modification
  impotence and, 405
  for PCOS, 424
  for type 2 diabetes mellitus, 32–33
Liothyronine (LT$_3$), 313
  clinical antidepressant response, 366
  for depression, 367
  hypothyroidism and, 361–362
Lipids, 92–98
  disorders, 92–99
    causes of, 95b
    treatment of, 98b
  in fetal growth, 67–68
  in GDM, 79
Lipoprotein(a), 94
  role of assessment of, 98
Lipoproteins, 92
  in bloodstream, 92
  lipase, 93t
  metabolism of, 92, 93f, 93t
Liraglutide, 107
Lispro, in pregnancy, 74
Lithium
  affecting pituitary-thyroidal axis, 364
  goiter and, 365
  hypercalcemia and, 152
Lithium carbonate, 364t
Liver
  disease, 165
  metastases, 525
Local osteolytic hypercalcemia (LOH), 161
  cancer and, 161
LOH. See Local osteolytic hypercalcemia
Longevity, increased, interventions and, 477
Long-term sequelae, of GDM, 80–81
Loop of Henle, 225
Lorcaserin, 107
Lovastatin, 96
Low-calorie diets, 104
Low-density lipoprotein (LDL), 92
  function of, 92
  metabolism of, 92
  reduction in, 103
Low-dose cosyntropin stimulation test, 282
Luteinizing hormone (LH), 500–501
17, 20-lyase, 377
Lymph node metastases, in differentiated thyroid
    cancer, 511
Lymphocytic hypophysitis, 196
Lymphomas, 547
Lyon, Mary, 372
Lyon hypothesis, 372

M
Macrosomia
  diabetes and, 70, 80f
  FFA and, 79
  triglycerides and, 79
Macrovascular disease, in diabetes mellitus, 20
Magar, Khagendra Thapa, 539
Magnesium, 171
Magnetic resonance imaging (MRI)
  for adrenal pathology, 518
  of aldosterone-producing adenoma, 260–261
  of Cushing's syndrome, 216
  of GH-secreting pituitary tumors, 210
  of hypopituitarism, 184
  of idiopathic hyperaldosteronism, 260–261
  of pheochromocytoma, 268
  in puberty disorders, 385
Malabsorptive surgery, 528, 529f

Male hypogonadism, 393–403
  affecting bone architecture, 397–398
  clinical symptoms in, 397
  defined, 393
  determining, 397
  diagnostic tests for, 398
  laboratory tests for, 398
Malignant gastrinomas, 464
Malignant pheochromocytomas, 277
  clinical features of, 278
  localization of, 278
  prognosis for, 279
  treatment of, 269, 279
Malignant pituitary tumors, 223
Malnutrition-related diabetes mellitus (MRDM), 532
Mannitol, 226–227
MAO inhibitors. See Monoamine oxidase (MAO) inhibitors
Marfan's syndrome, 251
Maternal-Fetal Medicine Units Network, 345–346
Matrix Gla protein, 146
Maturity-onset diabetes of the young (MODY), 78
Mbuti pygmies, 539
McCrary, Benny, 540
McCrary, Billy, 540
McCune-Albright syndrome, 210t, 385–387
  treatment of, 387
Meal replacements, 104
Mediastinal adenopathy, 239–240
Medullary thyroid cancer (MTC), 332–333, 333b, 549
  associated with MEN 2A, 458
    treatment of, 459
  defined, 332
  genetic syndromes associated with, 332
  preoperative evaluation of, 332–333
  staging of, 332, 333t
  surgical management for, 333, 511
  symptoms of, 458–459
  treatment of, 333
Meglitinides, 36
Melanocortin, 102
Melanocyte-stimulating hormone (MSH), 281
Melanopsin, 497
Melatonin, in circadian rhythms, 498f, 499
MEN syndromes. See Multiple endocrine neoplasia (MEN) syndromes
Menarche, 382
Menopause, 433–437, 435b, 436b
  in abdominal obesity, 476
  androgen supplementation for, 436
  bone health and, 474
  bone mineral loss and, 474
  diagnosis of, 433
  estrogen during and after, 434
  HRT during, 434–435
  male, 436
  PCOS affecting, 424
  physiologic changes during, 434
  references, 436–437
  symptoms of, 433
    duration of, 433
    management of, 436
    severity of, 433
    timing of, 433
Metabolic acidosis, 14
Metabolic syndrome, 10–11, 94
Metanephrines, OSA in, 504
Metformin, 410
  adverse effects of, 33
  for PCOS, 426
  pregnancy and, 70–71, 82
  for type 1 diabetes mellitus, 29
  for type 2 diabetes mellitus, 483

Methadone, 364t
Methimazole (MMI), 306
  breast-feeding and, 351
  placenta and, 347
    pregnancy, 349–350
Methylprednisolone, 151t
Metyrapone, 217, 277
Microsurgical testicular sperm extraction (micro-TESE), 400
Microvascular disease, in diabetes mellitus, 17
Mifepristone, 217
Mihavecz, Andreas, 540
Milk alkali syndrome, 549
Mineralocorticoid hypertension, differential diagnosis of, 258
Minimally invasive parathyroidectomy (MIP), 514
Minimally invasive radio-guided parathyroidectomy (MIRP),
    514–515
Minnoch, Jon Brower, 539
MIP. *See* Minimally invasive parathyroidectomy
MIRP. *See* Minimally invasive radio-guided parathyroidectomy
Mitotane, 217, 276
  adrenal function and, 276–277
  endocrine effects of, 277
MMI. *See* Methimazole
Modified radical neck dissection, 511
MODY. *See* Maturity-onset diabetes of the young
Monoamine oxidase (MAO) inhibitors, 365
Monogenic diabetes, 10
Monoglycerides, 93–94
Mood disorders, 360t*See also* Psychiatric disorders
  hyperthyroidism and, 360t
  hypothyroidism and, 360t
Moore, Mary Tyler, 535
Morrison, Adam, 535
Motivational interviewing, 103
MRI. *See* Magnetic resonance imaging
MSH. *See* Melanocyte-stimulating hormone
MTC. *See* Medullary thyroid cancer
Mucocutaneous candidiasis, treatment of, 453–454
Multiglandular parathyroid disease, 515
Multinodular goiter, 321
Multiple births, for single gestation, 540
Multiple endocrine neoplasia (MEN) syndromes, 150,
    455–461
  clinical presentations of, 460
  defined, 455
  prognoses of, 460
  type 1, 89, 210t, 458b
    associated gastrinomas, 456
    causes of, 457–458
    defined, 455
    diagnosis of, 455
    endocrine tumors associated with, 457
    enteropancreatic tumors in, 456
    hyperplasia of parathyroid glands affected by, 456
    incidence of, 455
    neuroendocrine tumors associated with, 457
    pancreatic islet cells in, neoplastic transformation
      of, 456
    pancreatic neuroendocrine tumors in, 524
    pituitary adenomas in, 457
    pituitary tumors in, 457
    primary hyperparathyroidism in, 455
    screening for, 458
  type 2A, 458, 460b
    defined, 455
    genetic basis for, 459
    hyperparathyroidism associated with, 459
    incidence of, 458
    MTC associated with, 458
    pheochromocytomas in, 459
    treatment of, 459–460

Multiple endocrine neoplasia (MEN) syndromes *(Continued)*
  type 2B, 458, 460b
    causes of, 460
    comprises of, 460
    defined, 455
    findings in, 460
    incidence of, 458
    mortality rate in, 460
    screening for, 460
    treatment of, 460
  type 4
    defined, 455
    description of, 460
Muresan, Gheorghe, 536
Musters, Pauline, 539
Myxedema, hypothyroidism *versus,* 314
Myxedema coma
  clinical manifestations of, 337–338, 337f
  defined, 337
  development of, 337
  diagnosis of, 338
  laboratory abnormalities in, 338
  scoring system, 338–339t
  treatment of, 339–340, 339t

N
Naltrexone plus bupropion sustained-release (SR), 107
NAMS. *See* North American Menopause Society
Nasal testosterone gel, 399t
Natal male/female, 439t
National Institutes of Health (NIH), 76
Near-total thyroidectomy, 510–511
Neck dissection, 511
Neonatal hyperthyroidism, 349
  fetal hyperthyroidism and, 349
Nephrocalcin, 171
  kidney stones and, 172
Nephrocalcinosis, 170
Nephrolithiasis, 170–180
  causes of, 170
  defined, 170
  drug therapy
    oral, 177t
    special considerations in, 178
  hyperoxaluria and, 173
  normocalciuric calcium, 170
  prevalence and etiology of, 172b
  thiazide diuretics for, 178
  treatment of, 176b
Neuroendocrine tumors (NETs), 467
  associated with MEN 1, 457
  liver metastases from, surgery for, 525
  metastatic, systemic therapy for, 525–526
Neurotransmitters, 405
Neutral protamine Hagodorn (NPH), 23
Niacin
  deficiency, 467
  for dyslipidemias, 96t
  role of, 98
NICE-SUGAR study. *See* Normoglycemia in Intensive Care
    Evaluation and Surviving Using Glucose Algorithm
    Regulation (NICE-SUGAR) study
Nighttime basal rate adjustments, 28–29
NIH. *See* National Institutes of Health
Nikzaban, Nik, 540
Nitric oxide (NO), 404
Nivolumab, 487
Nocturnal penile tumescence, 407
Nonendocrine diseases, 245
Nonendocrine toxicities, grade 4, 489
Nonexercise activity thermogenesis (NEAT), 102

Nonfunctional adenomas
    endocrine complications in, 192
    follow up of, 191
    hereditary, 190
    medical therapies for, 191
    presentation of, 188–190
    radiation therapy for, 192
    risks of regrowth, 192
    transsphenoidal surgery for, 191
    treatment options for persistent/recurrent, 192
    types of, 190
Nonfunctioning pituitary tumors, 188–195, 194b
    natural history of, 191
    treatment of, 191
Noninsulinoma pancreatogenous hypoglycemia syndrome
    (NIPHS), 89
Non-islet cell tumor hypoglycemia (NICTH), 90
Nonpancreatic GI neuroendocrine tumors, 524
Nonproliferative diabetic retinopathy (NPDR), 18
Non-rapid eye movement (NREM) sleep, 493–494
    nervous system in, 495–496
Nonthyroidal illness syndrome (NTIS), 341, 490, 545
Noonan's syndrome, 248
Norethindrone, 84
Normocalciuric calcium nephrolithiasis, 170
Normoglycemia in Intensive Care Evaluation and Surviving Using
    Glucose Algorithm Regulation (NICE-SUGAR) study, 61
North American Menopause Society (NAMS), 434–435
NREM sleep. *See* Non-rapid eye movement (NREM) sleep

O

OATP. *See* Organic anion transporting polypeptide
Obesity, 100–108, 104b
    abdominal, 476
    abnormal genes causing, 102
    adverse health consequences of, 100
    antiobesity pharmacotherapy for, 105
    assessment of, 100
    BMI in, 527
    defined, 100–108, 527
    diet and, 104
    disease model of, 101
    economic consequences of, 100
    energy expenditure and, 102
    hyperandrogenic anovulation and, 420–421
    medications for, 104–105
    nonsurgical treatment of, 527
    OSA and, 504
    PCOS and, 423
    prevalence of, 100–101, 103
    psychological complications of, 100
    sarcopenic, 473
    surgery for, indications for, 527
    treatment of, 103
Obstructive sleep apnea (OSA)
    abnormal glucose metabolism with, 505
    catecholamines and, 504
    CPAP in, 506
    endocrine diseases and, 504
    of GH excess, 504
    metanephrines and, 504
    PCOS and, 424
    prevalence of, 504
    sleep deprivation and, 504
    sleep disordered breathing and, 503
    testosterone in, 506, 506t
    of thyroid hormone deficiency, 504
OGTT. *See* Oral glucose tolerance test
1, $_2$5-(OH)$_2$ vitamin D (calcitriol), 168
100-g 3-hour oral glucose tolerance test, 76
ONJ. *See* Osteonecrosis of jaw

Ophthalmoplegia, 189
Oral contraceptives
    GDM and, 84
    hirsutism and, 431
Oral glucose tolerance test (OGTT), 8
    100-g 3-hour, 76
    75-g 2-hour, 76
Organic anion transporting polypeptide (OATP), 367
Organic impotence, 406t
Orlistat, 104
    dose of, 107
    side effects of, 107
OSA. *See* Obstructive sleep apnea
Osmolality, 226–227
    evaluating, 227
Osmolar free water clearance, 240
Osmoles, 226–227
Osteoarthritic pain, bisphosphonate therapy, 142
Osteogenesis imperfecta, 113
Osteomalacia, 134–139, 138b
    biochemical abnormalities in, 137
    causes of, 134
    conditions associated with, 135–136, 136t
    defined, 134
    histologic features of, 137
    important facts, 134
    radiographic findings with, 137
    signs and symptoms of, 136
    therapy for, 137–138
Osteonecrosis of jaw (ONJ), 126
    bisphosphonate and, 125
    bisphosphonate therapy and, 142
Osteopetrosis, 113
Osteopontin, 146
Osteoporosis, 109–115, 113b
    defined, 110
    diagnosis of, 110
    glucocorticoids cause, 113
    management, 123–131, 130f, 131b
        algorithm, 130f
        benefits of, 128
        BMD loss during, 129
        high-risk patients in, 128–131
        low-/ moderate-risk patients in, 128
        nonpharmacologic measures for, 123–128
        pharmacologic therapy for, 124
            BMD changes in, 129
            combination, 127–128
            drug holiday in, 128–129
            FDA-approved, 124–125t, 124–125
            optimal duration of, 128–131
        risks of, 128
        treatment failure to, 129
    in men, 112
    risk factors for, 110, 112
    screening, 443
    testosterone for, 127
Osteoporotic fractures
    complications of, 110
    factors contributing to, 110
Osteoprotegerin, 124
Osteosarcoma, 143
Overbasalization, 39
Overbeck, Carla, 537
Overt diabetes, 77t
Overweight
    assessment of, 100
    defined, 100–108
Ovotesticular DSD, 379
    sex assignment in, 380
Oxalates, 175t

P

Paget's disease of bone, 140–143, 143b, 549
  bones involved in, 140
  causes of, 140
  complications of, 142–143
  defined, 140
  diagnosis of, 140, 141f
  differential diagnosis of, 140
  histologic appearance of, 140–141
  imaging for, 141
  laboratory tests for, 141
  medications for, 142, 142t
    goals of, 142
    indications of, 142
    side effects of, 142
  osteosarcoma risk in, 143
  presentation of, 140
  radiologic appearance of, 140–141
Painless thyroiditis, 317
Palmar creases, 213–214
Pamidronate, 151t
Pancreas, 523–526, 526b
Pancreatic cholera, 465
Pancreatic islet cells
  gastrinomas from, 464
  neoplastic transformation of, in MEN 1, 456
Pancreatic neuroendocrine tumors (PNETs), 464b, 462–466.
    See also Gastrinomas; Insulinomas
  benign, 462
  defined, 462, 463f, 523
  endocrine disorders and, 462
  functional, 523
    imaging for, 524
    subtypes and syndromes of, 523
  glucagon-secreting, 545
  incidence of, 523
  malignant, 462
  in MEN 1, 524
  nonfunctional, 523
  types of, 465
Pancreatic tumors, 89
Pancreatitis, 165
Pan-gender, 439t
Papillary thyroid carcinoma (PTC), 323, 327, 536
Paraganglioma, 265–270
  cardiovascular manifestations of, 265
  diagnostic method for, 268
  genetic testing for, 268
  intracerebral symptoms related to, 265
  location of, 266
  malignant, 278
  metastatic, 266
  preoperative therapy for, 268
  prognosis for, 269
  syndromes associated with, 269–270
  treatment of, 268
Parathyroid adenoma, 158
Parathyroid cancer, 517
Parathyroid gland
  hyperplasia of, affected by MEN 1, 456
  localization studies, preoperative, 514
  "missing, management of, 515
Parathyroid hormone (PTH), 127, 156
  in absorptive hypercalciuria, 173
  effects on calcium metabolism, 146–147
  elevated, with normal serum calcium, cause of, 516
  recombinant human, 168
Parathyroid hormone-related peptide (PTHrP), 127,
    161
Parathyroid surgery, 510–517, 517b
  ioPTH assay in, 515

Parathyroidectomy
  minimally invasive, 514
    radio-guided, 514–515
  for primary hyperparathyroidism, 153–154, 513–514
    complications of, 516
  subtotal, 516
  total, 516
Paraventricular hypothalamic (PVH) nuclei, 497
Parenteral nutrition (PN), 64
Parveen, Siddiqa, 539
PCOS. *See* Polycystic ovarian syndrome
PCR. *See* Polymerase chain reaction
PD5. *See* Phosphodiesterase 5
Pegvisomant, 211
Pellagra, 467
Pemberton's sign, 321
Pembrolizumab, 487
Penile brachial index, 406–407
Penile prosthesis implantation, 408t
Penile tumescence, 501
Peptide receptor radioligand therapy, 469
Percutaneous biopsy, 519
Perimenopause, 433
Peripheral arterial disease, diabetes mellitus and, 20
Peripheral precocious puberty, 385
Peripubertal hypogonadism, 393
Peroxisome proliferator-activated receptor (PPAR) gamma-2,
    146
Perphenazine, 364t
Persistent hyperparathyroidism, 516
PET. *See* Positron emission tomography
Phenobarbital, 364t
  thyroid function test and, 365
Phenocopy, defined, 457
Phentermine, 105
  efficacy of, 105
  plus topiramate, 105, 107
  side effects of, 105–107
Phenytoin, 364t
  thyroid function tests and, 365
Pheochromocytoma, 167, 265–270, 269–270b, 272, 541
  blood pressure response in, 267
  cardiovascular manifestations of, 265
  diagnostic method for, 268
  genetic testing for, 268
  intracerebral symptoms related to, 265
  located of, 266
  malignant, 277
    clinical features of, 278
    localization of, 278
    prognosis for, 279
    treatment of, 269, 279
  in MEN 2A, 459
  metastatic, 266
  perioperative management of, 520
  preoperative therapy for, 268
  prognosis for, 269
  "rule of 10, " 265
  syndromes associated with, 269–270
  treatment of, 268
Phosphate
  calcium and, 147, 148t
  FGF 23 and, 145
  load, 165
Phosphodiesterase 5 (PD5), 407
  comparison of, 409t
  drug interactions associated with, 409
  side effects of, 409
Phosphorus
  in absorptive hypercalciuria, 173
  restricted diet, 173

Physical activity
  patient readiness for, 103
  weight loss and, 105
Physical activity energy expenditure (PAEE), 102
Pigmented nodular adrenal hyperplasia, 210t
Pitavastatin, 96
Pituicytoma, 201
Pituitary adenomas, 397
  classification of, 188
  evaluation of, 190
  incidence of, 188
  in MEN 1, 457
  nonfunctional, 188–190, 189f
  testing for, 190–191
Pituitary apoplexy, 184, 189
Pituitary carcinomas, 193–194
Pituitary fossa, 189f
Pituitary gland, 189f
  cancers in, 194
Pituitary hormone deficiencies, 188
Pituitary hyperplasia, 221
Pituitary incidentalomas, 188–195, 194b
  evaluation of, 190
  follow up of, 191
  treatment of, 191
Pituitary insufficiency, 181–187, 187b
  after traumatic brain injury, 184
  causes of, 182
  defined, 182
  diabetes insipidus and, 182
  functional causes of, 185
  long-term management of, 193, 193t
  physical examination, 182–183
  presentation of, 182
  radiation therapy and, 184
  treatment of, 185
Pituitary stalk
  abnormalities, 196
  inflammation, immunotherapeutic agents causing, 199
  lesions, 196–202, 202b
    biopsy of, 201, 201t
    evaluations of, 198–199
    imaging for, 198
    monitoring of, 201
    treatment options for, 201, 201t
  normal, 196
  pituicytoma, 201
  thickening, 196, 198f
    neoplasm causing, 200–201
Pituitary stalk interruption syndrome (PSIS), 196
Pituitary tumors
  in adults, 397
  causes of, 223, 223t
  hormones secreted by, 219
  malignant, 223
  in MEN 1, 457
  silent/plurihormonal, 190
  thyroid hormone resistance distinguished from, 220
Pituitary-thyroid axis, 221f
  lithium affecting, 364
Placenta
  hyperthyroidism and, 347
  medications crossing, 347
  methimazole and, 347
  propylthiouracil and, 347
  thyroid hormone and, 346–347
  thyroid-related antibodies and, 347
  TRH and, 346–347
  TSH and, 346–347
  TSI and, 347
Plasma cell (immunoglobulin G4) hypophysitis, 196

PNETs. *See* Pancreatic neuroendocrine tumors
POI. *See* Premature ovarian insufficiency
Polycystic ovarian syndrome (PCOS), 422–426, 426b
  affecting menopause, 424
  clinical manifestation of, 423
  conditions screened for, 424
  diagnosis of
    in adolescents, 423
    in adults, 422
  differential diagnosis for, 423
  fertility treatment options for, 425–426
  indications for, 425
  insulin sensitizers in, 425
  lifestyle modification for, 424
  long-term consequences of, 423
  manifestation of, 427–428
  metabolic screening needs, 423–424
  oral contraceptives in, 425
  pathogenesis of, 422
  pathophysiology of, 427
  patient with, 422
  pregnancy complications in, 424
  treatment of, 430–431
  treatment options for, 424
Polycystic ovary syndrome (PCOS)
  OSA and, 504
Polydipsia, 543–544
Polygender, 439t
Polygenic hypercholesterolemia, 95
Polymerase chain reaction (PCR), 293
Polyuria, 234, 543–544
  in diabetes insipidus, 234–235
POMC. *See* Proopiomelanocortin
Positron emission tomography (PET), 89
  "hot" thyroid nodule on, 513
Postgastric bypass hypoglycemia (PGBH), 88
Postmenopause, 479–480
Postoperative polyuria, 192
Postpartum management
  diet and, 81
  exercise and, 81
  GDM and, 82–83
  glucose monitoring during, 83
  Graves' disease in, 351
Postpartum thyroiditis, 356
  clinical course of, 316, 356
  phase 1, 356
  phase 2, 356
  prevalence of, 316, 317f
  risk for, 317
  subacute thyroiditis *versus*, 317t
  thyroid function in, 317
  treatment of, 316
  with type 1 diabetes mellitus, 84
Postpartum thyrotoxicosis, 546
Postprandial/reactive hypoglycemia, 87
PPAR- -2. *See* Peroxisome proliferator-activated receptor (PPAR) gamma-2
Prader's classification, 375t
Prader-Willi syndrome, 248
Pramlintide, 29
Pravastatin, 96
Precocious puberty, 383
  causes of, 390b
  evaluation of, 383, 384f
  hypothyroidism and, 387
  matter, 383
  peripheral, 385
Preconception counseling, 69
  ACE inhibitors and, 71
  window of opportunity for, postpartum period as, 84

Prednisone, 151t
Preeclampsia, 72
Pregabalin, 18–19
Pregnancy. *See also* Birth
  aspart in, 74
  beta-blockers during, 350
  CAH and, 295
  CGM in, 73–74
  coronary artery disease and, 71
  detemir and, 74
  diabetes in, 67–86, 75–76b
    White classification, 73
  diabetic nephropathy and, 72
  diabetic retinopathy and, 73
  DKA and, 75
    physician remember about, 75–76
  fetus well-being and, 69–70
  fibrates and, 72
  first trimester, 67
    diabetes management in, 68
  fuel metabolism and, 67–76
  glargine and, 74
  glucose control and, 69–70
    goals in, 73
    insulin pump in, 74
  glyburide and, 70–71
  glycemic patterns in, 67
  Graves' disease and, 348–349
    alternatives to, 351
    natural history of, 351
    treatment, 349–350
  hyperthyroidism and, 347
    diagnostic approach, 348
    subclinical, 349
    surgery for, 351
  hypoglycemia and, 70, 74
  ^{123}I scan, 351
  inpatient glycemic targets and, 61
  lispro in, 74
  metformin and, 70–71, 82
  methimazole in, 349–350
  preconception counseling, 69
  prolactin-secreting pituitary tumors and, 205–206
  PTU and, dosage, 349–350
  radioiodine therapy during, 351
  rapid-acting insulin analogues in, 74
  renal transplantation and, 72
  second trimester, 67
    diabetes management in, 68
  sleep in, 68
  smoking and, 72
  statins and, 72
  sulfonylureas and, 70–71
  third trimester, 67
    diabetes management in, 68
  thyroid disease and, 71, 354b
  thyroid gland volume, 346
  thyroid hormone in, 354
    requirements in, 354
    timing of, 355
  thyroid nodules during, 355
  thyrotoxicosis during, 308–309
  TSH in, 353
  type 1 diabetes mellitus and, 74
  type 2 diabetes mellitus and, 74–75
  weight and, 67
Premature ovarian insufficiency (POI), 433, 543
  diagnosis of, 419–420
  disorders coexisting with, 420
  treatment options for, 420
Preoperative parathyroid localization, 514

Primary adrenal hyperplasia (PAH), 261
Primary adrenal insufficiency, 453t, 549
  with immune checkpoint inhibitors, 490
Primary aldosteronism, 257–264, 263b, 542
  clinical manifestations of, 258
  defined, 258
  detection of, 259
  diagnosis of, 259
    confirmation, 260
  evaluation and management algorithm for, 263,
    263f
  forms of, 260, 263
  imaging study for, 260–261
  medications for, 262
  postoperative period of, 262–263
  prevalence of, 258
  screening for, 259
Primary amenorrhea, 391
  causes of, 417, 418t
  ovarian, 417
Primary dyslipidemias, 94
Primary hyperaldosteronism (PA), 519
Primary hyperparathyroidism, 153, 546
  age and, 153
  anatomic alterations in, 153
  causes of, 153
  CKD and, 154
  classic radiographic findings in, 154–155
  diagnosis of, 153
  differential diagnosis of, 154, 155
  familial hypocalciuric hypercalcemia *versus,* 154
  in MEN 1, 455
  normocalcemic, 159
  parathyroidectomy for, 513–514
  pathophysiologic changes in, 155
  prevalence of, 153
  surgery for, 514
  symptoms and signs of, 154, 155t
  therapeutic options for, 158–159
  treatment of, 514
Primary hypogonadism, 222, 394–395
  acquired causes of, 396
  aging and, 396
  congenital causes of, 394–395
  laboratory tests for, 222
  sperm production in, 400
Primary hypoparathyroidism, 544
Primary hypothyroidism, 313, 489
PRL. *See* Prolactin
Process-C, 496
Process-S, 496
Progestagen, 436
Progesterone, 103, 441
Programmed cell death ligand 1 (PD-L1), 491
Programmed cell death protein 1 (PD-1), 491
Prohormones, 449–450
Prolactin (PRL)
  abnormal production of, 204t
  bone metabolism and, 205
  carcinomas, 223
  deficiency, 182, 183
  gonadal dysfunction and, 203
  impotence and, 406–407
  secretion of, 203–206, 204f
  serum, 203
    elevated levels of, 204t
    in functioning prolactinoma, 190
    reducing, 206
    typical levels of, 203
  in sleep, 500
  24-hour profiles of, 498f

Prolactinoma, 547
  giant, 206
  hirsutism and, 429
  malignant, 206
  in MEN 1, 457
  tumor enlargement, 205
Prolactin-secreting pituitary tumors, 203–207, 205b
  differential diagnosis of, 203
  galactorrhea in, 203
  imaging techniques, 205
  in men, 203–205
  pregnancy and, 205–206
  radiotherapy for, 206
  secretion in, 203–206
  surgical removal of, 206
  treatment of, 205–206
    duration of, 206
  in women, 203–205
Proliferative diabetic retinopathy (PDR), 18
Proopiomelanocortin (POMC), 102, 281
Proprotein convertase subtilisin-like kexin type 9
    (PCSK9), 92
  inhibitors, 97–98
Propylthiouracil (PTU), 306
  placenta and, 347
  in pregnancy, 349–350
    management, 350
Prostaglandin E1 (PGE1), 404
Prostate, 400
Protein kinase A, 228–229
"Proximal" Roux-en-Y gastric bypass, 529, 529
Pseudohermaphrodite, defined, 398
Pseudohypoparathyroidism, 165
Pseudotumor cerebri, 250
Psychiatric disorders. See also Mood disorders
  abnormalities in, 363
  hypothyroidism and, 359
  PCOS and, 424
  T₄ values in, 365
  thyroid disease and, 359–370, 368b
  thyroid evaluation in, 368
  thyroid hormone for, 368
Psychogenic impotence, 406, 406t
Psychotropic medications, 364t
PTH. See Parathyroid hormone
PTHrP. See Parathyroid hormone-related peptide
PTPN11 mutation, 248
PTU. See Propylthiouracil
Puberty
  benign, 387
  delay, 388
    gonadotropin levels in, 388
    laboratory tests for, 388
    management of, 390–391
    physical examination of, 388
    radiographic studies in, 388
  disorders of, 382–392, 391b
    features of, 388
    MRI in, 385
  female pattern, 382
  first signs of, 382
  growth velocity
    before, 243–252
    after, 243
  male pattern, 382
  normal timing of, 417
  physiologic events, 382
  physiologic gynecomastia in, 388
  precocious, 383
    causes of, 390b
    evaluation of, 383, 384f

Puberty (Continued)
    hypothyroidism and, 387
    matter, 383
    peripheral, 385
  Tanner stages of, 383t
  underlying processes of, 417
Pyrophosphate, 171

R
Radiation therapy
  for acromegaly, 211
  for nonfunctional adenomas, 192
  pituitary insufficiency and, 184
  for prolactin-secreting pituitary tumors, 206
Radioactive iodine uptake (RAIU), 306t, 308
  for destructive thyroiditis, 318
  for differentiated thyroid cancer, 330, 330t
  thyroid scan versus, 306
  utility of, 302, 302t
Radiographic studies
  in ambiguous genitalia, 376–377
  in pubertal delay, 388
Radioiodine-refractory thyroid cancer, 331
Rainer, Adam, 539
RAIU. See Radioactive iodine uptake
Raloxifene, 124–125t
Randomized controlled trial (RCT), 61
RANK. See Receptor activator of nuclear factor κ
RANK-L. See Receptor activator of nuclear factor κ ligand
Rapid eye movement (REM) sleep, 493–494
  nervous system in, 495–496
Rapid-acting insulin analogues, 74
Rebound hyperglycemia, 29
Receptor activator of nuclear factor κ(RANK), 124
Receptor activator of nuclear factor κ ligand (RANK-L), 124
Recombinant human PTH (rhPTH), 168
Recurrent hyperparathyroidism, 516
Recurrent thyroid cancer, surgery for, 512
Rehnquist, William, 537
Reidel's struma, 318
REM sleep. See Rapid eye movement (REM) sleep
Renal calculi, 170
Renal disease, 165
Renal leak hypercalciuria, 173
Renal lithiasis, 170
Renal transplantation, 72
Renal tubular acidosis (RTA), 171
Renin, 146
Respiratory distress syndrome, 80
Respiratory effort-related arousal (RERA), 503
Respiratory events, 503
Restrictive surgery, 528
Reticular activating system (RAS), 496
Retina ganglion cells (RGCs), 497
Rhinorrhea, 190
Rickets, 134–139, 138b
  biochemical abnormalities in, 137
  causes of, 134
  clinical findings of, 137
  conditions associated with, 135–136, 136t
  defined, 134
  important facts, 134
  radiographic findings with, 137
Risedronate, 124–125t
Robinson, Jackie, 537
Romosozumab, 127
Rosuvastatin, 96
Rousimoff, Andre "The Giant, " 536
Roux-en-Y gastric bypass (RYGB), 529, 529f
RTA. See Renal tubular acidosis
RYGB. See Roux-en-Y gastric bypass

S

Saline therapy, 151t
  kidney and, 229
  mechanism of action, 151t
Santo, Ron, 536
Sarcopenic obesity, 473
Sateow, Hoo, 540
Schizophrenia, 239
Schmidt's syndrome, 452
Scoliosis, 250
Second trimester, 67
  diabetes management in, 68
Secondary amenorrhea, 542, 543
  causes of, 417–418
Secondary dyslipidemias, 95, 545
Secondary hypogonadism, 394, 395f
  causes of, 397
  sperm production in, 400
Seizure, 165
Selective androgen receptor modulators
  (SARMs), 450
Selective serotonin reuptake inhibitors (SSRIs), 365
Selenocysteine, 342t
Sellar mass, 188
Sertoli cell, 372
Serum album, 164
Serum calcium
  correcting levels, 164
  factors controlling, 148t
  hypercalciuria and, 172
  ionized, 164
  low, 164
  serum albumin and, 164
  sources of, 144, 145f
  vitamin D metabolism and, 164
Serum prolactin, 203
  elevated levels of, 204t
  in functioning prolactinoma, 190
  reducing, 206
  typical levels of, 203
Serum T$_4$, 219
Serum triglycerides, 440
Serum TSH values, 361
75-g 2-hour oral glucose tolerance test, 76
Sex assignment, 379
  factors in, 380
  in ovotesticular disorder, 380
  principles of, 380
  in undervirilized male, 380
  in virilized female, 379–380
Sex chromosome disorders, 375t
Sex hormone-binding globulin (SHBG)
  conditions associated with, 394, 394t
  hyperandrogenism and, 423
Sex hormones, 474
Sexual ambiguity, 376*See also* Ambiguous genitalia
  etiology of, 379
  evaluation of, 376
  multidisciplinary approach to, 379
Sexual differentiation
  disorders, 371–381, 373–374b
    classification of, 375t
  factors considered in, 379
  female, 373
  first level of, 372
  level of, 372
  male, 372, 373f
Sexual maturity, 382
Sexual orientation, 439t
SHBG. *See* Sex hormone-binding globulin
Sheehan's syndrome, 184

Short stature. *See also* Height
  endocrine causes for, 248
  familial, 245
  idiopathic, 251
  laboratory measurements, 248
Shoulder dystocia, 80
SIADH. *See* Syndrome of inappropriate secretion of antidiuretic
  hormone
Sildenafil citrate, 407
Simvastatin, 96
Sipple's syndrome. *See* Multiple endocrine neoplasia syndromes
Skeletal lesion, relative frequency of, 149
Sleep, 493–509, 508b*See also* Circadian rhythm; Obstructive
  sleep apnea
  abnormalities of
    associated with abnormal glucose metabolism, 505
    with fatigue, 507–508
  in AM testosterone, 501
  androgen replacement therapy on, 507
  deprivation, 504
    on ghrelin, 506
    in glucose tolerance, 505
    on leptin, 506
    sleep apnea and, 504
  hormones and, 500
  neurotransmitters in, 496
  non-rapid eye movement, 493–494
    nervous system in, 495–496
  penile tumescence and, 501
  processes controlling, 496
  rapid eye movement, 493–494
    nervous system in, 495–496
  stages of, 493–494, 494t
    in life span, 495, 495f
    progression of, 494, 494f
  systems in, 496
Sleep apnea, 208
Sleep disorders, 493
Sleep disordered breathing (SDB), 503
Sleep-wake cycles, 493
Sleep-wake homeostasis (SWH), 496
Sleeve gastrectomy, 528, 528f
Slipped capital femoral epiphysis, 250
Smoking, 72
Sodium, 172
Sodium-glucose cotransporter (SGLT)-2 inhibitors, 34t, 36, 484
Somatostatin analogues
  efficacy of, 211
  mechanism of action of, 211
Somatostatinomas, 523
  characteristics of, 464–465
  treatment of, 465
Sorbitol, 226–227
Sotomayor, Sonia, 537
Soto's syndrome, 251
Sperm production
  in primary hypogonadism, 400
  regulation of, 394
  in secondary hypogonadism, 400
Sporadic nonfunctioning pituitary tumors
  pathogenesis for, 190
SSRIs. *See* Selective serotonin reuptake inhibitors
Statins
  for dyslipidemia, 96t
  mechanism of action of, 96
  pregnancy and, 72
  side effects of, 97
Steroid-induced hyperglycemia, 64
Steroidogenesis pathway, 288–289, 288f
Stewart, Rod, 536
Stickler's syndrome, 251

Stratton, Charles Sherwood, 536
Stress, medically significant, 295
"Stress dose" glucocorticoids, 285–286, 285t
"Stuttering" impotence, 405
Subacute thyroiditis
    causes of, 315
    four stages of, 315
    management of, 316
    postpartum thyroiditis *versus*, 317t
    thyroid function during, 316f
Subclinical hyperthyroidism, 349
    in elderly, 483
    treatment of, 352–353
Subclinical hypothyroidism
    depression and, 359–360
    in elderly, 483
    treatment of, 361–362
Subclinical thyrotoxicosis
    defined, 304
    long-term consequences of, 304
    treatment of, 304
Subtotal parathyroidectomy, 516
Subtotal thyroidectomy, 510–511
Sulfonylureas, 34t, 35
    in GDM, 82
    pregnancy and, 70–71
Suprachiasmatic nuclei (SCN), organization of, 497–499
Syndrome of inappropriate secretion of antidiuretic hormone
        (SIADH), 232–234
    four patterns of, 234
    management of, 192–193
    treatment of, 234

T
T_3. *See* Triiodothyronine
T_4. *See* Thyroxine
Tadalafil, 407
Tamm-Horsfall protein, 171
Tamoxifen, 416
Tanner stages, 383t
TBG. *See* Thyroxine-binding globulin
TBS. *See* Trabecular bone score
TBW. *See* Total body water
TCAs. *See* Tricyclic antidepressants
TCW. *See* Transcellular water
TDD. *See* Total daily dose
TDF. *See* Testis-determining factor
Telotristat, for carcinoid syndrome, 469
Teratogenicity, 307
Teriparatide, 124–125t, 475
Tertiary hyperparathyroidism, 516
Testis-determining factor (TDF), 372
Testolactone, 416
Testosterone
    aging and, 477–478, 501
        decreases in, 478
    buccal, 399t
    estradiol and, 446
    gel, 399t
    laboratory values in, 442
    for older hypogonadal men, 484
    OSA and, 506, 506t
    patch, 399t
    pellets, 399t
    physical changes caused by, 442
    production of, 428f
    regulation of, 393
    serum, 394
    in sleep, 500, 501
    supplementation, 478–479
    synthesis pathway, 378f

Testosterone *(Continued)*
    topical solution, 399t
    transmen on, 442
Testosterone enanthate, 399t
Testosterone replacement therapy (TRT), 398–399
    adverse effects of, 399–400
    for androgen deficiency, 479
    for constitutional delay of growth, 245–248
    contraindications for, 401, 441–442
    parameters monitored in, 400–401
Testosterone undecanoate, 399t
Testotoxicosis, 387
TG. *See* Thyroglobulin
Thermic effect of food, 102
Thiazide diuretics
    for hypercalciuria-induced nephrolithiasis, 178
    for hypocalcemia, 168
Thiazolidinediones (TZD), 34t, 36, 103, 484
Third trimester, 67
    diabetes management in, 68
Thirst stimuli, 228
Thyroglobulin (TG), 302
Thyroglossal duct cysts, removal of, 513
Thyroid antibody testing, 305–306
Thyroid axis, 363
Thyroid cancer, 327–334
    anaplastic, 331–332, 332b
        defined, 331
        staging of, 331, 332t
        surgery for, 512
        treatment of, 331–332
    diagnostic challenges of, 534
    differentiated, 327–331, 331b
        lymph node metastases in, 511
        preoperative evaluation of, 328–329
        prognosis of, 330, 330t
        radioactive iodine for, 330, 330t
        recurrence of, 331
        risk factors for, 327
        staging for, 327, 328t
        surgery for, 329
        thyroidectomy for, 511
    follicular, 327
    immune checkpoint inhibitors for, 491
    incidence of, 327
    management of, 534
    medullary, 332–333, 333b, 549
        associated with MEN 2A, 458
            treatment of, 459
        defined, 332
        genetic syndromes associated with, 332
        preoperative evaluation of, 332–333
        staging of, 332, 333t
        surgical management for, 333, 511
        treatment of, 333
    papillary, 323, 327, 536
    presentation of, 327
    radioiodine-refractory, 331
    types of, 327
Thyroid crisis, 335
Thyroid cyst, aspiration of, 512
Thyroid cytology, interpretation of, 324
Thyroid disease
    in Africa, 533
    diabetes and, 71
    pregnancy and, 71, 345–358, 354b
        affecting, 345
        TSH levels change in, 345–346
    psychiatric disorders and, 359–370, 368b
Thyroid dysfunction
    ipilimumab and, 491

Thyroid dysfunction (Continued)
"labeling effect" with, 362
mild, 360
in psychiatric populations, 364
Thyroid emergencies, 335–340, 339–340b
Thyroid function tests, 345
within age-specific range, 361
antidepressants and, 365
carbamazepine and, 365
depression and, 367–368
genes, implication in, 367
for hypothyroidism, 312
in acutely ill inpatients, 312
during normal pregnancy, 346t
in older adults, 482
phenobarbital and, 365
phenytoin and, 365
for psychiatric patients, 364
psychotropic medications and, 364t
valproic acid and, 365
Thyroid gland
ablation, 220
fetal function of, 347
function of, screening for, 300, 300f
palpation of, 311
volume, 346
Thyroid hormone
for antidepressant response, 366
assay, 300–301
deficiency, 504
depression and, 366
fetal, 347
inhibiting, 335
levels of, elevated, 344
mechanisms of, 367
placenta and, 346
in pregnancy, 354
requirements, 354
requirements in, 354
timing of, 355
preparations of, 312
production, 346
reduction, treatments for, 307
resistance, 220
synthesis of, 335
therapy, 300
for euthyroid sick syndrome, 343
for psychiatric symptoms, 368
titration of, 362–363
Thyroid hormone-binding proteins, disorders of, 301, 301t
Thyroid nodules, 321–326, 325b
aging and, 482
biopsy for, 323, 324t
cold, 322
defined, 321
evaluating, 355
fine-needle aspiration of, 510
FNA for, 322
hot, 322
on PET, 513
indeterminate, management of, 325
initial approach to, 322, 322f
intraoperative frozen section on, 510
malignant, during pregnancy, 355–356
management of
benign cytology on FNA, 324
malignant after FNA, 325
molecular testing in, 325
molecular testing of, 510
in pregnancy, 355
prevalence of, 321

Thyroid nodules (Continued)
risk of cancer and, 323
ultrasonography of, 323, 323f
Thyroid peroxidase (TPO), 71
antibodies, 353–354
Thyroid scan, 302
radioactive iodine uptake versus, 306
Thyroid storm
clinical manifestations of, 335, 335f
conditions may mimic, 335
development of, 335
diagnosis of, 335
laboratory abnormalities in, 335
scoring system, 335, 336t
treatment of, 335, 337t
Thyroid surgery, 510–517, 517b
Thyroid testing, 299–303, 303b
Thyroidectomy
completion, in thyroid nodule, 510
complications of, 513
for differentiated thyroid carcinoma, 511
on Graves' ophthalmopathy, 513
for hyperthyroidism, 512
near-total, 510–511
subtotal, 510–511
total, 510–511
Thyroiditis, 315–320, 318b
acute, 315
management of, 315
after delivery, 317
amiodarone-induced, 318, 319t
cause of, 316
defined, 315
differential diagnosis for, 315
drugs inducing, 318
postpartum, 356
clinical course of, 316
prevalence of, 316, 317f
treatment of, 316
with type 1 diabetes mellitus, 84
prevalence of, 316
subacute
causes of, 315
four stages of, 315
management of, 316
thyroid function during, 316f
Thyroid-stimulating hormone (TSH), 71, 335
alpha subunit molar ratio, 220, 220t
carcinomas, 223
circadian rhythm, 363, 502
circulating thyroid hormone levels, 359
deficiency, 182, 183
laboratory tests for, 249
treatment of, 185
elevated, 219, 489, 548
heterophile antibodies, 219
jet lag and, 502–503
measurement of, 300, 300f
placenta and, 346–347
in pregnancy, 345, 354
in primary hypothyroidism, 313
pseudotumor secreting, 221
release of, factors influencing, 500t, 502
serum, 300
TRH and, 363
tumors secreting, 219
medical therapies for, 220
radiation therapy for, 220
thyroid gland ablation for, 220
treatment of, 220
24-hour profiles of, 498f

Thyroid-stimulating immunoglobulins (TSI), 347
Thyrotoxic periodic paralysis (TPP), 547
Thyrotoxicosis
  amiodarone-induced, 546
  biochemical, 542
  clinical, 542
  hyperemesis gravidarum and, 347–348
  hyperthyroidism *versus*, 304
  laboratory testing for, 305
  physical signs of, 305
  postpartum, 546
  pregnancy and, 308–309
  presentation of, 305
  subclinical, 304
    long-term consequences of, 304
    treatment of, 304
  ultrasonography for, 306
Thyrotropin, 220
Thyrotropin-releasing hormone (TRH)
  depression and, 363
  placenta and, 346–347
  TSH and, 363
Thyroxine (T$_4$), 300, 301f
  conversion to T$_3$, 307
  for depression, 365
  interpretation of, 312
  with psychiatric disorders, 363
Thyroxine-binding globulin (TBG), 219, 308–309
Thyroxine-binding prealbumin (TBPA), 219
Time-restricted feeding, 104
Titralac, 168t
TMNG. *See* Toxic multinodular goiter
Tonicity, 226–227
  evaluating, 227
Total body water (TBW), 226f
  decreased, 231
  increased, 231
Total daily dose (TDD), 62
Total parathyroidectomy, 516
Total parenteral nutrition (TPN), 64
Total thyroidectomy, 510–511
Total thyroxine (TT$_4$), 345
Total triiodothyronine (TT$_3$), 345
Toxic multinodular goiter (TMNG), 305
Toxic shock syndrome, 165
TPN. *See* Total parenteral nutrition
TPO. *See* Thyroid peroxidase
Trabecular bone score (TBS), 111, 119–120, 121f
Transcellular water (TCW), 225
Transgender, 439t
  gonadectomy in, 443
  health disparities in, 439–440
  medicine for, 438
  multidisciplinary approach to, care of, 444
Translocation hyponatremia, 238–239
Transman, 439t
  gender-affirming hormone therapy for, 441
  on testosterone, 442
Transsphenoidal surgery
  for acromegaly, 211
  for Cushing's syndrome, 216
Transwoman, 439t
  estrogen therapy for
    blood clots in, 441
    concerns for, 441
  gender-affirming hormone therapy for, 440
  progesterone in, 441
Traumatic brain injury, 184
TRH. *See* Thyrotropin-releasing hormone
Tricyclic antidepressants (TCAs), 365
Triglycerides, 67–68, 92
  elevated serum levels, 94
  function of, 93–94

Triglycerides *(Continued)*
  GDM and, 79
  macrosomia and, 79
  metabolism of, 93–94
Triiodothyronine (T$_3$), 300, 301f, 484
  reverse, 301, 484
Trousseau's sign, 165
Troyer, Vern, 535
TRT. *See* Testosterone replacement therapy
True hermaphroditism, 379
T-score, 111, 117
  abnormal, 117–118, 118t
TSH. *See* Thyroid-stimulating hormone
TSI. *See* Thyroid-stimulating immunoglobulins
Tumor lysis syndrome, 167
Turner's syndrome, 545
  clinical findings of, 386t
  defined, 390
  GH therapy and, 250
  prognosis, 250
  treatment of, 390
Tutankhamen, endocrine disorder of, 536
Two-spirited gender, 439t
Type 1 diabetes mellitus, 21–30, 453t
  Africans with, 532
  hypoglycemia and, 16, 74
  with immune checkpoint inhibitors, 490
  natural history of, 9
  noninsulin medications for, 29
  pathophysiology of, 8
  postpartum thyroiditis and, 84
  pregnancy and, 74
  treatment of, 21
Type 2 diabetes mellitus, 31–42, 41b
  in Africa, 533
  chronic kidney disease and, 39–40
  comprehensive evaluation of, 31
  glycemia in, 483
  glycemic control for, 31–32
  goals of therapy for, 31, 32t
  hypoglycemia and, 16
  interventions, 83
  ketosis-prone, 532
  lifestyle modifications for, 32–33
  management of, 31–41
  medical treatment of, 483–484
    first-line, 33
    general approach to, 37, 38t
    second-line, 33, 34t
    third-line, 36
  natural history of, 9
  in older adults, 485
  OSA and, 504
  pathophysiology of, 8
  pregnancy and, 74–75
  prevention of, 40–41
  SMBG for, 39
  water metabolism in, 238–239

U
UFC. *See* Urine free cortisol
UKPDS. *See* United Kingdom Prospective Diabetes Study
Ultrasonography
  for thyroid nodules, 323, 323f
  for thyrotoxicosis, 306
[U$_{Na}$ + U$_k$]/P$_{Na}$ ratio, 237–238
Undervirilized male
  assignment determined in, 380
  defined, 376
  sex assignment in, 380
Undiagnosed chronic illness, 248
United Kingdom Prospective Diabetes Study (UKPDS), 21, 31–32
Urinalysis, 176

Urinary citrate, 171, 174
Urinary crystals, 176–177
Urinary metanephrines, falsely elevated, medications causing, 267
Urinary osmolality, 235
Urinary pH, 174
Urine free cortisol (UFC), 215
Urine output, 228
Urodilatin, 226
Urolithiasis, 170
Uropontin, 171

V

VA Diabetes Trial (VADT), 20–21
Valproic acid, 364t
    thyroid function test and, 365
Van der Meer-Timmerman, Annie, 540
Vandross, Luther, 537
Vardenafil, 407
Vasodilators, 404
Vasopressin receptor antagonists (VRA), 238
Vassilyev, Valentina, 540
Ventrolateral preoptic (VLPO) nuclei, 496
Verner-Morrison syndrome, 465
Vertebra, excluded L-spine, 117
Vertebral fracture, 111–113
Vertical-banded gastroplasty, 528
Very-low-calorie diet (VLCD), 104
Very-low-density lipoproteins (VLDLs), 92
Veterans Affairs Diabetes Trial (VADT), 32
Villechaize, Herve, 535
VIPomas, 465, 523
Virilization, 427–432
    causes of, 429
    defined, 427
    diagnosis of, 431b
    female, 375, 376
        causes of, 375
        further evaluation of, 377
        infant, 377
    laboratory tests in, 430
Vision defects, 188
Vitamin D
    adequate intake, 123
    autonomic determinants of, 144–145
    in bone mineral density, 484
    calcium metabolism and, 146–147
    classic and nonclassic effects of, 146
    deficiency, 123–124, 548
    insufficiency, 134–139, 138b
        biochemical abnormalities in, 137
        diagnosis of, 138
        genetic disorders in, 135
    metabolism, 134, 135f
        diseases processes interfering with, 134
        FGF 23 and, 145, 145f
        serum calcium levels and, 164
    metabolites, 137, 167
    in older adults, 476–477
    physiologic determinants of, 144–145
    receptor, 146
    synthesis of, 134, 135f
VLCD. *See* Very-low-calorie diet
VLDLs. *See* Very-low-density lipoproteins
Voluntary weight loss, in elderly, 476
VRA. *See* Vasopressin receptor antagonists

W

Wadlow, Robert, 539
Waist circumference
    measurement of, 100
    in risk stratification, 100

Water
    composition, 225
        body weight and, 226t
        distribution of, 225
    dysfunction, 229b
    free water clearance, 239–240
        electrolyte, 240
        osmolar, 240
    input of, 228
    kidney and, 229
    metabolism, 225–242, 225b
        clinical problems in, 238
        main factors, 228
        schizophrenia in, 239
        in type 2 diabetes mellitus, 238–239
    output of, 228
    total body, 226f
        decreased, 231
        increased, 231
    transcellular, 225
Water restriction test (WRT), 234–235
    ADH values and, 236t
    interpreting, 235
    performing, 235
    values before and after, 235t
Watusi tribe, 539
Weight gain, 105*See also* Body weight
Weight loss, 103
    in bariatric surgery, 530
    exercise and, 105
    intentional, 476
    medication, 107–108
    obesity and, 484
    physical activity and, 105
    program, commercial, 104
    reduction percent in, 103
    surgery, incretin effect in, 530
Weight reduction, surgical options for, 528
Weight-bearing exercise, 474
Wermer's syndrome, 455
Werner-Morrison syndrome, 523
WHI trial. *See* Women's Health Initiative (WHI) trial
Whipple's triad, 462
    laboratory tests for, 88
White classification
    of diabetes in pregnancy, 73
    modified, 73t
    obstetrician use of, 73
WHO. *See* World Health Organization
Winfield, Don, 540
Wolff-Chaikoff effect, 307
Wolffian ducts, 373f
Women's Health Initiative (WHI) trial, 434, 434f
    limitations of data from, 434
World Health Organization (WHO), 117–118, 118t
WRT. *See* Water restriction test

X

Xanthomas, 548
Xanthomatous hypophysitis, 196
46, XX disorders, 375t
46, XY disorders, 375t, 377

Z

Zoledronate, 142
Zoledronic acid, 124–125t, 151t
Zollinger-Ellison syndrome, 463
Zona glomerulosa, 261
Z-score, 111, 117
    abnormal, 117